Handbook of Management of Zoonoses

Krishna Gopal Narayan
Dharmendra Kumar Sinha
Dhirendra Kumar Singh

Handbook of Management of Zoonoses

Springer

Krishna Gopal Narayan
Birsa Agricultural University
Ranchi, Bihar, India

Dharmendra Kumar Sinha
ICAR-Indian Veterinary Research Institute
Izatnagar, Uttar Pradesh, India

Dhirendra Kumar Singh
ICAR-Indian Veterinary Research Institute
Izatnagar, Uttar Pradesh, India

ISBN 978-981-99-9884-5   ISBN 978-981-99-9885-2   (eBook)
https://doi.org/10.1007/978-981-99-9885-2

This Springer imprint is published by the registered company Springer Nature Singapore Pte Ltd.
The registered company address is: 152 Beach Road, #21-01/04 Gateway East, Singapore 189721, Singapore

If disposing of this product, please recycle the paper.

Preface

We began working on our project of writing a book on Veterinary Public Health and Epidemiology during the COVID-19 lockdown. We were confined within the four walls of our respective abode but well connected with the world of literature. We have been teaching this subject, engaged in doing research, guiding master's and PhD students and contributing to the development of courses, syllabus and curricula. We have accumulated a wealth of information. We had a base material that covered literature up to the year 2023.

Mr Bhavik Sawhney of Springer at the interface of publisher-author suggested splitting the manuscript into following two books.

1. Veterinary Public Health & Epidemiology: Veterinary Public Health-Epidemiology-Zoonosis-One Health
2. Veterinary Public Health: Management of Zoonoses

The first book *Veterinary Public Health & Epidemiology (Veterinary Public Health-Epidemiology-Zoonosis-One Health)* published in May 2023 presents principles and application of Veterinary Public Health (VPH), Epidemiology, Zoonosis, One Health and a section on Foodborne illnesses.

We are happy to publish the second book Handbook of Management of Zoonoses devoted to zoonoses in form of a reference book as agreed to after due deliberation and consideration by the editorial board and the authors.

The origin of zoonosis is interesting. The journey of infectious agents emerging from animals and transformation into a specialized human pathogen (zoonotic agent) is complex. Tracing the origin of zoonoses reveals barriers that the infectious agents must overcome including the multiple events associated with progression to become a human pathogen.

Diverse wildlife, with a pool of various pathogens, is in a state of equilibrium evolved through dynamic natural ecological processes. The interaction of human-ecosystem is also dynamic but imperceptible till the balance (equilibrium) is altered. The wildlife, vectors and humans share the same space. Pathogens spill over from the natural niche in the forest—expansion of natural hotspot, to other hosts (bridge hosts) and finally to the target hosts (human) to cause pandemics. The vector population, development, activity and spread are dependent upon environmental temperature, rainfall, humidity, soil, type of terrain and vegetation around. Understanding the transmission of infectious agents between maintenance hosts, bridge hosts and target hosts requires the integration of ecological and epidemiological approaches.

Understanding what is happening or predicting changes at the interfaces and ecotones is necessary to avert pandemics. Surveillance is a tool. The health system uses this with intervention methods to prevent infection progressing through sporadic, endemic, outbreak, and epidemic stages to pandemics.

Most of the bacterial and parasitic zoonoses appear to have evolved along with agriculture beginning over thousand years ago. Fungi are ubiquitously spread in the environment, plants and animals threatening human health, e.g. angio-invasive mucormycosis and mycotoxicosis and Candidiasis in hospital setting. The changes in farming systems to suit mass marketing conditions are related to re-emergence of certain zoonoses, alteration in pathogens' characters such as virulence and drug resistance causing serious public health problems. Endemic status may progress to epidemic. Intensive dairy goat farming was linked to Q fever epidemic in the Netherlands.

Averting zoonotic pandemics is a matter of global concern. Available measures of averting zoonoses have been elucidated.

The responsibility to control and prevent zoonoses may be independent or joint. Disease like Rabies is illustrative of its control by VPH efforts only. Reducing dog rabies to zero eliminates deaths due to hydrophobia (except due to exposure from wildlife). Metazoonoses like West Nile and Rift Valley Fever require One Health approach. Viruses like DENV, SARS-COV-1 and SARS-COV-2 evolved from zoonoses to anthroponoses (human-human transmission) and require human health efforts (health sector) to reduce human suffering and deaths due to illness.

A number of viral (28), bacterial (26), mycotic (11) and parasitic (39) diseases have been dealt with. Diseases of wildlife, non-human primates and bats have been discussed in detail; they are important as "infections at the Interface". Swine, equine, dogs, rats all in "Synanthropic area" have been tabulated.

Ranchi, Bihar, India   Krishna Gopal Narayan
Izatnagar, Uttar Pradesh, India   Dharmendra Kumar Sinha
Izatnagar, Uttar Pradesh, India   Dhirendra Kumar Singh
November, 2024

Acknowledgements

Our family members solidly stood with us during the pandemic. They extended all services related to our protection like preparation and serving all protective and immunostimulant concoctions, steam, gargle, moral boosting during hardship, and soothing/calming during emotional setbacks. Often, they shared some such family responsibilities which otherwise were ours. It would not have been possible to prepare the text for the following two books without their affectionate and caring support. We gratefully acknowledge and sincerely thank them.

Being teachers, we are bestowed with academic ambience. We have been fortunate to have colleagues bubbling with knowledge and sharing it open-heartedly. Interaction with colleagues and students, as well as participation in seminars, presentations and academic discussions, is always educative. It offered opportunity to modify the content and presentation of our academic texts. We used this blessed situation profusely. We extend sincere thanks to our colleagues and students.

Management of outbreak/epidemic requires understanding the mode of infection, routes of transmission and the lifecycle of parasites, some of which are complex. Illustrations have been used to help the readers. We appreciate and sincerely thank Dr. M. Suman Kumar, Scientist, Division of VPH, ICAR-IVRI, for making some of the illustrations.

Clinical presentation of zoonoses is often baffling, as well as confusing. Diagnosis is challenging. Teaching a human disease (e.g. zoonoses) in a veterinary college where sick animals and not human case(s) are available is very difficult. It is important that teachers plan and organize practical classes, demonstrations and visits to medical colleges to make up such deficiencies. We experienced and prepared the text in a fashion that enables readers/students to comprehend and conceptualize a clinical case and pathology in the absence of live demonstration and pathological specimens. While writing *Epidemiology, Diagnosis and Management of Zoonoses, ICAR 2004* the first author had access to a book *Atlas of Infectious Diseases by David R Stone and Sherwood L Gorbach, (2000) published by W B Saunders Company of Philadelphia* from which some photos were reproduced with permission. Reproduction of such photos of clinical case/pathologies from published reports is not always possible. We have tried and have succeeded in some cases. We extend thanks to all such publishers/authors including WHO for extending permission for reproduction and to our publisher Springer for cooperation.

Unlike *intuitive knowledge* which sages gather by connecting themselves with God, we deal with *borrowed knowledge*. We have borrowed knowledge generated by scientists, researchers, meta-analysts and experts contributing to exhaustive specific reports on diseases. We have aggregated and shaped the *borrowed knowledge* as the "best-fit" for academics, postgraduate scholars, teachers, scientists and professional administrators. We have cited their contribution. It is not enough. We sincerely acknowledge their hard work and contribution.

Ranchi, India   K. G. Narayan
Izatnagar, India   D. K. Sinha
Izatnagar, India   D. K. Singh

Contents

55   African Tick Bite Fever 601
   55.1   Aetiology 601
   55.2   Epidemiology.. 602
       55.2.1   Distribution 602
       55.2.2   Vector...................................... 602
   55.3   Symptoms 603
   55.4   Diagnosis 603
   55.5   Treatment 603
   References 603

56   Epidemic Typhus.. 605
   56.1   Aetiology 606
   56.2   Epidemiology.. 606
       56.2.1   Epidemic Typhus 606
       56.2.2   Sylvatic Typhus 607
       56.2.3   Geographic Distribution....................... 607
       56.2.4   Lice, the Vector............................. 608
       56.2.5   Transmission 608
       56.2.6   Modes of Infection........................... 609
   56.3   Pathology... 609
   56.4   Symptoms 609
   56.5   Diagnosis 610
   56.6   Treatment... 610
   56.7   Prevention 611
   References 611

57   Indian Tick Typhus.. 613
   57.1   Aetiology 613
   57.2   Epidemiology.. 614
       57.2.1   Mode of Infection........................... 615
   57.3   Symptoms 615
   57.4   Diagnosis 616
   57.5   Treatment... 617
   57.6   Prevention 617
   References 617

58   Murine Typhus 619
   58.1   Aetiology 619
   58.2   Epidemiology.. 620
       58.2.1   Natural History/Maintenance of *R. typhi* 620
       58.2.2   Vectors 620
       58.2.3   Hosts....................................... 620
       58.2.4   Distribution................................. 621
       58.2.5   Season and Other Contributing Factors 621
   58.3   Modes of Infection................................... 622
   58.4   Symptoms 623
   58.5   Diagnosis 624

Abbreviations

AAS	Allergic aspergillus sinusitis
ABPA	Allergic broncho-pulmonary aspergillosis
ACA	Acrodermatitis chronica atrophicans
ACE2	Angiotensin converting enzyme II
ACIP	Advisory Committee on Immunization Practices
ADE	Antibody dependent enhancement
AE	Alveolar echinococcosis
AES	Acute encephalitis syndrome
AF	Aflatoxin
AFB	Acid-fast bacillus
AHD	Alveolar hydatid diseases
AIA	Aspergillus-induced asthma
AIDS	Acquired immune deficiency syndrome
AIV	Avian influenza virus
AKI	Acute kidney injury
ALT	Alanine amino-transferase
ANDV	Andes virus
ANT	Antiqua
AQF	Acute query fever
ARDS	Acute respiratory distress syndrome
ART	Antiretroviral therapy
AST	Aspartate amino-transferase
AT1R	Angiotensin type-1 receptor
ATA	Alimentary toxic aleukia
ATB	Aspergillus tracheobronchitis
ATBF	African tick bite fever
ATCC	American Type Culture Collection
ATS	American Thoracic Society
AVA	Anthrax vaccine adsorbed
AVP	Anthrax vaccine precipitated
BA	Bacillary angiomatosis

BAL	Broncho-alveolar lavage
BAYV	Bayou virus
BBB	Blood-brain barrier
BCCV	Black creek canal virus
BCG	Bacillus Calmette-Guerin
BCNE	Blood culture negative endocarditis
BCoV	Bovine coronavirus
BEBOV	Bundibugyo ebolavirus
BEN	Balkan endemic nephropathy
BHK	Baby hamster kidney fibroblasts
BPS	Barking pig syndrome
Brps	*Bartonella* Repeat Proteins
BSE	Bovine spongiform encephalopathy
BSL-4	Biosafety level 4
BTB	Bovine tuberculosis
BTM	Bulk-tank milk
CNA	Chronic necrotizing aspergillosis
CAT	Computed axial tomography
CATT	Card agglutination test
CCA	Cholangiocarcinoma
CCD	Cold cloud density
CCHF	Crimean-Congo haemorrhagic fever
CCHFV	Crimean-Congo haemorrhagic fever virus
CDC	Centers for Disease Control and Prevention, Atlanta
CE	Cystic echinococcosis
CEPI	Coalition for Epidemic Preparedness Innovations
CER	Chicken embryo reticulum
CEV	California encephalitis virus
CFIA	Canadian Food Inspection Agency
CFR	Case fatality rate
CFT	Complement fixation test
CHD	Cystic hydatid disease
CHIKV	Chikungunya virus
CIDRAP	Centre for Infectious Disease Research and Policy
CIEBOV	Côte d'Ivoire ebolavirus/Ivory Coast ebolavirus
CIEP	Counter-immunoelectrophoresis
CL	Cutaneous leishmaniasis
CLIA	Chemiluminescence immunoassay
CLSI	Clinical Laboratory Standards Institute
CNS	Central nervous system
CNVR	Catch, Neuter, Vaccinate and Release
COPD	Chronic obstructive pulmonary disease
CoV	Coronaviruses
COVID-19	Coronavirus disease 2019
COWP	Cryptosporidium oocyst wall protein

CPA	Chronic pulmonary aspergillosis
CPE	Cytopathic effect
CRCL	Chronic relapsing cutaneous leishmaniasis
CR-CoV	Canine respiratory coronaviruses
CSD	Cat scratch disease
CSF	Cat scratch fever
CSF	Cerebrospinal fluid
CT	Computed tomography
CTF	Colorado tick fever
CV	Chikungunya virus
CZS	Congenital Zika syndrome
DALY	Disability-adjusted life year
DAT	Direct agglutination test
DCL	Diffuse cutaneous leishmaniasis
DDT	Dichloro-diphenyl-trichloroethane
DEET	N,N-diethyl-meta-toluamide
DH	Definitive host
DHF	Dengue haemorrhagic fever
DIC	Differential interference contrast
DIC	Disseminated intravascular coagulation
DIVA	Differentiating infected from vaccinated animals
DKA	Diabetic ketoacidosis
DMP	Dimethyl phthalate
DNA	Deoxyribonucleic acid
DOBV	Dobrava virus
DoD-GEIS	Department of Defense-Global Emerging Infections Surveillance and Response System
DON	Deoxynivalenol
DOTS	Directly Observed Treatment, Short course
DRIT	Direct rapid immunohistochemical test
dsDNA	Double stranded deoxyribonucleic acid
DSS	Dengue shock syndrome
DV	Dengue fever virus
ECDC	European Centre for Disease Prevention and Control
ECM	Erythema chronicum migrans
ECSA	East, Central and Southern African
EEA	European Economic Area
EEA1	Early endosomal autoantigen 1
EEE	Eastern equine encephalitis
EF	Oedema factor
EFSA	European Food Safety Authority
EGF	Epidermal growth factor
EIA	Enzyme immunoassay
ELISA	Enzyme-linked immunosorbent assay
EMA	European Medicines Agency

EMJH Medium	Ellinghausen-McCullough-Johnson-Harris Medium
EMPRES	Emergency prevention system
EMPRES-i	EMPRES Global Animal Disease Information System
EMR	Electronic medical recording
EPA	Environmental Protection Agency
ERCP	Endoscopic retrograde cholangiopancreatography
ESP	Excretory-secretary product
ESR	Erythrocyte sedimentation rate
ETUs	Ebola treatment units
EU	European Union
EUCAST	European Committee for Antimicrobial Susceptibility Testing
FAO	Food and Agriculture Organization
FAVNT	Fluorescent antibody virus neutralization test
FB1	Fumonisins
FBT	Flea-borne typhus
FDA	Food and Drug Administration
FERG	Foodborne Disease Burden Epidemiology Reference Group
FHB	Fusarium head blight
FITC-C-Mabs	Fluorescein isothiocyanate-conjugated-monoclonal antibody
FNV	French neurotropic vaccine
GARC	Global Alliance for Rabies Control
GAVI	Global Vaccine Alliance
GBS	Guillain-Barré syndrome
GC	Gas chromatography
GC-ECD	Gas chromatography-electron-capture detector
GC-FID	Gas chromatography-flame ionization detector
GDP	Gross domestic product
GM	Genetically modified
GP	Glycoprotein
GWD	Guinea worm disease
H_2S	Hydrogen sulphide
HA	Haemagglutinin
HAART	Highly active antiretroviral therapy
HAI	Hemagglutination inhibition
HARSP	Haiti Animal Rabies Surveillance Program
HAT	Human African trypanosomiasis
Hbp	Hemin-binding proteins
HCPS	Hantavirus cardio-pulmonary syndrome
HCWs	Health care workers
HEPA	High efficiency particulate air
HeV	Hendra virus
HFRS	Haemorrhagic fever with renal syndrome
HGA	Human granulocytic anaplasmosis
HE	Human granulocytic ehrlichiosis
HIV	Human immunodeficiency virus

HME	Human monocytic ehrlichiosis
HP	High pathogenic
HPLC	High performance liquid chromatography
HPLC-DAD	High performance liquid chromatography with diode-array detection
HPLC-FLD	High performance liquid chromatography with fluorescence detection
HPLC-MS	High performance liquid chromatography with mass spectrometry
HPS	Hantavirus pulmonary syndrome
HRIG	Human rabies immune globulin
HTNV	Hantaan virus
IARC	International Agency for Research on Cancer
IB	Immunoblotting
IBCM	Integrated bite case management
IC	Immunochromatography
ICAM	International Companion Animal Management Coalition
ICMR	Indian Council of Medical Research
ICU	Intensive care unit
ID	Intradermal
IED	Immunoelectrodiffusion
IEP	Immunoelectrophoresis
IFA	Immunofluorescence assay
IFAb	Indirect fluorescent antibody
IFI	Invasive fungal infection
IgM	Immunoglobulin M
IH	Intermediate host
IHA	Indirect haemagglutination
IN	Intermediate
IP	Incubation period
IPA	Invasive pulmonary aspergillosis
IPC	Infection prevention and control
IPT	Immunoperoxidase test
ITC	International Commission on Trichinellosis
ITT	Indian tick typhus
IU/kg	International unit per kilogramme
JEV	Japanese encephalitis virus
KFD	Kyasanur forest disease
KUNV	Kunjin virus
LAC	La Crosse encephalitis
LACV	La Crosse virus
LA-MRSA	Livestock-associated methicillin-resistant *Staphylococcus aureus*
LAT	Latex agglutination test
LBRF	Louse-borne relapsing fever

LCL	Localized Cutaneous Leishmaniasis
LCV	La Crosse encephalitis virus
LCV	Large cell variant
LDH	Lactic dehydrogenase
LERG	Leptospirosis Burden Epidemiology Reference Group
LF	Lethal factor
LP	Low pathogenic
LP	Lumber puncture
LPS	Lipopolysaccharide
MAC	*Mycobacterium avium* complex
MALDI-TOF MS	Matrix-assisted laser desorption ionization–time of flight mass spectrometry
MAP	*Mycobacterium avium* subspecies *paratuberculosis*
MARV	Marburg virus
MAT	MICROSCOPIC agglutination test
MCL	Mucosal leishmaniasis
MDA	Mass drug administration
MDBK	Madin-Darby bovine kidney
mDCs	Monocyte-derived dendritic cells
MDR	Multidrug-resistant
MDV	Mass dog vaccination
MED	Biovar Medievalis
MERS	Middle East respiratory syndrome
MIC	Minimum inhibitory concentration
MIF	Merthiolate, iodine, formalin
MIR	Minimum infection rate
MIRU	Mycobacterial interspersed repetitive unit
Ml	Millilitre
MLST	Multilocus sequence typing
MMWR	Morbidity and Mortality Weekly Report
MOTT	Mycobacteria other than tuberculosis
MP	Milwaukee protocol
MRI	Magnetic resonance imaging
MS	Multiple sclerosis
MTB/RIF Test	Rapid molecular detection of tuberculosis and rifampin resistance test
MVEV	Murray Valley encephalitis virus
NA	Neuraminidase
NAT	Nucleic acid amplification test
NCDC	National Centre for Disease Control
NDVI	Normalized difference vegetation index
NGOs	Non-governmental organizations
NIAID	National Institute of Allergy and Infectious Diseases
NICD	National Institute of Communicable Diseases
NIH	National Institute of Health

NiV	Nipah virus
NO	Nitric oxide
NP	Nucleoprotein
Nsp	Non-structural proteins
NTD	Neural tube defect
NTDs	Neglected tropical diseases
NTM	Nontuberculous mycobacteria
NVBDCP	National Vector Borne Disease Control Programme
OB	Outbreak
OIE	Office International des Epizooties/World Organization for Animal Health
OLE	Oil of lemon eucalyptus
ONNV	O'Nyong-nyong fever virus
OR	Odd ratio
ORI	Orientalis
OT	Ochratoxin
PA	Protective antigen
PAH	Phenylalanine hydroxylase
PAHO	Pan American Health Organization
PAIR	Puncture, Aspiration, Injection, Re-aspiration
PAIRD	Puncture, Aspiration, Injection, Re-aspiration and Drainage
PAT	Patulin
PCR	Polymerase chain reaction
PE	Pestoides
PEP	Post-exposure prophylaxis
PHD	Polycystic hydatid disease
PKDL	Post Kala azar dermal leishmaniasis
PMD	Para-menthane-diol
POH	Presumed ocular histoplasmosis
POWV	Powassan virus
PP	Pneumonic plague
PPDC	Percutaneous puncture with drainage and curettage
PPE	Personal protective equipment
PrEP	Pre-exposure prophylaxis
PRES	Porcine respiratory & encephalitis syndrome
PRNT	Plaque-reduction neutralization tests
ProMED	Program for Monitoring Emerging Diseases
PTLDS	Post-treatment Lyme disease syndrome
PUO	Pyrexia of unknown origin
PUUV	Puumala virus
PVRV	Purified Vero cell rabies vaccine
Q fever	Query fever
RABV	Rabies virus
RABVV	Rabies virus variant
RAVV	Ravn virus

RBCs	Red blood cells
RBD	Receptor-binding domain
RDT	Rapid diagnostic test
REBOV	Reston ebolavirus
RFFIT	Rapid fluorescent focus inhibition test
RFLP	Restriction fragment length polymorphism
RGM	Rapidly growing mycobacteria
RIG	Rabies immunoglobulins
RITE	Rapid isolation and treatment of Ebola
RMSF	Rocky Mountain spotted fever
RNA	Ribonucleic acid
RRV	Ross River fever virus
RSSD	Remote sensing satellite data
RTCIT	Rabies cell culture inoculation test
RT-LAMP	Reverse transcription-loop-mediated isothermal amplification
RT-PCR	Real-time polymerase chain reaction
RT-PCR	Reverse transcription polymerase chain reaction
RVFV	Rift Valley fever virus
Sa	Sphinganine
SAAV	Saaremaa virus
SAPs	Secreted aspartyl proteinases
SARS	Severe acute respiratory syndrome
SAT	Slide agglutination test
SCID	Severely combined immunodeficient mice
SCV	Small cell variant
SDS-PAGE	Sodium dodecyl sulphate–polyacrylamide gel electrophoresis
SEBOV	Sudan ebolavirus
SEOV	Seoul virus
SHF	Simian haemorrhagic fever
SHPS	Severe pulmonary haemorrhage syndrome
SIV	Swine influenza virus
SIV	Simian immunodeficiency viruses
SLEV	St. Louis encephalitis virus
SLP	Spore-like particle
SN	Serum neutralization
SNP	Single nucleotide polymorphism
SNS	Smithburn neurotropic strain
SNV	Sin Nombre virus
So	Sphingosine
STARI	Southern tick-associated rash illness
STAT	Standard tube agglutination test
STCs	Sterigmatocystins
TAG-VE	Technical Advisory Group on Virus Evolution
TB	Tuberculosis
TbG	*Trypanosoma brucei gambiense*

TbR	*Trypanosoma brucei rhodesiense*
TBRD	Tick-borne rickettsial diseases
TCID50	Median tissue culture infectious dose
TCTC	Trichothecenes
TGR	Typhus group rickettsia
Th1	T-helper-1
THAIV	Thailand virus
TLC	Thin-layer chromatography
TLR	Toll-like receptor
TNF	Tumour necrosis factor
TPMV	Thottapalayam virus
TST	Tuberculin skin test
TULV	Tula virus
UCLA	University of California, Los Angeles
UNICEF	United Nations International Children's Emergency Fund
UNSIC	United Nations System for Influenza Coordinator
UPLC	Ultra performance liquid chromatography
USA	United States of America
UV	Ultraviolet
VECs	Vascular endothelial cells
VEE	Venezuelan equine encephalitis
VEGF	Vascular endothelial growth factor
VHF	Viral haemorrhagic fever
VL	Visceral leishmaniasis
VNT	Virus neutralization test
VP	Virion protein
VS	Veterinary services
VSG	Variant surface glycoprotein
wb-CATT	Whole blood-card agglutination test
WEE	Western equine encephalitis
WHO	World Health Organization
WNV	West Nile virus
WNVKUN	West Nile Virus–Kunjin
WSPA	World Society for the Protection of Animals
WW	World War
XDR	Extensively drug-resistant
YF	Yellow fever
YFV	Yellow fever virus
ZEA	Zearalenone
ZEBOV	Zaire ebolavirus
ZIKV	Zika virus
ZN	Ziehl-Neelsen

List of Figures

List of Tables

Part I
Management of Zoonoses

Abstract

Management of zoonoses suggests managing a patient of zoonoses which is the domain of clinical medicine. Clinical medicine is important to mitigate suffering due to illness/disease, pain, save life and reduce fatality. This part devotes to managing events preceding the precipitation of clinical illness/disease in population. Averting zoonotic pandemics is a matter of global concern. Available measures have been elucidated.

Journey of infectious agents emerging from animal to transformation into a specialized human pathogen (zoonotic agent) is complex. Tracing the origin of zoonoses reveals barriers which the infectious agents must overcome including the multiple events associated with progression to become a human pathogen. These events devote to natural abode of infectious zoonotic agents, their movements, ventures into other locations, interactions with new ecosystem in a framework of transmission through maintenance, bridge and target hosts.

Epidemiology is basic to the understanding of disease in herd or population and comprises studies dedicated to the diseases (a) in single host species or to a single target species (classical epidemiology) and those (b) caused by multi-host pathogens (ecology of diseases). Understanding of this complex multi-host system (ecology of disease) is a prerequisite to designing measures to prevent zoonoses in the target hosts, i.e. human population.

Diverse wildlife with a pool of variety of pathogens are in a state of equilibrium evolved through dynamic natural ecological processes. Interaction of human-ecosystem is also dynamic but imperceptible till the balance (equilibrium) is altered. The wildlife and human share the same space at the interface. Pathogens spill over from the natural niche in the forest to cause pandemics.

Understanding of what is happening or predicting the changes at the interfaces and ecotones is necessary in averting pandemics. Surveillance is a tool. Health system uses this with intervention methods to prevent infection progressing through sporadic, outbreak, epidemic to pandemic.

The five chapters are devoted to these.

Chapters

1. Origin, emergence and re-emergence of zoonoses
2. Wildlife zoonoses
3. Epidemiology of vector-borne diseases
4. Evolution of methods of managing/controlling zoonoses
5. Prevention of zoonotic pandemics

Chapter 1
Origin, Emergence, and Re-emergence of Zoonoses

Human pathogens emerge from animals. These are zoonoses. There exists 'infectivity continuum of pathogens' from animal to human. Transformation of an animal pathogen into a specialized human pathogen depends upon multiple variables that combine in a dynamic process that is not yet fully understood. The species of animal that harbours the pathogen, the nature and the frequency of human interaction with that animal modulate the risk of zoonotic transmission. In absence of these, phylogenetic proximity may be important, e.g. HIV and chimpanzee and human.

Wolfe et al. *(2007) explained the transit of an animal pathogen to human. They assembled a data base of 15 temperate and 10 tropical diseases (Box) that have/had the highest DALY/disease burden, studied origin of respective pathogens and geography and made ten analyses.*

Data base on these 25 diseases (boxes) were assembled.

The nine tropical diseases	The fifteen temperate diseases
Acquired immune deficiency syndrome (AIDS), Chagas disease, cholera, dengue haemorrhagic fever, East and West African sleeping sicknesses, falciparum and vivax malarias and visceral leishmaniasis AND *A disease that caused heavy burden*—yellow fever	Hepatitis B, influenza A, measles, pertussis, rotavirus A, syphilis, tetanus and tuberculosis [stage 5 diseases] *AND* *Diseases that caused heavy disease burden* = diphtheria, mumps, plague, rubella, smallpox, typhoid and typhus

Major infectious diseases of *temperate zones* arose overwhelmingly in the Old World (Africa, Asia and Europe) and from domestic animals. *Tropical diseases* too originated in the Old World. Reasons were different.

© Springer Nature Singapore Pte Ltd. 2024
K. G. Narayan et al., *Handbook of Management of Zoonoses*,
https://doi.org/10.1007/978-981-99-9885-2_1

1.1   Crowd Vs Sparse Population

1.1.1   Crowd Epidemic Diseases

The epidemic soon exhausts the local pool of susceptible potential victim. These sustain only in large human population and must have evolved with rising agriculture, about 11,000 years ago when there was a steep rise in population. Most human diseases in *temperate* zones are 'crowd-epidemic'. These are acute. Deaths or recovery occurs within one or several weeks. The immunity lasts long.

Domestic animals donated few tropical but many temperate diseases, because they lived in the temperate regions (high population density). Thus, the rise of agriculture starting 11,000 years ago played multiple roles in the evolution of animal pathogens into human pathogens, generated crowd of human and animals, and increased encounter/contact opportunities; domestic animal herds served as conduit (passage tunnel) for transfer from wild animals to humans, e.g. influenza A virus. The process of crowd disease might have evolved.

1.1.2   Sparse Population Diseases

Diseases that can persist in sparse population (a) occur in animal reservoir and human as well (e.g. Yellow fever), (b) produce incomplete or short-lived immunity so that individuals continue to be in pool of susceptible (e.g. Malaria), and (c) have slow or chronic course and the sufferers continue infecting new victims over years (e.g. Chagas disease).

1.1.3   Geographic Origin

More temperate diseases arose in the Old World (except Chagas disease) than in the New World, because domesticated livestock in the Old World harboured and made available ancestral pathogens. Thirteen of 14 major domesticated livestock species originated in the Old World. Humans come in close/closest contact with five species cow, sheep, goat, pig and horse.

The exchange of pathogen between Old (Africa, Asia, Europe) and New (Americas) Worlds was unequal.

1.1.4   Genetic Distance Between Human and the New World and Old World Monkeys

Nine tropical diseases and one temperate disease arose from these animal species in the Old World (and not in the New World) because the genetic distance between humans and the New World monkeys is almost twice the distance between humans and the Old World monkeys and is many times that between humans and Old World apes. The time available for evolutionary transfer from animals to humans was about five million years in the Old World compared to 14,000 years in the New World. The geographic origins of rotavirus, rubella, tetanus and typhus are not known and those of syphilis and tuberculosis are debatable.

1.2   Origin of Pathogen

Almost all of the animal-derived pathogens came from warm-blooded vertebrates, primarily mammals and in two cases (influenza A and ultimately falciparum malaria) birds:

- Diphtheria, influenza A, measles, mumps, pertussis, rotavirus, smallpox and tuberculosis from domestic animals
- Hepatitis B from apes
- Plague and typhus from rodents
- Rubella, syphilis, tetanus and typhoid from still-unknown sources

Temperate and tropical human diseases differ markedly in their animal origins. *Weak species barrier (phylogenetic closeness) for pathogens to cross*

This is measured by the following formula =

$$\frac{\text{Number of major human diseases contributed}}{\text{Number of animal species in the taxonomic group contributing those diseases}}$$

The values for apes, non-human primates other than apes, mammals other than primates and vertebrates other than mammals are approximately 0.2, 0.017, 0.003 and 0.00006, respectively.

Of all vertebrate species, primates account for 0.5% but contributed 20% of major human diseases. The 'species barrier' concept stands strengthened.

AIDS, dengue fever, vivax malaria, yellow fever (4/10 tropical diseases) and hepatitis B (1/15 temperate disease) originated from wild non-human primates. The reasons are (a) phylogenetic closeness (*weak species barrier for pathogens to cross*) between human and non-human primates and (b) vast majority of these live in the tropics.

1.3   Transformation of Animal Pathogens to Humans

Some of the historical human pathogens (stage 5 in Table 1.1) could have co-evolved. An ancestral pathogen already present in the common ancestor of

Table 1.1 Transformation of animal pathogens to humans

Stage	Detection/Transmission under natural condition	Examples
1	**Animal microbes** not detected in human (Except transfer by modern technologies - blood transfusion, organ transplants, or hypodermic needles). **Transmission None**	
2	Example: Rabies virus from bat to man **EBOLA ONLY FROM MONKEY** No human - human transmission **Primary transmission only**	Anthrax, Tularemia, Rabies, Nipah, West Nile
3	Example: Ebola virus from monkey; Monkey -human, limited outbreaks HUMAN – HUMAN FEW CYCLES **Secondary transmission (few cycles)**	Marburg, Ebola, Monkey pox
4	Animal pathogen with natural sylvatic cycle Example: Dengue virus DENGUE FROM MONKEYS TO HUMAN PRIMARY TRANSMISSION **Long sequences of secondary transmissions** between humans without the involvement of animal hosts. **Transmission from animals (sylvatic) and many cycles, human-mosquito-human**	Dengue
4a	Sylvatic cycle much more important than direct human-vector-human spread. Yellow fever exhibit more frequent secondary transmission	Chagas' disease, Yellow fever
4b	The greatest spread is between humans.	Influenza A, Cholera, Typhus and West African sleeping sickness.
5	*Historical* pathogens, exclusively human pathogens Example: HIV apes to man	Smallpox, Falciparum malaria, Measles, Mumps, Rubella, Smallpox, Syphilis, HIV

chimpanzees and humans could have co-speciated when the chimpanzee and human lineages diverged around five million years ago. Animal pathogens had to pass through progressive stages 1–5 to become exclusively human pathogens (Table 1.1).

Most pathogens fail to cross species barrier (stage 1–2, e.g. rabies virus) because of a number of factors. Animal pathogens transmissible to humans evolve the ability to sustain many cycles of human-to-human transmission (transmission efficiency), rather than just a few cycles before the outbreak dies out (e.g. Ebola outbreaks).

It is also related to the size of the human population. The number of encounters and phylogenetic distance is important. Chimpanzees being phylogenetically close to humans have donated a number of zoonoses, e.g. AIDS. Phylogenetically distant rodents have donated plague and typhus because of high, frequent encounters and sharing human dwellings. About 50% of established temperate diseases have been acquired from domestic livestock because of abundance and frequent encounter. Pathogens need to evolve and adapt in a new host or a new vector and overcome barriers to spread to a new host and other tissues. Rabid animals bite others, rarely does a rabid human. Prion (BSE) is restricted to CNS and lymphoid tissues.

Certain developments have augmented transmission between humans and also clusters of susceptible humans (elderly, compromised immunity, antimicrobial resistance). Examples are hepatitis C by blood transfusion and retroviruses through bushmeat trade, BSE through change in processing technology and anthrax and HIV among injectable drug addicts.

Understanding the 'human-animal interface' is important. It appears to be fluid, always in a dynamic state. The frequency and type of interaction with animals, particularly reservoirs of zoonotic pathogens, fluctuate in response to a number of factors and in turn influence the potential for transmission. Multiple variables must combine in a dynamic and as yet not fully understood process of cross-species transmission. Animal pathogens must evolve to be able to infect humans and also maintain long-term human-to-human transmission without the need for reintroduction from the original animal host. The route taken by an animal virus to reach human population varies, e.g. SARS from bats of the genus *Rhinolophus*, through intermediate hosts in the wet markets of southern China to humans.

Pike et al. (2010) observed that the traditional practice of keeping primate pets and hunting and butchering non-human primates continues to be a gateway for the zoonotic transmission of retroviruses among Central Africans. A wide array of primate T viruses was identified in them that had not previously been described as infecting humans. One per cent of 1000 rural Cameroonian villagers with reported exposure to primates had antibodies to simian foamy virus. Transmission of zoonotic viruses occurs on an astonishingly regular basis.

1.4   Drivers

It appears that the ability of an animal pathogen to infect human and reside increases with increased interaction/contact. Drivers could be exposed to animal reservoirs at the human-animal interface, wet market and trade, activities like hunting and butchering (of non-human primates led SIV switch over to HIV), socioeconomic pressure and nutritional requirement forcing bushmeat hunting and deforestation and climate change.

1.5   Prevention

Global alliance for early detection and alert considering the speed of spread through air and global trade is very important. Study of population with high level of exposure, say at the wild-domestic animal interface, e.g. hunters, butchers of wild game, wildlife veterinarians, workers in the wildlife trade and zoo workers for detection of pathogen and/or antibodies, will be able to detect primary transmission. Efforts to prevent secondary transmission should include awareness and behavioural modification campaign. This 'risk reduction' measure helped in the control of Lassa fever in Sierra Leone and was undertaken by Pike et al. (2010) for the Cameroonian bushmeat hunters.

References

Pike BL, Saylors KE, Fair JN, LeBreton M et al (2010) The origin and prevention of pandemics. Emerg Infect 50:1636–1640

Wolfe ND, Dunavan CP, Diamond J (2007) Origins of major human infectious diseases. Nature 447(7142):279–283

Chapter 2
Wildlife Zoonoses

2.1 Introduction

Forests are host to a highly diverse wildlife population with pathogens in a state of endemic equilibrium, which evolved and are maintained through natural ecological processes and homogeneity. A complex mixture of niches is naturally available in each landscape and habitat to support animals, insects and microscopic parasites. Diversity in the wild host population promotes a broad pool of pathogens and a source. Low diversity in the domestic animal host promotes the expansion of the pathogen after spillover. Disruption of the state of equilibrium causes the 'spillover' and emergence of zoonoses. Biodiversity and opportunities for contact are key to the transmission and emergence of diseases. Transferring from this huge store of insects and microbes in the natural habitat is possible. Nearly 72% of zoonoses originated in wildlife, including emerging and re-emerging ones. Zoonoses at the livestock-wildlife interface seriously threaten global health security and endangered wildlife species.

Human and wildlife share the same space. Bera, the Rabari pastoral region in the Aravalli hills in India, has one of the largest concentrations of leopards on earth. Rabaris are shepherds living in close proximity to them, without any attacks by leopards. They treat leopards with respect. *Ambe Devi*, the deity, has a leopard as her *vahan*. An example of grassroots-level wildlife conservation is to provide food to wildlife: Tigers venture out of the sanctuary and kills sheep/goats in villages. It is said it happens because tigers do not get their food—say deer. The new approach is to develop a sheep/goat/deer farm in the forest to meet the requirement. Wildlife volunteers work to prevent poaching. They are an auxiliary staff in the forest/sanctuaries.

© Springer Nature Singapore Pte Ltd. 2024
K. G. Narayan et al., *Handbook of Management of Zoonoses*,
https://doi.org/10.1007/978-981-99-9885-2_2

2.2   Wildlife as a Source of Zoonoses

Anthropogenic activities in the recent past have reduced the distance between humans and wildlife. These activities encroached on wildlife habitats and include agriculture and animal husbandry practices, wildlife trade, translocation of wild animals, consumption of bushmeat, wet market, exotic foods, ecotourism, wildlife safari, adventure sports, exotic pets, petting zoos and migration of wild animals. High-risk groups are biologists, field assistants, workers in forests, hunters, those who prepare meat and those who engaged in trade. Infection may be acquired either within a specific locality primarily or secondarily, occupationally and avocationally.

The similarity of human and non-human primates at the anatomical, cellular and molecular levels offers a field for seeding similar harmful and harmless microbes. Rodents share human habitation besides their natural holes in earth in fields, i.e. urban-rural-wild linkage. They have great adaptability. This bridge brings infectious agents to the synanthropic nidus. Bats and insects are naturally sylvatic. Their flying nature enable them to disburse infectious agents from their natural habitat and autochthonous nidii even beyond mosaic-penetrating villages adjoining forests.

Primates, rodents and bats harbour zoonotic viruses more than any other order of mammals. Bats have more zoonotic viruses than any other mammal group and birds in terms of viral diversity relative to host diversity because bats are the second most diverse order of mammals.

Luis et al. (2013) compared bats and rodents as reservoirs of zoonotic viruses. Bats are the natural reservoirs of a number of high-impact viral zoonoses. They observed that the rodent species are nearly twice the number of bat species. The number of viruses identified in bat hosts is 61 compared to 68 in rodents. Bats and rodents host many pathogens affecting humans. The former host more zoonotic viruses per species. The species of bats whose distribution is overlapping with a greater number of sympatric (same taxonomic order) species have smaller litters (one), more litters/year and greater longevity and generally host more zoonotic viruses. Interspecies transmission is more common than in rodents.

The health of wildlife, livestock, pets and humans must be protected. Pathogens know no barriers. At the same time, inclusive health system is so huge and wide that no single sector can handle it. Anthroponotic pathogens (affecting only humans) fall in the domain of the health sector. Livestock and pet animals' diseases are tackled by the veterinary sector. The veterinary sector and wildlife managers manage diseases in zoos and wild animals.

According to Bengis et al. (2004), zoonotic diseases emerging from wild animals appear to follow two patterns. In the first pattern, transmission of pathogens to humans is rare, but once it has happened, the pathogen is transmitted from human to human. The pathogen is subsequently maintained in humans temporarily or permanently. Examples are Marburg disease, SIV/HIV, influenza A, Ebola and SARS. The second pattern is exemplified by directly transmitted rabies and other lyssa viruses, nipah virus, leptospirosis, vector-borne west Nile virus, lyme borreliosis and plague. In these, the principal reservoir is a population of wild animals and man-to-man transmission is rare. Zoonoses increase the burden on the human healthcare system. The former pattern of transmission has almost always caused serious illness and pandemic and added considerably to the burden of nosocomial zoonoses. All these impact agricultural production, wildlife-based economies and wildlife conservation.

2.3   Wildlife-Associated Zoonoses

Avian influenza virus, West Nile virus, viral encephalitis, Hendra virus, viral haemorrhagic fever (e.g. Ebola), hantavirus (HPS, HRS/HFRS), monkeypox, Nipah virus, Rift Valley fever, mosquito-borne viral encephalitis, rabies, severe acute respiratory syndrome (SARS-coronavirus), Colorado tick fever, brucellosis, Streptobacillus moniliformis (rat bite fever), salmonellosis, tuberculosis, Lyme disease, rickettsial pox, murine typhus, Rocky Mountain spotted fever, leptospirosis, tularaemia, plague, psittacosis, ehrlichiosis, giardiasis, echinococcosis, trichinellosis, Baylisascaris procyonis (raccoon roundworm), histoplasmosis. (Sources: Dhama et al. 2013, McLean 1994).

Wildlife-associated zoonoses can be grouped as (a) contact-borne and (b) broadcast diseases.

2.3.1   Wildlife Contact-Borne Diseases

Mycobacteriosis: Old World monkeys are more susceptible to tuberculosis than New World monkeys: 74% *Mycobacterium tuberculosis* and 24% *M. bovis*. The rest of the reported infections are due to *M. africanum, M. kansasii, M. intracellulare, M. scrofulaceum* and *M. paratuberculosis*.

Chimpanzees, sooty mangabey, *Rhesus* and African green monkeys are infected with *M. leprae*. Pet marmoset causes TB in pet owners.

2.3.2   Wildlife Broadcast Diseases

These are rabies, avian influenza, severe acute respiratory syndrome (SARS), viral encephalitis and haemorrhagic fever, Hendra and Nipah viral infections, Rift Valley fever, monkeypox, Kyasanur forest disease (KFD), brucellosis, leptospirosis, Lyme disease, psittacosis, plague, tuberculosis and human monocytic or parasitic ehrlichiosis, alveolar echinococcosis. It is difficult to prevent their spread.

2.4   Animal Reservoirs

According to a study on wildlife-livestock interaction made jointly by the International Livestock Research Institute, Nairobi and Royal Veterinary College, London (Grace and Jones 2011), 82% of 292 zoonoses had a wildlife reservoir, 74% had a domestic animal reservoir and 60% had both a wildlife and a domestic animal reservoir. At the interface, 61 diseases (including some unproven zoonoses) were identified, impacting negatively on people, domestic animals, wildlife and the ecosystem. Nearly half of these adopted multiple contact routes of transmission, while others adopted different routes. Single transmission routes were direct, vector-borne or foodborne.

2.5   Opportunities of Contact and Transmission of Diseases

- *Livestock farming*—Badgers in the United Kingdom and brush-tailed possums in New Zealand are sources of infection for *M. bovis*. Intensification of animal farming without matching regulation, biosecurity and surveillance leads to spillover and spread of pathogens from wildlife to farmed animals and further to humans (mycobacteria, *Brucella*, hepatitis E, anthrax, *E. coli* O157:H7, *Salmonella*, *Campylobacter*, etc.). Scavenging birds (vultures) and carnivores may acquire infection from carcasses of domestic animals and human wastes improperly disposed of and spread these further. Infected livestock and human may transmit infection to wildlife.
- *Agricultural activities*—result in multi-species land use, or 'buffer zones'.
  Livestock-human-wildlife share the same space, resulting in increased contact and the chance of transmitting certain pathogens, e.g. Argentine haemorrhagic fever—corn plantations supported the main virus reservoir, the corn mouse. Nipah (RNA) virus switched (for bat and human isolates identical in some outbreaks, adaptation may not be necessary) from fruit bats to pigs and horses or from fruit bats to pigs to humans. Deforestation, ecological and landscape changes for intensive pig farming and fruit tree plantation forced bats to encroach in the agricultural zone, resulting in devastating economic loss in Malaysia.
- *Human habitat/agri-expansion—encroaching forest*
  Examples are Chikungunya, Kyasanur forest disease and Lyme disease (*Borrelia burgdorferi*). These are vector-borne. Human activities helped the abundance of vectors (and often also the density of hosts). Similarly, West Nile virus transmission required high mosquito density. The persistence of *Yersinia pestis* in established foci is related to the abundance of reservoirs and vectors.
- *Trade in livestock and live wild animals for exotic pets, zoos or consumption*
  Trade in livestock and poultry involves movement and congregation and is likely to disperse and disseminate infectious organisms, for example, live poultry market—HPAI; international trade in wild birds causes the spread of H5N1.

The cattle trade introduced the Rift Valley fever to Egypt from the Arabian Peninsula. Monkeypox spread by the trade of African rodent reservoirs from Ghana to prairie dogs and spread to humans in importing countries. Contact with infected parakeets caused psittacosis among customs officers in Belgium. A contact of even 2 h was 3× more risky than lesser contact time.

- *Wet/live animal market*
  Infected, susceptible and amplifying hosts, including wildlife, are put together, offering opportunity for cross-species transmission. A cycle of transmission is established in the wet market. Bats for foods or medicine—masked palm civet (*Paguma larvata*)-man cycle –resulted in SARS-CoV. A cycle of SARS-COVs (RNA virus)—bats-Himalayan palm civets and related carnivores and switching to humans with some adaptation for binding human ACE2 receptors—led to the pandemic.
- *Consumption of bushmeat*
  Hunting and butchering caused infection, e.g. *B. suis* from wild boars, Ebola from chimpanzees, trichinellosis from eating boar meat, and cross-species transmission of several retroviruses in humans, e.g. simian immunodeficiency virus (SIV) and simian T-lymphotropic virus (STLV) from nonhuman primate (NHP) bushmeat in wild or captivity.
- *Wildlife management for conservation or recreational hunting*
  This can increase the population size and density of wildlife species resulting in higher disease prevalence in wildlife and increased risk of spillover to livestock, for example, *Mycobacterium bovis*.
  Recreational hunting in southern Spain led to an intensive management system—translocation of animals such as wild boars and red deer; feeding, watering and fencing on private estates; and sharing of resources for livestock. European wild boar is a maintenance host for bovine tuberculosis in the Spanish Mediterranean ecosystem. High prevalence in cattle, wild boar and red deer in the same areas has been observed. There, humans are infected with the same genotypes of *Mycobacterium tuberculosis* complex (MTBC).
  An opposite situation in Michigan supports the relationship between recreational farms and bovine tuberculosis. Managemental changes in the recreational hunting of white-tailed deer with supplemental feeding and fencing led to a doubling of the population and a simultaneous increase in the prevalence of *M. bovis*. Bovine tuberculosis was eliminated from cattle in Michigan, but it re-emerged.
- *International trade and travel*
  Chikungunya virus—spread to several countries is attributed to the spread of *Aedes albopictus* from the western Pacific and South Asia to Africa and the Middle East, North and South America and Europe, mainly to the international trade in used tyres in which mosquito eggs have been laid. *Aedes* spp. feed on subclinically infected primates and lay eggs that are transovarially infected. Chikungunya caused major outbreaks in India, Malaysia and Sri Lanka.
- *Migratory birds*
  West Nile-vector-borne-polyhostal: Rapidly spread through infected migratory (American robins) and resident birds (sparrows, blue jays) and the competent

mosquito vector *Culex pipiens* to cause epidemics in humans and wild birds by
dispersing mosquitoes. Human activities also assist mosquitoes' spread.

- *Man and his animals encroaching on forest*
  Brucellosis and, most likely, bovine tuberculosis also infected wildlife—bison
  and white-tailed deer. After the two diseases have been controlled in the livestock, the wildlife source is also threatened. Kyasanur forest disease is a tick-
  borne disease affecting monkeys. Deforestation, wood cutting and cattle grazing
  under social forestry or otherwise caused epidemics in humans in India.
- *Climate change*
  It may lead to either an expansion or contraction of range or no overall change in
  an area.
  For example, in North America, the hispid cotton rat (*Sigmodon hispidus*), a
  reservoir of hantavirus, has undergone a northward and altitudinal expansion,
  and the white-footed deer mouse, a reservoir of lyme disease, human granulocytic anaplasmosis, babesiosis and hantavirus, has extended its range northwards. Climate change is likely to altering the distribution, composition and
  migration patterns of wild bird populations. They are reservoirs for avian influenza viruses. Transmission between wild bird species, wild birds and domestic
  poultry will be consequently affected.
  Intensification of livestock farming led to deforestation and related disturbance
  of ecological equilibrium and endemicity, carbon emission, climate change and
  related expansion or contraction of natural niches of infectious agents.

2.6   General Preventive Measures

- *General—anthropause*
  The coronavirus disease 2019 (COVID-19) caused a pandemic. Lockdown all
  over the world was adopted to prevent its spread. The related and astonishing
  side effect was a clean environment. It appears that nature's autocorrect mechanism repaired the damages done by anthropogenic activities. A valuable lesson
  was learnt—let the entire world observe a '2-month vacation with no outdoor
  activities'.
- *General education/awareness*
  Public awareness, especially for livestock farmers, and pastoralist communities,
  about forests, wildlife and conservation, poaching and trade, and related laws
  and regulations.
- *Surveillance* for zoonotic infections in wild animals and trade of wildlife and
  their products.
  Smith et al. (2012) observed that wildlife trade posed a health risk to the public,
  agricultural industry and native wildlife—monkeypox, exotic Newcastle disease
  and amphibian chytridiomycosis in wildlife imported to the United States were

cited as respective examples. They detailed the methods for surveillance of zoo-notic infections in confiscated wildlife products. Initial findings of screening at the airports of parts from rodents and national health mission (NHM) identified retroviruses (simian foamy virus) and/or herpesviruses (cytomegalovirus and lymphocryptovirus) in the non-human primate (NHP) samples.

- *Health services* to protect human infections with 'reverse zoonoses' like *M. tuberculosis* to protect wildlife.
- *Veterinary services* to protect wildlife from disease of livestock (e.g. *Brucella* spp.) and pets (e.g. *Toxoplasma*) spilling over.

2.7   Care of Occupational Exposure

- *Personal protection*
  Rangers and workers in forests and zoos are occupationally exposed. They need a vaccine protection against known diseases/sets of diseases identified on the basis of the species of animals they care for. For example, those caring canids need prophylactic protection against rabies.
  Sick animals essentially require approaching and handling. Extreme precaution has to be taken. Using masks and hand gloves helps protect against direct contact and airborne infections and respiratory and fungal infections. Basic hygiene, personal protective equipment—clothing/overall to protect against insects and rubber or plastic gloves—cleaning equipment such as dissecting/skinning knives, etc. are necessary. Safe disposal of carcasses or tissues and disposables and proper washing, cleaning and disinfecting of reusables need to be practised.
- *Location specific*
  Insecticide applications to control vectors like ticks, fleas and mosquitoes may be done in specific areas (refer to wildlife-associated diseases—rodents).
- *Accidental exposure*
  Immediately reporting to a physician after exposure/in case of developing/experiencing abnormal signs of health after exposure should be a part of standard operative procedure.
- *Diligent practice*
  A low level (3.7%) of wildlife health professionals had zoonotic disease. Despite near-optimal awareness of various hazards, preventive measures are minimally practised. Wildlife health professionals should diligently practice precautionary measures themselves and see their staff working with them also do so (Nigam and Shrivastav 2011).

2.8   Preventing Wildlife-Originated Zoonoses

• *Management of interfaces (e.g. wildlife-livestock-human)*
Human-ecosystem interaction is dynamic and has been happening since the
appearance of humans. The impact of dynamism on human health has been
imperceptible because of sustained balanced human-ecosystem interaction. It is
strongly believed that the altered balance of human-ecosystem interactions led to
the spillover of infectious agents from the natural niche in the forest at the
wildlife-human interface to cause pandemics.
An *interface* may be defined as a boundary across which parasites can be passed
between biological communities. Interface (e.g. human-livestock-wildlife) consists of the community of species on both sides of the boundary and the biotic
niches within which these communities exist.
Ecotone: edges or transitional zones between adjacent ecological systems
where biophysical factors, biological activity and ecological and evolutionary
processes are concentrated and intensified.
The emergence of several zoonoses, Lyme disease, Nipah virus encephalitis,
hantavirus and pulmonary syndrome has been associated with ecotones.
Natural or original biome gets fragmented due to anthropogenic activities (e.g.
land-use change) into patches of original biome and new matrices with 'interfaces' between the two and can be classed as ecotones with edges or transitional
zones between the two adjacent ecological systems. Anthropogenic activities,
such as farming, and human settlements shorten the distance between pathogens,
reservoir hosts (wildlife or domestic animals) and vectors increasing the risk of
transmission. Wild rodents at the interface may be attracted to farmland and
human settlements for resources and breeding.
Interfaces may be diverse, e.g. wildlife-human interface, wildlife-livestock-
human interfaces. The latter offers an opportunity of increasing contact between
humans, livestock and wildlife (both non-synanthropic and synanthropic species). Interfaces represent a critical point for cross-species transmission and the
emergence of diseases.
Understanding of the interfaces is necessary for defining suitable interventions to
prevent the emergence of diseases (Hassell et al. 2017). The following is an illustrative example:
An evolving urban landscape is seen increasing intensive farming, low biosecurity, backyard farming and large dumps of wastes ignoring the 'interfaces/eco-
tone'. There is a consequential increase in contact between humans, livestock
and synanthropic wildlife. There is every likelihood of the emergence and re-
emergence of zoonoses.

Conscious about the 'interface/ecotone', the urban landscape is managed, and animal farms have high biosecurity, and wastes and sewage are treated at plants. Parks, gardens and recreational facilities that are suitable habitats for wildlife are also managed. The opportunity of contact between human, livestock and wildlife is minimized.

- *Protection from animals*
  Multiple pathogens can originate from a single type of animal, e.g. *Mycobacterium bovis*, *Brucella suis*, *B. melitensis*, *B. abortus*, *Coxiella burnetii*, *Yersinia pestis* and *Leptospira* spp., among others from wild boars. Rodents are a source of 36 pathogens (Appendix A) and non-human primates to about 27 pathogenic species (Appendix C). Many factors influence the risk of zoonotic transmission from wildlife, such as density of wildlife, intensity of infection in wildlife reservoirs, nature of contact transmission and human encroachment in wildlife habitats. The following are contemplated intervention approaches:
  Reducing vectors, e.g. *ticks*
  Burning bushes, managing landscape and local ecology such as around water bodies to promote health in animals and manipulating stocking densities.
  Control of wildlife population
  Culling and birth control—Sustenance of rabies virus in wildlife niche required two foxes/sq m density. Gassing fox dens was once practised to control the spread of rabies from wildlife. Culling of badgers is effective in tackling bovine tuberculosis in England, Australia and Ireland. One culling was effective for 6.5 years.
  Managing disease in wildlife
  By vaccinations, oral rabies vaccination of foxes, skunks, raccoons, etc.

According to Karim (2021), there is a general agreement that 'the human-animal interface will continue to worsen with deforestation and climate change; sustainability in living habitats of human populations and wildlife is necessary to prevent further pandemics from occurring'.

References

A_Systematic_review_of_zoonoses_at_the_i.pdf Zoonoses (Project 1) Wildlife/domestic livestock interactions. A final report to the Department for International Development, UK. Submitted by: The International Livestock Research Institute, Nairobi & Royal Veterinary College, London. Report editors: Delia Grace and Bryony Jones. September 25th 2011

Bengis RG, Leighton FA, Fischer JR, Artois M, Mörner T, Tate CM (2004) The role of wildlife in emerging and re-emerging zoonoses. Rev Sci Tech 23(2):497–511

Dhama K, Karthik K, Chakraborty S, Tiwari R, Kapoor S (2013) Wildlife: a hidden warehouse of zoonoses—a review. Int J Curr Res 5(7):1866–1879

Hassell JM, Begon M, Ward MJ, Fèvre EM (2017) Urbanization and disease emergence: dynamics at the wildlife-livestock-human Interface. Trends Ecol Evol 32(1):55–67

Karim W (2021) Zoonoses, Human encroachments and trafficking in wildlife. Academia Letters 3858. https://doi.org/10.20935/AL3858

Luis AD, Hayman DT, O'Shea TJ, Cryan PM, Gilbert AT et al (2013) A comparison of bats and rodents as reservoirs of zoonotic viruses: are bats special? Proc Biol Sci 280(1756):20122753

McLean RG (1994) Wildlife diseases and humans. In: The handbook: prevention and control of wildlife damage 38. https://digitalcommons.unl.edu/icwdmhandbook/38

Nigam P, Shrivastav A (2011) Assessing occupational hazards among Indian wildlife health professionals. Vet Archives 81:731–741

Smith KM, Anthony SJ, Switzer WM, Epstein JH, Seimon T et al (2012) Zoonotic viruses associated with illegally imported wildlife products. PLoS One 7(1):e29505

Chapter 3
Epidemiology Vector-Borne Diseases (VBDs)

Vectors are living organisms that can transmit infectious pathogens between humans or from animals to humans. Generally, these are insects, in which most are blood-sucking. The pathogens are ingested during a blood meal from infected hosts, human or animal, suffering from a disease or asymptomatic. The pathogens multiply in their body and are transmitted to other hosts during another blood meal. The vectors can carry pathogens through the rest of their life.

Over 17% of all infectious diseases caused by parasites, bacteria, and viruses are vector-borne, causing >700,000 deaths yearly. For example, Anopheline mosquito-transmitted parasitic disease, malaria, causes an estimated 219 million cases and 400,000 deaths annually, mostly children of 5 years of age. *Aedes* mosquito trans-mitted dengue, a viral disease prevalent in >129 countries, with 3.9 million people at risk, 96 million cases and 40,000 deaths annually. Some encephalitic diseases are caused by tick-transmitted viruses. Other vectors of diseases are triatomes for Chagas disease, sandflies for leishmaniasis and snails for schistosomiasis. Vector-borne diseases (VBDs) like dengue, Chikungunya, Zika, yellow fever and malaria have caused major outbreaks since 2014. Vector-borne diseases are the major burden in tropical and subtropical countries, disproportionately affecting the poorest populations and causing worry to the health system. Diseases like leishmaniasis and lymphatic filariasis cause chronic suffering, lifelong morbidity, disability and occasional stigmatization. A WHO list of such diseases according to vector is reproduced (Table 3.1) (https://www.who.int/news-room/fact-sheets/detail/vector-borne-diseases).

© Springer Nature Singapore Pte Ltd. 2024
K. G. Narayan et al., *Handbook of Management of Zoonoses*,
https://doi.org/10.1007/978-981-99-9885-2_3

Table 3.1 Vector-borne diseases (non-exhaustive), according to their vector (WHO)

Vector		Disease caused	Type of pathogen
Mosquito	*Aedes*	Chikungunya	Virus
		Dengue	Virus
		Lymphatic filariasis	Parasite
		Rift Valley fever	Virus
		Yellow fever	Virus
		Zika	Virus
	Anopheles	Lymphatic filariasis	Parasite
		Malaria	Parasite
	Culex	Japanese encephalitis	Virus
		Lymphatic filariasis	Parasite
		West Nile fever	Virus
Aquatic snails		Schistosomiasis (bilharziasis)	Parasite
Blackflies		Onchocerciasis (river blindness)	Parasite
Fleas		Plague (transmitted from rats to humans)	Bacteria
		Tungiasis	Ectoparasite
Lice		Typhus	Bacteria
		Louse-borne relapsing fever	Bacteria
Sandflies		Leishmaniasis	Parasite
		Sandfly fever (*Phlebotomus* fever)	Virus
Ticks		Crimean-Congo haemorrhagic fever	Virus
		Lyme disease	Bacteria
		Relapsing fever (borreliosis)	Bacteria
		Rickettsial diseases (e.g. spotted fever and Q fever)	Bacteria
		Tick-borne encephalitis	Virus
		Tularemia	Bacteria
Triatome bugs		Chagas disease (American trypanosomiasis)	Parasite
Tsetse flies		Sleeping sickness (African trypanosomiasis)	Parasite

3.1 Introduction

Zoonotic agents are polyphagous, involving essentially humans and a single or more species of animals in the infection chain. The pathogen meets a dead end if the transmission does not proceed to another man, e.g. hydatidosis. Pathogens may use invertebrates, say insects, called vectors for further transmission. A vector may be mechanical or biological. A biological vector may be providing conditions only for the propagation (propagative), development (developmental) or both (cyclopropagative) of the infectious agent. Zoonosis-causing agents requiring a combination of vertebrate and invertebrate species for their maintenance in nature are called metazoonoses. Some require a combination of one species of each vertebrate, and invertebrates like JE are subclassed as I; those requiring one vertebrate and two invertebrate species are subclassed as II. Subclass III metazoonoses require two vertebrate and one invertebrate species, e.g. clonorchiasis. Infectious agents vertically transmitted in invertebrate hosts, transovarial transmission in ticks and requiring a vertebrate species for their maintenance in nature are classed as subclass IV.

3.2 Biotope, Biotic Community and Natural Nidii

A biotope is the smallest natural location providing uniform conditions of life for an infectious agent, vector/intermediate and reservoir/definitive host and is shared by all. The members are called the biotic community. Such a pristine home of an infectious agent is the 'natural nidus/focus' of infection. This constitutes the primary source of infection or epidemic. Locating a biotope is useful in concentrating intervention activities at the site. Identification of the reservoir species in these biotopes further makes the plan more specific. An autochthonous nidus is untouched by humans and is often located deep in the forest. The infectious agent is maintained in the enzootic state by a spiral travel from a wildlife reservoir to an insect vector which in turn transfers it to another host of the same species commonly. Russian epidemiologist E. N. Pavlovsky in 1966 coined and postulated the theory of natural nidality. It states that *the existence of the natural focus of a transmissible disease depends on a continuous interaction of the quintet (five) of its prerequisites associated with a specific geographic landscape. The quintet consists of (1) animal donors, (2) vectors, (3) animal recipients, (4) the pathogenic agent itself in an infective state, and (5) the influence of factors of the external environments contributing to an unhindered transmission of infection from one organism to another (circulation of pathogenic agent)*. A balanced state maintains the biotic community of wild donor and recipient animals, vectors and pathogens in the biotope. Various factors like changing climate or anthropological reasons challenge and alter the balanced state. Pathogens, vectors and natural reservoir hosts are under constant pressure as the ecosystem is challenged. They attempt to adapt for survival. Survival mechanisms are varied. Human beings are brought in proximity to biotope. Spillover of pathogens from the biotope and transmission to new hosts and humans is facilitated to cause disease or emerging disease (re-emergence or emergence).

The range of vector activity is determined by its capacity to crawl, hop and fly. Additionally, vertebrate hosts may carry a vector, e.g. cattle as a paratenic host for Kyasanur forest disease virus or migratory birds carrying the vector of Crimean-Congo haemorrhagic fever virus (CCHFV). The range is thus determined by the hosts' range of movement.

More than 300 infectious diseases, including VBDs, mostly viral, have emerged since 1940. Above 60% are zoonotic, and 52% of all emerging infectious diseases (EIDs) recorded in the last decade of the twentieth century were zoonotic. Wildlife represented the most significant threat, as 71.8% originated from these. VBDs are serious, and many are increasingly recorded, e.g. Rocky Mountain spotted fever (RMSF), human monocytotropic (or monocytic) ehrlichiosis (HME) and human granulocytotropic (or granulocytic) anaplasmosis (HGA) (formerly known as human granulocytotropic ehrlichiosis (HGE)) (Chapman et al. 2006).

The impact of these diseases is great in the form of annual morbidity and mortality in livestock; poultry (affecting animal industries); humans (absence from workplace and cost of treatment/control measures); wildlife-based economies such as ecotourism, bushmeat trade, etc.; and wildlife conservation.

Kilpatrik and Randolph (2012) grouped VBDs into two:

- Introduced and increased areas of occurrence and incidence—e.g. WN disease in the United States (identified by vet and med clinicians in 1999 in NY city spreading from east to west coast in 4 years), dengue in Australia and Chikungunya in India
- Endemic but increased disease incidence/burden, e.g. Lyme disease in North America, tick-borne encephalitis, plague in Africa and Crimean-Congo haemorrhagic fever (CCHF) in Turkey.

A study of the incidence of tick-borne encephalitis (TBE) by Randolph and on behalf of the Emerging diseases in a changing European environment (EDEN)-TBD sub-project team (2010) in selected European countries suggests that *human foraging activities* leading to exposure to tick bites rather than abundance and questing activities of ticks explained the increased incidence of TBE. TBE incidences peaked in the months of June to August in Germany, Slovenia and Switzerland, *matching the tick abundance profile*. Yet, the exposure to tick bites happened because of *outdoor activities (recreation) of people starting in May and continued till September*. In Latvia, the high TBE incidence continued later in summer and autumn even when tick activities declined markedly compared to its peak in spring because people visited the forest for food and to gather mushrooms.

3.3 Zoonoses Transmitted by Haematophagous Arthropods

3.3.1 Hard Ticks

1. African tick typhus (also called African tick bite fever): *Rickettsia africae*
2. Babesiosis: *Babesia microti*
3. Crimean-Congo haemorrhagic fever: *Crimean-Congo haemorrhagic fever virus (Nairo virus)* Human granulocytotropic anaplasmosis (HGA), also known as human granulocytic ehrlichiosis (HGE)
4. Sennetsu fever: *Anaplasma phagocytophilum*
5. Human ehrlichiosis: *Ehrlichia ewingii*
6. Human monocytic ehrlichiosis (HME): *Ehrlichia chaffeensis*
7. Lyme disease (European version called tick-borne encephalitis): *Borrelia burgdorferi*
8. Kyasanur forest disease (also known as monkey disease): *Kyasanur forest disease virus (Flavivirus)*

3.3.2 Soft Ticks

Tick-borne relapsing fever—*Borrelia hermsii, B. turicatae* and *B. parkeri.*

3.3.3   Lice

1. Trench fever (also called Wolhynia fever, shinbone fever, quintan fever, 5-day fever, Meuse fever, His disease and His-Werner disease): *Bartonella quintana*

3.3.4   Mosquitoes

1. Bagaza virus: Bagaza virus (*Flavivirus*)
2. Banna virus: Banna virus (*Seadomavirus*)
3. Barmah forest: *Barmah Forest virus* (*Alphavirus*)
4. California encephalitis (viral encephalitis): California encephalitis virus (*Orthobunyavirus*)
5. Chikungunya fever: *Chikungunya virus* (*Alphavirus*)
6. Dengue fever (also called dengue haemorrhagic fever, dengue shock syndrome): *dengue virus* (*Flavivirus*)
7. Eastern equine encephalitis (EEE): *Eastern equine encephalitis virus* (*Alphavirus*)
8. Filariasis (also called lymphatic filariasis or elephantiasis): *Wuchereria bancrofti*
9. Guama virus: Guama virus (*Orthobunyavirus*)
10. Japanese encephalitis (also known as Japanese B encephalitis): *Japanese encephalitis virus* (*Flavivirus*)
11. Leptospirosis: *Leptospira interrogans*
12. Malaria: *Plasmodium* spp.—*Plasmodium falciparum* and *Plasmodium vivax*
13. Mayaro virus fever: *Mayaro virus* (*Alphavirus*)
14. Murray Valley encephalitis (formerly known as Australian encephalitis): *Murray Valley encephalitis virus* (*Flavivirus*)
15. O'nyong nyong fever: *O'nyong-nyong virus* (*Alphavirus*)
16. Oropouche fever: *Oropouche virus* (*Orthobunyavirus*)
17. Rift Valley fever: *Rift Valley fever virus* (*Phlebovirus*)
18. Ross River epidemic polyarthritis (also known as Ross River fever): *Ross River virus* (*Alphavirus*)
19. Shigellosis: *Shigella dysenteriae*
20. Sindbis fever: *Sindbis virus* (*Alphavirus*)
21. St. Louis encephalitis (SLE): *St. Louis encephalitis virus* (*Flavivirus*)
22. Venezuelan equine encephalitis: *Venezuelan equine encephalitis virus* (*Alphavirus*)
23. Western equine encephalitis (WEE): *Western equine encephalitis virus* (*Alphavirus*)
24. Wesselsbron: *Wesselsbron virus* (*Flavivirus*)
25. West Nile illness, West Nile fever, West Nile neurological illness: *West Nile virus* (WNV) (*Flavivirus*)
26. Yellow fever (also called yellow jack, black vomit or *vomito negro* in Spanish or sometimes American plague): *Yellow fever virus* (*Flavivirus*)
27. Zika fever: *Zika virus* (*Flavivirus*)

3.3.5   Sandflies

1. Sandfly fever: Salehabad virus
2. Sandfly fever: Naples virus (*Phlebovirus*)
3. Leishmaniasis (visceral, cutaneous and mucocutaneous leishmaniasis, kala-azar, dumdum fever): *Leishmania donovani, Leishmania donovani infantum* and *Leishmania donovani chagasi*

3.3.6   Tsetse Fly/Reduviid Bugs

1. Sleeping sickness (also known as African trypanosomiasis, Nagana): *Trypanosoma brucei*
2. Chagas disease (also known as American trypanosomiasis): *Trypanosoma cruzi*

3.3.7   Deer Flies/Blackflies

1. Loa loa filariasis (also called loiasis and African eyeworm): *Loa loa* River blindness (also known as onchocerciasis): *Onchocerca volvulus*

3.3.8   Fleas

1. Cat-scratch fever (also called cat-scratch disease, cat-scratch adenitis, cat-scratch-oculoglandular syndrome, Debre's syndrome and Debre-Mollaret syndrome
2. Foshay-Mollaret cat-scratch fever, Foshay-Mollaret syndrome and Foshay-Mollaret cat-scratch
3. Fever syndrome, lymphadenitis (regional, nonbacterial), lymphoreticulosis (benign inoculation), maladie des griffes du chat, Parinaud oculoglandular disease and Petzetakis' disease): *Bartonella henselae* and *Bartonella clarridgeiae*
4. Murine typhus: *Rickettsia typhi, Rickettsia felis* and *Rickettsia prowazekii*
   Total = 43
   Source: Linda Vrbova et al. (2009) (Table 3.2)

Arthropods are cold-blooded (ectothermic) and, therefore, sensitive to weather and climate changes. Climate influences their habitat, survival, reproduction rate, capacity and competence.

Table 3.2 Summary of some tick-borne diseases (Source: Tick-borne diseases [http://www.emedicinehealth.com/ticks/article_em.htm, *Institutional animal care and use committee of University of California, Santa Barbara])

Disease	Infectious agent	Ticks	Non-human hosts	Reported in
Kyasanur forest disease	KFDV, a *Flavivirus*	*Haemaphysalis spinigera* and *Ixodes* spp.	Black-faced langurs (*Semnopithecus, earlier Presbytis entellus*), red-faced bonnet monkeys (*Macaca radiata*), rats (*Rattus blanfordi, Rattus rattus wroughtoni*), shrews (*Suncus murinus*) and bat (*Rhinolophus rouxii*). Experimentally KFDV infected and caused high viraemia in black-naped hare, porcupines, flying squirrel, Malabar giant squirrel, gerbil, mice, long-tailed tree mice and shrews	Karnataka, India, Saudi Arabia, China
Southern tick-associated rash illness (STARI)	*Borrelia lonestari*	*Amblyomma americanum*	White-tailed deer	Several southeastern and south-central states, including Georgia, Maryland, Missouri, North Carolina and South Carolina of the United States

(continued)

Table 3.2 (continued)

Disease	Infectious agent	Ticks	Non-human hosts	Reported in
Ehrlichiosis *Synonym: tick-borne fever	*Ehrlichia ewingii, E. chaffeensis, E. canis* Family Anaplasmataceae, genus Ehrlichia*	*Amblyomma americanum, R. sanguineus* Also mites: Leptotrombidium deliense, Liponyssoides sanguineus*	Deer, dogs	Worldwide* South-central and south-eastern states of America
Anaplasmosis (human granulocytic anaplasmosis (HGA))	*Anaplasma phagocytophilum* Family *Anaplasmataceae, genus Anaplasma*	*Ixodes* spp.	Deer, elk and wild rodents	New England and the north-central and Pacific regions of the United State
Lyme disease *Synonyms: **Lyme arthritis, Bannwarth's syndrome, tick-borne meningo-polyneuritis, erythema chronicum migrans (ECM), Steere's disease**	A spirochaete— *Borrelia afzelii* and *B. garinii* in Europe and *B. burgdorferi* sensu lato in America and other places	*Ixodes scapularis* in North America and *I. pacificus* in the west coast of the United States *I. ricinus* in Europe, *I. persulcatus* in China	Rodents	Europe, Russia, Mongolia, Japan, China, America, Canada, Brazil, Morocco, Algeria, Egypt, Tunisia, Kenya in Africa
Tick-borne relapsing fever *Synonyms: **spirochetal fever, vagabond fever, famine fever**	*Borrelia hermsii, B. turicatae, B. parkeri*	*Ornithodoros hermsii, O. turicata, O. parkeri*	Wild rodents-ground and tree squirrels, chipmunks, prairie dogs, burrowing owls	Spain, Saudi Arabia, Canada, Africa, the Americas (North, Central and South), Asia, parts of Europe
Tularemia *Synonyms: **Francis' disease, deer fly fever, rabbit fever, O'Hara disease**	*Francisella tularensis*	*Dermacentor variabilis, Amblyomma americanum*	***Rabbits, squirrels, muskrats, deer, bull snakes, sheep, wild rodents, cats and dogs**	

(continued)

Table 3.2   (continued)

Disease	Infectious agent	Ticks	Non-human hosts	Reported in
Babesiosis	*Babesia microti*, *B. divergens*	*Ixodes* spp.	*White-footed mouse, white-tailed deer	***Coastal and island areas of the northeast and mid-Atlantic states, as well as Wisconsin, Minnesota and California. *B. divergens* occurs in Europe. Other areas: China, Japan, Taiwan, Egypt, Mexico, South Africa**
Colorado tick fever	*Coltivirus* (RNA)	*Dermacentor andersoni*	Golden-mantled ground squirrel (*Citellus lateralis*)	Colorado, United States
Powassan encephalitis	RNA arbovirus	*Ixodes* spp., *Dermacentor andersoni*	Woodchuck (groundhog) and others like squirrels and chipmunks	United States, Canada
Rocky Mountain spotted fever *Synonyms: **American tick typhus, tick-borne typhus fever**	*Rickettsia rickettsii*	*Dermacentor variabilis*, *D. andersoni*, *Rhipicephalus sanguineus*, *Amblyomma cajennense*	*Dogs, wild rodents, rabbits	*USA, mostly south-central, south-Atlantic states
Q fever *Synonyms: **Query fever, Balkan influenza, Balkan grippe, pneumorickettsiosis, abattoir fever**	*Coxiella burnetii*	*R. sanguineus*, *Dermacentor andersoni*, *Amblyomma americanum*	*Wild animals with ticks, domestic animals—sheep, goats, cattle, dogs, chicken (+ Python Yadav's work)	Worldwide except New Zealand

(continued)

Table 3.2 (continued)

Disease	Infectious agent	Ticks	Non-human hosts	Reported in
Indian tick typhus	*R. conorii*	*Rhipicephalus sanguineus and also other ticks*	*Rodents (Rattus* spp., *Otomys irroratus, Rhabdomys pumilio or striped mouse), rabbits and dogs*	*Asia, including India, East and South Africa and the Mediterranean region*
Crimean-Congo haemorrhagic fever, Congo fever, Central Asian haemorrhagic fever, Hungribta (blood taking), Khunymuny (nose bleeding), Karakhalak (black death)	CCHFV group; family *Bunyaviridae*, genus *Nairovirus*	Principally *Hyalomma*, transovarial, transstadial and venereal. Other ticks: *Rhipicephalus, Boophilus, Dermacentor* and *Ixodes*	European hares, Middle African hedgehogs and multimammate rats are principal reservoirs Viraemia also occurs in cattle, sheep, goats, hares, hedgehogs, dogs and mice	Africa, Middle East, Asia and Southern Europe

3.4 Vector Competence

Vector competence is the ability to acquire, maintain and transmit infectious agents. A vector acquires a virus while feeding on a viraemic host. Demonstration of virus in the salivary glands of vector or transmission to a host through feeding demonstrates 'maintenance'. The number of successful transmissions determines the 'infection rate'. Vertical transmission of the virus from the mother vector to progenies is another maintenance mechanism. Besides, this is a mechanism of 'maintenance of the infectious agent in the biotope'. If the infected mother vector hibernates in winter, this is an 'overwintering' mechanism.

3.5 Vector Capacity

Vector capacity is similar to the 'contact rate' in directly transmitted infections. It depends upon (a) vector density relative to vertebrate hosts, (b) frequency of bites (biting rate), (c) biting preference such as anthrophilic (human)/zoophilic (other mammals)/ornithophilic (birds), (d) biting habits—day/night-time, (e) extrinsic incubation period (duration of replication of infectious agent in the vector) and (f) vectors' daily survival rate (ability to survive from one day to the next, expressed as 0–1).

3.5.1   Factors Determining Vector Capacity

3.5.1.1   Weather

Vectors and microbial survival, replication and development in them are greatly influenced by weather. For example, city-dwelling mosquitoes, such as *Culex pipiens* and *C. modestus*, multiply and increase in density around water sources where avian hosts abound when temperature and humidity are high; the latter is aggressive, as has been observed during the WNV epidemic period (Epstein 2001; Ludwig et al. 2005).

Knowledge of the geographical distribution of vectors is important for the application of control measures targeted/limited to that area. For example, *I. scapularis* is the tick vector in the East and Midwest states and *I. pacificus* in the Pacific Northwest, and *A. phagocytophilum* causes human granulocytic anaplasmosis (HGA). Outside the United States, in the temperate regions, *I. ricinus* and *I. persulcatus* are the primary vectors. The major mammalian reservoir for *A. phagocytophilum* in the eastern United States is the white-footed mouse, *Peromyscus leucopus.*

A single insect species may be a vector of more than one pathogen, e.g. a single tick specimen (*Dermacentor variabilis)* was found to carry *Rickettsia bellii, R. montanensis* and *R. rickettsii* (Carmichael and Fuerst 2010). In the same way, a single vertebrate species may simultaneously host more than one pathogen (Lee and Chae 2010; O'Guinn et al. 2010). About 10% of patients with HGA show serologic evidence of coinfection with Lyme disease (*Borrelia burgdorferi*), babesiosis or tick-borne meningoencephalitis in some endemic areas. Mixed infection presents a problem in treatment.

3.5.1.2   The Dynamism of the Vector-Pathogen-Host Relationship

The vector and host and their population are dynamic and responsive to changing climate and environment (driven by nature or human activities). The relationship between vector, host and agent is interrelated. If the maximum reproduction number (individuals likely to be infected) is R_0 and the effective pathogen reproduction number is R_{eff}, then *high vector population relative to host population (mosquito population during summer and rains and pathogens like Plasmodium, Dengue, Chikungunya, etc) and (b) high susceptible host population will result in the effective pathogen reproduction number (R_{eff}) close to the maximum (R_0).*

The resulting pattern of disease in the population would be rapid spread, a substantial number of cases appearing shortly after introduction. High Chikungunya virus viraemia in acute human cases and mosquito population result in increased R_{eff}. The transmission of VBPs is generally less efficient when vectors feed on several hosts compared to when they feed almost entirely on people (one host). There is a selective pressure on zoonotic pathogens (especially for those human beings who are dead-end hosts) to adapt to be efficiently transmitted by human specialist vectors like *A. gambiae* and *A. aegypti* to a slightly lesser extent *A. albopictus* (that feed sometimes on non-human mammals and birds) when human population is abundant. Increase in such human specialist vectors increases opportunities for transmission.

3.6 Drivers of VBDs

Extending the theory of natural nidality to the understanding of EIDs has led to the identification of the (a) causes or 'drivers' that challenge a 'balanced ecosystem/ landscape' and (b) bridges between pathogen and susceptible population. This understanding is needed to plan control measures (Daszak et al. 2001).

Drivers for VBDs could be either 'micro' or 'macro' (Chomel et al. 2007).

Micro, e.g. genetic change mutation in pathogens, vectors or both. Examples:

– *The "evolutionary convergence" occurring in nature driven directly as a consequence of human activities led to rapid adaptation of CHIKV to ecological perturbance. A mutation at residue 226 of the membrane fusion glycoprotein E1 (E1-A226V) was detected in more than 90% of Chikungunya virus isolates from Reunion Island after September 2005. This reduced the cholesterol dependence of the virus to infect mosquito hosts and facilitated and enhanced the replication and transmission of the virus by Aedes albopictus (de Lamballerie et al. 2008; D'Ortenzio et al. 2011).*
– *After introduction into new locations, the virus comes across new anthrophilic vectors and tends to mutate. The original WNV (NY99) was replaced by the new WNV (WN02), which differed—three consensus nucleotide changes enabling increased transmission efficiency in Culex pipiens and C. tarsalis.*

Macro drivers may be:

3.6.1 Modification of Habitats

• Deforestation—e.g. KFD
• Communities and settlement encroaching natural habitat—e.g. Lyme disease
• Water resource management—e.g. schistosomiasis

3.6.2 Human Behaviour

• Ecotourism—e.g. tick-borne infections like rickettsial infections
• Transport—e.g. transport of mosquito-larva like *Aedes aegypti* (dengue, yellow fever, Chikungunya virus, etc.)
• Socioeconomic—e.g. Plague in Africa vs plague in Asia and tick-borne encephalitis in Eastern (e.g. communist countries) vs Western Europe (historically free market)

3.6.3   Climate Change

Climatic change-derived warming has led to expanding areas of Lyme disease in Canada, and it is suggested by Leighton et al. (2012) that the range of the tick *I. scapularis* will expand by 46 km/year over the next decade.

Expansion of the existing areas of vector activity, e.g. of *Ixodes ricinus* and *I. persulcatus*, increased the burden of diseases like Lyme disease, ehrlichiosis, rickettsiosis and tick-borne encephalitis in Europe and Eurasia.

3.6.4   Anthropogenic Changes

Changes in land use and political unrest and socioeconomic conditions
Changes in land use bring about habitat changes of wildlife and vectors and often reduce the distance between these and domestic animals and the human population, thus increasing chances of exposure and disease emergence.

Reforestation in northeastern parts of North America led to recolonization by deer and consequential expansion of the range of *I. persulcatus* in the twentieth century. This is the reason considered for the emergence of Lyme disease.

CCHF cases rose sporadically from about 20 in 2002 to 1400 (epidemic) in 2008 in Turkey. Most cases occurred in agricultural workers through tick bites and direct contact with infected animals. The abundance of infected vectors and people's exposure may happen independently or synergistically. Rich people may construct a dwelling in woodlands or visit for recreation and thus get exposed. People driven by civil conflicts or natural disasters to woodlands are compelled to have close contact with people, vectors and animals. Such abrupt changes alter the status from endemic to epidemic. As a consequence of the democratization process in the 1990s, Tick-borne Encephalitis (TBE) increased by 2× in Czechoslovakia and 4–30× in the Baltic states. Latvia too was hit hard. But TBE incidence markedly declined from 1999 because people avoided tick bite exposure by reducing visits to forests as a result of the campaign.

Urbanization, on the other hand, reduces mosquitogenic conditions and controls associated diseases.

3.7   Control of VB Pathogens

Control and mitigation efforts require understanding the above-explained mechanism of VBD causation and increase. An integrated analysis at the landscape scale allows a better understanding of interactions between changes in ecosystems and climate, land use and human behaviour and the ecology of vectors and animal hosts of infectious agents (Lambin et al. 2010).

Kilpatrik and Randolph (2012) suggested the following methods of control:

1. Clinicians are the first line where a cluster of patients reports. Their empowerment for correct diagnosis and novel public health agencies for disease management (including rapid diagnostic facilities, epidemiologists' intelligence, risk assessment and prompt action) are required for control. An integrated effort—One Health approach—is desired.
2. Vaccination protects only individuals who are vaccinated/who can afford vaccination; transmission is dependent upon exposure to or contact with vectors. Vaccination of wildlife reservoirs is an option but is presently limited to a few viruses; administration is a problem.
3. Culling—Culling of wild/domestic reservoirs to reduce their population might increase transmission. Seeking remaining hosts would be relatively easy for vectors and hosts will be infected. Subsequently, feeding a greater number of vectors would get infected. This is likely to result in intensified epizootics and, consequently, human infections.
4. Zooprophylaxis—Diverting vector feeding away from people to protect them by using animals, actively or passively. This may sometimes increase vector densities as they find alternative hosts to feed upon. This may thus be counterproductive. There may be a 'dilution effect' if naturally occurring biodiversity diverts vectors from infectious hosts, with the desired effect. In any case, this method does not appear to be dependable.
5. Direct measures: target vectors directly—Elimination of mosquitogenic habitats, such as water pools, coolers and water containers (as in Rajasthan); tickicides on the pathways in forests/taiga.
6. Newer techniques include raising pathogen-resistant vectors.
7. Integrated approach.

Integrate efforts of clinicians, public health agencies and reversal of ecological drivers of disease emergence and transmission. The latter requires a holistic approach in the identification of drivers and stitching together each of the components of the 'drivers'.

- Disease intelligence (searchers of emergence and transmission—epidemiologists, diagnostic labs/agencies, disease reporters)
- Risk assessors
- Public health agencies (clinicians as disease identifiers and reporters) + those who initiate (active) or passively act (general cleanliness, hygiene, sanitation)
- Government/authorities—deciding and funding actions: critical decisions on land use/landscaping, altering conditions at recreational facilities, developmental activities and restoration activities after a disaster
- Public awareness for demanding/supporting action

In Latvia, there was an increased incidence of tick-borne encephalitis among children. Vaccination campaigns led to public awareness, reducing high-risk activities in tick-infested areas in forests and the incidence was reduced by 74% by 1999.

The World Health Assembly in 2017 approved the 'Global Vector Control Response (GVCR) 2017–2030'. WHO responds to vector-borne diseases by:

- Providing evidence-based guidance for controlling vectors and protecting people against infections
- Providing technical support to countries so that they can effectively manage cases and outbreaks
- Supporting countries to improve their reporting systems and capture the true burden of the disease
- Providing training (capacity building) on clinical management, diagnosis and vector control with support from some of its collaborating centres
- Supporting the development of and evaluating new tools, technologies and approaches for vector-borne diseases, including vector control and disease management technologies

3.8   Conclusion

Vector-borne zoonoses present a complex system. It consists of a reservoir-agent system, vector-agent system and factors intrinsic and extrinsic to both systems that influence transmission and ultimately to humans. Understanding epidemiology is basic to planning surveillance and response.

References

Carmichael JR, Fuerst PA (2010) Molecular detection of Rickettsia bellii, Rickettsia montanensis, and Rickettsia rickettsii in a Dermacentor variabilis tick from nature. Vector Borne Zoonotic Dis 10(2):111–115

Chapman AS, Bakken JS, Folk SM, Paddock CD, Bloch KC et al (2006) Diagnosis and management of tickborne rickettsial diseases: Rocky Mountain spotted fever, ehrlichioses, and anaplasmosis–United States: a practical guide for physicians and other health-care and public health professionals. MMWR Recomm Rep 55:1–27. http://www.cdc.gov/mmwr/preview/mmwrhtml/rr5504a1.htm Tickborne Rickettsial Diseases Working Group; CDC

Chomel BB, Belotto A, Meslin FX (2007) Wildlife, exotic pets, and emerging zoonoses. Emerg Infect Dis 13(1):6–11

D'Ortenzio E, Grandadam M, Balleydier E et al (2011) A226V Strains of chikungunya virus, Reunion Island, 2010. Emerg Infect Dis 17:309–311

Daszak P, Cunningham A, Hyatt A (2001) Anthropogenic environmental change and the emergence of infectious diseases in wildlife. Acta Trop 78:103–116

de Lamballerie X, Leroy E, Charrel RN, Ttsetsarkin K, Higgs S, Gould EA (2008) Chikungunya virus adapts to tiger mosquito via evolutionary convergence: a sign of things to come? Virol J 5:33

Epstein PR (2001) Climate change and emerging infectious diseases. Microbes Infect 3(9):747–754

Kilpatrik AM, Randolph SE (2012) Drivers, dynamics and control of vector-borne emerging zoonoses. Lancet 380:1946–1955

Lambin EF, Tran A, Vanwambeke SO, Linard C, Soti V (2010) Pathogenic landscapes: interactions between land, people, disease vectors, and their animal hosts. Int J Health Geogr 9:54

Lee MJ, Chae JS (2010) Molecular detection of *Ehrlichia chaffeensis* and *Anaplasma bovis* in the salivary glands from *Haemaphysalis longicornis* ticks. Vector Borne Zoonotic Dis 10(4):411–413

Leighton PA, Koffi JK, Pelcat Y, Lindsay LR, Ogden NH (2012) Predicting the speed of tick invasion: an empirical model of range expansion for the Lyme disease vector Ixodes scapularis in Canada. J Appl Ecol 49(2):457–464

Ludwig A, Bicout D, Chalvet-Monfray K, Sabatier P (2005) Modelling the aggressiveness of the *Culex modestus*, possible vector of West Nile fever in Camargue, as a function of meteorological data. Environ Risques Santé 4(2):109–113

O'Guinn ML, Klein TA, Lee JS, Richards AL, Kim HC et al (2010) Serological surveillance of scrub typhus, murine typhus, and leptospirosis in small mammals captured at firing points 10 and 60, Gyeonggi province, Republic of Korea, 2001-2005. Vector Borne Zoonotic Dis 10(2):125–133

Pavlovsky EN (1966) Natural nidality of transmissible diseases in relation to the landscape epidemiology of zooanthroponoses. Peace Publishers, Moscow

Randolph SE, on behalf of the EDEN-TBD sub-project team (2010) Human activities predominate in determining changing incidence of tick-borne encephalitis in Europe. Euro Surveill 15(27):24–31

Vrbova L, Stephen C, Kasman N, Boehnke R, Doyle-Waters M et al (2009) Surveillance systems for emerging zoonotic diseases. Vancouver. Zoonoses_Surveillance_May_2009.pdf. Appendix 1: Emerging and re-emerging zoonoses listed by agent

Chapter 4
Management of Zoonoses

Human population is the target population for infectious disease-causing agents including zoonoses. They are also the target population for management of diseases. *Zoonotic pathogens are polyphagous (infect more than one species of hosts) and are polyhostal.* The epidemiology is complex and contemporary compared to the classical epidemiology that targeted single species.

Coined by Rudolf Virchow, 'zoonoses' originated from two Greek words, *zoon* = animals and *noses* = disease. Zoonoses are diseases of animals including humans. Anthropozoonoses are disease-causing agents that are monophagous (infecting single host species) and adapted to human beings in the course of evolution and exist in them through uninterrupted chain of transmission, e.g. cholera and smallpox. Such human pathogens constitute only 40%. *The rest or 60% of human pathogens and 75% of emerging infections and diseases are hosted by animals that constitute zoonoses. Of animal diseases, 61% are zoonotic* (Taylor et al. 2001). *Some of human pathogens are capable of infecting animals also. These are classed as* zooanthropozoonoses or reverse zoonoses (transmission from humans to animals), e.g. *Corynebacterium diphtheriae*. Zoonoses are diseases and infections, the agents of which are naturally transmitted between other vertebrate animals and humans.

According to Haydon et al. (2002), 77% of livestock pathogens and 91% of domestic carnivore pathogens and also 57/70 animal diseases of international importance have multiple hosts. Outbreaks among endangered species and some recent pandemics were caused by pathogens that can infect a number of other species of hosts. Infectious agents make a species jump from animals to humans. The transformation to human pathogen depends upon multiple variables that combine in a dynamic process that is not yet fully understood. Some pathogens became adapted to transmission from human to human and evolved as predominantly or exclusively human infections (Ro >1 in human), e.g. measles originated from closely related morbilliviruses of cattle (rinderpest) and smallpox from poxviruses of either camel or cattle. Zoonotic pathogens like pneumonic plague, Ebola and Marburg continue human-to-human transmission. Certain pathogens (of established zoonoses) like

K. G. Narayan et al., *Handbook of Management of Zoonoses*,
https://doi.org/10.1007/978-981-99-9885-2_4

rabies and monkeypox viruses have non-human reservoir host(s) and are occasionally transmitted to humans. Blocking transmission from the wild reservoir hosts protects humans.

Zoonosis like *T. saginata* requires human beings for completion of its life cycle and is an example of true or obligate zoonosis. Measures directed to the target human population (such as specific treatment) or measures to interrupt transmission from infected cattle, like meat inspection, will eliminate this zoonosis. This approach may limit but would fail to eliminate non-obligate cyclozoonoses like *Echinococcus granulosus* because more than one vertebrate host is required for maintenance of such parasites. Man is incidentally/accidentally infected and suffers from hydatidosis and trichinellosis. Infections fail to proceed further and the pathogens meet a dead end.

Infectious agents may encounter invertebrate insects in the ecosystem and adopt these for mechanical/spatial spread or for their propagation and development. In the latter situation, the infectious agents take time to be able to infect others (extrinsic incubation period), e.g. plague bacillus. Although this appears to be an addition to multiple hosts and enhancement of complexity, it offers sites of and means of interventions, such as rodenticide and insecticide. Such zoonoses are classed as pherozoonoses or metazoonoses.

The ability of pathogens to infect a wide range of hosts may be a potential risk for emergence of diseases in humans and animals. The polyphagous pathogens are likely to encounter a number of host population, some of which may constitute reservoirs. Identifying reservoir host may be key to designing a control measure of a multi-host pathogen.

4.1 Management of Zoonoses

Management of zoonoses requires understanding of pathogens, hosts systems and transmission routes. Zoonotic pathogens are polyphagous and polyhostal, maintained and transmitted in multi-host systems.

The concepts of transmission function of maintenance hosts and bridge hosts contribute to a better understanding of disease ecology in multi-host systems. The operational framework for protection of target population requires demonstration of bridging (bridge hosts). This requires integration of ecological and epidemiological approaches (Caron et al. 2015). Surveillance should include both the target and bridge populations, because these serve as the epidemiological functions.

4.1.1 Epidemiological Functions of Hosts

The epidemiology of hosts is basic to the understanding of diseases in a herd or population. Classical epidemiology dedicated to the diseases is either in single host species or in single target species. Understanding diseases caused by multi-host pathogens requires studying the ecology of diseases.

4.1.1.1 Maintenance of Pathogen

The pathogens may employ population of different species of animals for survival. Any host complex in which a disease persists indefinitely is a reservoir. While Haydon et al. (2002) conceptualized only two components, reservoir (for maintenance M) and target (T) populations, Caron et al. (2015) realized three components—M, bridge (B) and T.

One or more epidemiologically connected populations or environments in which the pathogen can be maintained permanently, e.g. *anatids* for avian influenza virus world over are called Maintenance community/Maintenance host complex.

A population of brushtail possums maintains *Mycobacterium tuberculosis bovis* (bTB) in New Zealand even without transmission from other hosts, and such hosts are called *maintenance hosts* (M). The population (size) of the maintenance host community may be critical under which a pathogen fails to persist, e.g. white-footed mouse (*Peromyscus leucopus*) for Lyme disease in the United States. This approach may be used for control of infection by a pathogen.

Transmission function of the maintenance host system is the capacity to transmit infection to the target population. The maintenance host does not always have infectious contact with the target host.

4.1.1.2 Bridge Hosts

Such hosts act as link/bridge through which pathogens can be transmitted from *maintenance hosts' population or communities* to the *receptive (target) hosts* (whom we want to protect). Bridge host population must be competent for a pathogen, i.e. infection, replication and excretion. The reproductive number R_0 is <1, and infection cannot be maintained. Bridging is dependent upon the number of *infectious contacts along the maintenance-bridge-target hosts transmission chain*. Lack of infectious contact between the maintenance and target population is compensated spatially, temporally and behaviourally.

The bridge population of birds creates a spatial link for the spread of avian influenza virus between the separately located maintenance and target populations. Feral pigs (*Sus scrofa*) are spatial bridge host in the epidemiology of bovine tuberculosis in New Zealand between possums (M) and cattle (T).

The epidemiology of *M. tuberculosis bovis* in New Zealand in the multi-host system is represented as possum (M)-feral pigs and ferrets (B)-cattle (T or target) transmission chain. Control of possum (M) population prevents transmission between M and T, which is adopted to protect cattle population from bTB and prevent economic loss. But the path of transmission built by bridge hosts (B) thwarts the effect. Red deer (*Cervus elaphus*) and ferrets act as temporal bridge hosts and transmit *Mycobacterium tuberculosis bovis* to possums (Nugent 2011). The population of red deer is controlled to levels well under critical community size.

Wild carnivore (e.g. jackals/skunks) are M for rabies virus ($R_0 > 1$). Dogs are (B). Vaccinating dogs will break transmission of rabies from M to T (human).

The maintenance and bridge hosts contribute to emergence and re-emergence of infectious diseases. According to Jones et al. (2008), 60.3% emerging infectious diseases (EIDs) are zoonoses and 71.8% originated in wildlife. The origin of EIDs was significantly related with environmental, ecological and socioeconomical factors and provided the basis for identifying hotspots.

Surveillance and control programme must include both the bridge and the target hosts.

4.1.2   Application

4.1.2.1   Approach to Identifying Bridge Population

Caron et al. (2015) presented the steps to identify bridge population for avian influenza virus (AIV). The maintenance hosts (M) for low pathogenic AIV are waterfowls (ducks, geese, waders, gulls and terns). There is a spillover of LPAIV to poultry (target/T population) and high pathogenic strains (HPAIV) evolve in the target population 'poultry'.

M and T are spatially separated as wetland and dryland dwellers. Identify/detect bridge hosts (B) contributing to spillover. The summarized steps and methods were:

- Studying and collecting ecological data to gather information about the presence/abundance of potential bridge hosts in the ecosystem.
- Synthesizing ecological and epidemiological data to determine their likelihood acting as bridge host.
- Hosting competence (receptivity, replication and excretion) data from experimental, serological and virological studies.
- Identifying potential contacts with maintenance and target host (interface)— using satellite telemetry for contact between wild and domestic birds, capture-recapture technique, bird ringing and monitoring and bird counting for estimating population size.

4.1.2.2   Reservoir Hosts, Evidence and Control

If a disease disappears in a target population by ring-fencing, existence of a reservoir is most likely. Reservoir host population with respect to the target population has to be identified. Control measures need to be directed to target population but need to be extended to reservoir hosts to block the transmission from reservoir to target population.

4.1.2.3 Identifying a Reservoir

Epidemiological evidence of association—link between the T and a reservoir (R) is elusive if transmission from R to T is sporadic or rare, e.g. Ebola and Marburg. Epidemiological studies are required. Badger as risk for bTB in cattle in the United Kingdom was realized by a case-control study.

Evidence of natural infection in 'nontarget population' can be generated by active/passive surveillance using serological, virological, genome-sequencing techniques.

4.1.2.4 Methods of Control in Reservoir Hosts

Ring-fencing, population control by culling (possum in New Zealand for bTB), reducing vector density (West Nile fever, JE) and partitioning at the interface of forest-grazing land.

4.2 Domestic Animals, Pets and Birds as Sources of Zoonoses

The cost of zoonoses is higher than the loss in the livestock sector. Management of diseases in animals, particularly domestic animals and birds, is covered by the veterinary sector. Veterinary science is inherently a preventive animal medicine and is economical. Traditionally, ante-mortem and post-mortem meat inspection, prophylactic measures like regular and periodic vaccination, OIE regulations on animal movement, trade, disposal of dead animals, etc. are practiced to maintain healthy livestock, poultry and pets. Quoting FAO (2021): 'Disease in animals poses potential health threats in human'. The FAO has been building the capacity of veterinary services to forecast, prevent, detect and respond to infectious zoonotic diseases and AMR with an objective of stopping the emergence and spread of the potential epidemics and pandemics at source.

A rational grouping of animal diseases may be required to identify priority and the service sectors assign responsibilities of controlling diseases. The animal disease may be grouped as:

1. Causing serious illness in humans and animals, e.g. rabies
2. Causing serious economic loss in animals, e.g. anthrax, brucellosis
3. No apparent illness in animals, e.g. JE
4. Serious illness in humans and wildlife, e.g. SARS and Ebola

Another way to group the diseases would be according to host species: swine erysipelas, *Streptococcus suis* from pigs, *Brucella melitensis* from sheep and goats, anthrax from cattle and glanders from equines.

Veterinary public health and epidemiology professionals present the risk associated with these diseases. The veterinary services control these diseases. Human population is protected.

4.3   One Health Approach

Animals, human, plants and the environment are interrelated and interdependent. Rudolf Virchow realized this interdependence in relation to the health of humans and animals. This concept was furthered by Osler and later by Calvin W Schwabe (Box for chronology).

The principle of 'One World, One Health' was conceived on September 29, 2004. It was recognized that an interdisciplinary approach was required to combat threatening diseases like West Nile fever, Ebola, SARS, Mad cow disease, monkeypox and avian influenza. The concept was developed by, and is a trademark of, the Wildlife Conservation Society.

Contributing to One World, One Health. A strategic framework for reducing risks of infectious diseases at the animal–human–ecosystems interface (available at ftp.fao.org/docrep/fao/011/aj137e/aj137e00.pdf).

Birth of One Health
1. Hippocrates (c. 460 BCE—c. 370 BCE), Greek physician—*Public Health depended on Clean Environment*—"On Airs, Waters, and Places".
2. Giovanni Maria Lancisi (1654–1720), Italian physician - ***Physical environment** had role in the spread of disease in humans and animals-* "mosquito net for control of malaria, rinderpest control"
3. Louis-René Villerme (1782–1863) and Alexandre Parent-Duchâtelet (1790–1835)—***Public hygiene***—"human, animal, and environmental health are linked"
   Source: https://en.wikipedia.org/wiki/One_Health,
4. Rudolf Virchow (821–1902), German Physician and Pathologist—"*no dividing lines between animal and human medicine*"—coined the term ***Zoonosis***
5. William Osler (1849–1919), Canadian Physician, father of modern medicine—published—"*The Relation of Animals to Man*"; *organized a significant study of parasites in the pork supply of Montreal with one of his most brilliant veterinary students, Albert W. Clement.*
6. James H. Steele (1947) DVM, MPH, founded the Veterinary Public Health Division at CDC. "*Understood the important role of animals in the epidemiology of zoonotic diseases and recognized that good animal health is important for good public health*".
7. Calvin W Schwabe (1927–2006)—in his book "Veterinary Medicine and Human Health" coined the term ***One Medicine*** called for unified approach against Zoonoses.
   Source: https://www.cdc.gov/onehealth/basics/history/index.html
"One Medicine" is commonly referred to as "One Health" implied the crossing over between veterinarians and physicians.

'One Health' is defined as *a collaborative, international, cross-sectoral, multi-disciplinary mechanism to address threats and reduce risks of detrimental infectious diseases at the animal-human-ecosystem interface* (https://www.fao.org/ag/againfo/home/en/news_archive/2010 one-health.html).

One Health High-Level Expert Panel (OHHLEP) realized that the interpretations, scope and practice of this definition have been different. A revised definition *relevant to a much broader global audience was desired.* The revised definition is:

One health is integrated, unifying approach that aims to sustainably balance and optimize the health of people, animals and ecosystems. It recognizes the health of humans, domestic animals and wild animals, plants and the wider environment (including ecosystems) are closely linked and interdependent. The approach mobilizes multiple sectors, disciplines, and communities at varying levels of society to work together to foster well-being and tackle threats to health and ecosystems, while addressing the collective need for health food, water, energy, and air, taking action on climate change and contributing to sustainable development. (One Health High-Level Expert Panel (OHHLEP) et al. 2022).

One Health approach to avert outbreak and pandemic seeks 'drivers' of disease, design preventive and control measures and implement (Table 4.1).

One Health concept benefits greatest the low- and middle-income countries where extensive veterinary health and food safety frameworks are not developed. Absence of veterinary resource affects vaccine-preventable diseases, e.g. "reduction of 0.007 rabid dog cases/1000 (human) population for every $\log_{10}$ increase in per capita GDP (*95% CI −0.002 to −0.01; P = 0.004*) (RabNet. https://apps.who.int/globalatlas/default.asp; The World Factbook. https://www.cia.gov/library/publications/the-world-factbook/index.html; Lee and Brumme 2013).

Table 4.1 Examples of diseases, drivers and inter-sectoral team

Diseases	Drivers	Inter-sectoral team[a]	Remarks
Bird flu influenza virus H5N1	Ecological, evolution	Wildlife-poultry farmers-live animal traders	Waterfowl-domesticated birds-human interaction
Lyme disease and other wildlife-originated diseases	Deforestation (i.e. land-use change, extractive industries)	Departments of forest, mining, oil and natural gas, agriculture	Wildlife-human come close for hunting, recreation, search of foods, extractives like coal, iron, etc. (mining), oil and gas, agriculture and commercial agri-farming
Tuberculosis, deer; trichinellosis, wild boar; SARS, civets	Demand for wildlife for research, food, pets, etc. is increasing	Traders in wildlife and its meat, biomedical research laboratories, import-export control agencies, animal quarantine centres	The trade creates ideal conditions for pathogens to multiply

(continued)

Table 4.1 (continued)

Diseases	Drivers	Inter-sectoral team[a]	Remarks
Antibiotic resistance—spread with animal and animal produce trade, emergence of pathogens	Intensive farming		Deforestation, farming for feed, climate change—increased CH_4, CO, CO_2
Hantavirus cases in southwestern USA in 1991–1992 and 1997–1998	Ecological cascade initiated by climate change—El Niño	Environmentalist, predictive epidemiologist, research institutions	Rodent population increased unexpectedly
Surat plague, 1994	Disaster-like earthquake—Latur 1993	Disaster management team should have had a predictive epidemiologist	The rodent and flea population grew exponentially in the damaged houses used as granaries by survivors

[a]*Veterinary Services, Veterinary Public Health-Wildlife-Human medicine*

References

Caron A, Cappelle J, Cumming GS et al (2015) Bridge hosts, a missing link for disease ecology in multi-host systems. Vet Res 46:83

FAO (2021) Managing diseases in animals to prevent health crisis in humans—FAO supports Egypt to fight zoonotic diseases and antimicrobial resistance threats. Emergency Centre for Transboundary Animal Diseases (ECTAD) in Egypt (2007–2020). Cairo

Haydon DT, Cleaveland S, Taylor LH, Laurenson MK (2002) Identifying reservoirs of infection: a conceptual and practical challenge. Emerg Infect Dis 8(12):1468–1473

Jones KE, Patel NG, Levy MA, Storeygard A et al (2008) Global trends in emerging infectious diseases. Nature 451(7181):990–993

Lee K, Brumme ZL (2013) Operationalizing the One Health approach: the global governance challenges. Health Policy Plan 28(7):778–785

Nugent G (2011) Maintenance, spill over and spillback transmission of bovine tuberculosis in multi-host wildlife complexes: a New Zealand case study. Vet Microbiol 151(1–2):34–42

One Health High-Level Expert Panel (OHHLEP), Adisasmito WB, Almuhairi S, Behravesh CB, Bilivogui P et al (2022) One Health: a new definition for a sustainable and healthy future. PLoS Pathog 18(6):e1010537

Taylor LH, Latham SM, Woolhouse ME (2001) Risk factors for human disease emergence. Philos Trans R Soc Lond Ser B Biol Sci 356(1411):983–989

Chapter 5
Preventing Zoonotic Pandemics

Human beings are often sentinel population for zoonoses. Zoonoses emerge, spread and are potential cause of epidemics and pandemics, often with high case fatality rates, increased burden on the health system and significant economic loss.

Interaction between actual and potential host and reservoir species including vectors is complex and dynamic and depends upon ecological changes. Understanding the interaction and spillover is important for prevention and control. SAARS coronavirus and the recent SAARS COV-2 originated from bats (reservoirs). Some zoonotic agents sustain in human after spillover from animals, e.g. Japanese encephalitis virus. Detection of JEV/infection in animals (e.g. pigs) alerts health services on the hotspots. Other zoonoses like brucellosis and rabies require introduction from animals for human infection. Veterinary services control and eliminate these from animals. Brucella-free animals reduce the health burden of pyrexia of unknown origin. Elimination of rabies from canine population results into zero hydrophobia.

The policy makers and the financers consider financing only the 'post-spillover activities, diagnosis, vaccine and treatment' in the preparedness and response to pandemic and not 'prevention'. The 'pre-spillover or preventive activities' are economical. If prevention actions cut the economic loss in GNI (global national income) estimated at $212 billion by half, there would be a savings of $106 billion in addition to halving mortality costs. This estimate excludes major outbreaks in domestic livestock and crops. Preventing 'spillover/emergence' was suggested by Bernstein et al. (2022). They studied 28 novel viral outbreaks recorded since 1950. Most resulted from spillover from animals. These have been organized according to respective reservoirs, modes of transmission, vectors and biosafety requirement (Table 5.1).

© Springer Nature Singapore Pte Ltd. 2024
K. G. Narayan et al., *Handbook of Management of Zoonoses*,
https://doi.org/10.1007/978-981-99-9885-2_5

Table 5.1 *Novel* viral zoonotic outbreaks observe since 1950 (Source: Bernstein et al. 2022)

Virus	Reservoir	Transmission	Vector	Safety level required
Andes, South American Hanta, Lassa, Hantaan, Puumala, Sin Nombre, Hanta, Guanarito, Junin, Venezuelan equine encephalitis*, La Crosse*	Rodent	Direct, aerosol	*Mosquitoes	Most cause HFRS, HPS and HCPS and require BSL4
Monkeypox	Possibly rodents	Direct		?
Rift Valley fever	Mosquitoes	Direct from infected livestock	*Aedes* spp.	BSL4
West Nile	Birds		Mosquitoes	BSL3
SARS-corona	Bats	Direct	Human-human	BSL4
SARS-corona-2	Bats	Direct	Human-human	
Middle East respiratory syndrome (MERS)	Bats	Direct	Human-human	BSL4
Marburg	Bats	Direct, aerosol, close contact—caregiver, nosocomial	Human-human	BSL4
Nipah	Bats	Direct, ingestion		BSL4
Chikungunya, Zika, human Immunodeficiency[1]		Direct[1]	Mosquito	? HIV[1](BSL2)
Kyasanur forest disease	Monkey		Ticks	BSL4
Influenza viruses—Spanish flu, H1N1, H2N2, H3N2	Birds, Swine, Equine	Direct, airborne	Human-human	BSL2

Majority of the 28 viral zoonotic agents are highly pathogenic and virulent requiring BSL4 laboratories. Only 6 viral zoonotic agents out of 28 are vector-borne; the rest are contact-transmitted.

The agent-host relationship with reservoir hosts is generally innocuous. Three major reservoir hosts accounted for most of the pandemic zoonoses, viz. rodents, bats and primates. Birds are reservoir for influenza virus and West Nile virus.

Infections with Chikungunya, Zika and influenza viruses spilled over from the respective reservoirs like monkeys, birds and swine and become established in humans. These are more anthroponosis than zoonosis.

Kyasanur forest disease virus (KFDV) is a member of the family *Flaviviridae* and genus *Flavivirus*. It is highly infectious causing CFR of 2–20% and requires biosafety level 4 lab. There is no cure and vaccine is only partially effective. It has been expanding to new areas in India, from the single district of Shimoga, Karnataka, in 1957–1958 to 16 districts in three states during 1957–2017.

KFD had intermittent outbreaks: high number of cases during focal periods, 37 years had fewer than 100 cases, 16 years had cases between 100 and 399 and 8 years had 400 or more cases (Chakraborty et al. 2019).

The viruses like Ebola, SARS, SARS CoV-2, and MERS spilled over from wild-life and bats to humans and spread through human-human transmission which causes great sufferings in terms of cases and fatality, draining health services and inflicting huge economic loss. Human infection with MERS may be contracted by direct/indirect contact with camels (dromedaries), secretions, excretions, body fluids, infected milk and meat (exact route unclear). An unusual outbreak occurred in Riyadh during 2017 (Amer et al. 2018). A patient in Riyadh infected directly 16 and led to an outbreak infecting 44 in three health centres in the surrounding area *in a period of just over a fortnight*, in the year 2017. *Eleven patients died.* The following was the conclusion: 'In MERS-CoV endemic countries, there is an urgent need for developing rapid point-of-care testing that would assist emergency department staff in triaging suspected cases of MERS-CoV to ensure timely isolation and management of their primary illness and prevent major MERS-CoV outbreaks'.

5.1   Understanding 'Spillover' and 'Species Jump'

An infectious agent evolves as an established and genetically consolidated pathogen of an 'emerging disease of the novel host'. The process involves crossover events occurring between non-human species of animals including reservoir in nature (natural nidii) or between wildlife and domestic animals and transmission (spillover) to novel host population, including human. Most emerging infectious diseases are zoonoses. The events of emergence may be grouped.

According to Engering et al. (2013) the events of emergence are:

1. Pathogens showing up in a *novel host*, ranging from spillover to complete species jumps
2. Mutant pathogens displaying *novel traits* in the same host, including an increase in virulence, antimicrobial resistance and host immune escape
3. Disease complexes emerging in *a new geographic area*, either through range expansion or through long-distance jumps.

Each of these categories is characterized by a typical set of drivers of emergence, matching pathogen trait profiles, disease ecology and transmission dynamics. The underlying causal factors or 'drivers' of emergence may be climate change, intensification of agriculture to meet the demand of increasing population, increased travel, trade coupled with unmatching health systems and protection practices. The host-agent-environment interplay is modulated by driver(s).

"Spillover environment" offering opportunity of mixing of species of animals eventually progressive exposure of a 'new host species' to a 'new pathogen' (also new host species—'existing' pathogen) generates 'species jump' and sustained transmission in 'new host'. Examples (of spillover environment) are live animal market, hunting, dressing of wildlife and consumption of bushmeat, deforestation, wildlife-domestic animal interface, etc. Species jump resulted in influenza A and HIV epidemics. HEV and monkeypox with apparent pandemic potential failed to make human-human transmission.

Pathogen infecting only the reservoir hosts (spillover without subsequent transmission in the novel host) will have R_0 = nil (expected secondary cases per primary case), whereas a sustained novel host-novel host transmission will have R_0 = 1. Pre-adaptation to the novel host (like human) enables certain pathogen (H1N1 influenza virus outbreak in 2009) to jump from the reservoir (swine) to another host via ecological fittings during its circulation in swine. Successful adaptation depends upon several factors: number of primary infections, R_0, required genetic changes, evolvability, etc. (Engering et al. 2013). Successful emergence may require a number of times of repeated transmission in a novel host. It is suggested that Nipah virus was repeatedly introduced by bats into the same pig farm and produced a herd immunity supporting on-farm circulation of the virus followed by spread to other farms.

Emerging pathogens of livestock exploit the same routes to spillover as those that cause human pandemics. The mitigating effect of preventing spillover and related preventive action will have similar effect of disease of livestock.

5.2   Preventing Spillover/Emergence

Preventing spillover/primary prevention was included (Bernstein et al. 2022) in the five phases of infectious disease emergence. Modified forms of activities during the emergence of zoonoses are presented in Table 5.2. Intervention at a stage prevents the progression of zoonoses to the next stage, e.g. stopping spillover will stop emergence of an infectious disease in domestic animals, birds and/or humans (sporadic form). Primary pandemic prevention actions aim at detecting novel pathogens before these spread locally or globally in order to prevent the outbreak and pandemic. The speed of detection and issue of 'alert for action' have to be high.

5.2.1   Wildlife-Linked Viral Zoonoses

Certain viruses are more prone to periodic species jumps. Influenza type A viruses are avian, swine and equine influenza and include zoonotic viruses. Influenza A viruses underwent multiple species jumps in recent history, including from avian host sources to horses, humans and pigs, from horses to dogs, from pigs to human and from dogs to cats. Host switching from avian to human resulted in H5N1 virus which is capable of recognizing and binding to human receptor sites, and a few mutations would render it airborne transmissible.

Table 5.2 Phases of emergence of zoonoses

S. no.	Phases	What is happening	Preventive action
1	Pre-emergence (anticipated)	Evolution of pathogens in wildlife	Viral surveillance
2	Spillover (primary prevention)	In autochthonous nidus, the pathogen is maintained in mammal/bird-mammal/bird cycle or mammal/bird-vector-mammal/bird-vector cycle	(a) Detect drivers, e.g. deforestation for agriculture, animal trade, etc. and appropriate action (b) Detection, reduction and isolation of natural nidii of infection to prevent exposure
3	Emergence in domestic animals and birds	Sporadic to fulminant disease (e.g. RVF, WN, H5N3)	Preventive vet. Services and VPH actions: detection, containment, reverse tracing, quarantine, culling and safe disposal
4	Emergence in human	Sporadic cases	Early detection by syndromic surveillance
5	Outbreak	Localized transmission	Containment, contact tracing, quarantine
6	Epidemic	Number of cases exceeding expected number	Scaled-up health activities: close schools and business centres (lock-up), widespread testing, quarantine
7	Pandemic	Global spread	All containment activities enhanced to larger scale

Strategic actions in phase serial numbers 1–3 are 'pre-emptive' and can prevent a pandemic

Evolution processes, antigenic shift and drift and reassortment of genes in influenza viruses go on during circulation among animals and birds, resulting in variants such as influenza A(H1N1v) and A(H3N2v). These originated in pigs, are zoonotic and cause non-seasonal flu, spreading through direct human-human transmission, e.g. swine influenza 'A (H1N1) pdm09' virus appeared in 2009. The first pandemic, the 1918 Spanish flu, was caused by influenza virus H1N1 responsible for high mortality, >1000 deaths/million. The H2N2 Asian flu pandemic in 1957–1958 was reported first in Singapore in February 1957 and then in Hong Kong and coastal cities in the United States. It caused an estimated death of one to four million, with the WHO settling at 2.0 million with an overall mortality rate of 0.6%. The epidemic lasted till 1958 (https://en.wikipedia.org/wiki/Influenza_A_virus_subtype_H2N2). The H3N2 pandemic occurred in 1968–1969. The estimated basic reproduction rate (R_0) of 1.8. and attack rate of 28% were similar in pandemics of 1957 and 1968; the case fatality rate in 1918 was >10× than in 1957 and 1968.

The CDC Pandemic Severity index based on case fatality rates evaluates the pandemic: <0.1% for the seasonal flu/2009 swine flu, 0.1–0.5% Asian flu and Hong Kong flu and 0.5–1%, 1–2% and 2 or >2% 1918 influenza pandemic.

Preparedness for influenza pandemic: The origin of the 1918 Spanish flu virus is unknown; avian and swine origins have been proposed. Jester et al. (2018)

discussed the present preparedness as compared to those available during the 1918 pandemic. The tools used to deal with pandemics were limited, viz. surveillance, diagnostic, treatment and prevention. For nonpharmaceutical strategies*, guidelines were published by the CDC in 2007 and revised in 2017. Presently, vaccines are available for seasonal influenza and their effectiveness is continuously improving such as broad and long protection and quick availability (current time frame is about 12 weeks). Antiviral drugs and anti-influenza drugs are available, viz. oseltamivir given orally, zanamivir for oral inhalation in persons 7 years and above age group and peramivir for iv injection to children 2 years and above also.

*Nonpharmaceutical strategies: *Personal protective measures* for everyday use and pandemic use (face mask, face shield, etc.) and *community measures*— increased social distancing and environmental measures, such as surface-cleaning measures, to reduce the transfer of viruses. The revised guidelines include a section on community engagement principles, as well as links to six supplemental planning guides for specific community settings.

Spillover from wildlife to human is a complex process. For example, KFDV in the natural nidus depends upon combination of competent reservoir-vector and their density. The tick (*H. spinigera*) uses a variety of animals from rodents to cattle for the development of their eggs to infectious nymph and adult; surface areas offered by these are climate-dependent. There is no human-human transmission after spillover.

According to Chakraborty et al. (2019), displaced niche for monkeys due to shrinking forest, reducing the distance between humans and monkeys and decreasing precipitation (climate) possibly led to spillover of KFD from Karnataka to new areas like Maharashtra, Goa and Kerala.

5.2.1.1 Averting Pandemic of Wildlife-Linked Viral Zoonoses

These are primarily detecting spillover event early followed by appropriate action preventing the spread of the pathogen.

Viral surveillance: It is expected to detect any emerging pathogen. According to Bernstein et al. (2022), 'the rate at which novel viral pathogens are identified increases with increasing number of animals sampled'. Many related information is required, such as transmission efficiency for the desired host like human or livestock; connecting viral genomic information (library) with serological data would help in determining 'rates of spillover' and 'probable host'.

Sentinel surveillance: Detects viral presence and activity in a region.

Yellow fever is indicated by deaths in primates. Cyclic epizootics amplify the viral transmission. South American monkeys seem to be susceptible and often there is high fatality among marmoset (*Callithrix*), howler (*Alouatta*), spider (*Ateles*) and squirrel (*Saimiri*).

Vectors may also be used as sentinel. Mosquitoes are collected using specially designed traps baited with CO_2. SMACK (sentinel mosquito arbovirus capture kit) is used to detect arboviruses by PCR on honey-soaked nucleic acid preservation cards deployed in purpose-built CO_2-bated traps.

Veterinary public health and epidemiology: Detection of the avian influenza H5N3 outbreak prompts containment actions, isolation, quarantine, culling and safe disposal of carcasses. This has prevented the evolution of a variant of H5N3 capable of causing a pandemic. Oral rabies vaccination of wild carnivores prepares an immune-belt to prevent spillover of rabies virus from forest in countries it has been pushed to natural forest habitat. Bovine TB is endemic in badgers in the forest of Gloucestershire, Dorset and Somerset, England, and spills over to cattle. Culling of badger reduces incidence of B-TB in cattle for 6.5 years.

5.2.2 Rodent-Linked Viral Zoonoses

Eleven (>40%) viruses of the novel outbreaks (▸Table 3.1) have rodents as reservoir hosts. Spillover from rodents led to the emergence of these zoonotic outbreaks. Nine of the zoonotic viruses are transmitted directly from reservoir rodent species to human. These viruses caused HPS/HFRS/HCPS and required BSL4 facilities. Two (La Crosse virus and VEEV) are maintained in a mosquito-rodent cycle and infect human through mosquito bites (Fig. 3.1). The probable natural host for monkeypox virus is also rodents. This brings a total of 12/27 or 44.44% of the viral zoonoses spilled from rodent hosts.

Except for VEEV, all cause viral haemorrhagic fever, HFRS, HPS and HCPS. Multiple systems are affected. The vascular system is damaged and there is bleeding. Many are life-threatening, and only some are mild. These require BSL4 laboratory for handling. These RNA viruses belong to arena, filo, bunya and flaviviruses. These are maintained by natural reservoir rodent hosts with or without a vector (Fig. 5.1). The area of infection is restricted to the region of species of natural rodent reservoirs' habitat. Some may have wide distribution. Imported cases are responsible for reports from non-endemic area. Human infection occurs when they come in contact with reservoir host.

Exposure is likely through breathing in virus-laden air (aerosolized droppings and urine of rodents), touching of the eyes, nose or mouth with hands contaminated with rodents' excreta and nesting material, handling rats and their bite. de St Maurice et al. (2017) used the HPS surveillance data on >600 cases to determine the risk of exposure. Risk is linked to cleaning rodent-infested areas and dry dusty environment (inhalation-infection) and related works.

Outbreaks of HFS cannot be easily predicted and occur irregularly and sporadically. Vaccine is available for Argentine haemorrhagic fever only.

La Crosse virus (family, *Bunyaviridae*, genus, *Orthobunyavirus*): LACV is considered as the cause of 'rural encephalitis' and affects children less than 16 years old. The habitat of LACV—*Aedes triseriatus-chipmunk* cycle—is rolling terrain and dense oak trees with of plenty of food and water, predominantly the hardwood forest east of Rocky Mountains (Harding et al. 2019). Infection in mosquitoes is

PANDEMIC EMERGENCE MODELS

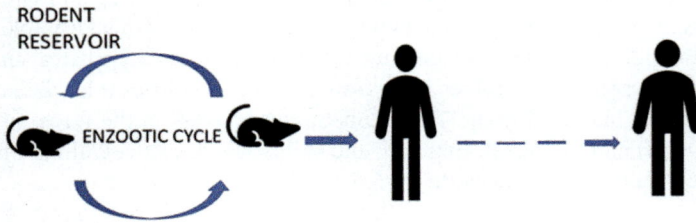

RODENT
RESERVOIR

ENZOOTIC CYCLE

Model 1. Rodent reservoir. Examples : Arena virus, Hanta virus and others.
Limited human-Human transmission (broken arrow)

Fig. 5.1 Natural reservoir rodent with or without a vector transmission to human

lifelong, and female mosquitoes transfer infection transovarially—a mechanism for amplification and maintenance. The flight range is 200 m from its breeding site. Experimental evidences suggest that *Aedes albopictus* and *Aedes japonicas* are also competent vectors. Exposure risk is during the months of June–August and October as the mosquito density is highest in August.

Understanding epidemiology is essential to prevent 'spillover'. The emergence and expansion of zoonotic diseases are particularly sensitive to ecological changes, population movements, and the intrusion of humans and domestic animals into sylvatic environments. Anthropogenic factors (e.g. deforestation, agricultural development, colonization and urbanization) have increasingly placed human and domestic animal populations at risk of many vector-borne diseases.

A high rodent density corresponds to and can be corelated with epidemics.

According to Mills (2005), the regulators of prevalence and transmission of viruses in rodents are the following:

- *Natural environmental*: Weather, habitat quality and food supply affect reproductive success and population densities.
- *Anthropogenic*: Human disturbance or alteration of habitat may help opportunistic species that may serve as reservoirs for zoonotic viruses.
- *Genetic*: Variation among individuals or populations influence susceptibility of mice to infection or capacity for chronic shedding and may be related to population cycling.
- *Behavioural*: Actions such as fight increase the risk of transmission. Communal nesting may help in overwinter transmission.
- *Physiological*: Influences rodents' response to infection and length or period of infectious state.

Deforestation and expanding and extensive agriculture disturbed rodent habitat favouring opportunistic or generalist species that may be reservoir of hantaviruses. Commonly environmental changes lead to reduction in rodent diversity, aggressive encounters and interactions among rodents, consequentially increasing the risk of spillover of rodents into areas of human activities (favouring greater hantaviral transmission among rodents and to humans).

5.2.2.1   Climate as Driver/Regulator

The Four Corner regions of the United States (the shared borders between the states of New Mexico, Arizona, Colorado and Utah) had suddenly higher rodent population than usual. There was drought for several years in this region. There was heavy snow and rainfall in early 1993 resulting in revival and growth of plants and animals in larger-than-usual numbers. Most HPS (SINV and reservoir deer mouse) cases in 1993 were related with high population density of deer mice ascribed to El Niño Southern Oscillation (ENSO) that brought heavy rainfall.

Apodemus agrarius-borne HFRS—incidences/cases relate with abundance of this field mice, which in turn is the result of abundance of seed crops and low rainfall and/or absence of flood in China.

Rodent population in temperate Europe peaks due to 'mast years'—the year when abundant nutrients for forest rodents are available in the form of abundant nuts of forest trees that accumulate on the ground. Only a modest rodent population occurs 'without masting phenomenon', transmission and efficient spread of virus are not enabled.

Observing 'high summer temperature for two consecutive years (flower buds develop) and high autumn temperature 1 year prior (actual seeds develop)', *high rodent density can be predicted.*

'More rain appeared to translate to more virus and higher risk' but it cannot be generalized.

5.2.2.2   Anthropogenic Activities as Driver/Regulator

Habitat structure (space in burrow, cover, etc.) can also influence the reservoir host population density. Anthropogenic activities such as deforestation, agricultural land cover conversions and recreational activities affect rodent habitat.

Rat-borne diseases/infections in urban areas have the following risk factors—hantaviruses cause aerosol infection. Non-aerated, closed and unused or less frequently used buildings have access to rodents, e.g. barns and cabins. Period of viral survival in excretions and secretions of rodents is an important factor, e.g. PUUV survive for about 2 weeks at room and cold temperature indoors (absence of radiation) in excreta of bank voles; PUUV infection in winter has been found to be associated with inhalation, indoor cigarette smoking and possibly also inflammation of airways. Professions linked to HFRS are farming, construction work, forestry and proximity to forest and wood cutting.

There may be relationship between density of rodent population and spread of virus among rodents, and after some time (lag period) to humans.

The pattern of interaction is complex. A simple increase in rodent population may not necessarily lead to infection.

5.2.2.3 Averting Pandemic of Rodent Linked Viral Zoonoses

Tools for Alert

- Satellite data on climate and elevation have been used to predict occurrence of PUUV infection in Scandinavia.
- Geographic information systems and remote sensing techniques—increased HFRS incidence correlated with elevation, NDVI, prairie temperature, semi-hydromorphic soils, timber forests and orchards in China.
- Rodent trapping and estimating changes in population density.
- Biogeographic properties of wildlife reservoirs such as range and intrinsic host traits related with reproductive output help predict hotspots where monitoring and surveillance should be made for an early detection (Han et al. 2015).

In a way, these are diagnostic/screening methods applied to climate and ecosystem which seek relationship with reservoir host-agent cycle or reservoir-vector-agent cycle to predict the spillover of pathogens to humans. These help in 'taking preventive measures, alerting health services to prepare for the possible outbreak and making the public aware of the outbreak'. A pandemic may be prevented.

5.2.2.4 Prevention-Awareness

HPS/HFRS infection may be prevented through awareness programmes for persons at risk such as farmers, ranchers, temporary labourers, forestry/outdoor recreation workers, oil drilling and cleaning industry workers, janitors and house cleaners in homes, residential settings, workplace and recreational parks. Rodent exclusion methods—'foam and wire mesh at the point of entry in living spaces'—and seasonal health alert network messages to public health staff and clinicians (when rodent population is increasing) may be used.

HPS surveillance has kept the rate of infection low in the United States. HPS is rare (i.e. typically 20–40 cases per year).

5.2.3 Livestock-Linked Viral Zoonoses

In order to meet the demand of feeding increasing human population, intensification and expansion of farming were resorted to. Livestock population and density increased. Wild animal farming came up. Environment and opportunity for spillover of pathogens was thus created by the density of livestock. Risk of emergence and re-emergence of pathogens of pandemic potentially increased, e.g. pandemic influenza in animal and bird incubators through genetic reassortment.

Integration of veterinary services, VPH and health service and other stakeholders is required to prevent a pandemic.

Nipah virus emerged in a large pig farm of Malaysia which was encircled by mango trees and located on the edge of a native forest. The reservoir is *Pteropus* spp. and several other species of bats.

Fruits punctured by bats and contaminated soil infect the scavenging pigs. Date palm sap (in Bangladesh), fruits (mango in Malaysia), vegetables and pork contaminated with saliva, urine and/or faecal matter of the reservoir bats caused human infection. Nipah virus spreads through contact with infected pigs and handling dead and slaughtered pigs and pork. Human-human transmission occurs among family members and healthcare workers caring patients.

Pigs and other domestic animals act as bridge/amplifying hosts of Nipah virus after its spillover from bats.

NiV has pandemic potential. Nipah virus spread is associated with pig farming, processing and trade.

Averting pandemic requires surveillance, identifying infected farms and destroying the whole flock. Syndromic surveillance and awareness about risks associated with hunting and consuming bats and fruits partially eaten by animals, palm-nectar collection is also required.

Understanding circulation pattern and potential transmission routes from bats to humans and identification of spillover and associated risks: Studies suggested intensified surveillance during March to May because circulation of Nipah virus increased when female bats were pregnant and lactating (Cappelle et al. 2020).

Rift Valley fever virus (RVFV) is a *Phlebovirus* in the order *Bunyavirales* which affects cattle, buffalo, sheep, goat and camel causing sweeping abortion storms and fatality of 100% among neonatal animals resulting in loss of animal produce, stock, weight and future stock and also zoonotic outbreaks associated with severe illness related with blindness, retinitis, encephalitis haemorrhagic fever, mortality and sequelae.

It is transmitted to humans through contact with body fluids, blood and tissues of infected animals and bites of infected mosquitoes, *Anopheles coustani*, *Mansonia africana* and *M. uniformis*. Consuming raw or undercooked animal product and inhalation (lab accident) also transmit infection. No human-human transmission occurs. It spreads through international trade of meat of animals.

RVFV is vertically transmitted to eggs of mosquitoes and remains infectious in the eggs of mosquitoes during dry conditions for several years. Outbreaks have occurred in areas where drought-resistant vectors (*Aedes* spp.) lay eggs that can survive for several years and require flooding events for hatching. Epizootics naturally follow heavy rains. Viraemia is high in infected animals infecting secondary vector species (*Culex* spp.). Persistent rains and environmental conditions favour mosquito breeding and density. Explosive epidemics occur in endemic areas in this way. Amplification of virus in livestock causes human infection collaterally.

The ecological niche of RVF vectors varies widely. Rainfall is an important predictor of RVF. Optimal environment for RVF includes a number of factors determining (1) the rehydration of desiccated mosquito eggs in soil; (2) soil type that retained water better (solonetz, calcisols, solonchaks and planosols), for example, clay or very clayey soil; (3) landing and resting areas for vector provided by dense bush vegetation cover (shrubbery grasses, occasional trees); (4) plain land forms better allowing formation of water pools for larval habitat than elevated or hilly land forms; and (5) areas having soils with both extremely slow and very slow drainage (Hightower et al. 2012).

Risk factors: living in rural areas, agri-related activities and livestock rearing (farming), butchering/handling raw meat, vets and lab workers and sleeping out—exposure to mosquito.

5.2.3.1 Averting Pandemic of Livestock Linked Viral Zoonoses

Mariner et al. (2022) described actions for averting epidemics of RVF. Three strategic options for action frameworks are as follows:

- Pre-emptive risk-based—actions initiated in response to climate warning designed to *interrupt* an evolving scenario of outbreak. Alarmed with climatic prediction (NDVI*, flooding and mosquito RVF warning system), procurement of vaccine is done. Targeted vaccination and vector control in risk-hotspots are done with the beginning of the downpour. A well-implemented plan has the highest cost-effectiveness and requires high level of management to implement interventions in a timely manner.
- Preventive actions to reduce the risk of an outbreak taken during inter-epidemic period. Required actions include primarily vaccination and One Health risk communication. Open-ended commitment and resource prioritization are required. Outbreak may be less severe or may even be prevented.
- Reactive approach—begins after the first diagnosis in humans and aims to contain and limit the impact of RVF epidemic on public health, livestock and trade. The reactive response is least effective and the costliest. Rapid case detection and prompt lab confirmation plus active 'rapid response teams' reduce human suffering and deaths as evidenced by 16 cases of whom 7 died were recorded in 10 independent outbreaks between March 2016 and June 2018 in Uganda (Nyakarahuka et al. 2019).

*The normalized difference vegetation index (NDVI) is an indicator that uses remote sensing to detect visible red and infrared spectral reflectance and thus determine whether or not an area of land contains live green vegetation. Simply put, in the context of arthropod vector activity, where ever there is green growth after rainfall, there will also be mosquito vectors.

Early warning models are based on broader range of indicators—e.g. sea surface temperature, remote sensing and satellite images. The FAO has developed a prototype RVF early warning system that allows 2 months (before the first sign of RVF is detected) to prepare and take action. It produces monthly risk maps and risk assessment for Africa.

The web-based RVF Decision Support Tool (DST) issues alerts and early warning messages to allow prevention and control in countries at risk of RVF occurrence well before the first signs of RVF infection in the countries are reported.

OIE regulations adequately intercept the spread through trade.

RVF surveillance: Syndromic surveillance, preferably participatory syndromic surveillance, reaches out to livestock owners and the public increase the number and timelines of case detection. Sentinel herd (surveillance) is an objective, evidence-based tool to document circulation of RVFV within a population. Data can be anchored to the overall RVF surveillance data base for response and trade-related decisions.

Sentinel surveillance is useful to other zoonoses also, e.g. West Nile fever—screening of American crows/ill and admitted raptors/sentinel domestic chicken and horses is tested means of detecting viral activity in advance; Japanese encephalitis—sentinel pigs/ducks/wild birds/mosquitoes detect JEV activity and its location.

5.3 One Health Approach

Zoonoses impact public health. One Health approach is the most appropriate approach. Prevention in animals is the most cost-effective way to protect the public from zoonoses. Veterinary services, especially veterinary public health and epidemiology, take care of preventing spillover of zoonotic agents to humans. One Health approach manages the risk –mitigation. Zoonoses like rabies, RVF, WN and Nipah occur in animal and human settings. Management of these diseases in livestock and poultry would be a part of comprehensive One Health.

5.4 Conclusion

Agriculture intensification and expansion have resulted into spillover of viruses such as influenza, bird flu H5N3 and Nipah virus from bats to pigs. It has led to the resurgence of old pathogens like anthrax, brucellosis and salmonellosis.

Global Animal Disease Intelligence Reports are issued quarterly, e.g. Issue No. 2/2015, FAO (a-i5199e Global Disease Report), including zoonoses. It reports the status (no change/increase/decrease), drivers, risk assessment and forecasting. Assessment of risk associated with each factor follows. Appropriate mitigation steps are initiated.

A robust veterinary service maintains endemicity and prevents outbreaks or re-emergence of diseases of livestock and birds.

More vets are required. Their capacity needs augmentation; one area is 'wild-life'. Veterinary science is inherently a preventive medicine, which is based on understanding the 'epidemiology'. Enrolment of veterinarian for public health responsibility is the best choice for 'pre-emptive' actions to avert pandemic (▶Table 3.2).

Veterinarians have been contributing to public health. Ante-mortem inspection eliminates sick animals and post-mortem-infected tissues from entering the food chain, thus preventing foodborne infections. Human trichinellosis and taeniasis are prevented by the action at the level of animals. Detection of bovine tuberculosis during post-mortem inspection and tracing down to the bovine TB-infected herd for effective control illustrates 'economic method of reverse tracing', enabling actions to eliminate bovine TB and consequently spread to humans. Veterinary science is a comparative pathology. Development of diagnostic methods has made detection of pathogens easy, rapid and specific.

Control of animal (and poultry) diseases including zoonotic diseases by vaccination and suitable anthelmintics reduces pathogen burden and consequential human infection. Good management practices in animal farming produce zoonotic pathogen-free food animals, e.g. stopping swill feeding eliminated vesicular exanthema and collaterally drastically reduced a zoonosis, trichinella infection in pigs.

'Livestock-inclusive One Health' agenda is recommended by the scientists of the International Livestock Research Institute to protect the world against pandemic diseases (https://www.news-medical.net/news/20220718/New-livestock-inclusive-One-Health-agenda-could-help-protect-the-world-against-pandemic-diseases. aspx). It is wise to invest into healthy and sustainable livestock systems and this will reduce the risk of spillover of zoonoses. About 75% of human infectious diseases have originated from livestock and wild animals. According to the scientists of the International Livestock Research Institute, 13 of 200 zoonotic diseases account for 2.2 million deaths/year mostly in developing nations.

References

Amer H, Alqahtani A, Alzoman H, Aljerian N, Memish Z (2018) Unusual presentation of Middle East respiratory syndrome coronavirus leading to a large outbreak in Riyadh during 2017. Am J Infect Control 46:1022–1025

Bernstein AS, Ando AW, Loch-Temzelides T, Vale MM et al (2022) The costs and benefits of primary prevention of zoonotic pandemics. Sci Adv 8(5):eabl4183

Cappelle J, Hoem T, Hul V, Furey N et al (2020) Nipah virus circulation at human–bat interfaces, Cambodia. Bull World Health Organ 98:539–547

Chakraborty S, Andrade FCD, Ghosh S, Uelmen J, Ruiz MO (2019) Historical expansion of Kyasanur Forest disease in India from 1957 to 2017: a retrospective analysis. Geo Health 3:44–55

de St Maurice A, Ervin E, Schumacher M, Yaglom H et al (2017) Exposure characteristics of hantavirus pulmonary syndrome patients, United States, 1993-2015. Emerg Infect Dis 23(5):733–739

Engering A, Hogerwerf L, Slingenbergh J (2013) Pathogen-host-environment interplay and disease emergence. Emerg Microbes Infect 2(2):e5

Han BA, Schmidt JP, Bowden SE, Drake JM (2015) Rodent reservoirs of future zoonotic diseases. PNAS 112(22):7039–7044

Harding S, Greig J, Mascarenhas M, Young I, Waddell LA (2019) La Crosse virus: a scoping review of the global evidence. Epidemiol Infect 147:e66

Hightower A, Kinkade C, Nguku PM, Anyangu A et al (2012) Relationship of climate, geography, and geology to the incidence of Rift Valley fever in Kenya during the 2006-2007 outbreak. Am J Trop Med Hyg 86(2):373–380

Jester B, Uyeki T, Jernigan D (2018) Readiness for responding to a severe pandemic 100 years after 1918. Am J Epidemiol 187(12):2596–2602

Mariner JC, Raizman E, Pittiglio C, Bebay C, Kivaria F et al (2022) Rift Valley fever action framework. FAO animal production and health guidelines, no. 29. Rome. https://doi.org/10.4060/cb8653en

Mills JN (2005) Regulation of rodent-borne viruses in the natural host: implications for human disease. Arch Virol Suppl 19:45–57

Nyakarahuka L, Balinandi S, Mulei S, Kyondo J et al (2019) Ten outbreaks of rift valley fever in Uganda 2016-2018: epidemiological and laboratory findings. Int J Infect Dis 79(Suppl 1):4. https://doi.org/10.1016/j.ijid.2018.11.02

Part II
Viral Zoonoses

Describing zoonoses cuts across microbiology, epidemiology, and ecological niches including reservoir hosts, vectors, and, more importantly transmission chains leading to infection of a range of hosts and spatial distribution impacting health and economy.

Most of the viral zoonoses are important causes of pandemics, for example, influenza, SARS-1, SARS-2, and serious and deadly hemorrhagic disease-causing viruses like Ebola and Marburg. Chapters cover a range of metazoonotic encephalitis causing viruses such as VEE, EEE, WEE, and JE.

Diseases like rabies are illustrative of their control by VPH efforts only. Reducing dog rabies to zero eliminates deaths due to hydrophobia (except due to exposure from wildlife). Metazoonoses like West Nile and Rift Valley fever require "One health" approach. Viruses like DENV, SARS-COV-1, and SARS-COV-2 evolved from zoonoses (animal-human transmission) to anthroponoses (human-human transmission) and require human health efforts (health sector) to reduce human suffering and deaths due to these illnesses.

Epidemiology of some viral diseases is presented in the following subsections:

1. Mosquito-borne viral zoonoses
2. Tick-borne viral zoonoses
3. Avian-borne viral zoonoses
4. Bat-borne viral zoonoses
5. Rat-borne viral zoonoses
6. Dog-borne viral zoonoses
7. Monkey-borne viral zoonoses
8. Human-to-human transmission

Chapter 6
Mosquito-Borne Viral Zoonoses

Mosquito-borne zoonotic infections may be classified according to the main pathology as follows:

(a) Encephalitis: EEE, WEE and VEE (*Togaviridae*), California encephalitis and La Crosse encephalitis (*Bunyaviridae*) and Japanese encephalitis, St. Louis encephalitis, Australian encephalitis and West Nile encephalitis (flaviviruses)
(b) Haemorrhagic fevers: Rift valley fever and dengue fever
(c) Others: Chikungunya fever, Ross River fever, o'nyong'nyong, yellow fever and Zika fever

This classification may be of some help for planning management of diseases caused by these arboviruses. Management of these zoonoses requires more information. Salient ones are tabulated.

Table 6.1 lists these diseases (column 1) with other related information. The endemic areas or regions from where outbreaks have been reported are shown in column 5. The reservoir hosts in the natural enzootic cycle are shown in column 4. The mosquito vectors for the respective viruses (column 2) are listed in column 3.

The journey of arboviruses (Go et al. 2014) has three important stations (Fig. 6.1). The home is forests where arboviruses are naturally maintained by enzootic cycle of transmission between reservoir hosts and mosquitoes (primary vector), hence also called sylvatic cycle. The reservoir or primary host can harbour a virus indefinitely with no ill effects and may be re-infected several times during their life. There is amplification of the virus in the vector.

The viruses spill out with primary or accessory vectors (bridge vectors) to rural areas to infect non-wild or domestic animals and birds. This can lead to outbreak/ epizootics in domesticated animals and birds in rural areas. The virus is amplified, as in the case of JEV and VEEV, and extends its infection to humans. Humans are viraemic and the source of infection to biting mosquitoes. Large numbers of humans are infected as in epidemic by mosquito vector (most of encephalitis, dengue, yellow fever, RVF and other diseases listed in Table 6.1).

© Springer Nature Singapore Pte Ltd. 2024
K. G. Narayan et al., *Handbook of Management of Zoonoses*,
https://doi.org/10.1007/978-981-99-9885-2_6

Table 6.1 Mosquito-borne zoonoses (mainly arboviruses)

Column 1	2	3	4	5
Disease	Infectious agent	Mosquitoes	Reservoir hosts	Reported from
Encephalitis	Eastern equine encephalitis virus (EEEV), Alphavirus, Togaviridae	Culiseta melanura, Coquillettidia perturbans, Aedes vexans, Culex erraticus	Birds Also mammals, reptiles and amphibians through bite by infected 'bridge mosquitoes'	North, East and South America, Caribbean
	Western equine encephalitis virus (WEEV), Alphavirus, Togaviridae	Culiseta melanura Culex tarsalis common in farming area	Songbirds (C. melanura—songbird cycle in nature) Finches and sparrows amplify	Endemic in states west of the Mississippi River, Western and Central United States Argentina, northern and western Canada
	Venezuelan equine encephalitis virus (VEEV), Alphavirus, Togaviridae	Mosquitoes. Culex spp. vector in enzootics Ochlerotatus taeniorhynchus—primary vector in epizootics	Sylvatic rodents are reservoir hosts. Equines are amplifying hosts	Central and South America
	Japanese encephalitis virus (JEV), Flavivirus, Flaviviridae	Mosquitoes. Culex spp.— C. tritaeniorhynchus, Anopheles, Mansonia	Birds, egrets, pond herons, cattle egrets and ducks act maintenance and amplifying hosts. Pigs (amplifier)	Asia—People's Republic of China, Korea, Japan, South East Asia, the Indian, Western Pacific countries, Australia
	St. Louis encephalitis virus (SLEV), Flavivirus, Flaviviridae	Culex salinarius, C. tarsalis, C. nigripalpus, C. quinquefasciatus and C. pipiens	Wild birds, Peridomestic birds and domestic fowl—geese—and domestic pigeons are amplifiers of virus; sparrows Ab+	Argentina to Canada, unknown outside Americas
	West Nile virus (WNV), Flavivirus, Flaviviridae	Culex pipiens, C. tarsalis, C. restuans	Wild birds	Europe, Middle east, parts of Asia, Australia, Canada—geographic areas expanding
	California encephalitis virus (CEV), La Crosse encephalitis virus (LEV) (Bunyaviridae)	Ae. triseriatus Ae. albopictus Ae. japonicus	Small wild animals—chipmunks, squirrels, rabbits and hares	United States, Canada, Europe- Russia, Yugoslavia

Column 1	2	3	4	5
Australian encephalitis syndrome (AES)	Ross River virus (RRV), Alphavirus, Togaviridae	Ae. camptorhynchus, Ae. vigilax, Cx. annulirostris, Ae. notoscriptus (eggs survive in dessication-resistant eggs of Aedes spp.)	Kangaroos, wallabies, possums, horses	Australia, Papua New Guinea, other South Pacific islands
	Murray Valley encephalitis virus, Flavivirus, Flaviviridae	Culex spp., Cx. annulirostris, Aedes spp.	Bird-mosquito/kangaroo- Mosquito-bird/kangaroo cycle maintains the virus; virus survives in mosquito eggs for two seasons Rufous night heron (Nycticorax caledonicus) and the cormorants/darters (Pelecaniformes)	Papua New Guinea, endemic in northern Australia, reported across Australia
	Kunjin virus (WNV$_{KUNJIN.}$) Flavivirus, Flaviviridae	Culex spp.—Cx. annulirostris. Aedes spp. occasionally	Bird-mosquito cycle Wading birds (particularly Nycticorax caledonicus)—an important natural reservoir	Northern Territory and Western Australia
Haemorrhagic fever	Rift Valley fever (RVF), Phlebovirus, Phenuiviridae	Mosquito: A. mcintoshi, Ae. dentatus, Ae. unidentatus, Ae. juppi	Mosquito, Aedes spp. of the Neomelaniconium group	Rift Valley stretching between eastern Africa and Mozambique Outbreaks in sub-Saharan Africa, Kenya, Somalia and Tanzania
	DENV, Flavivirus, Flaviviridae	Aedes aegypti, A. albopictus	Zoonotic 'sylvatic' cycles in Africa and Asia Non-human primates (monkeys) are asymptomatically infected by the dengue virus, which is efficiently transmitted by the mosquito.	Africa, the Americas, the Eastern Mediterranean, South East Asia and the Western Pacific

(continued)

Table 1 (continued)

Column 1	2	3	4	5
Other fever	*Yellow fever virus (YFV) Flavivirus, Flaviviridae*	*Aedes, Haemagogus*	All primates	Africa, Central and South Americas
	Zika virus (ZIKV), Flavivirus, Flaviviridae	*Ae. africanus, Ae. apicoargenteus, Ae. luteocephalus, Ae. aegypti, Ae. vittatus, Ae. furcifer*	Monkeys, Mosquitoes-monkey cycle	Africa (Uganda), Asia, Yap island
	Chikungunya (CHIKV), genus Alphavirus, family Togaviridae	*Aedes aegypti, Ae. albopictus, Mansonia, Culex*	Monkey, chimps, baboons, rodents, birds	Africa, Asia, South East Asian countries including India, islands of the Pacific Ocean
	O'nyong'nyong virus (ONNV), Alphavirus, Togaviridae	*Anopheles funestus, A. gambiae*	Not known	Uganda, Kenya, Tanzania, Zaire and others in sub-Saharan Africa

MOSQUITOBORNE ZOONOSES

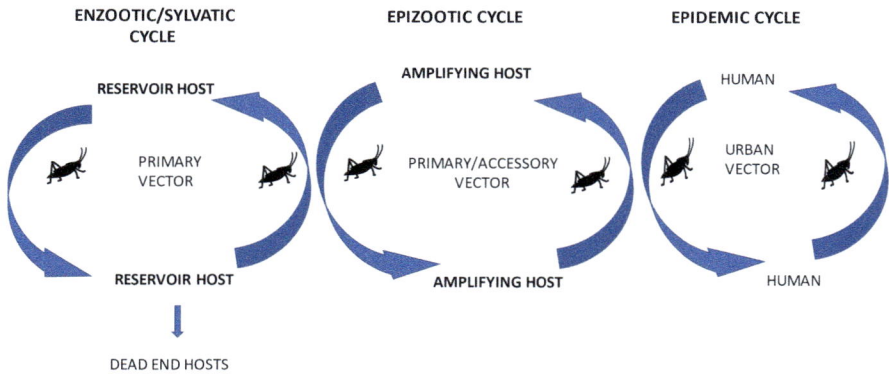

Fig. 6.1 Mosquito borne zoonoses

DENGUE VIRUS

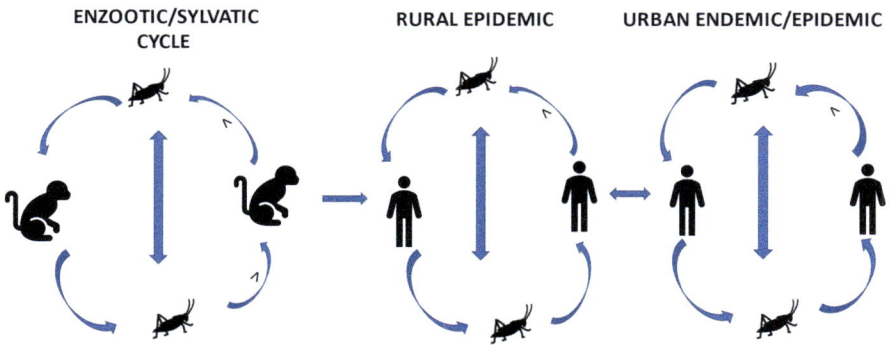

Aedes mosquito – DNV vertically transmitted to progeny mosquito

Fig. 6.2 Transmission of Dengue virus

This is explained with haemorrhagic fever caused by dengue virus (*DENV*), *Flavivirus, Flaviviridae* (Fig. 6.2).

Enzootic sylvatic DENV transmission cycle occurs in canopies in Malaysia, maintained by Ae. niveus group; these most probably use monkeys of genera Macaca and Presbytis as reservoir and amplification hosts. Aedes niveus group (Aedes pseudoniveus, Aedes subniveus, Aedes vanus, Aedes albolateralis, Aedes niveoides and Aedes novoniveus) is primatophilic and known to descend to ground level to feed on humans. This could facilitate the transfer of sylvatic DENV from the forest to peridomestic environments.

The 'zone of emergence' is where human population in the rural areas contact the sylvatic cycle which results in rural epidemic.

DENV persist in mosquito population by transovarial transmission on *Ae. aegypti* which is the principal vector. It is found in abundance close to human dwellings. It prefers to lay eggs in artificial containers commonly found in and around homes, for example, flower vases, old automobile tires, buckets that collect rainwater and trash in general. It prefers to feed during daytime and feeds on multiple persons in a short time. Several members of the same household become ill with dengue fever within a 24- to 36-h time frame, suggesting that all of them were infected by a single infective mosquito.

Certain terms need to be understood.

Amplifying hosts: Hosts developing high level of viraemia are amplifying hosts. These are important for transmission, e.g. nestlings and 'young-of-the-year birds' developed EEV-viraemia more and more rapidly than adults.

Dead-end hosts: Some secondary and incidental hosts develop low viraemia after infection. They have insufficient viruses to feeding vector for transmission. Therefore, transmission ends. Such hosts are dead-end hosts.

Bridge mosquito vectors: These species acquire infection from the reservoir and are responsible for infecting human and other mammals (secondary hosts), for example, *Coquillettidia perturbans*, *Aedes vexans*, *Ochlerotatus sollicitans* and *Oc. canadensis*. Vectors of EEV feed primarily on mammals and can also feed on birds and other hosts.

6.1   Management of Mosquito-Borne Viral Zoonoses

It requires the study of the vector mosquitoes, virus-mosquito interaction, virus-mosquito-host interaction and a number of factors surrounding and influencing these.

Mosquitoes look for sites to oviposit. Sunlit peri-domestic areas are preferred by *Ae. albopictus* and *Ae. japonicus*. Overwintering survival of *Aedes* eggs depends on minimum temperature and duration of exposure. *A. albopictus* eggs can tolerate up to -12 °C and -5 °C if the females oviposit in containers (e.g. disused tiers) that are not exposed to prolonged extreme cold exposure. Eggs of desiccation-resistant *Aedes* spp. carry virus like Rift Valley fever virus, DENV, Ross River, etc., which is a mechanism of protection of pathogen—persistence in nature—over seasons/years.

RVFV is vertically transmitted to eggs of mosquitoes and remains infectious for several years during dry conditions. Eggs hatch during rainy season. Optimal environment for RVF includes a number of factors determining (1) the rehydration of desiccated mosquito eggs in soil; (2) soil type that retained water better (solonetz, calcisols, solonchaks, and planosols), for example, clay or very clayey soil; (3) landing and resting areas for vector provided by dense bush vegetation cover (shrubbery grasses, occasional trees); (4) plain land forms better allowing formation of water pools for larval habitat than elevated or hilly land forms; and (5) areas having soils with both extremely slow and very slow drainage (Hightower et al. 2012).

The initiating vector "flood water *Aedes*" bred in these foci which were well away from human habitation but not from livestock. Infected mosquitoes bite transmits and spreads RVF in livestock and human. Livestock-to-human but not human-to-human transmission occurs.

The dispersal of mosquitoes, *Aedes* in particular, is greatly influenced by travel and trade routes. Progressive invasion of temperate regions could be also influenced by climate change (Go et al. 2014).

According to Leisnham and Juliano (2012), LACV is endemic in the Appalachian region in the Midwest. The emergence of cases in this region coincided with invasion and spread of the Asian tiger mosquito, *Aedes albopictus* (Skuse), and the Asian bush mosquito, *Aedes japonicus*, that cooccurs with *A. triseriatus* as larvae in water-holding containers. *A. albopictus* and *A. japonicus* invaded via used tiers.

Increased global population, deforestation, uncontrolled urbanization, unplanned construction of houses and development of small township, large suburbs and rural homes led to increased number of artificial water-holding containers and mosquito breeding sites.

Management of sewer and waste water accompanied with mosquito control measures is required.

References

Hightower A, Kinkade C, Nguku PM, Anyangu A, Mutonga D et al (2012) Relationship of climate, geography, and geology to the incidence of Rift Valley fever in Kenya during the 2006-2007 outbreak. Am J Trop Med Hyg 86(2):373–380

Go YY, Balasuriya UB, Lee CK (2014) Zoonotic encephalitides caused by arboviruses: transmission and epidemiology of alphaviruses and flaviviruses. Clin Exp Vaccine Res 3(1):58–77

Leisnham PT, Juliano SA (2012) Impacts of climate, land use, and biological invasion on the ecology of immature Aedes mosquitoes: implications for La Crosse emergence. Ecohealth. 9(2):217–228

Chapter 7
Eastern Equine Encephalitis (EEE)

Eastern equine encephalitis is a zoonotic arboviral illness. It has wide distribution—North, Central and South America and the Caribbean. Seventy horses died of encephalitis in 1831 in Massachusetts, USA. The epizootic was recognized as EEE. Regular epizootics followed. The causative agent was identified in 1933 from infected horse brain. In 1938, 30 children died of encephalitis in the same region of the north-eastern United States where epizootic in horses occurred establishing zoonoses.

EEEV infection occurs in horses accompanied by sporadic human cases commonly in summer in southeast states. Infection in both is highly virulent; CFR reaches 70% and most survivors have residual neurological disability. The average number of cases per year is six in the United States. However, there was an unusual and dramatic increase in human cases in the United States in 2019. Historically, the CDC reported 72 neuroinvasive cases in the United States from 2009 to 2018. During those 10 years, there was an average of seven cases of neuroinvasive disease each year, with a low case (3) in 2009 and a high case (15) in 2012. Most cases were reported from Florida, Massachusetts, Michigan, New York and North Carolina. In 2019, the number of human cases was five times higher than the average, involving eight states. Michigan and Massachusetts had the maximum human cases. There were nine cases as of October 2020 (CDC n.d.).

7.1 Aetiology

There are four lineages of EEEV antigenic complex, I, IIA, IIB and III. Group I caused most of human diseases endemic in North America and the Caribbean. The rest caused primarily equine illness in Central and South America (Virus | Eastern Equine Encephalitis | CDC).

© Springer Nature Singapore Pte Ltd. 2024
K. G. Narayan et al., *Handbook of Management of Zoonoses*,
https://doi.org/10.1007/978-981-99-9885-2_7

Modes of human infection other than vector-borne are contact with EEV in laboratory and exposure of the eyes, lungs or abraded/wounded skin to the brain and/or spinal cord of infected animals.

7.2   Epidemiology

EEE is distributed in North America, Central and South America and the Caribbean and the eastern seaboard states, the Gulf Coast and some inland midwestern areas of the United States. Since 1964, EEE seems to be in control and few cases are reported annually. Most cases have been reported from Florida, Massachusetts and New Jersey and Gulf Coast states. EEE seems to be re-emerging (http://www. news10.com/story/19135352/rare-deadly-virus-found-in-mosquitoes-in-pittsfield; http://www.boston.com/news/globe/city_region/breaking_news/2006/08/ middleborough_b.html).

Early studies in the southeastern United States suggested that *Culiseta melanura*, *Coquillettidia perturbans*, *Aedes vexans* and *Culex erraticus* had most of the blood meals during a brief period coincident with the breeding season and from nestlings of the targeted birds. The nestlings and 'young-of-the-year' birds developed viraemia more rapidly and in higher titre than adults. This led Unnasch et al. (2006) to study the effect of interactions between population of vectors and avian hosts. Four of the 11 parameters studied were related to vector interacting with 'young-of-the-year' birds. It was concluded that 'young-of-the-year' initiated and maintained the predicted enzootic outbreak and adult birds could not substitute for the 'young-of-the-year'. Abundance of mosquitoes and 'young-of-the-year' were important for the prevalence of EEEV. Breeding sites of mosquitoes are increased with rains. Summer heat accelerates the rate of growth of mosquito larvae. Longevity of individual mosquitoes is favoured by temperature and humidity; in turn, their availability for viral transmission is increased. Viral replication and activity are increased as more and more birds and mosquitoes are infected.

EEEV infects also mammals, reptiles and amphibians through bite by infected 'bridge mosquitoes', *C. melanura*. This also acts as the main epizootic vector. Mosquitoes primarily feed on mammals but can also feed on birds, mammals and other hosts. Mosquitoes like *Coquillettidia perturbans*, *Aedes vexans*, *Ochlerotatus sollicitans* and *Oc. canadensis* act as enzootic vectors in southeastern United States. The larvae of *C. melanura* are commonly found in pockets of water surrounding tree roots, fresh water and hardwood swamps. *Coquillettidia perturbans* lay eggs on shallow lakes and in heavy emergent vegetation. *Culex erraticus* larvae are found in the grassy shallow margins of ponds, lakes and marshes. Infection of reptiles, amphibians and mosquitoes seems to be the overwintering mechanisms of EEEV.

Infected birds are generally asymptomatic. There is high level of viraemia in passerine birds sufficient to infect enzootic and a variety of bridge vectors, such as *Aedes* and *Coquillettidia* that transmit the virus to humans and horses. Some infected birds suffer from diseases and deaths and high level of viraemia, such as chukar partridge, egrets, glossy ibises, doves, sparrows, ducks and cranes (Go et al. 2014).

Occasionally, mammals like cattle, alpacas, swine, llamas, cats, deer and goats can get infected and have this disease. Mammals-humans and horses do not develop enough viraemia to infect additional mosquitoes and hence act as 'dead-end'.

Movement of infected hosts and vectors spreads EEEV. Some of the mosquitoes travel to a long distance. For example, *Coquillettidia perturbans* has a flight range of nearly five miles. Others have less than a mile from the breeding area.

7.2.1   The Florida Outbreak of 1991–1992 Identified the Driver (Anonym 1992)

EEE is the rarest mosquito-borne encephalitis but with 30% CFR in the United States. EEEV is maintained in freshwater-swamp habitat in enzootic cycle involving birds (passerine birds are effective reservoirs)—*Culiseta melanura*. Heavy rains *(driver)* in Florida (1991) created ecological conditions leading to the outbreak of the 1991–1992 EEE. *C. melanura* population increased. EEV activity increased and was reflected in 70 cases in horses by July. *Ae. albopictus* was established as the epizootic and endemic vector. EEEV was isolated from *Ae. albopictus* collected from tire dump and detection of cases in equines in May and June in Polk County. Later studies (White et al. 2011) suggested highest endemicity in Florida with 'year-round' transmission of EEEV compared to other states in the United States. Clustering of the same phylogenetic strains from the north-eastern states and Florida suggested that Florida served as the centre from where EEEV periodically spread to north-eastern states.

7.3   Pathogenesis

EEEV is deposited in human/horse by bite of infected mosquitoes. There is endocytosis. It replicates in macrophages and neutrophils and in organs. It spreads through the lymphatics to lymph nodes. Immunologically active cells, neutrophils and macrophages infiltrate brain parenchyma and perivascular areas causing neuronal destruction, neuronophagia, focal necrosis and demyelination. Additionally, vascular inflammation and perivascular cuffing may also develop. Autopsy findings include diffuse cerebral atrophy, particularly of the cortex, oedema, leptomeningeal vascular congestion, haemorrhage and encephalomalacia. There seems to be minimal involvement of the spinal cord.

7.4 Symptoms

7.4.1 Horses

Disease in horses precedes human disease. This is an alert that EEEV is actively being circulated. The incubation period ranged between 1 and 3 weeks. Pyrexia (106 °F) and neurological symptoms appear gradually but fast. The initial symptoms are increased sensitivity to sound/noise, excitement and restlessness. The patient develops drowsiness, has droopy ears and presses their head against a hard object. It wanders aimlessly and moves in circle. The condition deteriorates further to weakness, ataxia and uncoordinated voluntary muscular contraction resulting in staggering gait. The horse is unable to raise its head, complete paralysis sets in and death occurs 2–4 days after the onset of symptoms. CFR ranges between 70 and 90%. Outbreaks in horses may occur during the summer and fall. EEEV in horses is indicative of viral activity in the region and alerts public health.

7.4.2 Human

Those aged <15 years and >50 years stand at greatest risk of neurologic disease. Human infection is asymptomatic in most; only 4–5% develop encephalitis. The resulting immunity lasts almost lifelong. Incubation period varies between 3 and 10 days. Symptoms may be mild flu-like fever, headache and sore throat. Severe (encephalitis) illness is manifested in sudden high fever, body ache, headache, irritation, restlessness, drowsiness, anorexia, nausea and vomiting, diarrhoea, photophobia, altered mental status, seizures, cranial nerve palsy and coma. Systemic cases have abrupt onset. Encephalitis signs and symptoms appear abruptly in infants and within few days in older children and adults. Duration of illness is 1–2 weeks. Cases with no involvement of CNS recover completely. Nearly one third to half of the severe cases dies, usually within 2–10 days, or may be later, of the onset of symptoms. Survivors suffer from mild to severe disability of varying nature such as personality disorder, minimum brain or nerve dysfunction, intellectual impairment and paralysis.

7.5 Diagnosis

Area chicken test (birds as sentinel) is used to detect viral activity. Blood samples taken every 2 weeks from 'area chicken' are examined to detect antibodies.

- Clinical presentation consistent with neuroinvasive EEE, electroencephalogram, CT scan and MRI reveal abnormality.
- EEEV isolation in Vero cell culture/suckling mouse brain followed by IFT.

- EEEV isolation or detection of nucleic acid (Lambert et al. 2003) by PCR in tissues-brain (autopsy) and CSF.
- EEEV-specific antibodies—IgM in serum or CSF, neutralizing antibody in acute and convalescent serum samples—IgM-capture enzyme-linked immunosorbent assay (ELISA), microsphere-based immunoassay or IgG ELISA.

EEEV is a potential bioweapon. High-risk groups include those living in/visiting endemic areas and those whose work necessitates outdoor activities including recreational activities.

7.6   Treatment

There is no specific treatment for Eastern equine encephalitis (EEE); rest and clinical management are supportive. Meningeal symptoms require medications for headaches and antiemetic therapy and rehydration for associated nausea and vomiting (CDC 2022).

7.7   Prevention

7.7.1   Vaccine

The Department Agriculture and Consumer Services reported the first case of EEE in Virginia in 2010 (http://www.examiner.com/pet-care-in-roanoke/eastern-equine-encephalitis-reported-va). Vaccine is available for horses and not for humans. Generally, horses are vaccinated at least 2 weeks before the expected exposure to virus and a booster is given 30 days later in the first year of vaccination. The vaccine is effective for 6–12 months and therefore annual vaccination in endemic areas is recommended. Most veterinarians recommend vaccination six-monthly in areas where EEE is most frequent, such as southeast and Tidewater Virginia (http://www.wpcva.com/articles/2010/08/19/chatham/news/news49.txt).

7.7.2   Mosquito Control

Protection against mosquito bites—mosquitoes are most active (peak biting time) during dusk, dawn and darkness. Use of repellents, covering most of the skin, use of nets while sleeping, etc. are recommended. Destruction of mosquito-breeding sites by treating with adulticides is also recommended.

References

Anonym (1992) Eastern Equine Encephalitis virus associated with *Aedes albopictus*—Florida, 1991. MMWR 41(7):115–121. http://www.cdc.gov/mmwr/preview/mmwrhtml/00016118.htm

CDC   (2022).   https://www.cdc.gov/easternequineencephalitis/symptoms-diagnosis-treatment/index.html

CDC Eastern equine encephalitis. https://www.cdc.gov/easternequineencephalitis/index.html

Go YY, Balasuriya UB, Lee CK (2014) Zoonotic encephalitides caused by arboviruses: transmission and epidemiology of alphaviruses and flaviviruses. Clin Exp Vaccine Res 3(1):58–77

Lambert AJ, Martin DA, Lanciotti RS (2003) Detection of north American eastern and western equine encephalitis viruses by nucleic acid amplification assays. J Clin Microbiol 41(1):379–385

Unnasch RS, Sprenger T, Katholi CR, Cupp EW, Hill GE, Unnasch TR (2006) A dynamic transmission model of eastern equine encephalitis virus. Ecol Model 192:425–440

White GS, Pickett BEE, Lefkowitz EJ, Johnson ALG et al (2011) Phylogenetic analysis of eastern equine encephalitis virus isolates from Florida. Am J Trop Med Hyg 84(5):709–713

Chapter 8
Western Equine Encephalitis (WEE)

Encephalitis is an inflammation of the brain and meninges produced by multiple causative agents. Western equine encephalitis (WEE) is a mosquito-borne viral disease that affects the central nervous system with severe complication and deaths.

Western equine encephalitis virus (WEEV) was isolated from a fatal case of equine encephalitis in Joaquin Valley of California in 1930. It caused widespread outbreaks between the 1930s and 1950s. An outbreak in 1941 affected several states of the United States and Canada. There were nearly 800 cases and 90 deaths in Minnesota (Minnesota Department of Health Vector borne Diseases Unit, www. health.state.mn.us).

This is followed by sporadic outbreaks with 209, 87 and 4 cases during the 1970s, 1980s and 1990s, respectively. Since 1998, no case has been reported in the United States and Canada. The virus has not been detected in mosquito pools since 2008.

8.1 Aetiology

WEEV, belonging to family *Togaviridae* and genus *Alphavirus*, possibly evolved from EEEV and Sindbis-like alphavirus such as Aura found in Brazil and Argentina through recombination. The epizootic strains are more virulent and neuro-invasive. WEE is enzootic in South America and strains are less virulent causing sporadic cases as compared to strains of North America. Exchange of epizootic and enzootic strains seems to be rare. WEE viruses are genetically diverse.

The Highlands J virus, Fort Morgan virus and Buggy Creek virus are closely related to WEEV. The Highlands J virus is less pathogenic and is maintained in nature by *Culiseta melanura* and songbirds in fresh swamps. It is pathogenic to turkeys and partridges and causes sporadic illness in horses and insignificant illness

© Springer Nature Singapore Pte Ltd. 2024
K. G. Narayan et al., *Handbook of Management of Zoonoses*,
https://doi.org/10.1007/978-981-99-9885-2_8

in human. These viruses and the four subtypes of Sindbis virus from Africa, Asia, Australia and Europe are regarded as members of WEEV complex.

The original California strain fell into group A lineage. WEEV is a highly conserved alphavirus. There are two lineages: A and B. The B group has three sublineages: B1, B2 and B3; two of these B went into extinction. Strains of group A and B1 were more virulent (Bergren et al. 2014). Searching the reason of 'submergence' of WEEV, Bergren et al. (2020) suggested ecological factors led to the decreased levels of enzootic circulation during the late twentieth century even in the face of adaptive evolution.

8.2   Distribution

It is endemic (primarily in states west of the Mississippi River) in the plains of the Western and Central United States. It is distributed further from the western half of North America to South America, including Guyana, Ecuador, Brazil, Uruguay and Argentina to northern and western Canada. A case was reported from Uruguay. WEE is relatively a rare disease, which occurs sporadically. Less than five cases per year are reported in the United States. Expansion of irrigated agriculture favoured the grain-eating birds and mosquitoes. Human travel has increased. These increased the opportunity of exposure.

8.3   Epidemiology

Birds act as reservoir of WEEV. Passerine birds (finches and sparrows) amplify the virus. It may cause fatal infection in sparrows and emus but asymptomatic in chickens.

The virus infects also equines and other domestic animals and humans. Infection in horses and humans is dead-end. Non-avian species of animals have been found seropositive for WEEV. These are rodents, rabbits, squirrels, ungulates, tortoise and snakes but do not amplify the virus. Strong evidences suggest involvement of blacktail jackrabbits in transmission cycle.

The natural transmission cycle of the virus involves the primary amplifying hosts, passerine birds, and the primary vectors, *Culex tarsalis*. The agriculture settings of western America are most suitable for both the birds and the vector. The epizootic reservoir and amplifying hosts are domestic and wild birds. Other cycle involves the blacktail jack rabbits as amplifying hosts and *Aedes melanimon* and *Ae. dorsalis* as vectors. *C. tarsalis* can infect also horses and humans. *Aedes melanimon* in California and *Ae. dorsalis* in Utah and New Mexico and *A. campestris* in New Mexico act as bridge hosts in epizootic transmission to horses and humans (Go et al. 2014).

8.3.1   Transmission to Horses and Humans

Emus show mild symptoms. Humans and horses suffer and are dead-end hosts. Other equids like ponies and burros suffer with moderate viraemia. These might contribute in amplifying the virus during epizootics. *C. tarsalis* are common in the farming areas and around irrigated fields. Horses are common in these regions and get infected. People in the endemic areas living/working in the farms/visiting/recreational or outdoor activities are likely to get infected. *C. tarsalis* increase (peak) in late summer and feed more on mammals compared to birds in spring; this varies with climatic factors and irrigation practices. In Minnesota, mosquitogenic months are from mid-July to mid-September. Most WEEV infections in humans and equines occur in summer and slightly later in temperate regions like Canada.

8.4   Disease

8.4.1   Human

All age groups are susceptible. The virus invades the central nervous system (brain and spinal cord) with severe neurological sequel. Infants and children are most susceptible and likely to develop encephalitis. The brain is damaged in about 50% of affected infants and 13% of older people. Fatality among encephalitis cases is approximately 5–15%. The incubation period varies, 1–2 weeks after mosquito bite (www.health.state.mn.us 3/9/2018).

Result of infection ranges from no symptom to fatal. There is a mild febrile illness, chills, nausea, vomiting, stiff neck and occasionally respiratory difficulties. Meningismus, weakness, tremor and alert mental status are seen in <10% of patients. This is followed by symptoms of aseptic meningitis, encephalitis, confusion, headache, drowsiness, irritability, seizures, disorientation, coma and death. Infants suffer from seizures. Patients with severe encephalitis die within 1 week of the onset of symptoms.

8.4.2   Equine

WEEV enters muscles after mosquito bite and then to regional lymph nodes and multiplies in macrophages and neutrophiles and later in endothelial cells. After concentrating in spleen and liver cells, the virus enters the vascular system for the second viraemia. Clinical signs begin; the central nervous system is invaded 3–5 days after the second viraemia. Incubation period varies between 1 and 3 weeks. Affected horses show in-coordinated movement, drowsiness, prostration, coma and death.

Fatality (or euthanasia) may be as high as 50% (usually 15–20%) (https://www.vet-stream.com/treat/equis/diseases/western-equine-encephalomyelitis#pathogenesis).

8.5   Diagnosis

Same as for EEEV, samples include also the spinal cord. CSF and serum are examined for IgM.

8.6   Treatment

No specific treatment is available. Symptomatic treatment is given to maintain vital functions of the body.

8.7   Prevention

8.7.1   *Vaccine*

No licensed vaccine is available for human use. Vaccination in horses may be carried out with a formalin-inactivated vaccine that is available in combination with EEEV (vaccination: two times in a year; Go et al. (2014)).

8.7.2   *Protection from Mosquitoes*

Use approved mosquito repellent and follow the manufacturers' direction on applying on the skin and clothing, e.g. products containing 20–50% DEET (N,N-diethyl-meta-toluamide). This is not for use in infants and children under 3 years old. Children over 3 may put their hands in their mouth; hence, do not apply it on their hands; also avoid contact with eyes, lips and broken irritated skin. This is water washable. Permethrin: Spray on fabric to prevent mosquito bite.

References

Bergren NA, Auguste A, Forrester NL, Negi SS et al (2014) Western equine encephalitis virus: evolutionary analysis of a declining alphavirus based on complete genome sequences. J Virol 88(16):9260–9267

Bergren NA, Haller S, Rossi SL, Seymour RL, Huang J et al (2020) "Submergence" of Western equine encephalitis virus: evidence of positive selection argues against genetic drift and fitness reductions. PLoS Pathog 16(2):e1008102

Go YY, Balasuriya UB, Lee CK (2014) Zoonotic encephalitides caused by arboviruses: transmission and epidemiology of alphaviruses and flaviviruses. Clin Exp Vaccine Res 3(1):58–77

Chapter 9
Venezuelan Equine Encephalitis

Venezuelan equine encephalitis is a mosquito-borne zoonotic disease in human often misdiagnosed as dengue fever and causing neurological and fatal infection among children.

VEEV was isolated in 1938 from a horse that died of encephalitis. In 1950, it was isolated from human cases during an outbreak of febrile illness in Espinal, Colombia.

VEEV was developed as a biological weapon by the United States and the former Soviet Union during the Cold War. It requires biosafety level 3 laboratory.

9.1 Aetiology

Venezuelan equine encephalitis virus is a single-stranded RNA alphavirus in the family *Togaviridae*. Alphaviruses are mosquito-borne pathogens. VEEV replicate in mosquitoes before transmission to vertebrate. Venezuelan equine encephalitis complex consists of antigenic subtypes I-VI. There are five antigenic variants (AB-F) under subtype I, VEEV, viz. I-AB, I-C, I-D, I-E and I-F. The variants I-AB and I-C are associated with epizootics (equine) and epidemics (human). The remaining three variants of subtype I (I-D, I-E and I-F) and the other five subtypes circulate in natural enzootic cycles.

Equids and humans are incidental hosts and also dead-end hosts.

According to Aguilar et al. (2011), Ecuador recorded 31,000 cases, 310 deaths in humans and nearly 20,000 equine deaths in the early part of 1969. In the late part of the year, it spread to El Salvador and Guatemala and to Central America and Mexico and an estimated 50,000 equines died; there were 52,000 human cases and 93 fatalities in Mexico only. Beginning from near the Guatemala border in summer of 1969, it spread to Pacific states of Chiapas and Oaxaca by 1970 and northwards to 17 states in Mexico, to the Gulf Coast and finally into southern Texas. It was controlled by vaccinating horses with TC-83 vaccine and vector control.

© Springer Nature Singapore Pte Ltd. 2024
K. G. Narayan et al., *Handbook of Management of Zoonoses*,
https://doi.org/10.1007/978-981-99-9885-2_9

9.2   Epidemiology

New World alphaviruses, VEEV, WEEV and EEV, causing encephalitis are distributed in Americas. Old World alphaviruses like Chikungunya causing fever and polyarthritis are found in Europe, Asia and Africa (Crosby and Crespo 2022). VEE outbreaks in humans and equids occur in at least 12 countries of Central and South America, Mexico and the United States reporting a sporadic occurrence. The VEE complex of alphaviruses including the epizootic subtypes I-AB and I-C is widely distributed throughout Americas.

Equine herd immunity induced by past outbreaks and vaccine and unusual rains accompanied with increased vector (mosquito) density determine major outbreaks.

The natural habitat is Neotropical forests. The ecotone habitat is rich in mosquitoes, including vectors of VEEV. There is continuous circulation of enzootic strains. It is suggested that vector mosquitoes cover 1–3 km by flying and can reach 82–97% of the total land areas. Humans and equids are exposed to VEEV and such exposure is likely to continue in the foreseeable future as encroachment and destruction of forests continue.

VEE and dengue cases present similar symptoms (except neurological in VEE and haemorrhagic in dengue); hence estimating incidence of either becomes difficult. An estimated one tenth of dengue cases are VEE suggesting a large burden in the Amazon basin (Aguilar et al. 2011). If a highly efficient vector of dengue, *Ae. Aegypti*, gets infected, major outbreaks of both endemic and epidemic VEEV may appear. A laboratory efficient vector, *Ae. albopictus*, that prevails in both temperate and tropical regions is likely to spread VEEV far and wide. There is high viraemia in humans after infection with both endemic and epizootic strains. Viraemia is sufficient for a human-mosquito-human transmission. This situation combined with urban vectors presents a possibility of creation of a stable urban VEEV cycle with a potential major public health problem.

9.2.1   Reservoir

The rodent reservoirs belong to genera *Sigmodon*, *Oryzomys*, *Zigodontomys*, *Heteromys*, *Peromyscus* and *Proechimys*. The viraemia is sufficient to infect mosquitoes *Culex (Melanoconion)*. The virus is maintained in rodent-mosquito-rodent cycle (Fig. 9.1). Rodents like cotton rats and spiny rats and opossums act as reservoir hosts. *Culex* spp. are the primary vectors. This enzootic or sylvatic cycle has limited distribution, e.g. tropical forests or swamps or humid regions.

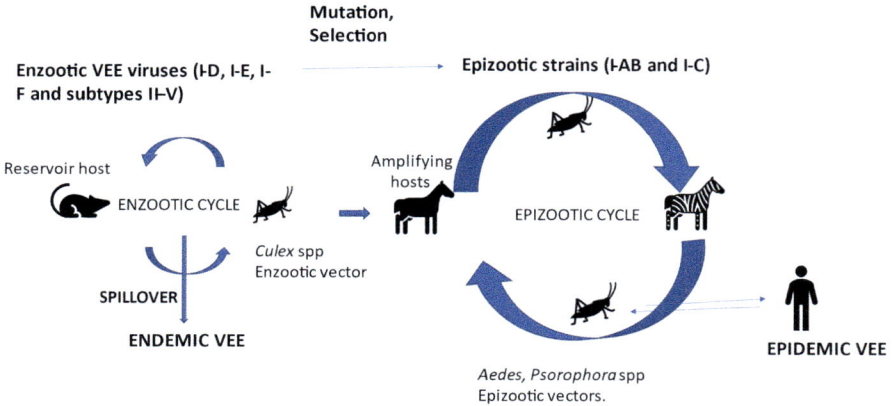

Fig. 9.1 Enzootic cycle and epizootic VEEV

9.2.2   Vector

The vectors in the equine-amplified epizootics/epidemic are *Aedes and/or Psorophora* species. Their density is high during periods of high rainfall. Surveillance in endemic areas suggested that the adult female mosquitoes of some enzootic vectors are abundant in agricultural habitat and also found in urban areas, even within areas of human habitation.

The enzootic strains (I-D, I-E and I-F and the other five subtypes) are maintained in tropical ecosystem primary reservoir, sylvatic rodents and perhaps birds with mosquito vectors. These are avirulent to equids (equid amplification-incompetent). Lowland tropical and subtropical forest, tropical wet forest, swampy areas and areas where rainfall occurs throughout the year are favourable for enzootic. Spillover from rodent-mosquito transmission cycle causes epidemic in humans, usually limited to the enzootic localities. The vectors' flight range is 1–3 km and covers large areas in enzootic regions. The enzootic viruses cause clinical disease in humans indistinguishable from those caused by epizootic strains. The enzootic viruses tend to cause clinical disease in equids with exception of I-E virus seen in 1993 and 1999 in Mexico.

9.2.3   Spillover to Human and Transmission

Spillover to human is determined by virulence of VEEV, high density of flying vector and number of enzootic cycles in rodents followed by cycles of epizootics in equid amplifying hosts (horses, donkeys, zebras). Viraemia is high and prolonged in equids. The large body size allows a wide range of mosquitoes not necessarily restricted to equids feed upon and get infected to spread infection. The epizootic, equid amplification-competent IAB and IC strains appear to have evolved from enzootic ID strains with an adaptive mutation in the E2 envelope glycoprotein gene. The mutation increased the ability to infect the epidemic vector, *Ae. Taeniorhynchus*, and replicate in equids. These circulate in the northern region of South America. Human-vector-human transmission spreads VEEV in human population.

VEEV-infected horses can shed virus in body fluids. Non-vector (direct, aerosol) transmission from equids and human-human transmission are not known (https://www.oie.int/app/uploads/2021/03/vee.pdf).

Epizootic strains of VEEV are I-AB and I-C. These occur in amplifying hosts, equines (horses, donkeys, zebras), and infect humans and occasionally other mammals with viraemia sufficient to infect mosquito, but without important epidemiological role. Horses are severely affected; about half of the infected develop encephalitis. Cattle, swine, chickens and dog seroconvert. VEEV has been isolated from cotton rats, opossums, grey fox, bats and many wild birds. Epizootic strains have been isolated from the genera *Aedes*, *Anopheles*, *Culex*, *Deinocerites*, *Mansonia* and *Psorophora* (https://www.oie.int/app/uploads/2021/03/vee.pdf). Dogs and pigs may be clinically infected and infection can be fatal. Infected dogs, pigs, cattle, birds and others can be a source of mosquito infection in addition to infected humans.

The epizootic strains continue for months to years only in the epizootic cycle and are thought to end with the outbreak as the supply of naïve horses gets exhausted due to mortality or developing herd immunity (Fig. 9.1). Rapid spread is determined by the VEEV subtype (causing high viraemia in equids), vector density and susceptible population.

9.3   Symptoms

9.3.1   In Human

The incubation period is 2–5 days. Fever, headache, myalgia, chills, arthralgia, retro-orbital pain, nausea, vomiting, cough, sore throat and prostration may or may not progress to neurological signs. Acute VEEV lasts for 3–4 days. Most patients recover in about a week. Illness is self-limited. The disease is more severe (encephalitis) in children than in adults. The case fatality rate is around 20% and is higher in children up to 5 years of age.

The serious neurological condition develops in 4–14% infected and manifest as convulsions, disorientation, drowsiness, depression and death. All genotypes of the subtype I-D cause neurological/fatal disease, principally in children reported in Bolivia, Colombia, Panama and Peru. In Panama, patients with haemorrhages have been observed. VEEV has been isolated from aborted and stillborn foetuses. Infection in pregnant women may lead to spontaneous abortion, preterm delivery, stillbirths and congenital disabilities. Fatality rates vary from 0.7 to 1.0%.

Neurological sequelae are common in children and include recurrent seizures, motor impairment, psychomotor retardation and changes in behaviour.

Symptoms resemble dengue fever. Surveillance on the Pacific coast of Mexico and the Gulf Coast showed that VEE was widespread and endemic and most often misdiagnosed as dengue.

9.3.2   In Equines

Infected equines suffer from encephalomyelitis. The IP is 1–5 days, there is high fever within 12–24 h and depression and the neurological signs and symptoms appear usually after 5 days to 4 weeks after infection.

Morbidity rates vary from 10–40% to 50–100%. Mortality rates in horses can be 50–70%.

The period of infectivity is 14 days.

Infected horses shed the virus in body fluids, and humans can then become infected by direct contact or aerosolized fluids (Crosby and Crespo 2022).

9.4   Diagnosis

Symptoms, disease and deaths in equids are strongly suggestive.

Laboratory diagnosis is based on virus isolation, PCR from serum and CSF and serological tests (VEEV-specific blocking ELISA to identify serotype).

9.5   Treatment

No specific drug is available.

9.6   Prevention and Control

Surveillance detects enzootic VEE. There is a constant threat of emergence of epizootic strains from the enzootic progenitors in many Latin American countries.

Sentinel mice and hamster and vector mosquito species have been used in Colombia. Isolation of VEEV and demonstration of antibodies have been made.

Early detection, mosquito control and vaccination of equids control outbreak and prevent large epidemic.

9.6.1 Vaccine

TC-83 is the FDA-approved vaccine. Live attenuated TC-83 is reactogenic, causes flu and may revert to wild-type virulent virus and only 80% vaccinated seroconvert. The formalin-inactivated TC-83 is used in those who fail to seroconvert with the live attenuated vaccine. It requires booster to maintain immunity.

Post-infection immunity is lifelong but serotype-specific.

TC-83—vaccinate animals >3 months of age, s/c in cervical region; booster every year. Reconstituted vaccine to be used within 4 h.

9.6.2 Drivers

Neotropical forest destruction/fragmentation may increase (a) exposure of equids and human to virulent VEEV; (b) the length of ecotone habitats that are species-rich for mosquitoes, including enzootic VEEV vectors; and (c) vector abundance. Climate change may affect enzootic areas, vector density and spread. Global warming may favour emergence of epidemic.

References

Aguilar PV, Estrada-Franco JG, Navarro-Lopez R, Ferro C et al (2011) Endemic Venezuelan equine encephalitis in the Americas: hidden under the dengue umbrella. Future Virol 6(6):721–740
Crosby B, Crespo ME (2022) Venezuelan equine encephalitis. [Updated 2022 Jul 4]. In: StatPearls [Internet]. StatPearls Publishing, Treasure Island. https://www.ncbi.nlm.nih.gov/books/NBK559332/
OIE Scientific and Technical Department (scientific.dept@oie.int). 2020.
Venezuelan equine encephalitis: aetiology epidemiology diagnosis prevention and control. https://www.oie.int/app/uploads/2021/03/vee.pdf

Chapter 10
St. Louis Encephalitis

St. Louis encephalitis (SLE) is a severe neuroinvasive viral disease spread through bite of mosquitoes. Older adults are most commonly affected. Others infected do not show any apparent symptom. Deaths (5–30%) and long-term disability occur in rare cases. It is an important disease because there is no availability of vaccine and specific treatment.

10.1 Aetiology

Phylogeographic investigation led Kopp et al. (2013) to infer that the current cosmopolitan lineage of St. Louis encephalitis virus (SLEV) emerged from the ancestor in a primary rainforest area of Palenque National Park, Mexico, Central America, in the seventeenth century when intense human invasion of primary rainforests occurred. Further spread followed major bird migration pathways over North and South America. Strains of SLEV can be divided into I–VIII genotypes. Genotypes I and II circulated mainly in North America and the rest in the Central and South America. Genotype V also is prevalent in Florida.

Ottendorfer et al. (2009) isolated SLEV from cloacal swabs of sentinel chickens and identified them as VA and VB lineage that circulated in Brazil in 1972 and 2006, suggesting importation.

10.2 Epidemiology

According to Ottendorfer et al. (2009), SLEV is active in the Western Hemisphere. It was detected in 1933 during an epidemic in St. Louis, Missouri. It has been active in the United States since then. It has been an important cause of epidemics of viral

© Springer Nature Singapore Pte Ltd. 2024
K. G. Narayan et al., *Handbook of Management of Zoonoses*,
https://doi.org/10.1007/978-981-99-9885-2_10

encephalitis before the introduction of West Nile virus in America in 1999. SLEV was detected almost every year till West Nile virus (WNV) entered (1998–2007), and then there was a natural decline and increased activity was coincident with reduced WNV activity. This suggested that these closely related flaviviruses exerted competitive pressure altering their natural transmission cycle. It was experimentally demonstrated that WNV immunity in wild birds limited subsequent SLEV infection.

SLE is distributed throughout North, Central and South America and the Caribbean and is a major public health problem in the United States. Periodic outbreaks and epidemics have occurred in the Mississippi Valley, Gulf Coast, western states and Florida. Occasionally, it is reported from Canada and Mexico. Episodic urban-centred outbreaks in eastern and central states and endemic in rural western states occur.

SLEV is maintained by horizontal transmission between birds and mosquitoes. Infected mosquitoes surviving winter and venereal and transovarial transfer of the virus in them constitute the overwintering mechanism.

Birds, abundant in the urban-suburban areas such as sparrows, finches, blue jays, robins, doves, and mosquito cycle maintain the virus in nature. Mosquitoes belonging to *Culex* spp., *Cx. pipiens* and *Cx. quinquefasciatus* in the east, *Cx. nigripalpus* in Florida and *Cx. tarsalis* and members of the *Cx. pipiens* complex in western states are important vectors. Mosquitoes remain infected for life. The virus is *amplified by the birds* including the peridomestic ones and transmitted to human beings by mosquito bites. In birds, viraemia develops after 1–2 days of mosquito bites and lasts for 1–3 days. Human and domestic animals are dead-end hosts. Chickens are susceptible, develop antibodies without manifesting any symptoms and are used as sentinels.

Climatic conditions trigger increase in mosquito population. SLEV transmission is favoured by a convergence of favourable rainfall, mosquito and birds' nesting activities. Cases cluster during late summer or early fall (August to October) in the temperate regions of the United States. In the milder climate of southern states, cases occur round the year.

Those who are participating in outdoor and recreational activities and low-income group are more prone to SLEV infection. Once infected, a person is immune for life.

10.3   Clinical Disease

Infections may lead to (a) asymptomatic form, (b) mild form, (c) aseptic meningitis and (d) encephalitis. Moderate form manifests as headache, fever and myalgia. Severity and risk of fatal form increase with age—milder in children than in older adults. Mild form and aseptic meningitis are seen in about 40% of children and young adults compared to 90% of elderly developing encephalitis.

Following bite by infectious mosquitoes, it takes about 5–15 days for symptoms to appear. Most of the infections (>99%) are silent. SLEV replicates at the site of inoculation. This is followed by viraemia. Cells of the RE system clear the infection and attempt to prevent the invasion of the CN system. Continued viral replication and secondary viraemia may foil this and invasion of the central nervous system, brain and spinal cord occurs. There is perivascular inflammation, neuronal degeneration and microglial proliferation. Pathogenesis is unclear. SLE manifests in fever, headache, nuchal rigidity, tremors, dizziness, stupor, disorientation, somnolence, coma and death. Infants show convulsion and spastic paralysis. Recovery is spontaneous in some cases. In others, irritability, memory loss and motor deficits of some type of movement disorder may be observed.

Population at risk: Outdoor activities expose to mosquito bite. Related with this probably is observation of more cases among males. Poor socioeconomic conditions are often related with less awareness and protection against mosquitoes. Children compared to adults suffer from mild illness. Case fatality rate increases with age. People with hypertension, cardiac disorder and atherosclerosis are more prone to the illness.

10.4 Diagnosis

- Brain and cerebrospinal fluid (CSF) are the ideal tissues for SLEV isolations.
- SLEV-specific IgM antibody in serum or CSF.
- Neutralizing antibody test on paired, acute and convalescent serum samples.

10.5 Treatment

There is no vaccine and specific treatment. Supportive therapy, hospitalization, respiratory support, intravenous fluids and prevention of other infections are made.

10.6 Prevention

Protection from mosquito bite is the best way to prevent SLE, for example, using insect repellent, wearing long-sleeved shirts and pants, treating clothing and gear, and taking steps to control mosquitoes indoors and outdoors. Standing water sites should be emptied and kept dry when not in use.

The Florida Sentinel Chicken Arboviral Surveillance Network enabled a targeted strategy for sampling 'sentinel chickens in hot zones of SLEV.' Serum samples are collected weekly from each chicken during July to December. Seroconversion is detected by HAI, IgM-capture ELISA and/or plaque reduction neutralization tests.

Sentinel chicken flocks and mosquito population surveillance provide basis for identifying emergence of infection.

References

Kopp A, Gillespie TR, Hobelsberger D, Estrada A, Harper JM et al (2013) Provenance and geographic spread of St. Louis encephalitis virus mBio 4(3):e00322–e00313

Ottendorfer CL, Ambrose JH, White GS, Unnasch TR, Stark LM, Isolation of genotype V St. (2009) Louis encephalitis virus in Florida. Emerg Infect Dis 15(4):604–606

Chapter 11
Australian Encephalitis

Synonyms

Murray Valley encephalitis, Kunjin virus, Ross River virus.

Acute encephalitis syndrome (AES) is a multi-aetiology condition. AES cases suffer from fever, headache and altered level of consciousness. AES increased from 47% (1979–1992) to 57.6% (1993–2006).

Huppatz et al. (2009a, b) observed that a high proportion (70%) of encephalitis with unknown aetiology occurred in Australia suggesting statutory notification of all hospitalized encephalitis cases and their investigation for aetiology. Paterson et al. (2011) suggested (a) investigating 'standard diagnostics and testing algorithm', (b) using 'sentinel surveillance of adult and paediatric in patients' and (c) improving the encephalitis surveillance at the animal-human-environmental interface in identification of pathogens and alerting and control of AES.

Higher rates of Barmah Forest virus, Kunjin virus, Ross River virus, Murray Valley encephalitis (MVE) were reported in 2011 and alerted the Department of Health and Surveillance. 'MVE and Kunjin viruses are associated with encephalitis while Barmah Forest and Ross River viruses with fever, headache, rash and joint pains. This plus full history of travel should be sent for laboratory examination. All travellers should be vigilant about mosquito bite avoidance and be aware of symptoms of MVE.' Visitors, tourists, new workers, babies and young children were advised to consult doctors immediately (Health Professionals 2012).

Encephalitis due to Murray Valley Encephalitis virus (MVEV) is potentially fatal and frequently causes long-term neurological sequelae.

© Springer Nature Singapore Pte Ltd. 2024
K. G. Narayan et al., *Handbook of Management of Zoonoses*,
https://doi.org/10.1007/978-981-99-9885-2_11

11.1   Aetiology

There are 70 arboviruses prevalent in Australia, and ten are associated with human infections. Murray Valley encephalitis virus (MVEV), Kunjin virus (KUNV) and Ross River virus (RRV) are the most important.

11.1.1   Ross River Virus (RRV)

It is a mosquito-borne alphavirus that causes infectious disease characterized by polyarthritis and pandemic in Australia and occurs in Papua New Guinea and other South Pacific islands.

RRV is an encapsulated and a positive-sense, single-stranded RNA alphavirus of family *Togaviridae*. It has a protein capsid, 700A in diameter, two glycoproteins E1 and E2 and a host-derived lipid envelop. The virus was isolated and identified in 1959 from mosquitoes trapped from around Ross River near Townsville, Queensland, Australia. Its association with 'epidemic polyarthritis' in Queensland was established by observing antibodies in patients' sera specific to this virus isolate; thus, the virus was so christened. This virus was later isolated from patients in a series of epidemic polyarthritis in Fiji, Samoa and Cook Islands during 1979 and also from an Australian patient in 1985.

The mean annual incidence rate of RRV per 100,000 is 117, 59 and 33 in Northern Territory (NT), Queensland and Western Australia (WA), respectively. The highest incidence rates were in remote rural regions. Largest number of cases occurred in densely populated semi-urban and urban areas of Queensland. RRV is active in tropical to temperate and occasionally arid climatic regions.

As many as 75% of infected may be clinically ill. Symptoms are fever, fatigue, malaise, pain in muscles and joints and generalized rash in 50–60%. Most (80–90%) of the patients develop swelling and joint pain persisting for months. Commonly affected joints were wrists, knees, ankles and small joints of extremities, fingers, toes, etc. Patients reported moderate fever and swollen face. Rarely glomerulonephritis develops in a severe case. The estimated average total burden is around AU$ 5500/patient.

Principal mosquito vectors, among 40, are *Aedes camptorhynchus* and *Ae. vigilax* (coastal regions), *Cx. annulirostris* (inland and coastal regions) and *Ae. notoscriptus* in urban areas. RRV persisted in the arid north-west of Western Australia in desiccation-resistant eggs of *Aedes* spp. mosquito, reappeared after rains and was associated with human infection. The amplifying hosts are kangaroos, wallabies, possums and horses. Other domestic and wild animals also have been implicated. Circumstantial evidence suggests human as the amplifying host introducing RRV to cause a major epizootic in south-west Pacific Islands nations in 1979–1982 and during an outbreak in metropolitan Perth in 2003–2004. RRV appear(s) to have been introduced by man to urban mosquito vectors and through them to urban reservoir hosts like possums and macropods. Human-urban wetlands-macropod interaction was implicated in a cluster of 111 cases in 2011–2012. Major outbreaks occur every

3–4 years in south-west Western Australia. *Ae. camptorhynchus* and grey kangaroo (*Macropus fuliginosus*) seem to maintain RRV in the region (Mackenzie et al. 2017).

The virus killed mice. Experimental infection in inbred mouse reproduces disease, hindlimb arthritis/arthralgia and pathology and inflammatory infiltrates; macrophages and serum C3 protein contribute to immunopathology.

11.1.2 Murray Valley Encephalitis Virus (MVEV)

MVEV spread out of enzootic areas very occasionally causing severe outbreaks. Outbreaks of X disease during 1917–1918, 1922 and 1925 might have been MVE. A patient of encephalitis died in the Murray Valley in Victoria and South Australia in 1951. The virus isolated was named as MVEV. The 1974 outbreak spread over all Australia. Since then, most cases occurred in Western Australia and the Northern Territory and sporadic cases in Queensland, central Australia and central regions of Western Australia. It is found across Australia, Papua New Guinea and Irian Jaya and is endemic in northern Australia with occasional outbreaks in south-eastern Australia.

11.1.3 Kunjin Virus

WNV has seven genetic lineages. Lineages I and II: Lineage I contains WNV$_{KUNJIN}$. It is further divided into clade Ia and Ib. Clade Ia contains WNV isolates from around the world. Clade Ib contains the Australian WNV$_{KUNJIN}$. Traditionally, it is associated with mild and rare diseases in horses and humans in Australia (Prow 2013). Sub-lineage 1a has caused epidemics of severe diseases in animals and humans during the past decade but has never been found in Australia.

West Nile virus-Kunjin (known prior to 2010) or (WNVKUN) was detected first in 1960 in northern Queensland. It has a wide distribution across the Northern Territory and Western Australia. Enzootic cycles involve *Culex* spp. mosquitoes and ardeid aquatic birds.

The important vector is *Cx. annulirostris*; occasionally, others like *Aedes* (*Ae.*) *tremulus, Cx. australicus, Cx. squamosus, Ae. alternans, Ae. nomenensis, Ae. vigilax, Anopheles amictus* and *Cx. quinquefasciatus* have been reported. Wading birds (particularly *Nycticorax caledonicus*, the rufous night heron) are considered an important natural reservoir.

Horses and humans are considered as dead-end hosts.

The endemicity is detected in south-eastern Australia without any human infection. There is great similarity with MVE in the natural history, detection by sentinel chicken flock testing, clinical manifestation, absence of drug and vaccine. A vast majority do not develop symptoms. About 20% may develop symptoms. Serious illness, sometimes fatal, occurs in about 1 in 150 infected people. Incubation period is 2–6 days, which is extendable to 14 days. The infection is mild and ends in complete recovery. Symptoms include fever, headache, muscle pain, swollen lymph nodes, fatigue, swollen and aching joints and rash. Encephalitis cases manifest as rigor, stiff neck, irritability, confusion, excessive sleepiness, fits and need hospitalization. According to Paterson et al. (2011), it accounted for 11% of encephalitis cases during the 1974 MVE outbreak, but during the last three decades, it caused only three non-fatal cases when MVEV caused 68.

According to the Western Australian Health Department, Murray Valley encephalitis (MVE) caused a death in 2008 in north-east Kimberley. Additionally, more than 25 cases of the milder Ross River, Kunjin and Barmah Forest diseases were reported in Kimberley and Pilbara (Promed 2009). MVE spread to areas of Pilbara. Those residing in Kimberley for over 3 years usually had natural protective immunity. Re-emergence of MVEV activity in the endemic regions in 2011 followed flooding and consequential increase in vector *Cx. annulirostris* density. It was detected by seroconversion in flocks of sentinel chickens that alerted the health department. Horses died and several human cases appeared with fatality.

11.2   Epidemiology

MVE is endemic in northern Australia and is a disease of public health concern for residents and travellers. MVE is a notifiable disease in Australia. Sentinel chicken flocks are used for early warning. Infection may be asymptomatic and symptomatic (1/150–1/1000). Characteristic symptoms include flaccid paralysis when the spinal cord is affected, cranial nerve palsy and tremor when the brainstem is involved, encephalitis, death in 20–30% and long-term neurological sequelae in about 30–50% survivors.

Floridis et al. (2018) presented a case report of 22 meningoencephalitis (2000–2015). Briefly, 6 died and 59% were males, 59% indigenous rest travellers and 41% children.

Cases were detected by observing diffuse leptomeningeal enhancement changes in left basal ganglia and bilateral thalami seen in MRI of the brain and confirmed by PCR, IgM in serum and CSF. The Department of Health launched a radio and social media awareness programme in 2015 following two cases and in February in 2016.

More cases occurred in 2000 and 2011 coincident with exceptionally high rainfall. Maintaining and amplifying enzootic activity of MVEV begin in the middle of wet season and peak towards its end. It required heavy rainfall and flooding. The onset of most cases was recorded between February and July. A correlation between high summer rainfall >100 mm, overnight adult mosquito traps ≥300, seroconversion in sentinel chicken and MVE disease cases was found in the earlier non-endemic Alice Springs region.

The enzootic is maintained by bird-mosquito-bird transmission. Heavy rainfall and flood increase the density of mosquito and also the viral activity. Infected mosquito bite transmits infection to humans resulting in sporadic cases or small outbreaks in a few years.

Infected native birds flying to or infected mosquitoes blown by wind spread MVEV from endemic to epidemic areas. The virus survived for one or two seasons, most likely in eggs of mosquitos and by unidentified mechanism. The common natural hosts are aquatic birds, egrets and heron (*Ardeiformes*), particularly the rufous night heron (*Nycticorax caledonicus*), and the cormorants/darters (*Pelecaniformes*). Many animals, wild and domesticated, show antibodies to MVEV. Rabbits and possibly grey kangaroos develop viraemia sufficient to support local transmission. Horses suffer from encephalitis but viraemia is probably insufficient to infect mosquitoes. The primary mosquito vector is *Culex annulirostris*. Other mosquitoes may also be involved—*Cx. australicus*, *Ae. normanensis* and *Ochlerotatus* spp. Eggs of *Aedes* spp. are desiccation-resistant. MVEV is believed to survive over several dry seasons in eggs of *Aedes* spp. in arid areas until sufficient rainfall occurs causing flooding. MVEV has been isolated from male *Aedes tremulus*. Low level of local transmission cycles might also be simultaneously operative (Mackenzie et al. 2017).

Human activities contributed to the spread of MVE in Western Australia. It is hypothesized that building dam and increasing irrigated agriculture areas attracted aquatic birds and mosquitoes and expanded enzootic focus of MVEV to south and southeast. Viraemic waterbirds moved following rainfall and flooding. In Alice Springs in Central Australia, effluent discharges from an adjacent sewage farm increased the breeding of mosquito vectors of MVEV and WNVKUN (anthropogenic) and re-emergence of MVEV encephalitis in 2000–2001, and drainage of effluent led to reduction in mosquito population and seroconversion in sentinel chicken.

Mackenzie et al. (2017) suggest understanding patterns of monsoon rainfall in the region (Kimberley), i.e. flooding, to predict increased MVEV activity and alert. One Health approach is recommended for control.

The 2011 outbreak was preceded by heavy rainfall, regional flooding during October–November and increased vector density of *Cx. annulirostris*. Mosquito-borne disease peaked during autumn months, from December to May. Horses with neurological symptoms and death were recorded in south-eastern Australia. Sixteen human cases and deaths (in bracket) were distributed across Australia—9 (1), Western Australia; 4 (1), Northern Territory; 2 (1), South Australia; and 1 (0), New South Wales and one suspected-unproven from Victoria. Gordon et al. (2012) described a case of MVE in a horse showing neurological symptoms of sub-acute nonsuppurative encephalitis, which is confirmed by immunohistochemistry, virus isolation in cell culture and sequence determination and PCR. The strain was identified as genotype 1 closely related to the previous Queensland isolate. Mann et al. (2013) studied 11 cases. Eleven horses from Victoria suffered from neurological symptoms before death. Five of the isolates were MVEV and six West Nile virus, subtype Kunjin. The genome sequences studied indicated that isolates were highly homogenous.

11.3 Clinical Presentation

Knox et al. (2012) reviewed MVEV in Australia. The ratio of clinical to subclinical cases was 1 to 800–1000. The case fatality rate was 25% and the other 25–50% recovered with permanent neurological disability. Most MVE infections are subclinical or mild. This may progress to involve brain-causing meningitis or even encephalitis of variable severity. MVE is characterized by fever, drowsiness, dizziness, nausea, headache and stiff neck and in severe cases fits and coma. The illness may end fatally or leave a permanent brain damage. Most cases occur between November and July.

The disease affects all ages. Incubation period ranges between 1 and 4 weeks (average 2 weeks). Infection leads to symptoms that may be (a) non-encephalitis, headache and fever, (b) mild encephalitis that passes off without hospitalization or (c) a full range of encephalitis. Initial symptoms are commonly febrile: fever >40 °C, nausea, vomiting, diarrhoea, headache, cough and mild neurological like lethargy, irritability and confusion. There may seizures common in children, but less so in adults. Neurological features may progress into one of the following four patterns: (a) relentless progression to death, (b) prominent spinal cord involvement causing flaccid paralysis, (c) cranial nerve/brainstem involvement and tremor and (d) encephalitis followed by complete recovery. Overlapping clinical features of flaviviral encephalitis do not allow differential diagnosis. JEV is likely to cause Parkinsonian features—cranial nerve, cerebellar and upper motor neuron signs. WNV is likely to cause polio-like symptoms (suggesting anterior horn sell process), seizures, cerebellar ataxia, brachial plexopathy and optic neuritis.

11.4   Diagnosis

- MRI/CT scan is useful within a week of the onset of symptoms.
- Cerebrospinal fluid examined for IgM to diagnose meningoencephalitis.
- Serum is examined for detection of IgM; fourfold rise in IgG titre between acute and convalescent (7–10 days) serum samples. HA/HAI, EIA and IFA are the tests; a check for ruling out cross-reactivity with other flaviviruses is essential. Serum-virus neutralization test and epitope-blocking ELISA are useful to detect specific antibodies.
- Isolation of virus.
- Identification of the MVEV-RNA.

11.5   Treatment

There is no specific treatment. Immediate hospitalization and supportive therapy are helpful.

11.6   Prevention

Several predictive models have been developed but not yet tested. Controlling mosquito population, lack of preventive measures and treatment are challenging. Directives (Health Professionals 2012) should be followed.

Early warning system—Sentinel chicken: these do not suffer but seroconvert and antibody detection alerts. Sentinel mosquito arbovirus capture kit (SMACK) detects arboviruses by PCR on honey-soaked nucleic acid preservation cards deployed in purpose-built CO_2-baited traps. It is a simple tool compared to traditional overnight mosquito traps. It may substitute sentinel animal programme.

References

Floridis J, McGuinness SL, Kurucz N, Burrow JN et al (2018) Case report Murray Valley encephalitis virus: an ongoing cause of encephalitis in Australia's North. Trop Med Infect Dis 3:49

Gordon AN, Marbach CR, Oakey J, Edmunds G et al (2012) Confirmed case of encephalitis caused by Murray Valley encephalitis virus infection in a horse. J Vet Diagn Invest 24(2):431–436

Health Professionals (2012) Murray Valley encephalitis and other mosquito borne diseases: advice for travellers to Australia—update. 12 January 2012. http://www.nathnac.org/pro/clinical_updates/mve_au_120112.htm

http://www.theaustralian.news.com.au/story/0,25197,25148291-26103,00.html

https://www.sahealth.sa.gov.au/wps/wcm/connect/public+content/sa+health+internet/conditions/infectious+diseases/kunjin+west+nile+virus+infection/kunjin+west+nile+virus+infection+-+including+symptoms+treatment+and+prevention

Huppatz C, Kelly PM, Levi C, Dalton C, Williams D, Durrheim DN (2009a) Encephalitis in Australia, 1979–2006: trends and aetiologies. Commun Dis Intell 33:192–197

Huppatz C, Durrheim DN, Levi C, Dalton C et al (2009b) Etiology of Encephalitis in Australia, 1990–2007. Emerg Infect Dis 15(9):1359–1365

Knox J, Cowan RU, Doyle JS, Ligtermoet MK, Archer JS et al (2012) Murray Valley encephalitis: a review of clinical features, diagnosis and treatment. Med J Aust 196(5):322–326

Mackenzie JS, Lindsay MDA, Smith DW, Imrie A (2017) The ecology and epidemiology of Ross River and Murray Valley encephalitis viruses in Western Australia: examples of One Health in Action. Trans R Soc Trop Med Hyg 111:248–254

Mann RA, Fegan M, O'Riley K, Motha J, Warner S (2013) Molecular characterization and phylogenetic analysis of Murray Valley encephalitis virus and West Nile virus (Kunjin subtype) from an arbovirus disease outbreak in horses in Victoria, Australia, in 2011. J Vet Diagn Invest 25(1):35–44

Paterson BJ, Mackenzie JS, Durrheim DN, Smith D (2011) A review of the epidemiology and surveillance of viral zoonotic encephalitis and the impact on human health in Australia. NSW Public Health Bull 22(5–6):99–104

Promed (2009) Murray Valley Encephalitis—Australia: (Western Australia), ALERT Archive no. 20090306.0936; 06 March, 2009; PRO/AH/EDR> Murray Valley encephalitis—Australia: (WA), alert. A ProMED-mail post. http://www.promedmail.org. The Australian online [edited]

Prow NA (2013) The changing epidemiology of kunjin virus in Australia. Inter J Environ Res Pub Hlth 10(12):6255–6272

Chapter 12
California Encephalitis

Synonyms

La Crosse encephalitis.

California encephalitis is a viral infection of the brain transmitted to humans by *Aedes triseriatus* endemic in Midwest USA, affecting primarily children 5–10 years of age. Most cases are caused by La Crosse virus.

Originally discovered in the USA, the California group of viruses causes human infections on five continents, seemingly because these are maintained and amplified in a wide variety of microclimates, such as tropical, coastal, temperate marshland, lowland river valleys, alpine valleys and highlands. Of all the arboviral illnesses recorded in 1993, California serogroup of viruses accounted for 71%. La Crosse virus (LACV) encephalitis was the most common (Rust et al. 1999), in which approximately 80–100 cases occurred annually.

California encephalitis virus was isolated in 1943 from mosquitoes. Three human cases were detected 2 years later. All these happened to originate in Kern County in California. Eldridge et al. (2001) reported the fourth case. Obviously, California encephalitis is a rare infection. The year 2002 recorded the highest number of California serogroup virus cases. However, 99% of the California serogroup virus neuroinvasive disease cases recorded by CDC during 2003–2007 were caused by LACV. Most cases during the 1960s and 1970s are confined to the states in the Upper Midwest. Since the 1980s, more cases occurred in Mid-Atlantic states for unexplained reasons, possibly vector ecology and better diagnosis and reporting (CDC 2010; http://www.cdc.gov/mmwr/preview/mmwrhtml/mm5928a2.htm). A neuroinvasive disease in a boy aged 8 years was diagnosed as LACV northwest Missouri. Environmental inspection identified multiple vector habitats including tree holes and discarded tires within 300 ft. radius of patient's home. Diagnosis was

© Springer Nature Singapore Pte Ltd. 2024   99
K. G. Narayan et al., *Handbook of Management of Zoonoses*,
https://doi.org/10.1007/978-981-99-9885-2_12

based on serological test-plaque-reduction neutralization with 90% cut-off value
and LACV-specific IgM and IgG capture ELISA (CDC 2010; http://www.cdc.gov/
mmwr/preview/mmwrhtml/mm5928a2.htm).

12.1   Aetiology

The California serogroup within family *Bunyaviridae* and genus *Orthobunyavirus*
has 16 viruses, causing arboviral encephalitis more frequently than WEE, EEE and
St. Louis combined.

It is an enveloped virus having negative-sense tripartite genome. The segments
are small (S), medium (M) and large (L). The envelope contains glycoproteins, G1,
that elicit neutralizing antibodies that block fusion of the virus with hosts' cells.

The California serogroup of viruses includes California encephalitis, La Crosse
encephalitis, Jamestown Canyon, Keystone, Snowshoe and Trivittatus.

LACV was isolated in 1964 from the brain of a 4-year-old girl who had died of
encephalitis in 1960 in La Crosse County, Wisconsin. CDC has been keeping record of
arboviral neuroinvasive diseases including the California serogroup of viruses since
then. Since 1995, the California serogroup of virus neuroinvasive disease is notifiable.

12.2   Epidemiology

Epidemiological factors influencing the incidence include season, geographic location, regional climatic conditions and the demographic—say age profile.

12.2.1   Maintenance and Transmission in Nature

LACV is naturally maintained in hardwood deciduous forest by transovarial, trans-
stadial and venereal transmission mechanisms within mosquitoes, and horizontal
transmission can occur via small daytime-active mammals (e.g. chipmunks and
squirrels) that act as amplifying hosts for blood-feeding mosquitoes. Chipmunks
(*Tamias striatus*), grey squirrels (*Sciurus carolinensis*) and fox squirrel (*S. niger*)
are the natural vertebrate hosts. Eastern tree hole mosquito (*Aedes triseriatus*) is the
vector. These mosquitoes are aggressive during both daylight and twilight periods
and feed on human. *Ae. triseriatus* lay eggs in water collected in natural tree holes
and artificial crevices, rock pools, spaces like clogged gutters and discarded tires,
buckets and pots. Larvae and pupae develop in these aquatic environments. These
breeding sites are within peridomestic environment and contribute to increased biting rates and risk of infection. Humans are incidental hosts. Viraemia is low and
insufficient for transmission through mosquito bites and hence human is considered

a dead end. *Aedes triseriatus* transovarially transmits LACV and the virus overwinters in diapausing *A. triseriatus* eggs.

This seems to the mechanism of overwintering; the virus emerges with the flying mosquitoes in the spring. There is also a venereal transmission (from male to uninfected female) in mosquitoes. Mosquito bite infects humans. *Ae. albopictus* and *Ae. japonicus* are also competent vectors. The principal vector is *Ae. triseriatus*. It is distributed throughout wooded regions east of the Rocky Mountains. LACV-associated encephalitis has a geographic distribution within the range of the native tree hole breeding mosquito—*Ae. triseriatus*.

Ae. japonicum is another vector and requires tree cover and is abundant at the edge of the forest like *Ae. triseriatus*. *Ae. albopictus* has field habitat and has high anthropogenic tolerance.

12.2.2   Season

Haddow and Odoi (2009) detected clustering in four geographic regions, shift from the earlier distribution and identified high risk areas for targeted intervention. Eighty-one per cent cases occurred in summer. Southern states significantly presented higher risk than northern states during June, July, August and October.

Lambert et al. (2010) isolated LACV from *Ae. albopictus* collected in Dallas County, Texas. *Ae. albopictus* was introduced in 1985 in Houston, Texas, apparently in shipment of used tires, spreading to most of southeastern United States. Concurrently, LACV encephalitis activity increased.

In the United States, most cases occur from late spring to early fall (July–September). Rare cases can occur in winter in subtropical endemic areas, e.g. Gulf states. LACV is endemic in rural central and midwestern states.

Outdoor activity in woodland areas is risky.

12.2.3   Geographic Areas

Historically, most cases occurred in the upper Midwestern (Ohio, Wisconsin, Minnesota, Indiana, Illinois, Iowa), mid-Atlantic and south-eastern states. Recently, new areas have reported cases, in north-eastern, mid-Atlantic and south-eastern states (North Carolina, Tennessee, West Virginia, Georgia, Virginia, Kentucky and Rhode Island; https://www.cdc.gov/lac/tech/epi.html) and in the south as far as Louisiana, Alabama and Florida.

During 2003–2012, paediatric neuroinvasive arboviral infection caused 1217 cases and 22 deaths in 48 contiguous states. La Crosse virus accounted for 55% and infected younger children <15 years (Gaensbauer et al. 2014), and an average of 68 cases are reported every year in the United States from late spring to early fall (https://www.cdc.gov/lac/tech/epi.html).

Byrd (2016) reported a case fatality <1% but the economic cost is high – long-term neurological sequelae causing chronic seizures, poor academic performance, impaired mental function and/or behavioural problems. Economic and social burden estimated at (a) $48, 775–3,090,798 as medical expenses plus and (b) DALYs −17.5–92% of productive life lost in severe cases and 54.8% timespan for convalescence period.

12.3   Pathogenesis

The surface glycoproteins of the virus are involved in the transmission of the virus, G1 for attachment to human cells and G2 for attachment to mosquito cells. The California group of viruses replicates at the site of entry after the mosquito bite to infect chondrocytes and reticuloendothelial cells mainly in the liver, spleen and lymph glands. The systemic infection and spread of the virus may end here in many cases. In others, the virus enters the CNS through vascular endothelial cells or choroid plexus and neuro-invasion and infection of neurons and glia occur. This is the proposed mechanism of La Crosse encephalitis. Post-mortem pathology reveals neurodegeneration with patchy inflammation and vasculitis. There is a reversible (vasogenic) cerebral oedema.

12.4   Symptoms

LACV is an important paediatric encephalitis, often underdiagnosed or confounded with other causes such as herpes simplex encephalitis and enteroviral meningitis (McJunkin et al. 2001).

Haddow and Odoi (2009) observed that LACV affected 83.3% children of ≤15 years, and most were males. The commonest pathology was meningoencephalitis (56.3%) followed by encephalitis (20.7%), meningitis (17.2%) and uncomplicated fever (5%). 1.9% of confirmed cases died.

Diseases in children are meningoencephalitis, encephalitis and seizures, whereas in adults are fever, headache and hyponatraemia. Hyponatraemia and increased intracranial pressure have also been observed (McJunkin et al. 2001). Some adults may have altered mental status but seizures are uncommon. Cerebral oedema with respiratory problem is a complication. Clinical manifestation of infection can stop after primary or secondary spread.

Primary spread: Infection is inapparent, mostly in adults. They end up with mild fever and are carriers. Nearly 4% manifest symptoms. Death occurs in <1%. Prognosis is favourable. The IP varies between 5 and15, with a minimum of 3–7 days. Fever lasts for 2–3 days and is often confused with 'flu' or 'summer cold'. Illness starts with fever, fatigue and headache, chills, nausea, vomiting, lethargy and abdominal pain lasting for 3–4 days progressing to vomiting, disorientation, lack of alertness and necessitating hospitalization.

Secondary spread: Severe form is a neuroinvasive disease showing seizure (in 50% of children), coma and paralysis. Most cases (80–90%) manifest headache, fever and vomiting for 1–3 days followed by improvement. Convalescence for over a week shows lethargy, behavioural changes and seizures—focal, generalized or epilepticus. Focal neurological findings include motor abnormalities and paralysis, abnormal and irregular reflexes in children (20%) and coma in 10%.

Duration of hospitalization is about 6 days. Duration of illness is generally between 10 and 14 days. Recovery is complete in most cases. Twenty per cent of those who recovered show behavioural changes and recurrent unprovoked seizures, especially those who had manifested seizures.

12.5 Diagnosis

- Detection of serum IgM and IgG against LACV by ELISA, fourfold increase in antibody titre in convalescent serum (paired samples of serum collected after 2 weeks), MIA (microsphere-based immunoassay) and IgG-ELISA (McJunkin et al. 2001).
- PCR on CSF.
- Histopathology and PCR of brain tissues after autopsy. Indirect IFT show strong fluorescence of neurons and capillary endothelial cells.

12.6 Treatment

There is no specific treatment and no vaccine. Supportive therapy is the mainstay. Prevention lies in measures to protect against mosquito bite.

12.7 Prevention

There is no vaccine and the best way to prevent LAC is to protect from mosquito bites by using insect repellent, wearing long-sleeved shirts and pants, treating clothing and gear and taking steps to control mosquitoes indoors and outdoors (CDC 2022).

References

Byrd BD (2016) La Crosse encephalitis: a persistent Arboviral threat in North Carolina. N C Med J 77(5):330–333

CDC (2010) Editorial note-La Crosse Virus Neuroinvasive Disease—Missouri, 2009. MMWR 59(28):869–871.http://www.cdc.gov/mmwr/preview/mmwrhtml/mm5928a2.htm

CDC (2022). https://www.cdc.gov/lac/prevention/index.html#

Eldridge BF, Glaser C, Pedrin RE, Chiles RE (2001) The first reported case of California encephalitis in more than 50 years. Emerg Infect Dis 7(3):451–452

Gaensbauer JT, Lindsey NP, Messacar K, Staples JE, Fischer M (2014) Neuroinvasive arboviral disease in the United States: 2003 to 2012. Pediatrics 134(3):e642–e650

Haddow AD, Odoi A (2009) The incidence risk, clustering, and clinical presentation of La Crosse virus infections in the eastern United States, 2003-2007. PLoS One 4.7(2009):e6145

Lambert AJ, Blair CD, D'Anton M, Ewing W, Harborth M et al (2010) La Crosse virus in *Aedes albopictus* mosquitoes, Texas, USA, 2009. Emerg Infect Dis 16(5):856–858

McJunkin JE, De Los Reyes EC, Irazuzta JE, Caceres MJ, Khan RR et al (2001) La Crosse encephalitis in children. N Engl J Med 344:801–807

Rust RS, Thompson WH, Mathews CG, Beaty BJ, Chun RWM (1999) Topical review: La Crosse and other forms of California encephalitis. J Child Neurol 14(1):1–14

Chapter 13
O'Nyong'Nyong Fever

The Acholi people of northwestern Uganda called 'O' 'nyong-nyong' to describe very painful weakening joints experienced in O'nyong'nyong fever. It is a mosquito-borne disease characterized by fever, headache, generalized joint pain, arthralgia and also maculopapular skin rash and lymph adenopathy endemic to sub-Saharan Africa.

O'nyong'nyong virus (ONNV) was isolated during the 1959 epidemic which began in Uganda and spread through Kenya and Lake Victoria's shores to southeastern Africa in 1962.

ONN fever is under-diagnosed and underestimated. Enzootic source and epidemic potential are not defined. Although the disease has remained limited to Africa, there is a risk of spread and potential epidemic because of increased air travel. Once introduced into a new area where *Anopheline* mosquitoes are available and competent, ONNV morbidity is likely to be high.

13.1 Aetiology

ONNV belongs to the genus *Alphavirus* of the family *Togaviridae*. Chikungunya (CHIKV) and ONNV form a monophyletic group within the Semliki Forest complex. There are two clades of ONNV. Strains isolated from Gulu, Uganda, in 1959 and from Senegal in 1963 are closely related. Strains from Nigeria (1966), Uganda (1996), and Chad (2004) cluster in a distinct clade. This suggested that these virus strains had their independent distribution within Africa (Rezza et al. 2017).

© Springer Nature Singapore Pte Ltd. 2024
K. G. Narayan et al., *Handbook of Management of Zoonoses*,
https://doi.org/10.1007/978-981-99-9885-2_13

13.2   Epidemiology

Transmission is by night-feeding anopheline mosquitoes (deviation from most mosquito-borne infections), *Anopheles funestus* and *Anopheles gambiae*. These are malaria vectors also. These mosquitoes are found in large clear and permanent water bodies like shores of lakes, rivers and swamps. Vector competence of *A. gambiae* appeared to be conditioned by its innate immune response and also strains of ONNV.

Large epidemics of ONNV have occurred interspersed with years of quiescence. The virus is probably maintained through an enzootic cycle. Natural reservoirs and enzootic vectors are not known.

The 1959–1962 epidemic, one of largest vector-borne epidemic, affected >2 million people in both eastern (Uganda, Kenya, Tanzania, Malawi and Mozambique) and western Africa (Democratic Republic of Congo, Central African Republic, Cameroon and Senegal).

The health officials in Rakai district of southwestern Uganda noticed in June 1997 increasing number of cases of acute febrile, crippling arthritis, skin rash, chest pain, reddening of eyes without discharge and lymphadenitis spreading to Mbarara and Malaka districts, confirmed as O'nyong'nyong (12 March 1997—O'nyong'nyong (ONN) fever in Uganda. https://www.who.int/csr/don/1997_03_12/en/). According to Rwaguma et al. (1997), it had started in June 1996 in Rakai district. Epidemic areas had a 60–70% infected and clusters in families. Four hundred people were affected. Large variation in the number of cases reported in different sites was observed. The number of cases reported in affected areas differed in 'sites – infection rates' (3–45%) and 'estimated attack rates' (3–29%). Increased risk of transmission among children and/or waning immunity among adults in coastal Kenya was suggested by a serological study. Rate of infection in Kano plain of Kenya was estimated at about 10% (Rezza et al. 2017).

During the gap of about 35 years between the two epidemics, ONNV was isolated from a pool of *A. funestus* in western Kenya in 1978. Seroprevalence studies suggested continued transmission.

ONNV caused several outbreaks in Kenya, Uganda, Tanzania, Zaire, Malawi and Mozambique in East Africa where virus isolation from sera of animals, humans and mosquitoes, *Anopheles funestus* and *A. gambiae*, was made. Nigeria, Ghana and Sierra Leone presented serological evidence of infection in humans and animals. An outbreak occurred in Cote d'Ivoire, West Africa (Posey et al. 2005). According to Bessaud et al. (2008), ONNV was isolated from sentinel mice in Senegal. They reported its isolation from peripheral blood mononuclear cells of a patient in Chad.

Prevalence of ONNV: Studies on alphavirus exposure in rural coastal area of Kenya were made by LaBeaud et al. (2015). The majority of alphavirus exposures were due to O'nyong'nyong virus (ONNV)—found by confirmatory PRNT testing in young children. Rezza et al. (2017) have mapped the distribution of ONNV in Africa. Evidence of viral activity has been found in Central African Republic, Gulu, Chad, Nigeria, Gabon, Democratic Republic of Congo, Cameroon, Liberia, Ivory

Coast, Senegal, Uganda, Kenya, Tanzania, Malawi and Mozambique. Studies suggested an increased risk of transmission in children in recent decades and/or waning immunity in adults.

Outside Africa: Travellers may carry the virus outside of Africa. A 60-year-old woman carried ONNV to Germany in 2013. She had a 7-week vacation in East Africa. She had to seek medical attention 2 days after reaching Heidelberg. The generic alphavirus, dengue and Chikungunya were ruled out. Virus neutralization test confirmed ONNV. The case recovered spontaneously after 10 days. There is a known invasive anopheline mosquito vector in Europe. The culicine mosquito species *Aedes aegypti* might be a competent vector and is found in some parts (Tappe et al. 2014).

13.3 Clinical Disease

Arthritogenic viruses are Chikungunya (commonest), O'nyong'nyong, Ross River, Mayaro and Sindbis. These have wide geographic distribution. A clinician should be aware.

The apparent to in-apparent ratio is estimated at 2:1 or more. Incubation period is estimated to be around 8 days. Symptoms include crippling arthritis affecting mainly big joints and myalgia. There is fever, general malaise, polyarthralgia, lymphadenitis, painful reddening of eyes without discharge, generalized rash, pruritus, chest pain and also miscarriages. Rarely, bleeding gums and nose may also occur. It is self-limiting. The duration of illness is few days. A patient is immobilized for about 4 days. The morbidity and loss of workdays are considerable.

It affected all age group with significant morbidity, but rare fatality. It seems to spread rapidly and outbreak covered as many as 60–80% with clusters in families.

13.4 Diagnosis

- Biological-intracranial inoculation in mice for isolating virus from serum collected in the first week of illness, preferably first 3 days of illness, and from mosquitoes.
- Molecular methods—RT-PCR.
- Serology-specific IgM antibodies, fourfold increase in IgG antibodies. Detectable levels of IgM appear during the second week of illness and lasts for 2 months or more.

Cross-reactivity with CHIKV and other co-circulating alphaviruses may pose a problem. Reciprocal plaque reduction neutralization tests (PRNT) are recommended to distinguish humoral immunity (typically IgG) from ONNV from CHIKV.

13.5   Treatment

None.

13.6   Prevention

Transmission is human-*Anopheles* mosquito-human. Vector is night-feeding. Prevention is challenging. Malaria control programme matches and would be very useful. No vaccine available. Candidate vaccine against Chikungunya may protect.

References

Bessaud M, Peyrefitte CN, Pastorino BAM, Gravier P et al (2008) O'nyong-nyong virus, Chad. Emerg Infect Dis 12(8):1248–1250

LaBeaud AD, Banda T, Brichard J, Muchiri EM, Mungai PL et al (2015) High rates of O'NyongNyong and Chikungunya virus transmission in coastal Kenya. PLoS Negl Trop Dis 9(2):e0003436

Posey DL, O'Rourke T, Roehrig JT, Lanciotti RS, Weinberg M, Maloney S (2005) Short report: O' Nyong-nyong fever in West Africa. Am J Trop Med Hyg 73(1):32

Rezza G, Chen R, Weaver SC (2017) O'nyong-nyong fever: a neglected mosquito-borne viral disease. Pathog Glob Health 111(6):271–275

Rwaguma EB, Lutwama JJ, Sempala SDK, Kiwanuka N et al (1997) Emergence of epidemic O'nyong-nyong fever in southwestern Uganda, after an absence of 35 years. Emerg Infect Dis 3(1):77

Tappe D, Kapaun A, Emmerich P, Campos R, Cadar D et al (2014) O'nyong-nyong virus infection imported to Europe from Kenya by a traveler. Emerg Infect Dis 20(10):1766–1767

Chapter 14
Chikungunya

Etymologically, Chikungunya means 'that which bends up.' The root verb *kungun-yala* in Makonde language spoken in south-east Tanzania and northern Mozambique means 'to dry up or become contorted.' *Buka-buka* in Congo means 'broken-broken,' all describing the condition of a patient.

Chikungunya disease is characterized by sudden onset of fever with severe arthralgia, rashes and other constitutional symptoms, self-limiting, high morbidity and rarely death.

14.1 Aetiology

Chikungunya virus (CHIKV) is a positive-sense, single-stranded RNA virus, of *Alphavirus* genus and *Togaviridae* family. The capsid is 60–70 nm diameter and has a phospholipid envelope. The West African and the East, Central and Southern African (ECSA) phylogroups are responsible for the epidemic in Africa. The third phylogroup is Asian. The isolates from the epidemic in India and the ongoing Indian Ocean outbreak represent a distinct clade within the ECSA phylogroup (E1:226A). The earlier isolates (1963–1973) were of Asian genotype (Mohan et al. 2010).

14.2 Epidemiology

Human is the reservoir host during epidemic with daytime biting vectors *Aedes albopictus* and *Aedes aegypti*. Viraemia is high in the beginning of acute infection and human-mosquito-human transmission is common. Chikungunya virus may circulate within a number of animals; non-human primates, e.g., monkeys, birds and small mammals as reservoirs; and mosquito vectors in sylvatic cycle. This sylvatic

© Springer Nature Singapore Pte Ltd. 2024   109
K. G. Narayan et al., *Handbook of Management of Zoonoses*,
https://doi.org/10.1007/978-981-99-9885-2_14

cycle spreads to cause outbreaks in humans in Africa. Chikungunya spread beyond Africa and was introduced to Asia in the nineteenth century or more recently. CHIKV was detected in 1952, was described in 1953 and caused initial epidemics in the Philippines, Thailand, Cambodia, Vietnam, India, Myanmar and Sri Lanka. It caused epidemics during 1963–1973 in some parts of India. During the following three decades, it was reported sporadically.

Pre-emergence: Chikungunya epidemics have occurred in Africa, Asia, South East Asian countries, like India and others in the islands of Pacific Ocean from 2003 onwards. In 2004, it re-emerged in Kenya and spread to Indian Ocean islands in February 2005, mainly French island of La Reunion, Seychelles, Mauritius and Mayotte (French), and later to Indonesia, Maldives, Sri Lanka, Malaysia, Thailand and Singapore (Chikungunya 2009).

Emergence: The emergence from 2006 drew international attention. It directly impacted economy. A very large epidemic occurred in Reunion Island in January 2006 and then in India with 1.3 million suspected cases. The estimated national loss in India in 2006 was 25,588 disability-adjusted life years (Krishnamoorthy et al. 2009).

Cases have been diagnosed in the United States, the United Kingdom, Australia, Belgium, Canada, Czech Republic, French Guiana, Germany, Hong Kong, Italy, Japan, Kenya, Malaysia, Martinique, Norway, Switzerland and Sri Lanka (Thiboutot et al. 2010). Major outbreak occurred in islands of Indian Ocean, starting in February 2005 and peaking in 2006. This was associated with a large number of imported cases in Europe. Besides India, large outbreaks also occurred in other South East Asian countries during 2006–2007. Europe earlier free from it, which recorded for the first time Chikungunya in a localized outbreak (WHO 2008).

Several factors are attributed for the resurgence: globalization, increase in the mosquito population, loss of herd immunity and the mutation of A226V in the E1 gene causing a significant increase in CHIKV infectivity for *Ae. albopictus* (Cecilia 2014). International travel spread it from endemic to non-endemic areas. Travellers act as transporters, transmitters and also sentinels. They introduced it to France, Italy, Australia and the United States. Transportation vehicles acted as mechanical vectors for entry and dispersal of *Ae. albopictus* and larvae of *Ae. aegypti* during trade and transport of goods.

Host-Aedes aegypti cycle: According to Chhabra et al. (2008), geographical genotypes differed in their transmission cycle. Monkeys and wild mosquitoes maintain a sylvatic cycle in Africa. 'Human-*Ae. Aegypti*' cycle maintains it in Asia. It is claimed that epidemics resembling Chikungunya occurred in India and elsewhere in 1824. It was first described in 1952 when an outbreak occurred in Makonde Plateau (Mohan et al. 2010). The virus is maintained in nature during the inter-epidemic period by an epizootic cycle that includes several vertebrates, monkeys, rodents, birds and mosquitoes (*Aedes* spp.) as vectors. The sylvatic cycle in Africa is 'chimpanzee, monkeys and baboons—*Ae. africanus*, *Ae. furcifer-taylori*, *Ae. dalziel* and others like *Mansonia* and *Culex*.' Once the virus spills over to humans, it is "human (reservoir)-mosquito-human" cycle and epidemic. Vertical transmission from affected pregnant women to foetus occurs, but transovarial transmission in mosquitoes does not. The epidemics are seasonal coincident with mosquito density. Cyclic and secular trends of epidemics also occur.

Quiescence: After explosive epidemics, the disappearance for years to few decades (quiescence) is difficult to explain, but in case of CHIKV, this has been documented in Bangkok and India. Outbreaks occurred in 1963 and 1964 in Kolkata and southern India and in 1973 in Solapur, Maharashtra, and after 32 years, since December 2005, it invaded 13 states including Andhra Pradesh, Karnataka, Maharashtra, Madhya Pradesh, Tamil Nadu, Rajasthan, Gujarat, Kerala, etc. (Chhabra et al. 2008). Studies by Yergolkar et al. (2006) showed that all earlier isolates (1963–1973) were Asian genotype, whereas the current and Yawat (2000) isolates were African genotype.

Factors like human susceptibility, vector population and efficiency may be responsible for periodic quiescence/emergence. A similar phenomenon occurred in Europe: 'Following an outbreak in 2007 in the Emilia-Romagna region, the outbreak in cities of Anzio and Rome in 2017 is the second event.' Other autochthonous transmission events were detected in France in 2010, 2014 and 2017. Such events happen in areas where *Ae. albopictus* is established and when environmental conditions are suitable for mosquito abundance and activity (European Centre for Disease Prevention and Control 2017a).

The principal vector *Aedes aegypti*: It breeds in stored fresh water, e.g. dessert cooler, flower vases and water tanks, and in household junk items like coconut shell, car/scooter tyres, bins and cans in urban and suburban areas. Their feeding time is day. Human beings resting in shady and cool areas and in park under shady tree are easy victims as the mosquitoes also prefer such environmental conditions. Adult females require blood meal and thus are the biting real transmitters of infection. *Aedes aegypti* is the vector for other pathogens also, such as dengue virus and *Plasmodium falciparum*. Multiple infections are thus possible.

New vector Ae. albopictus: According to Akiner et al. (2016), *Ae. aegypti* disappeared from the European continent in the Mediterranean, Black Sea and Macaronesian biogeographical regions for reasons not understood. The distribution of *Ae. albopictus* is wide and has already invaded large parts of the Mediterranean and has been recognized as an important vector. One of the viral envelope genes (E1) has mutated (E1-A226V, replacing alanine with valine at position 226) enhancing its infectivity for mosquitoes that facilitated transmission by *Ae. albopictus*. This seems to have happened after September 2005, and more than 90% of subsequent strains causing outbreaks in the Indian Ocean had incorporated the mutation (Thiboutot et al. 2010). *Ae. albopictus* was the main vector in the outbreaks in French metropolitan island of La Reunion of Indian Ocean (Delatte et al. 2008).

Ae. albopictus, the Asian tiger mosquito, is zoophilic which originated in the forests of South East Asia. It adapted to alternative blood sources (humans and domestic animals) and water sources. It occurs in rural and suburban areas of Asia. Like *Ae. aegypti*, it is exophilic (breeds outside) and a daytime feeder. It bred in small disposable containers, bamboo stumps and rock holes. CHIKV was isolated from pools of females and larvae, demonstrating vertical transmission. The consultation committee of ECDC on vector-related risk for CHIKV transmission in Europe

(ECDC 2007) considered that there was a possibility of survival of CHIKV through the winter diapause mechanism. The extrinsic incubation period was shorter than earlier known. It was 3–4 days at 26°C. It is assumed that CHIKV replicated at this or even lower temperature, at a low rate. The life of *Ae. albopictus* was >1 month if environmental temperature between 25 and 30°C persisted for several weeks. Eggs survived desiccation for several months depending upon the time they were laid (ECDC 2006). The biological cycle from egg hatching to adult may be completed in 6–7 days. Average rainfall of 500 mm/year, sufficient rains in summer and optimal temperature are required for development (larvae, pupae, adult). Dense human population provided enough of blood meal.

14.3   Pathogenesis

CHIKV appears to exhibit cell tropism for murine brain. Endothelial and epithelial cells, macrophages and fibroblasts exhibit susceptibility to the virus. Endocytosis is pH-dependent. Replication of CHIKV leads to apoptosis and cytopathy. The observed destruction and death of cells (apoptosis) or tissues may be due to over-secretion of toxic chemokines and antibody-dependent enhancement of pathogenesis. Long persistence of virus after primary viraemia and clinical recovery is indicated by detection of viral antigen in a patient who had relapsed some weeks after the onset of disease. Cell-mediated immune response seems to be affected. CD8+ and T-lymphocytes are either inactive or absent, resulting in viral persistence and chronic disease.

14.4   Symptoms

Clinical manifestations have been neatly described by Mohan et al. (2010). Attack rate varies between 40 and 85% in susceptible population. CHIKV shows no preference for any age or sex. Newborn, >65 years of age and those with comorbidities like hypertension are high-risk groups. Chikungunya may have three phases: acute, lasting for <3 weeks; sub-acute, 3 weeks to 3 months; and chronic, >3 months. Symptoms resolve in >90% in 7–10 days. Persistence of joint pain or stiffness with or without pain, called Chikungunya rheumatism, may be observed in some. Meningoencephalitis, hepatitis and haemorrhage are rare complications.

   The first stage is acute and the second, experienced by most, is chronic, characterized by persisting disabling polyarthritis. The incubation period is 3–12 (usually 3–7) days. The patient develops high level of viraemia lasting for 3–5 days, may even be 10 days enabling easy detection but also transmission.

   Acute: The onset is abrupt and sudden. Symptoms commonly observed are high fever (102–105°F), severe myalgia, arthralgia and skin rash. Others like abdominal pain and constipation, headache, conjunctivitis and cervical/generalized lymphadenopathy may also be observed. Polyarthritis, acute tenosynovitis, and swelling of small joints of the hands and wrist and shoulder and small joints of feet, ankles and knees cripple the patients who have painful sleepless nights. Movement exacerbates pain. Sometimes, sternoclavicular and temporomandibular joints are also affected. Skin lesions like morbilliform eruption, scaling, erythema, urticaria, hypermelanosis and petechiae are its mucocutaneous manifestations.

Chikungunya virus causes abortion in the first trimester. Amniotic fluid is PCR+. Vertical transmission occurs if the mother is affected during the perinatal (−4 to +1 day) period. Neonatal infection was associated with intra-partum viraemia in mothers owing to vertical transmission. The neonates showed fever, distal oedema, skin lesions, seizures, meningoencephalitis and echocardiographic abnormalities. Infected infants present constitutional symptoms like fever, lethargy, irritability and excessive cry and skin lesions, acrocyanosis and erythema. Patients may also show neurological, ocular and haemorrhagic symptoms, fulminant hepatitis and myocarditis. The course of the disease is short, resolving in 3–4 days. Some cases may show biphasic fever and febrile episode of 4–6 days followed by few days of afebrile phase and recurrence of mild fever lasting for few days.

Chronic: Most of the acute cases recover and joint pain resolves in 1–3 weeks. Arthritis persisting for 4 months, 20 months and even 3–5 years may be observed in 33%, 15% and 12% of cases, respectively. Patients experience unpredictable relapse of a fever, asthenia, enhanced arthralgia and stiffness. There is inflammatory polyarthritis and severe sub-acute tenosynovitis/bursitis. Pain in the previously injured joints is increased. Elderly and those having rheumatic and traumatic joint disorders appear more prone to suffer from severe Chikungunya fever. The national burden of Chikungunya in India during the 2006 epidemic was estimated at 25,588 DALYs of which persistent arthralgia accounted for 69%.

Majority of patients in India manifested the cardinal symptoms: fever, arthropathy and mucocutaneous lesions. Encephalitis, neuropathy, myelitis, myeloneuropathy, myopathy, peripheral neuropathy, entrapment neuropathy and muscle injury; altered mental functions, sensorineural hearing loss and eye infections like iridocyclitis, uveitis and neuroretinitis; and haemorrhagic manifestations like epistaxis, subconjunctival bleeding and petechial/purpuric rash were rarely observed (Mohan et al. 2010).

14.5 Diagnosis

- Clinical presentation.
- Viral culture in mosquito cell cultures (C6/36) and mammalian cell cultures (Vero cells). Specimens: blood/serum/blood from mosquito from viraemic stage (usually within 48 h of infective bite).
- Mice inoculation.
- It takes 1–2 weeks and requires a biosafety level 3 laboratory.
- RT-PCR is fast and can be used within the first week of the onset of disease.

- Serodiagnosis—IgM detected after a mean period of 2 days (acute phase) by ELISA and IFAT. IgG in convalescent patients; fourfold increase in paired serum samples (taken 3 weeks apart) by ELISA, indirect IFT, HAI and serum neutralization tests.

These tests can also be used to detect viral antigen in mosquitoes.

14.6   Treatment

Symptomatic and supportive; avoid aspirin, antibiotics and steroids. Trials with chloroquine are suggestive. No vaccine is available.

14.7   Prevention

Surveillance of vector-borne diseases is required for early detection and stopping transmission. The National Vector Borne Disease Control Programme (NVBDCP) in India is equipped with 347 sentinel centres in 35 states and 14 apex referral laboratories, where DENV- and CHIKV-specific IgM detection kits produced by the National Institute of Virology (NIV) are available. Diagnosis, data assimilation and analysis are done since 2007 (Cecilia 2014).

Preventive measures include the following:

- Avoid mosquito bites always, especially during outbreaks.
- Education of the community about disease, especially on vectors.
- Vector surveillance and control.
- Integrated vector management.
- WHO (2008) recommends proper clothing to minimize skin exposure to daytime biting vectors; repellents, DEET (*N*,*N*-diethyl-3-methylbenzamide), IR3535 (3-[*N*-acetyl-*N*-butyl]-aminopropionic acid ethyl ester) or icaridin (1-piperidinecarboxylic acid and 2-(2-hydroxyethyl)-1-methylpropylester; and mosquito coils or other insecticide vaporizers to reduce indoor mosquito bite.

References

Akiner MM, Demirci B, Babuadze G, Robert V, Schaffner F (2016) Spread of the invasive mosquitoes *Aedes aegypti* and *Aedes albopictus* in the black sea region increases risk of Chikungunya, Dengue, and Zika Outbreaks in Europe. PLoS Negl Trop Dis 10(4):s

Cecilia D (2014) Current status of dengue and chikungunya in India. WHO South-East Asia J Public Health 3(1):22–27

Chhabra M, Mittal V, Bhatacharya D, Rana U, Lal S (2008) Chikungunya fever: a re-emerging viral infection. Indian J Med Microbiol 26(1):5–12

Chikungunya (2009) Short epidemiological update, South-East Asia—15 July 2009

Delatte H, Pauoy C, Dehecq JS, Thiria J et al (2008) *Aedes albopictus*, vector of chikungunya and dengue viruses in Reunion Island: biology and control. Parasite 15(1):3–13

ECDC (2006) Meeting Report | Stockholm, 30.03.2006. Consultation on Chikungunya

ECDC (2007) Meeting Report | Paris, 22 October 2007. Consultation on vector-related risk for chikungunya virus transmission in Europe

European Centre for Disease Prevention and Control (2017) Cluster of autochthonous chikungunya cases in France—23 August 2017. ECDC, Stockholm

Krishnamoorthy K, Harichandrakumar KT, Krishna Kumari A, Das LK (2009) Burden of chikungunya in India: estimates of disability adjusted life years (DALY) lost in 2006 epidemic. J Vector Borne Dis 46:26–35

Mohan A, Kiran D, Manohar IC, Kumar DP (2010) Epidemiology, clinical manifestations, and diagnosis of chikungunya fever: lessons learned from the re-emerging epidemic. Indian J Dermatol 55:54–63

Thiboutot MM, Kannan S, Kawalekar OU, Shedlock DJ, Khan AS et al (2010) Chikungunya: a potentially emerging epidemic? PLoS Negl Trop Dis 4(4):e623

WHO (2008) Chikungunya Fact sheet no 327 March 2008. http://www.who.int/mediacentre/factsheets/fs327/en/index.html

Yergolkar PN, Tandale BV, Arankalle VA et al (2006) Chikungunya outbreaks caused by African genotype, India. Emerg Infect Dis 12:1580–1583

Chapter 15
Dengue

Synonyms

'Break-bone fever or bone-crusher disease' is the nickname suggestive of excruciating pain, 'Dandy' as was called by certain natives of East Indies because of the peculiar stiff gait of the patient, dengue haemorrhagic fever and dengue shock syndrome.

15.1 Definition

Dengue (DEN) fever (DF) is an infectious tropical mosquito-borne disease. The uncomplicated form is characterized by fever; pain in the head, muscle and joints; and measles-like skin rash. Some develop life-threatening severe forms: dengue haemorrhagic fever (DHF) or dengue shock syndrome (DSS). The patients of the former have low platelets, plasma leakage and bleeding. Dangerously low blood pressure, shock and death occur in the latter. Dengue fever has become very important because of the increasing number of cases, mostly requiring hospitalization and spreading to new areas.

15.2 Global Burden

There has been eightfold increase in DEN cases during the last two decades (505,430 in 2000 to 4.2 million in 2019). Mortality also increased. A large number of asymptomatic, mild and self-managed cases and also misdiagnosed cases may be additional burden. Estimated global burden is 390 million cases/year; 3.9

© Springer Nature Singapore Pte Ltd. 2024   117
K. G. Narayan et al., *Handbook of Management of Zoonoses*,
https://doi.org/10.1007/978-981-99-9885-2_15

million people in 129 countries are at risk. It is now endemic in more than 100 countries in the WHO regions of Africa, the Americas, the Eastern Mediterranean, South East Asia and the Western Pacific. Nearly 70% of global burden is located in Asia. Bangladesh, Brazil, Cook Islands, Ecuador, India, Indonesia, Maldives, Mauritania, Mayotte (Fr), Nepal, Singapore, Sri Lanka, Sudan, Thailand, Timor-Leste and Yemen report increasing number of cases. Risk of DEN in Europe: autochthonous cases appear almost every year in many European countries. Imported cases are also detected among travellers returning from low—and mid-dle-income countries (https://www.who.int/news-room/fact-sheets/detail/dengue-and-severe-dengue23rdJune2020). Uncomplicated and severe forms of dengue occur almost every year in India. It occurs between the early period of July and November.

Virologically proven epidemic occurred in 1963–1964 along the east coast. Hati (2009) studied the 2005–2007 epidemic in West Bengal. It was caused by DENV-3 and spread over 18 districts. Most cases recorded during post-monsoon peaking in September were young (11–20 years old) males. The primary cases were recorded mostly in the age group 1–10 years. The number of secondary cases was almost twice the primary. All the four serotypes of DENV co-circulated in Delhi (Gupta et al. 2006) and Tamil Nadu (Victor et al. 2007). Cases appeared post-monsoon, between September and November, with peak in the third week of October in Delhi and between June and December in Tamil Nadu. Kumar et al. (2010) observed a steady increase in the number of cases in Karnataka, India, during 2002–2007, with most cases clustering in post-monsoon month, September. The percentages of dengue fever, DHF and DSS were 82.8, 9.8 and 7.3, respectively.

15.3   Aetiology

Dengue virus is a single-stranded RNA *Flavivirus*, with icosahedral nucleocapsid and glycoprotein envelope. There are three structural protein genes: C or nucleocapsid/core, M or membrane and E or envelope and seven NS or non-structural protein (NS1, NS2a, NS2b, NS3, NS4a, NS4b, NS5) genes. There are four serotypes of DENV, 1–4. Genetic variability (i.e. genotypes/lineage) within each serotype occurs. The fifth serotype has been indicated (www.sciencedaily.com/releases/2015/09/150918132028.htm). Anti-E-Abs neutralize infectivity in vitro, protect mice on passive transfer against challenge with the same serotype of DENV and show variable cross-reactivity among other serotypes. The antibodies to non-structural proteins, NS1 and NS3, play important role in the lysis of virus-infected cells.

15.4 Epidemiology

Dengue virus is maintained in sylvatic biotope by monkey-mosquito cycle. Examples are *Presbytis obscura* and *Macaca fascicularis* in Malaysia and *Macaca sinica* in Sri Lanka with primatophilic species of *Ae. niveus* group found at the canopy level and *Ae. albopictus* found at the ground level in Malaysia and *Ae. furcifer taylori* group and West African monkeys in Africa. Infection is asymptomatic but monkeys are viraemic (De Silva et al. 1999). Infection may spill over to humans causing illness.

Aedes aegypti and *Ae. albopictus* are vectors. The former is considered as the primary vector because of its rural and urban habitat breeding in man-made containers. Feeding time is day, preferably dawn and dusk. Female feeds multiple times between each egg laying periods. DENV in infected blood meal is vertically transferred (transovarial). Eggs remain viable for months (even for a year of desiccation, WHO 1997), a mechanism of survival for the virus. Eggs hatch when they find contact with water. The climatic zones—tropical monsoon, equatorial, deciduous dry and wet climate zones—and sub-Himalayan foothills cover countries where dengue is prevalent and coincidentally favour *Aedes aegypti*.

Aedes albopictus is the secondary vector in Asia. Travelling in used tyres and other items like lucky bamboo (breeding habitat) under international trade, it has spread to more than 32 states in the United States and more than 25 countries in the European region. *Ae. albopictus* is highly adaptive to environmental conditions. Eggs and adults tolerate cold conditions. It has reportedly been primary vectors of dengue fever in places where *Ae. aegypti* is either absent or low in number.

Studies by Angel and Joshi (2008) revealed that (a) *Ae. Albopictus*, *Ae. aegypti* and *Ae. vittatus* are the common vectors in Rajasthan and vertical transmission occurred (b) Transovarial transmission was important for inter-epidemic survival and re-emergence of disease. (c) *Ae. albopictus* showed the maximum vertical transmitted virus during winter season (which is not the epidemic season), i.e. harboured the virus during the inter-epidemic period. (d) *Ae. aegypti* was the main vector transmitting the virus during summer and rainy seasons in the desert districts of Jodhpur, mainly because of the indoor breeding in the domestic water storage pots.

Factors favouring outbreaks have been overlooked. Scattered junks like tyres, coconut shells, broken earthenware, flower pots, etc. collect water and constitute mosquito breeding sites. Urbanization has not considered these in many places.

15.4.1 Transmission

DENV in infected blood meal by female mosquito replicates in the midgut and spreads to tissues including salivary glands in about 8–12 days (extrinsic incubation period (EIP)) at ambient temperature of 25–28°C. The mosquito is capable of transmitting the virus for the rest of its life. EIP is dependent upon multiple factors such as ambient temperature, daily temperature fluctuations, viral concentration and its genotype.

Human beings are the amplifying host and also the source of infection. Viraemia develops a little before the symptoms appear and continue for 4–5 days during which biting mosquitoes get infected. Patients with even insignificant symptoms may also transmit virus to biting mosquitoes, thus spreading with their movement. An infected *Aedes* can fly about 400 meters around, meaning infected man spreads infection more rapidly in community. *Infected humans in community burdened with mosquitoes sustain DENV.* Travellers from endemic countries to non-endemic countries/areas are important in spreading DF. However, secondary cases may not appear in the absence of a vector.

Transfusion of infected blood, plasma or blood products is another mode of transmission. Infected pregnant mother to her foetus and transplants from infected donors may rarely transmit the virus.

15.5   Dengue Infection

Infection may be asymptomatic and symptomatic. The symptomatic DEN are grouped into three. (i) DF or dengue (uncomplicated) fever is a milder form, symptoms of which may be confounded with influenza or other viral infection. (ii) Severe dengue or DHF (dengue haemorrhagic fever) is an unusual haemorrhagic syndrome, characterized by biphasic fever, myalgia, arthralgia, retro-orbital pain and generalized maculopapular rash. It affects older children and adults and is rarely fatal. DHF is further classified (I–IV) according to the grade of severity. (iii) DSS or dengue shock syndrome belongs to grades III and IV which affects mostly children and is fatal. The contributory host factors may be age, ethnicity and individual health status like asthma, chronic bronchitis, diabetes mellitus and sickle cell anaemia. DHF/DSS occurred less in blacks compared to whites and Asians and in those suffering from moderate to severe protein-calorie malnutrition. Few primary infections are severe. Primary infection of infants born of dengue-immune mothers regularly and young children are at high risk of getting the severe form.

15.6   Symptoms

Infected mosquito bite causes infection by any of the four serotypes. Primary infection produces immunity to the infecting serotype. The protection is lifelong against the infecting serotype and temporary, 2–3 months against other serotypes.

Secondary heterotypic infection causes severe dengue. The period of interval between primary and secondary infections also determines the severity—longer interval is often associated with higher fatality.

Dengue fever appears suddenly, 3–15 (commonly 5–8) days after infected mosquito bite (IP). The virus circulates in serum or plasma, circulating blood cells, and is found in selected tissues especially of the immune system for 2–7 days, coincident with febrile period. The febrile, critical and recovery phases are shown in Figure 15.1. Patients complain of retro-orbital pain while moving it (pain from behind the eyes), headache, myalgia in legs and arthralgias in the initial few hours, shooting up of temperature to 104°F, chills, bradycardia, hypotension and flushing of the face—pale to pink rashes appear and disappear. Patients continue in this state for 2–7 days. Defervescence (rapid drop in temperature) and profuse sweating and a feeling of wellness for a day occur. Body temperature rises (biphasic pattern) but is milder. This is accompanied with appearance of characteristic maculopapular rashes (measles-like) and thrombocytopenia. Rashes are bright red pinpoint spots appearing and spreading from extremities to all parts of the body except the face.

There is hepatomegaly with soft tender liver. The palm and sole may be red and swollen. Platelet count is low and there is leukopenia. There are non-specific constitutional symptoms like injected pharynx and gastritis manifested in some

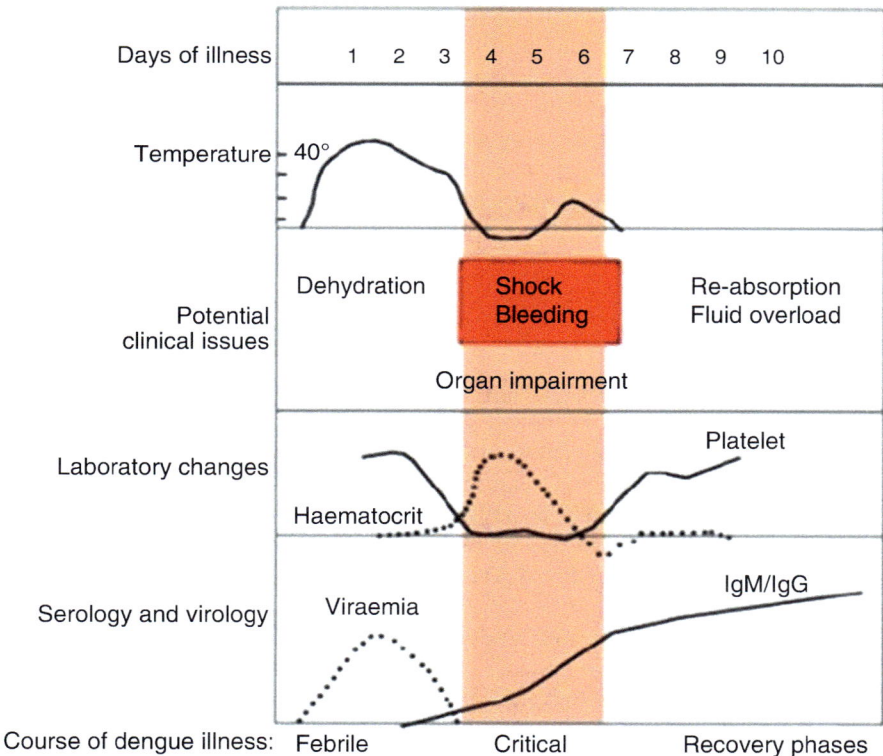

Fig. 15.1 Course of Dengue illness (Source: Handbook for clinical management of dengue, WHO 2012)

combination of abdominal pain, nausea, vomiting coffee-grounds-like congealed blood or diarrhoea. Atypical manifestations recorded are encephalitis/encephalopathy, myocarditis, hepatitis, etc. There is rapid uneventful recovery in most cases. Infection in pregnancy carries the risk of haemorrhage for both the mother and the newborn and also a serious risk of premature birth and foetal death. Dengue may affect infant of 2 months; the maternal antibodies to the first infection (of the mother) may form complex with the second infecting virus to make it serious. Vertically transmitted infection in baby caused fever, cold extremities, erythematous rash and hepatosplenomegaly (Singh et al. 2008).

15.6.1   DHF and DSS

There is vascular leak without morphological damage to the capillary endothelium, thrombocytopenia, altered leucocyte count and its function and haemostasis, haemoconcentration, reduced platelets (Fig. 15.1) and hepatomegaly. Humoral and cellular response, neutralizing antibodies, CD4+ and CD8 + T-lymphocytes and cytokines fight the virus.

There is extensive fluid leaking from blood vessels through the skin or into spaces around lungs, in the belly and into the pleura, peritoneum and pericardium. Patients bleed from any organ(s)—eyes, mouth, nose, ear, gut and skin pores. As a result of fluid loss and severe bleeding, blood pressure falls. Dengue grade III and IV patients may enter into shock. The patient may die of shock, called dengue shock syndrome (DSS). DSS has high mortality rate.

15.7   Pathogenesis

DHF/DSS occurs in cases of secondary infection by another serotype. There is an enhanced virus replication in macrophages. The cross-reactive antibodies fail to neutralize the virus; they instead form a DENV-Ab complex and may increase the number of monocytes which engulf the complex. The 'antibody-dependent enhancement' (ADE) hypothesis (WHO 2009) explains the severe dengue as observed in secondary infection and in infants with primary infection. ADE has been elaborated by Chaturvedi and Nagar (2008). The three landmark-related findings mentioned are the roles of (a) enhancing antibodies; (b) shift from Th-1 response in mild dengue to Th2 response in severe DHF, resulting in 'cytokine storm'; and (c) presence of cross-reactive memory T cells that induce a large amount of cytokine on a second exposure to DENV. DENV-specific memory lymphocytes have been detected 20 years after primary infection with the virus. The ultimate target is the endothelium.

Secondary DENV infection causes a transient and reversible imbalance of inflammatory mediators, cytokines and chemokines driven probably by a high early viral burden. This causes dysfunction of vascular endothelial cells, derangement of haemocoagulation system, plasma leakage, shock and bleeding (WHO 2009a).

The resulting pathophysiological changes are (a) increased vascular permeability resulting in plasma loss, haemoconcentration, low pulse pressure and signs of shock in case plasma loss is critical; (b) haemostasis, a disorder that involves vascular changes, thrombocytopenia and coagulopathy; and (c) platelet defects, both quantitative (low count, $<100,000/mm^3$) and qualitative; platelet is just non-functional (even when the count is $>100,000/mm^3$).

Biopsy of (a) the bone marrow presented depression of haematopoetic cells; (b) kidney, mild glomerulonephritis of immune-complex type; and (c) skin, perivascular oedema of terminal microvasculature of dermal papillae.

Autopsy shows some degree of haemorrhage in decreasing order, in the skin, subcutaneous tissues, mucosa of the gastrointestinal tract (may be severe), heart and liver, rarely cerebral and subarachnoid. Serous effusion is seen commonly in pleural and abdominal cavities but less often in pericardial. Dengue viral antigen is predominantly found in the liver, spleen, thymus, lymph nodes and lung cells although it may be detected in almost all organs.

15.8   Diagnosis

Specimen of blood from *febrile/viraemic/acute phase* (4–5 days after onset of illness) examined by 'direct methods': (a) isolation of virus in infant mice or tissue culture, (b) detection of NS1 antigen by ELISA, (c) detection of virus in situ by immunocytochemistry and (d) molecular diagnostic methods, like RT-PCR, nested PCR, real-time RT-PC and multiplex PCR may be used for confirmation after serodiagnosis.

In a primary infection (i.e. when an individual is infected for the first time with a flavivirus), viraemia develops from 1 to 2 days before the onset of fever until 4–5 days after.

Primary infections are characterized by high levels of IgM and low levels of IgG. Accordingly, anti-dengue IgM-specific antibodies can be detected 3–6 days after the onset of fever. On average, IgM is detected in 50% of cases by days 3–5 after the onset of illness; this figure increases to 95–98% for days 6–10. Thereafter, low levels of IgM are detectable around 1–3 months after the fever.

In addition, the primary infection is characterized by slowly increasing but low levels of dengue-specific IgG, which becomes elevated at days 9–10 (Fig. 15.2). Low IgG levels persist for decades, which is an indication of a past dengue infection.

Secondary heterotypic infection is characterized by a rapid and higher increase of anti-dengue-specific IgG antibodies and slower and lower levels of IgM. High

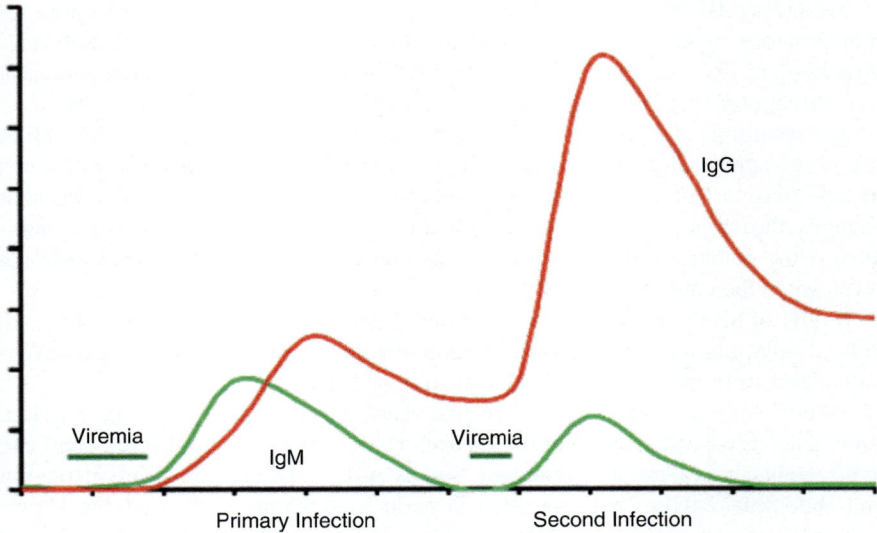

Fig. 15.2 Interpretation for primary and secondary infection (Source: Handbook for clinical management of dengue, WHO 2012)

IgG levels remain for 30–40 days. A short-lasting but higher viraemia level characterizes the secondary infection compared to the primary infection. Low levels of IgM with high levels of IgG characterize secondary infections.

Post-febrile phase by (indirect methods) detecting antibodies—IgM in early part (5–10 days) and IgG (after 2 weeks post onset of illness) in blood by capture ELISA.

Chaturvedi and Nagar (2008) developed a bedside test. Reusable microchip implanted with artificial NS1 receptors can capture DENV instantly.

15.8.1 Cross-Reaction: A Problem—Interpretation

The antibodies may cross-react with other flaviviruses and may give false-positive reaction after recent infections or vaccinations against Japanese encephalitis or yellow fever. Necessary precautions need to be taken, e.g. examination of paired sera samples for fourfold increase in titre. Infection with DENV in individuals with immunity against flavivirus from previous infection leads to anamnestic or secondary antibody response. The dominant antibody is IgG. Secondary infection is defined as low molar fraction of anti-DENV IgM and high molar fraction of IgG that is broadly reactive to flaviviruses.

Specimens for diagnosis may be serum, plasma, leucocytes washed of antibodies, CSF in case of patients and minced tissues-lungs, liver, thymus, spleen, lymph glands, pleural fluid, serum, plasma and CSF in case of autopsy and homogenized pool of vector mosquitoes.

15.9   Treatment

There is no antiviral drug for treatment. Careful management of patients saves life. Oral rehydration therapy before shifting patient to hospital and intravenous fluid/blood transfusion and paracetamol for controlling fever are given. Non-steroidal anti-inflammatory drugs and aspirin are not recommended.

15.10   Control

Vaccine—Three injections of CYD (sold as Dengvaxia 2019) is given over a year but has limitations. It increases the risk of severe dengue in those who have not been previously infected. As such, the recommendation by WHO states: 'Use only if the risk of severe dengue in seronegative individuals can be minimized either through pre-vaccination screening or recent documentation of high seroprevalence rates in the area (at least 80% by age 9 years)'.

15.11   Prevention

15.11.1   The Bi-Regional Dengue Strategy (2008–2015)

The Bi-regional Dengue Strategy (2008–2015) of the WHO South East Asia and Western Pacific regions to control and prevent dengue consists of six elements: (1) dengue surveillance, (2) case management, (3) outbreak response, (4) integrated vector management, (5) social mobilization and communication for dengue and (6) dengue research (a combination of both formative and operational research). The strategy has been endorsed by resolution SEA/RC61/R5 of the WHO Regional Committee for South East Asia in 2008. The integrated vector control has five elements (WHO 2009a). These are the following:

– Advocacy, social mobilization and legislation to ensure that public health bodies and communities are strengthened.
– Collaboration between the health and other sectors (public and private).
– An integrated approach to disease control to maximize use of resources.
– Evidence-based decision-making to ensure any interventions are targeted appropriately.
– Capacity-building to ensure an adequate response to the local situation.

There is a general agreement on 'dengue is one disease entity with different clinical presentations and often with unpredictable clinical evolution and outcome' (WHO 2009a). Individuals returning from dengue-endemic areas and developing fever within 2 weeks are suspected. This lays emphasis on defining a *probable case' and 'warning signs' in order to initiate rapid action to (a) save life and (b) to prevent transmission. Probable case requires strict observation and medical intervention.* A *'dengue probable case'* should have fever plus two of the following: nausea and vomiting, rash, generalized pain, low white blood cells and positive tourniquet test or any 'warning signs'. Warning signs are abdominal pain or tenderness, persistent vomiting, clinical fluid accumulation, mucosal bleeding, lethargy, restlessness, liver enlargement >2 cm and laboratory increase in haematocrit (HCT) concurrent with rapid decrease in platelet count.

Tourniquet test is conducted as a blood pressure cuff is applied at between the diastolic and systolic pressures for 5 min. The resultant petechial haemorrhages are counted. More than $10–20/2.5$ cm^2 is considered as positive.

15.11.2 Epidemiological Surveillance

The objective is early detection so that prompt intervention measures can be initiated:

- Sentinel hospitals in strategic locations in the high-risk areas should be monitoring febrile cases, referring to the identified hospitals for proper diagnosis and management.
- Detection of infected mosquitoes—Guedes et al. (2010) collected adult mosquitoes and eggs from houses where suspected dengue cases lived, extracted viral RNA and performed RT-PCR and detected DENV 1, 2 and 3 in both. It was concluded that these serotypes were circulating and transovarial transmission in mosquitoes was common in Brazil.

Entomological surveillance was considered sensitive for detection of circulating virus even before the occurrence of human cases and was thus useful for initiating early intervention.

- The GeoSentinel Surveillance Network (www.geosentinel.org)—information about dengue in travellers (WHO 2009a). It provides early alert to (a) assist clinicians to treat the cases on arrival, (b) stop the geographic spread to non-endemic areas and (c) 'alert' internationally with 'month-by-month dengue morbidity data' for such endemic countries where the reporting system is not available. This is also useful for 'outbreak alert'. This is arrived at by comparing the 'number of current/probable dengue cases per week/month with the average of those of the preceding 5–7 years'. A deviation of +2SD is considered 'endemic channel'. If the current/probable number of cases exceeds this, 'outbreak alert' is triggered.

15.11.3 Vector Control Measures

It aim at eliminating, reducing the density and longevity of female mosquitoes to reduce transmission. The methods include (a) elimination or management of larval habitats, (b) larviciding with insecticides and (c) the use of biological agents and the application of adulticides:

– Management of 'solids'—in use and waste.
– Weekly empty, scrub and clean—water storage tanks, water containers, animal water container, flower vase and potted plant with saucers.
– Clean and redesign/modify—water storage tanks, water containers, roof drains/ gutter and potted plant with saucers.
– Fill with sand, soil or concrete—flower vase, rock holes, tree holes, fence poles and used tyres.
– Collect, recycle and dispose (solid waste)—discarded broken food containers, used tyres, appliances and buckets; practice good solid waste management—collect weekly/twice weekly in sac and carry to disposal plants/incinerators.
– Larviciding with insecticides.

Perifocal spray is practised. The target areas consist of (a) such places where people congregate such as schools, hospitals, high-density houses and apartments, (b) house of dengue case (s) and surrounding 400 meters and (c) where the vector density is high. Handheld or power-operated equipment may be used. The spray must cover items such as broken tyres, bottles, drink containers, etc. and additional area of 60 cm around. It should leave a film of residual chemical. This kills the existing and also those mosquitoes landing later.

Follow the direction of the insecticide manufacturer; methoprene can be applied at dosages of up to 1 mg of active ingredient (a.i.) per litre (1 ppm); pyriproxyfen can be applied at dosages up to 0.01 mg a.i. per litre (0.01 ppm) and (*Bacillus thuringiensis israelensis*) Bti at 1–5 mg per litre can be used for drinking water. Other WHO-recommended chemicals are organophosphates, temephos and primiphos-methyl (1 ppm); insect growth regulators, diflubenzuron, DT, GR and WP (0.02–0.25 mg/l); novaluron (0.01–0.05 mg/l) and biopesticide, spinosad (0.1–0.5 mg/l).

Although the number of application and gap between (treatment cycle) depends upon factors—mosquito species, seasonal patterns of rainfalls and transmission, habitat and efficacy of the chemical—two to three annual applications should suffice especially in areas where the main transmission season is short.

Space spray—Rapid reduction in vector density, as may be warranted in emergencies, requires space treatment carried out ideally every 2–3 days for 10 days. To sustain the reduced density of adult mosquitoes, repeat spray once or twice a week.

Entomological and epidemiological monitoring provides useful guidance. Insecticide formulations may be oil−/water-based.

15.11.4   Supplementary Methods

Insecticide-treated materials such as bed nets, window/door/wardrobe curtains and sheets to cover water containers are useful.

Lethal ovitraps—Ovitrap or oviposition traps are used for surveillance of *Aedes* vectors. This may be modified into an additional vector control device by combining oviposition substrate with insecticide. Autocidal ovitraps allow oviposition but prevent emergence of adults. Sticky ovitraps trap mosquito as it lands.

Advantages are reduction in population density, shortening the life expectancy and thus reducing the number of mosquitoes becoming infective and thus reducing transmission.

15.11.5   Recent Approaches

Mosquito population suppression: sterile male mosquitoes raised in lab released— They carry genes lethal to females, and males left in the population do not bite and transmit disease, such as DEN. The offspring after mating with wild females are males with genetic quirk and dead females. The reproductive ability is thus cut down.

Mosquito population replacement—The *Wolbachia* symbiotic bacteria infecting about 70% of all known insect species is marked as the genetic trait that suppresses either the ability of insects to reproduce or spread pathogens and is programmed to hijack the insect's reproductive methods to spread itself through the species.

Within the last 8 years, scientists have worked with *Wolbachia*, taking the strain in fruit flies and passing them, as well as at least 1500 prerequisite genes, into mosquitoes that transmit dengue.

15.11.6   GM Mosquitoes to Fight Dengue

GM Mosquitoes to fight dengue: Scientists find way to cut lifecycle of virus, making it harmless. (Jupatanakul et al. 2017).

Johns Hopkins University scientists genetically engineered *Ae. aegypti.* Expression of either DOME or HOP in fat body tissue was turned on earlier in GM-modified mosquitoes immediately after ingesting blood to make more of these proteins. These mosquitoes were then infected with DENV. Mosquitoes had 78.18% DOME and 83.63% HOP; replication of DENV was adversely affected—fewer copies of the virus detected in the gut and significantly less virus in salivary glands. Mosquitoes had a normal life span but produced fewer eggs.

Mechanism of mosquitoes' fight with DENV infection passed through a molecular pathway—JAK/STAT to stop cycle of viral replication and development. Proteins DOME and HOP are involved in turning on the JAK/STAT when mosquitoes are infected with DENV.

It may be possible to achieve improved or total resistance to DENV or other viruses by expressing additional transgenes in multiple tissues that block the virus replication/infection.

This mechanism did not work with Zika and Chikungunya viruses suggesting JAK/STAT as DENV-unique/DENV-specific pathway.

References

Angel B, Joshi V (2008) Distribution and seasonality of vertically transmitted dengue viruses in Aedes mosquitoes in arid and semi-arid areas of Rajasthan. India. J. Vector Borne Dis. 45:56–59

Canyon DV (2008) Historical analysis of the economic cost of dengue in Australia. J Vector Borne Dis 45:245–248

Chaturvedi UC, Nagar R (2008) Dengue and dengue haemorrhagic fever: Indian perspective. J Biosci 33:429–441

Dengvaxia 2019 is a vaccine.

De Silva AM, Dittus WPJ, Amerasinghe PH, Amerasingh FP (1999) Serologic evidence for an epizootic dengue virus infecting toque macaques (*Macaca sinica*) at Polonnaruwa. Sri Lanka Am J Trop Med Hyg 60(2):300–306

Guedes DRD, Cordeiro MT, Melo-Santos MAV, Megalhaes T et al (2010) Patient-based dengue virus surveillance in *Aedes aegypti* from Recife. Brazil J Vector Borne Dis 47(2):67–75

Gupta E, Dar L, Kapoor G, Broor S (2006) The changing epidemiology of dengue in Delhi. India Virology J 3:92

Hati AK (2009) Dengue serosurveillance in Kolkata, facing an epidemic in West Bengal, India. J Vector Borne Dis 46(3):197–204

Jupatanakul N, Sim S, Angleró-Rodríguez YI, Souza-Neto J, Das S, Poti KE et al (2017) Engineered aedes aegypti JAK/STAT pathway-mediated immunity to dengue virus. PLoS Negl Trop Dis 11(1):e0005187

Kumar A, Pandit RK, Shetty S, Pattanshetty S et al (2010) A profile of dengue cases admitted to a tertiary care hospital in Karnataka, southern India. Trop Dr 40(1):45–46

Singh N, Sharma KA, Dadhwal V, Mittal S, Selvi AS (2008) A successful management of dengue fever in pregnancy: report of two cases. Indian J Med Microbiol 26:377–380

Victor TJ, Malathi M, Asokan R, Padmanaban P (2007) Laboratory- based dengue fever surveillance in Tamil Nadu. India Indian J Med Res 126:112–115

WHO (1997) Diagnosis, treatment, prevention and control, 2nd edn., World Health Organization, Geneva, Switzerland

WHO (2009) Dengue and dengue haemorrhagic fever fact sheet No. 117, March 2009. http://www.who.int/mediacentre/factsheets/fs117/en/

WHO (2009a) DENGUE: guidelines for diagnosis, treatment, prevention and control. A joint publication of the World Health Organization (WHO) and the Special Programme for Research and Training in Tropical Diseases (TDR) New edition. 9789241547871_eng-Dengue.pdf. (https://www.who.int/news-room/fact-sheets/detail/dengue-and-severe-dengue23rd June2020)

WHO (2012) Handbook for clinical management of dengue (ISBN 978 92 4 150471 3). World Health Organization, Geneva, Switzerland

Chapter 16
Zika Virus

Zika virus (ZIKV) is a flavivirus transmitted primarily by *Aedes* mosquito bites and is known to have caused alarming epidemics. ZIKV disease manifested in three different forms. The flu-like epidemics in Yap Islands (Federated States of Micronesia) in 2007 and in the French Polynesia in 2013 and other countries and territories in the Pacific is the first form. The March–October 2015 epidemic in Brazil was described as congenital Zika syndrome characterized by microcephaly. The July 2015 epidemic was associated with Guillain-Barré syndrome (https://www.who.int/news-room/fact-sheets/detail/zika-virus).

16.1 History

According to Hayes (2009), ZIKV was first isolated from one of 766 rhesus monkeys used as sentinel for yellow fever virus in Zika forest of Uganda. It had fever. Its serum was i/c inoculated in mice that fell ill and the isolate from mice was named after the name of the forest in 1947. It was isolated from *Aedes africanus* collected from the same forest in 1948. Artificially fed *Ae. aegypti* transmitted ZIKV to mice and monkeys establishing vector transmission. It was isolated from humans in 1968, from febrile children 10 months to 3 years old and from a 10-year-old boy who had fever, headache and body ache. It is distributed in Uganda, Tanzania, Egypt, Central African Republic, Sierra Leone, Gabon and parts of Asia including India, Pakistan, Malaysia, the Philippines, Thailand, Vietnam and Indonesia.

© Springer Nature Singapore Pte Ltd. 2024   131
K. G. Narayan et al., *Handbook of Management of Zoonoses*,
https://doi.org/10.1007/978-981-99-9885-2_16

16.2   Aetiology

ZIKV is a member of the Spondweni (SPOV) serocomplex in the genus *Flavivirus* and family *Flaviviridae*. Zika virus is enveloped and icosahedral with a non-segmented, +ssRNA genome. It is related to dengue (DNV), yellow fever (YFV), West Nile fever (WNV) and Japanese encephalitis (JEV).

Epidemic potential and pathogenicity of ZIKV lineages and strains are not fully understood. Lanciotti et al. (2008) studied the virus from the Yap epidemic. ZIKV belonged to a unique clade among the mosquito-borne flaviviruses and most closely related to SPOV. ZIKV and Spondweni viruses are the only two members of their clade. SPOV caused sporadic human infections in Africa, was isolated from *Culex* spp. and replicated in the placenta of pregnant mice (Salazar et al. 2019). There are three subclades—Senegal and Uganda subclades may represent West and East African lineages, respectively. The 2007 ZIKV is distantly related to these and may represent divergence from a common ancestor spreading throughout South East Asia and the Pacific. Human ZIKV cases occurred in 1980 in Malaysia. There are two lineages—the Asian lineage spread to the Pacific Islands and the Americas. This caused the 2018 outbreak in India. It caused congenital Zika syndrome (CZS), microcephaly and foetal death in women. The African lineage circulated for decades in Africa. Its effects on pregnancy and birth outcomes have not been reported. In vitro and animal model studies suggested the potential for causing foetal loss rather than foetal defects.

The surface of mature infectious flaviviruses is composed of envelope (E) proteins (of flat-lying conformation) which contain fusion peptide responsible for insertion into host cell membrane after infection. The progeny viruses bud into the lumen of the endoplasmic reticulum. The immature virions (with spike-like precursor membrane) reach the low pH environment of the trans-Golgi network where spikes rearrange into the flat-lying conformation. The neutral pH outside triggers the dissociation of E and pr rendering the virus infectious. pr remaining associated with E inhibits fusion with host cell membrane (Renner et al. 2021).

16.3   Vector

Mosquitoes are vectors—*Ae. africanus, Ae. apicoargenteus, Ae. luteocephalus, Ae. aegypti, Ae. vittatus* and *Ae. furcifer*. Although *Ae. hensilli* was the predominant species in the Yap epidemic, ZIKV could not be isolated from any of the mosquitoes during the outbreak.

The virus concentration was high in mosquitoes on the day of artificial feeding, dropped to undetectable level by 10 days after feeding and increased by 15 days and remained so from 20 to 60 days. The extrinsic incubation period was ~10 days. *Ae. albopictus* is a potential vector.

16.4   Reservoirs

It is thought that mosquito-monkey transmission cycle maintains the enzootic. In Uganda, cyclic epizootics occur in monkeys. ZIKV antibodies have been detected in elephants, hippos, impala, lions, kongoni, wildebeest, zebra, rodents, water buffaloes, sheep and goat. Humans may act as reservoir and amplifying hosts, if viraemia is sufficiently high and of long duration, in areas where non-human primates are absent (Haddow et al. 2012).

16.5   The Yap Outbreak

The outbreak occurred between 15 April and 14 July, peaked in late May and subsided in early July infecting about 75% population; an estimated over 900 were ill. The median age of patients was 36 years (1–76 years), highest among 55–59 years, 61% female. Attack rate was 114/1000.

The physicians on Yap Islands noted an outbreak of the illness characterized by headache, malaise, stomach ache, dizziness, anorexia, rashes, conjunctivitis, fever, arthralgia and arthritis. There was no death and hospitalization. A *Flavivirus* was detected in patient's serum, misdiagnosed as dengue because of clinical similarity and serologic cross-reactivity. Duffy et al. (2009) investigated it. Three patients tested dengue IgM positive. An estimated 73% of Yap residents of 3 years and older were recently infected with ZIKV. The viral DNA was identified in the serum samples collected within 10 days of the onset of acute illness. The predominant mosquito species identified was *Ae. hensilli*. Of the 185 identified cases of suspected ZIKV disease, 26% were confirmed and 32% probable.

The study revealed that ZIKV first time leapt out of Africa and Asia and has a potential to spread to other islands in Pacific Ocean and to Americas.

16.5.1   Clinical Feature

Incubation period ranged between 3 and 14 days and duration of the illness was 2–7 days. Signs and symptoms of ZIKV infections are not specific and mimic for other flaviviral infections like dengue and Chikungunya. Symptoms appear within 3–12 days post-infection; however, majority (80%) of cases remain asymptomatic. Symptoms include low-grade fever, headache, joint pain, body rash, conjunctivitis and gastrointestinal disturbance (Basarab et al. 2016). Acute cases are mild and self-limiting and recover within a week. Neonatal complication in cases of chronic ZIKV infections is seen such as increased number of neonatal microcephaly (Kleber de Oliveira et al. 2016).

Apart from neonatal complications, strong association of Guillain-Barré syndrome (GBS), an autoimmune condition, with ZIKV infections in the adult has been observed. Other associated complications include arthralgia and cardiovascular problems (Edupuganti et al. 2017; Minhas et al. 2017).

16.5.2   Pathogenesis

Generally, mosquito-borne flaviviruses multiply near the site of inoculation, in the dendritic cells, and then spread to lymph nodes and blood stream. Flaviviruses generally replicate in the cytoplasm. However, ZIKV antigen has been detected in cell nucleus. Infectious ZIKV has been detected on day 1 of the onset of the illness in the blood of human and the viral nuclei as late as 11 days after the onset. ZIKV was isolated from serum 9 days after inoculation in experimental monkeys.

16.6   Congenital ZIKA Syndrome: Microcephaly

ZIKV was identified in two cases suspected to have died of dengue and from an infant born with microcephaly by Brazil's Ministry of Health in November 2015 (recent deaths, microcephaly cases in Brazil linked to Zika virus infection. Zika Resource Centre, 30 November 2015). Microcephaly cases linked to Zika virus nearly tripled in Brazil. (Zika Resource Centre, 16 December 2015]. As of 26 December 2015, a total of 2975 suspected cases of microcephaly and 40 suspicious deaths were reported in 20 Brazilian states, including 656 municipalities.

Microcephaly was associated with infection in the first 3 months of pregnancy (Costello et al. 2016), and ZIKV was vertically transmitted at the end of first trimester of pregnancy. It was neurotropic and affected foetal brain tissues. Mothers had no symptoms during pregnancy and delivery and showed no serological evidence. Newborn had microcephaly and died within 20 h of birth (Martines et al. 2016; Mlakar et al. 2016). Children born to mothers with ZIKV infection during pregnancy but with no apparent disability are at risk of neurodevelopmental implications at older age.

ZIKV appears to be associated with adverse pregnancy outcomes, neurotropism and neuropathology. There is increased risk of preterm birth, foetal death and still-birth and congenital malformations collectively characterized as including microcephaly, abnormal brain development—severe neurodevelopmental delay, sensory organ dysfunction or both—limb contractures, eye abnormalities, brain calcifications and other neurologic manifestations (Lopes Moreira et al. 2018).

16.7 Guillain-Barré Syndrome (GBS)

Zika virus infection is also a trigger of Guillain-Barré syndrome, neuropathy and myelitis, particularly in adults and older children. ZIKV infection is complicated by GBS. Oehler et al. (2014) observed a French Polynesian patient. They detected neutralizing antibodies against ZIKV and the four DENV serotypes in the sera of the patient. The serological analyses indicated a recent infection by ZIKA. They hypothesized: 'a sequential arboviral immune stimulation responsible during concurrent circulation of ZIKA and two dengue serotypes' and suggested that clinicians should be made aware of the likelihood of GBS complications in DENV- and ZIKV-endemic areas.

16.7.1 Clinical Presentation

A Polynesian woman in her 40 s reported no past history of neurological deficits. She was hospitalized with ascendant muscular weakness/paraesthesia of four limb extremities suggestive of GBS. Disease progressed by day 3—tetraparesis in the lower limbs, diffuse myalgia and a bilateral but asymmetric peripheral facial palsy. Deep tendon reflexes were abolished. Chest pain is related to a sustained ventricular tachycardia and orthostatic hypotension—suggestive of dysautonomia. She was discharged after 13 days but had to use a walking frame. Facial palsy slowly disappeared. She was able to walk without help after 40 days.

16.8 Transmission

The main route of transmission for ZIKV is bite of infected mosquito. Other modes of transmission, such as infected blood transfusion, sexual and materno-foetal, have also been reported. Enzootic or sylvatic and epidemic or urban life cycles have been reported for ZIKV. The virus is maintained in nature in sylvatic cycle between *Aedes* mosquitoes and non-human primates like apes and monkeys. Man is an incidental host and carries the virus to the urban cycle where human-mosquito-human transmission is observed (Fig. 16.1). Humans are the main host and serve as amplifier and carrier of infection to uninfected mosquitoes in urban cycle. *Ae. aegypti* and *Ae. albopictus* are the main species involved in transmissions. *Ae. aegypti* is mostly confined to tropical and subtropical regions, while *Ae. albopictus* in temperate areas besides tropical and subtropical regions.

Zika is known to be transmitted through bites of *Ae. aegypti*, sex—men to women but also women to men; virus has been detected in blood, semen, vaginal fluid, saliva and urine, but non-sexual transmission from person to person has not been recorded (Fig. 16.1).

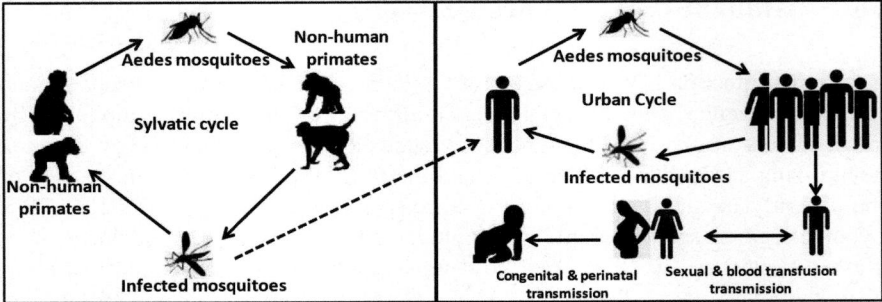

Fig. 16.1 Transmission of Zika virus

16.9   Diagnosis

Clinical symptoms such as rash, fever and conjunctivitis and patient history could be helpful in initial screening of symptomatic infections. But for confirmation of infection, RT-PCR and serological tools have been recommended by WHO (PAHO 2017).

Serum is the preferred specimen for diagnosis of ZIKV by serological or molecular methods. Sensitivity of molecular methods is compromised when there is low viraemia and serum is collected 10 days after symptoms appear (St. George et al. 2017; Theel and Hata 2018). Higher viral loads in urine have been reported. Body fluids such as amniotic fluid, saliva, cerebrospinal fluid, semen and placental tissue can also be used.

16.10   Public Health Implications

ZIKV has the potential to spread through travel and commerce and is considered an emerging pathogen. Zika virus illness is mild and self-limiting but it is not sure that it will remain the same in times to come. Symptoms are confounded with other illnesses like dengue. Its presence is likely to be masked by other cross-reacting flaviviruses. These demand 'One Health' approach for surveillance, control and prevention.

16.11   Epidemiology

ZIKV circulated predominantly in wild primates and *Ae. Africanus* and rarely spilled over to humans. ZIKV has a global distribution, affecting 87 countries with evidence of autochthonous mosquito-borne transmission in many territories (WHO 2019). Sixty-one countries and territories have evidence of established competent

Ae. aegypti vectors but without documented ZIKV transmission, i.e. are potentially at risk for ZIKV infection. In India, the first four reported cases were from Gujarat (3) and Tamil Nadu (1). There were 159 cases in Rajasthan, including 63 pregnant women, 130 from Madhya Pradesh and 1 from Gujarat.

Introduction and emergence of ZIKV epidemic with pandemic in progress are ascribed to travel, human density, behaviour and microperturbances in ecological balance favouring vector density.

Complication like Guillain-Barré syndrome and other neurological syndromes have been observed in some cases. ZIKV may mediate antibody-dependent enhancement of infection observed in vitro but of little clinical significance. It caused explosive Brazilian epidemic of microcephaly in 2014–2015. Neurotropic and teratogenic virus infections place high economic and emotional burden on society. Zika has long-term health and economic consequences (Fauci and Morens 2016). The symptoms of ZIKV, DENV and CHKV are similar, overlapping and confounding. ZIKV infection in areas where the latter two are already endemic is most likely to pass undetected.

Two lineages of ZIKV are African and South East Asian. The latter circulated for 50 years in South East Asia, entered the Yap Islands in 2007 and caused a paediatric case in Cambodia in 2010. This study highlights the danger of ZIKV introduction into new areas. *Ae. aegypti* and *Ae. albopictus* appeared to be the primary vectors in Asia, although others might also be responsible for maintenance and transmission of ZIKV. It is relatively less studied. Studies were required to understand tropism and pathogenesis. Surveillance is required to know more about distribution and spread of the virus and expansion of enzootic areas and range of vectors.

16.12 Treatment

Currently, no specific antiviral drug or vaccine is available against ZIKV infection. As such management is based on symptomatic care, which includes rest, fluid intake, analgesics and antipyretics. Non-steroidal anti-inflammatory drugs should not be given until dengue fever is ruled out.

In the absence of specific treatment, for protection against ZIKV, preventive measures for protection from mosquito bites and control of vector population should be practised. People travelling from endemic areas to non-affected regions should use mosquito repellent for 2–3 weeks to check transmission of the virus to the non-infected mosquitoes of areas. As sexual transmission of ZIKV has been reported, safe sex should be practiced by persons after visiting high-risk areas (Musso et al. 2015; Hills et al. 2016).

16.13 Vaccine

No vaccine is yet available for the prevention or treatment of Zika virus infection.

References

Basarab M, Bowman C, Aarons EJ, Cropley I (2016) Zika virus. BMJ. 352:i1049

Costello A, Dua T, Duran P, Gülmezoglu M, Oladapo OT et al (2016) Defining the syndrome associated with congenital Zika virus infection. Bull World Health Organ 94(6):406–406A

Duffy MR, Chen TH, Hancock WT, Powers AM, Kool JL et al (2009) Zika virus outbreak on Yap Island, Federated States of Micronesia. N Engl J Med 360:2536–2543

Edupuganti S, Natrajan MS, Rouphael N, Lai L, Xu Y et al (2017) Biphasic zika illness with rash and joint pain. Open Forum Infect Dis 4(3):ofx133

Fauci AS, Morens DM (2016) Zika virus in the Americas — yet another arbovirus threat. N Engl J Med 374:601–604

George J, Valiant WG, Mattapallil MJ et al (2017) Prior exposure to zika virus significantly enhances peak dengue-2 viremia in rhesus macaques. Sci Rep 7:10498

Haddow AD, Schuh AJ, Yasuda CY, Kasper MR, Heang V et al (2012) Genetic characterization of Zika virus strains: geographic expansion of the Asian lineage. PLoS Negl Trop Dis 6(2):e1477

Hayes EB (2009) Zika virus outside Africa. Emerg Infect Dis 15(9):1347–1350

Hills SL, Russell K, Hennessey M, Williams C, Oster AM et al (2016) Transmission of Zika virus through sexual contact with travelers to areas of ongoing transmission—continental United States, 2016. MMWR 65(8):215–216

Lanciotti RS, Kosoy OL, Laven JJ, Velez JO, Lambert AJ et al (2008) Genetic and serologic properties of Zika virus associated with an epidemic, yap state, Micronesia, 2007. Emerg Infect Dis 14(8):1232–1239

Lopes Moreira ME, Nielsen-Saines K, Brasil P, Kerin T, Damasceno L et al (2018) Neurodevelopment in infants exposed to Zika virus in utero. N Engl J Med 379:2377–2379

Lopes Moreira ME, Nielsen-Saines K, Brasil P, Kerin T, Damasceno L, et al. Neurodevelopment in Infants Exposed to Zika Virus In Utero. N Engl J Med. 2018; 379: 2377-79.

Martines RB et al (2016) MMWR. Morbidity and mortality weekly report, p 65. https://doi. org/10.15585/mmwr.mm6506e1er

Minhas AM, Nayab A, Iyer S et al (June 27, 2017) Association of zika virus with myocarditis, heart failure, and arrhythmias: a literature review. Cureus 9(6):e1399

Mlakar J, Misa Korva M, Tul N, Mara Popović M et al (2016) Emerging evidence strengthens association between Zika, microcephaly. N Engl J Med 374:951–958

Musso D, Roche C, Robin E, Nhan T, Teissier A, Cao-Lormeau VM (2015) Potential sexual transmission of Zika virus. Emerg Infect Dis 21(2):359–361

Oehler E, Watrin L, Larre P, Leparc-Goffart I, Lastère S et al (2014) Zika virus infection complicated by Guillain-Barré syndrome—case report, French Polynesia, December 2013. Euro Surveill 19(9):20720

Oliveira Melo AS, Malinger G, Ximenes R, Szejnfeld PO, Alves Sampaio S et al (2016) Zika virus intrauterine infection causes fetal brain abnormality and microcephaly: tip of the iceberg? Ultrasound Obstet Gynecol 47(1):6–7

Pan American Health Organization/World Health Organization. Zika suspected and confirmed cases reported by countries and territories in the Americas Cumulative cases, 2015-2017. Updated as of 05 October 2017. Washington, D.C.: PAHO/WHO; 2017. http://www.paho.org

Renner M, Dejnirattisai W, Carrique L et al (2021) Flavivirus maturation leads to the formation of an occupied lipid pocket in the surface glycoproteins. Nat Commun 12:1238

Salazar V, Jagger BW, Mongkolsapaya J, Burgomaster KE, Dejnirattisai W et al (2019) Dengue and Zika Virus Cross-Reactive Human Monoclonal Antibodies Protect against Spondweni Virus Infection and Pathogenesis in Mice. Cell Rep 26(6):1585–1597

Theel ES, Hata DJ (2018) Diagnostic testing for zika virus: a postoutbreak update. J Clin Microbiol 56(4):e01972-17

WHO (2019) Zika_epidemiology_update_July_2019.pdf

Chapter 17
Yellow Fever

Histotry of Yellow Fever

Yellow fever spread from Africa to South America probably at the time of Spanish conquest and subsequent slave trade in the sixteenth century. Several episodes were recorded in Africa, Americas and Europe since the seventeenth century. It was considered most dangerous in the nineteenth century. This disease killed over 30,000 labours engaged in digging the Panama Canal; work had to be stopped in Panama isthmus in 1889. In 1898, 6000 soldiers died in the Spanish-American war; 969 in the battle rest due to yellow fever.

Around 1881, Cuban doctor Carlos Finlay hypothesized that the disease was transmitted by mosquitoes.

Walter Reed committee was assigned to investigate this hypothesis. Of the three, Aristide Agramonte, Jesse Lazear and James Carroll, the latter two volunteered to be bitten by infected mosquitoes. Lazear died after 12 days of serious illness and Carroll survived. Finlay's hypothesis was proven. Henry Rose Carter observed 'extrinsic incubation period'. The summary of findings are as follows: (a) Stegomyia fasciata (old name of Ae. aegypti) was the vector; (b) patient's blood was infectious for the first 3 days, coincident with viraemic phase; (c) mosquitoes were able to transmit after 12 days of infectious blood meal (extrinsic incubation period); and (d) the causative agent was not a bacterium but a filterable agent.

Yellow fever (YF) is an acute dangerous haemorrhagic hepatonephritis. Patients are commonly jaundiced, hence the name. The case fatality rate is high in untreated severe cases, may be 50%.

YF is endemic in tropical areas, 34 countries of Africa, 13 countries of Latin America and the Caribbean. Asia is free. A modelling study based on African data sources estimated the burden of yellow fever during 2013 was 84,000–170,000 severe cases and 29,000–60,000 deaths.

© Springer Nature Singapore Pte Ltd. 2024
K. G. Narayan et al., *Handbook of Management of Zoonoses*,
https://doi.org/10.1007/978-981-99-9885-2_17

The world has largely forgotten the repeated epidemics in the port cities of Europe and North America during the eighteenth and nineteenth centuries. Death of 150,000 in the United States, including 10% of Philadelphia (then capital) in 1793, compelled the then American President George Washington and his government to flee. The virus was isolated in 1927. French neurotropic vaccine (FNV) and live attenuated 17D vaccine were developed. The latter is one shot conferring lifelong immunity and has excellent cost-benefit ratio. It is used even today. The former was discontinued in 1983 as it had severe neurological side effects. Vaccination leading to elimination of epidemic was demonstrated.

Outbreaks in urban settings of West Africa appeared in early years of 2000, which led to (a) global vaccine stockpile, (b) routine childhood immunization in endemic regions and (c) emergency mass vaccination in the face of outbreaks. YF epidemics have not appeared in West Africa since 2010. Central and eastern Africa still stand at risk.

The female of *Aedes aegypti* and other species transmit this *Flavivirus*. Non-human primates amplify the virus. Major epidemics have occurred in Americas, Africa and Europe since the seventeenth century. Annually, 2.0 lakh cases and 30,000 deaths in unvaccinated population occur: up to 5000 new cases in Africa and 300 in South America and over 90% in Africa. Declining population immunity, deforestation, urbanization, abandoning/stopping vector control programme, climate change and increased population movement are contributing to the increasing number of cases (http://www.who.int/mediacentre/factsheets/fs100/en/YellowfeverFact sheet N°100 May 2013). Since the 1980s, yellow fever seems to be re-emerging.

There is an increasing risk of introduction of yellow fever to North and Central Americas, the Caribbean, the Middle East, Asia, Australia and Oceania because the distribution and density of the vector *Ae. aegypti* are increasing simultaneously with international travel (Tomori 2004).

17.1   Aetiology

Yellow fever virus is the first arthropod-transmitted virus. It was isolated in 1927 in West Africa. It is a ribonucleic acid (RNA) virus belonging to the genus *Flavivirus*. West Nile virus, St. Louis encephalitis virus and Japanese encephalitis virus are antigenically related. Yellow fever virus is highly infectious and pathogenic. Less than one plaque-forming unit is the 50% lethal dose for monkeys.

17.2   Epidemiology

The spread of yellow fever from Africa to Americas occurred during the slave trade in the fifteenth and sixteenth centuries. The ecological conditions were favourable for the YFV and a sustained sylvatic cycle was created. The twin approach of vector control and vaccination kept YF under control for nearly 100 years. It re-emerged in many Latin American countries.

Ae. aegypti and *Ae. albopictus* fly for short distance and thus dependent upon passive transportation, especially humans or goods (e.g. waste tyres). Introduction of virus, naïve susceptible human population, presence of competent anthrophilic vectors and inadequate preventive and health management system allow emergence/re-emergence. Migration between endemic and epidemic regions, increasing contact with the sylvatic virus and poorly planned and uncontrolled urbanization favouring increased density of mosquitoes spread the infection.

17.2.1   Recent Outbreaks

The November–December 2020 YF outbreak in Nigeria—There were 172 deaths and 48 confirmed cases out of 530 suspected. The Rapid Response Team attended to it. Nigeria is already a high-risk YF country and priority for yellow fever epidemic (EYE) (https://www.afro.who.int/news/responding-yellow-fever-outbreak-nigeria-amidst-global-pandemic).

WHO reported outbreaks of yellow fever in Brazil in 2016. Last major epidemics occurred in 1935–1940. Human cases and epizootics increased rapidly due to persistent virus circulation in at-risk areas spreading to new not considered at-risk earlier, such as municipalities and near urban areas of São Paulo and Rio de Janeiro. The population was dense and non-immunized. Between 1 July 2017 and 28 February 2018, there were 723 confirmed cases and 237 deaths, higher than in the past (2016–2017). Confirmed cases included ten unvaccinated travellers from France, the Netherlands, Romania, Switzerland, Argentina and Chile.

The probable sites of confirmed cases corresponded with areas where epizootics in non-human primates were reported continuously through the pre-seasonal and seasonal period. This suggested that the ecosystem favouring YFV circulation is sustained and expanding. *Ae. aegypti* was not found linked to YF infection in 2016–2017. *Forest-dwelling Haemagogus* and *Sabethes* mosquitoes have been linked with all human cases in current outbreaks. Urban transmission (human-*Ae. aegypti*-human) in Brazil has not occurred since 1942. Intensification of vaccination was suggested. Adverse effects (including severe) following immunization also occurred (WHO|Yellow fever–Brazil 2018a, b). [(https://www.who.int/csr/don/27-february-2018-yellow-fever-brazil/en/) Yellow fever Brazil, 9 March https://www.who.int/csr/don/09-march-2018-yellow-fever-brazil/en/)].

Epidemics begin with introduction of infection by infected people (e.g. travellers/workers returning from endemic regions) into areas with dense population without immunity and high mosquito density. Person-to-person transmission by *Ae. aegypti* spread the disease.

Yellow fever impacts hugely socioeconomics, politics, travel and trade.

A combination of interacting factors results in yellow fever outbreaks. These are related to the virus, vectors, non-human primate hosts, humans and environment.

17.2.2   Yellow Fever Virus

There are seven genotypes geographically separated. Outbreaks are caused by particular genotypes in different regions (Barrett and Higgs 2007). Mutebi and Barrett (2002) observed five genotypes (Angola, Central/East Africa, East Africa, West Africa I and West Africa II) in Africa. Each genotype circulates in a defined geographical region. West Africa genotype I in Nigeria and surrounding areas cause frequent outbreaks; three genotypes in East and Central Africa cause sporadic outbreaks.

YFV originated in Africa. East African stain is the oldest, probably diverged from the ancestral flavivirus 3500 years ago. The Western African strains separated from the East African ones some 300 years before the alleged entry into Americas, and the American strains are closer to the East African ones (Chippaux and Chippaux 2018).

East Africa presents unpredictable focal periodicity but with a potential for large epidemics. The East African genotype remained quiescent for nearly 40 years. Two outbreaks occurred in Kenya (1992–1993) and Sudan (2003 and 2005) but not in urban areas (Ellis and Barrett 2008).

The natural history in *West Africa* is well described. Stock et al. (2013) studied strains isolated between 1973 and 2005 in West Africa. Various lineages of one genotype circulated. Their growth behaviour in the human liver and insect cells correlated with the source of isolation suggesting host adaptation.

South American genotypes I and II yellow fever virus appear to have originated from West Africa. Phylolineage studies (de Souza et al. 2010) showed that the South American genotype 1 clade 1 subclade designated as 1E included strains that caused symptomatic yellow fever in humans and monkeys in 2004 and 2008 in Brazil. Strains from the disease in 2000 and earlier also formed subclade 1D. Possible diversification of 1D into 1E started in 1975 and strains of 2004–2008 arose in 1985.

Bayesian phylogeography of isolates of yellow fever viruses from eight South American countries studied by Auguste et al. (2010) revealed that (a) YFV originated from Brazil and dispersed @ 182 km/year to surrounding countries, (b) ancestors of the 2008–2009 epizootics in Trinidad existed there some 4.2 years earlier and (c) Trinidad epizootic of 1995 was caused by the virus that evolved between 1979 and 1988–1989 epizootics. The authors made a complete sequence analysis of the Trinidad 2009 isolate of genotype 1.

17.2.3   Season

January to May is the period in South America. Yellow fever virus circulation is high. In West Africa, August to October is the period. These mosquitoes breed in water containers also, so viral activity/transmission may occur even in dry season.

17.2.4 Human

Cases cluster in villages in the savannah region contiguous with the forest in Africa. More children than older people are affected because the latter have acquired a natural immunity. Occupational (lumbering, forest clearing, etc.) exposure leads to infection of unvaccinated working age group in South America. *Ae. aegypti* breeds around home in urban areas and children and women are predominant victims.

17.2.5 Vectors

Mosquitoes require high temperature, humidity and rainfall for breeding. The extrinsic incubation period is 14 days at 28°C for *Ae. aegypti*. In order that yellow fever virus is transmitted, the vector must survive beyond this period and its anthropophily is maintained. It appears that the true reservoir is mosquito that remains infected throughout life and also transovarial and transstadial infection occurs.

Vector infection, extrinsic incubation period and transmissibility may be affected by certain subtle factors, such as simultaneous infection with more than one infectious agent. Parasites like malaria sporozoites damage the salivary gland 'barrier" allowing arboviruses which have reached haemocoel to enter the salivary gland and thus facilitate transmission. Similarly, microfilaria damage 'gut barrier', helping arboviruses to penetrate the gut. This results in shortening of the extrinsic incubation period and facilitating rapid dissemination, e.g. *Ae. albopictus* infected with *Dirofilaria immitis* facilitating dissemination of Chikungunya (Lecture notes on Tropical Medicine—Arboviruses-Yellow fever (http://itg.content-e.eu/Generated/pubx/173/arboviruses/yellow_fever.htm).

17.2.6 Reservoirs

Infection in monkeys is followed by viraemia and death or solid immunity and they do not appear to contribute to recrudescent virus activity in nature. Deaths in primates may be considered as a forewarning for the coming epizootics. The cyclic epizootics amplify the virus for transmission. Viraemia is for a maximum period of 9 days.

Susceptibility of non-human primates to yellow fever virus differs. South American monkeys seem to be susceptible and often there is high fatality among marmoset (*Callithrix*), howler (*Alouatta*), spider (*Ateles*) and squirrel (*Saimiri*) and to a lesser extent in Capuchin (*Cebus*) monkeys. Recovery of population takes a long time. On the other hand, African monkeys seem to be resistant. They do not

die. Once naturally infected, they become immune for their entire life. The susceptible population thus are the newborn and juveniles. These are *Cercopithecidae* like
Colobus monkeys, baboons (*Papio*), various guenons (*Cercopithecus* sp.) and
mangabeys (*Cercocebus*).

It appears that non-human primates, wild mammals and humans amplify the
virus (because of short duration viraemia, solid immunity and high fatality) and
play only a secondary role in the persistence of YFV. The eggs of mosquitoes seem
to play the role of reservoir. YFV is maintained eggs of *Aedes*. Infection of adult
mosquitoes is assured when these hatch out at the beginning of the following season.

17.2.7 Sentinel

The dependable means of detecting viral presence and activity in a region is its
detection in vector and non-human primates as most infections in humans are
asymptomatic. Further, cases may be detected at one place and then remain undetected for years.

17.3 Transmission

Yellow fever virus has three cycles of transmission—sylvatic or jungle, urban and
intermediate (Fig. 17.1).

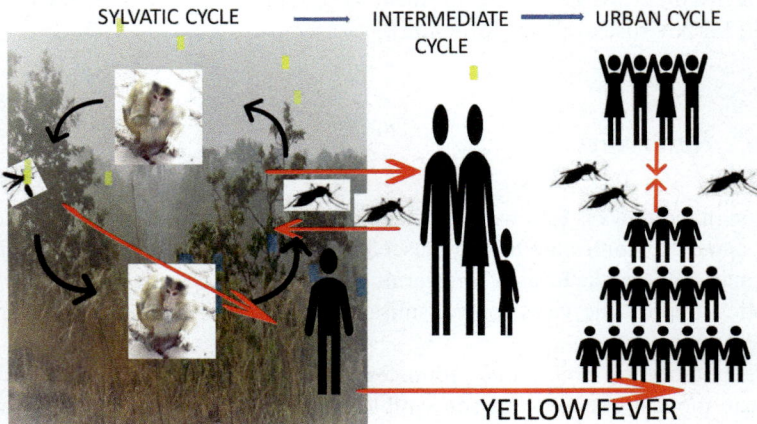

Fig. 17.1 Three cycles of transmission of Yellow fever virus—sylvatic or jungle, urban and
intermediate

17.3.1   Sylvatic/Jungle/Wild Cycle

Yellow fever virus infects non-human primates in the jungles of Africa and South America in the tropical rainforests. The female *Aedes africanus* is the vector in Africa and *Haemagogus* spp. and *Sabethes* spp. in South America. These vectors are canopy dwellers. They bite sleeping monkeys at night. There is no contact with people. Mosquitoes-monkeys-mosquitoes transmission maintains the virus naturally. Non-human primates do not suffer clinically. Humans exposed to this natural nidus in South America get infected. The incidence of human infections is low in this region.

17.3.2   Intermediate or Savannah Cycle

It is most common in humid and semi-humid parts of Africa. Mosquitoes that breed in wild and around human dwellings bite both humans and monkeys, e.g. *Ae. bromeliae*, *Ae. africanus* and *Ae. simpsoni* live near plantation in East Africa. *Ae. furcifer*, *Ae. vittatus*, *Ae. luteocephalus* and *Ae. africanus* are the semi-domestic vectors in West Africa. Infected humans in villages in the mosaic areas may be bitten by peri-domestic mosquito like *Ae. aegypti*, and human-to-human transmission leads to the spread of infection.

17.3.3   The Urban Cycle

'The urban cycle' is the most common and occurs in densely populated areas in Africa. *Aedes aegypti* is the vector. It transmits infection from infected to susceptible humans (human/monkeys-mosquito-human). The vector mosquito sucks blood of infected humans or non-primate hosts and along with it the virions. Virions reach the stomach, infect epithelial cells and replicate. These travel to salivary glands via the haemocoel. While feeding upon the next host, the infected mosquitoes pass on the infection. Viraemia is at the peak shortly before and 3–5 days after onset of fever in human beings. This is the period when the patient is infectious to mosquitoes.

17.3.4   Transovarially Infected Mosquito-Human Transmission

The infected female *Ae. aegypti* can transfer the virions to the eggs (transovarial) and also through the developmental (larval) stages to adult. This may also be the mechanism of persistence of yellow fever. The eggs survive several months of desiccation. Sudden outbreaks may be initiated by such mosquitoes, which transmit

infection even without a blood meal on infected host. *Aedes albopictus* can also act
as the vector.

The natural and epidemic cycles of YF begin from the sylvatic move to anthropogenic sylvatic (deforestation, plantation) cycle to village epidemic to peri-urban
and then urban cycles. There has been a change in sequence of transmission pattern,
from sylvatic directly to urban human-human.

17.3.5   Other Modes of Human Infection

It seems that blood transfusion and needle transfer can transmit infection. Laboratory
hazards may occur while handling infected blood, the liver and cerebrospinal fluid
from patients, infected monkeys, mouse and other laboratory animals and aerosols
of concentrated yellow fever 17D vaccine. Thirty cases with eight deaths are on
record till 1980 (Public Health Agency Canada 2010). Containment facility—biosafety level 3 is required.

Travellers from the United States and Europe have got the infection in South
America and West Africa (Fig. 28.3) as were unvaccinated (Barnett 2007).

17.4   Pathophysiology

Monocytes, macrophages and dendritic cells are invaded. The process involves
receptor binding, fusion of the endosomal membrane with viral envelope, entry of
virus into the endosomal vesicle and release of the genome. The virus replicates in
the endoplasmic reticulum. The immature virus particles are processed in the Golgi
apparatus and mature infectious virions are released. Lymph nodes are affected
initially. The virus moves out from the lymph glands to reach the liver. Hepatocytes
are infected. Cytokines are released. Councilman bodies and necrotic mass appear
in the cytoplasm of hepatocytes. Councilman body (named after William Thomas
Councilman, an American pathologist) is an eosinophilic globule surrounded by
normal parenchyma and represents hepatocytes undergoing apoptosis. This is
found in viral hepatitis, viral haemorrhagic fever, yellow fever and burn in the liver
(http://en.wikipedia.org/wiki/Councilman_body).

17.5   Signs and Symptoms

Most of infections in humans are asymptomatic. Incubation period is 7–10 days.
Symptoms may be mono—or biphasic. Clinical presentation in the first 'acute/red'
phase includes fever, anorexia, nausea, vomiting, chills, headache and pain in

muscles, especially the back, injected conjunctiva and red skin of the face and neck. These subside after 3–4 days. In some (about 15%) patients, it is biphasic. The second or toxic phase appears within 24 h and is serious. Generally, there is no viraemia in this stage.

There is high fever and abdominal pain, the liver is damaged and jaundice makes the patients appear yellow—hence the name 'yellow fever'. Yellow fever is a haemorrhagic fever as the patients tend to bleed from the mouth, nose, eyes, urinary tract (haematuria) and gastrointestinal tract. Ecchymoses, non-menstrual bleeding, petechiae, bleeding from gums and needle puncture are also present. Black vomit and faeces earned its Spanish name *vomito negro*. Kidney failure begins.

Examination may reveal sclera and dermal icterus and epigastric tenderness without enlarged liver. Death follows in 10–14 days. Cardiovascular shock, cytokine storm and multi-organ failure occur in severe cases ending fatally. Convalescence may last several weeks. Abnormal liver function test continues for months after recovery but healing of the liver and kidneys is complete. Death can occur at the end of convalescence due to cardiac arrythmia or myocardial damage.

Case fatality rate is 20% of the toxic phase. Severe epidemics may have high mortality, 50%. Survivors have lifelong protection.

17.6   Diagnosis

Symptoms are confounding and require differentiation from severe malaria, leptospirosis, hepatitis and other haemorrhagic fevers. Travel history may be helpful. Blood and urine tested in early stage for YF can sometimes detect the virus. Later, antibody detection is done:

- Liver biopsy is examined for Councilman body, apoptosis of hepatocytes and viral detection.
- Identification of yellow fever virus: cell culture—Vero (monkey kidney) or MOS 61 (*Ae. pseudoscutellaris*) cells.
- Intracerebral inoculation in baby mice.
- Intrathoracic inoculation in male *Ae. aegypti* and *Toxorhynchites* spp. monitor by FAT monoclonal antibodies-conjugate and specific antibodies (hyperimmune mouse-ascites fluid or monoclonal antibodies).
- Serum is collected during viraemic phase (first 2–3 days). Detection of specific IgM antibodies (from the fifth day) during acute phase and 4x increase in titre of IgG antibodies in serum collected later (convalescent). Cross-reaction with other flaviviruses is a possibility.
- Tests like complement fixation, haemagglutination inhibition and virus neutralization, antigen capture ELISA.
- Reverse transcription-polymerase chain reaction.

17.7   Treatment

There is no effective therapy. No specific symptomatic treatment is given. Cases need hospitalization and intensive care. Ribavirin given during the first 5 days of infection may be useful.

17.8   Prevention

YF cannot be eradicated but epidemic can be prevented. Strategy included (a) protect at-risk populations, (b) prevent international spread and (c) contain outbreaks rapidly.

17.8.1   Surveillance

The 'integrated surveillance and response system' should be effective. The surveillance should include (a) 'syndromic' and (b) sentinel surveillance. Supported with laboratory diagnosis, these are the first-line detection of YF.

17.8.2   Vaccination

Security threshold of 60–80%; >80% is required for interrupting human-mosquito-human transmission.

17.8.2.1   Vaccine Coverage in High-Risk Areas

Childhood vaccination—make YF vaccination a part of expanded immunization programme. Age of vaccination is 9 months in Africa and 12 months in LAC (Latin America and Caribbean). It takes 30 years to reach appropriate population immunity, which would be inadequate in the face of an outbreak earlier than 30 years.

Preventive mass vaccination campaigns rapidly increase population immunity and protection wanes, in 25–30 years almost to nil.

Catch-up campaigns to reach under-vaccinated cohorts or pockets are risk mitigation to close gaps in immunization.

17.8.2.2 Travellers

Unimmunized workers and eco-tourists can spread YF (Angola epidemic—unimmunized workers from China, Kenya and the Democratic Republic of the Congo (DRC)).

Two YF outbreaks (Luanda, Angola) and Kinshasa (DRC) in 2016 strongly indicated international spread and potential global threat. It is feared that YF may spill over to Asia, India and China, which are home to the vector *Aedes* spp.

The Eliminate Yellow Fever Epidemics (EYE) strategy was developed. WHO/UNICEF/Gavi (2017) identified 40 countries (27 in Africa and 13 in Americas) at the highest risk. A vaccine dose of 1.4 billion over 10 years is required to establish and maintain high level of immunity among children and adults. Rapid containment is required to prevent development of epidemic. Surveillance to detect cases early, community mobilization, vector control and reactive vaccination are responses to epidemic. Contain rapidly, protect at-risk population and prevent international spread because YF outbreaks can easily turn into public health emergencies on international concern.

Stockpile of 6.0 million doses of vaccine (attenuated chicken embryo live vaccine 17D) funded by Gavi guarantees rapid and effective response to outbreaks on time. Ninety-five percent develop protection in 10 days. Immunity lasts for 10 years (81% had for 30 years). It is expected to vaccinate 1.0 billion people by the end of 2026 (WHO 2019).

17.8.2.3 Adverse Events Following Immunization

Vaccine may affect the liver, kidneys or the nervous system of 0 and 0.21 cases per 10,000 doses in regions where yellow fever is endemic and 0.09–0.4 cases per 10,000 doses in populations not exposed to the virus. The risk is higher in >60 years, those suffering from chronic illness/allergies to egg protein, immunodeficient or those with disorder of the thymus and should not be vaccinated. Pregnant women and infants <9 months are also excluded, but need evaluation during outbreak (WHO 2019).

Mosquito Control and Prevention of Mosquito Bites.

17.8.3 Population at Risk and International Certification of Vaccination

Forty-five countries in Africa and Latin America covering 900 million people are listed where yellow fever is endemic (http://www.mfa.go.th/main/en/services/123/15384-List-of-countries-which-are-declared-Yellow-Fever.html Apr

10, 2012 20:33:05/Updated: Jun 30, 2012 19:33:26/Read 8295 Views). The distribution is 32 countries in Africa with 508 million and the remaining in 13 countries in Latin America, of which population at greatest risk reside in Bolivia, Brazil, Colombia, Ecuador and Peru. Estimated cases are 200,000 and deaths 30,000 per year. Ninety percent infections occur in the African continent (WHO estimates; http://www.who.int/mediacentre/factsheets/fs100/en/Fact sheet N°100.January 2011).

Some non-endemic countries, such as Asia, are ecologically potential to have yellow fever. These have host monkeys and vectors mosquitoes. If yellow fever virus makes an accidental entry, it is likely to invade the population. Imported cases occur. Outbreaks of yellow fever have occurred in the past (seventeenth to nineteenth centuries) in North America and Europe. Vaccination of travellers is thus important. The recommendations of the Advisory Committee on Immunization Practices include details of studies on vaccines and vaccination of yellow fever (2010). There are two vaccines—17DD YF manufactured in Brazil and other South American countries and 17D-204 outside Brazil including the United States. The virus strains share almost 100% homology. Both are equally effective. All travellers to YF-endemic countries need to be educated about the (a) risks and methods of personal protection, (b) vaccination, (c) those who should not receive the vaccines, and (d) side effects, and healthcare providers should consider precautions to be taken.

In order to prevent the entry of the virus, visitors/travellers passing through or coming from endemic countries must get vaccination.

International travel regulations and WHO guidelines are available.

Indian regulations (http://www.immigrationindia.nic.in/Health_regulation2.htm) stipulate the following:

1. Those without vaccination certificate of yellow fever arriving from endemic areas within 6 days of departure or transit from endemic areas will be quarantined for 6 days.
2. For those leaving for endemic countries, there is no regulation. In their own interest, they should get vaccinated and possess vaccination certificate.

Mosquito control—see chapter on dengue. Reduction of mosquito population to a level that virus transmission is not possible (Breteau index <5.0).

17.8.4 Vector Control vs. Virus Eradication

Vector control and strict vaccination almost eradicated the urban cycle from South America. A single urban outbreak occurred in Santa Cruz de la Sierra, Bolivia, since 1943. Virus eradication relying mostly on vaccination was largely unsuccessful in Africa. This failed to break the sylvatic cycle involving wild primates.

17.8.5   Risk/Drivers

The vector *Ae. aegypti* is common for Chikungunya, dengue and Zika viral infections. Therefore, areas where these diseases are endemic are most likely to be invaded by YFV. Risk activities are incursions into forest, deforestation, mining and oil extraction. Urbanization, peri-urbanization, large-scale speedy movement, internationally recruited workers, urbanization and climate change are risk-amplifying factors driving human for increasing exposure. Risks specific to urban transmission cycle are low immunity, crowding, dense population and plentiful breeding sites for mosquitoes around houses.

References

Auguste AJ, Lemey P, Pybus OG, Suchard MA, Salas RA et al (2010) Yellow fever virus maintenance in Trinidad and its dispersal throughout the Americas. J Virol 84(19):9967–9977

Barnett ED (2007) Yellow fever: epidemiology and prevention. Clin Infect Dis 44:850–856

Barrett AD, Higgs S (2007) Yellow fever: a disease that has yet to be conquered. Annu Rev Entomol 52:209–229

Chippaux JP, Chippaux A (2018) Yellow fever in Africa and the Americas: a historical and epidemiological perspective. J Venom Anim Toxins Incl Trop Dis 24:20

de Souza RP, Foster PG, Sallum MA, Coimbra TL, Maeda AY et al (2010) Detection of a new yellow fever virus lineage within the south American genotype I in Brazil. J Med Virol 82(1):175–185

Ellis BR, Barrett AD (2008) The enigma of yellow fever in East Africa. Rev Med Virol 18(5):331–346

Mutebi JP, Barrett AD (2002) Epidemiology of yellow fever in Africa. Microbes Infect 4(14):1459–1468

Public Health Agency of Canada (2010) Pathogen safety data sheet—infectious substances. Section infectious agent—yellow fever. http://www.phac-aspc.gc.ca/lab-bio/res/psds-ftss/yfv-vfj-eng.php

Stock NK, Laraway H, Faye O, Diallo M, Niedrig M, Sall AA (2013) Biological and phylogenetic characteristics of yellow fever virus lineages from West Africa. J Virol 87(5):2895–2907

Tomori O (2004) Yellow fever: the recurring plague. Crit Rev Clin Lab Sci 41(4):391–427

WHO/UNICEF/Gavi (2017) A Global strategy to eliminate Yellow Fever Epidemics (EYE) 2017–2026

WHO|Yellow fever–Brazil (2018a). https://www.who.int/csr/don/27-february-2018-yellow-fever-brazil/en/

WHO|Yellow fever–Brazil (2018b). https://www.who.int/csr/don/09-march-2018-yellow-fever-brazil/en/

WHO (2019) Yellow fever fact sheet. https://www.who.int/news-room/fact-sheets/detail/yellow-fever

Chapter 18
Rift Valley Fever

Rift Valley fever (RVF) is an emerging mosquito-borne zoonotic viral haemorrhagic infection of increasing global concern. It is associated with heavy rainfall. Generally, epizootic is followed by epidemic transmission in rural areas. Waves of a large number of abortions, neonatal mortality and death in young sheep, goats and cattle cause serious economic loss. Contact with infected animal body fluids leads to epidemic of serious haemorrhagic fever characterized by high fever, headache, retinitis, haemorrhages, encephalitis and death. Some cases present symptoms resembling dengue.

RFV is regarded as re-emerging disease (https://www.oie.int/en/animal-health-in-the-world/animal-diseases/rift-valley-fever/). It is a listed disease by the World Organization for Animal Health (the OIE *Terrestrial Animal Health Code* Chapters 1.1 and 8.15.). WHO considers it as a priority disease. It is considered category A priority disease for biodefense research by the National Institute for Allergy and Infectious Diseases, USA.

RFV is a disease of sub-Saharan Africa. 1.0 billion people are at risk. It has huge economic impact on agriculture, animal trade and human health through explosive outbreaks in livestock and human throughout Africa with potential to spread to the Middle East, Asia and Europe (WHO "Introduction to RVF" https://www.who.int/docs/default-source/documents/emergencies/rift-valley-fever/rvf-presentation.pdf?sfvrsn=9ab8f0d3_4).

The disease is named after the Rift Valley stretching between eastern Africa and Mozambique. Daubney et al. (1931) first described this disease after it had caused epidemic in sheep on a farm near Lake Naivasha in Kenya. In 1950–1951, it caused epizootic in Kenya—about 10,000 sheep died. Again, Garissa district of Kenya reported 170 haemorrhagic fever-associated deaths in December 1997 (Woods et al. 2002). Acute infection was detected in 18% of the enrolled cases tested by anti-RVFV IgM. An estimated 27,500 infections occurred in the district. Association between cases and contact with sheep body fluids was significant. Egypt experienced epizootic and also epidemic in 1977. The infection was probably introduced

© Springer Nature Singapore Pte Ltd. 2024
K. G. Narayan et al., *Handbook of Management of Zoonoses*,
https://doi.org/10.1007/978-981-99-9885-2_18

from Sudan with domestic animal trade. West Africa had the first epidemic in 1987, linked to Senegal River project wherein river flood altered the ecology and human-animal interaction. RVF spread out of Africa in September 2000 and caused outbreaks in Saudi Arabia and Yemen (Shoemaker et al. 2002). RVF was detected by RT-PCR, virus isolation (Vero E6 followed by IFA) and serologic tests (Ag-capture ELISA for IgM and ELISA for IgG) in Saudi Arabia and Yemen. Genetic analysis of selected regions of the virus RNA—S, M and L—confirmed the introduction into the Arabian Peninsula from East Africa. Animal trade from East Africa is active.

18.1   Aetiology

Rift Valley fever virus (RVFV) belongs to the genus *Phlebovirus* and family *Phenuiviridae*. Grobbelaar et al. (2011) made an elaborate genetic study on a number of RVFV strains collected from past and current outbreaks in different locations to conclude that RVFV was genetically stable. Neutralization with monoclonal antibodies suggested single serotype and that single vaccine was sufficient to control.

RVFV appears to have emerged from a natural reservoir in Africa at the time when large-scale farming of sheep and cattle was introduced. Present strains descended and dispersed through movement of infected animal (Ikegami 2012). Phylogenetic relationship of 198 RVFV strains from Saudi Arabia and 16 countries in Africa of 7 years (1944–2010) were studied by Grobbelaar et al. (2011). Results showed low diversity but wide geographical dispersal of the virus. The translocated virus initiated smouldering infections and remained undetected till suitable climatic conditions precipitated as it happened in the 2000–2001, 2006–2007 and 2010 outbreaks in the Arabian Peninsula, Kenya and South Africa, respectively.

Virus structures and functions are summed up from Boshra et al. (Boshra et al. 2011a, b). RVFV is enveloped and has three segments—small (S), medium (M) and large (L)—but single-stranded RNA; S segment encodes for two proteins—nucleocapsid protein (N) and non-structural filamentous nuclear protein (NSs)—which helps in viral replication and assemblage in the cytoplasm of infected cells and considered as a major virulence factor. Endocytosis is receptor-mediated. The virus replicates both in mammalian cells and insect vectors. The M segment encodes for proteins NSm (14 kDa and 78 kDa) and envelops glycoproteins Gn and Gc. L segments encode RNA polymerase for replication and viral transcription. Gn/Gc-gene segment M—mediated viral entry through receptors contributes to the assembly process and likely interacts with N protein. Virulence is associated with a single amino acid substitution in the ORF of Gc. Nucleotide substitution (G and A) at nucleotide 847 of the M segment can determine the virulence phenotype of the RVFV ZH 501 strain in mice. One of the two major subpopulations had a G residue at nucleotide 847 (rZH501-M847-G) and encoded glycine and others had A residue (rZH501-M847-A) that encoded glutamic acid in major viral envelope Gn protein. The latter caused rapid viral replication in the sera, liver, spleen, kidneys and brain and death of most of the mice within 8 days suggesting it to be virulent. Contrastingly, rZH501-M847-G seemed to be attenuated as it caused low viraemia and poor replication in these organs (Morrill et al. 2010). NSm1/NSm2 (78/14 kDa) M suppresses virus-induced apoptosis. N 27 S (segment S) induces humoral and T-cell immunity response. NSs (Mol. Wt. 31) S acts as an interferon antagonist: limits IFN-mediated host antiviral responses, inhibiting cellular transcription and degrading protein kinase PKR, and interacts with specific DNA regions of the host genome, inducing chromosome cohesion and segregation defects.

18.2   Epidemiology

RVF has not been reported in urban areas. It affects livestock, generally farmed in rural areas. Studies on sentinel sheep and goats in Eastern Africa by Lichoti et al. (2014) revealed that the inter-epizootic period was 5–15 years. Sporadic acute disease, seroconversion and undetected low level of virus transmission occurred during the inter-epidemic periods.

The 1950–1951 epizootic resulted into death of an estimated 100,000 sheep in Kenya. Dar et al. (2013) summarized major outbreaks since 1997–1998 in Kenya, Tanzania and Somalia to the latest outbreaks in South Africa in 2010 and Mauritania till December 2010. The 1997/1998 outbreak in Kenya and Somalia led to the ban of livestock export that affected the Middle Eastern countries, particularly Somalia. Saudi Arabia in particular imported a large number of ruminants for the annual Hajj pilgrimage and enforced ban. 2.8 million live animals were exported from the port Berbera of Somaliland a year before the ban was enforced. Livestock trade accounted for 65% of GDP of Somaliland in 1997. Civil war added to the loss. Loss for the first 16 months (February 1998–May 1999) was $109 million. The estimated and reported number of human cases and deaths were 33,9000, 4128 and 1210, respectively.

According to Kenawy et al. (2018), Egypt experienced four major outbreaks, 1977, 1978, 1993 and 2003, resulting in unpredicted human disease. Humans suffered from severe clinical manifestations and high mortality. Many abortions and deaths occurred in sheep, goats, cattle, water buffalo and camels. The vectors were *Culex pipiens* and *Cx. antennatus. Aedes caspius* was also suspected of disseminating the virus. Epidemiological studies identified continued introduction of RVFV-infected animals from Sudan, abundance of vectors, favourable environmental conditions and close proximity between humans and domestic animals contributed to epidemics.

RVF is capable of re-emerging after a long quiescence. Major outbreaks in humans re-emerged in Kenya, Somalia and Tanzania in 1997–1998 and 2006–2007 and in Mauritania in 1998 and 2010 (Dar et al. 2013). It has the capability of invading new territories. Outbreaks occurred in Sudan (2007–2008), Madagascar (2008) and South Africa (2010). An outbreak of RVF in humans and in livestock farms was reported (NICD Comm May10Vol09_Add1_Rift valley fever.pdf) (2010a).

RVF reappeared after 10 years in a French overseas department, Mayotte Island. Some seropositive cases were detected in Turkey, Tunisia and Libya. These raised the attention of the European Union for a possible incursion into neighbouring countries (EFSA J Scientific opinion, 06 March 2020). Seropositive cases in Korea and a single case imported from Angola to China seem alerting; RVF may enter Asia anytime (Bushra et al. 2020).

Tennant et al. (2021) studied the persistence mechanism of RVFV in the Comoros archipelago while developing a metapopulation model. RVFV sustained in the archipelago network. The ecosystem, host communities and meteorological factors presented favourable conditions for mosquito vectors to complete their life cycle and transmit the virus in the absence of explicit introduction events after early 2007.

The inter-epizootic/inter-epidemic period in Zambia is more than three decades. RVF is endemic in sub-Saharan Africa and reported at intervals of 5 to 15 years. Chambaro et al. (2022) studied epidemiological-related factors for this long persistence/quiescence. Retrospective analysis of RVF epizootics showed a positive correlation between above-normal rainfall (anomalous precipitation due to La Niña) and disease emergence. Pooled mosquitoes, sera from sheep, goats and wild ungulates covering a period from 2014 to 2019 were studied for RVFV by RT-PCR and for antibodies by ELISA. Viral genome could not be detected in pooled mosquito samples. Seroprevalence was high among wild ungulates compared to domestic ruminants. A silent circulation of RVFV, risk of emergence of disease in some areas and role of wildlife in maintenance of virus was evidenced.

18.2.1   Wild Animals

Olive et al. (2012) reviewed literatures on natural and experimental RVFV infections in wild animals covering at least ten orders. Wild ruminants, African buffaloes in particular and some domestic ruminants may be involved in maintenance. However, infection probably meets a dead end. *Carnivora* and *Perissodactyla* may not support RVFV replication.

18.2.2   Reservoir and Vector

Natural reservoir of RFVV is mosquitoes. The Peter's epauletted fruit bat (*Micropteropus pusillus*) and Aba round leaf bats (*Hipposideros abae*) from which the virus has been isolated are also believed to be reservoirs.

The initiating vector 'flood water *Aedes*' bred in these foci which were well away from human habitation but not from livestock. *Culex theileri* and *Culex zombaensis*, the former in particular, fed on a large number of vertebrate hosts, both men and animals, and bred in farm house refuges and watering troughs and were a possible source of human infection. These bred in large number in areas where flood water persisted for weeks or months (NICD CommMay10Vol09_Add1_Rift valley fever. pdf) (2010b).

RVFV can be transmitted by more than 53 species from eight genera of mosquitoes distributed widely. These can play different roles in sustaining the transmission. The dominant vector species varies in different regions.

Aedes spp. of the Neomelaniconium group is the main vector. These breed in temporary water pools, pans, vleis and floodplains which are common through the Rift Valley. These mosquitoes are commonly found in tropical forests, Guinea and Sudan, and arid and semi-arid zones associated with alluvial riverine floodplains. Flooding is dependent upon rainfall. RVFV-infected vector may emerge annually or biennially in bushed and wooded grasslands and semi-arid zones throughout the African continent but are missed because of the absence of disease-susceptible indicator hosts (http://www.fao.org/3/Y4611E/y4611e05.htm).

Transovarial transmission in mosquitoes, generation after generation, explains the continued presence of the virus (persistence) in enzootic foci. Eggs are laid on blades of grasses. Eggs of *Aedes* spp. have to undergo a dry spell before they can hatch. These survive for several months in dry condition and thus also the virus. The low-lying grasses and such habitat are flooded with water due to heavy rainfall or flood. The eggs hatch and there is a rapid increase in infected mosquito population that spread Rift Valley fever.

Some known species of *Aedes* are *A. mcintoshi* (*Ae. lineatopennis* sl.), *Ae. dentatus*, *Ae. unidentatus* and *Ae. juppi*. According to Miller et al. (2002), *Ae. vexans arabiensis*, *Cx. pipiens* complex and *Cx. tritaeniorhynchus* are considered the epidemic and epizootic vectors in Saudi Arabia. An isolate of RVFV from *Ae. vexans arabiensis* was closely related to strains from Madagascar and Kenya epidemics of 1991 and 1997, respectively, and was probably imported through the infected mosquitoes and livestock. Seufi and Galal (2010) detected RVFV by RT-PCR in female, male and larvae of *Anopheles gambiae arabiensis* and *Culex pipiens* complex in the 2007 Sudan outbreak.

Many secondary vectors—*Anopheles*, *Aedes* (*Stegomyia*), *Mansonia*, and *Eretmapodites* species—also play a role in the transmission of RVFV. *Culex*, *Eretmapodites*, *Mansonia*, *Mansonoides* and *Coquillettidia* mosquitoes also play a role. 'Bridge mosquitoes' (e.g. *Culex* spp.) population also bloom in the persistent rains and magnify an early outbreak by transmitting RVFV among amplifying vertebrate hosts, including cattle and goats they feed upon. Epizootics may result and epidemics may follow. Movement of infected animals to non-enzootic areas may introduce RVFV. New epizootics are thus likely. Severe and fatal cases occurred with haemorrhagic complications and hepatitis during the ongoing outbreak of RVF in South Africa between February and May 2010. The outbreak appeared to be associated with domestic/peri-domestic vectors that bred during major flooding. These vectors were restricted to sparsely populated agricultural areas with localized foci near pans, vleis or farm dams.

Stomoxys, *Phlebotomus*, *Simulium* and *Culicoides* spp. may act as mechanical vectors and be carried by winds over large distances, such as north and south trade winds. These winds converge in 'intertropical convergence zone' where low pressure area, rising air, cloud formation and heavy rainfall occur. This zone falls north and south of the equator depending upon the season.

Lake regions provided favourable ecological conditions for vectors in Gabon where higher seroprevalence was observed.

18.2.3   Movement of Animals and Vectors

Periodic expansion of mosquito vectors, the circulating virus and susceptible animals led to epizootics. It spreads with infected animals. Therefore, movement of animals is important, especially their health status. Epizootics cause heavy economic loss and seriously impact animals' trade.

The movement of live animals and vectors by ship, flights, containers and road transport is likely to spread globally. Globalization of arthropod vectors, mainly mosquitoes, *Aedes* spp., adds to the threat of introduction to other continents and spread.

18.2.4   Climate

Optimal environment for RVF favours the rehydration of desiccated mosquito eggs in soil and its water retention capacity and offers dense bush/grass shrubs for landing and resting of developing mosquitoes.

It is the climatic feature of the continent determined by the Intertropical Convergence Zone, characterized by convective activity which generates often vigorous thunderstorms. RVF may appear simultaneously in several countries at one and the same time. All the major outbreaks were preceded by heavy rainfall and/or flooding, possibly because huge number of vectors is required (http://www.fao.org/3/Y4611E/y4611e05.htm). RFV outbreaks in Africa, Saudi Arabia and Yemen are closely associated with periods of above-average rainfalls.

Climate change in the form of the warm phases of the *El Niño/Southern Oscillation* is accompanied with increased rainfall, floods and greenness of vegetation index (NDVI). The natural consequence is surge in mosquito population. The mosquito reservoir of RVFV vertically transmits it to progenies; virus remains viable for a number of years in eggs of mosquitoes; mosquito lays eggs in water and these eventually hatch into infective mosquito. Domesticated ruminants like sheep, goats, cattle and also camel suffer from epizootics.

18.3   Human Rift Valley Fever

Rift Valley fever virus has caused several outbreaks in sub-Saharan Africa since its first report in 1931. Livestock trade along the Nile irrigation system introduced it to Egypt resulting into an explosive outbreak in 1977. Extensive flooding, El Niño (climate effect) caused major outbreak in 1997–1998 in Kenya, Somalia and Tanzania. RVFV extended beyond the African continent in 2000 to islands in Indian Ocean, Madagascar, Comoros and Mayotte, invaded the Arabian Peninsula in 2000–2001 causing estimated 2.0 lakhs infections and 250 deaths in Saudi Arabia and Yemen (Javelle et al. 2020) and raised a concern about the possibility of invasion of Asia and Europe. The outbreaks and countries/regions affected are listed in Table 18.1.

An outbreak in Eldamar, Sudan, during May to July 2019 was reported by Ahmad et al. (Ahmad et al. 2020). A woman with spontaneous abortion was admitted to a hospital. Cases with high fever and headache poured in @ ~96/day, which peaked in June. 1129 cases and 19 deaths were recorded. There were more males than females mostly in the age group of 25–44 years. Most were animal farmers who reported abortion in their animals. Eldamar has animal market for sheep, goat and bovine. Vaccination of animals in dry season is recommended.

Human cases appearing after a 'storm of abortions' in animals are a characteristic feature (OIE Listed Diseases 2008). Protecting human from RVF is possible by controlling and preventing animal RVF.

Study of Rift Valley fever epizootic is related to heavy rainfall and floods. It is thought that successive and overlapping swarms of different mosquitoes infect and amplify infection in ruminants with subsequent transmission to humans resulting in

Table 18.1 Severe form of RVF in humans since 2000

Country/region	Year	Number of cases (deaths)
Sudan (Eldamar)[a]	2019 (May to July)	1129 (19)
Mayotte Island (France)	4 January 2019 (22 November–31 December 2018)	129
Republic of Niger: Tahoua region	As of 11 October 2016	105 (28)
Republic of Mauritania: six regions	16 September to 13 November 2012	36 (18)
Republic of South Africa: nine provinces	February to July 2010	237 (26)
Madagascar	December 2008–May 2009	23 (7)
Madagascar: four provinces	17 April 2008 (January to June)	47 (19)
Sudan	28 October 2008 (November 2007–January 2008)	738 (230)
Kenya	30 November 2006–12 March 2007	684 (234)
Somalia	19 December 2006–20 February 2007	114 (51)
Tanzania	13 January–3 May 2007	24 (109)
Egypt	2003	148 (27)
Saudi Arabia	2000	516 (87)
Yemen	2000	1087 (121)

https://www.who.int/news-room/fact-sheets/detail/rift-valley-fever
https://www.who.int/csr/don/13-may-2019-rift-valley-fever-mayotte-france/en/
[a]Ahmad et al. (2020)

epidemics. According to Bird and Nichol (2012), abortion storm in ruminants (cattle and sheep) and high neonatal (~70%) and adult mortality (20–30%) are characteristic features. Livestock provide a clear link between mosquito vector and human.

18.3.1   Modes of Transmission

- *Direct/indirect* with blood, body fluids (secretions and excretions) or infected tissues of livestock—cattle, sheep, goats, buffalo and camels.
- *Aerosol* inhalation, aerosol of blood from infected tissues such as foetuses/slaughtered infected animal laboratory accident.
- *Ingestion* of unpasteurized/uncooked milk and meat from infected animals.
- *Infected mosquito bite*—High viraemia in livestock may infect anthrophilic mosquito, *Culex* spp. and *Anopheles* spp. Blood-feeding flies also transmit infection to humans.

Human-to-human transmission does not occur. Vertical transmission of RVF has been observed (Arishi et al. 2006; Adam and Karsany 2008).

18.3.2   Risk Factors

Living in rural areas, agri-related activities and livestock rearing (farming), butchering/handling raw meat, vets and lab workers and sleeping out—exposure to mosquito.

Archer et al. (2011) made a cross-sectional epidemiological study in South Africa. Fifteen per cent had recent and 4% past exposure to RVF. Acute infection occurred in 21% veterinarians and 9% farmers. Direct contact was the mode of transmission. The risk of developing acute infection after performing autopsies was 16.3. After an incubation period (IP) of 4.3 days, symptoms like myalgia, headache and malaise appeared.

The most affected human age lies between 15 and 29 years old. This was followed by >45 years old, 30–44 years old and then 5–14 years old. Housewives followed by farmers, students, shepherds and workers were vulnerable to infection (Seufi and Galal 2010). In Gabon, more males were positive because of the exposure to vectors and animals while hunting and farming.

18.3.3   Clinical Presentation

RFV infection causes asymptomatic (98%) to severe (2%) diseases in humans. Overall case fatality rate is >1, mostly in haemorrhagic icteric form. The CFR is high during the epidemics, 18% in Saudi Arabia, 28% in Tanzania and around 22% in East Africa, West Africa, South Africa and Madagascar from 2006 to 2010.

Human asymptomatic infection is detected by serological tests. Pourrut et al. (2010) observed RVF-specific IgG antibodies in 10.3% of villages of Gabon indicating viral circulation.

Unknown haemorrhagic fever in humans and associated deaths in animals on the border regions of Saudi Arabia in 2000 were investigated and identified as RVFV. Investigation revealed 78% male and median age 46 years, 80% were Saudi and 20% Yemeni and 21% died (MMWR 2000).

RVF may appear as mild and severe. Absence of vaccine and antiviral treatment and difficult clinical diagnosis demand extra precaution. Often case detection is delayed.

1. *Mild form*: IP 2–6 days, asymptomatic; feeling feverish, pain in the head, muscle and joint; some show symptoms mimicking early stage of meningitis—stiff neck, anorexia, nausea and vomiting, duration 4–7 days; developing antibodies sanitize blood of the virus.
2. *Severe forms*: Appear in small percentage of cases. One of the three forms may appear—ocular (0.5–2%), meningoencephalitis (<1%) and haemorrhagic (<1%).

The mild form of the disease is accompanied with ocular symptoms (retinal lesions). The ocular form manifests usually 1–3 weeks after the appearance of the first symptoms. The patient reports blurred/reduced vision. Resolution takes 10–12 weeks. Nearly half the patients whose macula has the lesions lose vision permanently. Consultation with an eye specialist is recommended. Death is uncommon.

The meningoencephalitis form occurs 1–4 weeks after the appearance of the first symptoms. Patients report lethargy, severe headache, disorientation, vertigo, memory loss, confusion, hallucination, convulsions and coma. Neurological complications may appear after 2 months. The death rate is low but permanent damage like neurological deficit may be severe and is common. Emergency and intensive care in hospital is recommended.

The haemorrhagic form appears 2–4 days after the onset of the illness. It begins with severe liver dysfunction such as jaundice. Haemorrhagic signs follow: haemorrhagic liver, hematemesis, blood in faeces, menorrhagia, bleeding of gums and the nose and bleeding in the skin—purpuric rash, ecchymoses and sites of venepuncture. Duration is short: 3–6 days. Death follows, mostly in haemorrhagic icteric form. CFR is about 50%. Healthcare workers should protect themselves, preferring PPE. Cases require emergency and intensive care.

Confounding conditions in humans are many diseases causing fever, malaria, shigellosis, typhoid fever and yellow fever.

18.4   Animal Rift Valley Fever

Rift Valley fever has serious implications for livestock agriculture and trade. RVF may persist for years in endemic region with low prevalence during the inter-epizootic period. With rains, floods resulting in huge vector population and also turnover of susceptible livestock, epizootics occur (epizootic period).

Susceptibility depends upon breed and genotype of animals and those exotic to Africa or endemic areas are more susceptible.

RVF spreads in animals primarily by mosquito bites and not by contact. RVFV is able to infect many species of animals. It causes severe disease in domestic animals, such as sheep, goats, cattle and camels. Almost 100 per cent of pregnant ewe aborts. An explosive wave of unexplained abortion in livestock is observed at the beginning of epidemic. Young ones are more susceptible; >90% infected lambs die compared to 10% of adult sheep.

RVFV causes intense viraemia. The disease appears suddenly and dramatically in per-acute or acute form in domestic ruminants—sheep, goat and cattle. It is characterized by 'abortion storm' (80–100% abortion) in pregnant species and fever, weakness and sudden death in young postnatal period in all species. Nearly all (100%) of young lambs of susceptible species may die within 10–12 hours of hyperpyrexia (40–42°C). Older, 1–4 months suffer from acute fever, muco-purulent nasal discharge, haemorrhagic diarrhoea, generalized lymphadenitis, prostration and death in 1–2 days (fatality −10 to 40%). Adult sheep and cattle show excess salivation, nasal discharge, anorexia, weakness and diarrhoea with 20% and 10% mortality, respectively. Some deaths occur in all age groups. Milking cow suffer from agalactia. Sheep may die of acute hepatitis and jaundice. Dromedary camels suffer in-apparent infection but abortion rates may be as high as in cattle. Viraemia is brief. However, severe clinical signs, including haemorrhagic septicaemia and sudden death, have been observed among infected dromedary camels in Mauritania.

Recovery from natural RVFV infection results in long-lived cross-strain immunity conferred by neutralizing antibodies against the viral envelope glycoproteins, Gn and Gc.

18.5   Diagnosis

Whom to test? A suspected case is defined as 'the one having history of contact with hoofed animals/mosquito bites in an RVF endemic/potential area and presenting symptoms of fever, myalgia, arthralgia or headache', or with encephalitis, haemorrhage, hepatitis and/or ocular pathology (retinitis) or a person with unexplained encephalitis, hepatitis or haemorrhagic illness.

Approaches

1. Isolate/identify the virus or antigen.
2. Detect/titrate antibodies.

Isolation of virus/detection of antigen—RVFV—may be detected in blood in early phase of infection (up to 10 days in haemorrhagic icterus form) and in tissues/organs on post-mortem:

- RT-PCR.
- Isolation in suckling or weaned mice, or hamsters, by intraperitoneal inoculation (mice and hamsters die within 3–4 days).
- Xenodiagnosis—intra-thoracic inoculation into male mosquito, *Toxorhynchites*. It is safe and cheap. There is no chance for vertical and accidental transmission through bite.
- Grow in tissue culture and identify RVFV by IFT/IPT in 12–36 hours (e.g. Vero, BHK, CER (chicken embryo reticulum) and primary kidney or testis cells of calves and lambs).
- Cryostat sections of formalin-fixed tissues and staining for RVF by immuno-histochemical methods.
- Histopathology of the liver showing characteristic RVF hepatic necrosis with intracytoplasmic and intranuclear inclusion bodies.
- Detection of viral antigen by (a) agar-gel diffusion test using extract of the liver or spleen with RVFV-positive and RVFV-negative control antigens and immune sera and (b) antigen capture ELISA.

Detection of RVFV-specific antibody:

- ELISA system for IgM antibody.
- ELISA system for IgG antibody.
- Micro titre virus-serum neutralization tests in tissue culture.
- Plaque reduction tests in tissue culture.
- *Indirect immunofluorescent test
- *Indirect haemagglutination test.

*These tests may detect low titre cross-relationships with other phleboviruses, but high titre positives will be specific, i.e. 1/160 to 1/320 or greater.

RFVV is considered risk group 3 agent. Biosafety level 3 is required. Details may be found in OIE Terrestrial manual (2008).

18.6   Treatment

Use of antiviral ribavirin is not recommended. Antimalarial and antibiotics may be used in the beginning (to cover confounding diseases). Aggressive ICU: controlling blood pressure, electrolyte, rehydration, renal function and oxygen, use of blood component therapy to support coagulation system and use of painkiller, antiemetic and anxiolytic for agitation.

18.7   Prevention and Control

The Rift Valley fever action framework. FAO Animal Production and Health Guidelines, No. 29, is the recent document (Mariner et al. 2022). The action plan includes (a) pre-emptive risk-based action plan, and (b) preventive and (c) reactive approach is explained to control outbreaks and epidemics and avert pandemic.

Early warning/prediction includes study of climate and surveillance.

18.7.1   Monitoring Climate

A population of susceptible livestock, the virus RVF and massive build-up of vector population are prerequisite for an epidemic to occur. Assuming the presence of virus in the region, the other two factors become key to predicting early the RFVV activity.

Normalized difference vegetation index (NDVI) measures relative 'greenness' and 'brownness'. As the water table rises to the point where flooding may occur, the NDVI ratio approaches 0.43 to 0.45. Remote sensing satellite data (RSSD) enabled national and regional monitoring of rainfall and climatic patterns and their effects upon the environment. Cold cloud density (CCD) measurements are closely correlated with rainfall.

Surface sea temperature data about Indian and Pacific oceans combined with NDVI data are useful in predicting RVFV activity with 100% accuracy 2 to 5 months before virus activity occurs. A period of 2–6 weeks allows mobilizing and organizing adequate intervention measures like tele-epidemiology, geographic positioning system, etc., for proactive monitoring (LaBeaud et al. 2010). Intervention on time prevents RVF infection of livestock and cuts the link and protects humans.

RVF risk maps are updated monthly and edited by the US Global Emerging Infections Surveillance and Response System (DoD-GEIS).

The early Warning and Response System of the European Union reported five cases on Mayotte Island on 4 January 2019. Illegal animal movement possibly introducing RVFV caused 129 human cases and 109 animal foci (https://www.who.int/csr/don/13-may-2019-rift-valley-fever-mayotte-france/en/). The European Food Safety Authority (EFSA) performed a risk assessment and observed that the risk of introduction either by animal or mosquito to European Union was very low (Nielsen et al. 2020).

18.7.2 Surveillance

18.7.2.1 Sentinel Herds

Early detection of RVF is a prerequisite to effective control of the disease. Sentinel herds of small ruminants are located in geographically representative area that favour mosquito breeding, e.g. swamps, near dams, rivers, shallow water bodies and irrigation channels. Owners are informed, cooperation and participation are assured and incentives (animal health check-ups) are defined. Animals, say 30, that are identified, tested as RVFV-antibody negative and marked will be retained and not sold. Regular visit and collection of blood serum should be planned. Antibody detection is usually too late to be of any relevance control (http://www.fao.org/3/Y4611E/y4611e05.htm). Virus remained in mosquito-breeding site. Virus activity occurs even without eliciting any clinical disease and remains undetected. This calls for *active* surveillance to detect transmission between livestock and possibly humans in rural areas, e.g. livestock farmers (Lichoti et al. 2014).

18.7.3 Control

Controlling epidemic aims at reducing loss of life and suffering and cutting down transmission and spread. Epidemiology surveillance, laboratory diagnosis to detect active case and follow-up contacts are important. Triage, barrier nursing, infection control and organizing funeral are practised to cut down loss of lives and generation of new cases.

All efforts are directed to control disease in animals and prevent its spread to animals and humans. Quarantine and restriction of movement of animals should be introduced.

Coordinated sharing of information between animal health and public health services is essential.

Use of personal protective equipment (PPE), apron, gloves, mask and goggle by veterinarians, para-veterinarians and those who handle carcasses or aborted foetuses of infected animals and do necropsies. Hand hygiene: people must wash hands with soap immediately after every contact with any bodily fluid from an infected animal.

RVFV causes intense viraemia; vaccinating during outbreaks is likely to bring about a serial transfer of wild virus resulting in co-infection with wild and attenuated (vaccine) viruses. Natural vector transmission further increases this genetic interaction.

Protective vaccination of animals and control of mosquitoes which are both reservoirs and vectors are required.

Mass vaccination is done to control/prevent recurrence of RVF in animals. Kenya had outbreaks in 1998–1999 and again in 2002; 52,000 animals were vaccinated in

2002. National vaccination programme was introduced in January 2007 after the reported December 2006 outbreak. As many as 760,000 animals were vaccinated in Saudi Arabia after the 2004 outbreak. Egypt practices a regular vaccination of around 7.0 million animals yearly employing 50,000 vets and others; the last reported outbreak was in 1993 (Source—RVF_EN_DISEASE_CARD OIE.pdf).

18.7.4   Vaccines

18.7.4.1   Smithburn Neurotropic Strain (SNS) Vaccine

Routine vaccination of non-pregnant animals is recommended in endemic areas. SNS vaccine is safe for cattle. In the face of epizootic, vaccination is *not* recommended. It is too late. There is risk of needle propagation of RVFV.

The inactivated vaccines are often poorly immunogenic. A bovine virulent RVFV isolate adapted to cell culture has been used by Onderstepoort Biological Products in South Africa to produce an inactivated cell culture vaccine. It is suitable for pregnant ewes. Although antibody response in cattle is poor, vaccinated pregnant cows pass on colostral immunity to their calves. The booster dose is given 3–6 months after the first injection, followed by annual boosters (http://www.fao.org/3/Y4611E/y4611e05.htm).

18.7.4.2   Limitations of SNS Vaccine

It is a partially attenuated strain vaccine, approved as livestock vaccine in Africa and produces lifelong protection. Limitations are as follows: (a) induces abortion and exhibits pathogenicity in European cattle, (b) has limited use in areas threatened by imminent outbreak, (c) risk of reversion of vaccine virus to wild type and of teratogenicity and (d) can cause foetal pathology and abortion in pregnant sheep of susceptible genotypes.

Possibility of generation of recombinant and reassortment of genotypes thus exists. A number of new genotypes and lineages have emerged.

18.7.4.3   Developing Vaccines

A replication-deficient chimpanzee adenovirus vaccine, ChAdOx1-GnGc, has been co-developed and has a safety profile for both human and livestock. A single dose encodes RVFV envelope glycoproteins, elicits high-titre neutralizing antibodies, provides solid immunity and protects sheep, goats and cattle against challenges. It induces neutralizing antibody in vaccinated dromedary camel also. The authors proposed clinical trials in human. It has been tested in RFV-endemic setting and is

DIVA compatible*. This would be a 'One Health' vaccine, a single vaccine for human and multiple species (Warimwe et al. 2016).

*DIVA compatibility is particularly important for livestock disease surveillance and rapid effective control during epizootics. ChAdOx1-GnGc encodes RVFV envelope glycoproteins—the major target of protective immunity—making it compatible with commercially available serological DIVA kits that assign 'vaccinated' (only seropositive for RVFV envelope glycoproteins) or 'infected' (seropositive for all RVFV antigens) status with high sensitivity and specificity.

18.7.5 Vector Control

Mosquito population control programmes, using chemicals, larvicides, fogging, elimination of mosquito-breeding sites, etc.

Personal and community protection against mosquito bites—repellents, mosquito nets, full-sleeved shirts and trouser to cover most of the body parts.

18.7.6 Other Tactics

18.7.6.1 Control of Movement of Animals and Trade

RVF is considered a threat for Asia, Europe and America. Spread through trade route is a possibility. *FAO and the United Nations Development Programme held an expert consultation at FAO headquarters, Rome, on 15 and 16 May 2001.* It was considered that once a country was invaded by RVF, it is likely to be permanently infected. Recovered animals and those vaccinated 1 month earlier are safe for trade and consumption.

Each exporting and importing country is expected to take appropriate action in order to minimize the risk. Three levels of risk are envisaged—'high', 'potentially high' and 'low'. 'High level' of risk is associated with epizootic.

The exporting country is expected to (a) define the extent of infection through longitudinal monitoring (by clinical surveillance, isolation of virus, IgM antibody detection) and (b) return the viral activity to 'pre-epizootic' level.

The importing country stops all import and resumes only 3–6 months after the evidence of the last infection or when it considers that 'high risk' has disappeared.

When pre-epizootic conditions are identified, the risk of RVF is potentially high. The exporting country is expected to increase the monitoring in the RVF epizootic areas such as high floodplains by clinical surveillance in ruminants for abortion and disease in human and also serology in ruminants; vaccination of trade stock at least 1 month earlier may be considered.

The importing country has to institute vigilance at the entry ports—if any animal is recently infected, random check for IgM antibody, and if vaccinated animal is imported, random check for IgG antibodies.

Trade during the inter-epizootic period is associated with 'low risk'. The exporting country should check for infection in sentinel herds in 'high-risk' areas such as floodplains and consider vaccinating all trade animals of age 9–12 months. The importing country should make regular random check of trade animals for IgM antibodies (Empress Transboundary Animal diseases Bulletin (2001) EMPRES e-mail: empres-livestock@fao.org—Web   site: www.fao.org/empres NO. 17/2—2001/pages 1–5).

Good governance is required.

18.7.6.2   Breeding Resistant Animals

Susceptibility to RVFV depends upon genetic strain and breeds of animals. Developing RVF-resistant breed and rearing has been suggested (Dar et al. 2013).

Vaccination in endemic areas often gets hampered because of uncertainty about time and place where epizootic will occur. Predicting epidemic is thus important. Other disease prevention tactics are more effective in preventing spread during pre-epidemic and epidemic. These are public awareness and participation, quarantine and ban on slaughter.

References

Adam I, Karsany MS (2008) Case report: Rift Valley Fever with vertical transmission in a pregnant Sudanese woman. J Med Virol 80(5):929

Ahmad A, Ali Y, Elduma A, Eldigali MH, Mhmoud RA et al (2020) Unique Outbreak of Rift Valley Fever in Sudan, 2019. Emerg Infect Dis 26(12):3030–3033

Archer BN, Weyer J, Paweska J, Nkosi D, Leman P et al (2011) Outbreak of Rift Valley fever affecting veterinarians and farmers in South Africa, 2008. S Afr Med J 101(4):263–266

Arishi HM, Aqeel AY, Al Hazmi MM (2006) Vertical transmission of fatal Rift Valley fever in a newborn. Ann Trop Paediatr 26(3):251–253

Bird BH, Nichol ST (2012) Breaking the chain: Rift Valley fever virus control via livestock vaccination. Curr Opin Virol 2(3):315–323

Boshra H, Lorenzo G, Busquets N, Brun A (2011a) Rift Valley fever: recent Insights into Pathogenesis and Prevention. J Virol 85(13):6098–6105

Boshra H, Lorenzo G, Rodriguez F, Brun A (2011b) A DNA vaccine encoding ubiquitinated Rift Valley fever virus nucleoprotein provides consistent immunity and protects IFNAR (−/−) mice upon lethal virus challenge. Vaccine 29(27):4469–4475

Bushra A, Razzak KS, Hossain MN, Jain D et al (2020) Prevalence of Human Rift Valley Fever Virus as a Bio-threat in Asian Countries after COVID-19 lockdown. Bangladesh J Infect Dis 7(00):S72–S74

Chambaro HM, Hirose K, Sasaki M, Libanda B, Sinkala Y et al (2022) An unusually long Rift valley fever inter-epizootic period in Zambia: Evidence for enzootic virus circulation and risk for disease outbreak. PLoS Negl Trop Dis 16(6):e0010420

Dar O, McIntyre S, Hogarth S, Heymann D (2013) Rift valley fever and a new paradigm of research and development for zoonotic disease control. Emerg Infect Dis 19(2):189–193

Daubney R, Hudson JR, Garnham PC (1931) Enzootic hepatitis or Rift Valley fever. An undescribed virus disease of sheep, cattle and man from East Africa. J Pathol Bacteriol 34:545–579

Empress Transboundary Animal Diseases Bulletin (2001) Reducing the risk of Rift Valley Fever transmission in trade exchanges. EMPRES e-mail: empres-livestock@fao.org—Web site: www.fao.org/empres NO.17/2–2001/pages1-5

Grobbelaar AA, Weyer J, Leman PA, Kemp A et al (2011) Molecular epidemiology of rift valley fever virus. Emerg Infect Dis 17(12):2270–2276

Ikegami T (2012) Molecular biology and genetic diversity of Rift Valley fever virus. Antivir Res 95(3):293–310

Javelle E, Lesueur A, Pommier de Santi V, de Laval F et al (2020) The challenging management of Rift Valley Fever in humans: literature review of the clinical disease and algorithm proposal. Ann Clin Microbiol Antimicrob 19:4

Kenawy MA, Abdel-Hamid YM, Beier JC (2018) Rift Valley Fever in Egypt and other African countries: Historical review, recent outbreaks and possibility of disease occurrence in Egypt. Acta Trop 181:40–49

LaBeaud AD, Kazura J, King CH (2010) Advances in Rift Valley Fever Research: Insights for Disase Prevention. Curr Opin Infect Dis 23(5):403–408

Lichoti JK, Kihara A, Oriko AA, Okutoyi LA, Wauna JO et al (2014) Detection of rift valley Fever virus interepidemic activity in some hotspot areas of Kenya by sentinel animal surveillance, 2009-2012. Vet Med Int 2014:379010

Mariner JC, Raizman E, Pittiglio C, Bebay C et al (2022) Rift Valley fever action framework, vol 29. FAO Animal Production and Health Guidelines, Rome. https://doi.org/10.4060/cb8653en

Miller BR, Godsey MS, Crabtree MB, Savage HM, Al-Mazrao Y et al (2002) Isolation and Genetic Characterization of Rift Valley fever virus from Aedes vexans arabiensis, Kingdom of Saudi Arabia. Emerg Infect Dis 8(12):1492–1494

MMWR (2000) Outbreak of Rift Valley Fever — Saudi Arabia, August–October, 2000. MMWR Morb Mortal Wkly Rep 49(40):905–908. http://www.cdc.gov/mmwr/ preview/mmwrhtml/ mm4940a1.htm

Morrill JC, Ikegami T, Yoshikawa-Iwata N, Lokugamage N, Won S et al (2010) Rapid accumulation of virulent rift valley fever virus in mice from an attenuated virus carrying a single nucleotide substitution in the M RNA. PLoS One 5(4):e9986

NICD (2010a) Comm May: Preliminary report on an outbreak of Rift Valley fever, South Africa, February to 3 May 2010. https://www.nicd.ac.za/assets/files/NICDComm May10Vol09_Add1.pdf

NICD (2010b) Preliminary report on an outbreak of Rift Valley fever, South Africa, February to 3 May 2010. 9 (5): 1–5. NICD CommMay10Vol09_Add1_Rift valley fever.pdf

Nielsen SS, Alvarez J, Bicout DJ, Calistri P, Depner K et al (2020) Rift Valley Fever–epidemiological update and risk of introduction into Europe. EFSA J 18(3):e06041

OIE Listed Diseases (2008) Chapter 1.3 terrestrial animal health code. In: Rift Valley fever technical disease card. "Key Facts" RVF_EN_DISEASE_CARD.pdf

OIE Terrestrial manual (2008) 2.01.14_RVF_OIE.pdf chapter.2.1.14 Rift Valley fever

Olive MM, Goodman SM, Reynes JM (2012) The role of wild mammals in the maintenance of Rift Valley Fever Virus. J Wildl Dis 48(2):241–266

Pourrut X, Nikoghe D, Souris M, Paupy C, Paweska J et al (2010) Rift Valley fever virus seroprevalence in human rural population of Gabon. PLoS Negl Trop Dis 4(7):e763

Seufi AM, Galal FH (2010) Role of Culex and Anopheles mosquito species as potential vectors of Rift Valley fever virus in Sudan outbreak, 2007. BMC Infect Dis 10:65

Shoemaker T, Boulianne C, Vincent MJ, Pezzanite L, Al-Qahtani MM et al (2002) Genetic analysis of viruses associated with emergence of Rift Valley fever in Saudi Arabia and Yemen, 2000-01. Emerg Infect Dis 8(12):1415–1420

Tennant WSD, Cardinale E, Cêtre-Sossah C, Moutroifi Y et al (2021) Modelling the persistence and control of Rift Valley fever virus in a spatially heterogeneous landscape. Nat Commun 12(1):5593

Warimwe G, Gesharisha J, Carr B et al (2016) Chimpanzee Adenovirus Vaccine Provides Multispecies Protection against Rift Valley Fever. Sci Rep 6:20617

Woods CW, Karpati AM, Grein T, McCarthy N, Gaturuku P et al (2002) An outbreak of Rift Valley Fever in Northeastern Kenya, 1997-98. Emerg Infect Dis 8(2):138–144

Chapter 19
Japanese Encephalitis

Synonyms

Japanese B Encephaltis, Arbovirus B Encephalitis, Mosquito-Borne Encephalitis, Russian Autumnal Encephalitis, Brain Fever, Summer Encephalitis.

Japanese encephalitis is one of the neurological disorders characterized by rapid onset, high fever, meningitis and meningoencephalitis.

JE has worldwide distribution, especially in Asia, the Western Pacific countries and northern Australia. An estimated annual JE cases world over is 68,000 with mortality of 1000–15,000 in 24 countries.

Overt disease (encephalitis) appears much less than actual infections, 1 in 20 to 1000. Severe encephalitis ends fatally, 20–30%. Long-term residual neuropsychiatric sequelae appear in 30–50% cases. Only 20–50% of cases recover fully. JE is primarily a disease of children often ending in death. All age groups are susceptible. Adults in endemic countries have natural immunity after childhood infection.

JEV has been causing outbreaks in immunologically naive population in newer areas (emergence/re-emergence) in recent years. Twenty-four countries in the WHO South East Asia and Western Pacific regions have endemic JEV transmission, exposing more than three billion people to risks of infection (https://www.who.int/news-room/fact-sheets/ detail/japanese-encephalitis). Annual JE cases in the People's Republic of China, Korea, Japan, South East Asia, the Indian subcontinent and parts of Oceania account for most of the cases reported in the world. JE was first detected in India in 1955. Serologically positive cases admitted to CMC, Vellore originating from the North Arcot district of Tamil Nadu and the neighbouring districts of Andhra Pradesh were detected. The virus was isolated from mosquitoes and patients from the same area in 1958. Many states are affected since then.

© Springer Nature Singapore Pte Ltd. 2024
K. G. Narayan et al., *Handbook of Management of Zoonoses*,
https://doi.org/10.1007/978-981-99-9885-2_19

19.1   Aetiology

The Nakayama strain of JEV was isolated in 1935 from the brain of a fatal male patient of encephalitis and in 1938 from *Cx. tritaeniorhynchus* which breeds in paddy field. JEV is a single-stranded positive-sense RNA virus belonging to the genus *Flavivirus* of family *Togaviridae*. There are ~11,000 nucleotides, three structural and seven non-structural proteins. The virus replicates in the cytoplasm. The envelope gene E is the phylogenetic marker. There are five genotypes, GI–GV.

JEV seems to be genetically stable (Wang et al. 2009). Schuh et al. (2013) studied 487 viral sequences, sampled over 75 years and from 12 countries applying Bayesian phylogeographic, categorical data analysis and phylogeny-trait association techniques. The geographic distribution of JEV according to genotypes is tabulated (Table 19.1).

Table 19.1   Geographical distribution of 487 isolates according to genotypes (Schuh et al. 2013)

Genotype	Distribution	Sampled during (period)	Additional information
GI	Northern Australia[a], northern Cambodia, China, India, Japan, Korea, Laos, Malaysia, Taiwan, Thailand and Vietnam	1967–2013	
GII	Northern Australia[a], Indonesia, Korea, Malaysia, Papua New Guinea and southern Thailand	Sporadic, 1951–1999	
GIII	China, India, Indonesia, Japan, Korea, Malaysia, Myanmar, Nepal, Philippines, Sri Lanka, the former Soviet Union, Taiwan, Thailand and Vietnam	Annual epidemics, 1935–2013	GI displaced GIII in Thailand, South Korea, Malaysia, Vietnam. GIII maintained till the 1990s in China and Japan. G1 entered in Taiwan in 2008 and displaced completely in 2011[b]. GI and GIII co-circulating, GIII was dominant till 2007 in India[c,d]
GIV	Indonesia	Seven isolates only from mosquitoes, 1980–1981	
GV	Malaysia, China and South Korea	Only three isolates, 1952–2010	Re-emerged after 60 years, detected in Tibet in 2009, in South Korea in 2010

[a]JEV emerged in the Torres Strait in 1995. Its activity has been detected in almost all years since then and in Cape York on the Australian mainland in 1998 and 2004 (Paterson et al. 2011)
[b]Chen et al. (2011)
[c]Fulmali et al. (2011)
[d]Sarkar et al. (2012)

19.1.1   Genotype Distribution

Of the five genotypes, GI displaced GIII. GV has re-emerged after 60 years. GIII and recently emerged GIb are temperate genotypes. GIa and GII are tropical genotypes (maintained by mosquito-avian and mosquito-swine transmission). GV was isolated from a pool of *Cx. tritaeniorhynchus* collected from Tibet in 2009 and a pool of *Cx. bitaeniorhynchus* collected in South Korea in 2010. Possibly, GV was introduced into Tibet by infected migratory birds or wind-blown mosquitoes. According to Chen et al. (2011), the genotype GI was introduced in Taiwan in 2008. GIII was the dominant genotype without any ecological change—*Cx. tritaeniorhynchus* and swine maintaining and circulating the virus in Japan and China in the 1990s and in India till 2007. GI has replaced this in China and Japan and has entered India (Fulmali et al. 2011; Sarkar et al. 2012). GI and GIII are co-circulating in India.

19.2   Epidemiology

JEV is maintained by 'bird-mosquitoes' cycle with swine as the amplifying host. Human is a dead end. They have seldom high viraemia, enough to infect mosquitoes. Multiple factors affect JE epidemics. Climate and sociological factors, particularly agricultural practices, are important. Populations of natural reservoirs and vectors are determined by rainfall, temperature and relative humidity. Agricultural activities like intensive rice cultivation, switching over from wheat to paddy cultivation supplemented with canal or groundwater irrigation facilities in the absence of monsoon and animal (swine, ducks) farming support JE transmission. In areas where combined pig farming and paddy cultivation is operative, risk of Japanese encephalitis is enhanced. Other than pigs, aquatic birds (egrets, herons) and frogs are important risks for transmission of JEV to humans and horses especially in agricultural settings like paddy cultivation areas.

Flooding and local topography allowing water logging promote mosquito breeding. JE occurs commonly in peri-urban and rural settings where people reside near the reservoir/amplifying hosts. People at risk are generally agricultural workers.

Climate and environmental temperature influence the prevalence of genotypes of JEV. According to Schuh et al. (2013), GI and GIII viruses were collected mostly in temperate zones, while GII and GIV in tropical zones. In 2009–2010, GI and GIII were co-circulating in India as determined by analysis of isolates from CSF.

JE occurs in two patterns, epidemic and endemic. The endemic pattern occurs in the tropics and transmission occurs round the year. There are two seasonal patterns observed in India (Saxena and Dhole 2008). In temperate areas, such as northern regions of Asia (in north India), high incidences/huge epidemics occur during warm months and monsoon/rainy season—July to September. In tropical areas, such as southern tropical areas (in South India), JE is sporadic or endemic round the year and intensifies during the rainy season and pre-harvest period in rice-cultivating regions.

There are two types of epidemics in Karnataka in India, severe during April to July and mild during September to December. Murty et al. (2010) observed that southwest monsoon persisted between June and October, and agricultural practices were at the peak in Kurnool district of Andhra Pradesh. The temperature ranged between 22 °C and 34 °C and RH 42.7% and 69.6%. The density of vector *Culex* spp. increases when the temperature and humidity are 28°C and 50–55%, respectively. Higher prevalence of *Cx. gelidus* in urban than rural and just the opposite of *Cx. tritaeniorhynchus* was observed. Rainfall and temperature were correlated, whereas humidity was inversely correlated with per man hour density (PMH). The vectors adapted well to the prevailing temperature and humidity.

19.2.1   Maintenance of JEV in Nature

Inter-epidemic survival: JEV overwinters in the northern Asia, possibly in the hibernating mosquitoes, their eggs and progenies (vertical transmission) and cold-blooded vertebrates and/or bats. Supporting evidences are (1) isolation of JEV from overwintering *Culex* spp. in temperate Asia, (2) viral transmission by experimentally hibernating and progenies (vertical) of *Culex* spp., (3a) JEV antibodies in poikilothermic vertebrates, (3b) experimental infection of lizards that maintained the virus throughout winter and (3c) experimental transmission by infected mosquitoes (to uninfected lizards to mosquitoes to uninfected mice). JEV was isolated from several bat species in temperate Asia and also from China (Wang et al. 2009). Experimentally infected bats maintained viraemia during hibernation for over 100 days.

Maintenance and amplification: The birds like egrets, pond herons, cattle egrets and ducks act as both maintenance and amplifying hosts. They do not suffer from illness. Infection leads to detectable antibodies. Mosquito-birds transmission cycle maintains the virus in nature. Birds act as important sources of human infection especially in the absence of pigs. Migratory birds, particularly waterfowls, visit and stay during winter in and around large perennial lakes, ponds, swamp and rice fields. Migratory birds introduce and spread JEV (Fig. 19.1).

Pigs amplify the virus. The viraemia lasting for 3–4 days is high enough to infect the feeding mosquitoes. Their rural habitat, large body surface and sparse hair allow large number of mosquitoes to feed and become infectious. Pigs do not show symptoms, except sometimes abortion, but develop long-lasting antibodies. This makes them useful sentinels for human infection. Human cases began appearing 2–3 weeks after 50% of pigs are seropositive. Scientists of the Centre for Research in Medical Entomology, Madurai, Tamil Nadu, observed that goats were also sentinel animals (JAPANESE%20ENCEPHALITIS-ICMR document pdf).

Horse (may suffer with encephalitis), dogs and cattle are susceptible but experimental infection does not induce viraemia adequate enough for transmission.

JAPANESE ENCEPHALITIS

INTER-EPIDEMIC   MAINTENANCE, AMPLIFICATION OF JEV
                                              AND EPIDEMIC

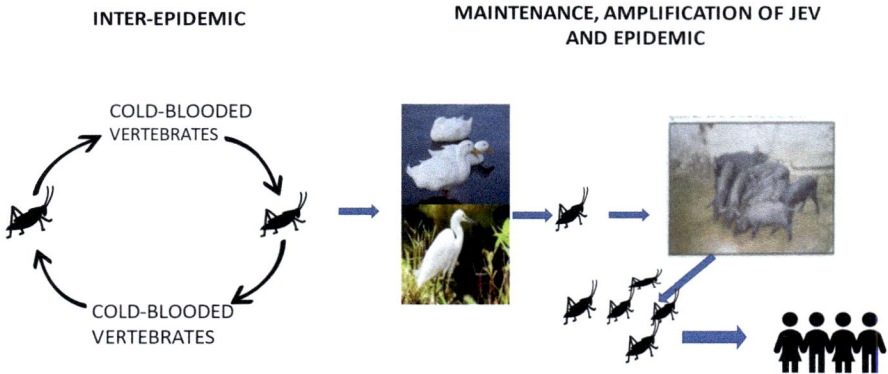

Fig. 19.1 Maintenance, amplification of Japanese Encephalitis Virus during epidemic and inter – epidemic period

The main vector is *Culex tritaeniorhynchus*. The extrinsic incubation period is about 2 weeks. Human infection follows 17–20 days after the peak isolation rate in mosquitoes. Mosquitoes develop resistance to insecticides. In India, 16 mosquito species of *Culex* (10), *Anopheles* (3) and *Mansonia* (3) are considered vectors. *Cx. tritaeniorhynchus*, *Cx. bitaeniorhynchus*, *Cx. vishnui*, *Cx. pseudovishnui*, *Cx. gelidus* and *Cx. quinquefasciatus* are the main vectors. *Cx. tritaeniorhynchus*, *Cx. bitaeniorhynchus*, *Cx. vishnui* and *Cx. pseudovishnui* transovarially transmit JEV to progenies. These breed in flood water, stagnant water, rice fields and marshes mostly in rural areas. The flight range of these mosquitoes is 5 km. These mosquitoes are outdoor, zoophilic. Only <2.0% female feed on humans, so high vector density is essential. Density is high in monsoon and post-monsoon and varies with season.

Other vectors may be *Cx. annulus*, *Cx. annulirostris* and *Aedes* mosquitoes.

19.3 Transmission

Infectious mosquito bite is the main mode of transmission. Transplacental transmission has been observed both in humans (Chaturvedi et al. 1980) and experimental mice leading to abortion. Boars transmit virus to progeny through infected semen to cause stillbirths.

19.4 Clinical Presentation

JE presents four different progressing stages. These are prodromal, acute and sub-acute lasting for periods in days 2–3, 3–4 and 7–10 and long period (4–7 weeks) of convalescence. The incubation period varies between 4 and 14 days. Motor abnormalities and unusual behavioural patterns appear during 2–3 days.

Illness begins with severe rigor and non-specific symptoms of fever (100–105°F), headache, lethargy, nausea or abdominal pain lasting for 1–6 days. Cerebral and meningeal manifestations—tremors, nuchal rigidity, confusion, disorientation and thick slurred speech –followed by choreoathetosis and other extra-pyramidal signs are evident in the second week of illness. Meningoencephalitis is the most important and serious ending fatally in most. Salient features include flat dull mask-like face, unblinking eyes, cogwheel rigidity and acute flaccid paralysis (more of legs) like in polio. Convulsion occurs more commonly in children than in adults. Most of the survivors (50–60%) suffer from long-term neurological sequelae—tremors, paralysis, ataxia, memory loss, deafness and impaired cognition. Convulsion and coma appear. Mortality is high in comatose patients. Kumar et al. (2008) described a case, a 4-year child who had fever and left hemiplegia and left facial weakness. The patient was conscious throughout the illness. Extra-pyramidal symptoms developed after the fifth day. CSF IgM ELISA titre was diagnostic.

JEV causes enhanced microglial activation, resulting in secretion of cytokines, neurotoxins, excitatory neurotransmitters and other soluble factors having toxic effects in the brain.

JEV strains vary in their neuro-virulence, e.g. strains from Malaysia and Indonesia are less neuro-virulent than those detected in Thailand (Schweitzer et al. 2009). Sarkar et al. (2012) identified 36/135 and 13/61 JE cases by Mac-ELISA and RT-PCR in West Bengal. ELISA negative <3-day febrile cases required RT-PCR for diagnosis. More cases are detected in paediatrics-adolescents than older people.

Age: Children 3–5 years are five to ten times more susceptible than adults >15 years; debilitated, chronically ill and immunosuppressed are more susceptible; the number of cases reduces with advancing age in endemic areas because of the natural immunity.

19.5 Diagnosis

Detection of changes under CT scan and electroencephalogram are suggestive; laboratory confirmation is required. The methods are the following:

- Genome detection—PCR. Dhanze et al. (2015) developed and compared three nucleic acid-based assays viz., reverse transcription-polymerase chain reaction (RT-PCR), reverse transcription-loop-mediated isothermal amplification (RT-LAMP) and real-time RT-PCR; all were 100% specific. The real-time RT-PCR reported here is the test of choice for reference laboratories, and the newly developed one-step RT-LAMP assay will be suitable for field-level testing.

- Virus isolation (from say brain suspension) by tissue culture—Primary cell cultures like chicken embryo, porcine or hamster kidney and cell lines Vero/MDBK/mosquito are further tested for viral genome or antigen.
- Infant (2–4 days old) mouse intra-cerebral inoculation.
- Mosquito inoculation.
- Antigen detection in serum or CSF by JEV-specific IgM, antigen capture ELISA [Mac ELISA kit—National Institute of Virology, Pune, India] and IFA.
- Serological tests—HA-HAI, IgM, IgG ELISA and neutralization.
- A fourfold increase in antibody titre is diagnostic. Paired (acute and convalescent) serum samples are examined. Check for the cross-reacting flaviviruses.

IgM antibodies are detectable 3–8 days after the onset of illness (serum collected within 10 days may not be positive) and persist for 30–90 days.

19.6 Treatment

There is no specific treatment. Supportive therapy and care help.

19.7 Prevention and Control

According to Verma (2012), there are three pillars of preventing and controlling JE. These are surveillance of JE cases, vector control and vaccine. Immunization strategy is based on regional experience. WHO recommends integrating in national vaccination schedules where JE is a public health issue. Sentinel pigs are used for JE surveillance to spot the site leads to targeted vector control. Confirmatory laboratory testing is often conducted in dedicated sentinel sites, and surveillance may be case-based and/or expanded to laboratory-based.

Available vaccines are (1) GIII virus based, SA14–14-2, (2) IXIARO, (3) JEEV (Biological E Limited/BEL) and (4) Chimeri Vax-JE (marketed as IMOJEV).

IXIARO is indicated for active immunization against Japanese encephalitis in adults, adolescents, children and infants aged 2 months and older. IXIARO should be considered for use in individuals at risk of exposure through travel or in the course of their occupation. IXIARO is an inactivated vaccine produced in Vero cells: two doses 0.5 mL each 28 days apart. Persons aged 18 to ≤65 years can be vaccinated in a rapid schedule.

The JE virus (SA-14-14-2) is a stable neuro-attenuated strain. It is licensed in the Peoples' Republic of China, India, South Korea and Nepal, presented as a lyophilized powder in five-dose vials. It is diluted in 2.5 mL; the dose is 0.5 mL (5.4 log

PFU of virus) administered subcutaneously for all ages. It is administered at ages 8 months and 2 years routinely.

International travellers health clinics in Asia—Vaccines for paediatric use in one or more of Asian countries are *inactivated mouse brain-derived* vaccine manufactured in South Korea, inactivated Vero cell culture-derived vaccines manufactured in Japan and India and live attenuated SA-14-14-2 vaccine manufactured in China.

Inactivated Vero cell culture-derived JE vaccine, JE-VC, JEEV.

JEEV is a one-time inactivated vaccine to be taken in two doses for both children and adults, licensed by the Drug Controller General of India. It is administered as 6 mcg/0.5 mL, two doses 28 days apart, travellers to get last dose 1 week before travel. For more information (including dosage for children), refer to vaccineinfo. us@novartis.com.

19.8   Reduction of JE Burden

India and the People's Republic of China account for about 95% of JE cases worldwide. A comprehensive plan should include the following:

– Hospital—and case-based surveillance for acute encephalitis syndrome (AES) supplemented with laboratory confirmation because encephalitis is a multi-aetiology disease, in dedicated sentinel sites. Early diagnosis of JE cases and management is important to save life.
– Population surveillance includes sero-conversion in (a) sentinel pigs/ducks/wild birds and (b) human (useful for estimation of prevalence and targeted vaccination) and (c) virus isolation and genotyping from mosquitoes and humans.
– Vaccination against JE in high-risk areas and incorporation into routine immunization for children should control outbreak and also further recurrence.
– Mosquito vector control, improvement in the living environment to protect against mosquito bites and health education are important, especially during a JE outbreak. Elimination of adult mosquito population by ultralow-volume fogging of malathion or fenitrothion and for the resistant mosquito population, synthetic pyrethroids like deltamethrin, 0.025%; permethrin, 0.25%; and lambda-cyhalothrin, 0.1%.
– Controlling viral amplification: by moving large-scale pig/duck farms away from rice paddies, (b) shifting from near human habitation, (c) vaccination and (d) increasing cattle to pig ratio.
– Education of pig/duck farmers and people.

Complete surveillance and JE immunization reduced cases to <30 annually after controlling epidemic—Japan, South Korea and Taiwan. Risk areas like Australia, Siberia and Singapore have reported less than three cases annually. One-time immunization and continued surveillance should maintain status quo (Wang and Liang 2015).

References

Chaturvedi UC, Mathur A, Chandra A, Das SK et al (1980) Transplacental infection with Japanese encephalitis virus. J Infect Dis 141:712–715

Chen Y-Y, Fan Y-C, Tu W-C, Chang R-Y et al (2011) Japanese encephalitis virus genotype replacement, Taiwan, 2009–2010. Emerg Infect Dis 17(12):2354–2356

Dhanze H, Bhilegaonkar KN, Ravi Kumar GVPPS, Thomas P et al (2015) Comparative evaluation of nucleic acid-based assays for detection of Japanese encephalitis virus in swine blood samples. Arch Virol 160:1259–1266

Fulmali PV, Sapkal GN, Athawale S, Gore MM et al (2011) Introduction of Japanese encephalitis virus genotype I. India Emerg Infect Dis 17(2):319–321

Kumar A, Shrivastava AK, Singh DK, Shukla S (2008) Case Report Hemiplegia with dysarthria: an initial manifestation of Japanese encephalitis in a 4-year old child. J Vector Borne Dis 45:328–330

Murty US, Rao MS, Arunachalam N (2010) The effects of climatic factors on the distribution and abundance of Japanese encephalitis vectors in Kurnool district of Andhra Pradesh. India J Vector Borne Dis 47:26–32

Paterson BJ, Mackenzie JS, Durrheim DN, Smith D (2011) A review of the epidemiology and surveillance of viral zoonotic encephalitis and the impact on human health in Australia. NSW Public Health Bulletin 22(5–6):99–104

Sarkar A, Taraphdar D, Mukhopadhyay SK, Chakrabarti S, Chatterjee S (2012) Molecular evidence for the occurrence of Japanese encephalitis virus genotype I and III infection associated with acute Encephalitis in Patients of West Bengal, India, 2010. Virology J 9:271–276

Saxena V, Dhole T (2008) Preventive strategies for frequent outbreaks of Japanese encephalitis in Northern India. J Biosci 33(4):505–514

Schuh AJ, Ward MJ, Leigh Brown AJ, Barrett ADT (2013) Phylogeography of Japanese Encephalitis Virus: Genotype Is Associated with Climate. PLoS Negl Trop Dis 7(8):e2411

Schweitzer BK, Chapman NM, Iwen PC (2009) Overview of the Flaviviridae with an emphasis on the Japanese Encephalitis Group Viruses. Labmedicine 40(8):493–499

Verma R (2012) Japanese encephalitis vaccine: need of the hour in endemic states of India. Hum Vaccin Immunother 8(4):491–493

Wang H, Liang G (2015) Epidemiology of Japanese encephalitis: past, present and future prospects. Ther Clin Risk Manag 11:435–448

Wang JL, Pan XL, Zhang Hl FSH, Wang HY et al (2009) Japanese Encephalitis Viruses from Bats in Yunnan, China. Emerg Infect Dis 15(6):939–942

Chapter 20
West Nile Virus Encephalitis

West Nile virus encephalitis is a very widely distributed mosquito-borne zoonosis. The West Nile virus (WNV) infects a very wide range of hosts. In 1937, a virus was isolated from a woman in the West Nile district of Uganda and was named after the place as West Nile virus. In 1953, it was isolated from birds, crows and Columbiformes in Nile Delta and was not considered a pathogen. In 1997, its virulent strain caused encephalitis, paralysis and deaths in birds in Israel. Circulating in Israel and Tunisia, it was imported in New York in 1999 causing epidemic. WNV caused largest outbreaks in Israel, Greece, Romania, Russia and the United States. Whole of Africa, parts of Europe, the Middle East, West Asia and Australia happened to be the original regions of WNV activity, and the disease is now endemic from Canada to Venezuela.

Importation of a vector-borne infection and establishment in a new location are exemplified by WNV. The NY99 strain was 99.8% homologous with the isolates from Israel, one from the brain of a goose (1998) and another from a human case (1999), and similarly related with strains from Romania, proving its remarkable adaptability. It spread from a small area in New York City in 1999 to across much of the Western Hemisphere from Central Canada to southern Argentina and is endemic in 48 of the continental US (Nasci 2013).

The recorded disease burden is high, 36,000 cases including 16,000 neuroinvasive and 1500 deaths in the United States. An estimated two to four million have been infected and 400,000 to one million had illness since 1999 (Petersen et al. 2013).

© Springer Nature Singapore Pte Ltd. 2024

K. G. Narayan et al., *Handbook of Management of Zoonoses*,

https://doi.org/10.1007/978-981-99-9885-2_20

20.1   Aetiology

WNV is a mosquito-borne flavivirus, belonging to the family *Flaviviridae* and the Japanese encephalitis virus serocomplex. It has been associated with morbidities and mortalities in birds, horses, sheep, reptiles, cats, rodents, crocodiles and alligators.

WNV is spherical. The capsid contains single-stranded RNA that encodes capsid (C), envelope (E), premembrane proteins (prM) and seven non-structural proteins possibly contributing to viral replication. West Nile viruses have been grouped into nine lineages. Lineages 1 and 2 are the most virulent and caused severe neuroinvasive diseases worldwide. Lineage 2 is less virulent. Isolates from sub-Saharan Africa, Madagascar and Europe belong to lineage 2 and have caused outbreaks in humans, horses and birds. Lineage 1 has wide distribution and has been isolated in Africa, the Middle East, Europe, Asia, India, Australia and North America. WNV lineage 1 has three sub-lineages. The isolates from Africa, Europe and the Middle East belong to sub-lineage 1a. The Australasian virus WNVKUN belonged to 1b sub-lineage. The Indian isolates of WNV belong to the sub-linage 1c, also known as lineage 5 (Habarugira et al. 2020). Isolates from both the lineages cause neuroinvasive diseases in humans and animals.

The capsid (C), envelope (E) and structural protein NS1 apparently play significant roles in the invasion of hosts' cell. The C protein shelters viral RNA, induces cytotoxic effect and activates cell apoptosis pathway leading to death. The envelope (E) protein plays a critical role in the virus entry to the host cell, is highly immunogenic, induces virus-neutralizing antibody that inhibits virion cell attachment, endocytosis or membrane fusion. The NS1 protein is critical to WNV replication, through evading hosts' immune system. It is a useful serological marker for differentiating vaccinated from infected.

20.2   Epidemiology

20.2.1   Geographic Distribution

According to Hayes et al. (2005a), geographic distribution of WNV is wide—Europe, the Middle East, India, parts of Asia and Australia (Kunjin virus) and in the Eastern Hemisphere in the Mediterranean Basin: (1) pre-1999 in Algeria, Morocco and the Czech Republic; (2) pre—and post-1999 in Tunisia, Romania, Israel and Russia; and (3) post-1999 in France. Enzootics involving horses were reported in Morocco in 1996 and 2003, Italy in 1998, Israel in 2000 and southern France in 2000, 2003 and 2004. In the Western Hemisphere, most diseases occurred in the United States.

In the summer of 1999, it was first detected in New York. In the United States, it spread from the Atlantic to the Pacific coast. It has been reported from Canada, Mexico, some parts of the Caribbean Basin, Central America and northern Columbia. The geographical area of infection is expanding (Cabre et al. 2006; Pupo et al. 2006; Morales et al. 2006).

Acute encephalitis syndrome (AES) was reported in May 2011 in Kerala, India. CSF from 208 patients from sentinel hospitals tested positive by IgM capture ELISA and RT-PCR. Cases were reported before and during early monsoon in JEV-non-endemic areas. Most were > 15 years. WNV neutralization was positive for 76.19% (32/42) cases. Virus isolated from clinical cases had 99% homology with Russian lineage 1 WNV.

Dehghani et al. (2020) have reviewed the epidemiology of WNF in Iran and neighbouring countries. Beginning the 1970s, WNV is prevalent in over 26/31 provinces in Iran in humans, horses and birds. The infection rate ranged from 10% to 26%. During 2004–2007, studies on 26 aquatic bird species revealed a seropositivity rate of 15%. In 2012, WNV was detected in *Ochlerotatus* (*Aedes*) *caspius* indicating its role in local transmission. During 2015 and 2016, mosquitoes of 25 species from five provinces were studied. *Cx. pipiens* biotype *pipiens* from Sepid site of Guilan province was found positive. 1.3% humans and 2.8% horses in the northern and central provinces were found seropositive in 2010–2011 and 67.4% of horses' serum from Albroz and Tehran in 2011 and 2012.

According to the European Centre for Disease Prevention and Control data (2018), seroprevalence of WNV was as follows: Iran, 0–30%; Iraq, 11.6–15.1%; Egypt, 1–61%; Djibouti, 0.3–60%; Jordan, 8%; Lebanon, 0.5–1.0%; Libya, 2.3%; Morocco, 0–18.8%; Pakistan, 0.6–65%; Sudan, 2.2–47%; and Tunisia, 5.3–15.9%.

Among animals tested, horses (100%) and dogs (96%) were found seropositive in Morocco. Tunisia had the highest seropositive birds (23%). WNV was found prevalent in domestic animals including dogs in Morocco, Pakistan, Israel and Iraq. Seroconversion in dogs occurred 6 weeks before the emergence of human cases, suggesting sentinel potential.

In Europe, WNV infection is nonrecurrent and sporadic. According to Martinet et al. (2019), *Culex* mosquitoes are the principal vectors of WNV in Europe. *Cx. modestus* was introduced in metropolitan France in 1962. No human case was reported for 40 years. Low seropositivity was found in humans and equines in the 1970s. WNV resurgence in humans and horses occurred in 2000 followed by only sporadic seropositivity for 15 years. Epidemic occurred in 2015 in southern France, and 3 years later in Germany. *Cx. pipiens* biotype *pipiens*, *Cx. pipiens* biotype *modestus* and *Cx. torrentium* are competent vectors in Europe for WNV lineages 1 and 2. Recently, *An. plumbeus* has been found switching from natural breeding sites to man-made sites and is considered a potential vector for WNV.

The Ebro Delta is a wetland in Catalonia, northeast of Spain, where human infection was reported (Bofill et al. 2006). Seropositive migratory birds stop over while migrating between regions of Africa and Europe. Different vectors and reservoirs of WNV have been identified in this area. García-Bocanegra et al. (2011) described WNV infection in both horses and humans in Spain. The first case was reported on

10 September 2010; the number of cases peaked at 17 in mid-September, and then tapered and the last case was recorded on 15 December. It seems that the virus over-wintered and re-emerged during summer in the western Mediterranean and circu-lated silently or was introduced putatively from Africa. *Culex pipiens* population increased during June and September. Environmental conditions in general are favourable for establishment and seasonal circulation. WNV lineage 2 has been spreading further west in the Mediterranean region. It caused sporadic cases in birds in Spain and outbreak between July and September 2020 in southern provinces affecting humans and horses. WNV lineage 1 strain has been detected both in humans and animals. The event-based surveillance and weekly reporting of West Nile virus (WNV) infections in Europe (Bakonyi and Haussig 2020) recorded out-breaks in Spain and the Netherlands in 2020. The 2018 outbreak that spread to over 11 countries recorded 1548 cases of locally acquired mosquito-borne infections. WNV cases exceeded the cumulative number of all reported infections between 2010 and 2017 and also the highest number of newly affected areas ($n = 45$). Greece continued to report high number of infections. The 2019 recorded a drop by 73% but the total number was still high. The distribution of cases in 2020 seemed to be unchanged suggesting overwintering and local circulation of the virus. This is sup-ported by genetic data also. Once established, the likelihood of maintenance and the risk of re-emergence of WNV infections in the affected areas are high.

In the United States, the 2012 outbreak reported the highest number of cases since 2003. It spread to over 48 states. The outbreak remained restricted spatially and focally. Almost 75% cases occurred in ten states. Texas had the maximum and over 50% in its four counties. There were 5245 cases including 236 deaths as of 27 November 2012 and 51% were neuroinvasive (Nasci 2013). The following year (2013), WNV was again the leading viral infection with 2469 cases. Illness began during July and peaked in September. The median age was 55 years and 58% were male. Sixty-one per cent were hospitalized, 5% died and 51% were neuroinvasive of which most had encephalitis (53%), meningitis (38%) and flaccid paralysis (9%) (Lindsey et al. 2014). In the United States, WNV virus accounted for 94% of cases caused by arboviruses in 2018 and continues to be the leading cause. Compared to the median incidence of WNV neuroinvasive disease during 2008–2017, there was an increase by 25% in the year 2018. Two cases of WNV occurred through solid organ transplant from a common donor. Transmission through organ transplant was repeated after 2013. Median age of cases was 59 years and 62% were males. Of the neuroinvasive cases, 55% were encephalitis, 33% meningitis and 4% acute flaccid paralysis. The peak season has been consistently from April to September when arboviral diseases occurred. Factors influencing the outbreak included weather, vec-tor abundance, zoonotic host and human behaviour (McDonald et al. 2019). As of 5 January 2021, there were 557 diseased cases in the United States. WNV infections in people, birds and mosquitoes were reported in 44 states (https://www.cdc.gov/westnile/statsmaps/preliminarymapsdata2020/activitybystate 2020.html).

Epidemics of WNV fever in humans have occurred nearly every 10 years since the 1950s in many African, Middle Eastern and some Mediterranean countries. WNV infection persists, as observed in experimental hamsters and monkeys.

Persistence of infection in sparrows for 12–18 weeks occurs. WNV has been detected in urine samples of human months to a maximum of 6 years post-infection (Habarugira et al. 2020). Recovered will not be reinfected because of lifelong immunity.

20.2.2   West Nile Virus Infection in Commercial Flocks

An outbreak of WNV infection in commercial flocks of exotic and domestic ducks and geese in Wisconsin was confirmed with RT-PCR. Kidney, spleen and oral and cloacal swabs were tested and 84.1% of 88 dead birds were positive (Meece et al. 2006). Death occurred within a day of onset of signs. Fourteen of 30 asymptomatic and recovered birds randomly sampled and tested had neutralizing antibodies. WNV causes economic loss and is a potential occupational hazard. No human case occurred but earlier workers of a turkey breeding farm had reported suffering from clinical infection. Non-vector routes of transmission of WNV in this setting were suspected because of (1) cluster of deaths in small number of housing pens (each pen housed <200 birds) in late July and early August, (2) high seroconversion rate among asymptomatic and recovered birds, (3) behavioural traits like pecking of sick birds by others who also cannibalize, (4) congregation on ponds at night, (5) virus shedding in common water source, (6) high virus concentration in feather pulp and (7) susceptibility of these birds as they were young.

20.2.3   Infection Cycle

West Nile virus (WNV) is a zoonotic pathogen. 'Virus and ecology and transmission' on the one hand and 'virus and immune response and pathology' on the other hand should be understood. WNV infects cells of vertebrate hosts by cell receptor-mediated endocytosis. Optimal fusion of viral membrane with cell endosomes/liposomes occurs at pH 6.3–6.9, and nucleocapsid and viral RNA are released into host cell cytoplasm to initiate replication. Viral components are acquired during exocytosis and release from cell. Virus spreads throughout the hosts' body.

   Wild birds-mosquitoes-wild birds cycle maintains the virus in nature. *Cx. pipiens* and *Cx. restuans* are the primary vectors in prairie ecosystems. WNV is maintained in mosquito populations through vertical transmission (adults to eggs). The natural reservoirs are birds (Fig. 20.1). Different species of birds may have different potential for maintaining the transmission cycle. WNV is highly pathogenic for birds in the Americas but rarely so for birds in Africa, Europe, the Middle East and Asia. Members of the family Corvidae in particular are highly susceptible. The virus has, however, been isolated from some 250 species of dead or dying birds. Instances of disease in commercial flocks of domestic or exotic birds have been reported

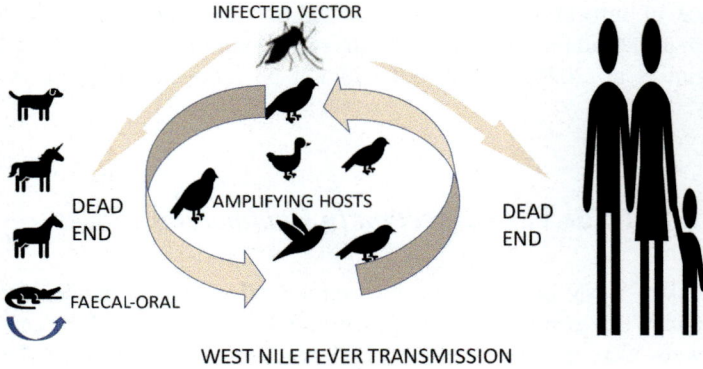

Fig. 20.1 West Nile Virus transmission

sometimes. In North America, WNV has been associated with death in >198 species of birds, including >33 species of raptors (Komar 2003).

In the absence of the preferred 'bird host', the ornithophilic mosquitoes seek mammals for meal to cause epidemic in humans. This happens during late summer and fall.

Birds can be infected by a variety of routes other than mosquito bites, most likely oral-cloacal route observed in experimental geese. Infection of horses, just like humans, is a 'dead end' for the virus. Infection in horses is asymptomatic, mild and neuroinvasive including fatal encephalomyelitis.

20.2.3.1   Vectors

The abundance of competent and infected mosquitoes (prevalence) determines the intensity of transmission. The prevalence of WNV infection in mosquitoes is measured by the minimum infection rate (MIR) needed to produce epidemic.

WNV enters the vector mosquito during blood meal, reaches the midgut, replicates there and in other tissues, spreads via haemolymph to the salivary gland and aggregates before the subsequent blood meal on final or incidental hosts. The infective dose is $>10^4 TCID_{50}$/mL of saliva. The infection in final hosts is dead end except crocodilian hosts. Mosquito probes blood vessels with the help of saliva before sucking blood meal. Saliva has anticoagulant and a protein that interferes host's T-cell response, thus evading host's cell-mediated immune response facilitating virus spread.

Mosquitoes are reservoir, intermediate host and amplifying host.

Ornithophilic mosquitoes, particularly *Culex* spp., are the main vectors in Africa, Europe and Asia. WNV has been detected in about 150 mosquito species, and their competency varies. The key vector species in the United States are *Cx. pipiens*, *Cx. tarsalis* and *Cx. Quinquefasciatus* (Table 20.1).

Table 20.1   Species of mosquitoes important in epizootic/epidemic (Hayes et al. 2005a; Dehghani et al. 2020; Habarugira et al. 2020)

Species of mosquito	Countries	Remarks
Cx. vishnui, *Cx. Vishnuicomplex,* *Cx. fatigans,* *Cx. tritaeniorhynchus,* *Cx.bitaeniorhynchus,* *Cx. univittatus, and* *Cx. Pipiensfatigans,* *Ae. albopictus*	Asia, mainly India and Pakistan	*Ae. albopictus is a potential competent vector*
Cx. modestus and Cx. pipiens, Cx. molestus, *Ochlerotatus caspius,* *Cx. torrentium,* *Anopheles maculipennis,* *Coquillettidia richiardii,* *Cx. pipiens, Cx.* *antennatus, Cx.* *univittatus*	Europe	Listed are main vectors. *Cx. modestus* involved in transmission to human*; Cx. Pipiens* amplifying among birds and transmission to humans in urban areas. Both are involved in sylvan and urban transmission cycles
Culex pipiens pipiens L.	Djibouti, Egypt, Iran and Tunisia	
Cx. pipiens, Cx. *perexiguus, Ae. caspius*	The Middle East countries, including Israel, Turkey, Jordan, Iran and Lebanon	Associated with WNV transmission
Cx. tritaeniohynchus, *Cx. theileri,* *Aedes caspius*	Iraq	*March to December have various larval habitats, annual spring floods in Tigris and Euphrates*
Cx. antennatus, *Cx. univittatus, Cx.* *theileri, Cx. neavei, Ae. caballus, Ae.* *circumluteolus,* *Coquillettidia spp.,* *Cx. poicilipes,* *Ae. albocephalus,* *Cx. quinquefaciatus,* *Mansonia spp.*	South Africa, Egypt, Senegal and Sudan	These play significant roles
Cx. pipiens, *Cx.tarsalis,* *Cx. quinquefasciatus,* *Cx. restuans,* *Cx. salinarius,* *Cx. nigripalpus*	United States	*Cx. Pipiens* is the most common and moderately efficient transmitter in eastern states in birds and mammals. *Cx. Quinquefasciatus* is common in the south, moderate to low efficient. *Cx. Tarsalis* lab-evaluated is the most efficient in western states. *Culex quinquefasciatus* and *Culex nigripalpus* are important in the South-Eastern United States

(continued)

Table 20.1 (continued)

Species of mosquito	Countries	Remarks
Cx. nigripalpus, *Cx. interrogator*	Mexico and other parts of Latin America	
Cx. univittatus. Cx. pipiens, Cx. tritaeniorhynchus, Cx. antennatus	Africa	Abundant and competent vectors for transmission to human
Cx. Annulirostris *Less competent vectors—* *Ae. nomenensis,* *Ae. tremulus, Ae. vigilax,* *Cx. australicus,* *Cx. squamosus,* *Anopheles amictus,* and *Cx. quinquefasciatus*	Australia	Is a freshwater mosquito, competent vector

Table 20.2 Mosquito spp. and minimum infective rate (MIR)

Mosquito species	MIR (%)	Epizootic/epidemic area
All *Culex* sp.	0.3 (0.07—5.7)	New York, 1999
Cx. pipiens/restuans mix	0.5-1.6	Staten Island, 2000
Cx. salinarius	0.3—1.2	Staten Island
Cx. restuans	0.2	Connecticut, 2000, intense epizootic, apparently low risk to humans
Cx. salinarius	0.1	Same
Cx. pipiens	0.1	Same
cx. quinfasciatus	0.5	Florida, 2001
Cx. nigripalpus	1.1	Florida, 2001

A total of 31,215 mosquitoes representing 25 species collected between 3 and 15 August from the patients' residences in south-eastern Louisiana using gravid traps and CO_2 baited light traps were examined for WNV. Infected mosquitoes were found in 5/11 confirmed sites and from 1/3 non-WNV confirmed site.

Vertical transmission of WNV has been experimentally demonstrated in *Cx. pipiens, Cx. quinquefasciatus* and *Cx. tarsalis*. In hibernating female mosquito, WNV has been detected. The persistence of the virus in colder latitudes through the winter and re-emergence of transmission in the spring are thus explained.

Minimum infection rates/1000 mosquitoes (MIR) ranged between 0.8 and 10.9 (Table 20.2). WNV was detected from nine pools of mosquito that included *Culex quinquefasciatus* (seven), *Cx. salinarius* and *Coquillettidia perturbans*—the first was considered to play a primary role and others a secondary role in the epizootic/ epidemic (Godsey Jr et al. 2005). MIR needed to produce epidemic is uncertain.

Minimum infective rate (MIR) observed in United States since 1999 in some outbreak was 15% (Hayes et al. 2005a).

The level of viraemia and transmission: Viraemic level of 107.1 PFU/mL infected 74–100% of *Cx. tarsalis* and with a lesser level 104.9 PFU/mL, 0–36% was infected. Maximum WNV concentration observed in blood of a donor was 103.2 PFU/mL. Hayes et al. (2005a) consider that humans have viraemic levels that may be insufficient to infect mosquito.

Other arthropods: Both hard and soft ticks can be infected. These may not be playing any significant role but have the potential to transmit WNV (Lawrie et al. 2004). These are (a) hard ticks, *Hyalomma marginatum*, *Rhipicephalus sanguineus* and *R. turanicus*; (b) soft ticks, *Ornithodoros maritimus* and *Argas reflexus hermanni*; (c) chicken mite, *Ornithonyssus sylviarum*, *Dermanyssus gallinae* and *Dermanyssus marginatus* (in Caucasus); and (d) swallow bugs, *Oeciacus hirundinis*.

20.2.3.2 Hosts

Reptiles may amplify the virus and transmit to other hosts in nature. Studies on WNV infection in crocodile have been made in Mexico, Israel and America. Prevalence of 41% in the healthy wild crocodile, 30% in captive Morelet's crocodile (*C. moreletii*) and 86% in farmed crocodile was reported from Mexico. In Israel, 70% of *C. niloticus* were found positive. Experimentally infected snakes developed viraemia of 10^5 PFU/mL enough to infect the mosquito vector and remained viraemic for 11 days and therefore may be playing a significant role in epidemiology. Seasonal sampling of six wild snakes showed a prevalence of 1.62% and more important viral RNA in oral swab samples, suggesting potential role in transmission to other hosts.

Most mammals do not develop enough viraemia to infect mosquitoes. Other animals—rats, wild ruminants, monkeys, Barbary ape and horses—are also infected with WNV. Infection of horses result in 10–20% clinical disease with 28 to 45% mortality.

Fox squirrel (Sciurus niger) appears to maintain WNV and spread to the final host. Seroprevalence in raccoons (*Procyon lotor*) has been found.

Birds are reservoirs, amplifying hosts and sources of transmission to dead-end hosts. WNV has been detected in >190 bird species, including neotropical migratory species and exotic zoo specimens, e.g. domestic geese (*Anser anser domesticus*), domestic Impeyan pheasants, Gruidae (cranes), Pelecanidae (pelicans), cormorants (*Phalacrocorax* spp.), American crows (*Corvus brachyrhynchos*), etc.

Observation of epizootic/epidemic revealed that common grackles (*Quiscalus quiscula*), various corvids (crows, jays, magpies), house finches (*Carpodacus mexicanus*) and house sparrows (*Passer domesticus*) were highly infectious to mosquitoes and had mortality rates of >40%. Allison et al. (2004) observed the level of viraemia in rock pigeons. Rock pigeons were abundant and common in all cities in the United States. House sparrows are also abundant and frequently infected with WNV. These may act as amplifying hosts in the urban setting.

Experimental studies showed that Passeriformes (song birds), Charadriiformes (shore birds), Strigiformes (owls) and Falconiformes (hawks) had viraemia sufficient to infect mosquitoes for transmission. Columbiformes (pigeons), Piciformes (woodpeckers) and Anseriformes (ducks) did not have viraemia sufficient to infect mosquitoes.

American alligators, saltwater crocodiles and lake frog (*Rana ridibunda*) amplify WNV sufficiently high titre in their blood to potentially infect mosquitoes for transmission. Alligator handler got infected (Klenk et al. 2004).

As stated above, mosquitoes are reservoirs, intermediate hosts and amplifying hosts.

20.2.4   *Extrinsic Factors*

A number of *complex interrelated factors* appear to modulate epidemic. Hosts' immunity and environmental temperature play an important role. A low level of population immunity (<5%) may not modulate epidemic (Hayes et al. 2005a).

American crows are very susceptible and often die before seroconversion can be detected. But crows in the Red River Valley survived WNV infection during 2002–2005. This was attributed to the environmental temperature and hosts' immunity by Bell et al. (2006). The viral activity was low during 2002 even with favourable conditions such as warm temperature and high vector activity, possibly because of (a) recent introduction of WNV, (2) insufficient number of infection nidi and (3) insufficient time to promote extensive amplification of the virus. In the year 2003, there were increased MIR and human cases—thus an epidemic—further contributed by the susceptible passerines. The environmental temperature in the year 2004 was low and led to the prolonged vector larval development, adult emergence and the arboviral extrinsic incubation period. The duration of the transmission season was observed to be nearly half that in the preceding seasons. WNV activity was thus low (similar to the one observed in 2002) as inferred from reduced vector abundance, number of human cases and seasonal MIR. In the year 2005, the passerine population presented a high level of immunity as a result of the epidemic in the year 2003. This prevented a repeat of the epidemic of 2003, even when the environmental temperature, length of transmission season and vector abundance were similar to those prevailed in the epidemic year. WNV activity however was not eliminated from the central Red River Valley.

Spread of WNV is determined by movements of human beings, nonmigratory birds and long-range travel of migratory birds, and availability of suitable vectors would determine the spread of WNV. A flock of white storks migrating southwards along their route of migration in Europe were forced landed in Israel because of hot strong westerly winds. Most were < 1-year-old fledglings. Thirteen dead and 11 live birds were examined. WNV was isolated from brains of dead and serum-neutralizing antibodies from the live birds strongly suggesting that migrating birds spread WNV

(Malkinson et al. 2002). Birds have been implicated in spreading WNV during migratory events in Europe, Asia, Africa and the Middle East.

Season and environmental temperature influence the ecology, vectors and enzootic foci. Abundance, feeding pattern of infected mosquitoes and local ecology determine the transmission. The incidence of WNV disease is seasonal in the temperate zones of North America, Europe and the Mediterranean Basin, with peak activity from July to October. Human illness has also been observed in late December 2003 and in April 2004 (Hayes et al. 2005a). Transmission of WNV in southern Africa and of Kunjin virus in Australia increases in the early months of the year after heavy spring and summer rainfall. In June 2002, WNV cases appeared in south-eastern Louisiana. The peak reached in July and then declined rapidly (Godsey Jr et al. 2005). Surveillance in winter of 2003–2004 suggested that WNV was active round the year in the Gulf Coast region, Texas and Louisiana (Tesh et al. 2004).

Environmental requirements for maintenance of enzootic focus are high temperature, dense avian population and *Culex* sp. mosquitoes. Tropics ensure this condition. Geographic connectivity in populations of migratory birds between winter and summer may provide a continuum of transmission. Epidemiologist needs to know the sites where the migratory birds spend winter and summer and the routes of transit in order to identify the routes of transmission. Capture, mark, release and recapture of birds interspersed with sampling for laboratory testing is the method available. This approach suggested that birds from the north-eastern United States tended to winter in the south-eastern United States and Greater Antilles (e.g. Puerto Rico, Jamaica), whereas birds from the western United States migrate to Mexico and Central America. In response to the potential introduction of WNV in tropical America during the fall migrations, Dupuis et al. (2003) established a network of monitoring sites on the overwintering grounds of neotropical migratory birds in Jamaica, Puerto Rico and Mexico. Plaque reduction neutralization test results indicated specific neutralizing antibodies to West Nile virus in 11 resident species from Jamaica out of >1600 specimens from resident and non-resident neotropical migratory birds in spring of 2002.

20.3   Transmission

- Infected mosquito bite.
- Contact with infected animals and their blood, tissues, excretions and secretion (veterinarians, para-veterinarians, laboratory workers).
- Breast milk.
- Transplacental.
- Blood transfusion, haemodialysis and needlesticks.
- Organ transplant—solid organ transplant from sero-negative donor.
- Oral-faecal route in alligators and saltwater crocodiles via contaminated water.
- Airborne among animal handlers and laboratory workers (hypothesized).

No human-to-human transmission has been reported. Occupationally, infection is acquired through percutaneous, aerosol and conjunctival routes while the animal control officer collected sick and dead corvids without personal protectives (Fonseca et al. 2005). Laboratory-acquired infection through percutaneous injuries involving blue jay and mouse has occurred.

20.4   Pathology and Pathogenicity

20.4.1   Pathology

WNV appears to cause apoptotic or necrotic cell death in parenchymal cells of the brain, heart and pancreas in birds and mammals. The lesions show demyelination, gliosis, loss of neurons, endoneural mononuclear inflammation of cranial nerves and spinal nerves, granulocytic meningitis, lymphoplasmacytic-histiocyte perivascular cuffing and lymphoplasmacytic meningoencephalomyelitis in humans, equines, alligators and birds. The spinal cord in flaccid paralysis patients is inflamed and shows perivascular lymphocytic infiltration, microglial nodules and loss of anterior horn cells.

Attempts to explain observed pathology have been made by relating and connecting the observation and outcome of experiments (Hayes et al. 2005a; Habarugira et al. 2020).

20.4.2   Pathogenesis

During the incubation period of 2–14 days, virus replication and immune modulation occur. There is an expression of DC-SIGN (also called CD219) by dendritic cells which are considered as early target cells. WNV replicates in keratinocytes and cells of Langerhans (dendritic cells) of the epidermis at the site of inoculation. Mosquito saliva modulates hosts' immune response favouring enhanced viral replication in cells of Langerhans which migrate to draining lymph nodes where replication continues. Virus enters blood stream and spread haematogenously to other organs. Macrophages pick up infected cells and free virus particles in an effort to clear the infection. Virus replication continues in dendritic cells in lymph nodes. Replication in B—and T-lymphocytes observed in vitro suggest these are also targeted by the virus. The virus has a wide range of tissue tropism.

A cascade of proinflammatory cytokines and protein genes are upgraded following infection resulting in the release of chemicals to initiate and maintain inflammation to control infection, including WNV. Continued upregulation and overexpression enhance severity of inflammation/infection and cause death, morbidity and chronic or permanent immunopathology.

Three clinical forms of WNV are neuroinvasive, skin and gastrointestinal. Multiple factors determine the form and severity, e.g. virus lineage, strain, tissue tropism coinfection, host species, intrinsic and extrinsic susceptibility such as the environment and resistance.

20.4.3 Neuroinvasive

Neurons in the deep nuclei and grey matter of the brain, brainstem and spinal cord are infected. Bystander nerve cells are also destroyed. The possible routes and mechanism of crossing the blood-brain barrier (BBB) by WNV could be (a) haematogenous; (b) passive migration, due to increased vascular permeability; (c) 'Trojan horse' or infected macrophages invading the brain parenchyma; and (d) transneuronal, WNV to the spinal cord to the brain or vice versa via motor neuron, olfactory nerve, astrocyte, microglia, motor neuron and transmigrating macrophage.

Most considered routes of invasion are haematogenous and transneuronal.

WNV antigen has been detected in enterocytes of the proventriculus and duodenum of goshawks. *Alligator mississippiensis* fed with infected mice displayed clinical and pathological picture of gastrointestinal infection and 84% cloacal samples were positive for WNV. The oesophagus showed ulcerative-proliferative changes and the liver and pancreas showed necrotizing inflammation, and there was haemorrhagic and proliferative enteritis and necrotizing colitis.

20.5 WNV Disease in Human

The incubation period varies between 3 and 14 days. Infection may result in (a) asymptomatic (80%), (b) WN fever (20%) and (c) severe/neuroinvasive West Nile fever in 1 in 150 which may be encephalitis, meningitis or poliomyelitis. Gastrointestinal form WNV infection has been reported in up to 30% of human cases. The infection of skin epithelial cells is believed to be the cause of skin rash in 25–45% of the neuroinvasive cases in humans.

Hayes et al. (2005b) studied the 1999–2004 epidemics of WNV in North America. Most experienced a self-limiting acute onset of fever (>38 °C) with headache, myalgia, fatigue, malaise and weakness. Some showed gastrointestinal symptoms, nausea, vomiting, transient rash on the trunk and extremities, lymphadenitis and hepatosplenomegaly. Those seeking medical help reported pain/stiff neck and muscle weakness, photophobia, difficulty in concentrating, depression, lethargy and altered personality lasting for a month or so. These are signs of neuroinvasive illness which could be due to meningoencephalitis, encephalitis and asymmetric flaccid paralysis (spinal motor neuron involvement).

Thirty-one per cent of 98 patients had to be hospitalized for neuroinvasive illness. Illness without neurologic manifestation led 79% of patients to be absent from their jobs or from school for a median period of 60 days. Chorioretinitis was the commonest non-neurological manifestation.

Post-recovery sequelae from neuroinvasive form range from lifelong physical morbidity to severe mental condition. These are tremors, poliomyelitis, cognitive disorders, anxieties, depression, hearing loss and chronic retinopathy.

Non-neurological manifestations occur but less frequent.

The optic nerve involvement may be considered as extension of infection of the brain, chorioretinitis, vitritis, optic neuritis and retinal haemorrhage. Kidney (renal) and heart (myocarditis) failure and rarely myositis, hepatitis, orchitis and pancreatitis may be seen.

20.6   Disease in Birds and Animals

Primarily birds and also eastern cotton tail rabbits, fox squirrels and alligators infect mosquitoes and hence important in the maintenance and transmission of the virus. WNV has the potential to infect and cause pathology in a wide range of vertebrates with some commonality, neurotropism, mononuclear inflammation, neuronal necrosis, gliosis and renal and ocular tropism (Byas and Ebel 2020).

20.6.1   Horses

About 20% infected develop neurological symptoms. Horses become listless and their limbs become weak. Fever, loss of appetite, difficulty in swallowing, depression, hyperexcitability, behavioural change, muscular twitching, stumbling, lack of coordination, inability to stand and death are present. Mortality (including euthanasia) varies between 30 and 50%. Permanent sequelae are seen in about 10 to 20% of recovered horses.

20.6.2   Birds

Birds are lethargic, are unable to fly or even hold upright and show ataxia, ruffled feather, unusual posture, leg paralysis, nystagmus and seizures.

20.6.3 American Alligators

American alligators suffer from gastrointestinal and neurologic forms of the disease. Bloating and anorexia are the signs of the former. Loss of leg control, spasm in the neck, head tilting and muscle tremor cause swimming sideways or in circle and inability to submerge underwater. Nearly 2000 alligators have died between 2001 and 2003.

20.6.4 Crocodiles

WNV caused clinical illness in Nile crocodiles (*C. niloticus*). Symptoms such as anorexia, bloody diarrhoea and scoliosis plus leg weakness, swimming in circles like in alligators and pathologies like pulmonary congestion, haemorrhagic intestines and trachea and hydropericardium are seen. In Australia farmed healthy crocodile, *C. porosus*, was positive for WNV.

20.7 Diagnosis

Examination of serum and/or CSF from patients by any of the following methods:

IgG-ELISA/IgM-antibody capture method/haemagglutination inhibition tests/serum neutralization (confirmatory) and IgG antibody sero-conversion (or significant increase in antibody titres) in two serial specimens collected at a 1-week interval by ELISA. IgM may persist for more than 1 year. Virus neutralization test is the golden test, which takes care of the cross-reacting flaviviruses. Immunohistochemistry on pathological tissue may be used.

- Western blot (is fast and specific).
- Nucleotide amplification/reverse PCR.
- African green monkey kidney cells (Vero cells, American Type Cell Culture #81-CCL, Manassas, VA, USA) for virus isolation.
- Combination of viral isolation and serological testing.

    RT-PCR, quantitative qRT-PCR and in situ hybridization are commonly used.

20.8 Risk Factors

WNV does not spare any age. Children, old age, comorbidities (diabetes, cardiovascular diseases and cancer) and immunosuppressed status may predispose and develop a severe disease. Risk of acquiring the disease increases by 1.5 for every

10 years. The number of deaths increases with age (60–89 years). More males than females die. The median ages of patients with neuroinvasive and febrile forms were 64 and 49 years, respectively, as the median age at death. CFR in the neuroinvasive form is 9%. Adults suffer from this disease. The neuroinvasive form of WNV occurred also in age group <19 years (34%), with 30% in age < 10 years and even in infants (Hayes et al. 2005a).

Peri-urban settings that favour mosquito vectors are risky. For example, *Cx. quinquefasciatus* and *Cx. pipiens pipiens* are urban vectors found indoors. Domestic fowl and scavenging birds may maintain and spread the virus in urban settings.

In rural settings, agricultural activities like irrigation are exposed to mosquito breeding sites. Activities like landscaping, construction workers and summer camp workers enhance opportunities of exposure. Occupationally, healthcare workers, laboratory workers, animal handlers, slaughterers and veterinarians also stand at risk.

20.9   Management of Cases and Preventive Measures

20.9.1   Treatment

No specific treatment is yet available. Therefore, management of cases through supportive therapy and intensive care is required to save lives. Hayes et al. (2005b) suggested supportive therapy for severe illness and controlling headache, dehydration and vomition for cases with symptoms of meningitis.

Severe encephalitis cases require monitoring for development of intracranial pressure and seizures. Encephalitis or paralytic cases must be observed for 'inability to protect airways' as acute neuromuscular respiratory failure may rapidly develop.

Drugs that have been used without rigorous clinical trial are ribavirin, interferon-alpha, anti-WNV immunoglobulin and antisense gene-targeted compounds. Specific immunoglobulin may be useful.

20.9.2   Prevention

WNV has a complex life cycle. A number of mosquitoes—wide vertebrate reservoirs and final hosts—are interacting within themselves and also with dynamic environment in the total infection dynamics in endemic areas. Ambient temperature and rainfall are fundamental drivers of mosquito abundance and amplification of WNV. There could be a variety of modes of spread to non-endemic areas: birds' migration and trade of birds, reptiles and other animals, human movement and transport of mosquitoes. Joint surveillance and/or sharing data on WNV activity in mosquitoes, avians, animals and humans is required.

WNV infection occurs in both medical and veterinary settings. One Health approach is the most appropriate approach, which makes a better comprehensive flaviviral infection control programme. The National Reference Centre for Dengue and Arboviral Diagnosis, Argentina, has implemented laboratory surveillance for WNV in birds, equines and humans (Morales et al. 2006).

Screening of blood donors and donors is useful for preventing nosocomial transmission.

Stopping activity of WNV at the point of detection is required to protect the population from infection. Early warning system enables preparation for the fight against the imminent outbreak. Nasci (2013) considers that surveillance and currently available indicators of WNV provide 2–4-week lead time in advance of human cases.

20.9.2.1   Veterinary Setting and Participatory Epidemiology

Screening of American crows/ill and admitted raptors/sentinel domestic chicken and horses is tested as means of detecting viral activity in advance.

Horses suffering with WNV manifest a characteristic triad, paralysis of limb, photophobia and nasal discharge. Observing clinical manifestation of WNV infection in horses, training equine vets/para-vets about the clinical patterns of WNV infection in unvaccinated horses and also an optimized surveillance design would be useful for participatory epidemiology and passive surveillance. Unvaccinated horses could be used as a relatively cheap system of 'alert' in form 'sentinel horses' (Saegerman et al. 2014)

Horses can be protected by vaccination. The following two vaccines are available:

1. Formalin inactivated vaccine (*Innovator, Fort Dodge, Princeton, NJ, USA*) confers immunity in 94% of vaccinated horses. The other is *Vetera (Boehringer Ingelheim)*. Following initial 2 injections 4–6 weeks apart a booster every 6 months is required.
2. Recombinant live attenuated vaccine (*Recombitek, Merial*): recombinant live canarypox virus expressing prM and E transgenes from WNV$_{NY99}$ strain—two doses at 5-week interval protects 100% for horses for 1 year and also tested as useful for cats and dogs.

Vector control of WNV needs to be comprehensive and integrated and has to be based on surveillance for identifying mosquitoes locally important for transmission; bridge mosquitoes for animal-birds-human transmission; breeding sites, mosquito population and vector index; appropriate action—pesticide and biological and habitat management (management of water).

WHO is intensively supporting the surveillance and outbreak response activities through its international partners in Europe, North America, Latin America and the Caribbean   (https://www.who.int/news-room/fact-sheets/detail/west-nile-virus,   3 October 2017).

References

Allison AB, Mead DG, Gibbs SEJ, Hoffman DM, Stallknecht DE (2004) West Nile virus viremia in wild rock pigeons. Emerg Infect Dis 10(12):2252–2255

Bakonyi T, Haussig JM (2020) West Nile virus keeps on moving up in Europe. Euro Surveill 25(s):pii=2001938

Bell JA, Brewer CM, Mickelson NJ, Garman GW, Vaughan JA (2006) West Nile virus epizootiology, Central Red River Valley, North Dakota and Minnesota, 2002–2005. Emerg Infect Dis 12(8):1245–1247

Bofill D, Domingo C, Cardeñosa N, Zaragoza J, de Ory F, Minguell S et al (2006) Human West Nile virus infection, Catalonia, Spain. Emerg Infect Dis 12(7):1163–1164

Byas AD, Ebel GD (2020) Review, comparative pathology of West Nile virus in humans and non-human -animals. Pathogens 9:48. https://doi.org/10.3390/pathogens9010048. www.mdpi.com/journal/pathogens

Cabre O, Grandadam M, Marié J-L, Gravier P, Prangé A, Santinelli Y et al (2006) West Nile virus in horses, sub-Saharan Africa. Emerg Infect Dis 12(12):1958–1960

Dehghani R, Kassiri H, Kasiri N, Dehghani M (2020) A review on epidemiology and ecology of West Nile fever: an emerging arboviral disease. J Acute Dis 9(3):93–99

Dupuis AP II, Marra PP, Kramer LD (2003) Serologic evidence of West Nile virus transmission, Jamaica, West Indies. Emerg Infect Dis 9(7):860–863

Fonseca K, Prince GD, Bratvold J, Fox JD, Pybus M et al (2005) West Nile virus infection and conjunctival exposure. Emerg Infect Dis 11(10):1648–1649

García-Bocanegra I, Jaén-Téllez JA, Napp S, Arenas-Montes A et al (2011) West Nile fever outbreak in horses and humans, Spain, 2010. Emerg Infect Dis 17(12):2397–2399

Godsey MS Jr, Nasci R, Savage HM, Aspen S, King R, Powers AM et al (2005) West Nile virus–infected mosquitoes, Louisiana, 2002. Emerg Infect Dis 11(9):1399–1404

Habarugira G, Suen WW, Hobson-Peters J, Hall RA, Bielefeldt-Ohmann H (2020) Review: West Nile virus: an update on pathobiology, epidemiology, diagnostics, control and "one health" implications. Pathogens. 2020(9):589

Hayes EB, Komar N, Nasci RS, Montgomery SP, O'Leary DR, Campbell GL (2005a) Epidemiology and transmission dynamics of West Nile virus disease. Emerg Infect Dis 11(8):1167–1173

Hayes EB, Sejvar JJ, Zaki SR, Lanciotti RS, Bode AV, Campbell GL (2005b) Virology, pathology, and clinical manifestations of West Nile virus disease. Emerg Infect Dis 11(8):1174–1179

Klenk K, Snow J, Morgan K, Bowen R, Stephens M, Foster F et al (2004) Alligators as West Nile virus amplifiers. Emerg Infect Dis 10(12):2150–2155

Komar N (2003) West Nile Virus: epidemiology and ecology in North America. Adv Virus Res 61:185–234

Lawrie CH, Uzcátegui NY, Gould EA, Nuttall PA (2004) Ixodid and argasid tick species and West Nile virus. Emerg Infect Dis 10(4):653–657

Lindsey NP, Lehman JA, Staples JE, Fischer M (2014) West Nile Virus and other Arboviral diseases -US 2013. MMWR Morb Mortal Wkly Rep 63(24):521–526

Malkinson M, Banet C, Weisman Y, Pokamunski S, King R et al (2002) Introduction of West Nile virus in the Middle East by migrating white storks. Emerg Infect Dis 8(4):392–397

Martinet JP, Ferté H, Failloux AB, Schaffner F, Depaquit J (2019) Mosquitoes of North-Western Europe as potential vectors of arboviruses: a review. Viruses 11(11):1059

McDonald E, Martin SW, Landry K et al (2019) West Nile virus and other domestic nationally notifiable Arboviral diseases—United States, 2018. MMWR 68:673–678

Meece JK, Kronenwetter-Koepel TA, Vandermause MF, Reed KD (2006) West Nile virus infection in commercial waterfowl operation, Wisconsin. Emerg Infect Dis 12(9):1451–1453

Morales MA, Barrandeguy M, Fabbri C, Garcia JB et al (2006) West Nile virus isolation from equines in Argentina, 2006. Emerg Infect Dis 12(10):1559–1561

Nasci RS (2013) Monitoring and controlling West Nile virus: are your prevention practices in place? J Environ Health 75(8):42–44

Petersen LR, Carson PJ, Biggerstaff BJ, Custer B et al (2013) Estimated cumulative incidence of West Nile virus infection in US adults, 1999-2010. Epidemiol Infect 141(3):591–595

Pupo M, Guzmán MG, Fernández R, Llop A, Dickinson FO et al (2006) West Nile virus infection in humans and horses. Cuba Emerg Infect Dis 12(6):1022–1024

Saegerman C, Alba-Casals A, García-Bocanegra I, Dal Pozzo F, van Galen G (2014) Clinical sentinel surveillance of equine West Nile fever, Spain. Transbound Emerg Dis 63(2):184–193

Tesh RB, Parsons R, Siirin M, Randle Y, Sargent C, Guzman H et al (2004) Year-round West Nile virus activity, Gulf Coast region, Texas and Louisiana. Emerg Infect Dis 10(9):1649–1652

Chapter 21
Powassan Viral Encephalitis

Powassan viral encephalitis is a fatal neuroinvasive disease of humans characterized by rapid onset of fever, body ache, disorientation, tremor, convulsion and paralysis.

21.1 Aetiology

The disease is caused by Powassan virus (POWV), which is a flavivirus. It was first identified as a human pathogen in 1958 after isolation from the brain of a young boy who died of encephalitis in the town of Powassan, Ontario (McLean and Donahue 1959).

21.2 Epidemiology

The incidence of Powassan viral encephalitis appears to be increasing.

Powassan viral encephalitis has been reported from the United States, Canada, Russia and warm areas across Eurasia (Hermance and Thangamani 2017). It is endemic in the United States with increasing infection rate. Powassan virus has emerged as a disease of public health concern as it has been found to be potentially affected by climate change and urbanization (Gould and Higgs 2009).

In nature, POWV is maintained by ixodid ticks and mammalian hosts. *Ixodes cookei, Ix. marxi, Ix. spinipalpus* and *Dermacentor andersoni* are the ticks from which the virus has been isolated in North America. *Ix. scapularis* has been found to carry a variant of Powassan virus. Thirty-eight mammalian species, mainly woodchuck, have been found infected with this virus.

The virus seems to be maintained in nature in a sylvatic cycle consisting of *I. cookie* and small mammals—woodchuck (groundhog) and others like squirrels

© Springer Nature Singapore Pte Ltd. 2024
K. G. Narayan et al., *Handbook of Management of Zoonoses*,
https://doi.org/10.1007/978-981-99-9885-2_21

and chipmunks. The ticks are found in or near the burrows and nests of small mammals. Another tick-host system consists of *I. scapularis*—white-footed mouse and white-tailed deer. Human is an incidental host. Ticks can survive feeding upon the natural host; feeding on human is not essential. Each stage, larva, nymph and adult needs blood meal to progress to the next stage in life. Nymph stage bites human. The virus is transferred to human within 15–30 min of attachment.

Most human cases of POWV have occurred in the Great Lakes and Northeast regions of the United States and eastern Canada (Corrin et al. 2018). In the United States, human cases of POWV have occurred primarily from northeastern states and the Great Lake region. The reported number of cases have increased in recent years (CDC 2023).

Transmission to humans occurs when they venture in the biotope, for example, gardening close to the burrows of woodchuck, although infected ones are unaware and do not report tick bite. The occurrence is seasonal, from May to December with peaks from June to September when ticks are most active.

21.3 Symptoms

Powassan viral infection is rarely diagnosed as encephalitis and by the time it is diagnosed, it has become acute disseminated encephalitis. It manifests in two forms: mild and severe. The former presents as a slight fever, body ache and/or headache. In the latter, the onset is rapid; fever is high with headache and disorientation—tremor, convulsions, paralysis, coma and death. Neurologic sequelae are common. There is a long-term neurological problem and disability. Case fatality rate is 10–15%.

21.4 Diagnosis

- Encephalitis and history of exposure to ticks or habitat of small-sized mammals are suggestive.
- Encephalitis is confirmed by laboratory examination such as CSF has elevated WBC—mainly lymphocytes and protein—supported with EEG findings.
- >Fourfold increase in antibody titre in paired serum samples.
- Confirmation is achieved by detection of Powassan virus-specific IgM and neutralizing antibody by IFA and plaque reduction test.
- Detection of virus-specific nucleic acid.
- Virus culture.

21.5 Prevention

In the United States, testing for arboviral encephalitis has been made comprehensive since the detection of West Nile encephalitis in 1999. Powassan virus is also included in the list of viruses looked for. Detection and reporting of Powassan viral encephalitis is thus more frequent and precise.

There is no vaccine. Protection against ticks is thus the most significant preventive measure, which needs sanitary practices like the following:

- Careful removal of rodent nests by avoiding direct contact with nesting material and with ticks is important.
- Environmental control—bush, weeds, trash, etc. supporting small-sized mammals around the house should be removed.
- Personal protective measures to prevent tick bites and continued encephalitis surveillance. (CDC 2001, http://www.cdc.gov/mmwr/preview/mmwrhtml/mm5035a4.htm)

References

Centres for Disease Control and Prevention (CDC) (2001) Outbreak of Powassan encephalitis—Maine and Vermont, 1999–2001. MMWR Morb Mortal Wkly Rep 50(35):761–764

CDC (2023). https://www.cdc.gov/powassan/statistics-data/historic-data.html

Corrin T, Greig J, Harding S, Young I, Mascarenhas M, Waddell LA (2018) Powassan virus, a scoping review of the global evidence. Zoonoses Public Health 65:595–624

Gould EA, Higgs S (2009) Impact of climate change and other factors on emerging arbovirus diseases. Trans R Soc Trop Med Hyg 103(2):109–121

Hermance ME, Thangamani S (2017) Powassan virus: an emerging arbovirus of public health concern in North America. Vector Borne Zoonotic Dis 17:453–462

http://www.cdc.gov/mmwr/preview/mmwrhtml/mm5035a4.htm

McLean DM, Donahue W (1959) Powassan virus: isolation of virus from a fatal case of encephalitis. Can Med Assoc J 80:708–711

Chapter 22
Colorado Tick-Borne Relapsing Fever

Synonyms

Mountain fever, American mountain fever, Mountain tick fever.

Colorado Tick-borne Relapsing fever is an acute febrile tick borne viral infection affecting mostly campers, foresters, and rangers on high altitudes (4000–10,000 ft) (CDC 2021).

22.1 Aetiology

Colorado tick fever virus belongs to the genus *Coltivirus*, family *Reoviridae* and subfamily *Spinareovirinae*. It is 80 nm in diameter, lacks a lipid envelope and has two protein coats and a double-stranded RNA genome having ~20,000 base pairs divided into 12 segments. It invades and replicates in haematopoietic cells, erythrocyte precursor cells and the infected immature cells. The virus matures simultaneously. The virus may be found in erythrocytes for 120 days from the onset of symptoms.

22.2 Epidemiology

Fifty-nine cases were reported to CDC, USA, from 2010 to 2019 (https://www.cdc.gov/coloradotickfever/statistics.html). The disease is endemic in the western parts of Canada and western United States, notably Colorado, Utah, Montana, Wyoming, Idaho, New Mexico, South Dakota and Oregon. This region is consistent with the range of activity of the tick *Dermacentor andersoni* (wood tick) [medlineplus (n.d.)].

© Springer Nature Singapore Pte Ltd. 2024
K. G. Narayan et al., *Handbook of Management of Zoonoses*,
https://doi.org/10.1007/978-981-99-9885-2_22

The mammalian reservoir host is primarily golden-mantled ground squirrel (*Citellus lateralis*) which is a part of life cycle of ticks. Usually, ticks are found attached to their hosts. Ticks may hide in cracks, crevices and soil and overwinter in case they fail to find a host to attach and resume the search of host in the following spring. Adult ticks tend to climb the top of grasses and low shrubs and wait for the hosts wandering by so as to attach them. The ticks are active during late spring and summer. The disease occurs in the Rocky Mountain region of the United States during February through October, 90% of cases during April and July. The case-fatality ratio for CTF is quite low.

Yendell et al. (2015) identified and studied 95 possible cases from 2002 to 2012 from the reports of the state health department and laboratory testing performed at the CDC Arbovirus Diagnostic Laboratory. During the period 2002–2012, the number of reported cases remained <15/year. An increase in the number of cases among travellers and in the proportion of cases diagnosed by RT-PCR testing was observed though the incidence, and distribution of cases remained unchanged during 2002–2012. Sixty-four per cent of cases were males and 65% were adults ≥40 years. Trends in the demographic characteristics occur over decades due to changes in care-seeking behaviour, testing and surveillance practices.

22.3   Transmission

Modes of transmission are bite of ticks and sometimes blood transfusion.

22.4   Symptoms

The incubation period (time of bite by infected ticks to appearance of symptoms) varies between 3 and 6 days, or may be up to 20 days. The duration of acute illness is 5–10 days generally. In about half of the cases, usually there are two clinical episodes, each lasting for 1–3 days with an interval of afebrile period of 24–72 hours when cases report anorexia and malaise. The patients experience fever; chills; pain in the head, muscles and behind their eyes; photophobia; injected conjunctiva; lymphadenopathy; pharyngeal erythema; general malaise; abdominal pain, nausea and vomiting; and flat or pimply, maculopapular or petechial rash in 5–12% cases. The second episode may be more pronounced. Children (especially under 10) suffer from severe disease. Rarely, complications like aseptic meningitis, encephalitis and haemorrhagic fever may be seen.

22.5   Diagnosis

This disease should be included in febrile cases for differential diagnosis:

- Clinical signs and symptoms and history of possible exposure to ticks are indicative.
- Clinical laboratory test results showing leukopenia, thrombocytopenia and mildly elevated liver enzymes are suggestive of Colorado tick fever.
- RT-PCR and cell culture during the first 2 weeks of the illness.
- Serological tests like IgM capture EIA, indirect fluorescent antibody and plaque-reduction neutralization on convalescent samples.

Samples taken from the first 2 weeks of the illness are often RT-PCR positive. Samples obtained from cases of 2–3 weeks of the illness are more likely to test positive by IgG or neutralizing antibodies.

22.6 Treatment

Often the disease is self-limiting. There is no specific treatment. Patient should be given supportive treatment. Aspirin and salicylates should not be given.

Removal of ticks from the skin fully and carefully: Put Vaseline over ticks, ticks will retract from the skin, grab it with tweezers and remove them; your hands should be protected with gloves and subsequently wash hands and the tick-infested site thoroughly with soap and water and apply antiseptic.

22.7 Prevention

- Patients with confirmed CTF should defer blood and bone marrow donation for at least 6 months after recovery because viraemia is prolonged. There is sequestration of CTFV in red blood cells.
- Check the pets and oneself for ticks. Ticks are easily visible on light clothes. Insect repellents may be useful.
- Reduce tick densities—(a) application of acaricides, (b) control of tick habitat (littered leaves, bush, crevices, cracks in floor), (c) application of acaricides to rodents by using baited tubes, boxes and feeding stations in endemic areas and (d) biological control measures—parasitic fungi, nematodes and wasps.

References

CDC (2021) https://www.cdc.gov/coloradotickfever/transmission.html
Medlineplus (n.d.) Colorado tick fever http://www.nlm.nih.gov/medlineplus/ency/article/000675.htm
Yendell SJ, Fischer M, Staples JE (2015) Colorado tick fever in the United States, 2002-2012. Vector Borne Zoonotic Dis 15(5):311–316

Chapter 23
Kyasanur Forest Disease

Synonyms

Monkey disease, Monkey fever.

Kyasanur forest disease (KFD) is a tick-borne viral haemorrhagic fever, first identified in 1957 in Shimoga district of Karnataka state, India.

Work and Trapido (1957) described Kyasanur forest disease that caused high mortality in monkeys in March 1955 in this forest and also some humans in the neighbouring village. The virus was isolated from a sick monkey from the Kyasanur forest in Karnataka (formerly Mysore) state, India. KFD is characterized by fever and signs of neurological manifestations, such as severe headache, mental disturbances, tremors and vision deficits.

23.1 Aetiology

Kyasanur forest disease virus (KFDV) is a member of the tick-borne encephalitis complex of the genus *Flavivirus* (formerly group B arbovirus) and family *Flaviviridae*. It is a part of a group of tick-borne viruses of mammals causing haemorrhagic fever—*Alkhurma* of Saudi Arabia and Egypt, *Omsk haemorrhagic fever* of Siberia and *Powassan* of the United States and Russia.

It has a single-stranded positive-sense RNA genome. It is a spherical, enveloped virion of about 45 nm in diameter. KFDV has three structural and seven non-structural proteins. The structural proteins are capsid (C), premembrane (prM) and envelope (E). The seven non-structural proteins are NS1, NS2a, NS2b, NS3, NS4a, NS4b and NS5. The KFDV genomes are highly conserved. The genetic diversity is considerably low (Yadav et al. 2020). The virus is sensitive to 70% ethanol, 1%

© Springer Nature Singapore Pte Ltd. 2024
K. G. Narayan et al., *Handbook of Management of Zoonoses*,
https://doi.org/10.1007/978-981-99-9885-2_23

sodium hypochlorite, contact time of 30 min, 2% glutaraldehyde and freezing and heating at 56 °C for 30 minutes.

23.2   Epidemiology

KFDV is a highly infectious tick-borne virus that causes Kyasanur forest disease (KFD) with no cure and a partially effective vaccine. The case fatality rate is 2–20%. It requires biosafety level 4 laboratory.

The KFDV is enzootic in India and causes epizootic in primates with high mortality. It has been expanding to new areas in India.

23.2.1   Outbreaks

According to Chakraborty et al. (2019), KFD had intermittent outbreaks and high number of cases occurred during focal periods. Over a study period of 61 years, 37 years had fewer than 100 cases; 16 years had cases from 100 to 399 and 8 years had 400 or more cases. The estimated number of KFD cases from 1957 to 2017 was 9594, distributed in 16 districts in India. Four significant outbreaks occurred in years 1957–1958, 1983–1984, 2002–2003 and 2016–2017 that recorded respectively 681, 2589, 1562 and 809 cases. The reported outbreak in 2015 in Goa was followed by detection in Dodamarg and Sawantwadi talukas of Sindhudurg district, Maharashtra, in 2016. Samples of human serum, monkey autopsy and tick were positive. New hotspots identified were talukas Kankavli, Kudal and Vengurla of Sindhudurg.

KFDV was reported from only five districts of Karnataka, namely, Shimoga, Chikkamagaluru, Uttara Kannada, Dakshina Kannada and Udupi. Recently, KFD has spread to Maharashtra, Goa, Tamil Nadu and Kerala stretching from north to south of Western Ghats (Tandale et al. 2015) presumably through the movement of animals carrying ticks.

The evolution and spatiotemporal transmission dynamics were studied by Yadava et al. (2020). Phylogenetic analysis of strains of KFDV isolated from different regions during 1957–2017 by whole genome sequence and 28 E-gene sequence was made. The mean rate of evolution based on E-gene was slightly higher than whole genomes. Strains (2006–2017): A subgroup of KFDV differed from early Karnataka strains (1957–1972) by 2.76% in their whole genomes and represented those that diverged around 1980 and spread to different regions. Strains dispersed from Karnataka to Goa and Maharashtra and the latter became a new source for transmission of KFDV since 2013. Cashew nut workers got infected with KFD during cashew nut harvesting which affected villages in Goa. Karnataka is most likely the earliest source and route of KFDV to Kerala, Maharashtra and Tamil Nadu.

23.2.2 Enzootic Cycle

KFDV is maintained in *Haemaphysalis spinigera* ticks (which are the main vectors) and monkeys (main host) cycle. *H. spinigera*, the primary vector of KFDV, is a hard tick prevalent in India and Sri Lanka. At least 16 tick species and different mammals are involved in natural cycle.

Some of the tick species are *Haemaphysalis turturis*, *Haemaphysalis kinneari*, *Haemaphysalis kyasanurensis*, *Haemaphysalis wellingtoni*, *Haemaphysalis minuta*, *Haemaphysalis cuspidata*, *Ixodes petauristae*, *Ix. ceylonensis*, *Dermacentor auratus* and *Rhipicephalus haemaphysaloides* and soft ticks of the *Ornithodoros* genus. These are distributed in almost all states of India.

KFDV has been isolated from black-faced langurs (*Semnopithecus* earlier *Presbytis entellus*), red-faced bonnet monkeys (*Macaca radiata*) and they are fatally infected. Rats (*Rattus blanfordi*, *Rattus rattus wroughtoni*), shrews (*Suncus murinus*) and bats (*Rhinolophus rouxii*) maintain the virus and have the potential to infect ticks. Experimentally KFDV infected and caused high viraemia in black-naped hare, porcupines, flying squirrel, Malabar giant squirrel, gerbil, mice, long-tailed tree mice and shrews. These animals, thus, were important in the maintenance and dissemination of the virus in enzootic areas. The virus latently persists in organs, particularly the brain, in experimentally infected rodents like spiny mouse, porcupines and long-tailed tree mouse. Virus-neutralizing antibody has been observed in cattle, buffalo, goats, boars and a variety of birds.

The first cases among human were from dead infected monkeys. When infected monkeys die, ticks drop from the body, creating a 'hotspot' of infectious ticks that can latch on to humans. Once infected, a tick stays infected for its lifetime. The original focus of infection was Sagar Taluk of Shimoga district.

It is thought that increasing human population in Sagar Taluk and associated deforestation, grazing areas, cattle grazing and extension of paddy fields led to the emergence of KFDV in 1957 from a cryptic enzootic cycle in this previously heavily forested area.

Trans-stadial transmission is common and transovarian transmission occurs only in *I. petauristae*. *H. spinigera* is the main vector and is highly anthrophilic.

KFDV is carried by infected *H. spinigera* through all stages of its development. *H spinigera* takes 118–160 days to complete its life cycle under lab conditions at temperature ranging from 18 °C to 35 °C. Adults feed on cattle for 8–13 days, engorge and drop down; females oviposit 2–5 days after dropping (number of eggs vary with the species of host, e.g. number is large if fed on calf, less if fed on rabbit); hatch after 25–30 days; usually after 5–7 days begin feeding on small mammals, monkeys and birds; and detach and moult into nymphs within 13–16 days after detachment. Nymphs feed for 25–30 days on a range of animals, monkeys, small mammals and birds, and humans. The transovarially transmitted virus is carried to nymphs. Infection picked by nymphs is carried to adults and females transfer to progenies transovarially.

The natural history of KFDV is complex which involves various stages of life cycles of ticks. Cattle carry adult stage of *H. spinigera* and all stages of other spp. of *Haemaphysalis* shown to be infected with this virus. Thus, cattle are most likely to increase tick population in cleared forest areas frequented by human beings. Though the viraemia in cattle is insufficient for dissemination, they act as paratenic hosts, bringing infected ticks to barn/cowsheds often shared by the owner. With the onset of monsoon in June, adult ticks become active, and population peaks during July and August and declines in September. The fed female ticks lay a large number of eggs. The population of larvae builds up in monsoon. These feed on small animals, like rodents, shrews, etc. (Fig. 23.1) and thus get infected. These drop off the hosts and hibernate under forest litter to become active post-monsoon (October to December) to develop into nymphs, which are active during January to May, coincident with the epidemics and hence considered the most important for transmission to humans (see time line, Fig. 23.1).

Zaki (1997) isolated a strain of KFDV, later known as the *Alkhurma* variant, from blood of six male butchers, two of whom died and four recovered, and later four additional cases were also confirmed as KFD. Eight of ten cases worked with sheep. Wang et al. (2009) isolated the *Nanjianyin* virus from serum of a patient in Yunan, China. The birds' role in maintenance of virus in enzootic areas is unclear even though high percentage of birds in the enzootic areas shows antibodies to KFDV. Infected birds and migrating viraemic ones are possibly responsible for the spread of KFDV to distant places, such as Saudi Arabia (Mehla et al. 2009).

Chakraborty et al. (2019) consider that the following influenced the occurrence of KFD:

Mechanism of persistence and spread of KFDV are not clear. Yet demographic, socioeconomic, political and environmental factors seem to act as 'drivers'.

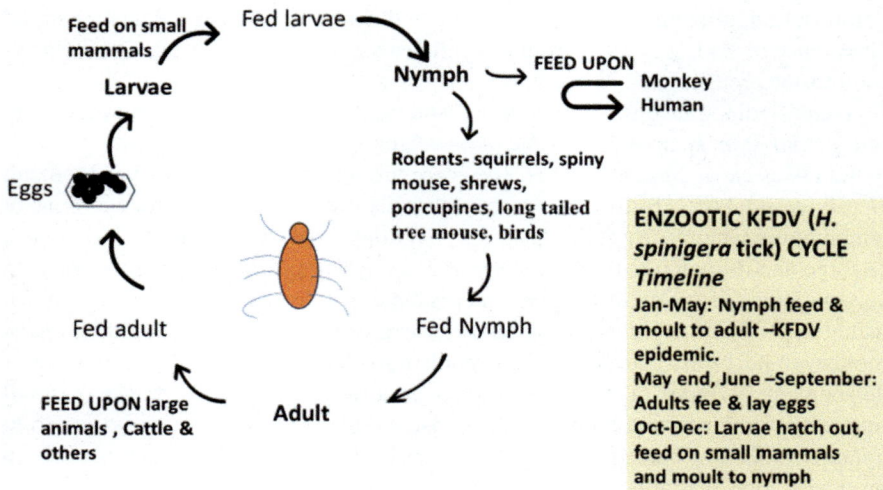

Fig. 23.1 Lifecycle of *Haemophysalis spinigera* and KFDV transmission

Deforestation force monkeys to move (displaced niche) and monkeys-humans distance is reduced. A large number of outbreaks during the 1980s coincided with large-scale deforestation. Deforestation and climate interaction may create conditions favourable for 'ticks-monkeys' interaction, leading to diseases in monkeys and subsequent interacting humans getting infected.

Increasing human population in Shimoga district from 46,524 in 1951 to 1755, 512 in 2011 might have led to migration/encroachment into forest enhancing opportunity of contact with KFDV-infected ticks. Shimoga district—taluks of Sagar and Sorab—experienced increase in population and number of cases.

Climate and climate change are factors that influence the occurrence of KFD, as evidenced by 'decreasing precipitation in all KFD-affected states (-0.71, -3.82, -0.05 and -1.43 mm/year, respectively, in Maharashtra, Goa, Karnataka and Kerala). Most cases occurred following the end of monsoon (December and May).

23.2.3 Population at Risk

Foresters; campers apart from those visiting forests to gather grass, firewood and other forest products; and laboratory workers are populations at risk.

23.2.4 Modes of Infection

- Bite by nymphal stage of ticks.
- Contact with infected, sick or dead monkeys.
- Aerosol—generated in the laboratory while working.

23.3 Symptoms

Incubation period varies between 2 and 8 days. There is high-titre viraemia lasting for the first 3–6 days or more (10–12 days). Fever is biphasic. There is sudden onset of high fever (40 °C), frontal headache, myalgia, persistent cough, vomiting, abdominal pain, gastroenteritis and haemorrhage. Fever continues for 12 days. The patients have abnormally low blood pressure, plate count, red cells and white blood cells and bleeding problems. There is long convalescence period. After 1–2 weeks, there is relapse of fever. This second phase is manifested by encephalitis-like symptoms: stiff neck, mental disturbance, giddiness, photophobia and abnormal reflexes. Most cases are in the age group 10–40 years. Male to female ratio is 2.6:1. These reflect the outdoor (in forest) activity-relatedness. Reported figures on the annual number of cases and mortality vary.

23.4 Diagnosis

- Virus isolation.
- Molecular methods—PCR.
- Serological—IF, SN, HAI and ELISA.

23.5 Treatment

There is no specific treatment available. Supportive treatment should be directed to manage symptoms, dehydration and bleeding.

23.6 Prevention

Early detection and supportive care.

Vaccination: Formalin-inactivated chick embryo tissue culture vaccine protects ≈70% of vaccinees. It has remained the key strategy for preventing KFD in Karnataka. Vaccination with formalin-inactivated tissue culture vaccine has been the primary strategy for controlling KFD in affected areas and mass vaccination has been done in areas reporting KFD activity (i.e. laboratory evidence of virus in monkeys, humans or ticks) and in villages within a 5 km radius of such areas. Two doses are administered at least 1 month apart to persons 7–65 years of age. As vaccine-induced immunity is short-lived, the first booster is recommended within 6–9 months after primary vaccination; thereafter, annual booster doses are recommended for 5 years after the last confirmed case in the area (Kasabi et al. 2013).

Search for hotspots: Apart from this, a search for hotspots and control strategy may be applied where three-level surveillance in humans, monkeys and ticks for early detection of hotspots and institution of control measures may be applied. This may be even insecticide spraying—lindane @ 1 kg/ha on either side of tracks in a forest or in 50 m radius with monkey death spot as the centre.

Repellents—dimethyl phthalate (DMP), DBP, DEET and N, N-diethyl-toluamide provide 90–100% protection against tick bite.

References

Chakraborty S, Andrade FCD, Ghosh S, Uelmen J, Ruiz MO (2019) Historical expansion of Kyasanur Forest disease in India from 1957 to 2017: a retrospective analysis. Geo Health 3:44–55

Kasabi GS, Murhekar MV, Sandhya VK, Raghunandan R, Kiran SK et al (2013) Coverage and effectiveness of Kyasanur Forest disease (KFD) vaccine in Karnataka, South India, 2005–10. PLoSNegl Trop Dis 7:e2025

Mehla R, Kumar SRP, Yadav P, Barde PV, Yergolkar PN et al (2009) Recent Ancestry of Kyasanur Forest Disease Virus. Emerg Infect Dis 15(9):1431–1437

Tandale BV, Balakrishnan A, Yadav PD, Marja N, Mourya DT (2015) New focus of Kyasanur Forest disease virus activity in a tribal area in Kerala, India, 2014. Infect Dis Poverty 4:12

Wang J, Zhang H, Fu S, Wang H, Ni D, Nasci R, Tang Q, Liang G (2009) Isolation of Kyasanur Forest disease virus from febrile patient, Yunnan, China. Emerg Infect Dis 15(2):326–328

Work TH, Trapido H (1957) Kyasanur Forest disease: a new infection of man and monkeys in tropical India by a virus of the Russian spring summer complex. In: Proceedings of the IX Pacific science congress, vol 17. Public Health and Medical Science. http://icmr.nic.in/pinstitute/niv/KYASANUR%20FOREST%20DISEASE.pdf

Yadav PD, Patil S, Jadhav SM, Nyayanit DA, Kumar V et al (2020) Phylogeography of Kyasanur Forest disease virus in India (1957-2017) reveals evolution and spread in the Western Ghats region. Sci Rep 10(1):1966

Zaki AM (1997) Isolation of a flavivirus related to the tick-borne encephalitis complex from human cases in Saudi Arabia. Trans R Soc Trop Med Hyg 91(2):179–181

Chapter 24
Crimean-Congo Haemorrhagic Fever

Synonyms

Congo fever, Central Asian haemorrhagic fever, Hungribta (blood taking), Khunymuny (nose bleeding), Karakhalak (black death).

Crimean-Congo haemorrhagic fever (CCHF) is a severe haemorrhagic fever with rapid onset and high case fatality rate. The annual incidence ranges from sporadic to high in different regions. It is an important tick-borne zoonosis with domestic and wild animal hosts. It has a bioterrorism potential (US select agent list—CDC/NIAID category C).

In the 1940s, soldiers reoccupying abandoned farmland in Crimea fell ill with a haemorrhagic disease. The causative agent was later considered similar to the causative agent of a haemorrhagic disease in the Belgian Congo (Democratic Republic of Congo). The disease was thus named Crimean-Congo haemorrhagic fever.

24.1 Aetiology

Crimean-Congo haemorrhagic fever virus belongs to the CCHFV group: family *Bunyaviridae* and genus *Nairovirus*. The genus *Nairovirus* includes 34 viruses. Three of these, the *Dugbe, Nairobi sheep disease and CCHF* viruses cause human diseases. CCHFV is the most important human pathogen (WHO 2001). *Ganjam* virus is considered as a variant of Nairobi sheep disease virus and causes diseases in humans in India (Yadav et al. 2014). The genome plasticity of the virus is surprisingly high for an arthropod-borne virus and there is extensive genetic diversity, particularly between virus strains from different geographic regions. Accumulation of mutations, frequent reassortment of RNA segment and even RNA recombination explains this genetic diversity. It has epidemic potential with fatality rate of 10–40%. It requires biosafety level 4 laboratory.

© Springer Nature Singapore Pte Ltd. 2024
K. G. Narayan et al., *Handbook of Management of Zoonoses*,
https://doi.org/10.1007/978-981-99-9885-2_24

24.2 Epidemiology

24.2.1 Distribution

It is an emerging disease. Its geographic range is increasing since it was first recognized. It has caused about 140 outbreaks with over 5000 cases in almost 52 countries. The distribution of CCHF mirrors the distribution of *Hyalomma* ticks and occurs in Africa; the Middle East; southern Europe, particularly southern portions of the former USSR (Crimea, Astrakhan, Rostov, Uzbekistan, Kazakhstan, Tajikistan), Turkey, Bulgaria, Greece, Albania and Kosovo; and Asian countries south of the 50th parallel north (WHO 2013). It is also distributed throughout the Mediterranean, in north-western China and the Indian subcontinent (CDC 2013). According to Maltezon and Papa (2010), newer foci emerged in several Balkan countries, southwest Russia and Turkey since 2000 because of changing climate that affected the rate of reproduction of the vector tick, *Hyalomma*, and also the anthropogenic factors related to agriculture and hunting.

Yadav et al. (2014) reviewed the CCHF status in India. The National Institute of Virology, Pune, India, detected antibodies against CCHFV in livestock serum samples from Gujarat, Rajasthan. In January 2011, a nosocomial outbreak occurred in Ahmedabad, Gujarat. The viral activity during and after the outbreak was evidenced serologically among buffalo, cattle, sheep and goat in Gujarat. CCHFV was reported from humans and animals in Gujarat state again in 2012. According to Mourya et al. (2019), males, close contacts and neighbours were at high risk. Tick screening and animal sero-survey detected hotspots.

Analysis by the Federal Health Agency 'Stavropol Research Institute Against Plague' of the epizootic situation during the past 2 years reports that the climate anomaly facilitated the increase of numbers of ticks, which caused changes in the development cycle of *Hyalomma marginatum*; mass activation of larvae started by the end of July and extended the new territories in the west, north-west and central parts of Stavropol Krai. According to Papa et al. (2011), the first CCHF case in Greece was reported in 2008; the strain was Rodopi, different from AP92. These authors conducted sero-epidemiological study and found that age, sex, prefecture, occupation and contact with goats and sheep, slaughtering and history of tick bite were significantly related.

Knust et al. (2012) defined 'suspected', 'confirmed' cases and made 'tick bite register' for surveillance. Temporal and spatial association between reported tick bites and CCHF during 2009–2010 in Kazakhstan emerged clearly. 'Precise' public health efforts like 'public awareness about tick bites, prevention and CCHF control practices at hospital' could also be planned.

24.2.2   Life Cycle

CCHFV usually circulates between asymptomatic animals and ticks in an enzootic cycle. This virus has been found in at least 31 species of ticks, including seven genera of the family *Ixodidae* (hard ticks). Principal vectors seem to be the members of the genus *Hyalomma.* Infection of ticks may be transovarial, trans-stadial and venereal.

CCHFV is naturally circulated as 'tick-tick' cycle transovarially, transstadially and so-called 'non-viraemic transmission' in addition to 'tick-vertebrate-tick' cycle (Fig. 24.1). In the 'non-viraemic transmission', the virus can be transferred between infected and uninfected ticks during co-feeding on a host (OIE 2018).

Ticks of the genera *Rhipicephalus*, *Boophilus*, *Dermacentor* and *Ixodes* also act as biological vectors. Other invertebrate species, such as midges (*Culicoides* spp.) and soft ticks (Argasidae), are not biological vectors, although CCHFV may sometimes be isolated from these as they might have fed on viraemic hosts (CCHF_H2007_2009 OIE) (OIE 2009).

Small mammals, particularly European hare, Middle-African hedgehogs and multimammate rats, are the main reservoirs (tick-vertebrate-tick cycle). Ixodid ticks, particularly those of the genus *Hyalomma*, get infected while feeding on viraemic animals or humans not showing any symptoms.

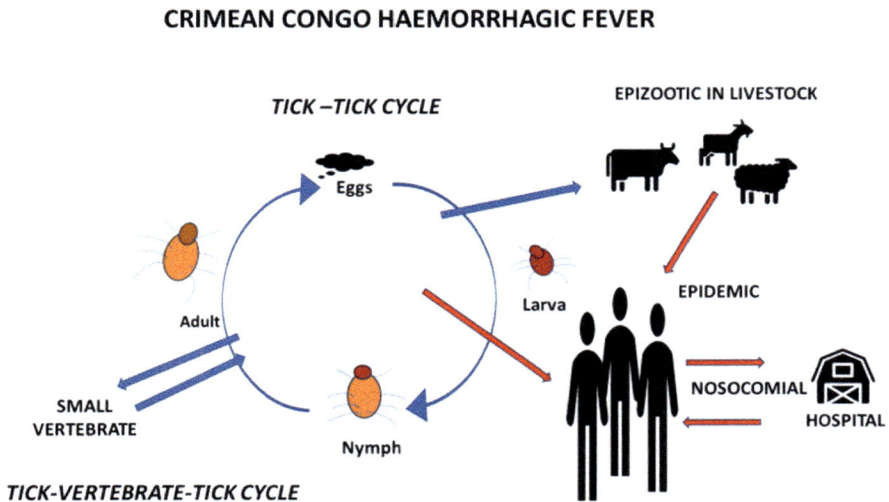

Fig. 24.1 Life cycle and transmission of Crimean Congo Haemorrhagic Fever Virus

24.2.2.1   Animals as Source of Human Infection

There is viraemia in infected mammals of many species: cattle, sheep, goats, hares, hedgehogs, dogs and mice (*Mastomys* spp.). Newborn rodents die of infection. Experimental infection revealed that cattle, sheep and goat remained viraemic for 1 week and ostriches for 1–4 days. Ostriches show high prevalence in endemic areas and have been at the origin of human cases, such as an outbreak at an ostrich abattoir in South Africa (WHO 2013).

Immature ticks attach to small vertebrates such as hares and hedgehogs. These animals act as *CCHFV* amplifying hosts. These infected ticks remain so through their developmental stages and mature ticks attach to large vertebrates, like cattle, to transmit infection to them.

Humans may get infected through (a) the skin (bite, contact with crushed infected ticks, infected animal blood or tissues), (b) ingestion (drinking unpasteurized milk) and (c) aerosol (suspected). Animal-to-human and human-to-human transmissions occur through the skin or mucous membrane exposed to blood or tissues, either during slaughter and processing of infected meat animals or haemorrhage/surgery in humans. Horizontal transmission from mother to child is known.

Aerosol nosocomial fatal infection in one of eight healthcare workers who were engaged in providing medical care to a patient in Russia was reported by Pshenichnaya and Nenadskaya (2015) demonstrating airborne transmission. This emphasized using standard precautionary procedure when a patient is on ventilator.

24.2.3   Spread

In general birds, with a few exceptions, seem to be refractory to infection. They may act as paratenic hosts transporting infected ticks to newer areas (Lindeborg et al. 2012). Palomar et al. (2013) observed that CCHFV circulated in north-western Africa and can be introduced to Europe by migratory birds. Trade and transport may be other means.

The seroprevalence in adult livestock is high (>50%) in endemic areas. Horses, donkeys, pigs, rhinoceroses, giraffes, buffalo and other mammalian species have been found seropositive. CCHF infection in animals is asymptomatic.

Tick bites/exposure to tick habitat results in sporadic cases. Exposure from treating/slaughter/eating infected livestock, ruminant or ostrich results in a cluster of cases. In the health facilities, exposure to blood and fomites from patients causes outbreaks.

24.2.4   Persons at Risk

Those occupationally close to animals and exposed to tick habitat, mainly rural communities comprising shepherds and animal herdsmen, veterinarians, slaughterhouse workers, healthcare workers, laboratory workers, foresters and travellers, are the persons at risk.

24.2.5   Season

CCHF is seasonal in many countries—it occurs during August–September in Iran and March–May and August to October in Pakistan.

24.3   Pathogenesis

According to Patil et al. (2020), the primary targets of CCHFV are monocyte-derived dendritic cells and macrophages. Infection of these cells induces alpha interferon response, activation of secretion of interleukin-6 and interleukin-8 and moderate chemokine response. *Dugbe* virus induced higher cytokine/chemokine response in macrophages.

There is vascular dysfunction in CCHF. It leads to haemorrhage, loss of fluid and disseminated intravascular coagulation.

24.4   Symptoms

Infection may be rarely subclinical. Mild cases do not show haemorrhages. The disease progresses through four stages, incubation, pre-haemorrhagic, haemorrhagic and convalescence.

The incubation period varies from 1 to 13 days. It depends upon the route of infection. The shortest is 1–3 days, with a maximum of 9 days through tick bite and 5–6 days or a maximum of 13 days following contact with infected blood or tissues (WHO 2013).

The onset of high fever is sudden. The pre-haemorrhagic symptoms are non-specific, which include chills, severe headache, dizziness, photophobia, neck pain, myalgia and arthralgia. Gastrointestinal form shows abdominal pain, nausea, vomiting and diarrhoea. Cardiovascular form manifests in bradycardia and low blood pressure.

Within 3–5 days of the onset of the illness, the haemorrhagic form appears suddenly and lasts for 2–3 days only. Initially, mood instability, agitation and mental confusion are present. Rash appears on the skin and mucous membranes and changes to petechiae, ecchymoses and large bruises. The patient bleeds from sites of venipuncture; haematemesis, haemoptysis, epistaxis, haematuria and melaena (bleeding from the upper bowel, passed as altered blood in the faeces) internally and in other organs, say brain. Decimated intravascular coagulation may occur. Some patients may show hepatomegaly and jaundice and splenomegaly. Death occurs after the fifth day of the illness from hepato-renal, pulmonary or cardiovascular failure.

The surviving patients show signs of recovery 10–20 days after the onset of the illness. Recovery is slow but complete, which may take a year. During convalescence, generalized weakness, weak pulse, tachycardia, laboured breathing, sweating, headache, dizziness; poor memory, vision and hearing; polyneuritis; anorexia; and total loss of hair in some are present.

24.5   Diagnosis

Cases presenting symptoms and history compatible with CCHF require laboratory confirmation:

* Virus isolation—During the first 5 days of the illness when virus concentration is high, isolation of *CCHFV* from blood, plasma, and tissues (lung, liver, spleen, kidney, brain and bone marrow on autopsy) on cell lines—SW-13, Vero, LLC-MK2 and BHK-21—is carried out in BSL4 labs.
* Newborn mice inoculation is more sensitive and can detect the virus in samples taken for a longer period.
* Detection of viral antigen by IF or EIA (immunohistochemical on tissues from fatal cases).
* Indirect IFA and antigen capture ELISA—to detect CCHF-specific IgM or rise in IgG titre; the IgM and IgG antibodies can be detected after 7–9 days of the illness. Antibody detection methods are less useful, mainly because antibodies are detectable only after 7 days and most deaths occur earlier. These tests may be useful for sero-epidemiological/retrospective studies as IgM and IgG antibodies remain detectable for 4 months and 5 years, respectively.
* RT-PCR (reverse transcription-polymerase chain reaction).
* Real-time (RT)-PCR detects viral variants, which is important in the study of epidemiology.

A combination of methods to detect viral antigen (antigen capture ELISA) and viral RNA sequence is useful for diagnosing an acute case presenting clinical history suggestive of CCHF.

24.6   Treatment

- Supportive therapy, in the form of replacement of volume and blood component.
- Ribavirin, oral or intravenous.
- Hyperimmune serum/serum from recovered patients with controversial results.
- No vaccine is available in most countries; inactivated mouse brain vaccine has been used in former USSR and Bulgaria.

24.7   Prevention

- Avoiding exposure to ticks and their bite.
- Tick repellents (containing DEET (N,N-diethyl-m-toluamide) and acaricides.
- Personal protective measures while attending cases of CCHF.
- Barrier nursing, isolation and the use of gloves, gowns, face shields and goggles with side shields.
- Ribavirin—prophylactic.
- Safe burial of dead bodies.
- Terminal disinfection.

CCHFV is sensitive to lipid solvents, boiling, autoclaving and formalin or beta-propiolactone.

Infectivity remains for few days at ambient temperature in serum.

24.8   Surveillance

CCHF is a veterinary public health problem. The animals do not become clinically ill and the infection causes no economic burden. CCHFV is amplified; viraemic livestock pose threat to the human health. The duration of viraemia in wild and domestic animals may be 2 weeks. These animals and/or ticks may be used as sentinel and may be examined for viral antigen, genome in ticks and antibodies in animal hosts. Identification of areas of vial activity is crucial for targeted preventive action.

De-ticking domestic animals reduced the risk of tick bites among animal handlers. Repellents used on animals before slaughter could reduce the infection among slaughterhouse workers (OIE 2018).

References

CDC (2013) Crimean-Congo haemorrhagic fever. https://www.cdc.gov/vhf/crimean-congo/ index. html. Page Last reviewed September 5, 2013

Knust B, Medetov ZB, Kyraubayev KB, Bumburidi Y, Erickson BR et al (2012) Crimean-Congo hemorrhagic fever, Kazakhstan, 2009–2010. Emerg Infect Dis 18(4):643–645

Lindeborg M, Barboutis C, Ehrenborg C, Fransson Jaenson TGT et al (2012) Migratory birds, ticks, and Crimean-Congo hemorrhagic fever virus. Emerg Infect Dis 18(12):2095–2097

Maltezon H, Papa A (2010) Crimean-Congo haemorrhagic fever: risk for emergence of new endemic foci in Europe? Travel Med Infect Dis 8(3):139–143

Mourya DT, Yadav PD, Gurav YK et al (2019) Crimean Congo hemorrhagic fever serosurvey in humans for identifying high-risk populations and high-risk areas in the endemic state of Gujarat, India. BMC Infect Dis 19:104

OIE (2009). Crimean_congo-hemorrhagic-fever.pdf. CCHF_H2007_2009 OIE, the Centre for Food Security and Public Health and Institute for International Cooperation in Animal Biologics

OIE (2018) OIE Terrestrial Manual 2018. Chapter 3(1):5

Palomar AM, Portillo A, Santibáñez P, Mazuelas D et al (2013) Crimean-Congo hemorrhagic fever virus in ticks from migratory birds. Morocco Emerg Infect Dis 19(2):260–263

Papa A, Tzala E, Maltezou H (2011) Crimean-Congo Haemorrhagic fever virus. Northeastern Greece Emerg Infect Dis 17(1):141–143

Patil S, Panigrahi P, Yadav MP, Pattnaik B (2020) Crimean–Congo Haemorrhagic Fever (CCHF): a zoonoses. Int J Curr Microbiol Appl Sci 9(09):3201–3210

Pshenichnaya NY, Nenadskaya SA (2015) Probable Crimean-Congo hemorrhagic fever virus transmission occurred after aerosol-generating medical procedures in Russia: nosocomial cluster. Int J Infect Dis 33:120–122

WHO (2001) World Health Organization. Communicable disease surveillance and response (CSR). Crimean-Congo haemorrhagic fever in Kosovo—update 5. http://www.who.int/csr/don/2001_06_29e/en/

WHO (2013). https://www.who.int/news-room/fact-sheets/detail/crimean-congo-haemorrhagic-fever. Accessed 31 Jan 2013

Yadav PD, Raut CG, Patil DY, Majumdar D, T, Mourya DT. (2014) Crimean-Congo hemorrhagic fever: current scenario in India. Proc Natl Acad Sci India Sect B Biol Sci 84(1):9–18

Chapter 25
Influenza Viruses: Avian and Swine Influenza

25.1 Influenza Virus: Some Basics

Influenza virus belongs to the family *Orthomyxoviridae* and genus *Influenza*. Influenza viruses are types A, B and C and cause flu in humans. Type A influenza viruses of pigs, horses and birds are important causes of seasonal, zoonotic and pandemic influenza. Seasonal influenza viruses are adapted to humans and are transmitted from human to human annually.

Influenza type A viruses are classified on the basis of combination of surface proteins, haemagglutinin (HA) and neuraminidase (NA). There are 18 different haemagglutinin subtypes and 11 different neuraminidase subtypes. Subtypes A (H17N10) and A(H18N11) are found in bats. Most others have been found in birds as low pathogenic (LP) and some high pathogenic (HP). Bird is almost a natural reservoir.

Influenza type A viruses are avian, swine and equine influenza and include zoonotic viruses. Swine flu viruses H1N1, H3N2 and H1N2 are not efficient in causing human-to-human transmission. The 'variant' viruses, e.g. A (H1N1v) and H3N2v, which originated in pigs are zoonotic and non-seasonal and infect humans through direct contact. Infected persons generally are not expected to be protected with vaccines for seasonal viruses, like H3N2. Zoonotic avian influenza viruses A (H5N1), A(H5N6), A(H7N7), A(H7N9) and A(H9N2) that originated in birds are rarely transmitted from human to human.

© Springer Nature Singapore Pte Ltd. 2024
K. G. Narayan et al., *Handbook of Management of Zoonoses*,
https://doi.org/10.1007/978-981-99-9885-2_25

25.2   Evolution

Influenza viruses circulate in animals and birds. Antigenic 'shift' and 'drift' and 'reassortment' are dynamic evolutionary phenomena. Swine, human, and/or avian-origin influenza viruses (as well as all influenza A viruses) can adapt or swap genes within a number of species, including pigs, potentially resulting in a mammalian-adapted influenza virus of public health concern.

The HPAI viruses seriously impact animal health and welfare, agricultural productivity, food security and the livelihood of poor farming communities, especially in poor and developing countries. The avian and equine viruses seriously affect the respective species. The swine viruses generally are mild. These viruses have a tendency to evolve into pandemic strains—the 1918 pandemic, H5N1 and 'A (H1N1) pdm09'.

Antigenic shift: *Swine influenza 'A(H1N1) pdm09' virus*—A new virus appeared in 2009 when H1N1 virus genes from North American swine, Eurasian swine, humans and birds emerged to infect people and caused a pandemic. Most people had little or no immunity.

Host switching: *Avian influenza virus-H5N1*—Haemagglutinin (HA) protein of avian influenza virus (AIV) binds to the receptor molecule 'sialic acids linked to galactose by *alpha-2,3 linkage*' which are located on the intestinal cells in birds. HA of human influenza virus recognizes *alpha-2,6-linked sialic acids* expressed on epithelial cells of human trachea.

For AIV to infect humans (switching of host), the HA protein is preferentially required to recognize the receptors of human influenza virus. Only limited H5N1 virus is capable of recognizing and binding to human receptor sites. Distribution of cells with receptors for AIV in different organs of humans explains the pathology in a man in zoonotic infection. Efficient human-to-human transmission seems to require additional molecular determinants.

25.3   Avian Influenza

25.3.1   The Hong Kong (H5N1) Virus (1997)

The virus H5N1 was first isolated as A/Chick/Scotland/59/H5N1 and it seems to be circulating in birds for decades. It has infected domestic, wild and migratory birds, mammals and human beings in 36 countries in Asia, Europe, Siberia, the Middle East and Africa (reviewed in 2005). In May 1997, an infant died of infection in Hong Kong. Later, the attending doctor died but had no known direct contact with chickens. Eighteen human cases with six deaths were reported. The event coincided with epidemic in a poultry in China and a mass slaughter of birds controlled it. The epidemic restarted. Two persons from Hong Kong visiting China died in February 2003 and the endemicity in ducks in southern China was realized. Bouts of fresh outbreaks started in 2003. Between 2003 and May 2020, there were 861 cases and

445 deaths reported in 17 countries (https://www.who.int/influenza/human_ animal_ interface/2020_MAY_table H5N1.pdf).

25.3.1.1 Virus

The avian H5N1 virus invades cells of the respiratory system from the nose to lungs. It binds to a type of galactose receptors that are virtually absent in human cells except in and around the alveoli. The site being deep in lungs, which can be expelled by coughing and sneezing, and consequential transmission is not easy. The virus H5N1 genotype Z emerged in 2002 through reassortment from highly pathogenic genotypes that infected birds in China in 1996 and infected humans in Hong Kong in 1997. It is endemic in birds in South East Asia, spreading in birds across the globe. Further mutations are increasing pathogenicity and transmissibility and the birds shed the virus for longer period.

25.3.1.2 Disease in Birds: Fowl Plague

The incubation period in fowl plague (fowl influenza/flu) varies from few hours to 3 days. The disease manifests in loss of appetite, reduced feed consumption and egg production and mild to severe respiratory symptoms like sneezing, coughing, lachrymation and cyanosis of combs and wattles. The case fatality rate varies between 50% and 90%.

The post-mortem lesions are very conspicuous—sinuses and trachea filled with catarrhal serofibrinous exudates; peritonitis; enteritis; petechiae on the mucosa of the trachea, inside the sternum; serosal and body cavity fat; and haemorrhage on the mucosa of the proventriculus-gizzard junction, gizzard and intestine. High case fatality rate in chicken leaves many birds dead. Surviving birds excrete the virus for 10 days orally and in faeces, thus increasing the period of risk of transmission.

Source of Infection

The virus is excreted in lachrymal secretion, faeces and nasal discharges and is aerosolized; thus, it is present in the environment. Domestic ducks can excrete large quantities of highly pathogenic virus *without showing any clinical sign of the illness*. The role of peri-domestic birds like pigeon and untreated bird faeces for fertilizer is unknown. Experimental infection in pheasants and chukar (quail) was studied by Humberd et al. (2006). The results suggested that pheasants can serve as a reservoir of influenza virus because of their continuous asymptomatic infection and longer stay in the markets. Pheasants are ideal carriers of all 15 subtypes of influenza A virus. The excreted virus is alive in their faeces for 14 days or longer. Transmission is mainly faecal-oral. Quail was less susceptible and the virus was isolated for 7 days mainly from the respiratory tract.

Bird flu transmission to human from poultry

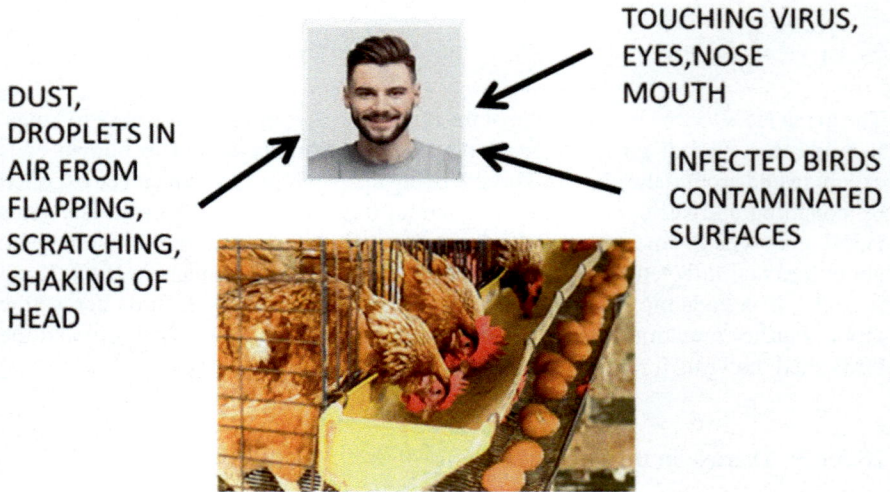

DUST, DROPLETS IN AIR FROM FLAPPING, SCRATCHING, SHAKING OF HEAD

TOUCHING VIRUS, EYES,NOSE MOUTH

INFECTED BIRDS CONTAMINATED SURFACES

Fig. 25.1 Transmission of Bird flu

Wild ducks, waterfowls and ducks are relatively resistant and considered as reservoirs. The virus survives well at low temperature and low relative humidity in aerosols. In liquid manure, it may survive for 105 days. The faecal matter may be infective for 30–35 days at 4 °C and for 7 days at 20°C. One gram of contaminated soil can infect a million birds.

Transmission and Spread

Modes of infection are oral, inhalation and direct or indirect contact. Broken contaminated eggs in incubators; movement of fomites like contaminated equipment, egg trays, feed trucks, clothing and shoes of employees; and garbage flies transmit the virus. A migratory infected bird can carry infection miles away to other flocks of wild or domesticated birds (Fig. 25.1).

25.3.1.3   Disease in Humans

Infection

H5N1 influenza appears to be a systemic infection in humans, birds and animals. Primarily lungs are infected but it may extend to other organs like the trachea, brain and intestines extending to other organs like the kidney and liver. This extra-pulmonary dissemination may be the result of viraemia or of infected immune cells transporting the virus to other organs. The interaction of host cells—H5N1 virus—at the cellular level and the resulting pathology have been discussed in detail by Korteweg and Gu (2008). The virus replicated in pneumocytes of alveolar alveoli, lymphocytes, macrophages, mononuclear cells and neurons and are demonstrated in organs like the lungs, trachea, intestine, liver, brain and placenta, foetus (vertical transmission) and body fluids such as cerebrospinal fluid, secretions, stool, serum and plasma (alerts: for handling these and possible transmission).

Pathogenesis

The epithelial cells in conjunctiva and ciliated nasal epithelial cells of human beings have receptors recognized by the avian influenza virus haemagglutinin. Replication of the H5N1 virus results in cell and organ damage either by cytolytic or apoptotic mechanisms. Highest viral loads have been detected in fatal cases. H5N1 viruses induced significantly higher expression of several cytokines and chemokines in human macrophages and respiratory epithelial cells than human influenza viruses. 'Dysregulation' of cytokines and chemokines may be one of the key mechanisms. Additional factors contributing to cell deaths and pathology may be 'up-regulation' of tumour necrosis factor-related apoptosis-inducing ligand and reduced cytotoxicity of $CD8^+$ lymphocytes.

Pathology

Uiprasertkul et al. (2005) described the pathology of H5N1 in a case. Autopsy showed interstitial pneumonia and proliferative, diffuse alveolar damage; pneumocytes showed reactive hyperplasia without cytopathy, focal haemorrhage and bronchitis. Lesions in lymph nodes and the spleen and bone marrow hyperplasia; the brain had oedema and small foci of necrosis. H5-specific RNA was detected in the lung, spleen and small and large intestines by RT-PCR. Immunohistochemical analysis detected virus antigen-positive alveoli-lining cells. Pneumocyte type II was infected (Fig. 25.2).

25.3.1.4 Symptoms

The avian influenza (H5N1) virus causes a more aggressive, rapidly deteriorating (3–5 days in Turkey, 6 days in Thailand) disease causing failure of multiple organs—notably the kidney and heart—usually ending fatally. Most cases were observed in healthy young and adults. The incubation period may be 2–8 days or longer up to 17 days, compared to 2–3 days for ordinary flu. Initial symptoms include a high fever (> 38 °C) and influenza-like symptoms affecting the lower respiratory tract, chest pain, diarrhoea, vomiting, abdominal pain and bleeding of the nose and gums

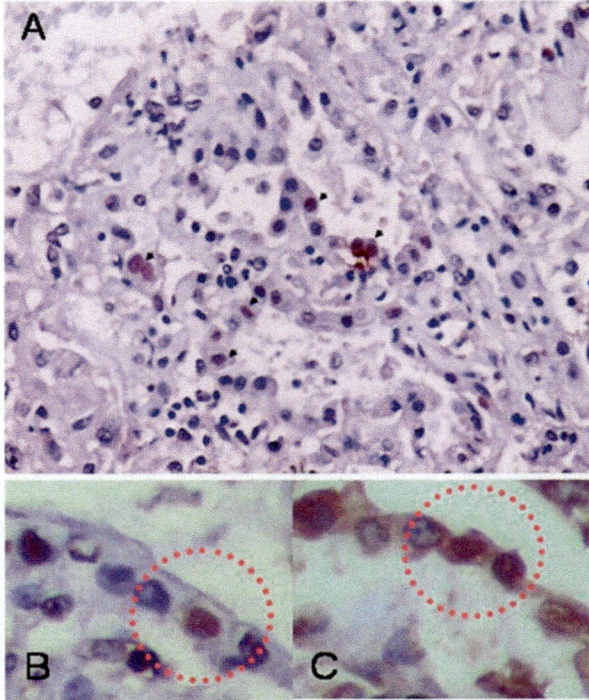

Fig. 25.2 Immunohistochemical analysis [Source: Uiprasertkul et al. (2005)]

in some patients. Watery diarrhoea without blood with or without respiratory symptoms and difficulty in breathing develop around 5 days following the first symptoms. Respiratory distress, a hoarse voice and a crackling sound when inhaling are also commonly seen. Sputum production is variable and sometimes bloody. Acute encephalitis without respiratory symptoms was seen in two Vietnamese patients. Common laboratory abnormalities include lymphopenia, leukopenia, elevated aminotransferases and mild-to-moderate thrombocytopenia with some instances of disseminated intravascular coagulation.

25.3.1.5 Epidemiology

Migrating waterfowls like wild ducks, geese, gulls, shore birds and swan naturally carry H5N1 without falling sick. Incidence is highest among juveniles and in fall of the year. The virus probably spilled from the natural reservoirs over to domestic ducks. The 1997 epizootic in birds in Hong Kong coincided with human infections; the virus possibly jumped directly from poultry. Humans may get also infected indirectly from surfaces contaminated with poultry excreta or fertilizer dust. Culling of poultry prevented panzootic but the virus continued spreading to cause outbreaks in

2003. The genotype Z of H5N1 emerged in 2002 and caused a pandemic. Migratory birds, movement of infected poultry, poultry products, poultry manure, contaminated feed and equipment spread the infection. The virus survives even when temperature is low. Several domestic species, including cats, dogs, ferrets, pigs, and birds, have been infected with and have shown symptoms of H5N1 viral infection. The pandemic impacted the economy seriously. Over 50 million birds had to be killed in Vietnam only. Economic loss in South East Asia was estimated to be around US$ 10 billion. Backyard poultry is labour intensive, employed women and is livelihood for many—all seriously affected. Trade and export temporarily reduced. It resulted in loss of protein in diets (20% came from poultry) and consumers' confidence. Backyard poultry—raised under extensive conditions free range between multiple households—were frequently impacted in the early part of the pandemic. Intensively raised commercial flocks of homogeneous stock with poor biosecurity were later found to pose a threat, which contributed for the virus to spread fast and wide.

A number of migratory birds died, *bar-headed geese*, Pallas's (great black-headed) gull (*Larus ichthyaetus*), brown-headed gull (*L. brunnicephalus*), ruddy shelduck (*Tadorna ferruginea*), great cormorant (*Phalacrocorax carbo*), swan and flamingo, in which the infection is possibly picked from domestic birds. Infection was detected among birds in international trade or/smuggled birds.

Domestic cats, tigers and leopards are infected, suffered and died. Horizontal transmission was evidenced (Keawcharoen et al. 2004). This finding has important implications for wildlife conservation and influenza virus epidemiology. First, H5N1 virus infection may threaten the survival of endangered felids. There is no evidence that domestic cats are reservoirs or can play a part in the transmission, nor there is any report of human case linked to cats (Rimmelzwaan et al. 2006).

25.3.1.6 Control and Eradication

Control

Vaccination with H5N2—This was done in 2002 in Hong Kong and in 2004 in some South East Asian countries, the People's Republic of China, Indonesia, El Salvador, Guatemala, Mexico and the United States. The advantages are (a) protection from low to high grade of challenge exposure, (b) protection from diverse field viruses within the same HA subtype, (c) increases resistance, (d) reduction of virus shedding and (e) reduction of contact transmission. The method of vaccination, DIVA (differentiating between vaccinated and infected animals) and other complimentary measures and strong scientific support to poultry farmers is useful. *(DIVA: (a) leaving sentinel birds unvaccinated in each flock and monitor these for possible infection with the field virus (in this case H5N1) and (b) monitoring vaccinated birds for infection with the field virus. The test used is neuraminidase inhibition.)*

The disadvantage is that the virus is still capable of infecting and replicating in the vaccinated.

International organizations agreed upon generic protocol for early detection, containment and eradication as 'any human case apart from serious disease represents potential for virus reassortment that could produce a variant transmissible between humans'. All cases of HPAI found in any domestic or wild bird must be notified to the OIE by the country's competent authorities (veterinary services). Low pathogenic AI viruses of subtypes H5 and H7 in poultry are also notifiable because they have the potential to mutate readily into highly pathogenic viruses or to infect other species (OIE *Terrestrial Animal Health Code*).

Eradication

Two approaches are the following:
Culling infected and contact animals is normally used to rapidly contain, control and eradicate the disease. Restocking is permitted 21 days after eradication. Requirements are described in the OIE *Terrestrial Animal Health Code*. Detecting outbreaks and stamping out are applied at the level of the infected farm or within a short radius around the infected premises in conjunction with active surveillance.

Vaccination can be implemented when culling policies alone cannot be applied in situations like endemicity and infection is widespread or detection in animals is very difficult. Policies and recommendations from the World Organisation for Animal Health (OIE) and the OIE-FAO network of expertise on animal influenza (OFFLU) on vaccinations and vaccines must be closely followed.

Early detection was very important. Participatory epidemiology—training farmers/people to report was economical and useful. A generic biosecurity protocol is available.

Epidemiology of bird flu in Mekong sub-region (GMS) and its control reviewed by Pfeiffer et al. (2012) present a comparison of the two protocols. The H5HPAI outbreak impacted direct loss to producers and all connected with poultry production and marketing, cost of disease and deaths in poultry, restarting farming, etc. The basic reproduction rate (R_0) ranged between 2 and 5 in Thailand. Spatial cluster analysis defined hotspots in the Red and Mekong river deltas that sustained transmission. Live markets drew a variety of birds from different sources, as if a farm/cluster of birds with low biosecurity, posing a high risk of exposure among producer, handlers and buyers. Transmissibility from poultry to human is low, but mortality is very high. Thailand and Vietnam had 2000 and 3000 outbreaks, respectively, in 2004, which reduced to 200 and 2000, respectively, in 2005. There were 59/119 (deaths/cases) in Vietnam between 2003 and 2011, 17/25 in Thailand and 16/18 in Cambodia.

Containment, control and eradication started.

Thailand is one of the largest poultry meat producers in the world. Thailand adhered closely to the recommendations of FAO, WHO and OIE disease containment policy: culled all susceptible birds in and around 5 km of the epicentre, paid compensation, restricted movement within 50 km and banned export of poultry for 90 days from affected areas. Reduction in outbreaks began from mid-2004; any outbreak was dealt with culling of birds within 1 km radius. Active surveillance using diagnostic support covered samples from farms, movement and markets of birds. Disease-free compartments were made surrounding industrial poultry farms. *Intensive surveillance in a 2 km buffer zone around the compartmentalized farms* and other measures is a part of biosecurity protocol. This procedure appeared to eliminate infection and prevent outbreaks.

Vietnam resorted to a wide range of control measures, large-scale culling (1 km ring culling), closure of live poultry markets, education, etc., which was very expensive. Then it began targeting culling of birds immediately adjacent to infected farms and later extended this in some areas. *Comprehensive nationwide vaccination* was adopted from 2005. It reduced R_0 within the flock significantly, but not <1 suggesting coverage less than the desired. Vaccination prevented outbreaks for 12 months and a human case for 18 months in Vietnam. Cambodia used culling within 3 km (protection zone) and 10 km surveillance zone (Pfeiffer et al. 2012).

Factors that may cause vaccine failure may be insufficient dose, concurrent immunosuppression in population, antigenic variants and poor antigenic match with existing vaccine. H5HPAI has diversified into multiple clades. Agro-ecological conditions, mobile free-ranging ducks, low biosecurity of backyard/small-scale production and poor bio-secure live bird market contribute to the emergence of clades (Nguyen et al. 2019).

Vaccines for humans are not available for civilians but stockpiled for emergency.

25.3.2 Avian Influenza H7N9 Virus

(H7N9_5NOV2013_WHO.pdf (Avian influenza Response: an investment in Public Health Preparedness)

25.3.2.1 Evolution of H7N9 Subtype

H7N9 is a subgroup of H7 viruses earlier isolated only from birds and caused outbreaks in the Netherlands, the United States and Japan. Avian influenza A H7 viruses in humans are uncommon and are restricted to those having direct contact with infected birds, manifesting mild conjunctivitis and upper respiratory symptoms. The human strain is a result of recombination of genes between several parent viruses noted in poultry ducks and wild birds in Asia and has not acquired a genetic sequence allowing a sustained efficient transmission in humans.

25.3.2.2 Outbreak

The first report was of pneumonia of unknown aetiology in an 87-year-old man and his two sons, later laboratory confirmed as H7N9. The Shanghai CDC, China, sent the respiratory samples for laboratory examination on 24 March 2013. Four family

Total reported cases

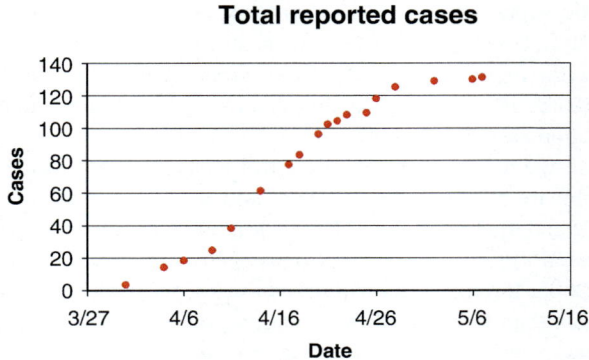

Fig. 25.3 Outbreak of H7N9 strain of avian influenza in human

clusters were identified. The median age of cases was 62 years (range: 2–91 years). The majority of cases (73%, 97/133) were male and 54% (71/132) were aged 60 years or older. Case fatality proportion was 32%. The strain of the H7N9 virus found on pigeons was highly congenic with those found on persons infected with H7N9 virus.

H7N9 influenza virus infection in humans appears to be a directly transmitted infection from pigeon, ducks and poultry in poultry market or farm. The disease appeared in China and has been reported from Shanghai, Beijing and five other provinces. No human-to-human transmission has occurred. It has caused 22 deaths and 109 laboratory confirmed cases (April 2013). Generally, a mixture of mammal and bird flu hybrid is likely to be milder than pure bird flu strains [Human infection with avian influenza A (H7N9) virus—update http://www.who.int/csr/don/2013_04_25/en/index.html?goback=%2Eanb_1503767_*2_*1_*1_*1_*1_*1]. The number of cases declined by the end of May 2013. The last cases were reported on 29 May. The total number of cases reached 132, with 37 deaths, and covered the two municipalities and eight provinces in China (Fig. 25.3). One case was reported from Taipei's Centre for Disease Control, Taiwan, China.

The outbreak caused a loss of $2.7 billion.

Investigation of the Outbreak

Three surveillance systems were used.

*Event-based surveillanc*e detected H7N9. Information about events that are potential risk to public health is captured in an organized manner. Daily monitoring of acute public health events by screening media revealed that Shanghai authority had reported an unusual event of a family cluster of cases of severe acute pneumonia of unknown aetiology.

Indicator-based surveillance collected data from healthcare provider. Data are routinely collected on predefined diseases (influenza-like illness). This helped in generating baseline data, assessing risk and no sustained human-to-human transmission. Majority (2/3) of patients were aged ≥50 years.

Individual case-based surveillance: Epidemiological relationship was sought. Spread was related with movement of live poultry.

Action by the Health Ministry of Shanghai:

• Culling of birds at the Huhuai wholesale agricultural products market in Songjiang District on 4 and 6 April 2013,
• Temporary closure of live poultry trading zones in Hangzhou, Minhang and Shanghai.
• Awareness about the spread of avian influenza.

25.4 Swine Influenza Pandemic Variants

First detected in April 2009, pH1N1 (2009) infections were reported in several species of animals, particularly pigs, and in almost all cases, it was linked to exposure to infected humans. WHO declared on 11 June 2009 that a pandemic was underway and on 10 August 2010 it ended and took the features of seasonal flu. Available seasonal influenza vaccines are protective. The virus continues to be circulating in pigs and endemic in some herds. '(H1N1) 2009 pandemic' refers to the event and 'A(H1N1) pdm09' to the name of the virus. The pandemic caused an estimated number of cases of 700 million to 1.4 billion and 284,000 deaths. This is primarily a human infection, transmitted from human to human. Animals have no significant epidemiological role and do not appear to impact animal health. Therefore, culling of pigs and trade restrictions are not warranted.

25.4.1 Swine Influenza Virus (SIV)

Swine influenza is a respiratory disease of pigs characterized by fever, depression, cough, off feed, sneeze, tachypnoea and laboured abdominal breathing and discharge from the nose and eyes. Mild infection may go unnoticed. Once introduced in a pig farm, it spreads rapidly affecting almost all, i.e. 100% morbidity. Mortality rate is low. Uncomplicated cases recover rapidly. Co-infection with either bacteria or viruses causes complication. The impact is low: reduced reproductive performance or may be abortion and reduced weight gain. Swine influenza is endemic in North and South America, Europe and Asia. The common influenza A virus subtypes affecting swine are H1N1, H1N2 and H3N2. Transmission among pigs continues round the year, but outbreaks occur with beginning of winter.

25.4.2   SIV Variants: Human

Human infection is caused by 'variants'—H1N1v, H3N2v and H1N2v. Limited human-to-human transmission has occurred with the variant (v) strains. Children may get infection when exposed in pig fair. Exposure to sick pigs may result in more people falling sick. Modes of infection are *direct contact*—touching contaminated surface and then the mouth, nose and eyes, *aerosol* (from cough and sneezes of pigs) and inhalation of drop and droplets.

Sickness manifests as fever, loss of appetite, malaise, eye irritation, coughing, sore throat and nasal discharge. Patient may also show nausea, vomiting and diarrhoea. Severe cases showed rapid deterioration around 3–5 days of onset, progressing to respiratory failure within 24 h. Immediate transfer to ICU for respiratory support/mechanical ventilation is required.

The virus is shed during 4–5 days post illness and respiratory specimen is good for diagnosis. Shedding of the virus may be longer especially in children. Recommended drugs for treatment are oseltamivir, peramivir, zanamivir and baloxavir.

25.4.3   Swine Influenza a (H3N2)

This is a novel virus isolated from pigs in 2010 and from humans in July 2011.The transmission from person to person is not easy (CDC's Dr. Joseph Bresee). A lot of very close contact with pigs over relatively long period have led to infection, mostly in children engaged in exhibiting or helping to exhibit pigs, such as fairs and markets.

According to the weekly influenza surveillance report of the Influenza Division, CDC (http://www.cdc.gov/flu/weekly/), 288 H3N2 infections that spread in ten states were recorded from July to 30 August 2012. Of these, 15 had to be hospitalized and one died. Three instances of person-to-person transmission were identified, two living in the same household, each linked to exposure to pigs at an agricultural fair. Illness associated with this virus so far continues to be mostly mild with symptoms similar to seasonal flu. Serious illness with H3N2v infection is possible like in seasonal flu. Those aged <5 (specially 2 years) and > 65 years and suffering from underlying health conditions like pregnancy, chronic diseases like asthma, heart diseases, weak immune system, neurological or neuro-developmental conditions and diabetes stand at high risk. They need to avoid exposure to/contact with pigs as 90% of cases had exposure to pigs. Transmission from pigs to people and people to pigs occurs but not through eating pork. However, no community transmission has been observed.

The H3N2v virus is susceptible to the influenza antiviral drugs oseltamivir (Tamiflu®) and zanamivir (Relenza®).

25.5   Epidemiology, Diagnosis and Prevention

Pandemic avian influenza H5N1 and other pandemics lead to international initiatives.

FAO, OIE, WHO and UNICEF in collaboration with the United Nations System Influenza Coordinator (UNSIC) and the World Bank (2008) developed a joint strategy addressing risks associated with emerging and re-emerging infectious diseases. The concept of One Health was born and strategies are developed to tackle the continuing influenza virus H5N1 followed by pH1N1, Mexico (2009). 'One Flu' has been identified as an example and a model for the 'One Health' approach (ISIRV 2011).

Accordingly, the animal health sector monitors influenza viruses in animals and birds and analyses and shares data/information with public health and other related agencies. Two major sub-agencies should devote respectively to the following areas:

(a) *Surveillance*—for early detection of animal and bird disease, allowing rapid containment and/or control in affected populations. This included epidemiology, detection of reservoirs and study risk factors, assessment of immune response to vaccination and detection of infected animals in vaccinated population.
(b) *Antigenic analysis* to detect 'drift' or 'shift'—sharing data with the public health sector to detect viruses circulating simultaneously in humans and animals so as to detect potential emerging human pandemic virus and match the field and vaccine strains to contribute to new vaccine preparation and relevant diagnostic reagent.

The document (OIE, FAO 2011) outlines surveillance of swine influenza viruses at *the animal-human interface* to check for 'antigenic shift' and 'genetic reassortment' leading to emergence of potential pandemic virus. Pigs are susceptible to avian, human and swine influenza viruses. This susceptibility has the potential to induce an antigenic shift which can produce potential pandemic strains. Pigs can be infected with A (H5N1) virus. Pigs would be then an ideal mixing vessel for emergence of avian/mammalian novel virus with pandemic potential.

25.5.1   Animal Health

- Epidemiology of endemic and emerging SIV—altering risks to animal and human health.
- Detection of genetic and antigenic evolution/reassortment of genomes from H1N1 and other endemic SIV. Methods to use include *serology*, HAI and NA (neutralizing antibody) titres and antigen detection, *virus isolation* and *genetic*, RT-PCR and sequencing. The non-subtypeable virus is considered potentially new and emerging. Reference laboratory has to be approached.
- Selection of isolates for relevant diagnostic reagent and vaccine.

25.5.2 Public Health

- Identification of new and emerging SIV for human and risk assessment on time.
- Assessment of reassortment and mutation events in pigs and other animals that might signal a public health concern.
- Monitoring of important molecular markers of resistance to antiviral drugs and pathogenicity.
- Preparedness for pandemic—stocking vaccines/vaccine seed stock, diagnostic reagent, etc.

During the pandemic, occasional cases of infection in turkeys occurred. Attempts to experimentally infect poultry including turkeys through respiratory route with pH1N1 failed. Quails were infected but onward transmission failed. There is no evidence of natural circulation in turkeys or endemicity.

25.5.3 Targeted Surveillance

It is an efficient way of detecting active influenza infection.
It should be carried in any of the following:

- Herds identified with cases (conforming definition)/with serological evidences/ vaccinated swine herds/farms.
- Population with *acute outbreaks of respiratory illness or illness in unexpected age/having* epidemiological link to or contact with known infected animals/ herds/caretakers or contact with human or animals showing ILI (influenza-like illness).
- Age targeted population: 8–12 weeks when maternal antibodies are waning; animals may be shedding virus without manifesting any sign and symptom of illness.

A combination of all or some of these may be used as a customized approach. Choice depends upon geographic disease history, swine management practices and resources available.

25.5.4 Sampling and Sampling Protocol

Nasal swab from symptomatic cases (consistent with ILI/fever) and pen-mates— tracheal swab and pieces of the lung from post-mortem/sacrificed pigs/slaughterhouse, following guidelines on handling, preservation and transport of samples to diagnostic laboratory.

Basic information for epidemiological interpretation is required to be collected—location/demography, association with suspected ILI in humans or other animals, birds, etc.

Sharing data/receiving response from veterinary service provider, stakeholder, human health/public health service provider, etc.

Wider/relevant scientific institution and community in case new or emerging subtype/a variant associated with significant morbidity or mortality or a virus with zoonotic potential is detected (*OIE Terrestrial Animal Health Code*).

25.5.5 Risk Communication

A joint veterinary and public health risk communication strategy needs to be developed for a rapid and coordinated response. It should maintain a level of awareness among key stakeholders and general public without creating any panic and adverse consequences to pork producers.

25.5.6 Response

Endemic swine influenza is not a notifiable disease. Any response should be decided in proportion to the risk and considering scientific principles of influenza infection. Accordingly, culling is not recommended. General principle such as no ill pigs should be shipped for slaughter, recovered and healthy ones can be sent for slaughter and as a part of good biosecurity practices, temporary restriction on movement of pigs may be implemented.

References

Humberd J, Yi G, Webster RG (2006) Comparison of the replication of influenza a viruses in Chinese ring-necked pheasants and Chukar partridges. J Virol 80(5):2151–2161

ISIRV (2011) Isirv_Respiratory_Virus_Rep_Summer_2011.pdf. International Society for Influenza and other Respiratory Virus Diseases –Respiratory Virus Report Summer 2011

Keawcharoen J, Oraveerakul K, Kuiken T, Fouchier RAM, Amonsin A et al (2004) Avian influenza H5N1 in tigers and leopards. Emerg Infect Dis s(12):2189–2191

Korteweg C, Gu J (2008) Pathology, molecular biology, and pathogenesis of avian influenza a (H5N1) infection in humans. Am J Pathol 172(5):1155–1170

Nguyen LT, Firestone SM, Stevenson MA et al (2019) A systematic study towards evolutionary and epidemiological dynamics of currently predominant H5 highly pathogenic avian influenza viruses in Vietnam. Sci Rep 9(1):7723

OIE, FAO (2011) OFFLUsurveillancepH1N1_180110.pdf (OFFLUsurveillancepH1N1_180110. pdf Contact OFFLU Secretariat at secretariat@offlu.net OFFLU strategy document for surveillance and monitoring of influenzas in animals; OIE FAO

Pfeiffer DU et al (2012) A one health perspective on HPAI H5N1 in the greater Mekong sub-region. Comp Immunol Microbiol Infect Dis 36(3):309–319. https://doi.org/10.1016/j.cimid.2012.11.005

Rimmelzwaan GF, van Riel D, Baars M, Bestebroer TM, van Amerongen G et al (2006) Influenza A virus (H5N1) infection in cats causes systemic disease with potential novel routes of virus spread within and between hosts. Am J Pathol 168:176–183

Uiprasertkul M, Puthavathana P, Sangsiriwut K, Pooruk P, Srisook K et al (2005) Influenza a H5N1 replication sites in humans. Emerg Infect Dis 11(7):1036–1041

Chapter 26
Bat-Borne Viral Zoonoses

There are over 1300 species of bats, making up about 20% of the biodiversity of mammalian species, only second to rodents. More than 70% are insectivorous. These fall under two suborders, *Micro*—and *Megachiroptera* under the order Chiroptera, which represent biologically and ecologically diverse species with global distribution. *Microchiroptera* have 963 widely diverse species and are widely spread in the tropics. These are largely insectivorous; some have diverse diets. *Megachiroptera* have 187 species and are Old World bats, with the exception of 1 species; do not echo-locate; are larger in size, commonly 'fruit bats'; and eat fruits and nectar. These occur in tropical and subtropical regions of the Old World, from eastern Mediterranean and Arabian Peninsula across Africa to Asia, Australia and the islands in the Pacific. Of the mammals, bats are the second most widespread order of mammals, only next to primates.

Bats are useful in many ways. These regulate the population of insects (natures' pest control); disperse seeds and pollinate over large areas, thus supporting vegetative habitats and nutrients (bat meat); regenerate cleared areas; and help maintain forests (guano as fertilizer).

26.1 Bat—Natural Reservoir of Virus

A widely diverse group of viruses are associated with bats, referred to as bat virome. (https://en.wikipedia.org/wiki/Bat_virome). Certain unique life traits make bats a natural reservoir of viruses.

Longevity varies greatly with species. Small rodents live in the wild for about 1–2 years. A similar body sized bat can live for over 30 years.

High longevity is conducive for replication and multiple, horizontal and vertical transmission through several generations. Bats are capable of asymptomatically harbouring and disseminating a wide array of highly pathogenic viruses. The

© Springer Nature Singapore Pte Ltd. 2024
K. G. Narayan et al., *Handbook of Management of Zoonoses*,
https://doi.org/10.1007/978-981-99-9885-2_26

immune system of bats lacks several inflammasomes naturally enabling the pathogens to invade and settle down. The inflammasomes activate other mammals' inflammatory response and interferon stimulator genes to fight out invading pathogens. Viruses survive and the source of infection persists for long. Maternity and maternity colonies favour amplification of viruses. Female aggregates may be in few millions. There is increased viral transmission and circulation in the young susceptible population. Majority of bats show cycle of summer maternity roost and winter hibernacula in the temperate zone. Their immune system is affected. These affect bats' density and host contact and transmission of infection. Seasonality in the prevalence of rabies (RABV), coronavirus and astrovirus has been observed. Reproduction season and type of roosts affect RABV exposure in the case of *Tadarida brasiliensis*. Cave colonies harbour millions, mostly actively reproducing female bats, nearly doubling the population after reproduction. Transmission of RABV increases because contact between adult and newborn increases during early lactation. George et al. (2011) observed that the perpetuation of RABV in brown bats (*Eptesicus focus*) was affected by the timing of the annual birth pulse and the prolonged incubation period of RABV due to torpor. RABV perpetuated throughout the hibernation period. Infection and mortality reduced till crop of susceptible population from annual birth pulse was available to continue the cycle. It was seasonal in temperate Colorado. It could be different in warm temperate and tropical areas. Roosting in manmade structures increased opportunities for contact with humans and exposure for infection by aerosol and contact with saliva, urine and excreta. In caves a large number of bats co-roost throughout the year. The assemblages, social behaviour, mating, grooming and fighting facilitate high rates of intra—and inter-species transmission of viruses. They can travel long distances 10–15 km, *Microchiroptera* venturing up to 80 km, while *Megachiroptera* 87.5 km from their day roost during foraging. Migration offers opportunity for a long-distance dissemination of virus (e.g. the *Egyptian rousette* has been recorded to migrate as far as 500 km in South Africa) spreading infection to other animal species. Echolocation represents a sneeze and expulsion of droplets of oropharyngeal fluids, mucus or saliva that could act as a mechanism of virus shedding and spread. Partially eaten fruits, insects and droppings on the ground indicate the items they eat and may also be linked to emerging zoonotic viruses.

Heterothermy in some species and torpor (reducing rate of replication of pathogens and increasing length of incubation period) help overwintering of pathogens in bats. Hibernation and torpor are hypothesized to aid in viral persistence and subsequent viral reactivation due to decreased metabolic and immunological activity. Climate change may influence the distribution of bat species and viruses.

Bats are a reservoir of viruses and harbour them without any clinical signs and symptoms. It appears that bats have developed an ability to co-exist with a number of viruses over millennium through evolution, many of which are highly pathogenic to other mammals including man. Anthropogenic activities provide opportunities for the spillover events leading to deadly epidemics such as Nipah.

According to Moratelli and Calisher (2015) one cannot yet confidently link bats with emerging zoonoses. Over 200 viruses have been detected in bats including some deadly zoonotic. The connection between bats, bat viruses and human diseases is speculative in most cases although bats have been proven competent hosts for few zoonotic viruses.

26.2 Bat as Reservoir of Zoonotic Pathogens

About 9.8% or 108 species of bats act as reservoir of zoonotic agents. The hotspots appear to be located in Central and South America (wet regions east of Chile, north of Paraguay and Uruguay), South Brazil, Southeast Asia and Equatorial Africa and the pattern of bat biodiversity is generally consistent. In many ways, bats act as a perfect reservoir for emerging zoonotic pathogens. Often, they are found in large colonies or roosts and travel long distances to spread and disseminate zoonotic viruses over large areas besides their remarkable longevity. Anthropogenic activities provide increased opportunities for their interaction with livestock and man, thereby resulting in the spillover and transmission of viruses. Because of this, bats represent a potential source of emerging infectious diseases.

26.3 Searching Association of bat Viruses with Disease

Calisher et al. (2006) report 66 viruses that have been isolated from or detected in the tissues of 74 species of bats—some single species and 1 from as many as 14 species. Literature hunt seeking for the association of bat viruses with disease in animals and human led to arranging these into following groups:

1. Bat viruses—with no known history of transmission to wildlife and/or human (Table 26.1).
2. Bat viruses—evidence of transmission and expanding range of hosts and disease (Table 26.2).
3. Bat viruses—emerging infectious diseases.

Virus may take either of the two routes from reservoir bats—*spillover* or via *intermediate host*. Intermediate hosts harbour the pathogen only for a short transition period or a system 'reservoir>intermediate host>host'. Hosts retain the spilled-over virus and disseminate. Man may get infected from either of the sources through bite or contact with aerosolized saliva and excreta.

26.3.1 Viruses with no Known History of Association with Disease

Table 26.1 lists 36 viruses with no known history of transmission from bats. Inoculation into laboratory animals like mice, rats and monkeys established five bat viruses as potential pathogens, again without known history of natural transmission

Table 26.1 Viruses have been isolated/detected in bats but with no history of transmission to either wildlife or human and some proving pathogens (Source: Calisher et al. 2006; Moratelli and Calisher 2015; Blitvich and Firth 2017) and others like virus (https://wwwn.cdc.gov/arbocat/VirusDetails.aspx?ID=328&SID=5) (https://en.wikipedia.org/wiki/Bat_virome)

Virus	Bat species	Suggested potential pathogen
Flaviviruses with no known vector Batu cave virus	*Cynopterus brachyotis* (lesser short-nose fruit bat), *Eonycteris spelaea* (dawn bat)	
Flavivirus—Rio Bravo	Mexican free-tailed bat (*T. brasiliensis mexicana*)	
Cuevavirus—Lloviu	Little collared fruit bat (*Myonycteris torquata*) Schreiber's long-fingered bat (*Miniopterus schreibersii*)	
Bat adenovirus 2	Common pipistrelle (*Pipistrellus pipistrellus*)	
BtAdV 4	Leschenault's rousette (*Rousettus leschenaultii*)	
Mamastroviruses	Many genera and species	
Ryukyu	Ryukyu flying fox (*Pteropus dasymallus yayeyamae*)	
Hantavirus—-Araraquara	Tailed tailless bat (*Anoura caudifer*). Hairy-legged vampire bat (*Diphylla ecaudata*)	
Hantaan	Common serotine (*Eptesicus serotinus*)	
Huangpi	Japanese pipistrelle (*Pipistrellus abramus*)	
Longquan	Horseshoe bats (*Rhinolophus affinis, Rhinolophus sinicus, Rhinolophus monoceros*)	
Magboi	Hairy slit-faced bat (*Nycteris hispida*)	
Mouyassué	Banana pipistrelle (*Neoromicia nanus*)	
Xuan son	Pomona leaf-nosed bat (*Hipposideros pomona*)	
Bukalasa bat virus	*Chaerephon pumilus* (little free-tailed bat), *Tadarida (mops) condylurus* (Angolan free-tailed bat)	
Carey Island virus	*Cynopterus brachyotis* (lesser short-nosed fruit bat), *Macroglossus lagochilus* (lesser long-tongued fruit bat)	
Montana myotis leukoencephalitis virus	*Myotis lucifugus* (little brown bat)	
Phnom Penh bat virus	*Cynopterus brachyotis* (lesser short-nosed fruit bat), *Eonycteris spelaea* (dawn bat)	
Sokoluk virus	*Pipistrellus* spp. bats, *Argasidae* spp. ticks	
Yokose virus	*Miniopterus fuliginosus* (eastern bent-winged bat)	

Table 26.1 (continued)

Virus	Bat species	Suggested potential pathogen
Picornaviridae, genus undetermined Juruaca virus	Unidentified bat	
Mount Elgon bat virus	*Rhinolophus hildebrandtii eloquens*	
Mojui dos Campos virus	Unidentified bat	
Yogue virus	*Rousettus aegyptiacus* (Egyptian rousette)	
Agua Preta virus	*Carollia subrufa* (grey short-tailed bat)	
Parixa virus	*Lonchophylla thomasi* (Thmams's nectar bat)	
Pulao virus	*Pteropus hypomelanus* (variable flying fox)	
Fomede virus	*Nycteris nana* (dwarf slit-faced bat) *Nycteris gambiensis* (Gambian slit-faced bat)	
Genus *Orthoreovirus*— Nelson Bay virus	*Pteropus poliocephalus* (grey-headed flying fox)	
Toscana virus	*Pipistrellus kuhlii* (Kuhl's pipistrelle)	
Genus unassigned Kaeng Khoi virus	*Chaerephon plicatus* (wrinkle-lipped free-tailed bat)	
Bangui virus	*Scotophilus* sp., *Pipistrellus* sp., *Tadarida* sp.	
Reoviridae, genus Orbivirus Ife virus	*Eidolon helvum* (straw-coloured fruit bat)	
Japanaut virus	*Syconycteris australis* (southern blossom bat)	
Aravan lyssa virus (non-rabies virus)	*Myotis blythii* (lesser mouse-eared bat)	
Khujand lyssavirus non-rabies virus	*Myotis mystacinus* (whiskered bat)	
Kern canyon virus	*Myotis yumanensis* (Yuma bat)	
Potential pathogens—experimentally		
Uganda S virus Mosquitoes—*Aedes* spp. may be vector	*Rousettus* spp., *Tadarida* spp.	Neurotropic in experimental mice
Oita rhabdovirus *296/1972).* Zoonotic potential	*Rhinolophus cornutus* (little Japanese horse shoe bat)	Experimentally lethal encephalitis in mice. Mice susceptible until 3 weeks of age
Mapuera virus	*Sturnira lilium* (yellow epauletted bat)	Fatal intracranial infections of mice
Entebbe bat virus	*Chaerephon (Tadarida) pumilus* (little free-tailed bat)	i/c adult mice—ill
Tamana bat virus	*Pteronotus parnellii* (Parnell's mustached bat)	s/c white-faced capuchin monkey—ill. i/c—killed mice, rat

Bat viruses have been so arranged in the table to present an 'expanding range of hosts of bat viruses', although it may not be so. Table 26.2 lists 37 bat viruses. It appears viruses are seeking hosts other than bats. The first three viruses Rio Bravo, Dakar and Sosuga appear to have directly been transferred to human to cause disease. The two Jugra and Saboya viruses (in Table 26.2) infected mosquitoes and mouse, respectively. The host range seems expanding as the reader proceeds further in the table. The table lists viral infections and disease in wildlife, vectors and vertebrates including human. For example, genotype 1 rabies virus, the type species of the genus and the vampire bat variant confined to Latin America are the significant veterinary and public health problems. Major natural hosts are carnivores, dogs, foxes, mongoose, skunks, etc., and vampire bats, *Desmodus rotundus*, for genotype 1, and insectivore such as shrews for Mokola. Bats are major natural hosts of all but Mokola lyssaviruses. Bat lyssaviruses, EBLV 1 and 2 and ABLV rarely cause rabies in animals and humans, except the vampire bat variant. In the USA, insectivorous bat bite-associated rabies deaths are recorded to be 1–4 per year.

Table 26.2 Bat viruses, evidence of transmission and expanding range of hosts (Source: Calisher et al. 2006; Moratelli and Calisher 2015; Blitvich and Firth 2017) and others like virus (https://wwwn.cdc.gov/arbocat/VirusDetails.aspx?ID=328&SID=5)

Virus	Bat species	Intermediate host	Human infection
Rio Bravo virus	*Eptesicus fuscus* (big brown bat), *Molossus rufus* (black mastiff bat), *Tadarida brasiliensis mexicana* (Mexican free-tailed bat)	Mice—Paralysis on i/c inoculation	Febrile, CNS involvement
Dakar bat virus	*Chaerephon pumilus* (little free-tailed bat), *Scotophilus nigrita* (giant house bat), *Tadarida (mops) condylurus* (Angolan free-tailed bat), *Taphozous perforatus* (Egyptian tomb bat)		Febrile illness, lymphadenopathy, orchitis/oophoritis, CNS involvement
Sosuga virus, a paramyxovirus	Egyptian rousette bats Amman et al. (2015)		Severe non-fatal febrile disease in a field biologist
Jugra	*Cynopterus brachyotis* (lesser short-nosed fruit bat)	Mosquitoes	
Saboya	*Nycteris gambiensis* (Gambian slit-faced bat), isolated from blood of gerbil	House mouse	
Catu virus	*Molossus obscurus*; possibly *Molossus currentium* (Thomas's Mastiff bat)	Mouse, rodents	Fever, myalgia, headache

Table 26.2 (continued)

Virus	Bat species	Intermediate host	Human infection
Guama virus	Unidentified	Mosquitoes, wild animals, non-human primates, wild rodents, mice and mosquitoes	Febrile illness, myalgia, headache, leukopenia
Nepuyo virus	*Artibeus jamaicensis* (Jamaican fruit-eating bat), *A. Lituratus* (great fruit-eating Bat)	Mosquitoes, rodents, monkeys	Febrile, myalgia, headache
Lagos bat virus (5 bat species)	*Eidolon helvum* (African straw-coloured fruit bat), *Micropteropus pusillus* (Peters' lesser epauletted fruit bat)	Conspecific reservoirs, occasional spillover to dogs, cats, and humans By bite and aerosol	Paralysis, convulsions, coma, death
Duvenhage virus (3 bat species)	*Miniopterus* sp., *Nyctalus noctula* (noctule), *Vespertilio murinus* (parti-coloured bat), *Nycteris thebaica* (Egyptian slit-faced bat)	Do	Paralysis, convulsions, coma, death
Australan bat lyssavirus	Megachiroptera (multiple *Pteropus* spp.), Microchiroptera sp.	Do	Paralysis, convulsions, coma, death
European bat lyssavirus 1 (bite, aerosol)	*Eptesicus serotinus* (serotine bat), *Rousettus aegyptiacus* (Egyptian rousette)		Paralysis, convulsions, coma, death
European bat lyssavirus 2	6 bat species (transmission: Bite, saliva, urine and faeces)		Paralysis, convulsions, coma, death
Irkut lyssavirus, Ozernoe virus Leonova et al. (2010), from a human after exposure to a bat, appears to cluster with IRKV	*Murina leucogaster* (greater tube-nosed bat) West Caucasian bat virus *Miniopterus schreibersii* (Schreiber's bent-winged bat)	Dog Teng et al. (2018)	Paralysis, convulsion, coma, lethal infection
Rabies virus Rhabdoviridae; lyssavirus	Numerous bat species; Transmission: bite, aerosol	Foxes—Red, Arctic, grey; raccoon, striped skunk, coyote, Raccoon dog, black-backed jackal; mongoose—Small Indian, yellow, slender	Paralysis, convulsions, coma, death

(continued)

Table 26.2 (continued)

Virus	Bat species	Intermediate host	Human infection
Orthomyxoviridae, genus Orthomyxovirus, Influenza A virus	*Nyctalus noctule*	Domestic and aquatic birds	Febrile, flu
Parainfluenza— Undermined genus	*Rousettus leschenaultia* (Leschenault's rousette)	Vertebrates	
Nipah virus	*Pteropus hypomelanus* (variable flying fox), *Pteropus vampyrus* (large flying fox), *Pteropus lylei* (Lyle's flying fox)	Pigs	Encephalitis, fatal
Menangle virus	*Pteropus poliocephalus* (grey-headed flying fox)	Fatal deformities in pigs	Neurological
Paramyxoviridae, genus Henipa, Hendra virus	*Pteropus alecto* (black flying fox), *Pteropus poliocephalus* (grey-headed flying fox), *Pteropus scapulatus* (little red flying), *Pteropus conspicillatus* (spectacled flying fox)	Horse, livestock	Respiratory, fatal
Tioman virus	*Pteropus hypomelanus* (variable flying fox) Virus excreted in urine	Clinical illness in animals	Clinical illness
Coronaviridae, SARS coronavirus	*Rhinolophus sinicus* (Chinese horseshoe bat), *Rhinolophus pearsonii* (Pearson's horseshoe bat) *Rhinolophus macrotis* (big-eared horseshoe bat) *Rhinolophus ferrumequinum* (greater horseshoe bat)	Palm civet	Man to man transmission. Febrile, flu-like, cough, breathlessness, distress, death
Chikungunya virus	*Scotophilus* sp., *Rousettus aegyptiacus* (Egyptian rousette), *Hipposideros caffer* (Sundevall's leaf-nosed bat), *Chaerephon pumilus* (little free-tailed bat)	Mosquitoes, Birds, rodent	Flu, body ache, joint pain
Sindbis virus	*Rhinolophidae* spp., *Hipposideridae* spp.	Birds, mosquitoes	Arthralgia, malaise, rash
Venezuelan equine encephalitis	*Desmodus rotundus* (vampire bat), *Uroderma bilobatum* (tent-making bat), *Artibeus phaeotis* (pygmy fruit-eating bat)	Equids, Mosquitoes, mammals Without symptoms	Flu-like, Dangerous for elders Myalgias typically in the thighs or lumbar, back, occipital or retro-orbital headache, fever and chills, encephalitis

Table 26.2 (continued)

Virus	Bat species	Intermediate host	Human infection
Central European encephalitis	Unidentified bat	Small mammals, also birds, ticks	Fever, nausea, vomiting, severe headache and backache, focal epilepsy, flaccid paralysis, may be permanent, may be fatal
Japanese encephalitis	*Hipposideros armiger terasensis* (great roundleaf bat also known as Formosan leaf-nosed bat) *Miniopterus schreibersii* (Schreiber's long-fingered bat), *Rhinolophus cornutus* (little Japanese horseshoe bat)	Mosquitoes, birds, mammals	Febrile, illness, encephalitis, fatal
Kyasanur forest disease	*Rhinolophus rouxii* (rufous horseshoe bat), *Cynopterus sphinx* (greater short-nosed fruit bat)	Ticks, monkeys, rodents, shrews, porcupines, squirrels	Biphasic fever, high fever, frontal headache, gastroenteritis. Second-phase neurological
St Louis encephalitis	*Tadarida brasiliensis mexicana* (Mexican free-tailed)	Birds, mammals, mosquitoes	Encephalitis
Rift Valley fever	*Micropteropus pusillus* (Peter's pygmy epauletted fruit bat) *Hipposideros abae* (aba leaf-nosed bat) *Miniopterus schreibersii* (Schreiber's long-fingered bat), *Hipposideros caffer* (Sundevall's leaf-nosed bat), *Epomops franqueti* (Franquet's epauletted bat), *Glauconycteris argentata* (common butterfly bat)	Mosquitoes, livestock	Fever, headache, muscle ache; severe: Brain infection, loss of sight, severe headache confusion; liver problem, bleeding
A cytomegalovirus	*Myotis lucifugus* (little brown bat)	Mammal contact with urine, saliva	Skin blisters, incurable— Inapparent, latent; reactivation
Family *Arenaviridae*, Tacaribe virus	*Artibeus jamaicensis* (Jamaican fruit-eating bat), *A. Lituratus* (great fruit-eating bat)	Rodents, mosquitoes, man, monkeys	Febrile, myalgia, headache
Genus Nairobi Issyk-Kul	*Nyctalus noctula* (noctule)	Ticks infesting bats	

(continued)

Table 26.2   (continued)

Virus	Bat species	Intermediate host	Human infection
Yogue	Egyptian rousette (*Rousettus aegyptiacus*)	Ticks-vertebrate-human transmission	
Kasokera	*Eptesicus serotinus* (common serotine)		Severe illness in a lab worker
Gossas	*Pipistrellus pipistrellus* (common pipistrelle)		
Keterah viruses	*Myotis blythii* (lesser mouse-eared myotis) (14 bats)		
Yellow fever virus	*Epomophorus labiatus* (little epauletted fruit bat)	Mosquito-primate transmission	Biphasic fever; second phase—High fever, abdominal pain, jaundice, haemorrhagic— Haematuria, black vomit and faeces, CFR 20%
West Nile virus	*Eptesicus fuscus* (big brown bat)	Mosquito-bird transmission	Fever, myalgia, severe/neurological form— Meningoencephalitis, paralysis
Hepatitis B virus	*Uroderma bilobatum* (common tent-making bat); *Hipposideros* cf. *ruber* (Noack's leaf-nosed bat); *Rhinolophus alcyone* (halcyon horseshoe bat)		Hepatitis and liver cancer
Hepa C virus (hepatitis C virus) different clades	*Otomops martiensseni* (large-eared giant mastiff bat); *H. Vittatus* (striped leaf-nosed bat)[a]		Hepatitis and liver cancer

[a]https://www.publichealth.columbia.edu/public-health-now/news/hepatitis-c-viruses-identified bats-and-rodents

26.3.2   The Emergence of Bat-Associated Infectious Diseases

Emergence required agent and epidemiological bridge connecting/facilitating spillover from natural to susceptible host. Deforestation/wildlife consumption for various reasons may facilitate contact between agent reservoirs and human or agent-intermediate host-human. The impact of bat-originated viral epidemics, Ebola and SARS-corona, is huge. Most connections between bat-borne viruses and diseases have been established based on the detection of the same or similar viruses in bats. Evidence supporting the direct role of bats is limited (Markotter et al. 2020). The greatest share of viruses identified as of 2020 is of type IV of Baltimore classification system, family *Coronaviridae* (https://en.wikipedia.org/wiki/Bat_virome).

Coronaviruses are known to frequently undergo recombination and mutation events, conferring fitness advantages to new variants.

26.3.2.1   SARS-Corona Virus

SARS-corona virus emergence and infection in human followed the mechanism of host switching from fruit bats to Himalayan palm civets or related carnivores (unidentified specific reservoirs) and adaptation for binding ACE2 receptors in human. It was believed that eating the animal (known colloquially as the 'fruit fox' or 'flower fox') provided the same health benefits as eating fruit and they are more health-giving (and taste better) than their grain-fed farmed counterparts. This led to SARS-CoV in masked civet and then to human infection.

26.3.2.2   Hendra Virus (HeV)

Hendra virus (HeV) did not seem to have switched over and adapt. Although seasonal incidence in horses during May to July suggests biological and ecological relationship with the spillover of HeV from bats, it is difficult to predict high-risk period.

26.3.2.3   Nipah Virus

Deforestation, fruit-bearing tree plantation and pig farming appeared to be the epidemiological bridge between *Pteropus* bat species reservoir and pigs and human. Outbreak of Nipah disease in pigs and human in 1999 in Malaysia suggested host switching. Isolates from both bats and humans were identical in some outbreaks. Adaptation to human may not be a necessary mechanism. Direct transmission from bat to pigs and from pigs to man occurred. In Bangladesh, mode of transmission from bat to food (date palm sap contaminated with bat faeces and urine) to human and horizontal human to human was observed.

26.3.2.4   Ebola Virus

Deforestation is linked with Ebola virus epidemic. The virus is maintained in an enzootic cycle with fruit bats (*Hypsignathus monstrosus*, *Epomops franqueti* and *Myonycteris torquata*) as reservoir. The direct contact of mucous membranes or open wounds with excreta, bites and consumption of or contact with fruit and other objects contaminated with bat excreta cause human infection. Man gets infected also by contact with the infected wild animals and several species of monkeys such as baboons, great apes, chimpanzees and gorillas. This is followed by human-to-human transmission and an epidemic of fatal haemorrhagic fever.

26.3.2.5   Marburg Virus

Marburg virus causes viral haemorrhagic fever of human and non-human primates. The natural host is Egyptian fruit bats (*Rousettus aegyptiacus*) as experimentally confirmed. Relatively long period of viremia in experimental bats could possibly also facilitate mechanical transmission by blood-sucking arthropods. Outbreaks in human have been linked to gold mining activities and entering of caves with potential contact with faecal excretions or aerosols. Exposure to man and non-human primates effects direct transmission. Trade of monkeys from Uganda to Europe brought infected monkeys in contact with human and caused the first outbreak of Marburg disease.

26.3.2.6   Two New Distinct Lineages of Influenza a Virus

H17N10 in the little yellow-shouldered bat (*Sturnira lilium*, family Phyllostomidae), in Guatemala, and H18N11, the flat-faced fruit-eating bat (*Artibeus jamaicensis planirostris*, family Phyllostomidae), in Peru have been discovered. Bats constitute migratory reservoirs. These may have potentiality to cause human infection. Transmission of influenza viruses into a new host and subsequent adaptation for sustained replication occurs through a combination of mutations to individual viral genes and reassortment of the entire gene segments (Mehle 2014).

26.3.2.7   Paramyxovirus

Sosuga virus (*Pararubulavirus* genus, *Rubulavirinae* subfamily). The most likely reservoir bat is the Egyptian rousette from which spillover occurred. It caused a severe non-fatal febrile disease in a field biologist handling these bats (Amman et al. 2015).

26.4   Prevention

Understanding/identifying the route of transmission '*spillover* or via *intermediate host/system* reservoir>intermediate host>host' enables planning of preventing measures. Improving biosecurity on farm and farm gate and rapid detection and diagnosis are necessary to control and prevent the spread of EIDs. Physical contact with bats and getting a nick from bat's tooth or claw can transmit rabies. Pre—and post-exposure prophylactic vaccination against Australian bat lyssavirus is required. Animal Health Australia (2011) provides essential guidelines for protection against bat-borne infections, especially lyssavirus.

The aspects of bat ecology critical to the dynamics of the emergence of infectious diseases need elucidation. It is important to study infection/disease dynamics in populations of bats (wildlife in general). Increased bat-human contact is a prerequisite for human infection. Hayman et al. (2013) proposed a combination of field and laboratory studies of ecology to create a well-validated data-mechanistic model. Studies on infectious agents, their bat hosts, anthropogenic changes affecting bats' ecology, drivers of pathogens and integration of these may be helpful in developing plans for mitigating the emergence of infectious diseases under One Health concept.

Health of wildlife, livestock, pets and humans needs to be protected. Pathogens know no barriers. At the same time inclusive health system is so huge and wide that no single sector can handle. Anthroponotic pathogens (affecting only human) fall in the domain of health sector. Livestock and pet animals' diseases are tackled by veterinary sector. Veterinary sector along with wildlife managers manages diseases in zoo and wild animals.

References

Amman BR, Albariño CG, Bird BH, Nyakarahuka L, Sealy TK et al (2015) A recently discovered pathogenic paramyxovirus, Sosuga virus, is present in *Rousettus aegyptiacus* fruit bats at multiple locations in Uganda. J Wildl Dis 51:774–779

Animal Health Australia (2011) Disease strategy: rabies (version 3.0). In: Australian veterinary emergency plan (AUSVETPLAN), 3rd edn. Primary Industries Ministerial Council, ACT, Canberra

Blitvich BJ, Firth AE (2017) A review of Flaviviruses that have no known arthropod vector. Viruses 9:154

Calisher CH, Childs JE, Field HE, Holmes KV, Schountz T (2006) Bats: important reservoir hosts of emerging viruses. Clin Microbiol Rev 2006(19):531–545

George DB, Webb CT, Farnsworth ML, O'Shea TJ, Bowen RA et al (2011) Host and viral ecology determine bat rabies seasonality and maintenance. Proc Natl Acad Sci USA 108(25):10208–10213

Hayman DTS, Bowens RA, Cryan PM, McCracken GF, O'Shea TJ et al (2013) Ecology of zoonotic infectious diseases in bats: current knowledge and future directions. Zoonoses Public Health 60:2–21

Leonova GN, Belikov SI, Kondratov IG, Krylova NV, Pavlenko EV et al (2010) A fatal case of bat lyssavirus infection in Primorye territory of the Russian Far East. Rabies bulletin. Europe 33(4):5–8

Markotter W, Coertse J, De Vries L, Geldenhuys M, Mortlock M (2020) Bat-borne viruses in Africa: a critical review. J Zool 311:77–98

Mehle A (2014) Unusual influenza a viruses in bats. Viruses 6:3438–3449

Moratelli R, Calisher CH (2015) Bats and zoonotic viruses: can we confidently link bats with emerging deadly viruses? Mem Inst Oswaldo Cruz, Rio de Janeiro 110(1):1–22

Teng C, Miao FM, Liu Y, Zhang SF, Zhang F et al (2018) Possible transmission of Irkut virus from dogs to humans. Biomed Environ Sci 31(2):146–148

Chapter 27
Marburg Haemorrhagic Fever

Synonyms

Green Monkey Disease

Marburg haemorrhagic fever is characterized by fever, myalgia, chills, headache, maculopapular rash on trunk, progressing further to abdominal pain, diarrhoea and in severe case massive haemorrhages, multiorgan failure and death. CFR is 30–90%.

27.1 Aetiology

Marburgvirus (MARV) belongs to the family *Filoviridae*, genera *Marburgvirus*, *Ebolavirus*, *Cuevavirus*, *Striavirus* and *Thamnovirus*. Viruses in the genera *Ebolavirus* and *Marburgvirus* cause haemorrhagic and often lethal disease in human and non-human primates (NHPs).

Filoviruses are non-segmented RNA negative sense and encode for seven open reading frames: nucleoprotein NP, virion protein (VP) 35, VP40, glycoprotein GP, VP40, VP24 and viral polymerase L. The filovirus genome is packaged into a unique filamentous virion, approximately 790–97 nm in length and 80 nm in width.

MARV and Ravn virus (RAVV) are two members of the genus *Marburg*. Ravn virus (RAVV) is represented by the Ravn isolates from 1987, one isolate from the DRC outbreak in 1998–2000 and one human and several bat isolates from infections that took place in Uganda in 2007.

© Springer Nature Singapore Pte Ltd. 2024
K. G. Narayan et al., *Handbook of Management of Zoonoses*,
https://doi.org/10.1007/978-981-99-9885-2_27

27.2   Epidemiology

Fruit bats *Rousettus aegyptiacus* are reservoirs and humans and NHPs are spillover hosts. The bat is a cave dweller and distributed in Africa. Outbreaks were reported in male mine workers of the Kitaka gold mine in the Kamwenge district in June–September 2007. They acquired infection in the bat-infested mines and spread it to their community. The virus was isolated from bats in the Kitaka cave, Uganda. A Dutch woman tourist got infection while visiting Python cave harbouring fruit bats in Maramagambo Forest, Uganda in 2008. She died after return to the Netherlands. MARV poses risk to tourists; on their return, they are likely to import the virus and spread it in their country.

Primates including human are susceptible. The first outbreak in Germany and Yugoslavia (Serbia at present) was caused by African green monkeys (*Chlorocebus aethiops*) imported from Uganda.

Sporadic outbreaks of Marburg HF have occurred in Uganda, the Democratic Republic of the Congo, Zimbabwe, Kenya, South Africa and Angola. Considering the distribution of bat species, there is a potential risk of Marburg HF in far and wide region. The virus is not known in North America.

Following their discovery in 1967, MARV has been associated with several small to serious outbreaks, compiled by the WHO (Table 27.1).

27.2.1   High-Risk group

Family members of patients and HCWs in hospital are high-risk groups, particularly in the absence of barrier nursing. Others include veterinarians, laboratory and quarantine workers and travellers to endemic areas, especially caves and mines.

Table 27.1 Chronology of major Marburg virus disease outbreaks

Year	Country	Cases	Deaths	CFR (%)
2014	Uganda	1	1	100
2012	Uganda	15	4	27
2008	Netherland (ex-Uganda)	1	1	100
2008	USA (ex-Uganda)	1	0	0
2007	Uganda	4	2	50
2005	Angola	374	329	88
1998–2000	Democratic Republic of the Congo	154	128	83
1987	Kenya	1	1	100
1980	Kenya	2	1	50
1975	South Africa	3	1	33
1967	Yugoslavia	2	0	0
1967	Germany	29	7	24

27.2.2   *Transmission*

Aerosol and/or unprotected contact with bat excreta and tourists visiting bat-infested caves got infected, contributed to cases outside Africa. Contact while handling/dressing infected primates and tissues infect handlers. Human-to-human transmission occurs after the virus has jumped to man from bat through direct contact with infectious blood and body fluids or indirectly from contact with contaminated objects and equipment. Infection of HCWs and nosocomial transmission is common.

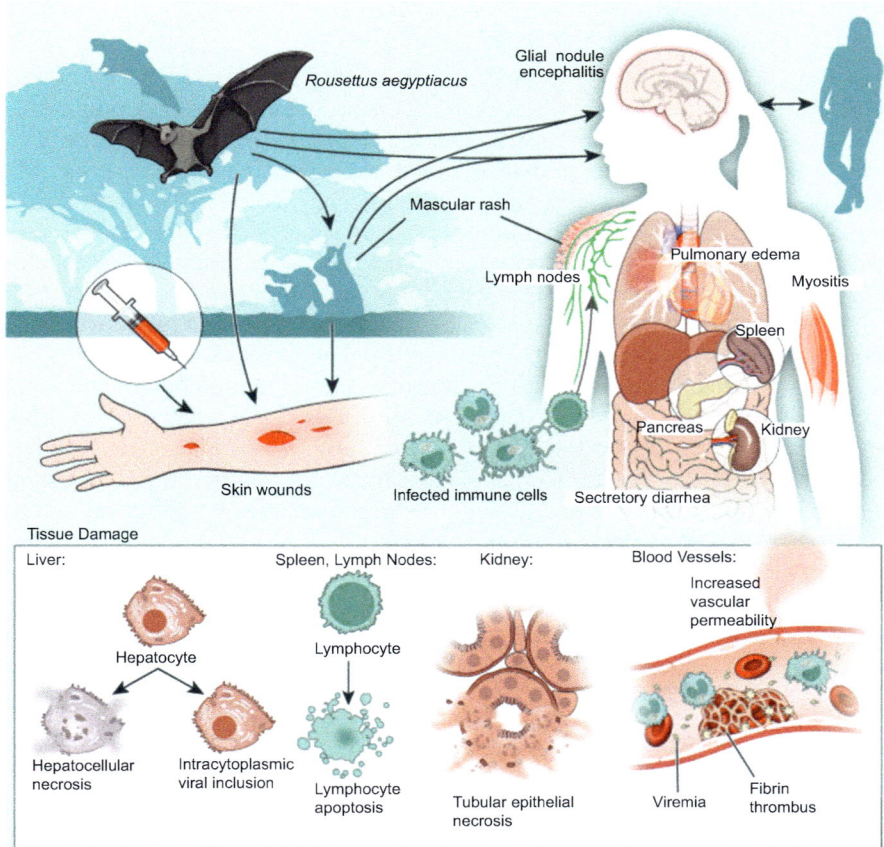

Fig. 27.1   Marburg virus pathogenesis [Source: Shifflett K, Marzi A (2019)]

27.3 Pathogenesis (Fig. 27.1)

MARV enters through small skin lesions and the mucous membrane and invade mononuclear phagocytes, macrophages and dendritic cells. Virus replicates in 24 h in macrophages and monocytes. Primary human monocyte-derived dendritic cells (mDCs) and endothelial cells support MARV replication. Lymph nodes, liver and spleen are the virus replication sites. Infected monocytes and macrophages transport and help virus dissemination via lymph or bloodstream to multiple organs.

27.4 Symptoms

Incubation period varies from 2 to 21 days (typically 5–10 days). Disease begins with high fever, severe headache and malaise, cramp and myalgia; beginning on the third day—severe watery diarrhoea, nausea and vomiting—patients look ghost-like, with sunken eyes and extreme lethargy, and are expressionless. Non-itchy rash within 2–7 days at the onset of symptoms was observed in the 1967 outbreak. Small dark spots around the hair follicles of the trunk and upper arm become diffuse, dark and erythematous and cover the face, neck, chest, and arms. Pathological features like lymphadenopathy, leukopenia and thrombocytopenia appeared.

Haemorrhagic manifestation appears between 5 and 7 days; in fatal cases fresh blood in vomitus is accompanied by bleeding from multiple areas: nose, gums and vagina; spontaneous bleeding at venepuncture site is troublesome. Confusion, increased sensitivity, irritability and aggression and coma, indicative of CNS involvement, appear in later stage.

Severe blood loss due to internal haemorrhage, dehydration, organ failure or some combination of these and dysregulated immune response result into death usually in 8–9 days at the onset of symptoms.

Orchitis occurred generally after 15 days. Survivors generally do not suffer from late stage symptoms but experience arthritis, conjunctivitis, myalgia and psychosis during and after. Blood picture indicative of hepatic and kidney damage, disseminated intravascular coagulation, lymphopenia, and thrombocytopenia.

27.5 Pathology

Pathological changes in organs autopsied fit with the course of disease and sequelae observed in cases of MARV and RAVV (Shifflett and Marzi 2019). The pathological changes observed are summed up:

27.5.1   RAVV

The heart, brain, spleen, kidneys and lymph nodes show evidence of swelling; haemorrhage of the mucous membranes, soft tissues and various other organs; and haemorrhage and focal necrosis in almost all organs, especially the liver, lymph glands, testis and ovaries. Histopathology: *Liver*—hepatocellular inflammation, degeneration, eosinophiles showed cytoplasmic basophilic inclusion and viral antigen near areas of necrosis. *Spleen*—moderate necrosis in red and white pulp of spleen with evidence of lymphoid depletion in white pulp, haemorrhage and severe necrosis in the germinal centres; viral antigen seen in macrophages and in red pulp. *Kidneys*—swollen, pale, haemorrhagic, tubular necrosis, parenchymal damage. *Lungs*—alveoli congested, haemorrhages, alveolar macrophages surrounded by fibrin occasionally positive for viral antigen. *Lymphatic organs* and mucous membranes of the stomach and intestines presented a high number of plasma cells and monocytes. Macrophages in the intestines and kidney contained what looked like viral inclusions.

27.5.2   Marburg

Three of five autopsies from the outbreak in Germany showed glial nodule encephalitis spread throughout the brain.

The virus persists in immune-privileged sites, testicles and inside of the eyes. Women infected after pregnancy have the virus persisting in the placenta, amniotic fluid and foetus, and when infected while breastfeeding, it persists in the breast milk. Male survivors' semen is positive for the virus with up to 7 weeks of recovery and they have to practise safe sex and hygiene for 12 months from the onset of symptoms or until semen tests negative twice.

Those who recovered may relapse to symptomatic illness, but rarely.

27.5.3   Pathology in Laboratory Animals

In search of animal models for MARV, especially for trial of drugs and vaccines, hamster, guinea pig and mouse, cynomolgus and rhesus macaque have been studied.

Non-human primates (NHP), cynomolgus and rhesus macaques have responded similar to human and develop disease with comparable pathology. Cynomolgus and rhesus macaques experience a more accelerated disease course. There is no difference between strains. MARV-Angola caused a more rapid onset. Increasing doses led to shorter course and lethal ending. Overall outcome did not differ with routes of challenge.

Summary of events: 4–6 dpi fever appears; 6–7 dpi anorexia, rash; haemorrhagic symptoms, bleeding from gums and venepuncture sites; dpi 7–12 (humane endpoint) lethargy, expressionless, loss of response, diarrhoea, dehydration, drop of temperature.

Pathology: There is viremia; the virus is detected in most tissues including the brain; the highest load is observed in the blood, liver and spleen.

Changes: 6–7 dpi lymphocytes reduced; spiked leucocytes due to lymphocytosis and neutrophilia; thrombocytopenia in mid-phase; evidence of damage of liver and kidney; increase in blood clotting time; cytokine response—indicated that MARV causes a dysregulation of the host immune system, similar to that of septic shock in bacterial infections. A similar dysregulated immune response contributed to the pathology and severity of EBOV haemorrhagic fever.

27.6   Diagnosis

Rule out confounding conditions like malaria and typhoid and confirm by the following methods in high-containment biosafety level 4 laboratories:

- Antibody-capture enzyme-linked immunosorbent assay (ELISA)
- Antigen-capture detection tests
- Serum neutralization test
- Reverse transcriptase polymerase chain reaction (RT-PCR) assay
- Electron microscopy
- Virus isolation by cell culture
- Immunohistochemistry of tissues in dead

27.7   Prevention

Marburg is a rare but dangerous disease. Two sites for preventive efforts are animal-human interface and human-human interface. Detection in sentinel should be looked for at the first interface and transmission to human should be intercepted.

In the absence of a defined sentinel in animals, bats and monkeys in the wild and pigs (recommended for surveillance during the outbreak for suspected amplification of virus) among domesticated animals may be under surveillance. Bats show viremia and hepatocellular necrosis and shed virus detected in oral swab and excreta. Experimentally infected cynomolgus and rhesus macaques respond like humans. [Summary of observation: fever appears 4–6 dpi, anorexia, rash; haemorrhagic symptoms, bleeding from gums and venepuncture sites 6–7 dpi; dpi 7–12 (humane endpoint) lethargy, expressionless, loss of response, diarrhoea, dehydration and drop of temperature].

Pathology: viremia, detection in most tissues including the brain; highest load in the blood, liver and spleen. Changes—lymphocytes reduced 6–7 dpi; spiked leucocytes due to lymphocytosis and neutrophilia; thrombocytopenia in mid-phase; evidence of damage of liver and kidney; increase in blood clotting time; cytokine response—indicated that MARV causes a dysregulation of the host immune system, similar to that of septic shock in bacterial infections. A similar dysregulated immune response contributed to the pathology and severity of EBOV haemorrhagic fever.

Detection of a suspected case (second interface: human-human), procedure for confirmation and actions to follow including IPC are available: Guidelines from the WHO (case definitions recommendations for Ebola or Marburg virus diseases (WHO/EVD/CaseDef 14.1)).

27.7.1   A Suspected Case of Marburg

A suspected case of Marburg should manifest fever without response to treatment PLUS one of the following: bleeding eyes/gum/skin or blood in urine/faeces, which should be confirmed by IgM antibodies/PCR/isolation of virus. Add to these, sudden death makes an ALERT case for the community—based surveillance in a pre-epidemic phase or during an outbreak. This should be used by volunteers and in participatory epidemiology. A suspected case/deceased suspected case having epidemiologic link with a confirmed case is a PROBABLE case for hospitals/surveillance team. A laboratory test-negative suspected or probable is a NON-CASE.

27.7.2   Contacts

(a) Community setting—exposed to suspect/probable/confirmed HUMAN or ANIMAL during <21 days of identification by surveillance team as suspected contact; exposure may be sleeping in the same household with a case/direct contact with dead or alive case or body fluids, clothes and linen/breastfed baby. Additional route of exposure is eating bushmeat.

(b) Hospital setting—exposure to hospital dedicated for Ebola or Marburg disease; injection/vaccination within 21 days of onset of symptoms.

(c) Laboratory setting—in less than 21 days of identification as a contact by the surveillance team for exposure to: (i) biological material, (ii) specimens from suspected patients and (iii) contact with specimens while collecting.

Contact person is observed/followed for 21 days for the appearance of symptoms and released if healthy.

27.7.2.1   Experience of the Uganda Outbreak 2017

A 50-year-old woman died due to laboratory-confirmed Marburg disease and the Ugandan Ministry of Health notified the WHO of the outbreak on 17 October 2017. Three people died in the outbreak that spread to two districts in eastern Uganda bordering Kenya. Health workers followed 316 close contacts of the patients and ensured they did not fall ill. The contacts of the last patient were followed for 21 days (the IP) for absence of illness and additional 21 days of intensive surveillance in the affected districts did not find any case.

The World Health Organization said on 8 December 2017 that the exemplary response by health authorities and partners controlled the spread within weeks. Response included early detection, deploying rapid response team (https://www.who.int/news/item/08-12-2017-uganda-ends-marburg-virus-disease-outbreak) within 24 h, surveillance, lab-testing support, search for new cases and contacts, IPC and engaging with the community. The following WHO documents are useful:

- Ebola and Marburg virus disease epidemics: preparedness, alert, control, and evaluation
- Infection prevention and control guidance for care of patients with suspected or confirmed Filovirus haemorrhagic fever in health-care settings, with focus on Ebola

27.8   Treatment

None as specific; maintain fluid, electrolyte, blood oxygen, and blood pressure; replace blood and clotting factors and check for complications.

References

Shifflett K, Marzi A (2019) Marburg virus pathogenesis—differences and similarities in humans and animal models. Virol J 16(165):1–12

Chapter 28
Severe Acute Respiratory Syndrome-Coronavirus (SARS-CoV)

Coronaviruses have crown-like spikes on their surface. Severe acute respiratory syndrome (SARS)-CoV-like virus occurs in animals and does not cause disease in them and is not transmitted to humans.

A new member, SARS-CoV, has >99% nucleotide homology with SARS-CoV isolated from palm civet and other animals found in live animal markets in Guangdong, China. The isolates from the early phase of outbreak were more closely related to animal isolates than the isolates from middle and late phases. The early evolution may have led to transmissibility from animals to human, followed by human-human transmission causing sporadic mild disease subsequently local and global outbreaks with high mortality.

Coronaviruses are Alpha, Beta, Gamma and Delta. CoVs of mammals, poultry and fish belong to Gamma and Delta. Alpha and Beta CoVs infect bats and other mammals. Evolution and emergence occur at the human-animal interface that offers new ecological niches. Species jump from bats to other mammals is considered due to combination in the Spike gene. Middle East Respiratory Syndrome-coronavirus (MERS-CoV) and 2019-novel coronavirus (2019-nCoV) are subsequently evolved to new human pandemic causing viruses.

28.1 Human Coronaviruses (https://www.cdc.gov/coronavirus/types.html)

Seven coronaviruses can cause human infections:

1. 229E (Alpha coronavirus)
2. NL63 (Alpha coronavirus)
3. OC43 (Beta coronavirus)
4. HKU1 (Beta coronavirus)

© Springer Nature Singapore Pte Ltd. 2024
K. G. Narayan et al., *Handbook of Management of Zoonoses*,
https://doi.org/10.1007/978-981-99-9885-2_28

5. MERS-CoV—the beta coronavirus that causes Middle East respiratory syndrome, or MERS
6. SARS-CoV—the beta coronavirus that causes severe acute respiratory syndrome, or SARS
7. SARS-CoV-2—the novel Beta coronavirus that causes coronavirus disease 2019, or COVID-19

Coronaviruses (CoV) cause respiratory illness and intestinal problems in animals and humans. NL63 and 229E cause mild-to-moderate respiratory infections and HCoV-OC43 and HCoV-HKU1 common cold and lower respiratory tract infections.

Disease in human beings ranges from mild flu-like to fatal severe acute respiratory syndrome (SARS), Middle East respiratory syndrome and severe pneumonia pandemic or the coronavirus disease (COVID-19).

According to Vijaykrishna et al. (2007) CoVs identified in bats are older than any other CoVs identified in other animals and have great genetic diversity, suggesting they are the natural hosts of all known CoVs. These viruses are endemic in bats. Epidemic-like conditions in all other animals indicate their interspecies transmission and occasional establishment. Positive selection pressure has been observed in SARS-CoV identified in masked palm civet and humans. These support the hypothesis—SARS-CoV diverged some 17 years before the SARS-CoV outbreak in 1986 from closely related SARS-like CoVs in bats and resided in some unknown intermediate hosts before infecting masked palm civets and humans.

28.2 SARS-CoV

28.2.1 Epidemiology

Animal origin of SARS-CoV was considered on the basis of the following: (a) detection of antibodies is more among animal market traders during 2002–2003, (b) detection of antibodies is more among the early case patients than later case patients who lived near a produce market and almost half of them were food handlers with probable animal contact, (c) virus isolates from animals in the market and human were almost identical, (d) early-phase isolates were more closely related to the animal isolates and (e) human isolates from the 2003–2004 outbreaks had higher sequence identity.

Two of the four patients of SARS identified in 2003–2004 were waitresses at a restaurant in Guangzhou, China. This restaurant served palm civet as food. All six palm civets caged a short distance from the customers were positive for SARS-CoV (Wang et al. 2005). Human SARS-CoV is capable of infecting domesticated animals particularly pigs; pigs were infected through virus-contaminated animal feed (Chen et al. 2005).

Detection of SARS-CoV in three palm civets (*Paguma larvata*) and one raccoon dog (*Nyctereutes procyonoides*) and neutralizing antibodies in two Chinese ferret badgers (*Melogale moschata*) was the first laboratory-confirmed infection in animals (Guan et al. 2003). According to Wang et al. (2006), >10 mammalian species are susceptible to SARS-CoV or related viruses. Most probably rats played a role in the transmission and spread of SARS in the well-publicized outbreak in Amoy Gardens apartment block in Hong Kong. Experimentally infected rats showed no symptoms but serologic evidence supported viral replication.

Abdullah et al. (2003) have summed up the experience with SARS control. SARS-CoV in aerosolized faecal waste is stable in faeces and urine at room temperature for at least 1–2 days, up to 4 days in patients' (with diarrhoea) stool and 48 h after drying on plastic surface; commonly used disinfectants are effective.

SARS presents complex factors of risk of transmission. Signs and symptoms are non-specific, IP is long, hospitalization is delayed, and the median period from onset of symptoms to admission to hospital was 6 days (range 0–9 days); there is a lack of reliable diagnostics for detection in the early phase; in elderly patients primary disease phase may be muted without evident fever.

SARS patients constitute the immediate source of infection. Steroid or other immunosuppressing drugs increase viral load and prolong virus shedding potentially increasing chances of transmission and duration of patients' infectivity. *Super spreaders* are patients with depressed immune system; cases undergoing haemodialysis are associated with high viral loads and shedding. For example, the Hong Kong index patient is thought to have infected persons who transmitted the virus worldwide, subsequently resulting in outbreaks of >300 patients in Amoy Gardens in Hong Kong and >60 cases in Singapore, and these 2 outbreaks may have been started by 2 persons undergoing haemodialysis.

In the hospital setting, certain medical procedures are associated with risk of spreading novel infectious agents like SARS-CoV. These are ventilators, nebulized bronchodilators, cardiovascular resuscitation, positive airway pressure devices, bronchoscopy, airway and sputum suction and endotracheal intubation.

28.2.2   Symptoms

It is interesting to note that index patients for Singapore, Vietnam and Canada outbreaks probably got infection from a physician from southern China while they stayed on the ninth floor of a hotel in Hong Kong. In Singapore the outbreak broke out in the middle of March 2003. The Singaporean patient was in the general ward of the hospital without barrier for 6 days, thereby spreading infection. The following contacts got infected: most were 1/8 physicians +9/30 nursing staff, 1/12 patients on adjacent beds and 9/30 visitors, family members and friends. All these 20 were hospitalized, isolated and treated. The profile of these 20 is as follows: median age 28 years, smoker 1, diabetes and end-stage renal failure 1, history of childhood asthma 1, and had single exposure 7 (Hsu et al. 2003).

The index patient and initial contacts: The index case had headache, dry cough, temperature 37.6 °C, dullness and clear chest on auscultation. Blood examination revealed reduced TLC, lymphocytes and platelets. Chest X-ray showed patchy consolidation in upper and lower lobes of her right lung. Blood culture was sterile. Nasopharyngeal aspirate was negative for influenza A and B, parainfluenza and adeno- and respiratory syncytial viruses. As the disease progressed there were rising temperature (40 °C), persistent cough and breathlessness and by the fifth day the patient required supplemental oxygen. Sequential chest X-ray showed progressive extensive lung involvement, infiltration extending also to left lung and elevated liver enzymes. On the seventh day electron microscopy of nasopharyngeal aspirate (NPA) showed viral particles of <100 nm with widely spaced, club-shaped surface projections characteristic of coronaviruses. On the ninth day onwards, the condition improved.

28.2.2.1 Symptoms in the Contacts

IP 2–10 days, median 4–5 days fever, myalgia, headache, dry cough, chest pain developed 2–4 days after onset of fever, shortness of breath in the second week; interstitial infiltration at the base of lung, acute respiratory distress requiring supplemental oxygen in six patients.

Lymphopenia and thrombocytopenia are characteristic in early phase. Neutrophils, platelets and lactate dehydrogenase rise as the disease progresses. The latter indicates tissue necrosis related to immune hyperactivity and poor outcome. If these are observed at the time of admission to hospital, heavy viral exposure or delay in seeking hospitalization is suggested. Advanced age, high neutrophil count at the time of admission and elevated initial lactate dehydrogenase level were independent correlates of an adverse clinical outcome.

Suggestions for healthcare workers: High-risk procedures include intubation, nasopharyngeal aspiration, chest physiotherapy and handling of excreta and even feeding. Wear N-95 masks, face shields, caps, gowns and surgical gloves.

28.2.3 Pathology

SARS is predominantly a respiratory infection. Spread to extrapulmonary sites may be through the mucosal lumen or bloodstream. Viral replication at these sites leads to respiratory manifestations. Prognosis is poor in cases of (a) high viral load in naso-pharyngeal aspirate and (b) presence of viral RNA in multiple sites.

Host-virus interaction was studied by Hung et al. (2004). There is dynamic interaction between virus and body defence system. Viral load peaked around 10 days after onset of symptoms accompanied by a rapid decrease and concomitant normalization of lymphocyte count and rise in serum antibodies. Mean peak viral load in NPA and stool on day 10 were 5.8 $\log_{10}$ copies/mL and 7.0 $\log_{10}$ copies/mL, respectively, suggesting respiratory droplets and indirect contact with faeces are important mechanisms of transmission. 10–15 days post onset of symptoms, nasopharyngeal or serum viral load was associated with oxygen desaturation, mechanical ventilation, diarrhoea, hepatic dysfunction and death. Stool viral load was associated with diarrhoea and urine viral load with abnormal urine analysis. According to Lau et al. (2005) IgG antibodies begin rising by day 11 after onset of symptoms; by the third week almost all patients show antibodies that persist through 100 days. Viral load begins to decline rapidly after 9–10 days after onset of disease.

28.2.4   Diagnosis

1. Cultivation of SARS-CoV in cell line (Vero cells—E6, E76).
2. Reverse transcription (RT)-PCR) and quantitative real-time PCR are standard diagnostic techniques. Useful for early detection.
3. SARS immunoassays (using antigen from whole virus, various recombinant proteins): ELISA (Che et al. 2004; Lau et al. 2004).

   (a) Polyclonal antibody-based sandwich ELISA detected nucleocapsid protein in 83% of nasopharyngeal aspirate collected 11–15 days post onset of symptoms.
   (b) Monoclonal antibody-based sandwich ELISA detected nucleocapsid protein in 85% of serum collected during the first 10 days of onset of symptoms.

Cultivation of SARS-CoV is useful for early detection and is relatively insensitive and difficult. Viral load begins to decline rapidly after 9–10 days after onset of disease.

qRT-PCR was more sensitive (80% of faecal and 25% of urine specimens) than polyclonal (50% and 5%) and monoclonal (35% and 8%) antibody-based sandwich ELISA. Whole virus and various recombinant proteins are used as antigen in Western blot and Immunofluorescence assay on slide.

Synthetic antigens taken from S, M and N proteins of the virus provide highly specific ELISA for detecting IgG antibodies. Standardization, convenience, freedom from biohazards, ease of scale-up production and usage in retrospective surveillance are advantages (Hsueh et al. 2004).

All recombinant tests require biosafety level 3 labs and are time consuming.

28.2.5   Vaccine

According to Jiang et al. (2005), for inactivated SARS-CoV vaccine under clinical trial in China, safety is a major concern. Vaccine using strain from late SARS strains (from 2002–2003 epidemic) is associated with the possibility of enhanced infection by early human strains (from late 2003 to early 2004 epidemic) and animal strains. S (spike)-protein is a major inducer of neutralizing antibodies. The receptor-binding domain (RBD) in the S1 subunit of S protein contains multiple conformational neutralizing epitopes. RBD sequences are relatively conserved. Recombinant RBD or vectors encoding RBD may be safe and effective.

28.2.6   Treatment

Effective antiviral agents administered in early stages (<10 days) are useful. Viral load is reduced and also shedding and risk of transmission; severity of symptoms is controlled and patients' conditions improve.

28.2.7   Control and Prevention

Pandemic control is a global problem and concern and not of one or few nations. Active collaboration/participation of all is necessary. An outbreak response and enhanced infection control unit is crucial to combat any future outbreak (Abdullah et al. 2003). Guidelines for travellers, screening of travellers at the entry through health declaration or thermal scanning at international borders and border screening to deter the travel of ill persons are useful.

Traditional public health interventions worked well (Bell 2004): early case detection and isolation, quarantine, increase 'social distance', wearing masks in public places, dissemination of health information and guidelines to all, especially patients' relatives, friends and visitors.

Quarantine and contact tracing contributed significantly in the control as it enabled screening potentially infective persons for swift diagnosis and hospitalization after onset, thereby indirectly reducing infections (Hsieh et al. 2005). According to the WHO:

- *Suspected case* as documented fever (temperature >38 °C), lower respiratory tract symptoms and contact with a person believed to have had SARS or history of travel to an area of documented transmission.
- *Probable case* is a 'suspected case with chest radiographic findings of pneumonia, acute respiratory distress syndrome (ARDS), or an unexplained respiratory illness resulting in death, with autopsy findings of ARDS without identifiable cause.'

References

Abdullah ASM, Tomlinson B, Cockram CS, Thomas GN (2003) Lessons from the severe acute respiratory syndrome outbreak in Hong Kong. Emerg Infect Dis 9(9):1042–1045

Bell DM (2004) World Health Organization working group on prevention of international and community transmission of SARS. Public health interventions and SARS spread, 2003. Emerg Infect Dis 10(11):1900–1906

Che XY, Qiu LW, Pan YX, Wen K, Hao W, Zhang LY et al (2004) (2004) Sensitive and specific monoclonal antibody–based capture enzyme immunoassay for detection of nucleocapsid antigen in sera from patients with severe acute respiratory syndrome. J Clin Microbiol 42:2629–2635

Chen W, Yan M, Yang L et al (2005) SARS-associated coronavirus transmitted from human to pig. Emerg Infect Dis 11(3):446–448

Guan Y, Zheng BJ, He YQ, Liu XL, Zhuang ZX, Cheung CL et al (2003) Isolation and characterization of viruses related to the SARS coronavirus from animals in Southern China. Science 302:276–279

Hsieh YH, King CC, Chen CW et al (2005) Quarantine for SARS, Taiwan. Emerg Infect Dis 11(2):278–282

Hsu L-Y, Lee C-C, Green JA, Ang B, Paton NI, Lee L et al (2003) Severe acute respiratory syndrome (SARS) in Singapore: clinical features of index patient and initial contacts. Emerg Infect Dis 9(6):713–717

Hsueh PR, Kao CL, Lee CN et al (2004) SARS antibody test for serosurveillance. Emerg Infect Dis 10(9):1558–1562

Hung IFN, Cheng VCC, Wu AKL, Tang BSF, Chan KH, Chu CM et al (2004) Viral loads in clinical specimens and SARS manifestations. Emerg Infect Dis 10(9):1550–1557

Jiang S, He Y, Liu S (2005) SARS vaccine development. Emerg Infect Dis 11(7):1016–1020

Lau SK, Woo PC, Wong BH, Tsoi HW, Woo GK et al (2004) Detection of SARS coronavirus nucleocapsid protein in SARS patients by enzyme-linked immunosorbent assay. J Clin Microbiol 42:2884–2889

Lau SK, Che XY, Woo PC et al (2005) SARS coronavirus detection methods. Emerg Infect Dis 11(7):1108–1111

Vijaykrishna D, Smith GJ, Zhang JX, Peiris JS, Chen, Guan Y (2007) Evolutionary insights into the ecology of coronaviruses. J Virol 81(8):4012–4020

Wang M, Yan M, Xu H, Liang W, Kan B, Zheng B et al (2005) SARS-CoV infection in a restaurant from palm civet. Emerg Infect Dis 11(12):1860–1865

Wang L-F, Shi Z, Zhang S, Field H, Daszak P, Eaton BT (2006) Review of bats and SARS. Emerg Infect Dis 12(12):1834–1840

Chapter 29
Middle East Respiratory Syndrome Coronavirus (MERS-CoV)

Middle East respiratory syndrome coronavirus (MERS-CoV) infection is acute respiratory disease with high case fatality rate. Human-to-human transmission is sustained and cases are amplified in healthcare settings.

29.1 Aetiology

MERS-CoV is a single-stranded RNA *beta-coronavirus* derived from bats. It was identified in a patient from Saudi Arabia in June 2012 and over 85% of cases were reported from this country and the rest from countries in or near the Arabian Peninsula. There are two phylogenetic clades A and B. Early cases were caused by clade A clusters (EMC/2012 and Jordan-N3/2012).

29.2 Epidemiology

29.2.1 Distribution

MERS-CoV has been identified in dromedaries in several countries in the Middle East and South Asia. Serological evidence of infection in dromedary camels in Nigeria, Tunisia and Ethiopia suggests circulation of virus across broad areas of Africa and indicates that MERS-CoV infection is currently underdiagnosed (Chantal et al. 2014).

MERS cases have been reported since 2012 from 27 countries, including the USA, Europe, North Africa, Middle East and Southeast Asia. Approximately 80% of human cases have been reported by Saudi Arabia (WHO 2019).

© Springer Nature Singapore Pte Ltd. 2024
K. G. Narayan et al., *Handbook of Management of Zoonoses*,
https://doi.org/10.1007/978-981-99-9885-2_29

From 2012 until 31 January 2020, the total number of laboratory-confirmed MERS-CoV infection cases reported globally to the WHO is 2519 with 866 associated deaths. The global number reflects the total number of laboratory-confirmed cases reported to the WHO under the International Health Regulations (IHR 2005) to date (WHO 2020).

Study of cases reported since 2012 showed a peak of 760 cases in 2014 followed by a decline to 423 in 2015 (WHO 2015).

Major epidemics occurred in Saudi Arabia and South Korea; the rest of 23/26 countries reported cases—mainly travel-related spread. This could happen anywhere again.

29.2.2   Epidemics

The first case in Saudi Arabia happened to be male of 60 years old. He suffered from acute pneumonia and ultimately died of renal failure in June 2012. The epidemic involved 1037 cases with a fatality rate of 44%. Most cases (65%) were males and the median age was 50 years (range 9 months to 99 years). Females' veils cover mouth and nose and thus reduced the chances of exposure.

The epidemic in the Middle East, its transmission and spread are largely under control.

The Republic of Korea (South Korea) reported another outbreak. A 68-year-old man returned from the Middle East. He sought medical help and was diagnosed MERS-CoV positive on 20 May 2015. Instances of defying intervention measures in the South Korea epidemic were observed. Patients and/or their relatives paid no notice to doctor's advice and did not observe 'self-quarantine' order and travel restrictions of the government; students were forced to remove masks. The disease spread and as of July 2015, 186 cases of MERS-CoV and 36 related deaths (fatality rate 19.4%) have been reported in South Korea. The epidemic impacted life and economy seriously through temporary closure of schools, absenteeism in the workplace, keeping consumers at home and tourists cancelling trips, in addition to direct health cost. South Korea finally declared it is effectively out of danger from Middle East respiratory syndrome (MERS) more than 2 months after the first case was reported (28/07/2015 Reuters).

According to the WHO (2018), human-to-human transmission is most efficient in healthcare settings and documented in several countries during 2012–2016 including Saudi Arabia. The number of cases per outbreak (size of outbreak) varied between 2 and 180 cases.

The overall reproduction number (R0) of MERS-CoV is <1; in outbreaks it is >1 and can be brought down to <1 with application of infection prevention and control measures and early isolation of subsequent cases.

29.2.3 Reservoir

MERS originated from animals like SARS. Mode of zoonotic transmission is not understood. Sabir et al. (2016) studied the viruses prevalent during 2014 and 2015 in Saudi Arabia. They observed that viruses of the MERS-CoV species and a human CoV 229E-related lineage co-circulated at high prevalence, with frequent co-infections in the upper respiratory tract of dromedary camels. Dromedary camels share three CoV species with humans. Camels harboured several lineages of MERS-CoV including a recombinant lineage that has been dominant since December 2014 and that subsequently led to the human outbreaks in 2015.

Experimental inoculation of MERS-CoV in three adult camels set up a benign, transient, primarily upper respiratory tract (nasal turbinates) infection and a short period (7 days pi to 35 days) of excretion, suggesting efficient camel-to-camel and camel-to-human transmission, through direct contact, droplet or possibly fomite. Virus was not detected in urine or faeces. Neutralizing antibodies were detected 14 days pi and peaked (titre 640) after 35 days. High titre observed in field samples indicated repeated exposure (Adney et al. 2014).

Studies on camels made by Wernery et al. (2015) confirmed the period of viral excretion and suggested that (a) virus can be maintained in flocks for several weeks or months and (b) avoiding contact with camels <2 years of age may reduce camel to human transmission.

There is a direct zoonotic risk for MERS-CoV infection among persons occupationally in contact with camels. Virus has been isolated from camels in Egypt, Oman, Qatar and Saudi Arabia but not from goats, sheep, cows, water buffalo, swine and wild birds. Humans without clinical disease seem to contribute least to transmission and spread of disease.

Sero-epidemiological surveys suggest that MERS-CoV has been circulating in camels for decades, ≥ 20 years. Sero-positivity correlated with density of camels; high density helped maintenance and spread of the virus. Camels serve as an important reservoir for the maintenance and diversification of the MERS-CoVs and are the source of human infections.

How and why human cases appeared/detected in 2012 is unknown. Early cases had exposure to dromedary camels from which virus has been isolated.

Epidemiological observations in 2015 suggested multiple introductions from animals to human and secondary transmission in health settings, thus making a strong case for stopping zoonotic transmission. Possibly transmission does not occur easily unless there is close contact and so sustained human-to-human transmission has not been documented.

Alraddadi et al. (2016) observed that exposure to dromedary camels during 2 weeks before the onset of illness, diabetes mellitus, heart disease and smoking were independently associated with illness. More severe disease was seen in people with weakened immune systems, older people and those with such chronic diseases as diabetes, cancer and chronic lung disease.

Asymptomatic MERS-CoV infection after exposure to sick camels, i.e. zoonotic transmission, has been reported from UAE (http://www.cidrap.umn.edu/news-perspective/2015/08/new-findings-build-case-camel-human-mers-transmission).

Camel farmers and slaughterhouse workers stand at risk.

29.2.4   Transmission

MERS-CoV is transmitted through direct/indirect contact with infected dromedary camels and camel-related products. Virus is shed in nasal secretion, milk and faeces. Raw camel milk is positive for viral RNA and drinking it infects. Virus may survive for 3 days in milk. Milk is also positive for antibodies, therefore useful for screening. Farmers, slaughterhouse workers and market workers are occupationally exposed. Azhar et al. (2014) isolated MERS-CoV from dromedary camel suffering from rhinorrhoea and a patient who had close contact and fatal exposure from it; the genetic sequences were identical.

Human-to-human transmission is most common in healthcare settings such as close contact with patients as in the case of nurses/family members caring without personal protective equipment. Cluster of asymptomatic seropositives and cases in health settings appear. Pilgrims travelling and living in close quarters stand at risk of exposure.

MERS-CoV appears in the secretions from the lower respiratory tract in human beings, peaking after a week of illness. Respiratory droplet infection seems to be the common mode of transmission, although faecal-oral route too may be possible.

29.3   Symptoms

Average incubation period is 5.5–6.5 days, maximum of 14 days. Infection results to asymptomatic to severe pneumonia leading to acute respiratory distress syndrome (ARDS).

Symptoms observed are fever, cough and/or shortness of breath, pneumonia, severe acute hypoxemia and myalgia. Acute respiratory failure requires ICU and mechanical ventilation. Extrapulmonary dysfunction, especially of kidney resulting in failure, may occur. Other serious conditions include disseminated intravascular coagulation, septic shock and pericarditis.

Gastrointestinal symptoms include abdominal pain, diarrhoea and nausea/vomiting. Those showing mild symptoms recover. The death rates are high (30–40%).

SARS and MERS-CoV have been compared for **virus shedding** (http://www.cidrap.umn.edu/news-perspective/2015/11/study-notes-mers-sars-virus-shedding-similarities). The average and peak lower airway excretion was similar. Unlike for SARS, tests rarely found MERS-CoV RNA in urine or stool samples. Sero-conversion occurred during the second and third week after onset of symptoms in both the viruses. Neutralizing antibodies were insufficient to clear either of the viruses from lower airways. Immunoglobulin A develops too late to stop viral replication in infected mucosa. Super shedders had extra-ordinary high viral load unaccompanied with life-threatening or more severe symptoms thus likely to continue social and other engagement. Onset of symptoms to lab positivity was 8 days as was in early cases of SARS in Hong Kong. Time of respiratory shedding and virus concentration were similar but failed to explain differences in transmissibility.

29.4 Diagnosis

A suspected MERS-CoV case is subjected to laboratory tests for classifying 'confirmed' and 'probable' case. Useful tests are:

- Virus isolation—it replicates efficiently in cell lines originating from goats and camels.
- RT-PCR.
- IFT and neutralizing antibody tests.

A *confirmed* case is a person with a positive lab test—'PCR on at least two specific genomic targets or a single positive target with sequencing on a second'. RT-PCR—amplify the upE target for screening assays as it is highly sensitive (WHO); and if positive, confirm with ORF 1A assay or RdRp or N gene sequence assay. If both an upE and secondary assays are positive, it is considered a confirmed case.

A seropositive case is considered '*probable* MERS-CoV' in the absence of PCR testing. Immunofluorescence assay (IFA)—cross-react within the genus. Specific microarray-based assay did not show cross-reactivity.

Samples are taken from the lower respiratory tract via bronchoalveolar lavage (BAL), sputum sample or tracheal aspirate and also upper respiratory sampling via nasopharyngeal swab.

Clinical tests—X-ray shows bilateral patchy infiltration consistent with viral pneumonia and ARDS. Interstitial infiltration is seen on CT scan. Reduced white blood cell count particularly lymphocytes is observed.

29.5 Treatment

There is no specific treatment. Usefulness of interferon, chloroquine, loperamide, lopinavir, mycophenolic acid and camostat is being investigated.

According to Corti et al. (2015), the antibody protein LCA60 obtained from MERS-CoV recovered patients' immune cells latched onto the virus, preventing it from infecting cells in experimental mice. Administering this protein a day before and a day after infecting mice led to the total clearance of virus in 5 days.

In the process of developing a drug, researchers have detected an inhibitor of the enzyme 3C-like protease that is vital for replication of MERS-CoV ["Researchers successfully target 'Achilles' heel' of MERS virus." Science Daily, 22 June 2015. <www.sciencedaily.com/releases/2015/06/150622124711.htm>.].

29.6   Vaccine

Almazán et al. (2013) generated a number of rMERS-CoV deletion mutants using reverse genetic system. One mutant with E gene deleted replicated well and could be a candidate vaccine virus strain capable of inducing mucosal immunity.

Another laboratory-engineered strain of MERS-CoV has altered envelop protein. This strain is able to infect a cell, replicate and produce enough antigen but not able to spread to other tissues and cause disease (Tomar et al. 2015).

29.7   Prevention

The approach to contain this potential global threat includes essentially targeted investigations, information sharing and coordination. Joint and coordinated investigations into human cases and a systematic search for source of infection in animals and environment are required. The Qatar meeting concluded with the 'Doha Declaration', which calls for more joint animal/human investigations of cases and recommended that all animals that test PCR positive for MERS-CoV, regardless of an epidemiologic link to humans, be reported immediately to OIE and to national health authorities (WHO 2015). High level of awareness and rapid intervention to limit exposure are required to restrict sporadic cases turning into outbreaks. Early isolation of cases and adequate measures to prevent and control infection have brought the reproduction number of cases under one in Saudi Arabia, UAE, China and Thailand.

The duration for which a case is infective is unclear. In the epidemic of SARS, the virus could not be isolated after resolution of symptoms. The current recommendation is 'a case is considered safe (unable to infect others) 24 h after the resolution of symptoms'.

Contact tracing is done to prevent transmission. The exposed ones are watched closely for these symptoms: (a) Fever - Take temperature twice a day, (b) Coughing, (c) Shortness of breath, and (d) Other early symptoms like chills, body aches, sore throat, headache, diarrhoea, nausea/vomiting, and runny nose. They are cared and treated if required for 14 days post last date of exposure.

Three steps for contact tracing are:

1. Identification of contacts—once a case is confirmed—enquiries about activities and roles in caring a patient help in identifying contacts.

2. List contacts and educate them about preventive measures and of the importance of early care if they develop symptoms and quarantine in home or hospital in the case of high-risk cases (persons with co-morbidities), if required.
3. Follow up the contacts daily.

Identification of case is difficult as symptoms are common febrile and confusing. History of travel is an important adjunct in all cases of respiratory infections. Standard prevention and cure facilities in hospital are important.

Health workers caring all cases with symptoms of acute respiratory infection and suspected/confirmed cases of MERS-CoV are required to protect themselves from droplet infection, particularly eyes (use goggles), and from aerosol infection in laboratory or aerosol-generating procedures such as intubation. Close contact is defined as contact with cases approximately within 6 feet/2 m or within the room or care area and without recommended personal protective equipment.

Practise regular hand washings for everybody visiting farms and animal markets before and after touching animals.

Avoid contact with animal excretion, especially sick animals.

Use facial protection shield (wherever feasible) and protective clothing, leave these and shoes in the place of work; do not carry to house to protect family members.

Careful handling of meat in the kitchen is required to avoid cross-contamination. Cooked and pasteurized camel meat or milk is safe. Raw milk, urine or meat is unsafe.

References

Adney DR, van Doremalen N, Brown VR et al (2014) Replication and shedding of MERS-CoV in upper respiratory tract of inoculated dromedary camels. Emerg Infect Dis 20(12):1999–2005

Almazán F, DeDiego ML, Sola I, Zuñiga S, Nieto-Torres JL et al (2013) Engineering a replication-competent, propagation-defective Middle East respiratory syndrome coronavirus as a vaccine candidate. MBio 4(5):e00650–e00613

Alraddadi BM, Watson JT, Almarashi A et al (2016) Risk factors for primary Middle East respiratory syndrome coronavirus illness in humans, Saudi Arabia, 2014. Emerg Infect Dis 22(1):49–55

Azhar EI, El-Kafrawy SA, Farraj SA, Hassan AM, Al-Saeed MS et al (2014) Evidence for camel-to-human transmission of MERS coronavirus. N Engl J Med 370(26):2499–2505

Chantal BEMR, Lilia M, Ashenafi F et al (2014) Geographic distribution of MERS coronavirus among dromedary camels, Africa. Emerg Infect Dis J 20(2014):1370

Corti D, Zhao J, Pedotti M, Simonelli L, Agnihothram S et al (2015) Prophylactic and postexposure efficacy of a potent human monoclonal antibody against MERS coronavirus. Proc Natl Acad Sci USA 112(33):10473–10478

International Health Regulations (2005) – 2nd ed. WHO Press, World Health Organization, 20 Avenue Appia, 1211 Geneva 27, Switzerland

Sabir JS, Lam TT, Ahmed MM, Li L, Shen Y, Abo-Aba SE et al (2016) Co-circulation of three camel coronavirus species and recombination of MERS-CoVs in Saudi Arabia. Science 351(6268):81–84

Tomar S, Johnston ML, St John SE, Osswald HL, Nyalapatla PR et al (2015) Ligand-induced dimerization of Middle East respiratory syndrome (MERS) coronavirus nsp5 protease (3CLpro): implications for nsp5 regulation and the development of antivirals. J Biol Chem 290(32):19403–19422

Wernery U, Corman VM, Wong EY et al (2015) Acute middle east respiratory syndrome coronavirus infection in livestock dromedaries, Dubai, 2014. Emerg Infect Dis 21(6):1019–1022

WHO (2015) Middle East respiratory syndrome coronavirus (MERS-CoV) summary of current situation, literature update and risk assessment. WHO/MERS/RA/15.1

WHO (2018) WHO MERS global summary and assessment of risk.. WHO/MERS/RA/August18 Global summary Between 2012 and 30 June 2018, risk-assessment-august-2018.pdf (who.int)

WHO (2019) Middle East respiratory syndrome coronavirus (MERS-CoV). https://www.who.int/en/news-room/fact-sheets/detail/middle-east-respiratory-syndrome-coronavirus-(mers-cov)

WHO (2020) Middle East respiratory syndrome coronavirus (MERS-CoV)—The Kingdom of Saudi Arabia. Disease Outbreak News: Update 24 February 2020. WHO | Middle East respiratory syndrome coronavirus (MERS-CoV)—The Kingdom of Saudi Arabia

Chapter 30
Nipah Virus Encephalitis

Synonyms

Porcine respiratory and neurological syndrome, Porcine respiratory and encephalitis syndrome (PRES), Barking pig syndrome (BPS).

Nipah viral infection is an emerging zoonotic viral encephalitis with marked neurological and respiratory symptoms accompanied with high fever, headache and lowered consciousness in man with high fatality and sudden death in animals, especially pigs. It has pandemic potential.

Nipah virus (NiV) has occurred in Malaysia, Singapore, Philippines, India and Bangladesh.

30.1 Aetiology

The causative agent is Nipah virus (NiV), a paramyxovirus of genus *Henipavirus*, subfamily *Paramyxovirinae*, family *Paramyxoviridae*, order *Mononegavirales*. It was isolated from a human patient with encephalitis by Dr. Chua of the University of Malaya on 18 March 1999 (Chua et al. 1999) and named after Sungai Nipah village of Malaysia from where it was first isolated (Lee et al. 1999; Middleton et al. 2002). It grows quite well in cell lines such as Vero and BHK.

Molecular analysis of the Nipah virus isolates from pigs indicates that the Malaysian outbreak was caused by at least two major strains of Nipah viruses in pigs (Abu Baker et al. 2004). According to Singh et al. (2019), there are two major clades of NiV in circulation. The clades are based on currently available complete N and G gene sequences. The NiV-MY clade viruses circulate in Malaysia and Cambodia. The viruses circulating in Bangladesh and India belong to NiV-BD clade. Viruses in Thailand represent a mixed population of sequences of NiV.

© Springer Nature Singapore Pte Ltd. 2024
K. G. Narayan et al., *Handbook of Management of Zoonoses*,
https://doi.org/10.1007/978-981-99-9885-2_30

Nipah virus (NiV) is closely related to but distinct from the Hendra virus (HeV), another new member of the family *Paramyxoviridae*, first isolated in Hendra, Brisbane, Australia, in 1994 (Murray et al. 1995). *Henipavirus* is a new genus in the family *Paramyxoviridae*, order *Mononegavirales* with a large genome and a wide host range. The Pteropid fruit bats (flying foxes) act as a natural reservoir of henipaviruses (Sawatsky 2008).

The members of the genus are pleomorphic (variably shaped), with a diameter ranging from 40 to 600 nm (Hyatt et al. 2001). The viral matrix protein is covered with a matrix membrane. The core is formed by a single helical strand of genomic RNA which is tightly bound to N (nucleocapsid) protein. This is associated with the L (large) and P (phosphoprotein) proteins which provide RNA polymerase activity during replication.

The F (fusion) protein trimers and G (attachment) protein tetramers are embedded within the lipid membrane. While the G protein helps in attachment to the surface of a host cell via ephrine B2, a highly conserved protein present in many mammals (Bonaparte et al. 2005; Negrete et al. 2005), the fusion of the viral membrane with the host cell membrane is mediated by F protein, thereby releasing its contents into the cell.

The virus particle varies from 120 to 500 nm in size with a typical 'herringbone' nucleocapsid structure of approximately 1.67 ± 0.07 µm long having an average diameter of 21 nm (Chua et al. 2000). Surface projections (10 nm long) are seen sporadically in thin EM sections. The nucleoprotein (N), phosphoprotein (P) and matrix (M) genes of NiV share 70–78% nucleotide homology with the HeV (Chua et al. 2000). The P gene of the virus encodes three non-structural proteins (C, V, W) besides the P. The V and W proteins appear to be the virulence factors. The L protein contains six linear domain structures. The fusion (F) protein contains a single basic amino acid. Attachment protein (G) differs from N or HN glycoproteins of other paramyxoviruses in that they do not have hemagglutinin or neuraminidase activities. It binds to an unidentified cellular receptor which allows F protein to mediate fusion with host cell membrane (Singh et al. 2019).

30.1.1   *Pathogenesis*

In a comprehensive review Singh et al. (2019) have described the pathology, immunobiology and vaccine in the making.

NiV suppresses antiviral cytokine production in the early phase. Release of inflammatory cytokines causes increased vascular permeability and spread of the virus. The innate and adaptive response to infection appears inadequate to prevent invasion of organs.

NiV-host interaction begins with the virus attaching receptors (B2/3) on host cells through its glycoprotein G and the fusion (F) protein makes fusion of virus-cell membranes for cellular entry. The epithelial cells in bronchi and alveoli are the initial target cells. The immune system cells are recruited; inflammatory cytokines are induced, inflammatory mediators; IL6, IL8, G-CSF and CXCL10 are activated.

Respiratory tract epithelial cells followed by endothelial cells of lungs are invaded, resulting in respiratory distress. NiV free in the bloodstream or leucocyte bound spread to other organs: spleen, kidney and brain. CNS invasion leads to neurological signs. Entry to the brain may be through olfactory nerve, as olfactory epithelium of nasal turbinate of experimental animals is found infected with the virus.

30.1.2 Persistence

The persistence of henipaviruses under various environmental conditions was studied by Fogarty et al. (2008). Henipaviruses survived for more than 4 days at 22 °C in pH-neutral fruit bat urine but were sensitive to higher temperatures and pH changes. The half-life of NiV is 18 h. On mango flesh, survival time varied depending on temperature and pH of fruit, ranging from 2 h to more than 2 days. It survived (Singh et al. 2019) for 7 days at 22 °C on artificial date palm sap (13% sucrose and 0.21% BSA in water, pH 7.0). Heating at 100 °C for >15 min, soap, detergents and sodium hypochlorite inactivate.

Nipah virus is relatively stable in the environment. Desiccation reduced survival time. A close contact with hosts is desired for transmission to occur. Henipaviruses appear to persist for extended periods facilitating vehicle-borne transmission.

30.2 Epidemiology

30.2.1 Distribution

More than 600 cases of Nipah virus human infections were reported during 1998–2015. Subsequent outbreaks in India and Bangladesh have occurred with high case fatality (WHO 2018). Cambodia, Ghana, Indonesia, Madagascar, the Philippines and Thailand may be at risk as evidence of the virus has been found in the known natural reservoir (*Pteropus* bat species) and several other bat species.

30.2.2 Natural Host

Fruit bats of the genus *Pteropus* have been identified as a natural reservoir host of Nipah virus (Johara et al. 2001; Yob et al. 2001). These Pteropid bats are commonly called as 'flying foxes' and occur across Southeast Asia. The world distribution of flying foxes (genus *Pteropus*) extends from the west Indian Ocean islands of Mauritius, Madagascar and Comoro, along the sub-Himalayan region of Pakistan and India, through Southeast Asia, the Philippines, Indonesia, New Guinea, the Southwest Pacific Islands (to the Cook Islands) and Australia. There are about 60 species of flying foxes in total. All flying fox species eat fruits, flowers or pollen and roost communally in trees (Hall and Richards 2000). Flying foxes are nomadic, known to travel over considerable distances up to 600 km (Eby 1991).

Studies on the immune response of bats to NiV infection suggested that clearance from body is delayed, minimum replication is retained and consequently persistence is enhanced. Virus-induced pathological changes are prevented. Virus is present in urine and saliva.

P. vampyrus, *P. hypomelanus*, *P. lylei* and *P. medius* (formerly *P. giganteus*) were associated with outbreaks of the Nipah viral disease in various countries of South and Southeast Asia, including Bangladesh, Cambodia, East Timor, Indonesia, India, Malaysia, Papua New Guinea, Vietnam and Thailand.

Epstein et al. (2020) described spatiotemporal patterns of NiV dynamics in *P. medius* in Bangladesh. Transmission occurred round the year and throughout the country. The local transmission dynamics were modulated by a number of factors, such as density, state of acquired immunity and recrudescence. Loss of humoral immunity, turnover of population and declining seroprevalence over multiple years increased transmission.

Pigs are the intermediate hosts. Other animals found infected are dogs, cats, horses and goats.

30.2.3   Transmission

30.2.3.1   Ingestion

Soil and fruits punctured by bats and date palm sap are naturally contaminated by bats' excretion. Pigs eating contaminated fruits or scavenging in area with contaminated soils get infected. A man drinking contaminated date palm sap (in north eastern India and Bangladesh) gets infected.

30.2.3.2   Direct Contact

Direct contact with infected pigs or consuming pork, vegetables, fruits (mango in Malaysia) or water contaminated with saliva, urine or faecal matter from infected bats cause infection. Human-to-human transmission occurs in hospitals (nosocomial) among healthcare workers and family members caring patients.

30.2.4   Spread

Domestic animals other than pigs may play a role in bridging/amplifying hosts in major spillover from bats. Such spillovers occurred during winter in Bangladesh, the number varied with temperature.

It is believed that the epidemic started in the northern Malaysian State of Perak. This led to panic sale, 'fire sales' causing wide dispersal of pigs across the country. The movements of pigs between farms and regions were the primary means of spread as suggested by the epidemiological evidences. It was believed that oro-nasal route was the mode of transmission. Dog, cat and boar semen (though the virus has not been identified in semen) might be considered as secondary modes of spread between farms within the localized farming communities. Pig-transporting lorries might have introduced the infection to otherwise non-infected farms.

Retrospective studies of the epidemic in Perak suggested that Nipah virus caused sporadic disease in pigs in the Peninsular Malaysia since late 1996. Detection was missed because morbidity and mortality were not remarkable and the clinical presentation was not markedly different from those of several endemic diseases (Aziz et al. 1999; Bunning et al. 2000).

Thus, the spillover of the NiV from its natural reservoir flying foxes to pigs remains a subject of speculation and ecological factors are widely thought to be the cause. It is believed that the intentional deforestation in the area coupled with El Niño during the period led to ecological imbalance, leading to the transmission of NiV from the fruit bats to pigs and pigs to human in Malaysia which was facilitated by the change in density and management of pigs (Chua, 2003). Additionally, the practice of growing fruit trees adjacent to the piggeries, too, aided the introduction of the virus into the pigs (Halder and Chakrabarty 2006).

Epidemiologic studies during the Malaysia and Singapore epidemic have established that direct contact with pigs or fresh pig products is responsible for viral transmission to humans, confirming preliminary observations (Chua et al. 1999). Among 110 NiV-infected patients, a significantly higher number of 59% versus 24% of community farm controls reported increased numbers of sick or dying pigs on the farm (Parashar et al. 2000). Also, the patients were found significantly more likely compared to the controls (86% versus 50%) to perform activities resulting in direct contact with sick animals. Infections among abattoir workers and pork sellers have also been reported (Chew et al. 2000; Premalatha et al. 2000; Sahani et al. 2001).

Among 1412 army personnel involved in culling of infected pigs and might possibly have physical contact with these animals, only 6 had antibodies to NiV. Of these, two soldiers were reported to have developed NiV encephalitis (Ali et al. 2001). Possible viral transmission to humans from other animals, e.g. cats and dogs, has also been suggested in a small number of patients (Tan et al. 1999; Parashar et al. 2000). While in Malaysia, the epidemic was controlled by culling of sick pigs (CDC 1999); in Singapore it was controlled by suspending imports of pigs from Malaysia and closure of abattoir (CDC 1999; Chew et al. 2000).

Viral transmission to healthcare workers was thought to be generally low (Mounts et al. 2001). In a large survey of 288 health workers, only 3 were found to have IgG antibodies but IgM and serum neutralization tests were negative, and thus these cases were thought to be false positives. However, there was a report of a nurse who had previously cared for a NiV-infected patient and who subsequently seroconverted but remained asymptomatic. The magnetic resonance (MR) scan of her brain showed a few discrete lesions like those seen in typical acute NiV encephalitis (Tan et al. 2000; Tan and Tan 2001). That human-to-human transmission is possible as exemplified by this case, and the fact that virus could be isolated from patients' secretions (Chua et al. 2000) was subsequently established during the outbreak in Bangladesh (Gurely et al. 2007) and India (Chadda et al. 2001; Halder and Chakrabarty 2006). During the Indian outbreak that occurred in Siliguri, the nosocomial spread was also established (Chadha et al. 2006). It is no surprise that there was a higher prevalence in males, especially from the Chinese ethnic group, as this group more than others was traditionally involved in pig farming (Goh et al. 2000). The 2018 outbreak in Kerala, India, was rapidly controlled. There were 16/18 deaths.

30.2.5   High-Risk Group

Pig farmers, veterinarians, para-veterinarians, abattoir workers and healthcare workers are directly exposed to sick pigs and human and consumers of palm sap.

30.3   Clinical Signs in Pigs

Pigs could be infected orally and by parenteral inoculation. The disease in pigs is highly contagious and can spread quickly to the in-contact pigs. Neutralizing antibodies are detectable 10–14 days post-infection.

Clinical disease in pigs can be very subtle and a large proportion of pigs in a farm may not exhibit any clinical signs. No pathognomonic signs and symptoms of Nipah virus infection in pigs are seen. However, severe respiratory and neurological symptoms, with or without increased mortalities in sows, are observed. Pigs of all ages are susceptible. In the Malaysian outbreak, different clinical picture in different classes of animals was seen. The sows show primarily neurological syndrome, while in porkers, the respiratory syndrome predominated. Majority of pigs on a farm may be infected without showing any symptoms. The incubation period in pigs is estimated to vary from 7 to 14 days (Nor et al. 2000).

30.3.1   Weaners and Porkers

Infection may be asymptomatic, mild or fulminant with low mortality varying from <1% to 5% but morbidity may reach 100%.

Acute cases show high fever with respiratory signs ranging from rapid and laboured breathing to harsh non-productive coughing. In severe cases, there may be blood-tinged mucous discharge from nostrils and open-mouth breathing in less severe cases. Neurological signs include trembling, twitching, muscular spasms and rear leg weakness with varying degree of lameness or spastic paresis.

30.3.2 Sows and Boars

Affected sows and boars may be found dead overnight (Nor et al. 2000), or there may be acute febrile (≥39.9 °C) illness with laboured breathing (panting) and increased salivation with serous, mucopurulent or blood-tinged nasal discharge. Neurological signs including agitation and head pressing, tetanus-like spasms and seizures, nystagmus, champing of mouth and apparent pharyngeal muscle paralysis are also seen. Pregnant sows may abort. Mortality may go up to 40%.

30.3.3 Suckling Pigs

Most of the infected piglets show symptoms of open-mouth breathing, weakness in leg with muscle tremors and neurologic twitches.

30.3.3.1 Necropsy Findings in Pigs

The post-mortem findings due to Nipah virus infection are relatively non-specific. Mild to severe lung lesions with varying degrees of consolidation, emphysema and petechial-to-ecchymotic haemorrhages and blood-tinged exudates in the airways are seen. On the cut surface, the interlobular septa may be distended. There may be generalized congestion and oedema in the meninges.

Nipah virus infection may cause disseminated microinfarction due to thrombosis induced by vasculitis in brain. Similar lesions may be found in the respiratory tract, kidney and heart. There are congestion and oedema. Small and medium blood vessels showed vasculopathy. Generalized vasculitis, fibrinoid necrosis and mononuclear cell infiltration appear in the brain, kidney and lungs.

30.4 Other Susceptible Domestic Species

Some farmers reported deaths in dogs at the same time as in pigs during the Malaysian outbreak. Two such animals exhibiting a distemper-like syndrome were examined. Nipah virus was isolated from the tissues of one and Nipah virus antigen demonstrated in both by immunoperoxidase staining of tissue sections (Chua et al. 2000). Lungs and kidneys seem to be affected. Serological surveys of dogs in infected areas showed that up to 50% of clinically normal dogs had anti-Nipah virus antibodies by ELISA. Some farmers reported that cats also were clinically affected. The susceptibility of cats was confirmed by experimental infections (Middleton et al. 2002). The lesions suggested endothelial syncytia and vasculopathy in multiple organs.

NiV appears to have spilled over to horse from the surrounding infected pig farms. All three horses were from a single property surrounded by infected pig farms.

30.5   Clinical Signs in Man

Nipah virus causes severe rapidly progressing disease. Incubation period in man is estimated to be 4–14 days. The temperature is high, accompanied by severe headache initially. Sore throat, coughing, acute respiratory distress and pneumonia follow. There may be septicaemia and renal and gastrointestinal involvement. In 1–2 days, signs of CNS involvement begin. The predominant clinical syndrome in humans is encephalitic rather than respiratory, with clinical signs including fever, headache, myalgia, drowsiness, disorientation and seizures sometimes proceeding to coma within 48 h (Chua et al. 1999; Goh et al. 2000). The surviving encephalitis cases may suffer nervous sequel. The case fatality is high (40–75%). Besides causing acute infection, it can also cause clinical relapse months and years after infection. A small number of patients—about 8% of the total number of survivors—suffer a second or even third neurologic attack after apparently complete recovery (Tan et al. 2002). However, majority of the recovered patients did not suffer any serious sequelae (Goh et al. 2000).

Nipah Virus infection may result in (a) asymptomatic or mild and (b) acute encephalitis, which may or may not be associated with pneumonia. A small number (3%) of asymptomatic or mildly infected may show relapse/late onset of encephalitis and recover with/without neurological deficiency. Of the acute cases about 30–40% may die. Symptoms among the rest subside. Very rare of them may suffer from massive cerebral haemorrhage and die. The rest of them recover with or without neurological deficiency directly or after manifesting a relapse of encephalitis.

30.6   Diagnosis

Laboratory diagnosis of NiV is challenging in many ways. There are no pathognomonic signs and symptoms. BSL-4 safety laboratory is required.

NiV isolation can be made in Vero cell and the isolate is identified by immunostaining, VNT, PCR or electron microscopy (Daniels et al. 2001). The brain, lungs, kidneys and spleen should be cultured. The CPE usually develops within 3 days but two 5-day passages should be done before the attempt is discontinued. A PCR targeting M gene of NiV (Daniels et al. 2001) and RT-PCR are available and being used routinely in CDC (Halder and Chakraborty 2006). PCR targeting N gene is also available.

Serological tests—Diagnosis of NiV in pigs can be made by serological tests, histopathology, immunohistochemistry, isolation of the virus, electron microscopy and polymerase chain reaction (PCR). The recommended initial tests are ELISA and immunohistochemistry (FAO 2002). ELISA is one of the most useful diagnostic tests and surveillance tools. An ELISA using a recombinant NiV G and M protein has been reported (Daniels et al. 2001). The CDC uses a NiV-specific IgG-based ELISA (Halder and Chakrabarty 2006). The High Security Animal Diseases Laboratory in Bhopal, India, developed a recombinant N protein-based ELISA.

Other options have been mentioned (Singh et al. 2019).

Virus neutralization test (VNT) is an accepted serological test but biosafety considerations require the test to be performed under PC4 facility and limit its use to certain specific laboratory (Daniels et al. 2001). The SNT is also an accepted reference standard for serology.

Immunohistochemistry using monoclonal or polyclonal sera is a very useful test which can be used for retrospective study, too, on a formalin-fixed tissue. It is also one of the safest tests and highly recommended for initial diagnosis.

A negative contrast electron microscopy can be performed on NiV grown in cell culture and supplemented with immunoelectron microscopy (Georges-Courbot et al. 2006).

30.7   Treatment

There is no specific treatment available for the NiV infection. Treatment is essentially supportive. However, ribavirin has been shown to reduce mortality in cases of acute NiV encephalitis (Chong et al. 2001).

Fully humanized monoclonal antibody m102.4 has shown success in treating experimental animals.

30.8   Prevention and Control

In Malaysia during the 1998–1999 outbreak a total of 901,228 pigs from 896 pig farms were destroyed in infected areas from 28 Feb to 26 April 1999. Subsequently, when an indirect ELISA targeting IgG was developed, a total of 889 pig farms were tested from 21 April to 20 July 1999, of which 50 were found positive. These farms were considered as infected and 172,750 pigs from these farms were destroyed by the end of July 1999. On an average 5.6% farms were found positive for NiV infection in Peninsular Malaysia (Nor et al. 2000). In Singapore, where the NiV encephalitis occurred because of the import of the infected pigs from the outbreak areas of Malaysia, it was controlled by banning the import of pigs from Malaysia and closure of the abattoir (Wong et al., 2002).

The Kerala (India) outbreak in 2018 started on 17 May 2018 with the admission of a critically ill patient into Kozhikode's Baby Memorial Hospital, Kerala, that was laboratory confirmed. Isolating patients, using personal protective equipment and decontaminating surfaces, contact tracing and surveillance in Kozhikode and

Malappuram where cases were reported plus neighbouring districts prevented further human-human transmission. Communication channels were open including countering rumours. Two thousand five hundred contacts were detected and monitored. Laboratory-confirmed cases were 18, out of which 16 died. The outbreak was contained by mid-June 2018. The WHO appreciated the effective, strong and connected health systems in close cooperation with animal health and wildlife sectors all that are vital to preparedness and fast reaction.

Nipah virus has pandemic potential because there are more than one strain of virus, error-prone nature of RNA virus replication, human-human transmission, large susceptible population, dense population as in Southeast Asia, global trade and transport and the possibility of spillover.

A recent study in Cambodia (Cappelle et al. 2020) suggested (a) testing of encephalitis patients for NiV, particularly in the case of severe infection and (b) intensifying surveillance during March to May and when female bats are pregnant and lactating and Nipah virus circulation was increased.

The integrated intervention measures to limit exposure to bats should include (a) risk awareness, (b) hunting and consuming bats and fruits partially eaten by animals, (c) palm-nectar collection, (d) using bamboo skirts on trees to prevent bats from accessing and contaminating palm sap, (e) dissociating pig and fruit farming, (f) control of infection in pigs by identifying infected farms and destroying the whole of the flock and (g) use of protective clothing by persons working in farms in endemic areas.

30.9   Vaccines

Vaccination of pigs in endemic areas can prevent pig-human transmission but not contaminated date-palm ingestion-caused disease. The Coalition for Epidemic Preparedness Innovations (CEPI) aims at developing safe, efficacious and affordable vaccines against pandemic potential diseases like Nipah, Lassa virus and MERS-CoV (Singh et al. 2019).

References

AbuBakar S, Chang LY, Ali AR, Sharifah SH et al (2004) Isolation and molecular identification of Nipah virus from pigs. Emerg Infect Dis 10:2228–2230
Ali R, Mounts AW, Parashar UD et al (2001) Nipah virus among military personnel involved in pig culling during an outbreak of encephalitis in Malaysia, 1998–1999. Emerg Infect Dis 7:759
Aziz J, Olson J, Lee OB, Daniels P, Adzhar AB et al (1999) Nipah virus infections of animals in Malaysia. In: Abstract book, XIth international congress of virology. International Unions of Microbiological Societies, Sydney, Australia, p 38
Bonaparte M, Dimitrov A, Bossart K et al (2005) Ephrin-B2 ligand is a functional receptor for Hendra virus and Nipah virus. Proc Natl Acad Sci 102:10652–10657

Bunning M, Jamaluddin A, Cheang H, Kitsutani P, Muhendren, et al (2000) Epidemiological trace-back studies of the Nipah virus outbreak in pig farms in the Ipoh district of Malaysia, 1997–1999. In: Proceedings of the 16th international pig veterinary society congress (ed. McOrist CCaS). International Pig Veterinary Society Congress, Ocean Grove, USA, p 551

Cappelle J, Hoem T, Hul V, Furey N et al (2020) Nipah virus circulation at human–bat interfaces, Cambodia. Bull World Health Organ 98:539–547

CDC (1999) Outbreak of Hendra-like virus—Malaysia and Singapore, 1998–1999. MMWR 48:265

Chadha MS, Comer JA, Lowe L, Rota PA, Rollin PE et al (2006) Nipah virus-associated encephalitis outbreak, Siliguri, India. Emerg Infect Dis 12(2):235–240

Chew MH, Arguin PM, Shay DK, Goh KT, Rollin PE et al (2000) Risk factors for Nipah virus infection among abattoir workers in Singapore. J Infect Dis 181:1760–1763

Chong HT, Kamarulzaman A, Tan CT, Goh KJ, Thayaparan T et al (2001) Treatment of acute Nipah encephalitis with ribavirin. Ann Neurol 49:810–813

Chua KB (2003) Nipah virus outbreak in Malaysia. J Clin Virol 26(3):265–275

Chua K, Bellini W, Rota P, Harcourt B, Tamin A et al (2000) Nipah virus: a recently emergent deadly paramyxovirus. Science 288:1432–1435

Chua KB, Goh KJ, Wong KT, Kamarulzaman A, Tan PSK et al (1999) Fatal encephalitis due to Nipah virus among pig farmers in Malaysia. Lancet 354:1256–1259

Daniels P, Ksiazek T, Eaton BT (2001) Laboratory diagnosis of Nipahand Hendra virus infections. Microb Infect 3:289–295

Eby P (1991) Seasonal movements of Grey-headed flying foxes, *Pteropus poliocephalus (Chiroptera: Pteropodidae)*, from two maternity camps in northern New South Wales. Wildl Res 18:547–559

Epstein JH, Anthony SJ, Islam A et al (2020) Nipah virus dynamics in bats and implications for spillover to humans. Proc Natl Acad Sci USA 117(46):29190–29201

FAO (2002) Manual on the Diagnosis of Nipah virus infection in animals. Food and Agriculture Organization of the United Nations Regional Office for Asia and the Pacific, APHCA. RAP publication no. 2002/01

Fogarty R, Halpin K, Hyatt AD, Daszak P, Mungall BA (2008) Henipavirus susceptibility to environmental variables. Virus Res 132(1-2):140–144

Gorges-Courbot MC, Contamin H, Faure C, Loth P, Baize S et al (2006) Poly(I)-poly(C12U) but not ribavirin prevents death in a hamster model of Nipah virus infection. Antimicrob Agents Chemother 50:1768–1772

Goh KJ, Tan CT, Chew NK, Tan PS, Kamarulzaman A et al (2000) Clinical features of Nipah virus encephalitis among pig farmers in Malaysia. N Engl J Med 342(17):1229–1235

Gurley ES, Montgomery JM, Hossain MJ, Bell M et al (2007) Person-to-person transmission of Nipah virus in a Bangladeshi community. Emerg Infect Dis 13:1031–1037

Hall L, Richards G (2000) Flying foxes: fruit and blossom bats of Australia. University of New South Wales Press Ltd, Sydney

Hyatt A, Zaki S, Goldsmith C et al (2001) Ultrastructure of Hendra virus and Nipah virus within cultured cells and host animals. Microbes Infect 3:297–306

Johara M, Field H, Rashdi A, Morrissy C, Van der Heide B et al (2001) Serological evidence of infection with Nipah virus in bats (order *Chiroptera*) in peninsular Malaysia. Emerg Infect Dis 7:439–441

Lee KE, Umapathi T, Tan CB, Tjia HT, Chua TS et al (1999) The neurological manifestations of Nipah virus encephalitis, a novel paramyxovirus. Ann Neurol 46:428–432

Middleton D, Westbury H, Morrissy C, Van der Heide B, Russell G et al (2002) Experimental Nipah virus infection in pigs and cats. J Comp Pathol 126(2–3):124–136

Mounts AW, Kaur H, Parashar UD et al (2001) A cohort study of health care workers to assess nosocomial transmissibility of Nipah virus, Malaysia, 1999. J Infect Dis 183:810

Murray K, Selleck P, Hooper P, Hyatt A, Gould A et al (1995) A morbillivirus that caused fatal disease in horses and humans. Science 268:94–97

Negrete OA, Levroney EL, Aguilar HC, Bertolotti-Ciarlet A et al (2005) EphrinB2 is the entry receptor for Nipah virus, an emergent deadly paramyxovirus. Nature 436:401–405

Nor M, Gan C, Ong B (2000) Nipah virus infection of pigs in peninsular Malaysia. Rev Sci Off Int Epiz 19:160–165

Parashar U, Sunn L, Ong F, Mounts A, Arif M et al (2000) Case-control study of risk factors for human infection with a novel zoonotic paramyxovirus, Nipah virus, during a 1998-1999 outbreak of severe encephalitis in Malaysia. J Infect Dis 181:1755–1759

Premalatha GD, Lye MS, Arokiasamy J et al (2000) Assessment of Nipah virus transmission among pork sellers in Seremban, Malaysia. Southeast Asian J Trop Med Public Health 31:307

Sahani M, Parashar U, Ali R et al (2001) Nipah virus infection among abattoir workers in Malaysia, 1998–1999. Int J Epidemiol 30:1017

Sawatsky (2008) "Hendra and Nipah viruses", animal viruses: molecular biology. Caister Academic Press

Singh RK, Dhama K, Chakraborty S, Tiwari R, Natesan S et al (2019) Nipah virus: epidemiology, pathology, immunobiology and advances in diagnosis, vaccine designing and control strategies—a comprehensive review. Vet Q 39(1):26–55

Tan CT, Tan KS (2001) Nosocomial transmissibility of Nipah virus. J Infect Dis 184:1367

Tan KS, Sarji SA, Tan CT et al (2000) Patients with asymptomatic Nipah virus infection may have abnormal cerebral MR imaging. Neurol J Southeast Asia 5:69

Tan KS, Tan CT, Goh KJ(1999) Epidemiology aspects of Nipah virus infection. Neurol J Southeast Asia 4:77–81

Tan CT, Goh KJ, Wong KT, Sarji SA et al (2002) Relapsed and late onset Nipah encephalitis. Ann Neurol 51:703–708

WHO (2018) Effective containment of the Nipah virus outbreak in India highlights the importance of a strong health system. https://www.who.int/news/item/30-07-2018-effective-containment-of-the-nipah-virus-outbreak-in-india-highlights-the-importance-of-a-strong-health-system. Accessed 30 July 2018

Yob JM, Field H, Rashdi AM, Morrissy C et al (2001) Nipah virus infection in bats (order Chiroptera) in peninsular Malaysia. Emerging Infect Dis 7(3):439–441

Chapter 31
Hantaviruses

Haemorrhagic fever with renal syndrome (HFRS) and haemorrhagic fever with pulmonary syndrome (HFPS) and cardiopulmonary syndrome are a group of haemorrhagic fever caused by hantaviruses. Korean haemorrhagic fever (haemorrhagic nephroso-nephritis) is characterized by renal failure, generalized haemorrhage and shock and 10% fatality. During the Korean War of 1951–1953 more than 3000 soldiers suffered from it. Investigation resulted into isolation of a virus from the lungs of striped field mice—Hantaan/hantavirus in 1976 named after river Hantan.

HFRS includes diseases such as Korean haemorrhagic fever, epidemic haemorrhagic fever, and nephropathia epidemica. The viruses that cause HFRS include the Old World hantavirus and are Hantaan (HTNV), Dobrava (DOBV), Saaremaa, Seoul (SEOV) and Puumala (PUUV).

In 1993 the outbreak of Four Corners disease (Four Corners region of the USA) occurred. This is now called hantavirus pulmonary syndrome (HPS)/hantavirus cardiopulmonary syndrome (HCPS). Death is attributed to cardiac failure in the latter. Although more than 40 hantaviruses are known, 21 are human pathogens and most are restricted to a single reservoir host species. Almost all pathogenic hantaviruses have rodent reservoirs. These are considered emerging and re-emerging zoonoses with biowarfare potential. These viruses caused nearly 200,000 human infections annually. PUUV and DOBV are common in Europe and Asia and cause HFRS with CFR <1–15% varying with the virus. SEOV is widespread and rodent reservoir *R. norvegicus* has worldwide distribution. The New World viruses, Andes and Sin Nombre, predominant in the Americas and Choclo in Central America cause HPS with case fatality of 40%.

Outbreaks of HFRS were reported in China (>878 by 20 Nov 2017) in Shaanxi province and in Germany (672 by 14 June 2017) (Dong et al. 2019). A cluster of 99 cases was reported in Los Santos Province in Panama in 2019. Of the 99 cases 51 were hanta fever virus without pulmonary syndrome and 48 hantavirus pulmonary syndrome, 4 of which died (https://www.who.int/csr/don/04-January-2019-hantavirus-panama/en/67% aged). Between 28 Oct 2018 and 20 Jan 2019, 29

© Springer Nature Singapore Pte Ltd. 2024
K. G. Narayan et al., *Handbook of Management of Zoonoses*,
https://doi.org/10.1007/978-981-99-9885-2_31

lab-confirmed HPS including 11 deaths were reported in Epuyen, Chubut province of Argentine Republic. Index case had environmental exposure. Against this, an average of 100 cases per year and 114 deaths had occurred during 2013–2018 (https://www.who.int/csr/don/23-January-2019-hantavirus-argentina/en/).

The development of disease is attributed to the host-related cellular immune response. HFRS and HCPS are uncommon in children. Chandy et al. (2008) reviewed hantaviruses as an emerging threat to public health in India.

Geographical distribution appears distinct. HFRS occurs in Asia and Europe, HPS/HCPS in the Americas and so also the viruses HTNV in Asia, PUUV and DOV in Europe and SEOV worldwide.

Hanta viral infections have become endemic in many countries and sporadic events of human-to-human transmission suggest pandemic potential.

31.1   Aetiology

Hantaviruses are enveloped, spherical-shaped negative-sense single-stranded RNA viruses with a diameter of 80–120 nm. These belong to the family *Bunyaviridae*, genus *Hanta*. The virus particle has three nucleocapsids, each containing one RNA segment complexing with N and RdRp RNA-dependent polymerase proteins. The three RNA segments are L (large), M (medium) and S (small). The L genome encodes L proteins that function as viral transcriptase/replicase (RNA-dependent RNA polymerase), M for polyprotein-glycoprotein precursors (GPC) that process two envelop glycoproteins, Gn (former G1) and Gc (former G2) and S for N nucleocapsid protein that forms ribonucleoprotein complexes with segmented RNA.

Hantaviruses have been grouped as (a) phylogenetic, (b) antigenic and (c) areas of activity—Old (Asia and Europe) and New World (the Americas). There are two major **phylogenetic lineages**: (a) Hantaan virus (HTNV), Seoul (SEOV), Thailand (THAIV) and Dobrava (DOBV and (b) Puumala (PUUV), Sin Nombre (SNV) and other New World hantaviruses. SEOV is genetically the most homogenous. HTNV is known to be stable. PUUV isolates are the most variable. Thottapalayam virus (TPMV) is the most divergent and shows greater genetic relatedness to HTNV-like virus group.

Antigenic cross-reactivity is great. Cross-reactivity is greater with N protein antigens than glycoproteins (G1, G2) between members belonging to the three groups of hantaviruses, namely:

1. HTNV-like viruses (HTNV, SEOV, DOBV, THAIV carried by *Murinae* rodents (Old World rats and mice))
2. PUUV-like viruses (PUUV, Tula virus (TULV) carried by *Arvicolinae* rodents (voles and lemmings))
3. SNV-like   viruses   (SNV)   and   Andes   virus   (ANDV)   carried   by *Sigmodontinae* rodents

The **Old World** hantaviruses include species which cause HFRS in Asia and Europe and are associated with rodents of the subfamilies *Murinae* and *Arvicolinae*. The majority of cases have been reported from Europe and Eastern Russia, China and Korea. The prototype virus is HTNV. The associated mouse species *Apodemus agrarius* is found in the fields. About 10,000 HFRS cases are seen in China every year, while in Korea about 300–900 cases occur annually. Thottapalayam virus (TPMV) is the Indian hantavirus isolated from an insectivore shrew (*Suncus murinus*) in 1966 in Vellore. It is quite distinct from other hantaviruses antigenically and phylogenetically.

The **New World** hantaviruses cause HCPS in the Americas. Sin Nombre virus was the first New World hantavirus isolated during the outbreak in the Four Corners region of south western USA in 1993. Subsequently many pathogenic New World hantavirus species have been added, Andes and Sin Nombre being predominant in the Americas and Choclo in Central America. These hantaviruses are associated with rodents belonging to the *Sigmodontinae* subfamily.

Andes virus (ANDV) is the only transmitted human-human.

31.2 Epidemiology

Hantaviruses are also called roboviruses because these are maintained in nature by reservoir rodent species. The distribution of the viruses coincides with the vector rodent species in a particular geographic region. Persistent infections in the rodent host provide opportunity of the two mechanisms—genetic shift and genetic drift—responsible for virus evolution. It appears that the hantavirus species and their rodent reservoirs co-evolved as there is amazing congruence of phylogenetic trees of the two. This has geographic and clinical correlations also. For example, viruses of the Old murine rodents including Hantaan, Seoul and Dobrava are associated with HFRS in Eurasia, whereas viruses of the New World Sigmodontinae rodents including SNV, Black Creek Canal virus (BCCV) and Bayou virus (BAYV) are associated with HPS in the Americas (http://www.cdc.gov/hantavirus/technical/hanta/virology.html). Isolation from a non-rodent host species may be considered as spillover and their role in transmission of hantaviruses is not clear.

Hantavirus infection in rodents is asymptomatic and persistent. Infection spills over to other species like human beings. The infection meets a dead end in humans.

31.2.1 Modes of Transmission

According to Tian and Stenseth (2019) the spillover of hantavirus to human from natural hosts may be an ecological process influenced by environmental forces, behavioural determinants of exposure and dynamics at the animal-human interface.

Rodents allow infection, amplification and perpetuation of the virus through an efficient transmission cycle. Infectious fresh droppings, urine and saliva of rodents contaminate soil that is aerosolized to cause infection through inhalation. The virus is transmitted among rats through bites and contamination of scratches. Human beings are also infected by exposure to these. Indirect transmission may also probably occur through hands and foods contaminated with rodents' excreta. Human-to-human transmission is uncommon, except the report from Argentina that was incidentally also nosocomial.

The period of shedding of virus varies with hantaviruses and type of excreta. For example, Old World HNTV is shed longest in the urine of *Apodemus* and the New World BCCV for 70 days to months after infection; PUUV is detected with a life span of maximum 2 years in tissues of bank vole but its most efficient transmission through excreta occurs during the first 2 months after infection.

PUUVA survive and remain infectious for 2 weeks in droppings of bank vole indoor (lack of sunshine/UV radiation) at cold or at room temperature. Therefore, barns and cabins/rooms abandoned for long but having free access to rodents aerosolize virus and may lead to infection.

31.2.2   Occupation/Risk Groups

Hanta virus infection is occupational in nature. People who live or work in close contact with infected rodents are at increased infection risk such as animal trappers, forest workers, farmers, laboratory workers handling experimental rodents and these viruses.

Risk factors in urban settings are different. Human settlements, their occupation and activity influence hantavirus transmission.

SEOV is cosmopolitan in nature and known to cause urban cases of HFRS. This virus circulates in domestic rats who take international shipping routes to get distributed worldwide.

31.2.3   Season

The distribution of human infection and also the seasonal variation are dependent upon rodent population and human activities. Infection during summer, spring and peak during fall in Asia is related with greater contact between rodents and man during agricultural operations. In the USA deer mouse, white-footed mouse, rice rat and cotton rats carry hantavirus.

Lundkvist et al. (2013) detected Seoul hantavirus in a pet rat's lung in Sweden following reports of association of infected pet and wild rats with human cases of HFRS in England and Wales.

Jonsson et al. (2010) discussed the relationship of rodent population and HFRS epidemics. Factors affecting rodent population thus would influence the epidemic.

These factors differ according to settings—such as forest, rural, urban, etc.—and climate.

31.2.3.1   Forest Setting

In the forest settings, rodent population peaks due to 'mast years' in temperate Central Europe, in the Balkans and in Scandinavia. Nuts of forest trees accumulate and are available as rodent food in abundance in certain years—called 'mast year'. Flower buds develop in summer (consecutive 2 years) and this is followed by the year of high autumn temperature necessary for seed development. Availability of abundant nuts follows.

Cold snowy winter is typical of northern Europe. Predation of rodents by certain specialist species, like weasel, results into alternate abundance of prey and predators. A regular cycle of 3–4 years of bank vole population density is observed. Bank vole population is high in two consecutive autumns (increase) and winters (peak) followed by a crash in the next spring. This is seen in Finland and northern Sweden. Southern Sweden is temperate, bank vole population is stable, and hantavirus infections are rare. However, a sudden warm spell in January in northern Sweden pushed bank vole population close to human dwellings and resultant exposure. Satellite data also showed dependence of rodent ecology on climate and prediction of PUUV in Scandinavia has been attempted.

31.2.4   *Climate*

Climate is considered to have determined the 1993 outbreak of HCPS (most cases occurred in late spring and summer) caused by Sin Nombre virus (SNV) in the USA. The prolonged El Niño effect led to the increased rain that promoted the abundance of deer mice (*Peromyscus maniculatus*), aggressive interaction among them and transmission of SNV.

Tian and Stenseth (2019) reviewed studies on dynamics of rodent population in relation to climate and human activities. Transmission of hantaviruses between rats is horizontal. A threshold population is essential, below which transmission will stop. Winter and food limitations affected the survival of rodents. A study of 50 years' data showed that low summer temperature and high precipitation favoured the transmission of HTNV from the striped field mouse to human and caused outbreaks of HFRS in Central China, and the relationship was highly correlated. Conversely, a population of striped field mouse *Apodemus agrarius*, main reservoir host of HTNV, was reduced during hot summer and extreme drought because of shortage of food (reduced farm crop production). The population density of bank voles, main reservoir for PUUV, was associated with summer and autumn temperature that favoured seed development.

Human activities cause habitat loss/change and affect reproduction and survivability.

31.2.4.1   Rural Setting

In rural settings of China the population of field mice increases when there are good seed crops, low rainfall and absence of flooding. Higher incidence of *Apodemus agrarius*-borne HFRS is predicted. HFRS and HPS are considered rural diseases.

31.2.5   Other Factors

Factors such as deforestation, extensive agriculture and climate change affect rodent population and lead to aggressive interaction within a single rodent species resulting into great transmission among rodents and greater risk of spread to humans.

31.3   Pathogenesis

The virions attach to hosts' cellular receptors and enter cells through endocytosis. Nucelocapsids are introduced and three actions seem to be initiated by L protein transcription, replicase and possibly also endonuclease that cleaves cellular mRNAS for the production of 'capped primers' to initiate transcription of viral mRNAs (called 'cap snatching'). Free ribosomes are thought to translate the viral N and mRNAs. The M mRNAs are translated in the endoplasmic reticulum to form glyco-proteins. These are transported to Golgi complex where hantaviruses are assembled and bud into Golgi cisternae. Nascent virions are carried in secretary vesicles to plasma membrane and released by exocytosis.

N protein forms in the host cell cytoplasmic inclusions and is filamentous in structure. It is multifunctional—(a) protects the RNA genome by encapsidation, replication and virus assembly, (b) interacts with cellular macromolecules to inhibit important cellular regulatory pathway and (c) is highly antigenic causing rapid and strong immune response and hence antibodies are detectable early in infection. Recombinant N protein is currently used in diagnostic assays. The glycoproteins mediate cell attachment and fusion.

Hantaviruses are typically airborne and infect lung parenchymal cells, phagocy-tosed and drained to the nearest lymph nodes. Further dissemination transports these to the target cells—endothelial cells of lungs, heart, lymphoid tissues, spleen, gall bladder and kidney in the case of HFRS. Cytopathy is related to immune mech-anisms that lead to massive vascular dysfunction and plasma leakage and reduced blood pressure. In the case of HPS there is heavy capillary leakage in the lungs (non-cardiogenic pulmonary oedema). This may progress rapidly to cardiogenic shock (HCPS).

31.4   Haemorrhagic Fever with Renal Syndrome (HFRS)

Synonyms: Porcine respiratory and neurological syndrome, Porcine respiratory and encephalitis syndrome (PRES), Barking pig syndrome (BPS).

HFRS occurs in Asia, Europe, Africa, China, the Korean peninsula and Russia and is commonly caused by three viruses—Hantaan, Puumala and Seoul. Pathogenic hantaviruses in Europe causing HFRS are Seoul, Dobrava, Saaremaa (SAAV) and Puumala. The respective reservoirs are *Rattus norvegicus* (the Norway rat), *Apodemus flavicollis* (yellow necked mouse), *A. agrarius* (striped field mouse) and *Clethrionomys glareolus*, currently known as *Myodes glareolus* (bank vole). SAAV is closely related to DOBV. SEOV has worldwide distribution because of the spread of reservoir through world trade (Lundkvist et al. 2013). DOBV, SAAV and PUUV have reducing virulence—as is observed by reducing case fatality rates in this sequence. PUUV causes nephropathia epidemica, a mild form of HFRS (Engler et al. 2013). Seoul virus (designated as strain Humber) was detected from *Rattus norvegicus* collected from a property in Yorkshire and Humber, UK, and from a patient of acute kidney injury. This is the first report of isolation from wild rodent in the UK (Jameson et al. 2013). The UK Public Health has undertaken a study to assess the risk of infection in (a) the general population, (b) owners and breeders of domesticated "fancy" rats, (c) those with occupational exposure to pet rats: breeders who supply pet shops and (d) those with occupational exposure to wild rats—small animal vets, pest control workers, sewage workers and farmers.

HFRS is a serious public health problem in the People's Republic of China. According to Zhang et al. (2010), there are >100 species of rodents and several dozens of insectivores widely distributed in HFRS-endemic areas in China. Hantavirus-specific antibodies and/or antigens have been identified in at least 38 rodent species. The seven geno-/serotypes of hantaviruses are HTNV, SEOV, Da Ble Shan, Hokkaido, Khabarovsk, Vladivostok and Yuanjiang and yet unknown hantavirus species may be circulating in China. Of these, Hantaan virus (*Apodemus agrarius* mice) and Seoul virus (*Rattus norvegicus*) only caused diseases. There were 155,622 cases between 1950 and 2007 with 3% mortality distributed in 29/31 provinces. Through comprehensive preventive measures including vaccination, the number of cases has drastically reduced and mortality brought down to less than 1% during the past 8 years. Yet China continues to report the maximum number of cases and deaths in the world.

According to Chandy et al. (2008), serological investigation in India revealed IgM antibodies in 14.7% of pyrexia patients and in 5.7% of healthy blood donors. The tribe *Irula* lives in close proximity to rodents and also patients with chronic renal disease show significantly higher frequency of seropositivity. The prevalence is 4% among the high-risk group (proximity to rodent). In another study in Cochin and Chennai area, of the patients presenting leptospirosis-like symptoms, 12% had SEOV-like and 5% had PUUV-like infections. Hantavirus infection presenting ocular involvement in Western India is reported. These authors have observed that hantaviruses like THAIV-like and HTNV-like/SEOV-like are prevalent in India. Nine of 54 rodent sera were positive for HTNV and 6/9 reacted with THAIV antigens.

31.4.1 Symptoms

Infection with different hantaviruses may manifest differently. Chandy et al. (2008) described the manifestation into the following five phases: febrile (lasting 3–5 days), hypotensive (few hours to few days), oliguric (3–7 days), diuretic and finally convalescent. However, a patient may present only three phases—fever with shock and multiorgan failure, fever with oliguric acute renal failure and fever without renal failure.

Febrile phase presents symptoms resembling influenza. These are nausea, vomiting, backache and abdominal pain. On the third to fifth day proteinuria appears suddenly and in severe HFRS (common in endemic areas) may be albuminuria. The febrile phase ends with flushing of face and suffusion of conjunctiva. The patients enter in hypotensive phase characterized by thrombocytopenia and most (about 1/3rd) die due to shock. Survivors enter into oliguric phase. Proteinuria may persist. Nearly 50% die due to renal failure. The disease progresses into diuretic phase lasting for a few days to a few weeks, during which there is renal recovery and patients convalesce and finally recover.

31.4.2 Laboratory Diagnosis

- Haematology—haemoconcentration, leucocytosis, thrombocytopenia, marked polymorphonuclear leucocytosis with left shift and CD8+ activated cells (appear as atypical leucocytes)
- Urine-proteinuria, haematuria, pyuria
- Enzymes—*elevated alanine aminotransferase, aspartate aminotransferase, lactate dehydrogenase and creatine kinase enzymes*
- Additional tests as for HPS

31.5   Hantavirus Pulmonary Syndrome/Cardiopulmonary (HPS/HCPS)

HPS/HCPS occurs in America. A 20-year's surveillance in the USA was reported by Knust and Rollin (2013). Most of the cases of hantavirus pulmonary syndrome (HPS) occurred in the states west of Mississippi River. This region continues to be endemic even in 2020, accounting for 94% of cases. There were 833 cases of hantavirus disease (HPS 807 and non-pulmonary 26) with 35% mortality at the end of 2020: median age 37.5 years (range 5–84 years), male (62%), female (38%); 73% of cases were white; 64% were not Hispanic/Latino (CDC 2022). Sin Nombre virus was the commonest. Indigenous cases of Seoul virus caused haemorrhagic and renal syndrome. Other viruses recorded were Bayou, Black Creek Canal, Monongahela and New York. The authors suggested that a case of pulmonary infection—presenting differently or not linked to deer mouse—exposure or exposed to other rodents and are from outside the Western United States must be investigated. Imported cases in the USA are military personnel returning from the Korean War (from Korea), others from China (caused by Seoul virus) and infection acquired in Brazil detected serologically (HPS) in Florida and acquired in Germany and detected in Florida (Puumala virus). *Rattus rattus* and *R. norvegicu*s are rodent hosts.

HPS has been reported from six countries in South America since 1993—Argentina, Bolivia, Brazil, Chile, Paraguay and Uruguay. According to Vicente Bayard et al. (2004), several hantaviruses have been isolated, and included in these are Andes virus (Argentina, Bolivia, Chile, and Uruguay), Bermejo virus (Bolivia), Juquitiba virus (Brazil), Laguna Negra virus (Bolivia, Paraguay), Lechiguanas virus (Argentina), Oran virus in Argentina and Choclo virus in Panama (Central America). Martinez et al. (2010) reported six lineages of hantaviruses in Argentina occurring during 1995–2008.

Travassos da Rosa et al. (2010) concluded from their serological and phylogenetic studies that Anajatuba virus caused HPS in Brazil. The reservoir rodent was *Oligoryzomys fornesi*. Infection in *N. lasiurus* rodent was considered as spillover. Cases of HPS were rare. The Baixada Maranhense region had HPS in common.

Hantaviral infections were reported from various parts of Argentina. Human-to-human transmission is suggested in an outbreak of HPS that occurred in Epuyen, Chubut province of southern Argentina between 28 October 2018 and 20 January 2019. There were 29 cases including 11 deaths confirmed by ELISA IgM *u*-capture or by polymerase chain reaction (PCR).

The index case had environmental exposure on 2 November. He participated in a get-together on 3 November. Six of the participants had an onset of symptoms between 20 and 27 November 2018. Another set of 17 cases were epidemiologically linked to previously confirmed cases. They reported onset of symptom between 7 December and 3 January 2019. Further 98 asymptomatic contacts identified by 17 January 2019 were being monitored.

A health worker from Los Lagos Region, Chile, travelled to Epuyen and cared for a case in her prodromal phase. She was a laboratory-confirmed case of HPS (https://www.who.int/emergencies/disease-outbreak-news/item/23-January-2019-hantavirus-argentina-en).

31.5.1   Symptoms

Incubation period varies as 1–6 weeks, usually 3–5 days. Illness is often confused with influenza—fever, severe muscle ache, fatigue, headache, dizziness, chills, nausea, vomiting, diarrhoea or stomach pain. HPS is characterized by fever, headache and pain in muscles—thigh, hip, back and shoulder—followed by dyspnoea, non-cardiogenic pulmonary oedema, hypotension and shock. Chandy et al. (2008) described two phases of illness: prodromal and cardiopulmonary. The former presents fever, headache, chills and myalgia, confused with influenza or other viral illness. The latter presents pulmonary oedema, dyspnoea and hypoxemia, usually 10 days later. Cardiac depression, respiratory failure and acidosis leading to fatal arrhythmias are seen in severe cases. Untreated cases experience short of breath, cough as lungs fill with fluid (non-cardiogenic pulmonary oedema), hypotension and shock. Increased haematocrit, leucocytosis with the presence of immunoblast cells and thrombocytopenia are common laboratory observations.

Hantaviruses infect every age group of both sexes. Case fatality rate can be as high as 52% (Bayard et al. 2004).

A study of Martinez et al. (2010) on 710 cases occurring during 1995–2008 in Argentina provides insight into the hanta viral infection. Prodromal phase was followed by varying degree of rapid and acute respiratory distress. Antibody response in 11.6 days after the onset of illness was mainly IgM but 85.6% had also IgG. The case fatality rate was 25.8% (maximum was 40.5%). The seasonal distribution of cases was spring followed by summer, autumn and winter, with eco-regional differences. HPS affected 0–77 years with maximum in the age group of 21–30 and 9.35% in the age group <14 years. The sex distribution of cases was males to females 3.7:1.0. Mortality was higher among females (34%) than males (21%). Higher mortality among those patients without IgG than with IgG was recorded. Platelet count was high and may be considered an indicator. Most cases occurred among those engaged in agricultural farm-related activities like tilling, planting, weeding, harvesting and cleaning barns and buildings. In the peridomestic settings high-risk group included housewives, children and those working with recreational and tourism, truck, sanitization and security. Activities that put one in contact with rodents and their environments directly expose those engaged in such activities.

31.6   Diagnosis

Symptoms are confounding, viremia is short lived, and cross-reactivity presents a problem. Diagnosis therefore depends upon the correlation of history of exposure to rodents, clinical and laboratory findings and serology. Use of homologous antigens is far more sensitive than heterologous antigens and is advisable in areas where circulating serotypes are known. A suspected HPS case is defined as (a) having fever >38.3 °C and unexplained acute respiratory distress requiring supplemental oxygen, (b) with radiograph support, (c) X-ray showing bilateral interstitial pulmonary infiltrates and (d) death from unexplained respiratory illness and post-mortem showing non-cardiogenic pulmonary oedema.

Rapid specific diagnosis is essential as the case may progress to unmanageable state. HPS (also HFRS) is confirmed by any of the following:

1. Detection of hantavirus-specific IgM antibodies in acute-phase serum
2. Hantavirus by RT-PCR

The preferred method for diagnosis of acute infections is detection of virus-specific IgM by the capture ELISA. Detection of virus-specific IgG and IgM in non-endemic areas should be used. IgG response is delayed sometimes.

Nested reverse transcription-polymerase chain reaction (RT-PCR) assay for detection of hantavirus genome using genus and species-specific primers (Bayard et al. 2004) from blood, serum, organ fragments.

3. Isolation of hantaviruses from clinical specimens is difficult and hazardous. A biosafety level 3 or 4 is required for animal studies. Vero E6 cell line (African green monkey kidney cell line) is used for growing hantaviruses. In the absence of cytopathic effect, IFA is used to detect the virus.

31.7 Treatment and Control

Antipyretic, analgesics and broad-spectrum antibiotics are used.

Hanta viral infection demands aggressive intervention in the form of 'intensive cardiopulmonary care' with a focus on maintaining blood pressure, oxygenation with measures like mechanical ventilation and extracorporeal membrane oxygenation. These control the progression of disease.

No effective drug is available. Ribavirin (1-ß-D-ribofuranosyl-1,2, 4-triazole-3-carboxamide) has shown reduction in fatality in HFRS cases in China, but was ineffective in treating HPS.

Post-hantavirus infection prophylactic treatment, as is practised for rabies, has been suggested.

According to Liu et al. (2020) there are no drugs and approved vaccines. A combination of antiviral, immunomodulator and supportive therapies should be strategically used. Antiviral therapy is effective if used prophylactically and in early stage and not after acute phase when uncontrolled immune response predominated pathogenesis. They have reviewed vaccines (DNA, subunit and whole virus inactivated) under different stages of studies and trials.

31.7.1   Vaccines

There is no approved vaccine. Inactivated vaccines, including bivalent (HTNV and SEOV grown in Vero cells), have been used in HFRS endemic areas. The protective response is short lived. Nucleic acid vaccines are being researched. Baculovirus and vaccinia-expressed hantavirus glycoproteins confer protection in animal models.

31.7.2   Prevention

Detection, investigation, reporting and case management are recommended for prevention and control. Travellers including eco-tourists returning from affected areas might suffer and introduce the infection, hence the need for special attention. Early detection followed by medical care on time is clue to positive clinical outcome.

Surveillance should be comprehensive and inclusive of clinical, laboratory and environment components.

Prevention of exposure to rodent excreta is the best way to avoid infection. Deratization to reduce rat population density may be done in high-risk areas. Predation by barn owl may be a method of controlling hanta viral infection as *Necromys lasiurus*, the main reservoir in the Cerrado biome, Brazil, and was the second most preferred prey (Margini and Facure 2008).

Avoiding all wild mice and rats and safely cleaning up their burrows/nests and droppings and urine is the best preventive measure.

References

Bayard V, Kitsutani PT, Barria EO, Ruedas LA, Tinnin DS et al (2004) Outbreak of hantavirus pulmonary syndrome, Los Santos, Panama, 1999-2000. Emerg Infect Dis 10(9):1635–1642

CDC (2022). https://www.cdc.gov/hantavirus/surveillance/index.html. Accessed 6 May 2022

Chandy S, Abraham P, Sridharan G (2008) Hantaviruses: an emerging public health threat in India? A review. J Biosci 33:495–504

Dong Y, Ma T, Zhang X, Ying Q, Han M, Zhang M et al (2019) Incorporation of CD40 ligand or granulocyte-macrophage colony stimulating factor into Hantaan virus (HTNV) virus-like particles significantly enhances the long-term immunity potency against HTNV infection. J Med Microbiol 68:480–492

Engler O, Klingstrom J, Aliyev E, Niederhauser C, Fontana S et al (2013) Seroprevalence of hantavirus infections in Switzerland in 2009: difficulties in determining prevalence in a country with low endemicity. Euro Surveill 18(50):20660

Jameson LJ, Logue CH, Atkinson B, Baker N, Galbraith SE et al (2013) The continued emergence of hantaviruses: isolation of a Seoul virus implicated in human disease, United Kingdom, October 2012. Euro Surveill 18(1):20344

Jonsson CB, Figueiredo LTM, Vapalahti O (2010) A global perspective on hantavirus ecology, epidemiology and disease. Clin Microbiol Rev 23(2):412–441

References   303

Knust B, Rollin PE (2013) Twenty-year summary of surveillance for human hantavirus infections, United States. Emerg Infect Dis 19(12):1934–1937
Liu R, Ma H, Shu J, Zhang Q, Han M, Liu Z, Jin X, Zhang F, Wu X (2020) Vaccines and therapeutics against hantaviruses. Front Microbiol 10:2989
Lundkvist Å, Verner-Carlsson J, Plyusnina A, Forslund L, Feinstein R, Plyusnin A (2013) Pet rat harbouring Seoul hantavirus in Sweden, June 2013. Euro Surveill 18(27):20521
Margini L, Facure KG (2008) Barn owl (*Tyto alba*) predation on small mammals and its role in the control of hantavirus natural reservoirs in a periurban area in southeastern Brazil Braz. J Biol 68(4):733–740
Martinez VP, Bellomo CM, Cacace ML, Suárez P, Bogni L, Padula PJ (2010) Hantavirus pulmonary syndrome in Argentina, 1995–2008. Emerg Infect Dis 16(12):1853–1860
Tian H, Stenseth NC (2019) The ecological dynamics of hantavirus diseases: from environmental variability to disease prevention largely based on data from China. PLoS Negl Trop Dis 13:e0006901
Travassos da Rosa ES, Sampaio de Lemos ER, de Almeida Medeiros DB et al (2010) Hantaviruses and hantavirus pulmonary syndrome, Maranhao, Brazil. Emerg Infect Dis 16(12):1952–1955
Zhang Y-Z, Zou Y, Fu ZF, Plyusnin A (2010) Hantavirus infections in humans and animals, China. Emerg Infect Dis 16(8):1195–1203

Chapter 32
Rabies and Related Viruses

Rabies or hydrophobia (in man) is an acute rapidly progressing severe encephalo-myelitis almost always ending in death. It is a *direct anthropozoonosis* caused by rabies virus which infects all warm-blooded animals. Hydrophobia is preceded by frightening and painful bite by a vicious rabid dog, discomfort, anxieties and risk of uncertainties and characterized by terrifying and agonizing bouts of intense sufferings.

Rabies is known to occur in the Arctic regions, temperate and tropical regions of both the hemispheres. It does not occur in Antarctica. Australia maintains freedom from rabies; only three cases of bat-associated rabies have been reported.

32.1 Human Rabies

Human rabies is either dog-mediated or bat-mediated. About 99% of human rabies in endemic areas is caused by dog bite.

32.1.1 Dog Mediated Rabies

According to the WHO/FAO/OIE (2018), a country is defined as free of dog rabies if no indigenously acquired dog-mediated rabies cases have been confirmed in humans, dogs or any other animal species for at least 2 years. Western Europe, Canada, the United States of America (USA), Japan and some Latin American countries and many Pacific Island nations are free from rabies. Such countries may report imported cases and bat- or wild animal-associated rabies.

Rabies is endemic in Latin America and the Caribbean, Asia, Africa, Central Asia and the Middle East. Rabies was reported in Bolivia, Brazil, the Dominican

© Springer Nature Singapore Pte Ltd. 2024
K. G. Narayan et al., *Handbook of Management of Zoonoses*,
https://doi.org/10.1007/978-981-99-9885-2_32

Republic, Guatemala, Haiti, Honduras, Peru and Venezuela between 2013 and 2016.

Rabies caused 59,000 deaths annually, 40% among children <15 years and 3.7 million DALYs. The vast majority (>99%) of DALYs lost (3.68 million) were due to the premature death of rabies victims (Hampson et al. 2015). About 80% of cases occur in rural areas. Global burden of rabies is estimated at US$ 8.6 billion per year. Its breakdown is as follows: loss of human life (54%), income during period of treatment (15%), due to deaths in livestock (6%), cost of dog vaccination and population control (4%) and cost of rabies surveillance (0.01%) and direct cost (on vaccines and immunoglobulins) (20%) (WHO/FAO/OIE 2018). The rabies burdens according to endemic regions are:

Asia: Rabies is a major burden, particularly for the poor. It accounted for 59.6% of global deaths and 2.2 million DALYs/year (59.9%) due to dog-mediated rabies. 35% of global deaths occurred in India. It is approximately 20,800 deaths more than in any other country (Hampson et al. 2015).

Africa: It accounted for 34.6% of global deaths and loss of 1.34 million DALYs.

Central Asia: 1875 human deaths and 14,310 DALYs loss/year.

Middle East: 229 human deaths and 1875 DALYs.

India, the world's second most populous country (with close to 18% of the global population), accounts for over 35% of the global rabies burden.

32.1.2 Bat Mediated Rabies

A small proportion of human rabies worldwide is due to bat rabies. Most cases occur in the Americas. More Americans sought PEP for exposure to terrestrial carnivores than bat; however, more rabid bats than rabid raccoons were recorded in 2015. Rabid bats were reported from every state in the USA except Hawaii. Majority of bats do not carry RABV but one cannot tell just by looking which bat is carrying the virus. Bats accounted for about 70% of locally acquired infection over the past 70 years. An average of 55,000 Americans received PEP each year in 2017 and 2018. Seventy percent of those who died from rabies in the USA were infected by bats (Infectious Disease News, June 12, 2019—CDC: Bats are leading cause of rabies infection in US). Vampire bat rabies caused loss of livestock in Argentina, Uruguay and northern Mexico. In Africa, Asia and Oceania, bat rabies is rare.

In the USA, Kunkel et al. (2022) reported three human deaths during 28 September–10 November 2021. They had direct contact with bats species commonly associated with rabies. The exposure was attributed to a bat roost in one of the patient's home. The other two had picked up bats with their bare hands. One had vaccine phobia and the others did not realize it was needed. While symptoms appeared 3–7 weeks after exposure, deaths occurred 2–3 weeks after the onset of symptoms. The bats were silver-haired (*Lasionycteris noctivagans*), Mexican free-tailed (*Tadarida brasiliensis*) and big brown bat (*Eptesicus fuscus*), commonly attributed to rabies deaths in the USA. Nearly 70% of 89 human rabies cases during 1960–2018 were due to exposure to bats; 5.8% of 24,000 bats screened in 2020 were positive for rabies virus. About two-third of the estimated 60,000 receiving PEP had bat exposure. Human-bat contact increased in late spring to early fall; bat activity is low during winter.

32.2 Aetiology

Rabies virus comes under the genus *Lyssavirus*, family Rhabdoviridae, order Mononegavirales. The International Committee on Taxonomy of Viruses named the genus after the Greek goddess 'Lyssa'—goddess of rage, fury related with pain, distress, frenzy and madness. Lyssaviruses are defined according to genotypes. The 14 species have been placed into three genotypes I–III. Isolates having >80–82% nucleotide identity for the nucleotide N gene (threshold value) belonged to the same species. Additional data are useful, such as antigenic pattern, pathology, reaction with nucleocapsid mAbs, ecology and geographic distribution.

The virus is bullet-shaped, enveloped single-stranded negative sense RNA and has approximately 12,000 base pairs, and its genome encodes five monocistronic genes: nucleoprotein (N protein), phosphoprotein (P), matrix protein (M), glycoprotein (G) and RNA-dependent RNA polymerase (RdRp) L protein. Together with the RNA, the N, P and L proteins form an inner ribonucleoprotein core, or nucleocapsid. The outer G protein forms spikes that project through the virion membrane. The M protein links the inner nucleocapsid and the outer membrane-bound G protein. Most variants arise through genetic drift—survival of mutations, because rabies virus does not have proof and reading ability during replication.

G protein carries main host cell receptor-binding and antigenic sites. Lyssaviruses of the same phylogroup cross-neutralize. The strains used in available vaccine belong to RABV virus species in phylogroup I. The vaccine is ineffective against infection with lyssaviruses of phylogroups II and III.

The antigenic cross-reactivity at the level of nucleocapsid (N protein) is broad and similar reagents can be used in diagnosis by immunofluorescence.

Currently known 14 viruses have been listed (Table 32.1). Gannoruwa bat lyssavirus isolated from *Pteropus medius* in Sri Lanka is closely related to RABV and Australian bat virus and likely to be phylogroup I. Lleida bat lyssavirus from bent-winged bat in Spain is highly divergent, likely to fall in group III. Taiwan bat lyssavirus and Kotalahti bat lyssavirus from Finland require more studies.

Genotype 1 rabies virus is the type species of the genus. This and the vampire bat variant confined to Latin America are the significant veterinary and public health problem.

Table 32.1 Summary of lyssaviruses (Barett, 2011 and WHO Technical Report Series No. 1012, 2018)

Antigenic phylogroup	Genotype	Lyssavirus	Maintenance host	Location	Number of human cases
I	1	Rabies virus	Carnivore and multiple species of insectivorous and hematophagous bats	Carnivores on all continents except Australia and Antarctica Insectivorous and hematophagous bats in the Americas	59,000/year
III	2	Ikoma lyssavirus	*Civetictis civetta*	United Republic of Tanzania	None
II	3	Lagos bat	Unconfirmed—a few isolates from Megachiroptera (*Epomophorus wahlbergi*—Wahlberg's epauletted fruit bat) and Microchiroptera	Central African Republic, Ghana, Kenya, Nigeria, Senegal, South Africa; travellers returning to France from Egypt or Togo	None
II	4	Mokola	Unconfirmed—a few isolates from shrews (*Crocidura* spp.), rodents and domestic cat. No bat isolates	Cameroon, Central African Republic, Ethiopia, Nigeria, South Africa, Zimbabwe	2 (both 1970)
I	5	Duvenhage	Egyptian slit-faced bat	Zimbabwe	3
I	5	Duvenhage	Unconfirmed—a few isolates from insectivorous bats (*Miniopterus* spp. and *Nycteris thebaica*)	Kenya, South Africa	3 (1970, 2006, 2007)
I	6	European bat lyssavirus (EBLV-1)	Insectivorous bats—typically *Eptesicus serotinus* (serotine bat)	Europe	2 (1977, 1985)[a]
I	6	EBLV-2	Insectivorous bats—typically *Myotis daubentonii* (Daubenton's bat)	Western Europe	2 (1985, 2002)[a]
I	7	Australian bat lyssavirus	Flying foxes (*Pteropus* spp.) and at least one species of insectivorous bat (*Saccolaimus flaviventris*—yellow-bellied sheath tail bat/black flying fox and related spp. and yellow-bellied sheath-tailed bat	Australia	3

Antigenic phylogroup	Genotype	Lyssavirus	Maintenance host	Location	Number of human cases
I	8	Aravan[b]	Unconfirmed—single isolate from *Myotis blythii* (lesser mouse-eared bat) 1991	Central Asia (Kyrgyzstan)	None
I	9	Khujand virus[b]	Unconfirmed—single isolate from *Myotis mystacinus* (whiskered bat) 2001	Central Asia Tajikistan	None
I	10	Irkut virus	Unconfirmed—single isolate from *Murina leucogaster* (greater tube-nosed bat) 2002	Eastern Siberia	1 (2007)
III	11	West Caucasian bat virus[b]	Unconfirmed—single isolate from *Miniopterus schreibersii* (Schreiber's bent-winged bat) 2002	Western Caucasus mountains	None
II	12	Shimoni[b]	Unconfirmed—single isolate from *Hipposideros commersoni* (Commerson's leaf-nosed bat) 2009	Africa	None
I	13[c]	Bokeloh bat lyssavirus (BBLV)	Fatal infection in Natterer's bat (*M. nattereri*) single isolate, antigenically atypical-not typable by 10 mAB against 7 other lyssaviruses, also phylogenetically different	Bokeloh, Lower Saxony, Germany	None
III	14	Lleida bat lyssavirus[b]	Common bent-winged bat	Spain	None
		Kotalahti bat lyssavirus[d]	Brandt's bat	Finland	None
I	15	Gannoruwa bat lyssavirus	Indian flying fox bat	Sri Lanka	None
		Taiwan bat lyssavirus[d]	Japanese house bat	Taiwan	None

[a]There are accounts of a few (<5) human rabies deaths following bat bites from which no virus has been retained for genotyping, but that are considered likely to be EBLV-1, EBLV-2, West Caucasian bat virus or other yet-to-be identified lyssaviruses. Janine Barrett (2011)

[b]Single isolate only

[c]Freuling et al. (2011)

[d]Serological evidence of infection in Kenya

32.3   Sources

32.3.1   Bats

Lyssaviruses appear to have originated in bats. Except for Mokola or Ikoma lyssavirus all (15/17) originated from bats. Bat lyssaviruses rarely cause rabies in animals and humans, except the vampire bat variant. It has significant impact on human and cattle health. It caused 1–5.0 lakhs cattle deaths and a number of poorly documented human deaths, costing >42 million USD loss/year. In the USA, for insectivorous bat bite-associated rabies 1–4 deaths per year are recorded. In Africa too, carnivore variant rabies is relatively common.

Bat lyssaviruses appear to be rare causes of rabies in man and animals. EBLV 1 and 2 caused rabies in Europe. Australia was free from rabies until the detection of Australian bat lyssavirus in *Pteropus* spp. and one species of insectivorous bat in 1996. Only three human and no animal rabies have been recorded.

European bat lyssaviruses 1 and 2 are distributed in Europe. Moving east, Russia and Kyrgyzstan have so far unclassified three bat viruses having some resemblances to EBLV but phylogenetically distant from the known genotypes. Surveys are made in East Asian countries: (1) Bangladesh, bat—*Pteropus giganteus* positive for Arvan and Khujand; (2) Thailand, bats positive for Arvan, Khujand, Irkut and Australian bat lyssavirus (ABLV); (3) Philippines, *Miniopterus schreibersii* bat positive for ABLV; and (4) Australia, home to ABLV.

Lyssaviruses spread *aerially* by bats and terrestrially by wild carnivores. The ecological support system of this agent is both comprehensive and complex. There is a suggested evolution of host cycles of rabies virus variant (RABVV) in sylvatic setting from Chiroptera to Carnivora (Leslie et al. 2006). There is a regular spillover of bat rabies virus among and between bats and a variety of mesocarnivores (Ellison et al. 2013). Area of viral activity is expanding; newer viruses are being added. The peripheral pathogenicity of LBV had been underestimated in previous studies. Available evidence indicates that LBV is likely persistently maintained in *Megachiroptera* populations in South Africa and other African countries.

Bat-mediated transmission occurs in North, Central and South America. Bats in Europe, Africa, Asia and Australia are reservoirs of different lyssavirus species (Table 32.1). Rabies virus is widespread in Latin American bat species; 22.5% of bat species have been confirmed as rabies positive. These are recognized as natural reservoirs of RABV variants (Escobar et al. 2015). Spatial distribution of RABV requires study on ecology of bat species, landscape changes and effect of rabies epidemiology. Epidemiological surveillance showed a decrease in canine rabies (RABV variants 1 and 2) by 95% by 2013 compared to earlier years and bat rabies (vampire and non-vampire bats together) maintained a stable status. Brazil, Mexico and Argentina had more bat rabies. Brazil had the most rabies-positive (43) species, but hematophagous (*D. rotundus*) played the most significant role in human and livestock rabies. Rabies-positive bats are distributed according to 'diet type'—hematophagous (100%), carnivorous (60%), insectivorous (27%), nectar-ivorous (19%), frugivorous (13%) and omnivorous (11%).

The Alaska State Virology Laboratory, Canada, reported five rabies-positive bats (till July 2015) after examining 165 bats. All bats had abnormal behaviour or were found dead (State of Alaska Epidemiology Bulletin No. 9, April 20, 2016).

32.3.2 Animals

Bats are natural reservoirs of RABV. Rabies virus is maintained by transmission cycle in wild carnivores, i.e. sylvatic rabies. Transmission cycle in domestic carnivores occurs worldwide. Major natural hosts are carnivores, dogs, foxes, mongoose, skunks, vampire bats *Desmodus rotundus*, for genotype 1, and insectivore such as shrews for Mokola.

The Chinese ferret badger (*Melogale moschata*) have been associated with human rabies and considered as a primary host. According to Chiou et al. (2014), outbreak of ferret badger associated rabies occurred during 2012–2013 after Taiwan was free from rabies for >50 years. They isolated the virus from three dead Taiwan ferret badgers (*M. subaurantiaca*) and characterized the virus. They opined that RABV was cryptically circulating.

32.4 Epidemiology: Classical Rabies Virus (RABV Genotype 1) and Variants

32.4.1 The Classical Rabies Virus

The classical rabies virus (genotype 1) is distributed worldwide. It has a very wide host range—terrestrial animals as well as bats. Strains of RABV (genotype 1) undergo genetic adaptation to particular animal hosts so that within specific areas the disease is manifested and transmitted predominantly by one host species. The canid, or dog, biotype of RABV is the most widely distributed in the world.

Studies on regional host cycles, phylogenetic and antigen typing of virus strains are significant to determine (1) the extent of spread and persistence, (2) interspecies transmission and evolution of new host cycle and (3) evolution of virus strain— called RABVV (V = variant). McCollum et al. (2012) observed that a bat rabies variant caused notable outbreaks in carnivore species in 2001, 2004, 2005, 2008 and 2009. Canine rabies virus variant stands eliminated and transmission involved skunks and foxes and human exposure in the last epizootic. Investigation revealed that otherwise knowledgeable community had gaps in knowledge about routes of exposure and potential hosts. Over 90% of rabies in the USA is in wild carnivores—raccoons, skunks and foxes in addition to many bat species—and responsible for 2–4 human cases and 35,000–38,000 post-exposure prophylaxis. Vampire (*Desmodus rotundus*) bat or AgV3 in Brazil and *Tadarida brasiliensis* or AgV4 in Chile are other variant viruses.

Messenger et al. (2003) observed a variant maintained and transmitted by *small insectivorous silver-haired bats*, *L. noctivagans* and *P. subflavus*, that accounted for 57% and 63% of bat-associated cases in terrestrial mammals and 80% and 89% of bat-associated cases in humans. This variant virus replicated to higher titres in fibroblast and epithelial cells, particularly at low temperatures 34 °C, probably facilitating successful infection after a superficial bite. In the USA, among the rabid house bats, 2 of 117 *E. fuscus* and 4 of 15 *M. lucifugus* were found infected with this variant. Small bat species such as Eastern Pipistrelles bites often go unnoticed, possibly leading to the impression that a bite has not occurred.

A white tufted-ear marmoset *(Callithrix jacchus jacchus)* [saguí] is a primate and primary source of rabies infection. It lives in a restricted geographic area in Brazil (Favoretto et al. 2001). It is a small diurnal and feeds on insects, fruits and tree exudates. These are commonly captured and kept as pets and can be found on plantations and in urban parks; population density is high in coastal area and 7/8 human cases occurred there. The distribution of cases according to exposure is as follows: attacked and bite on leg of the owner of the house after entry (1), handling a pet (1), during capture (4) and bite on the ear in one case. Genetic homology of the rabies viruses and surveillance data demonstrated epidemiologic linkage between the viruses and also an independent endemic cycle. The infection of *C. j. jacchus* with this distinct RABV genetic variant could be the result of spillover from an unknown reservoir.

32.4.1.1   RABV and Its Variants Kill Endangered Wildlife Species

Randall et al. (2004) report on a rabies outbreak in a subpopulation of endangered wolves in Ethiopia. The Ethiopian Wolf Conservation Programme staff monitored them. In the middle of August 2003 to 30 January 2004, 38 wolf carcasses were found. Additionally, 36 wolves were missing. Population study revealed that the mortality clearly increased during this period. It was possible to observe 10 sick wolves, and they manifested depression, severe weight loss, poor coat, restlessness, unusual ranging behaviour, aggression, loss of fear of humans or other wolves and excessive salivation at death. 13 of 15 brain samples were rabies positive.

A possible spillover of RABV killed >32 domestic dogs and 20 cattle exhibiting clinical signs consistent with rabies were reported in adjoining areas and at least three human beings were bitten by suspected rabid dogs.

Phylogenetic study showed the isolates were identical to the Ethiopian hyena (*Crocuta crocuta*) strain isolated in 1987 and belonged to canid type (domestic dog group prevalent throughout North and Central Africa). Domestic dogs are the reservoirs. It was suggested that unvaccinated immigrant dog accompanying man and animals in search of food introduced the infection. As this wolf species is rare and endangered, the Ethiopian Wildlife Conservation Organization decided to intervene. Wolf trapping and vaccination was done.

Sympatric rabid domestic dogs are recognized as a major threat to endangered African wild dogs (*Lycaon pictus*) which are a major attraction for tourists in South Africa National Park and cause an annual loss of an estimated $9000 (Lembo et al. 2010).

Matsumoto et al. (2011) identified a rabies virus variant that possibly diverged from Sri Lankan canine rabies viruses around 1933. It posed a danger to the endangered palm civets in Sri Lanka.

32.5 Modes of Transmission

Human infection occurs commonly through:

1. Rabid animal bites
2. Inhalation of aerosolized virus in high density of infected bats in caves or accidentally in laboratory
3. Human to human through organ transplant

Tears, saliva, urine and nervous tissues of hydrophobia patients carry rabies virus and can be theoretical risk of transmission but this does not hinder care of patient. There is a single case of likely perinatal transmission but breastfeeding is unlikely. Oral transmission through meat or milk from infected animal does not occur.

Example of transplant-linked rabies taken from Global Alliance for Rabies Control News 32, April 2013: In 1997 a corneal transplant case died. Four recipients of organs died in 2004. In 2013, interestingly a donor died of encephalitis, not tested for rabies but his kidney stored for transplant tested rabies positive. Of the recipients, one died and others given five doses of PEP were safe.

Learning points: (a) donor's status for rabies should be known; (b) organs for transplant should be tested for rabies. The viability time for organs is a point for consideration. Rabies detection time is 4 h. (c) PEP to be given to recipients should be known.

Rabies virus has been recovered from saliva 5, 3 and 1 day before the appearance of clinical signs in skunks, dogs and cats, respectively. Naturally infected vampire bats can transmit infection for 106 days to other bats and bovines. Insectivorous bats excrete virus for as long as 16 months. Aerosolized bat saliva containing virus infects fox or other carnivores sharing cave with bats. Spread from this natural nidus depends upon the extent of movement of these animals (i.e. vectors) and their density (e.g. two foxes/mile^2 supports epizootics). Rabies epizootics have been spreading at a rate of about 40 km/year from Poland westward.

32.6   Epidemiology

Epidemiologically two types of rabies are recognized—sylvatic and urban. Rabies in wildlife involves animals like foxes, skunks, wolves, jackals, raccoons, coyotes, mongooses, weasels and bats. The virus maintains itself in the forest by circulating in the wild animals. The origin of the urban rabies is often the sylvatic rabies. Both types of rabies may exist simultaneously. Once the urban rabies is controlled, the existence and significance of sylvatic rabies is realized, as in the USA.

Most rabid animals are excited and aggressive and bite. Virus is excreted in their saliva and is deposited in the tissues of the bitten animals at the site of bite. Extremely high and highly susceptible animals are infected with relatively small number of virus particles. Since most of such animals are wild, sylvatic rabies is enzootic in many countries.

Different species of wild carnivores are important in different geographical locale for rabies epizootics, e.g. red fox in Europe, jackals in some part of Africa and skunk, raccoon and fox each with distinct regions in North America. Similarly, each bat species seems to maintain epidemiological independent cycle (Streicker et al. 2010). Dog RABV of same lineage seems to be common in a locality, as in Chinese provinces (Tao et al. 2009).

Rabies is primarily a sylvatic infection in animals. Man is an accidental yet common victim. It occurs in all ages but is most common in 5–45 years age group. The opportunity of exposure is great in this age group because of outdoor activities. The possibility of bite on the upper parts of the body like face, neck and head is more in young children. Although all warm-blooded animals are susceptible, wild carnivores commonly act as reservoirs. Certain species of animals is more common for different geographical locale, for example, fox for Western Europe, skunks and raccoons for America, vampire bats for South America, jackals for India, etc. Man's entry to sylvatic habitat of rabies virus or infected wild animals wandering into mosaic areas leads to bite exposure, infection and death of man.

A rabid dog spreads the virus, as it may wander about 50 km in a short time, inflicting bite injuries to 60–100 animals and man. The author observed 24 bite victims of 1 rabid dog in 3 days. Appearance of rabies in an area is indicated by a cluster of dog bite cases, panic-stricken parents of dog-bitten children and hydrophobia deaths.

Almost 99% of human rabies cases in India and other endemic countries are transmitted from dogs. Jackals are important wild carnivore reservoir in India. It is thought that jackals are evicted out of their water-logged burrows during monsoon. In search of foods, they cross mosaic, enter human habitations, encounter dogs and transmit rabies virus and dog-dog chain of transmission continues.

Wild animals like foxes, wolves, jackals, racoons, skunks, mongoose and bat account for a small fraction of transmission.

32.6.1 Rabies in India

Rabies is endemic in India except for Andaman and Nicobar and Lakshadweep islands. Dog population in India has shown a steady growth. There are 30 million dogs. The distribution is not uniform. States like Nagaland, Manipur and Sikkim have a wide dog-human ratio. The effect is reflected in a very low incidence of hydrophobia in Sikkim, Arunachal, Nagaland and Mizoram. According to Rahman (1997) *rabies in animals was increasing even when there was increasing awareness, vaccination and stray dog control.*

Narayan's (2004) *suggestion of enlisting vaccine manufacturers' participation in vaccination programmes should boost vaccination with quality vaccine.*

32.7 Pathogenesis

Virus can enter through the mucosa and wounds and cannot cross intact skin. RABV along with saliva is deposited at the site of bite by a rabid animal. Period of localization at the site is variable and may be 18 days. There is no viremia. Primary multiplication in the muscle occurs before the virus particles find their way to motor endplates and motor axons; nerve cells bind to the postsynaptic nicotinic acetylcholine receptor. Viruses can enter motor axons in peripheral nerves directly during penetrating injury; also when the number of virus particles is available, nerve cells are high (Fig. 32.1).

Furious form is characterized by greater viral load in the cerebrum and minimal inflammation; inflammation of brainstem is relatively prominent in paralytic form.

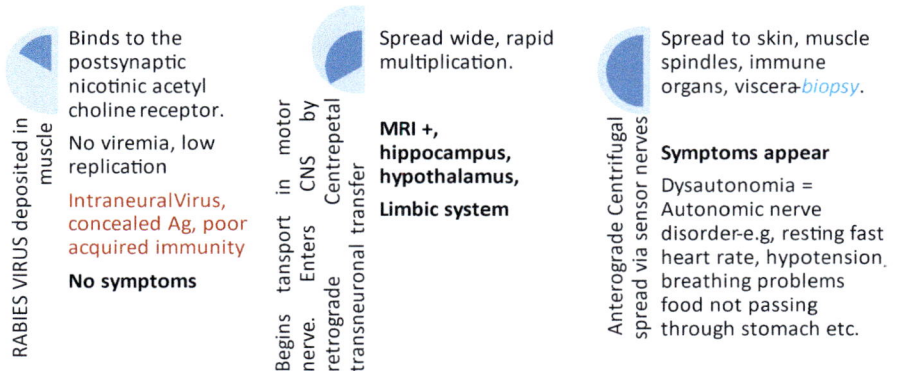

RABIES VIRUS-HUMAN HOST INTERACTION

RABIES VIRUS deposited in muscle — Binds to the postsynaptic nicotinic acetyl choline receptor. No viremia, low replication. IntraneuralVirus, concealed Ag, poor acquired immunity. **No symptoms**

Begins transport in motor nerve. Enters CNS by retrograde Centripetal transneuronal transfer — Spread wide, rapid multiplication. **MRI +, hippocampus, hypothalamus, Limbic system**

Anterograde Centrifugal spread via sensor nerves — Spread to skin, muscle spindles, immune organs, viscera-*biopsy*. **Symptoms appear** Dysautonomia = Autonomic nerve disorder-e.g, resting fast heart rate, hypotension, breathing problems food not passing through stomach etc.

Ab not detected until 2 weeks or before symptoms appear; RESULT- virus invades CNS; although host's immune response is active.

Fig. 32.1 Pathogenesis of rabies virus [Source: de Souza A, Madhusudana SN. 2014]

Longer survival in paralytic form may be due to brainstem inflammation impeding viral spread towards the cerebrum. Apoptosis is not prominent in infection with wild type, while it is common with fixed strain given i/c. Defective neurotransmission and oxidative damage may play a role in ultimate fatality.

In December 2015, the WHO, the World Organisation for Animal Health (OIE), the Food and Agriculture Organization (FAO) and the Global Alliance for Rabies Control (GARC) endorsed a global framework to eliminate human deaths from dog-mediated disease by 2030. The decision was reinforced by the OIE in May 2015.

Once RABV reaches exoplasm, it moves towards the CNS at an estimated speed of 3 mm/day. The transport is active and spread is centripetal. It is estimated that 30, 40 and 60 days may be taken by RABV to reach the CNS in man from the sites of bites on face, arms and legs, respectively. RABV invades the brain, multiplies extensively and damages the entire brain, especially the amygdaloid nucleus, hippocampus (cause of agitation, aggressive behaviour, hydrophobia), hypothalamus (cause of hypersalivation, etc.) and the limbic system. Clinical neuropathic symptoms appear. Death occurs approximately 3 weeks from the beginning of viral transport in motor nerves.

The centrifugal (anterograde) spread from CNS is passive diffusion. RABV spreads via slow axoplasmic flow in motor axons to ventral roots and nerves and peripheral sensory axons of the infected dorsal ganglia. The virus particles are dispersed through the nerves to muscle, salivary glands and other organs like lungs, adrenal glands, kidneys, bladder, ovaries, testicles, sebaceous glands, cells of hair follicles, cornea, tongue papillae (useful biopsy materials for diagnosis), intestinal walls and interscapular brown fats in bats (where the virus is thought to remain hidden for long).

According to de Souza and Madhusudana (2014), caudal-rostral polarity of viral antigen is seen in both furious and paralytic forms of rabies. Viral antigen load is more in the cerebrum in the furious form. The inflammation of the brainstem is prominent in the paralytic form and this possibly impedes viral migration towards the cerebrum resulting into longer survival of patient in the paralytic form. Oxidative damage and defective neurotransmitter function might contribute to death. Wild-type viral infection is not associated with apoptosis unlike the fixed viruses produced in experimental animals by intracerebral inoculation.

There is no neuronal death or immunosuppression. Virus is intraneuronal during infection and hence protected from immune surveillance. Viral replication is highly unaccompanied with neuronal loss. Inflammation of the brain is insignificant/variable. Virus is generally not cleared from the CNS by the immune effector cells. The immune response outside the CNS may be strong but inconsequential as damage has already been done. Antibody response is not detected until the second week of infection and often not until symptoms have appeared. Exceptional patients may respond appropriately to natural infection and clear the virus from the CNS.

A very small fraction (15) of infected humans survived after treatment since 1972. de Souza and Madhusudana (2014) attempted to explain. All of 12 cases discussed were rabies-confirmed by detection of antibodies and virus was isolated or RNA detected in 3. Recovery was complete, nearly complete and good in four. The rest had sequelae, mild (2), moderate (1), persistent headache without deficit (1) and severe (4).

32.8   Clinical Manifestation

Consequences of an infected dog bite depend on several factors like severity of bite/wound, location, virus load in saliva, RABV variant and time when PEP vaccination was started. On an average, the probability of bite converting into rabies was 55%, 22%, 9% and 12% if site of bite was head, upper extremity, trunk and lower limb, respectively. Viral load in saliva varies during the course of the disease.

The incubation period (IP) is dependent upon concentration of virus in the saliva, volume of infective saliva, severity of bite, virulence and the distance of the site from the CNS. It ranges between 21 and 80 days in 85% and >90 days in 14%. Over 1 year of IP is observed in 2–3% with an exceptional case of 8 years (WHO/FAO/OIE 2018). The IP in dogs may be short or long, 1 year; 4–8 weeks in horse and cattle; 3–6 weeks in sheep; and 6–18 months in pigs. Death occurs within 15–50 days of the rabid bite regardless of species. Death in dogs occurs within 10 days of the onset of symptoms.

32.8.1   Symptoms in Man

The feeling is numbness or itching turning into neuropathic pain at the site of bite due to viral replication in the corresponding dorsal root ganglion and inflammation. The patient is melancholic, depressed and anorexic. Gradually their voice changes, and swallowing is difficult and painful and agonising because of the spasms of throat muscles. Sight of water induces painful spasm—hence hydrophobia. Spasm extends to respiratory muscles causing dyspnoea. Such symptoms last for about 2 days, following which paralysis sets in. Patients enter into coma and death follows due to neuronal dysfunction without or with minimal signs of inflammation. Atypical symptoms and/or neuroimaging occurs but reasons are unknown; possibilities are atypical variant strain of virus and inoculum of a large number of viruses (in the case of organ transplant plus reduced host's immune response). Patients die usually in 7–10 days in the absence of intensive care.

32.8.2 Symptoms in Dogs

Diagnosis on the basis of observing clinical presentation of infected dogs/animals is important to advise the bite victims. According the WHO/FAO/OIE (2018), a *rabies-suspected* case would be manifesting hypersalivation, paralysis, lethargy, unprovoked aggression (biting two or more people/animals and/or inanimate object), abnormal vocalization and diurnal activity of nocturnal species. A suspected case with reliable history of contact with suspected/probable/confirmed rabid is considered a *probable* case. A suspected animal killed/died/disappeared within 4–5 days of illness is also treated as *probable*. Laboratory confirmation by OIE/WHO test of suspected/probable case makes it a *confirmed case*. Unconfirmed by laboratory or epidemiological investigation (i.e. the animal is alive after appropriate quarantine period) is *not* a case.

The course lasts for 4–7 or maximum of 10 days. Two clinical forms are known—furious and dumb.

Furious form may have three stages—prodromal, excitement and paralysis. Prodromal stage lasts for a few days. The symptoms are non-specific. It is dangerous for those who attend, care and handle them. Fly catching (bites at the air) and without reason, becoming attentive and then restless, may or may not attend to their master's call, stops eating and drinking, hiding in a corner are few of the symptoms. Hallucination and behavioural changes, frequent urination, penile erection, red conjunctiva and lachrymation may appear.

The second—stage of excitement—presents the classical symptoms of a 'mad dog'. The dog is unusually alert, gets excited readily, tries to come out of the cage/kennel, is aggressive, runs aimlessly if let loose and attacks anything moving—man, animals or vehicle. It salivates. The mad dog tends to eat anything, even non-edibles—stone and sticks; bark changes to howl and shrill as the laryngeal nerves are affected. An exhausted patient pants and remains quiet for some time to repeat the bout of madness. After a day or two, the dog enters into paralytic stage.

In the paralytic stage, the dog is dull and morose. Paralysis sets first in the lower jaw and then in other parts of the body. The dog is not able to swallow as throat muscles are paralyzed. This 'dropping jaw' often misleads—foreign body/piece of bone lodging in teeth or throat prompts the master or doctor to put his hand into the mouth. Saliva drools. Paralysis sets in limbs leading to staggering/stumbling gait and dragging of limbs. Paralysis is followed by coma and death.

In the 'dumb form' the stage of excitement is absent. The course is short; usually the dog dies in 3 days. The dropping of jaw, saliva dribbling and paralysis, coma and death are seen.

32.8.3 Symptoms in Cats

Cats are more furious than dogs, are ferocious, jump on a person, scratch viciously and grab with teeth. The normal voice is changed to hoarse mewing.

32.8.4 Symptoms in Foxes and Jackals

Infected foxes and jackals retain their basic/native cunning but lose fear of their enemies, like man, dog and other animals. They may stalk man or animal, attacking from rear. They may invade public places and houses and attack people in the open. Like the cats, they may grab or hang on until choked to death.

32.9 Diagnosis

Rabies case presents symptoms of acute encephalitis dominated by hyperactivity in furious form and signs of paralysis in the paralytic form. The disease progresses to coma and death usually due to cardiac or respiratory failure within 7–10 days of the first sign. Predominant signs are phobias—hydrophobia, aerophobia, photophobia—localized weakness, nausea, vomiting, dysphagia, paraesthesia or localized pain.

A case conforming to the above signs and symptoms plus a history of contact with suspected/probable/confirmed rabid animal is a 'probable case'. Differential diagnosis and laboratory confirmation is necessary to decide the line of action, more so for the exposed ones who have not yet shown any sign of clinical disease.

The following are the diagnostic methods:

- Histopathology.
- Seller's staining.
- Mouse inoculation.
- PCR and RT-PCR for detection of viral RNA.
- Fluorescent antibody test, immunoperoxidase test and ELISA.
- DRIT (direct rapid immunohistochemical test) and rabies tissue culture infection test (RTCIT).
- Lateral flow test is a rapid immunodiagnostic test useful with specimens from live and dead and does not require equipment.

Laboratory confirmation of rabies infection enables authentic data and decisive action.

Specimens and tests: Specimens are collected from those who have had suspected animal or bat bite before/after the appearance of symptoms and finally after death in human, dog or any animal.

Skin, hair follicle from nape of the neck, tear/corneal impression, saliva, serum and CSF are the specimens collected from the live victim. Storage at −20 °C or less is ideal. Serum and CSF samples from early course of illness are less likely to be positive, but if positive, it is most valuable as the probability of saving the life is more. Three saliva samples collected at intervals of 3–6 h and skin biopsy including hair follicles have the highest diagnostic sensitivity and should be preferred. RTCIT is sensitive and the preferred test for tears, saliva and CSF. Antibody in serum is most likely be detected by rapid fluorescent focus inhibition test (RFFIT)/fluorescent antibody virus neutralization test (FAVN).

Brain specimen from suspected dog/animal/human is the most preferred specimen collected post-mortem. FAT, DRIT and RTCIT are the most sensitive tests.

Strengthening diagnosis of rabies in animals in India is the mandate of Karnataka Veterinary, Animal and Fisheries Sciences University (KVAFSU), College of Veterinary Science—Crucell Rabies Diagnostic Laboratory, Hebbal, Bengaluru, in India, twinned under OIE Twinning Programme in 2016, with the Animal and Plant Health Agency (APHA), Weybridge, UK, and Centers for Disease Control and Prevention (CDC), Atlanta, USA. It has ISO 17025/2017 accreditation and OIE recognition as reference laboratory for rabies. Networking of rabies diagnostic laboratories in India has been done. This promotes submission of increased number of samples for testing and reporting. Sero-monitoring of vaccinal antibodies for evaluation of rabies control programme, international travel of pets and immune surveillance are possible with RFFIT/FAVN/ELISA.

32.10 Vaccines, Immunoglobulins, and Prophylactic (Pre-exposure) Vaccination (WHO/FAO/OIE 2018)

32.10.1 Vaccines

The vaccines should meet WHO recommendations which apply only to inactivated in embryonated eggs, cell culture or purified Vero cell and human diploid cell culture. CCEEVs are concentrated, purified cell culture and embryonated egg-based rabies vaccines. Other vaccines are Duck embryo vaccine, Nerve tissue vaccine. These are safe and effective in preventing rabies and are useful for prophylactic and post-bite vaccinal therapy. Many countries have stopped the production and use of nerve tissue vaccine. The WHO also recommends it because it is less immunogenic and causes severe adverse reaction.

CCEEVs have ≥3 years shelf-life at 2–8 °C when protected from sunlight. Post-reconstitution life is 6 h if kept at 2–8 °C. The minimal acceptable potency is 2.5 IU per intramuscular dose/0.1 mL intradermal dose and potency ≥0.25 IU, as determined in the mouse protection potency test. Intramuscular and intradermal inoculations provide equivalent immune response and the latter saves the vaccine for inoculation of more people, thus cutting the cost.

These vaccines are safe. Reactions (likely in 35–45%) include minor transient erythema or swelling at the site of injection, more likely after booster dose is given intra-dermally. 5–15% of vaccinees may report systemic effects like transient fever, dizziness and gastrointestinal symptoms. Serious effect like Guillain-Barre syndrome or allergy is rare.

Response to booster is seen within 7 days even among those who received the PEP/PrEP decades earlier regardless of the presence or absence of detectable RABV-specific antibodies. Periodic booster is not required. Nevertheless, previously vaccinated and exposed to suspected rabid bite must receive abbreviated schedule of vaccination.

These vaccines may not protect against lyssaviruses other than those in phylogroup I.

These are available in various brand names such as purified Vero cell rabies vaccine (PVRV)—Abhayrab-Indian Immunological and Indirab, Bharat Biotech, and PCEV—Vaxirab-Zydus-Candila (chick embryo cell).

32.10.2 Rabies Immunoglobulins (RIG)

Bite victims under exposure category III, those who have not received earlier PEP or PrEP and immunocompromised/immunodeficient people (AIDS, transplant cases) with exposure category II should receive rabies immunoglobulins. Immunoglobulin is infiltrated in and around the bite wound to neutralize the virus. Three forms of immunoglobulin are available—human, equine and highly purified F(ab')2 fragments from equine globulin. The maximum dose is 20 IU/kg and 40 IU/kg body weight for human and equine originated immunoglobulins, respectively. Most of the new equine immunoglobulin preparations are highly purified and safe, are potent and cause few adverse reactions. Serum sickness can occur 1 week after administration in 1–3% of cases. Chance of anaphylactic reaction is 1/150,000 and is generally treatable. Skin test before injection is not recommended for RIG.

The dose of RIG is weight based. In paediatric patients it is likely to be insufficient because of low body weight. There is higher susceptibility and rabies burden in this age group (paediatric). A trial on suspected or confirmed rabies exposure patients aged <17 years was conducted to study safety, tolerability, efficacy and immunogenicity of HRIG150, rabies immunoglobulin (human) and KEDRAB 150 IU/mL (Kedrion Biopharma Inc.) as part of PEP. The trial was a phase 4, prospective, 2-centre, open-label, single-arm clinical. **Results:** Thirty participants received 20 IU/kg HRIG150 infiltrated into the detectable wound site(s), with any remainder injected intramuscularly, concomitantly with the first of a 4-dose series (days 0, 3, 7 and 14) of rabies vaccine. No serious adverse effect for 84 observation periods; mild treatment emergent adverse events were observed within 14 days; rabies virus neutralization antibodies ≥0.5 IU/mL in 93.3% are observed (Nicholas Hobart-Porter et al. 2021).

32.10.3   Vaccination

32.10.3.1   Pre-exposure Prophylactic (PrEP) Vaccination (WHO/FAO/ OIE 2018)

High-risk group needs to be protected prophylactically. The occupational group includes animal healthcare workers, medical professionals and laboratory workers. Mass vaccination may be considered in remote settings where dog bite incidence exceeded 5% or if vampire bat exposure is prevalent.

32.10.3.2   PrEP Schedule

Intradermal two-site 7-day schedule (2-0-2) on 0, 3rd and 7th day 0.1 mL.
  Intramuscular 7-day schedule (1-0-1) on 0, 3rd and 7th day 1.0 mL.
  Immunocompromised/HIV should be given a third vaccine on 21–28th day. HIV patients on treatment respond like a healthy man.
  Special circumstance, e.g. before travel—demanding single visit—two sites intradermal or single intramuscular; second dose is administered on return or as soon as possible.
  In case of an exposure in less than 7 days of receiving vaccine, a full PEP schedule is required as development of immunity is not expected in this short period.

32.10.3.3   Post-exposure Prophylaxis (PEP)

PEP is highly effective as the long incubation period of rabies offers time. It eases psychological burden. PEP consists of (a) thorough *washing and flushing out* of the virus from site of bite injury/wound by washing withsoap/detergent and water for 15 min and *virucidal* agents, (b) infiltration of RIG to *neutralize the virus at the site* injected up to 7 days after the first vaccine dose, and (c) series of vaccine injection to induce antibody production to reduce RABV entering the peripheral nerves after bite by rabid animals and rabies illness and death can be prevented. It is estimated that post-exposure prophylaxis prevented about 327,000 deaths from rabies in Africa and Asia each year (WHO 2010).
  PEP should be initiated if history of biting animal is suspected, probable or confirmed for rabies and also if no history is available. Probable, suspected and confirmed rabid animal should be humanely killed and post-mortem examination done for rabies diagnosis. If laboratory test is negative for rabies, PEP vaccination may be discontinued. Suspected but apparent healthy dogs, cats and domesticated ferrets may be kept under observation for 10 days by trained veterinarian and PEP delayed only when advance surveillance (facility for post-mortem examination and rabies diagnosis) is in place till symptoms of rabies appear or the animal dies or escapes.

WHO-Recommended PEP Vaccination Schedule

Site of intradermal injection: deltoid, lateral thigh, supra-scapular. Deltoid muscle in adult and children ≥2 years old; anterolateral thigh for children <2 years for intramuscular injection.

Intradermal 1-week, two-site, 0.1 mL vaccine (2-2-2) on 0, 3rd and 7th day.

Intramuscular 2-week 1.0 mL (1-1-1-1) on 0, 3rd, 7th and 14th day.

Intramuscular 3-week 1.0 mL (2-0-1-0-1) on 0, 3rd, 7th, 14 and 28th day.

For immunocompromised/HIV patients: RABV neutralizing antibody response to vaccination should be monitored 2–4 weeks after vaccination to assess if additional doses of vaccine are required.

Recipients of PrEP/PEP full course or at least two doses: one site intradermal on 0–3rd day/four sites on 0 day. In the case of intramuscular, entire vaccine in vial on 0–3rd day. RIG is not required.

All unprovoked bites should be considered as rabies—suspect unless proven as negative on laboratory test. Anti-rabies vaccine should be given for category II and III exposures as soon as possible (Table 32.2). Anti-rabies immunoglobulin (anti-body) should be applied for all category III exposures and for immunosuppressed patients of category II exposures. Suturing (closing the wound) should be postponed, but if it is necessary immunoglobulin must first be applied. Where indicated, anti-tetanus treatment, antimicrobials and drugs should be administered to control infections other than rabies.

In case of human exposure to animals that are suspected of having rabies, immediate attempts should be made to identify, capture or kill the animal involved. In case of a category III exposure, post-exposure treatment should start immediately and can be stopped if the animal is a dog or cat and remains healthy after 10 days. Brain tissue samples should be taken from dead animals and sent to competent laboratories for diagnosis. The responsible veterinary services should be notified and information obtained on the epidemiological situation in the area.

Table 32.2 Category of exposure in enzootic areas and guidelines for PEP (WHO/FAO/OIE 2018)

Class of bite	Description	Treatment
I	Touching/feeding/fondling leading to animal lick on healthy skin without open wound, no evidence of contact of mucous membrane with dog saliva	No treatment
II	Nibbling of uncovered skin, superficial scratch without breaking skin/bleeding; licking over broken skin, open wound; situation under class I but with unreliable history. If exposure is of bat, treated as class III	Immediate vaccination
III	Single or multiple transdermal bite on face, head, neck, fingers. Scratches, broken skin, mucous membrane contamination with saliva from licks, Licks by bats of broken skin, direct contact with bats Severe exposure PEP indicated with vaccine and RIG	Immediate vaccination + antiserum

32.11   Dog Rabies Control

32.11.1   OIE Support

The Veterinary Service has the authority and responsibility to implement animal health and welfare programmes in coordination with other government agencies and institute. It includes control of endemic zoonoses like rabies and echinococcosis. A member country is guided by OIE.

There is a global network of 311 OIE Reference Laboratories and Collaborating Centres which offer policy advice, strategy design and technical assistance for the diagnosis, control and eradication of rabies.

OIE distributed 12.5 million anti-rabies vaccines till September 2016.

The WHO procures canine rabies vaccine through the OIE Rabies Vaccine Bank under the framework of Tripartite Alliance (WHO, OIE, FAO), e.g. as of September 2016, 11 million doses of rabies vaccines were purchased by the WHO through the OIE Rabies Vaccine Bank for delivery to the Philippines, South Africa and Tanzania.

The OIE develops through consensus by all 180 member countries and publishes regularly updated, scientific standards regarding (a) the prevention and control of rabies, (b) stray dog population control, (c) the international movement of dogs and cats originating from rabies-infected countries (ch. 8.10) and within the country and (d) diagnostic methods and the production of standard vaccines.

32.11.1.1   Vaccines for Dogs

The WHO/FAO/OIE (2018) lists currently ten rabies oral vaccines. Nine have licence for wildlife. Oral vaccine may be administered by a trained vaccinator for those aggressive, hard to reach and unapproachable for parental inoculation. It does not guarantee high seroconversion. The bait is required to attract the dog. It chews and breaks the sachet or blister and the vaccine is deposited in the correct amount onto the oral mucosa. The vaccines are modified live or recombinant.

Contact with orally vaccinated dogs should be avoided or minimized for at least 1 h and preferably longer. Probability of a human death due to contact with oral rabies vaccine distributed by hand-out method was 0/1 billion. Rate of contact was 1.4% compared to none when distributed by door to door (equal to hand out), observed in Tunisia (WHO/FAO/OIE 2018).

Direct contact with the vaccine and recently vaccinated animals should be reported. Surveillance in area covered with ORV should use molecular epidemiology to detect reversion of vaccine strain to virulent form.

In December 2015, the WHO, the World Organisation for Animal Health (OIE), the Food and Agriculture Organization (FAO) and the Global Alliance for Rabies Control (GARC) endorsed a global framework to eliminate human deaths from dog-mediated disease by 2030. The decision was reinforced by the OIE in May 2015.

Loss of human life is certain after rabies infection. There is no medicine and the health sector has only one answer, PEP. Mortality and loss of economic productivity due to premature human death are the most serious effects of canine rabies. How to quantify 'anxiety' is unknown. Hampson et al. (2015) suggested adding 10% of total burden. Only 6% is the loss of livestock caused by rabies.

The problem of rabies continues to hang between the two sectors working in silo and remained neglected for years. Rabies (hydrophobia) death rate is high in areas/regions where dog vaccination is either not implemented or is limited.

Rabies is possibly the only zoonosis that demonstrates the direct and definite effect of control of infection in animals and decisively establishes the role of veterinary public health. Establishing an independent veterinary public health seems necessary.

Control of dog rabies requires:

1. Regulatory authority—rabies is a notifiable disease (inherent is 'rabies surveillance' i.e. designating a laboratory for confirmation, decision making and authority to act)
2. Responsible pet management
3. Mass dog vaccination at an accelerated speed
4. Habitat (environment) control
5. Awareness, people participation
6. Research on wildlife rabies

Adoption of all 1–6 simultaneously assures achieving the goal. This is based on OIE support (vide supra).

32.11.2 Mass Dog Vaccination (MDV)

Vaccinating dogs against rabies cuts transmission among dogs, controls dog rabies and ultimately prevents transmission to human.

32.11.2.1 Cost-Effective

Investment in dog vaccination is the single most effective way of reducing the disease burden. It is cost-effective. According to Hampson et al. (2015), the economic burden is <1.5%. Sustained investment in dog vaccination in the Americas is ~0.11$/person/year resulting into low rabies burden <200 deaths/year.

The cost of PEP in dollars is averted, DALYs are saved, and these are calculated in terms of the country's GDP; 'an incremental cost-effectiveness' has been used for the evaluation of mass dog vaccination programmes by Bilinski et al. (2016). Canine vaccination is cost saving compared to no vaccination.

32.11.2.2   Level of Vaccination

In 2013, the World Health Organization (WHO) called for a renewed focus on rabies control in sub-Saharan Africa, advocating annual vaccination campaigns to achieve coverage of 70% in canine populations. Vaccination target of 70% should maintain population immunity above the critical levels (25–40%) required to interrupt rabies transmission, and this additional coverage above the critical level covers increase in susceptibility (turnover of population or introduction) and loss of immunity (Hampson et al. 2009).

32.11.2.3   Effect-Cuts 'Dog-Dog' Transmission

Canada, the USA, Japan, Western Europe and 28/35 Latin American countries have successfully eliminated rabies by mass vaccination. Great efforts are going on in Bangladesh, the Philippines, Sri Lanka, Tanzania, Vietnam and South Africa, to mention a few (Document 'United Against Rabies'). Annual mass vaccination of dogs is in practice for the past 60 years in Japan. Watanabe et al. (2012) studied the protective antibody levels. Dogs receiving single dose had lower mean virus neutralizing titres (O.61 IU/mL) than those who received at least two shots (7.86 IU/mL). Most of the latter retained protective levels into the second year of the last vaccination. The system of registration and vaccination schedules required improvement to ensure vaccination of an increasing number of dogs.

32.11.2.4   Action Has to Be Fast

One of the essential requirements of control of infectious contagious disease is to adopt a *measure that works faster than the speed of transmission.* In the USA, control of urban rabies was achieved by mass vaccination of pet dogs at a very fast speed (thousands of dogs were vaccinated in a week). One-time concerted effort pushed rabies from urban locale to its sylvatic habitat. This reduced the laboratory-confirmed cases of rabies from 6949 in 1947 to 117 in 2003 (Anonym 2005). It is the wildlife rabies and not the urban rabies that is observed occasionally in the USA. In 2003, for the first time South America recorded more of bat- and wildlife-associated human rabies than dog-associated after control measures were adopted.

The Worldwide Mission Rabies of UK (Report 2015) vaccinated over 300,000 community dogs in some of the world's worst hotspots in 18 months. Nobivac Rabies, MSD Animal Health, was administered at 40 s/dog in Ranchi. Jharkhand,

India. The vaccination exceeded 70% of population in 94 days. WHO certification of freedom from rabies was achieved. Mass dog vaccination (MDV) works faster as experienced in Bangladesh than ABC-AR (Animal Birth Control-Anti rabies vaccination).

32.11.3   Dog Population Management

Mass vaccination of domesticated and healthy dogs and education of dog owners about their responsibility have eliminated rabies in many regions, where there is no or minimal stray roaming dog population.

The not-owned dogs roam in search of food and shelter. These are not accessible for vaccination and have to be trapped for it. Dogs fight for food, sex or territory, when these are limited in relation to their population. Such endemic dog rabies regions are detected when a man gets infected and dies of hydrophobia. Dense human population in such regions experience frequent dog chase, bites and even fatal mauling by dogs and may be exposed to other more than 50 dog-associated zoonoses. In regions where dog-human ratio is wide, dog bite incidences and dog bite-associated rabies are low, e.g. the Indian states like Manipur, Meghalaya and Nagaland in contrast to the rest of the states, suggestive of dog density being a factor. A study by Bilinski et al. (2016) showed that dog rabies appeared *sporadically* in Ngorongoro where dog density was 1.5 dog/km^2. It was *endemic* in Serengeti, a smaller district with dog density of 9.5 dogs/km^2. Predicted numbers of canine cases over 10 years were 0.2 and 6.8 per km^2, respectively, for the two regions and the corresponding human health burden was 0.2 and 6.2 DALYs per km^2 over the decade. The budget over 10 years for PEP was also higher for Serengeti.

The study used three parameters: (a) sporadic vs endemic, (b) canine cases/km^2 and (c) human health burden, and results suggested that dog density did matter.

Reduction in population density reduces the number of dogs that need vaccination and also the cost of vaccine and vaccination. Reduction of population either by culling or sterilization should impact the subsequent rate of transmission.

Culling of free-roaming (stray) dogs has often been undertaken alongside mass vaccination programme as a means to reduce the number of animals needed to be vaccinated, as has been done with raccoons in Wolfe Island in Ontario. In Bhutan, the 2008 rabies outbreak appeared to follow the road networks, towns and areas of high human density associated with large, free-roaming dog population. Culling of such dogs was necessary to be included in the measures to control the outbreak (Tenzin et al. 2010).

The *Catch-Neuter-Vaccinate and Release (CNVR)* project in India vaccinates and controls dog population. It is expensive, slow but useful for owned dogs. The 'Help in Suffering street dog and rabies control programme' that started in 1999 continues to keep rabies and the street dog population under control in Jaipur. Jack Reece, a British vet, has been working since 1999. Seventy percent bitches in Jaipur have been spayed and vaccinated, covering >75% of population with a consequential drop in hydrophobia cases.

Guidance on humane dog population management is available on the website of World Society for the Protection of Animals (WSPA) and the International Companion Animal Management Coalition (ICAM Coalition) and also the OIE chapter Terrestrial Anima Health Code 7.7 (stray dog population control).

It should be noted that culling or any method of controlling dog population does not control rabies. *Culling spares RABV and kills the potential victim. Culling* vs *vaccination is compared in Korea, Israel and Indonesia—the latter succeeded* (Morters et al. 2013).

Controlling dog population is essential to protect the increasing incidences of dog bites, some of which are fatal, especially when infants, children, old and infirm are aggressively attacked by ferocious stray dogs.

32.11.3.1   Habitat Control

Stoppage of garbage dumping and management of wastes from hotel and eateries contributes to control of street dog population and dog bites and rabies.

Dog demography, management and roaming behaviour across four countries: Chad, Guatemala, Indonesia and Uganda were studied by Warembourg et al. (2021). It was suggested that these differed from region to region and also the use of dogs like shepherd dogs, hunting dogs and family pets. This in turn is controlled by owners' occupation, cultural background, knowledge about dog keeping and responsibilities and perception of animal welfare. Free-roaming dogs are potential disease transmitters, particularly rabies and cause of bite injuries. Free-roaming dogs are not completely under human control. Yet they strongly depend upon human for a habitat (home range).

Dogs use home range for activities like foraging and breeding and movement around it. Dogs' behaviour plays an important role in the spread of rabies. Dog population management is an important component of control strategies in endemic areas.

Availability of food is a consistent determinant of dogs' behaviour. The density was high in areas with potential sources of food such as university restaurants in Brazil or garbage dumps in India or from commercial food outlets.

Removal of left-over foods and wastes or recycling prevents dog assembly and density around these sites. The municipality in one of the cities in India practised removal of wastes from food outlets immediately after dumping past midnight when food outlets were closing. No stray dogs were seen around in this locality compared to other where it was not practised.

32.11.4 One Health Approach

The WHO, FAO, OIE and GARC united against rabies aimed at eliminating rabies by 2030. It is a coordinating, catalytic and country-centric programme under model of One Health. It is aligned to UN Sustainable Development Growth three plan 'to ensure healthy life and promote wellbeing for all age group', targeting neglected tropical diseases and to 'achieve universal health coverage and access to safe, effective, quality and affordable essential medicines and vaccines for all' (Zero 30. Doc United Against Rabies).

32.11.4.1 Integrated Bite Case Management (IBCM)

It aims at reducing the cost of treatment and risk of transmission control of rabies in dog population through channels of communication between proposed active rabies surveillance by VET SERV and PEP centre (HLTH. SERV).

Procedure: The VET SERV (active vet surveillance) examines the biting animal (rabies suspect) to assess the risk of rabies and considers rabies epidemiology: rabies endemic, extent and site of bite exposure; clinical features matching with rabies; vaccination status of the biting animal; and laboratory testing and results. It communicates findings to the PEP centre (HLTH. SERV).

Example:

The Haiti Animal Rabies Surveillance Program (HARSP) is an active surveillance that began in three communes. An estimated 130 rabies deaths in a year are recorded in Haiti, considered as the highest burden of rabies in the Western hemisphere. The tabulated (Table 32.3) data of 2 years from HARSP-IBCM compares a situation wherein there is NO integration of Passive Animal Rabies Surveillance with Health Service (NBCM).

It is apparent that 'comprehensive dog vaccination and communication' offered an effective approach to prevent human rabies.

Table 32.3 Cost-effectiveness of IBCM (based on $N = 2289$ exposed to rabies in the study area in 2014–2015). Undurraga et al. (2017)

Parameters	HARSP (IBCM)	NBCM
Overall costs	(Range: $39,568–80,290)[a]	($15,988–26,976)
Annual death averted	11 (2014), 9 (2015)	
Yearly life gained	654 (2014), 535 (2015)	
US$/death averted in 2014	$2891–4735	$5980–8453
In 2015	$3534–7171	$7298–12,284

[a] Diagnostic laboratory development, training of surveillance officers, operational costs

32.11.5   Awareness

Dr Bernard Vallat, Director General, OIE, had observed 'Animal disease-related events have covered the front pages of newspapers frequently during the past 15 years. Rabies, however, is rarely found on the front pages despite being one of the oldest and best-known zoonotic diseases. Rabies is still responsible for an unacceptable number of preventable deaths in humans due to exposure to infected animals, mainly dogs'.

Introducing a course in school curriculum/periodic educational lectures and enlisting print and electronic media should be done. Enlisting higher education, extension education and social institutions as platforms is important. These will be organizing in their own way discussions, lectures and fair to educate communities in their respective areas.

The Global Alliance for Rabies has done a commendable job and can be approached for educational materials.

32.11.6   Research in Wildlife Rabies and Control

OIE has nearly 100 years of experience working at the human-animal-ecosystems interface, wildlife in particular, to reduce disease threats and has the mandate to 'improve animal health worldwide' and in representing the interests of the National Veterinary Services in 182 member countries (OIE 2019).

Considering the aerial and terrestrial routes of movement of reservoirs (several species of bats and wild carnivores, respectively), it is essential to monitor rabies viral transmission among these. This is all the more required because rabies virus spills over to new hosts and evolves into new variants frequently. Control of wildlife rabies is required to check its possible spillover to domestic and pet animals and also to humans, besides protecting some endangered wildlife species.

Tischendorf et al. (1998) have cited literatures indicating that continuous vaccination for 5 years of about 70% of fox population (18–20 vaccine-filled baits/km^2 in spring and autumn distributed with aircraft) in Eastern Germany in about 108,000 km^2 area drastically reduced rabies incidence. Simulation model used by them suggested that at least 6 years of 70% mean immunization rate is required to guarantee a likely success. Oral vaccination eliminated wildlife rabies in Switzerland in 1999, France in 2000, Belgium and Luxemberg in 2001 and the Czech Republic in 2004.

32.12   Treatment

Post-bite (post-exposure) vaccination, integrated bite case management dealt with earlier.

32.12.1 Critical Care Milwaukee Protocol

In 2004, a non-vaccinated rabies case was treated by an approach later named as the Milwaukee Protocol (MP). This is based on the premises that rabies virus is minimum cytolytic and poor inflammatory. The pathology is disorder of neurotransmission. The clear candidate neurotransmitter or signalling pathway has not been identified. Treatment requires sedating the patient for prevention of dysautonomia until the patient generates a natural immune response to the rabies virus. The MP has been applied 43 times, with five additional young survivors and a significant increase in survival times. The five rare rabies cases had received vaccine prior to development of symptoms. O'Sullivan et al. (2013) used H NMR spectroscopy combined with multivariate statistical analysis to study fatal and survivors. The protocol was improvised around ketamine, a neuroprotective anaesthetic with putative activity against the rabies virus in vivo. The cluster analysis indicated that the metabolomic profiles of CSF samples collected from the two rabies survivors differed from those for whom rabies was fatal.

Hydrophobia cases need a comprehensive and compassionate patient management. It includes efforts to alleviate (a) thirst, (b) anxiety and (c) epileptic fits using infusions, diazepam or midazolam and antipyretic drugs via intravenous or intrarectal routes and to prevent respiratory failure.

References

Anonym (2005) National Association of State Public Health Veterinarians Committee. Compendium of animal rabies prevention and control, 2005. J Am Vet Med Assoc 226(8):1304–1310

Bilinski AM, Fitzpatrick MC, Rupprecht CE, Paltiel AD, Galvani AP. Optimal frequency of rabies vaccination\campaigns in Sub-Saharan Africa. Proc Biol Sci 2016; 283(1842): 20161211

Chiou HY, Hsieh CH, Jeng CR, Chan FT et al (2014) Molecular characterization of cryptically circulating rabies virus from ferret badgers, Taiwan. Emerg Infect Dis 20(5):790–798

de Souza A, Madhusudana SN (2014) Survival from rabies encephalitis. J Neurol Sci 339(1–2):8–14

Ellison JA, Johnson SR, Gilbert KA, Carson WC et al (2013) Multidisciplinary approach to epizootiology and pathogenesis of bat rabies viruses in the United States. Zoonoses Public Health 60(1):46–57

Escobar LE, Peterson AT, Favi M, Yung V, Medina-Vogel G (2015) Bat-borne rabies in Latin America. Rev Inst Med Trop Sao Paulo 57(1):63–72

Favoretto SR, de Mattos CC, Morais NB, Alves Araújo FA, de Mattos CA (2001) Rabies in marmosets (Callithrix jacchus), Ceará, Brazil. Emerg Infect Dis 7(6):1062–1065

Freuling C, Beer M, Contraths FJ, Finke S, Hoffmann B, Keller B et al (2011) Novel lyssavirus in Natterer's bat, Germany. Emerg Infect Dis 17(8):1519–1522

Hampson K, Dushoff J, Cleaveland S, Haydon DT, Kaare M, Packer C et al (2009) Transmission dynamics and prospects for the elimination of canine rabies. PLoS Biol 7(3):462–471

Hampson K, Coudeville L, Lembo T, Sambo M, Kieffer A, Attlan M et al (2015) Estimating the Global Burden of Endemic Canine Rabies. PLoS Negl Trop Dis 9(4):e0003709

Hobart-Porter N, Stein M, Toh N, Amega N, Nguyen HB, Linakis J (2021) Safety and efficacy of rabies immunoglobulin in pediatric patients with suspected exposure. Hum Vaccin Immunother 17(7):2090–2096

Janine Barrett J. Lyssaviruses; in the manual by Amman BR, Barrett J, Jong CE, Epstein JN, et al (2011) Investigating the role of bats in emerging diseases. Balancing ecology, conserving and public health interest. FAO ANIMAL PRODUCTION AND HEALTH i2007eOO1 [BATECO. EID].pdf. pp 80–101

Khan CM, Linn S (2006) Merck veterinary manual. Merck & Co. Inc., Whitehouse Station, NJ

Kunkel A, Minhaj FS, Whitehill F et al (2022) Notes from field: three human rabies deaths attributed to bat exposures-United States, August 2021. MMWR 71:31–32

Lembo T, Hampson K, Kaare MT, Ernest E, Knobel D et al (2010) The feasibility of canine rabies elimination in Africa: dispelling doubts with data. PLoS Negl Trop Dis 4(2):e626

Leslie MJ, Messenger S, Rohde RE, Smith J, Cheshier R et al (2006) Bat-associated rabies virus in skunks. Emerg Infect Dis 12:1274–1277

Matsumoto T, Ahmed K, Wimalaratne O, Nanayakkara S et al (2011) Novel sylvatic rabies virus variant in endangered golden palm civet, Sri Lanka. Emerg Infect Dis 17(12):2346–2349

McCollum AM, Blanton JD, Holman RC, Callinan LS, Baty S et al (2012) Community survey after rabies outbreaks, flagstaff, Arizona, USA. Emerg Infect Dis 18(6):932–938

Messenger SL, Smith JS, Orciari LA, Yager PA, Rupprecht CE (2003) Emerging pattern of rabies deaths and increased viral infectivity. Emerg Infect Dis 9(2):151–154

Morters MK, Restif O, Hampson K, Cleaveland S et al (2013) Evidence-based control of canine rabies: a critical review of population density reduction. J Anim Ecol 82:6–14

Narayan KG (2004) Epidemiology, diagnosis and management of zoonoses. ICAR, New Delhi, pp 83–93

O'Sullivan A, Willoughby RE, Mishchuk D, Alcarraz B, Cabezas-Sanchez C et al (2013) Metabolomics of Cerebrospinal Fluid from Humans Treated for Rabies. J Proteome Res 12:481–490

OIE (2019) The OIE Wildlife Health Framework-Protecting wildlife health to achieve One health. https://www.woah.org/fileadmin/Home/eng/Internationa_Standard_Setting/docs/pdf/WGWildlife/A_Wildlifehealth_conceptnote.pdf

Rahman (1997) India: rabies prevention and control—a veterinary prospective. In: Dodet B, Meslin F-X (eds) Rabies control in Asia. Elsevier, Oxford, pp 146–152

Randall DA, Williams SD, Kuzmin IV et al (2004) Rabies in endangered Ethiopian wolves. Emerg Infect Dis 10(12):2214–2217

Streicker DG, Turmelle AS, Vonhof MJ, Kuzmin IV et al (2010) Host phylogeny constrains cross-species emergence and establishments of rabies virus in bats. Science 329(5992):676–679

Tao XY, Tang Q, Li H, Mo ZJ, Zhang H et al (2009) Molecular epidemiology of rabies in Southern People's Republic of China. Emerg Infect Dis 15(8):1192–1198

Tenzin SB, Dhand NK, Timsina N, Ward MP (2010) Reemergence of rabies in Chukha district, Bhutan, 2008. Emerg Infect Dis 16(12):1925–1930

Tischendorf L, Thulke HH, Staubach C, Muller MS et al (1998) Chance and risk of controlling rabies in large scale and long term immunized fox populations. Proc R Soc Lond 265:839–846

Undurraga EA, Meltzer MI, Tran CH, Atkins CY, Elheart MD, Millien MF et al (2017) Cost–effectiveness evaluation of a novel integrated bite case management program for the control of human rabies, Haiti 2014–2015. Am J Trop Med Hyg 96:1307–1317

Warembourg C, Wera E, Odoch T, Bulu PM, Berger-González M et al (2021) Comparative study of free-roaming domestic dog management and roaming behavior across four countries: Chad, Guatemala, Indonesia, and Uganda. Front Vet Sci 8:617900

Watanabe I, Kentaro Yamada K, Aso A, Suda O et al (2012) Relationship between virus-neutralizing antibody levels and the number of rabies vaccinations: a prospective study of dogs in Japan. Jpn J Infect Dis 66:17–21

WHO (2010) Rabies vaccines: WHO position paper. Wkly Epidemiol Rec 85:309–320. http://www.who.int/wer

WHO/FAO/OIE (2018) Zero by 30: the global strategic plan to end human deaths from dog-mediated rabies by 2030. ISBN 978-92-4-151383-8 (WHO) ISBN 978-92-5-130461-7 (FAO) ISBN 978-92-95108-76-9 (OIE) WHO (2018) expert committee technical report series 1012. https://doi.org/10.1016/S2214-109X(18)30302-4

Chapter 33
Ebola Virus

Ebola is a highly infectious and contagious disease. It is characterized by a sudden onset of fever, sore throat, headache, muscle ache, extreme weakness progressing to diarrhoea, vomiting, internal and external bleeding, multiorgan failure and high CFR.

Severe viral haemorrhagic fever (VHF) appeared in 1976 simultaneously in Nzara, Sudan, and in a Yambuku village near Ebola River in the Democratic Republic of the Congo. The virus is named after the name of the river. Case fatality rate may be as high as 90%. The Ebola virus is transmitted from wild animals to human and spreads from man to man. Fruit bats are considered natural reservoirs.

33.1 Aetiology

Ebola and *Marburg* are two genera in the family *Filoviridae*. Genetic changes are slow and the two genera separated 1000 years ago.

The five chronologically detected Ebola viruses are:

1. Zaire ebolavirus (ZEBOV) Aug. 1976—first case a school teacher; reused needle suspected for transmission.
2. Sudan ebolavirus (SEBOV) 1976—first case exposed to potential natural reservoir and absence of 'barrier nursing' (bedside isolation) led to the spread to cotton factory workers.
3. Reston ebolavirus (REBOV) was isolated from an outbreak of simian haemorrhagic fever (SHF) in macaques in Reston, Virginia, in 1989. Subsequent three isolates were from non-human primates imported from the same facility in the Philippines. REBOV infected pigs also but not human beings even when exposed in laboratory.

© Springer Nature Singapore Pte Ltd. 2024
K. G. Narayan et al., *Handbook of Management of Zoonoses*,
https://doi.org/10.1007/978-981-99-9885-2_33

4. Côte d'Ivoire ebolavirus (CIEBOV) or 'Ivory Coast EBOV' first detected in chimpanzee from Tai Forest in Côte d'Ivoire, Africa, in 1994—scientist performing autopsy on infected chimpanzees got infected, had to be hospitalized for 2 weeks and recovered 6 weeks after infection. The natural reservoir is believed to be Western red colobus monkeys upon which chimpanzees prey.
5. Bundibugyo ebolavirus (BEBOV)—The 2007–2008 outbreak of Ebola virus in Bundibugyo was caused by this new species as confirmed by the CDC and the WHO.

33.2   A Comparison Between ZEBOV and REBOV

REBOV is not a human pathogen or at least does not cause a serious disease. It is genetically distinct among EBOVs with >40% nucleotide sequences for glycoprotein gene divergent from ZEBOV and these are responsible for pathogenesis. Infectivity is low; endothelial cell damage and lymphocyte apoptosis are less; immune response is good (reduction in the 'down-regulation of immune response') and antibody-dependent immunity enhanced. Only 15 of 800 exposed developed antibody. Replication was delayed and cytopathogenic effect was mild. The rate of cleavage of glycoprotein necessary for virus activation and pathogenicity was decreased.

There are six members of the genus *Ebola*: Zaire (EBOV), Tai Forest (TAFV), Sudan (SUV), Reston (RESTV), Bundibugyo (BDBV) and Bombali virus.

Weingartl et al. (2012) consider that response to EBOV infection between pigs and primates seems to differ. The respiratory system of pigs is primarily affected while primates develop a systemic infection. Ebola viruses endemic in Africa cause severe often fatal haemorrhagic fever in non-human primates and humans. REBOV, the Asian ebolavirus, was isolated from swine in the Philippines, induced antibodies in pig farmers and caused fatal infection in cynomolgus macaques. ZEBOV experimentally infected pigs, caused disease and transmitted to in-contact pigs.

The Ebola virions are approximately of 80 nm size. There are seven genes and seven structural proteins. The genomes of the five Ebola viruses differ in sequence and the number and location of gene overlap also antigenically. The centrally located nucleocapsid has helically wound genomic RNA complexed with proteins—NP, VP35 (polymerase co-factor), VP30 (transcription activator) and L (RNA-dependent RNA polymerase). The ribonucleoprotein is embedded in the major viral protein (VP40) and minor viral protein (VP24) matrix. These are surrounded by the lipid membrane of host cell membrane origin. The glycoprotein (GP) is anchored on the membrane in the form of spikes.

33.3   Host Cell Invasion and Viral Replication

Filoviruses (*Ebola* and *Marburg*) require a cholesterol transport protein, NPC1, for binding directly to the viral envelope glycoprotein. This suggests that NPC1 may be a target for potential anti-filovirus drug. Following binding, virus is endocytosed into macropinosomes of the host cell. The nucleocapsid is released into the cytoplasm. Viral proteins are synthesized using host cell machinery. Replication of viral RNA follows and rapid encapsidation occurs. Newly formed nucleocapsids and envelope proteins self-assemble at the host cell plasma membrane. Budding releases new virions and simultaneously destroys host cells. The released new virus particles invade other cells to repeat the cycle.

33.4 Pathogenesis

Ebola viruses target endothelial cells, mononuclear phagocytes and hepatocytes. Secreted glycoprotein (sGP) and the Ebola viral proteins including viral GP are synthesized. Host immune system is overwhelmed. The viral GP binds the virus to the endothelial cells lining blood vessels. The sGP interferes signalling of the neutrophils that are not activated and thus the virus succeeds in evading the initial host's defence. The invaded cells spread the virus throughout the body and post the virus to tissues like lymph nodes, liver, spleen and lungs. Release of cytokines (like TNF-alpha, IL-6, IL-8) is triggered. This is manifested in inflammation and fever. Invasion and destruction of endothelial cells lining blood vessels cause leakage and internal haemorrhage. The viral GP causes loss of natural integrins responsible for cells adhesion to intercellular structure. Cellular integrity is lost. Liver is damaged. Coagulopathy results.

33.5 Modes of Infection

Those handling infected or dead wild animals like chimpanzees, gorillas, monkeys, fruit bats, forest antelopes and porcupines in rain forest of Africa have been infected. Weingartl et al. (2012) brought out experimental evidences of aerosol transmission from pigs to macaques.

Transmission in human: Direct contact is the mode of transmission—blood, body fluids of patients, semen and breast milk of asymptomatic are infectious; indirect contact with surfaces contaminated with these also transmits the virus. The virus has been detected in breast milk; saliva and semen; amniotic, cerebrospinal and ocular fluids; and viral RNA in vaginal and rectal swabs. Exposure to these body fluids poses a durable risk of infection. The virus enters through broken skin, mucous membrane and placenta. Healthcare workers and mourners are commonly infected and suffer from Ebola virus haemorrhagic fever (EVHF).

33.6 Signs and Symptoms

The incubation period varies as 12.7 ± 4.3 days, maximum of 25 days. All cases of EVHF show evidence of damaged circulatory system and coagulopathy. Puncture sites and mucosa like gingiva bleed. Bleeding of the digestive system mucosa is manifested in hematemesis, haemoptysis and melena. The symptoms are varied depending upon the system/organs affected. Skin may present maculopapular rash, petechiae, purpura, ecchymoses and bleeding. Initial signs and symptoms are confounding. General malaise, fever and chill are confused with general flu. Pain in muscle and joints leads one to think of dengue. When the digestive system is affected, abdominal pain, anorexia, diarrhoea and vomiting may be seen. Pharyngitis, sore throat, cough and dyspnoea indicate respiratory involvement. Severe headache, confusion, fatigue, depression, seizures and coma indicate CNS involvement. Death in EVHF is considered to be due to multiple-organ/system failure caused by disseminated intravascular coagulation, fluid redistribution, focal necrosis and hypotension.

Prognosis is generally poor (see the table for CFR). Survivors may recover completely and promptly. Others may take time to recover with conditions like arthralgia, myalgia, orchitis, alopecia; photophobia, hyperlacrimation, iritis, choroiditis and blindness.

33.7   Epidemiology

EBOVs have restricted distribution, near rain forests in villages of Central and West Africa, though evidences of extension are appearing. Possible natural hosts in Africa are fruit bats of species of the genera *Hypsignathus monstrosus*, *Epomops franqueti* and *Myonycteris torquata*, family Pteropodidae. Distribution of Ebola virus may overlap the distribution of fruit bat reservoirs. Wild animals are incidental rather than reservoir hosts. However, Zaire and Ivory Coast viruses have caused outbreaks since 1994 in chimpanzees and gorillas. Gorillas seem to get infected with multiple Ebola viral strains. Contact with viral reservoirs seems to be the mode of transmission. Chimpanzees transmit through meat consumption rather than by direct contact and outbreaks of Ebola virus disease cause a decline in their population. Nidom et al. (2012) detected Zaire, Sudan, Côte d'Ivoire and Bundibugyo Ebola viruses in Indonesian orangutans. These viruses have so far been found only in Africa. Serum samples from 353 healthy Bornean orangutans were examined and 18.4% and 1.7% were positive for EBOV and MARV (Marburg virus), respectively. REBOV is recognized as Asian filovirus. Reston virus has been the cause of severe viral haemorrhagic fever among farmed monkeys (*Macaca fascicularis*) in the Philippines and those exported from here to the USA in years 1989, 1990 and 1996 and to the USA and Italy in 1992. This monkey facility was closed in 1997 and REBOV vanished.

Among domestic animals, dogs and pigs get infected. Dogs do not manifest symptoms. Pigs tend to suffer from clinical disease. Barrette et al. (2009) observed that it resurfaced in 2008 in domestic pigs on two farms within few 100 miles of the closed monkey breeding facility, possibly got infection from fruit bats. Pigs were co-infected with porcine reproductive and respiratory syndrome virus, but the histo-pathological findings resembled pigs experimentally infected with ZEBOV. Six workers on pig farms were seropositive but denied any contact with bats or monkeys—indicative of possible transmission to human. Kobinger et al. (2011) experimentally infected domestic pigs with ZEBOV through nasogastric mucosa; virus replicated in the upper respiratory tract and was shed in the secretion to spread to naïve pigs and macaques. Bausch (2011) argues that hunters, butchers of gorillas and chimps in Central Africa got infected with ZEBOV, most likely through ingestion of undercooked meat because the virus lipid envelope made it unstable to environmental conditions. REBOV infecting farmed pigs suggested the likelihood of transmission through eating undercooked pork and use of porcine products used for medical and cosmetic purposes. If that happened, REBOV could be the cause of serious economic loss through culling as was caused by Nipah and swine influenza pandemic in 2010. He advises not to press the panic button at this stage but keep vigilance. Weingartl et al. (2013) suggested that the role of pigs and macaques in Ebola outbreaks in Africa need to be clarified and detection of viral RNA should be the basis of diagnosis.

Olival et al. (2013) found 3.5% of *Rousettus leschenaultii* fruit bats were seropositive for ZEBOV and REBOV, although no virus was detected by PCR. Since excreta of fruit bats *Pteropus giganteus* has been earlier found to contaminate date palm with Nipah virus and caused outbreak in humans in Bangladesh, this finding is suggestive of further vigilance. The summary of outbreaks, case fatality rates and the causative viruses are tabulated (Table 33.1).

33.8 Epidemic and Control

Epidemics in West Africa (2014–2016) and subsequently in the Democratic Republic of the Congo are reported. As on 31 May 2020, there were 3436 cases and 2280 deaths (SITREP_EVD_DRC_20200606_eng.pdf).

The 11th Ebola outbreak in the Democratic Republic of the Congo was declared over on 18 November 2020 (https://www.afro.who.int/news/11th-ebola-outbreak-democratic-republic-congo-declared-over). There were 119 confirmed cases, 11 probable cases and 55 deaths. Over 40,000 were vaccinated. The COVID-19 pandemic and remote hard-to-access outbreak areas made tackling very difficult. The WHO Director for Africa Matshidiso Moeti attributed the success to the combination of science and solidarity. The 11th outbreak of Ebola in the Democratic Republic of the Congo (1 June–18 November 2020) is linked to the eight flare-ups linked to 'survivors becoming persistent subclinical cases' 11 months after the WHO had declared Ebola-free status in May 2015. EBOV persisted in the semen of the survivor for 18 months (Subissi et al. 2018). Undiagnosed/undetected survivors may also contribute.

Table 33.1 Number outbreaks: year, viruses, countries and CFR (%)/cases given in bracket

Ebola viruses	1976–1979	1994–1996	2000–2005	2007–2008	2011	2012
Zaire (EBOV)	2 (88–100%/319)	5 (60–100%/459)	5 (53–90%/314)	2 (47–71%/296)		
Sudan (SUDV)	2 (53–65%/318)		2 (41–53%/442)		1 (100%/1)	1 (71%/24)
Tai Forest (TAFV)/Côte d'Ivoire ebolavirus (CIEBOV)		2 (0%/1)				
Bundibugyo (BDBV)				1 (25%/149)		1 (44%/72)

Countries—Democratic Republic of the Congo 6, Congo 4, Gabon 4, Sudan 3, Uganda 4, Côte d'Ivoire 1, South Africa (ex-Gabon) 1. Total 23 + 3 lab. accidental—1988 (UK), Russia (1996, 2004)

Note: EBOV—highest infectivity and virulence; next is SUDV (number of outbreaks, cases and deaths) followed by BDEV and TAFV; current names are boldfaced. EVD is VHF indistinguishable from MVD (Marburg viral disease)

Sources: Ebola haemorrhagic fever. Fact sheet N0. 103, Aug. 2012 http://www.who.int/mediacentre/factsheets/fs103/en/index1.html; http://www.who.int/csr/don/2012_11_30_ebola/en/index.html; http://www.who.int/csr/don/2012_10_26/en/index.html

33.9 Fighting Epidemic: Experience of the West Africa Epidemic, 2014–2016

The economic effects Ebola epidemic (West Africa, 2013–2016) has on the three countries—Guinea, Liberia, and Sierra Leone—in 2015 are estimated to be more than \$1.6 billion, over 12% of their combined GDP (World Bank Group 2015). The scenario is as follows: on 9 Feb 2014 Liberia reported 3147/8864 lab-confirmed cases. The Liberia Ministry of Health and Social Welfare (MOHSW), supported by the CDC, the World Health Organization (WHO) and others, began the fight early, 20 August. Although the number of confirmed cases peaked in September 2014, it markedly dropped by the end of the year. Chain of transmission could be stopped and outbreaks ended in May, November and December 2016, respectively (WHO Ebola Response Team 2016).

There were 23 outbreaks reported in 1976 in equatorial Africa, in forested, sparsely populated areas with slow and infrequent connection by river/road (in contrast with the epidemic in interconnected population). A village boy of 2 years in the forest region of southeast Guinea fell ill on 26 Dec 2013 and died 2 days later due to *Zaire ebolavirus* species. Its origin remains uncertain, possibly a bat. The primary source is presumably the bat and mammals (primates) as alternate/secondary reservoirs and antelopes eaten as bush meat. Phylogenetic studies indicated that there was only one introduction of virus from an animal reservoir. The virus was introduced to Sierra Leone as two genetically distinct lineages: apparently from attendants at a single funeral, around Feb 2014, who repeatedly entered in Guinea and exported to Mali on two separate occasions during October and November 2014, demonstrating how fast the virus spread with men carrying it. The Ebola virus is nearly stable and does not undergo mutation during epidemic.

Salient features: Incubation period—9.4 ± 7.4 days; duration of illness—5 ± 4.7 days; male/female ratio almost even; cases—lowest in children 10–14 years; almost 3–4× in age group 15–44 years and less in female. Transmission of infection is most from cases in advanced stage or near about death. CFR 70% reducible with prompt hospitalization and supportive care. The $R_0 = 1.71$–2.02 and the generation time is 15.3 ± 9.1 days and sustained reduction of transmission by 50% can eliminate Ebola from the human population.

Nearly 20% of cases can be considered as 'super spreaders', being sources of infection for about 80% of cases in the following generation. Rapid intervention in the beginning is important.

33.9.1 The Strategy

Community engagement, early case detection and diagnosis, comprehensive contact tracing, prompt patient isolation, supportive clinical care and rigorous infection control, including safe burial, early case detection and stoppage of transmission, prevented conversion of minor outbreak into major outbreak or epidemic in mobile populations.

Ebola patients and excretions and secretions are the primary source of infection; exposure to these is the mode of transmission. Therefore, infection prevention and control (IPC) practices are essential in healthcare settings for the healthcare workers. They are on the frontline and exposed. Lack or oversight of IPC, poor waste management procedures, a lack of triage and isolation protocols, frequent lack or misuse of personal protective equipment (PPE) and inadequate standard infection control precautions can lead to outbreaks among healthcare workers (HCWs) and patients. The recommended PPE for Ebola patient care was a gown, gloves, eye protection and facemask; additional PPE (e.g. shoe covers, leg covers, double gloving and respirator) for HCWs was recommended if the HCW anticipated contact with copious body fluids or would be performing aerosol-generating procedures. It is essential for containment and prevention of re-emergence.

Innovative combinations of components of strategy control the epidemic fast. Examples: Kateh et al. (2015) planned RITE (Rapid Isolation and Treatment of Ebola) in October 2014, for controlling 15 outbreaks. Nyenswah et al. (2015a, b) used RING-IPC on 29 December 2014 for the last cluster of 22 cases in Liberia.

33.9.2 Process

1. Define:

    A suspected case—(1) disease in a living person with history of contact with a person who had laboratory-confirmed or probable EVD and (2) red eyes, unexplained bleeding or sudden onset of high fever or >3 of the following signs and symptoms: headache, anorexia/loss of appetite, lethargy, aching muscles or joints, breathing difficulties, vomiting, diarrhoea, stomach pain, difficulty swallowing and hiccups.

    Probable cases—disease in deceased persons who had an epidemiologic association with EVD but no laboratory testing.

    Laboratory confirmed—disease in any persons, dead or alive, who proved positive to real-time reverse transcription PCR/serologic positive samples tested >10 days after symptom onset and for PCR-negative samples.

    Outbreak—an outbreak is defined as one or more epidemiological linked cases.
2. Engaging community through County Health Teams (CHT); capacity building for RITE; delegated power to decide and mould according to community needs; coordinate response activities of 'response partners/team'– mobilize resources.
3. Activities of response team:

    • Rapidly isolate and treat Ebola patients, either in situ (establishing isolation and treatment facilities in the community)/safely transporting patients to existing Ebola treatment units (ETUs).

- Collection and safe transportation of samples for laboratory confirmation.
- Ascertain the index case—'first person in the transmission chain who entered the community from another county' to better understand importation and transmission patterns.
- Quarantine of asymptomatic high-risk contacts at home or in designated quarantine facilities.
- Identify all generations of cases by improving case finding and contact tracing to ensure no cases were missed.
- Train teams in safe burial procedures.
- Observe contacts for 21 days from the death or ETU admission of the last case to ensure interruption of transmission.

4. Infection prevention and control (IPC) include:

- Prompt triage (= assigning degree of urgency to decide the order of treatment of a large number of patients or casualties)
- Facilities for screening of suspected cases at entry points by trained staff; personal protective equipment for the screening staff (e.g. minimum gloves)
- IPC improvements in waste management, hand hygiene, environmental decontamination and other critical facilities
- Sustaining the education, training and competency of HCWs
- Innovation and improvement on IPC practices

5. Results

RITE: The median duration of outbreaks reduced from 53 to 25 days; number of generation of cases from 4 to 2; proportion of patients isolated increased from 28 to 81% and survival percentage rose from 13 to 50. CFR improved over time, from 87% of early to 50% in later outbreaks. All the outbreaks ended as of 8 January 2015 and no case identified within 21 days of exposure to the last patient.

RING-IPC: It is a focused infection prevention and control approach for target facilities that are at increased risk for exposure. It provided rapid, intensive and short-term IPC support to healthcare facility in areas of active Ebola transmission. Eight patients of a cluster of 22 received care from 10 non-Ebola HCFs before admission to ETU—thus, there was a risk of Ebola transmission in these 10. Three of such HCFs were recognized. Ring IPC was applied. The time interval from onset of illness to admission to an ETU decreased with each generation of cases—6, 4.7 and 1.5 days, respectively; case fatality rates were 100%, 60% and 50%. Contact tracing identified 745 contacts, of which 166 were HCWs from 10 HCFs. No case in healthcare workers from public or private health facilities was identified.

Last cases were admitted to ETU on 18 February 2015, and on May 19, the WHO declared Liberia free from Ebola.

Additional cases continued after the control of epidemic as the EV persisted in the tissues of the survivors. Semen is infective till 7 weeks after clinical recovery and 61 days in a lab-acquired case.

33.10   Diagnosis

Patients' history is helpful. History of possible exposure to bats and their excrements and wildlife and visit to endemic countries are suggestive.

Detection in blood and/or serum during acute phase:

1. EBOV antigen by IFT
2. Genome RNA
3. Subgenomic RNA by RT-PCR
4. Isolation EBOV in cell culture (e.g. Vero E6, MA-104, SW-13) and confirmation by observing cytopathic effect and IFT
5. Electron microscopy

Biosafety level 4 laboratory is required to handle specimens. Laboratory workers must strictly use the personal protective equipment.

33.11   Treatment

Supportive therapy includes countering dehydration, electrolyte loss, haemorrhage and disseminated intravascular coagulation, secondary infection.

Specific therapies are being developed.

- Recent novel method—Antisense therapy is promising. Small interfering RNAs (siRNAs) and phosphorodiamidate morpholino oligomers (PMOs) targeting the EBOVA genome could prevent disease in non-human primate (Geisbert et al. 2010).
- Receptor protein (TIM-1) for Zaire Ebola and Lake Victoria Marburg viruses has been identified and antibodies binding this receptor protein block the infection. The epithelial cells of mucosal surfaces of the respiratory tract and eyes – portals of entry of EBV, besides various tissues express TIM-1. Antibody ARD5 to TIM-1 effectively blocked Ebola and Marburg viruses from entry to cells. However, TIM-1 protein is not expressed by all cells that are infected by these viruses (Kondratowicz et al. 2011).
- Clomiphene is an FDA drug used to treat female infertility. It blocks also Ebola virus effectively. The virus is not allowed to deliver its RNA into the host's cell cytoplasm, degraded and removed quickly from the body as observed in a 'mouse model' (http://medicalxpress.com/news/2013-06-fda-approved-medications-unexpected-deadly-ebola.html).
- Ebola viral protein VP35 interacts with cellular protein PACT and blocks it, thus deactivating the host's innate immune system allowing the virus to infect the cells and replicate (Basler et al. 2013).
- James Pettitt, scientist at the US Army Medical Research Institute of Infectious Diseases, reported the results of MB-003, a drug under development. It prevented

symptoms in cent percent of experimental monkeys when administered i/v 1 h after exposure and cured 40% of monkeys that had developed the symptoms. MB-003 targeted a protein on the outer surface of EBOV stimulating the person's immunity that killed the infected cells (Africa: New Compound Holds Great Promise As Ebola Treatment; BY JESSICA BERMAN, 21 AUGUST 2013 http://allafrica.com/stories/201308220526.html).
• ZMapp might help treat Ebola virus.

33.12 Prevention

The absence of suitable therapy and vaccine demands a multiple approach to prevent transmission. This has been detailed by the WHO (Ebola haemorrhagic fever. Fact sheet N0. 103, August 2012 http://www.who.int/mediacentre/factsheets/fs103/en/index1.html).

Ebola virus can persist for years in bodily fluids. The WHO advises to test the survivor's semen samples till two consecutive tests are negative and heightened vigilance (active surveillance and post-mortem testing) for at least 6 months after 42-day period of 'without a new case' and passive surveillance indefinitely.

Epidemic/transmission—refer to above 'Fighting Epidemic'.

Controlling REBOV in domestic animals:
• Sodium hypochlorite and other detergents to clean and disinfect pig and monkey farms.
• Quarantine premises with suspected outbreak and restriction on the movement of animals from such premises.
• Culling of infected animals, burial and incineration of carcasses under supervision.
• Establish 'active animal health surveillance system' to detect new cases—it is an early warning system for both vet and human health, as Ebola Reston outbreaks in pigs and monkeys have preceded human infections.

Reduction of transmission:
• Awareness of the risk factors of Ebola infection and death.
• Reduce wildlife-human transmission—contact with fruit bats, monkeys/apes, consumption of their raw meat, handling with proper protective clothing/gloves, etc.
• Reduce human-to-human transmission—avoid/careful contact with patients and their body fluids and regular hand washings.
• Avoid/take precautions in pig farms; pigs in Africa get infected through contact with fruit bats.
• Educational messages about risks involved—(a) pig-human, (b) animal husbandry practices, (c) slaughtering and unsafe meat consumption, (d) tissues that

can transmit infection, (e) patient and dead body contacts and contact with their secretions and excretions, (f) Ebola-specific standard precautionary measures and (g) standard precautionary measures for laboratory workers.

- The WHO supports are available.

33.13   Vaccine

Johnson & Johnson's Ad26.ZEBOV/MVA-BN vaccine is preventive for population/ area at risk with no active transmission; two doses were given at an interval of 56 days (Burki 2020).

The European Medicines Agency (EMA) is the European regulator recommending a conditional marketing authorization for the rVSV-ZEBOV-GP vaccine. The WHO welcomed it. More than 236,000 have been vaccinated in the Democratic Republic of the Congo in the current outbreak including more than 60,000 health and frontline workers in the Democratic Republic of the Congo and in Uganda, South Sudan, Rwanda and Burundi. The vaccine will continue to be used in the country under a research protocol (also known as 'expanded access' or 'compassionate use') and with the ring vaccination strategy (https://www.who.int/news/item/18-10-2019-major-milestone-for-who-supported-ebola-vaccine).

References

Barrette RW, Metwally SA, Rowland JM et al (2009) Discovery of swine as a host for the Reston Ebola virus. Science 325:204–206

Basler et al (2013) Cell host and microbe July 2013 issue. Source Ebola virus Research Print. Researchers identify vulnerabilities of Ebola virus. http://www.infectioncontrolto-day.com/news/2013/07/researchers-identify-vulnerabilities-of-ebola-virus.aspx?utm_source=feedburner&utm_medium=feed&utm_campaign=Feed%3A+ICTSiteWideFeed+%28Infection+ Control+ Today+ Site + Wide+ Content+Feed%29

Bausch DG (2011) Ebola virus as a foodborne pathogen? Cause for consideration, but not panic. J Infect Dis 204(2):179–181

Burki T (2020) Ebola virus disease in DRC Congo. Lancet Infect Dis 20(4):418–419

Geisbert TW, Lee AC, Robbins M, Geisbert JB, Honko AN et al (2010) Post-exposure protection of non-human primates against a lethal Ebola virus challenge with RNA interference: a proof-of-concept study. Lancet 375(9729):1896–1905

Hageman JC, Hazim C, Wilson K et al (2016) Infection prevention and control for Ebola in health care settings—West Africa and United States. MMWR Suppl 65(Suppl-3):50–56

Kateh F, Nagbe T, Kieta A et al (2015) Rapid response to Ebola outbreaks in remote areas—Liberia, July–November 2014. MMWR 64:188–192

Kobinger GP, Leung A, Neufeld J et al (2011) Replication, pathogenicity, shedding, and transmission of Zaire Ebola virus in pigs. J Infect Dis 204(2):200–208

Kondratowicz AS, Lennemann NJ, Sinn PL, Davey RA, Hunt CL et al (2011) T-cell immuno-globulin and mucin domain 1 (TIM-1) is a receptor for Zaire Ebolavirus and Lake Victoria Marburgvirus. Proc Natl Acad Sci U S A 108(20):8426–8431

Nidom CA, Nakayama E, Nidom RV, Alamudi MY, Daulay S et al (2012) Serological evidence of Ebola virus infection in Indonesian Orangutans. PLoS ONE 7(7):e40740

Nyenswah T et al (2015a) Controlling the last known cluster of Ebola virus disease—Liberia, January–February 2015. MMWR 64(18):500–504

Nyenswah T, Massaquoi M, Gbanya MZ et al (2015b) Initiation of a ring approach to infection prevention and control at non-Ebola health care facilities—Liberia, January–February 2015. MMWR 64:505–508

Olival KJ, Islam A, Yu M, Anthony SJ, Epstein JH et al (2013) Ebola virus antibodies in fruit bats, Bangladesh. Emerg Infect Dis 19(2):270–273

Subissi L, Keita M, Mesfin S, Rezza G, Diallo B et al (2018) Ebola virus transmission caused by persistently infected survivors of the 2014-2016 outbreak in West Africa. J Infect Dis 218:S287–S291

Weingartl HM, Embury-Hyatt C, Nfon C, Leung A et al (2012) Transmission of Ebola virus from pigs to non-human primates. Sci Rep 2:811

Weingartl HM, Nfon C, Kobinger G (2013) Review of Ebola virus infections in domestic animals. In: Roth JA, Richt JA, Morozov IA (eds) Vaccines and diagnostics for transboundary animal diseases, vol 135. Karger, Basel, pp 211–218

WHO Ebola Response Team (2016) After Ebola in West Africa—unpredictable risks, preventable epidemics. N Engl J Med 375(6):587–596

World Bank Group (2015) The economic impact of Ebola on sub-Saharan Africa: updated estimates for 2015 January 20, 2015]-World Bank Group no 93721

Chapter 34
Monkeypox

Monkeypox (mpox) is characterized by an initial febrile prodrome and a centrifu-
gally distributed maculopapular rash developing often on the palms of hands and
soles of feet. The presentation is similar to smallpox in humans with additional
distinguishing symptom of lymphadenopathy. Monkeypox and smallpox viruses
belong to Variola virus. The WHO declared it as a global health emergency on 23
July 2022. From 1 January through 22 August 2022, 41,664 laboratory-confirmed
cases of monkeypox and 12 deaths have been reported to the WHO from 96 coun-
tries/territories/areas in all six WHO regions. A total of nine laboratory-confirmed
cases of monkeypox and one death were reported in India by 22 August 2022
(https://www.who.int/emergencies/situation-reports).

34.1 Aetiology

The 1958 outbreak in two colonies of monkeys maintained for research was investigated and the virus isolated was identified as monkeypox. Monkeypox virus is a
double-stranded DNA virus belonging to the genus *Orthopoxvirus*, family
Poxviridae. There are two clades of monkeypox virus: the Congo Basin (Central
African) and the West African, the former more virulent and transmissible reflected
in epidemiological and clinical features. Cameroon has both the clades.

34.2 Epidemiology

Monkeypox is a sylvatic zoonosis with incidental human infections that usually
occur sporadically.

© Springer Nature Singapore Pte Ltd. 2024
K. G. Narayan et al., *Handbook of Management of Zoonoses*,
https://doi.org/10.1007/978-981-99-9885-2_34

Monkeypox virus is endemic in several countries in Central and Western Africa. Sporadic cases associated with travel to endemic countries have been reported outside Africa, in the USA, England, Singapore and Israel.

34.2.1 Reservoir

There is no natural reservoir. Rodents are most likely reservoirs. Susceptible animals are rope squirrel, tree squirrel, Gambian poached rats, dormice, shrews, anteaters, hedgehogs, rabbits, American prairie dogs and non-human primates (monkeys). The virus has been isolated once each from rope squirrel (*Funisciurus anerythrus*) and sooty mangabey (*Cercocebus atys*) in Côte d'Ivoire (Durski et al. 2018).

34.2.1.1 Monkeypox in Animals

Symptoms in infected animals are not documented. Rash does not appear in all infected animals. Febrile symptoms such as lethargy, appetite loss, nasal secretions or crust, pimple or blister are likely. Small mammals may show no apparent symptoms of monkeypox infection. Non-human primates may get sick and manifest symptoms of infection like in man.

Infected animals can transmit monkeypox virus to human and it is possible that human can pass it to animals while petting, cuddling, hugging and sharing sleeping areas. There is no report of sick human transmitting monkeypox to animals.

In May and June 2003 outbreak of monkeypox occurred in the USA. Epidemiological investigation traced back the source as domesticated prairie dogs. They had shared bedding and caging with Gambian pouched rats and dormice imported from Ghana. The Texas animal distributor imported approximately 762 African rodents from Ghana. These included rope squirrels (*Funisciurus* spp.), tree squirrels (*Heliosciurus* spp.), Gambian giant pouched rats (*Cricetomys* spp.), brushtail porcupines (*Atherurus* spp.), dormice (*Graphiurus* spp.) and striped mice (*Hybomys* spp.). Some suffered from monkeypox as confirmed by laboratory testing. Several rodent species, including two Gambian giant pouched rats, nine dormice and three rope squirrels, were infected with monkeypox. Of the 762 rodents from the original shipment, 584 were traced to distributors in six states.

The 2003 outbreak of human monkeypox in the six Midwestern states of the USA happens to be the first outside Africa and zoonotic. There were 72 cases traced to the native prairie dogs (*Cynomys* spp.). These were housed at a pet distributor's facility along with wild rodents imported from Africa. Nine cases had exposure to two ill prairie dogs. Kile et al. (2005) observed that the risk of symptomatic infection correlated with the amount of exposure to prairie dogs, extensive direct contact among family members (100%), moderate exposure among veterinarians and nonfamily childcare attendees (19%) and limited exposure among schoolchildren (0). Guarner et al. (2004) diagnosed monkeypox in prairie dogs by PCR and electron microscopy. The pathological lesions observed were ulcers on tongue, conjunctivitis and necrotizing bronchopneumonia. Monkeypox virus antigen was demonstrated in abundance on the surface epithelium of lesions and less in adjoining connective tissues, fibroblasts and macrophages. This suggested that routes of exposure between rodents and human were respiratory and direct mucocutaneous exposures. Exposure to prairie dogs caused 37 human infections among exotic pet dealers, pet owners and veterinarians.

According to Bunge et al. (2022) monkeypox has appeared in 10 African countries and four countries outside of Africa since 1970. The number of cases has increased by tenfold. The median age of cases used to be 4 years in the 1970s. It has changed to 21 years in 2010–2019, possibility related with the stopping of smallpox vaccination. Monkeypox is gradually evolving to become of global relevance.

In May 2022 the unexpected rise in the number of human monkeypox cases began.

34.2.2 Source and Transmission

These infected animals and human are the two main sources of the virus. A patient is infective (can spread) from the time symptoms appear and it remains so until rashes have healed, scabs fallen off and fresh skin layer has appeared.

The routes of transmission in Africa are animal bites, scratch, touch and consumption of infected bushmeat. Human-to-human transmission occurs through respiratory droplets and close contact:

- Direct contact with monkeypox rash, scabs or body fluids from a person with monkeypox
- Close contact including skin to skin (during oral, anal, vaginal sex or touching genitalia); hugging, kissing, massage
- Touching contaminated surface and objects like bedding, towel and clothing used by a person who had/has monkeypox
- Contact with fomites, respiratory secretions (saliva from coughing)

Morgan et al. (2022) examined samples from commonly used objects within the household occupied by a patient diagnosed positive for MPXV-WA by the US CDC on 16 July 2021. Porous (e.g. bedding, clothing) and non-porous (e.g. metal, plastic) surfaces examined were positive by MPXV-WA PCR. Isolation in cell culture of monkeypox West African strain from seven samples was indicative of viable virus contaminated bedding, clothing, etc. Viable virus was detected even after at least 15 days. The titre was low ($\leq 10^2$ PFU). Risk of indirect transmission appeared to be low.

Sexual transmission was evidenced by finding primary genital, anal and oral mucosal lesions (inoculation sites) and supported by finding monkeypox virus DNA in seminal fluid in 29/32 cases (Thornhill et al. 2022). A study group from the National Institute for Infectious Diseases 'Lazzaro Spallanzani' (IRCCS), Rome, Italy, elucidated that semen from a patient might be infectious. All semen samples during the 5–19 days post onset of symptoms were positive of DNA virus. The semen specimen on the sixth day inoculated in Vero E6 cells showed growth and replication of monkeypox virus and cytopathy. The patient was PCR confirmed. He had fever, clustered itchy papular lesions in the anal region and single lesion on the head, thorax, legs, arms, hand and penis and was followed for virus shedding. The patient declared he was MSM, was a sex worker and had several condomless sexual intercourse with several male partners during the previous month (Lapa et al. 2022).

Vertical transmission via the placenta from mother to foetus (congenital monkeypox) and foetal deaths have been described (Mbala et al. 2017).

Community transmission involving six to nine successive person to person transmission has been observed in the recent years (WHO 2022).

34.2.2.1 Risk

- Those who had contact in the past 2 weeks with someone with monkeypox, e.g. relatives, friends, health workers, sexual partners
- Laboratory workers testing, handling cultures, animals with orthopox viruses and some designated health workers

Many of the cases in the outbreak in 2022 are gay, bisexual and other men who have sex with men (MSM) had close contact with a person (monkeypox case) regardless of his sex and sexual orientation.

34.2.3 Drivers of Infection

Drivers of infection are presumably contact with live/dead animal during hunting and preparation of bushmeat, animal-human contact due to increased movement of human activities, deforestation, demographic change, climate change and expanding geographic range. Smallpox was eradicated in 1980. The smallpox vaccine cross-protects against monkeypox. The waning smallpox vaccine-induced protection of population and turnover of susceptible population contributed to increasing cases of monkeypox.

34.2.3.1 Endemic Regions: Central Africa and Western Africa

Monkeypox was first reported in a 9-month-old boy admitted to a hospital in the Democratic Republic of the Congo in 1970. It occurs in rainforests in Central Africa and Western Africa. Communities of diverse backgrounds and ages in West Africa are affected. Secondary attack rate among contacts not vaccinated against smallpox is estimated at 10% and case fatality rate ranging between 1 and 11% in the endemic regions, Central and West Africa. Scarring and other sequelae are common (Beer and Rao 2019).

The number of confirmed human cases and also the countries has increased since 2016 compared to the earlier 40 years. Monkeypox cases have been reported in Central African Republic, Democratic Republic of the Congo, Liberia, Nigeria, Republic of the Congo and Sierra Leone and in captive chimpanzees in Cameroon. Eighty confirmed cases appeared in Nigeria (Kara et al. 2018). The number increased during September 2017 and 10 July of 2022 to 800. Majority were males 31–40 years of age. The case fatality ratio was 3%. The geographical pattern reported in the Nigeria outbreak suggests a possible new and widespread zoonotic reservoir requiring further investigation and research (Beer and Rao 2019).

The increasing number of cases in the endemic region is worrisome [Temporary recommendations: International Health regulations (https://www.who.int/news/item/23-07-2022-second-meeting-of-the-international-health-regulations-(2005)-(ihr)-emergency-committee-regarding-the-multi-country-outbreak-of-monkeypox)].

34.2.3.2   World Situation (23 July 2022)

International Health Regulations: Emergency committee—Presentation, deliberation. Proceedings of the meeting 23-07-2022.

The situation of monkeypox cases reported the world over during 1 January to 20 July 2022 was reviewed and deliberated.

There were 14,533 probable and laboratory-confirmed cases including three deaths in Nigeria and two in Central African Republic from 72 countries; 47 countries reported >3040 cases, the highest number from the WHO European region and the region of the Americas. Majority were males and 99% identified themselves as gay and bisexual men (MSM) with multiple partners. Sex parties or saunas, international travel and gatherings linked to sex-onsite activities may explain the global spread amplified through sexual networks.

Nigeria recorded a little over 800 cases, majority in males 31–40 years of age between September 2017 and 10 July 2022 with no evidence of sexual transmission. The case fatality ratio was 3%.

There is no clue as to how monkeypox virus spread outside the endemic region and has invaded the urban setting. It seems the virus has been circulating silently. Cases appeared among healthcare and sex workers. Community exposure, secondary transmission to some children and women and limited transmission to immunosuppressed and pregnant women were recorded. Patients reporting severe pain were hospitalized for pain management and secondary infection. Two cases required ICU and five died. Mathematical models estimate values of R, as >1 among MSM population and <1 in other settings (e.g. Spain 1.8, the UK 1.6 and Portugal 1.4).

The monkeypox virus is a West African clade strain. Some divergence observed in the genome is being studied. There is no evidence of circulation of the virus clade present in Central Africa outside the usual settings. There is no evidence of spill-back from human (anthropozoonotic transmission).

Evidence of anthropozoonotic transmission was published online on 10 August 2022 by Sophie Seang et al. (2022). *Two men who have sex with men—Latino age 44 years and a White of 27 years—lived together as non-exclusive partners and also had co-slept with their male Italian greyhound aged 4 years. They reported to Pitié-Salpêtrière Hospital, Paris, France, on 10 June 2022. Anal ulcer appeared 6 days after sex with other partners. Vesiculopustular rash followed on the face, ears, legs (patient 1) and legs and back (patient 2) associated with asthenia, headache and fever 4 days later. Monkeypox virus was detected in lesions by real-time PCR.*

The dog presented mucocutaneous lesions, abdominal pustules and a thin anal ulceration 12 days later. Samples tested positive for monkeypox virus. DNA sequencing of monkeypox virus from dog and patient 1 had 100% sequence homology. Monkeypox virus caused a real disease in the pet dog.

Both contained hMPXV-1 clade, lineage B.1, that has been reported in non-endemic countries since April 2022 and had infected >1700 in France as on 4 August 2022.

34.2.3.3   Non-endemic Region (29 July 2022)

According to Technical Report: Multi-National Monkeypox Outbreak, United States (2022) and monkeypox response (2022) CDC (https://www.cdc.gov/poxvirus/monkeypox/response/2022/world-map.html), in newly affected countries largely men are affected; most are MSM, i.e. gay, bisexual or who had sex with other men. Infection or cases in women and children are very limited. The number of cases recorded world over upto July 2022 was 22, 121 in 72 countries which did not reported cases historically, majority of cases reported from US (4,906), Spain (4,298), UK (2,546), Germany (2,595), France (1,955), and Brazil (978).

Summary of US case data includes those who tested positive for MPX (monkeypox) or OPX (orthopox) virus: as of 25 July, there were 3487 cases reported in 45 states, District Columbia and Puerto Rico: median age 35 years (range 18–76 years), 99.1% male, 1 transgender, 99% of male patients reported MSM contact. Their ethnicity is as follows: 38% white/non-Hispanic, 26% black and 32% Hispanic.

Epidemiological study in England indicated that MPXV transmission occurred in international sexual networks of gay and bisexual men since April 2022. Sexual health services should target sex on premises venues and geospatial dating to control the outbreak (Vusirikala et al. 2022).

34.3   Symptoms

Incubation period is less than 3 weeks. The outbreak in 2022 in many countries offered studying the time between exposure and onset of symptoms. 95% of individuals developed rash within 17.7 days. The mean IP was 7.6–9.2 days in the UK in the 2022 outbreak.

Monkeypox symptoms may be divided into two distinct periods: (a) invasion and (b) cutaneous eruption. The invasion period (0–5 days) is characterized by febrile symptoms and lymphadenopathy. The cutaneous eruption usually begins within 1–3 days of appearance of fever. Lesions appear on face, palms of hands and soles of feet.

A case of monkeypox reported fever, chill, exhaustion, pain in head, muscles, sore throat, cough, nasal congestion and rashes on the skin which may appear as painful or itchy pimples or blisters. Examination shows swollen lymph nodes. Rashes appear prior to lymphadenopathy, fever, malaise and pain associated with lesions. Rash may be flat and red. These may be popular (raised) and vesicular (small filled with fluid) and pustular (bulged and filled with fluid). The distribution of rashes may be localized, discrete or confluent or generalized. Sites where rashes have been recorded are peri-oral, near genitalia, peri-anal, hands, feet, chest, face and mouth. Rashes look like deep-seated, firm or rubbery papules, vesicles, pustules or scabs, surrounded by well-defined round borders; sometimes lesions show a dent in the middle (umbilicated). A patient may present a few of the symptoms, while most have rash; some show only flu-like symptoms. Rash appears in some before other symptoms. Generally rash appears 1–4 days after flu-like symptoms. Recovery follows. Some patients suffer from secondary bacterial infections. Sequelae include respiratory distress and bronchopneumonia, gastrointestinal involvement and dehydration, encephalitis and ocular infection leaving permanent scar.

A 22-year-old man from Kerala, India, tested monkeypox positive in UAE on 19 July 2022 and returned to India on the 21st. He was hospitalized in Thrissur on 27 July and died on 30 July 2022. He had no health problem. NIV Pune detected monkeypox virus, the variant of which not highly virulent and contagious.

The duration of illness is 2–4 weeks. It is a self-limiting disease.

34.4   Diagnosis

Confounding diseases are smallpox, varicella and several febrile rash illnesses. Therefore, laboratory confirmation is essential. Specimens for laboratory tests are swabs or crusts of lesions, swabs from throat and nasopharyngeal region and anal/rectal swabs from cases reporting anal pain or proctitis.

- Isolation of monkeypox virus, detection of orthopox DNA by PCR
- Detection of IgM antibody during the period of 4–56 days of onset of rash

34.5   Prevention

- Avoid touching rash, scab, genitalia; kiss, hug, huddle; have sex (oral/vaginal, anal), handle or share beddings, towels, etc. Frequent hand washing with soap
- Prophylactic vaccination of the risk group
- Intervention vaccination

Smallpox vaccines provided protection against monkeypox. MVN BN (modified vaccinia Ankara) is a third-generation vaccine, has better safety profile and is administered in 2 doses separated by 28 days. Newer vaccines have been developed, of which one has been approved for prevention of monkeypox (WHO 2022).

Reporting monkeypox is not mandatory through the Integrated Disease Surveillance and Response system across Africa. The Democratic Republic of the Congo has made it mandatory and systematic reporting has increased. Diagnosis, implementation of control measures like strict isolation and contact tracing are challenging.

If one thinks he has monkeypox infection, he should self isolate himself, recover at home and contact health worker; if condition worsens medical advice must be sought to prevent spread. Isolation of cases for 21 days and contact tracing could be effective in controlling the outbreak, though challenging. In most cases reported among males with MSM, there is a fear of stigma on health-seeking behaviour. Detection of case and contact tracing are difficult because of multiple anonymous contacts.

Search and reverse tracing required contacting and sexual health clinic/services. The dynamic sex networks connect some gay and bisexual in cities and countries and may become route of intercity and international spread. Some conscious gay or bisexual consult sexual health services/clinic for fear of HIV. Others may consider HIV or presently monkeypox as stigma and try to suppress. They need attention of outreach health services.

34.6   Treatment

Treatment is symptom-based. There is no approved anti-viral treatment. Antiviral agent developed for the treatment of smallpox has also been licensed for the treatment of monkeypox (WHO 2022). Thornhill et al. (2022) reported that a small number (5%) of patients received cidofovir or tecovirimat. Reports suggested these may be active in animals. These may be used for those severely ill or with weak immune system.

References

Beer EM, Rao VB (2019) A systematic review of the epidemiology of human monkeypox outbreaks and implications for outbreak strategy. PLoS Negl Trop Dis 13(10):e0007791

Bunge EM, Hoet B, Chen L, Lienert F, Weidenthaler H, Baer LR et al (2022) The changing epidemiology of human monkeypox—a potential threat? A systematic review. PLoS Negl Trop Dis 16(2):e0010141. https://doi.org/10.1371/journal.pntd.0010141

Durski KN, McCollum AM, Nakazawa Y, Petersen BW, Reynolds MG et al (2018) Emergence of Monkeypox—West and Central Africa, 1970-2017. MMWR 67(10):306–310

Guarner J, Johnson BJ, Paddock CD, Shieh WJ, Goldsmith CS et al (2004) Monkeypox transmission and pathogenesis in prairie dogs. Emerg Infect Dis 10(3):426–431

Kile JC, Fleischauer AT, Beard B, Kuehnert MJ, Kanwal RS et al (2005) Transmission of monkeypox among persons exposed to infected prairie dogs in Indiana in 2003. Arch Pediatr Adolesc Med 159(11):1022–1025

Lapa D, Carletti F, Mazzotta V, Matusali G, Pinnetti C et al (2022) Monkeypox virus isolation from a semen sample collected in the early phase of infection in a patient with prolonged seminal viral shedding. Lancet Infect Dis 22(9):1267–1269

Mbala PK, Huggins JW, Riu-Rovira T et al (2017) Maternal and fetal outcomes among pregnant women with human monkeypox infection in the Democratic Republic of Congo. J Infect Dis 216:824–828

Morgan CN, Whitehill F, Doty JB, Schulte J, Matheny A et al (2022) Environmental persistence of Monkeypox virus on surfaces in household of person with travel-associated infection, Dallas, Texas, USA, 2021. Emerg Infect Dis 28(10):1982–1989

Seang S, Burrel S, Todesco E, Leducq V, Monsel G, Le Pluart D, Cordevant C, Pourcher V, Palich R (2022) Evidence of human-to-dog transmission of monkeypox virus. Lancet 400(10353):658–659

Technical Report: Multi-National Monkeypox Outbreak, United States (2022). https://www.cdc.gov/poxvirus/monkeypox/clinicians/technical-report.html. Accessed 28 July 2022

Thornhill JP, Barkati S, Walmsley S, Rockstroh J, Antinori A et al (2022) Monkeypox virus infection in humans across 16 countries—April–June 2022. N Engl J Med 387:679–691

Vusirikala A, Charles H, Balasegaram S, Macdonald N, Kumar D et al (2022) Epidemiology of early Monkeypox virus transmission in sexual networks of gay and bisexual men, England, 2022. Emerg Infect Dis 28(10):2082–2086

WHO (2022) Monkeypox, fact-sheet. https://www.who.int/news-room/fact-sheets/detail/monkeypox. Accessed 19 May 2022

Chapter 35
Human Coronaviruses (COVID-19)

Severe pneumonia disease emerged in Wuhan city, China. The World Health Organization (WHO) declared it as the public health emergency of international concern on 30 January 2020 and on 11 March 2020 as pandemic. The emergence and spread of the virus were associated with seafood from Wuhan wet market, Hubei Province, China. The WHO designated COVID-19 as the official name of the disease. 'The International Committee on Taxonomy of Viruses' Coronavirus Study Group proposed the name of the virus *SARS-CoV-2*, referred to as *2019-nCoV*. Travellers spread it from Wuhan to Shanghai and Shenzhen in China and Thailand, South Korea and Japan initially. Globally, the death toll from the COVID-19 on 22 August 2022 reached at 6,471,931 and confirmed cases at 600,901,669 worldwide. In the global scene, the top five countries reporting the total number of cases are USA, India, Brazil, France and Germany (Anonymous 2022). Severe acute respiratory syndrome (SARS-CoV2) caused pandemic often ending fatally particularly in the elderly and people with comorbidities like hypertension, diabetes mellitus, coronary artery disease, etc. It caused panic and associated fear, anxiety, depression, panic attacks and a general decrease in overall wellbeing in the population for over 2 consecutive years (2019–2021).

35.1 SARS-CoV-2

Virus isolated from bronchoalveolar lavage samples of a patient of pneumonia of unknown aetiology was identified by real-time PCR (RT-PCR) assays as *pan-Betacoronavirus*—2B lineage. It was closely related with the bat SARS-like coronavirus strain *Bat Cov RaTG13*, identity 96%. Electron microscopy showed typical crown-like particles. Isolate grown in airway epithelial cells, Vero E6 and Huh-7, produced cytopathic effects 96 h after inoculation and CPE was neutralized with convalescent serum. Intranasally challenged transgenic human ACE2 mice and

© Springer Nature Singapore Pte Ltd. 2024
K. G. Narayan et al., *Handbook of Management of Zoonoses*,
https://doi.org/10.1007/978-981-99-9885-2_35

rhesus monkey suffered from multifocal pneumonia with interstitial hyperplasia and the virus was isolated from these tissues.

SARS-CoV-2 has a novel short putative protein within the ORF3 band, a secreted protein with an alpha helix and beta-sheet with six strands encoded by ORF8. Nucleocapsid protein and single-stranded positive sense RNA surrounded by lipid bilayer and major structural proteins, spike (S), membrane (M), envelope (E) and nucleocapsid (N) constitute the anatomy of the virus. The spike 'S glycoprotein' lies in a trimer on the virion surface, giving the virion a corona or crown-like appearance. It is a large, multifunctional class I viral transmembrane protein, required for the entry of the infectious virion particles into the cell through interaction with various host cellular receptors. The receptor binding motif (RBM) binds directly to the human angiotensin-converting enzyme II (ACE2).

M protein gives definite shape to the viral envelope, binds to the central nucleocapsid and is the central organizer of the virus. E is the smallest of the structural proteins but is important in pathogenesis, assembly and release of virus. N protein has multiple functions including augmenting efficiency of transcription.

The *SARS-CoV-2* genome contains 15 non-structural proteins (nsp) and 8 accessory proteins. These play a vital role in viral replication.

SARS-CoV-2 has five clades/strains—types O, B, B1, A1a and A2a. Type O is the original Wuhan strain, B in England, B1 in part of the USA and Singapore, A1a in Italy and A2a in India. Diversity of the virus increased and then decreased in each country. The ancestral virus was replaced by the viruses that belonged to the evolved type A2a in the most of the affected countries and also globally. In China the virus does not seem to have evolved and the original type O remained dominant, although virus diversity has increased over time. Sequence diversity remained low in Italy, with A2a being dominant. The pattern in the USA was interesting as sequence diversity decreased frequency of ancestral type O diminished remarkably and the A2a type seemed to be replacing the B1 type.

The Delta Plus, or Delta-AY.1 variant, is a mutated version of the B.1.617.2 variant or strain. This strain is characterized by the K417N mutation in the spike protein of the SARS-CoV2 virus that causes the COVID-19 disease. According to reports, the K417N mutation has been associated with 'immune escape', which basically means that the virus is less susceptible to—or less responsive to—any drug therapy. The Delta Plus variant is said to be resisting the monoclonal antibody cocktail—casirivimab and imdevimab—treatment given to high-risk COVID-19 patients in the early stages of this disease. This treatment recently got the nod in India from the drug regulator.

Scientists, however, are not certain if this resistance means that the new variant has a higher transmission rate or that it causes more severe infection compared to the other predominant strains.

It is believed to be 60% more transmissible than the B.1.1.7 variant (or the alpha variant) and may be associated with an increased disease severity such as hospitalization risk.

The WHO has created new system to name COVID-19 variants (Table 35.1), getting away from place-based names.

Table 35.1 New system to name COVID-19 variants

S. no.	Variant	First identified	New name
1	B.1.1.7	UK, September 2020	Alpha
2	B.1.351	South Africa, May 2020	Beta
3	P.1	Brazil, November 2020	Gama
4	B.1.617.2	India, October 2020	Delta
5	B.1.427/B.1.429	USA, March 2020	Epsilon
6	P.2	Brazil, April 2020	Zeta
7	B.1.525	Multiple countries, December 2020	Eta
8	P.3	Philippines, January 2021	Theta
9	B.1.526	USA, November 2020	Iota
10	B.1.617	India, October 2020	Kappa
11	B.1.1.529	South Africa, November 2021	Omicron

On 26 November 2021, the WHO designated the variant B.1.1.529 a variant of concern, named Omicron, on the advice of the WHO's Technical Advisory Group on Virus Evolution (TAG-VE). This variant has a large number of mutations. Preliminary evidence suggests an increased risk of reinfection with this variant, as compared to other variants of corona. The first known confirmed B.1.1.529 infection was from a specimen collected on 9 November 2021. The number of cases of this variant appears to be increasing in almost all provinces in South Africa, indicating its more infectivity. Current SARS-CoV-2 PCR diagnostics continue to detect this variant. Several labs have indicated that for one widely used PCR test, one of the three target genes is not detected (called S gene dropout or S gene target failure), and this test can therefore be used as marker for this variant, pending sequencing confirmation. Using this approach, this variant has been detected at faster rates than previous surges in infection, suggesting that this variant may have a growth advantage.

35.2 Virus-Host Cell Interaction

Exposure results into infection ranging from asymptomatic to fatal acute respiratory disease. Nasal mucosa is the first site of SARS-CoV-2 replication and the viral load reaches maximum at the onset of symptoms. On entry, S glycoprotein of the virus attaches cells (ACE-2 receptors) in the upper respiratory tract, virus releases its nucleic acid, and virus replicates. With the progress of infection, new copies of virus are assembled and invasion of cells proceeds. Immune system of host is triggered; antigen-processing cells present viral peptides to processing cells. T, B and cytotoxic T cells are activated. The S protein plays a significant role. Replication in the lower respiratory tract leads to secondary viraemia, which follows invasion of other organs, heart, kidney and gastrointestinal tract.

35.3   Pathophysiology

The distribution of ACE2 receptors in the body determines pathophysiology. Surface of nasal passages, throat, lung cells, blood vessels and intestines contains ACE2 receptors. Fewer ACE2 receptors in children possibly explain them at low risk.

SARS-CoV-19 exploits the ACE2 receptors on the surface of cells of host's cells to invade. The binding of viral spike S protein with angiotensin-converting enzyme 2 (ACE-2) receptor on the host's cell and endocytosis is facilitated by transmembrane protease serine 2. Nasal mucosal cells, bronchial epithelial cells, type I and type II alveolar pneumocytes and capillary endothelial cells are infected. Inflammatory response begins. Monocytes, macrophages and T cells rush to the site of infection, promoting further inflammation, resulting in alveolar interstitial mononuclear inflammatory infiltrate and oedema. Later (late stage) develop thickened interstitium, hyaline membrane, increased vascular permeability and influx of monocytes and neutrophils as seen in the early phase of acute respiratory distress syndrome. Excessive immune response leads to cytokine flush. SARS-CoV-19 induced increased amounts of IL1B, IFNγ, IP10 and MCP1, probably leading to activated T-helper-1 (Th1) cell responses. Patients requiring ICU admission had higher concentrations of GCSF, IP10, MCP1 and MIP1—indicative of association of cytokine storm with severity (Huang et al. 2020). Studying pathology on 522 patients in Wuhan, Diao et al. (2020) observed dramatic T-cell depletion, and surviving T cells appeared functionally exhausted—possibly cytokine storm prompted this; useful suggestion emerged—'non-ICU patients showing <800 T cells/ul required urgent intervention'.

35.4   Epidemiology

COVID-19 appeared as a travel disease in the beginning and later recognized as spreading to families and congregation in closed environment such as meeting, public transport, entertainment/ceremonies and long-term care units and prisons. Web-based surveillance was used for cross-sectional studies in the initial phase of pandemic. The outbreaks were initially linked to travel-related transmission (as in China, Italy, Iran.) followed by 'close contacts' and 'community spread'. Later studies detected that socioeconomic status, test strategies and reporting systems also affected the spread (Yilmaz and Aygün 2021).

The pandemic is characterized by higher transmissibility (R_0 2–2.5) with low fatality. Compared to the incubation period of 2 days for flu, it is about 10 days (range 3–14). Assuming it takes 6 days for an infected person to become infectious, flu will spread fast—1–2 in 2 days, 2–4 in 4 days, 16–32 in 10 days compared to SARS-CoV-2 as it will take 6 days for 1 case to spread to 2, 12 days from 2–4 and 16–32 in 30 days.

35.4.1   Transmission

Virus is shed for 5–6 days (high viral load during 2–3 days) before the onset of symptoms in a patient, i.e. period of infectiousness. Viral RNA may be recovered months after infection. Patients with mild to moderate disease are not infectious for longer than 10 days after onset of symptoms. Those with severe disease or immuno-suppression are not infectious for longer than 20 days after onset of symptoms (CDC 2019).

The most important means of transmission in human are droplets and aerosols generated in healthcare facilities around patients; fomites spread to the immediate environment of sick people and cause contact transmission. Mete et al. (2021) enlisted important modes of transmission as below:

- Primarily transmitted via respiratory droplets (>5 μm, **not** more than 1–2 m).
- Air-borne/aerosol by droplet nuclei (<5 μm travelling **more than** 1–2 m) may be considered as outbreaks occurred in crowded and poorly ventilated areas such as restaurants and buses. Loud speech, shouting, sneeze/cough and high-powered nebulizer generate aerosol. Viral RNA (not necessarily viable virus) remains suspended for 3–16 h in high-powered nebulizer, ventilation system or air of patients' room.
- Direct, indirect or close contact with infected respiratory secretions or droplets generated by coughing, sneezing, singing or talking to people in a close-range contact by patients.
- Faecal-oral route of transmission, sewage, waste water treatment plant management and waste-water-based epidemiology need to be studied. Blood transfusion and organ transplant and perinatal routes of transmission need to be determined.
- Fomite transmission, indirect contact transmission via contact with a contaminated object/surface and then spreading the virus to the eyes, nose or mouth by touching. Virus viability in fomite depends upon temperature, humidity and types of contact surface. The virus remained viable for 3, 4, 24 and 72 h in aerosols, on copper, cardboard, plastic and stainless steel, respectively; titre reduced over time.

SARS-CoV-2 RNA has been detected in urine, faeces, semen and ocular secretions—important as biological specimens for diagnosis. Viable virus has been reported only in some studies.

In February 2020, a Chinese newborn was diagnosed with the new coronavirus just 30 h after birth. The baby's mother tested positive before she gave birth. It is unclear how the disease was transmitted—in the womb or after birth. In March 2020, another newborn tested positive for the coronavirus in London, marking what appears to be the second such case as the pandemic worsens (International Pulmonologist's Consensus on CoVID-19.pdf).

35.4.2   *Origin and Zoonotic Transmission*

It is suggested that SARS-CoV originated from the reservoir host, bat. It jumped to civets and incorporated changes within the receptor binding domain enabling binding to civet ACE2. Subsequent exposure to human in live market of wild animals promoted further adaptation, leading to the outbreak and pandemic. Direct bat-to-human transmission may also occur. Frequent interspecies transmission from bats to animals and humans may occur because of high plasticity in receptor usage, adaptive mutation and recombination.

Of the six CoVs that infect human, SARS-CoV and MERS-CoV are zoonotic with civet cats and camels, respectively, as non-human hosts. HCoV-OC43 is a more prevalent cause of common cold. Although it is closely related to canine respiratory (CR-CoV) and to bovine coronavirus (BCoV), there is no evidence of cross-infection. COVID started as zoonosis and spread as anthroponosis.

SARS-CoV-2 has 96.2% similarity to a virus detected in bat faeces in a cave in Wuhan. It is suspected that it jumped to human through an animal host not yet identified as had SARS-CoV jumped from bat through palm civet to human.

Non-human primates, cats, ferrets, hamsters, rabbits, bats, puma, gorillas and snow leopard can be infected. The viral RNA has been detected in felids, mink and dogs in the field. Experiments suggested that ferrets, cats, raccoon dogs (*Nyctereutes procyonoides*), white-tailed deer (*Odocoileus virginianus*) and several species of non-human primates can harbour the virus. Infected and sociable ones can transmit infection to human. Transmission from convalescent humans to their pet ferrets was not observed in a study (Mallapaty 2021).

Pet cats and dogs got infected from their respective owners who were clinically ill with COVID-19. Infected cats show symptoms and can spread to other cats. Studies suggest that cats are most susceptible. Lions and tigers in zoo have been found infected. Ferrets have been experimentally infected and showed detectable antibodies.

Minks of two farms suffered from respiratory disease and increased mortality. Post-mortem showed interstitial pneumonia. Organs and swabs proved positive for SARS-CoV-2 by qPCR. Inhalable dust in mink houses was positive for the virus, suggesting exposure to farm workers. One worker from each farm also tested positive, which indicate zoonotic transmission from man to mink (because of pandemic) and back to man. Disease is spreading to more farms like wild fire probably through infectious droplets, on feed or bedding, or in dust containing faecal matter. Oude Munnink et al. (2020) demonstrated that SARS-CoV-2 is a zoonosis, two-way transmission on mink farms in the southeastern Netherlands. Further, outbreaks on 16 mink farms were investigated. Whole-genome sequencing studies included humans living and working on farms. It was revealed that the virus was initially introduced by human and evolved during widespread circulation among minks before detection. Early warning surveillance, enhanced biosecurity and immediate culling of affected minks did not stop transmission. Sixty-eight percent of humans who had contact with minks were found infected. Mink-to-human transmission was evidenced.

35.5   Disease and Symptoms

COVID-19 is a contagious disease commonly affecting people of average age of 46.7 years with female-male ratio 49.2–51.8%. Older age group, those in long-term care facilities and their care giving staff and comorbidity like diabetes and hypertension stand high risk. Healthcare workers linked with deficiencies related with hospital organization, mistakes in the use of personal protective equipment and non-compliance with hand washing and social distance are more likely to get infected.

The mean incubation period is 5–6 days, range from 1 to 14 days. According to Yilmaz and Aygün (2021), the clinical course of SARS-CoV-2 infection can be divided into three stages: the viraemia stage, the acute stage (immune response stage) and the progression or recovery stage. There is effective and sufficient immune response in those with normal immune function to suppress the virus in the first and second stage.

COVID-19 is a multisystem affecting infection. Symptoms vary accordingly and range from non-specific, none to severe pneumonia and death. Typical signs and symptoms observed in Wuhan in reducing order are fever, dry cough, fatigue, sputum production, shortness of breath, sore throat, headache, myalgia or arthralgia, chills, loss of smell (anosmia) and taste (ageusia), vomiting, nasal congestion, diarrhoea, haemoptysis and congestion of conjunctiva. Among the hospitalized patients, fever, cough and dyspnoea were the most common symptoms. Anosmia and ageusia are common before the start of symptoms and are indicators of COVID-19, demonstrate no severe disease and are common among young men and women requiring no hospitalization.

Children were hospitalized in the ICU in several counties for a rare multisystem inflammatory syndrome or paediatric inflammatory multisystem syndrome, manifesting as persistent fever, inflammation and organ dysfunction following exposure to SARS-CoV-2.

In the USA, Kawasaki disease-like syndrome was observed among children. Red eyes and/or rash and multisystem inflammatory syndrome were observed among children of African origin.

Children and those under 19 years did not suffer or had mild disease. Highest risk groups include those over 60 years of age and comorbidity such as hypertension, diabetes, cardiovascular disease, chronic respiratory disease, cancer, chronic kidney disease, obesity and smoking. Old persons suffered from immunosenescence (weakening of immune system) have high risk. Most cases were among males. Advanced age and presence of comorbidity, alone or combined, are marked risk factors for severe disease and mortality.

Disease is classified as mild to moderate, severe and critical. Most (nearly 80%) laboratory confirmed cases showed mild to moderate disease manifesting fever without and with pneumonia. Severe disease characterized by dyspnoea, respiratory frequency ≥ 30/min, blood $O_2 \leq 93\%$, $PaO_2/FiO_2 < 300$ and/or lung infiltrate >50% of the lung filled within 24–48 h was observed in 13.8% cases. Critical cases had respiratory failure, septic shock and/or one or the other organ failure or dysfunction. They constituted 6.1%. Period of recovery for mild cases was 2 weeks, for severe cases 3–6 weeks, and varied with age and comorbidity. Fatigue, dyspnoea, joint pain and chest pain are common persistent symptoms.

Most fatalities are associated with acute respiratory distress (ARD syndrome) and sepsis. Lymphopenia, cytokine flush, increased ferritin and D-dimer have been observed in most fatalities, i.e. indicative of poor prognosis.

Crude fatality ratio (death among laboratory confirmed cases) of COVID-19 is 3.8%, higher among males than in females (4.7% vs. 2.8%) and highest among the elderly (21% in ≥80 years) and those with comorbidity (1.4% no comorbidity vs. 13.2% with cardiovascular; 9.2% diabetes; 8.4% hypertension; 8.0% chronic respiratory disease; 7.6% cancer). CFR has varied in different countries; however, the WHO set it as 2.0%.

35.5.1   Precautions When Pets Get Infected

Pets' sick with the COVID-19 usually have mild illness and may have fever, coughing, difficulty breathing or shortness of breath, lethargy (unusual lack of energy or sluggishness), sneezing, running nose, eye discharge, vomiting and diarrhoea.

If a COVID-19 patient finds his pet has contracted sickness, he should not himself take his sick pet to a veterinary doctor; instead, he should have telecommunication with veterinarian seeking guidance. The 'home isolation protocol with good medical care' for human and pets is the same and should be followed. The owner should protect himself while caring sick pet by following the same precautions recommended for people caring for an infected person at home. The home isolation of pet ends when the pet has not shown symptoms for at least 72 h without medical care; AND it has been at least 14 days since the pet's last positive test; OR all follow-up tests for current infection are negative (CDC, https://www.cdc.gov/healthypets/covid-19/pets.html). Cat tested positive for the virus that causes COVID-19 should be kept inside, not allowed to roam outside. Cats tested positive for the virus that causes COVID-19 should be kept inside and not allowed roaming outside.

35.6   Diagnosis

Clinical test—According to Chaolin Huang et al. (2020), ICU patients showed leucopenia, lymphopenia, high prothrombin time and D-dimer level and increased aspartate aminotransferase. Patients with cardiac injury had increased troponin I (hs-cTnI).

Chest CT images detected bilateral ground-glass opacity with multiple lobular and sub-segmental areas of consolidation.

Virus detection—Isolation of virus from clinical specimen and inoculation on Vero E6 and Huh-7 cell line, cytopathic effects (CPE) are seen 96 hours post inoculation and CPE was neutralized with convalescent serum.

Nucleic Acid Extraction from clinical specimen and Real-time Reverse Transcription–Quantitative Polymerase Chain Reaction targeting the S gene to detect 2019-nCoV.

Electron microscopy showed typical crown-like particles.

Serology—Lateral flow tests, automated chemiluminescence immunoassay systems (CLIA), ELISA and other formats. Antibodies are detectable from the seventh day of the disease. IgM can be detected from the second week and IgG from the third week of infection. Antigen detection is rapid and less costly but less sensitive than molecular tests. Use of monoclonal antibodies improved the sensitivity.

Laboratory animals—Intranasally challenged transgenic human ACE2 mice and rhesus monkey suffered from multifocal pneumonia with interstitial hyperplasia and the virus was isolated from these tissues.

Histopathology—Acute respiratory syndrome is evidenced by desquamation of pneumocytes and hyaline membrane formation, bilateral alveolar damage and fibromyxoid exudates, pulmonary oedema and interstitial mononuclear inflammatory infiltrates, dominated by lymphocytes. No viral inclusions are seen. Inter-alveolar space showed viral cytopathic changes, and multinucleated syncytial cells with atypical large pneumocytes have prominent nuclei and nucleoli and amorphous cytoplasm.

Specimen for diagnosis—Bronchoalveolar lavage, nasopharyngeal, nasal and oropharyngeal swab, sputum (lower respiratory tract specimen—only 20% patients produced), saliva (best specimen; 91.7% of specimens positive), fibrobronchoscopy brush biopsy, faeces, blood, urine.

COVID-19 antibody test is unreliable. A good quality test kit becomes reliable if the rate of infection in population is high. The reliability percent increases with the increase in infection: rate—1% infection (I) vs. 47.2% reliability (R), 5% I vs. 82.3% R; 10% I vs. 90.8% R; 25% I vs. 96.7% R and 50% I vs. 8.8% R.

Requirement for handling COVID-19 specimen: Biosafety level 3 facility.

The National Research Centre on Equines, Hisar (Haryana), under the Indian Council of Agricultural Research (ICAR) has also developed a diagnostic kit for testing COVID in animals. The CAN-CoV-2 ELISA kit is a sensitive and specific nucleocapsid protein-based indirect ELISA kit for antibody detection against SARS-CoV-2 in canines.

35.7 Treatment

Initially symptomatic treatment is advocated. The timeline of cases after onset of symptoms—to first hospital admission 7 (4–8) days; to shortness of breath 8 (5–13) days; to acute respiratory distress 9 (8–14) days; to mechanical ventilation 10 (7–14) days; to ICU admission 10 (8–17) days (Chaolin Huang et al. 2020). ICU-admitted patients required high-flow nasal cannula or higher-level oxygen support measures to correct hypoxaemia. A combination of lopinavir and ritonavir had been useful in the treatment of SARS-CoV and may be combined with interferon beta, convalescent plasma and monoclonal antibodies (MAbs).

Remdesivir, a prodrug of adenosine nucleotide analogue, is an antiviral with a broad spectrum of activity that was tested on SARS and Middle East respiratory syndrome infections. Remdesivir became the first FDA-approved antiviral agent for the treatment of hospitalized patients with COVID-19. Despite the revealed beneficial effect of remdesivir in SARS-CoV-2 in animal and in vitro studies, clinical trials showed conflicting results in which some clinical trials did not show significant effect of remdesivir in the treatment of COVID-19 patients, while others showed promising results in terms of recovery time, oxygen need, mortality rate and clinical improvement (Tahaa et al. 2021).

Patients recovering from SARS showed robust neutralizing antibodies against this CoV infection. Passive immunotherapy using convalescent plasma is another strategy.

The binding of SARS-CoV-2 with ACE2 leads to the exacerbation of pneumonia as a consequence of the imbalance in the renin-angiotensin system (RAS). The virus-induced pulmonary inflammatory responses may be reduced by the administration of ACE inhibitors (ACEI) and angiotensin type-1 receptor (AT1R).

The plasma angiotensin 2 level was found to be markedly elevated in COVID-19 infection and was correlated with viral load and lung injury. Hence, drugs that block angiotensin receptors may have potential for treating COVID-19 infection.

35.8   Control

SARS-CoV-19 is said to have originated in the live-animal markets, Huanan South China Seafood Market—that mimics 'animal-human-ecosystem interface' in nature. This interface offers opportunity of interspecies contact of wildlife with domestic birds, pigs and mammals. This substantially increases the probability of interspecies transmission of CoV infections and could result in high risks to humans due to adaptive genetic recombination in these viruses. One health approach for control seems to be the right option.

Intervention methods included aggressive identification of cases and contacts, isolation and management, social distancing, personal protective measures like wearing personal protective equipment (PPE) and masks and personal hygiene like frequent hand wash with soap and use of sanitizers. Face masks not only protect from infectious aerosols but also prevent the transmission of disease to other susceptible individuals.

A national programme has to be worked out and implemented. A multi-sectoral team is essential to fight the epidemic. Intense disease surveillance is central.

Stopping/controlling the introduction/importing of infection is done through stoppage of incoming transport systems such as flight, railways, land and surface transport systems.

Lockdown and social distancing (plus noncontact greetings, cocooning the elderly and those with comorbidity, restricting gatherings and hand washing) were imposed by affected countries to reduce transmission and control the negative impact but large-scale movement of the people resulted into radiating spread. Period and intensity of restriction need to be weighed considering that COVID-19 is likely to stay long. Two broad policy options are moderate and strict. Sweden followed more or less the first wherein an average person's social interactions were reduced to 40%; if possible, they worked and studied from home but most went to work and school and other interactions were curtailed. Strict policy required 75% reduction of social interaction and closure of offices and schools—somewhat like in Italy. The latter cannot be pursued for long, especially in developing countries. The Imperial College model shows that sustained moderate social distancing can save up to 1.9 million lives in India against 6.0 million if nothing was done in India at an estimated cost of Rs. 96–231 trillion (Bibek Debroy, Chairman PM's Economic Advisory Council, and Bjorn Lomborg, President Copenhagen Consensus I. Times of India, Patna, dated June 23, 2021).

Large-scale screening programmes to identify infected (asymptomatic or active) are tracing and tracking contacts followed by isolation and quarantine; identification of epicentre, hotspots and cluster of cases; and cordoning followed by aggressive action.

Follow-up of infected patients by telephone on day 7 and day 14 prevented any further unintentional spread. At the same time, not all the households meet the needs of isolation of asymptomatic and initial stages of infection. Home environment for protection is inadequate in most developing countries.

Medical staffs are at highest risk, and prompt control of nosocomial transmission is required. Management of COVID-19 cases requires dedicated hospital facilities. Careful collection, transportation and handling of specimens for diagnosis are very important.

Proper disposal of dead bodies is important.

Terminal disinfection of wastes from laboratories and hospitals should be carried out sincerely.

Civil societies, volunteers and non-governmental organizations silently play a significant role in responding to the consequences/fallout of the pandemic—such as loss of livelihoods, hunger, starvation, exploitation, abuses and violence.

Newspaper and social media play an important role in analysing and reporting the implementation of control plan and this enables us to review and amend.

Selection and combination of tools would vary by situation. However, aggressive proactive efforts are required.

Example—Dharavi in Mumbai, India, is an overcrowded locality and densely populated, $227,136/m^2$—eight to ten persons sharing a room of 10×10 feet, community toilet and narrow lanes. Physical distancing of 6 feet and in-house quarantine are impossible. Proactive house-to-house screening using mobile vans and oximeters, opening fever centres, screening of high-risk group like the aged and those with comorbidity enabled separating those requiring quarantine, isolation and treatment and brought down case/incidence rate from 12% in April to 4.3% in May and 1.02% in June. Promptly removing probable cases from the rest of population by sending to institutional quarantine centres made in schools, community halls and dedicated hospitals checked transmission to the rest of the population and reduced mortality. Aggressive testing, tracing, tracking and treatment helped control the epidemic.

Animal reservoirs (free-roaming animals in particular) of SARS-CoV-2 could pose a problem. The virus could evolve in these. Global efforts include survey in animals from home, zoos, shelters, vet clinics, farms and their surroundings, detecting spillover as early as possible and immediately notifying the OIE.

35.9 Prevention

Does infection result into protective antibody and can a person get infected two times? Yes, it may be. During the third wave of the pandemic, those fully vaccinated or previously affected also got infected and few of them were even hospitalized. Since this malady is caused by RNA virus, which frequently mutate, previously acquired immunity either by infection or vaccination may not work. No doubt the severity of disease will be less and only few require hospitalization. Protective antibody most probably lasts for 6 months. However, the following measures need to be applied for prevention:

- Closing live animal markets like Huanan South China Seafood Market.
- Regulating wild animal trade.
- Screening, identification, isolation and characterization of CoVs in wildlife species, particularly in bats—isolating the natural nidus.
- Humans must follow COVID protocol, i.e. hand washing, use of mask and social distancing.

35.10 Vaccines

35.10.1 For Human

The WHO and authorities of different countries approved the use of the following vaccines (Table 35.2) as on emergency basis.

35.10.2 For Animals

Zoetis, the US-based company, has developed a subunit recombinant vaccine and uses a synthetic version of the SARS-CoV-2 spike protein and a proprietary adjuvant. It's administered in two doses, 3 weeks apart, and the magnitude of dose does

Table 35.2 Different types of human vaccines for COVID-19

S. no.	Name	Company	Type	Dose	Storage	Remarks
1.	Covaxine/ BBV₁₅₂	Bharat Biotech, India	Inactivated virus vaccine	0.5 mL i/m, 2 doses—28 days apart	+2 to 8 °C	SARS-CoV2 chemically inactivated by β-propiolactone. Virus cannot replicate but all of its proteins remain intact
2	Novavax (NVX-CoV 2373)	USA	Viral-like particle vaccine	0.5 mL i/m, 2 doses—21 days apart	+2 to 8 °C, 6 months; −20 °C, 2 years	Nanoparticles are coated with synthetic spike proteins. An adjuvant is added to boost immune response
3	Sputnik V (Gam-COVID-Vac)	Gamaleya (Sputnik, Russia)	Viral vector vaccine	0.5 mL, 2 doses—21 days apart	+2 to 8 °C, 6 months; −20 °C, 2 years	dsDNA encoding for the spike protein in adenoviruses. The infected cell expresses the spike protein which leads to an immune response
4	mRNA1273	Moderna, USA	Encapsulated mRNA vaccine	0.5 mL, 2 doses—28 days apart	+2 to 8 °C, 1 month; −20 °C, 6 months	mRNA encoding for spike protein protected in a lipid nanoparticle. Once absorbed, the cell expresses the spike protein resulting in immunity
5	Covishield	Oxford/AstraZeneca/ Serum Institute of India	Viral vector vaccine	Two doses—12 weeks apart	+2 to 8 °C—6 months	dsDNA encoding for the spike protein is protected in a safe virus. The infected cell expresses the spike protein which leads to an immune response
6	BBIBP-CorV	Sinopharm, China	Inactivated virus vaccine	Two doses—28 days apart	+2 to 8 °C	SARS-CoV2 chemically inactivated by β-propiolactone. Virus cannot replicate but all of its proteins remain intact
7	JNJ-78436735/ AD26.COV2.S	Johnson & Johnson, USA	Viral vector vaccine	One dose	+2 to 8 °C—3 months; −20 °C—2 years	dsDNA encoding for the spike protein is protected in a safe virus. The infected cell expresses the spike protein which leads to an immune response
8	CoronaVac	Sinovac, China	Inactivated virus vaccine	Two doses—14 days apart	+2 to 8 °C	SARS-CoV2 chemically inactivated by β-propiolactone. Virus cannot replicate but all of its proteins remain intact

not need to be adjusted depending on the size or weight of the animal receiving a jab. The vaccine is stored at regular fridge temperatures and, once opened, must be used within 24 h.

Another COVID-19 vaccine intended for use in animals (dogs, cats, foxes and mink) was developed in Russia, and there is a further, forthcoming vaccine made by Applied DNA Sciences and Evvivax. The two companies initially intended the vaccine to be used for cats but are now reported to be focused on inoculating mink instead.

The National Research Centre on Equines, Hisar (Haryana), under the Indian Council of Agricultural Research (ICAR) has developed the country's first COVID vaccine—Ancovax—safe for dogs, lions, leopards, mice and rabbits. Ancovax is an inactivated SARS-CoV-2 Delta (COVID-19) vaccine for animals. The immunity induced by Ancovax neutralizes both Delta and Omicron variants of SARS-CoV-2. The vaccine contains inactivated SARS-CoV-2 (Delta) antigen with Alhydrogel as an adjuvant. It is safe for dogs, lions, leopards, mice and rabbits.

References

Anonymous (2022). Animal disease outbreaks and news—Asia, 23 August 2022; vol 185

CDC (2019) Symptom-based strategy to discontinue isolation for persons with COVID-19: decision memo. https://www.cdc.gov/coronavirus/2019-ncov/community/strategy-discontinue-isolation.html

Diao B, Wang C, Tan Y, Chen X, Liu Y et al (2020) Reduction and functional exhaustion of T cells in patients with coronavirus disease 2019 (COVID-19). Front Immunol 11:827

Huang C, Wang Y, Li X, Ren L, Zhao J, Hu Y, Zhang L et al (2020) Clinical features of patients infected with 2019 novel coronavirus in Wuhan, China. Lancet 395(10223):497–506

Mallapaty S (2021) The hunt for Corona virus carriers. Nature 591:26–28

Mete B, Kurt AF, Aygün G (2021) Chapter 2. Transmission of SARS-CoV-2 and prevention strategies. In: Coronavirus disease. Yildiz Dincer © 2021 Nova Science Publishers, Inc.. ISBN: 978-1-53619-296-4

Oude Munnink BB, Sikkema RS, Nieuwenhuijse DF et al (2020) Transmission of SARS-CoV-2 on mink farms between humans and mink and back to humans. Science (New York, NY) 371(6525):172–177

Tahaa HR, Keewana N, Slatia F, Al-Sawalha NA (2021) Remdesivir: a closer look at its effect in COVID-19 pandemic. Pharmacol 106:462–468

Yilmaz SS, Aygün G (2021) Chapter 1. Epidemiology and pathogenesis of COVID-19. In: Coronavirus disease. Yildiz Dincer © 2021 Nova Science Publishers, Inc.. ISBN: 978-1-53619-296-4

Part III
Bacterial and Rickettsial Zoonoses

Epidemiology of 26 bacterial and rickettsial diseases is described.

Bacterial zoonoses have caused pandemic, for example, plague. Most of the bacterial zoonoses appear to have evolved along with agriculture beginning over 1000 years ago. The changes in farming systems to suit mass-marketing conditions are related to re-emergence of certain zoonoses, alteration in pathogens' characters such as virulence and drug resistance causing serious public health problems. Endemic status may progress to epidemic. Intensive dairy goat farming was linked to Q fever epidemic in the Netherlands.

These pathogens also impact productivity and cause consequential economic loss. Farmers' livelihood may be affected due to morbidity, mortality and mass slaughter to control the epizootics. They may get infected and suffer because of close contact, for example, brucellosis, anthrax. Consumers of animal produce are at risk of getting infected with *Salmonella*, *Yersinia* and other enteric pathogens (see also our book *Veterinary Public Health and Epidemiology*). Disease-like leptospirosis seriously affect people engaged in a wide range of activities like rice field workers, fruit harvesters, veterinarians, slaughterhouse, soil diggers, plumbers, electricians, etc. Rickettsiae are transmitted by insects such as hard or soft ticks, fleas, mosquitoes, mites, lice, and fleas. Scrub typhus is an acute febrile to life-threatening multiorgan disease driven by anthropogenic activities like deforestation, unplanned urbanization.

Domestic animals and pets also served as conduit for transfer of pathogens from wild animals to human, for example, TB from badgers to cattle; Lyme disease (*Borrelia*) infected ticks with dogs to pet owners' house.

These infections and diseases are managed by *Veterinary Public Health and Epidemiology*.

Chapter 36
Anaplasmosis

Anaplasmosis or human granulocytic anaplasmosis (HGA) is a disease caused by the bacterium *Anaplasma phagocytophilum* transmitted to persons by bites of tick, primarily the blacklegged ticks (*Ixodes scapularis*) and the western blacklegged tick (*Ixodes pacificus*). It is often confounded with human granulocytic ehrlichiosis (HGE).

36.1 Aetiology

Anaplasma phagocytophilum is an obligate intracellular bacterium of neutrophils, which is Gram-negative. The expression of genes of the invaded cells is altered, extending their life. The average reported annual incidence in the USA was 1.6 cases per million during 2001–2002. It has increased steadily from 348 cases in 2000 to 5762 in 2017. Incidence increases with age, highest in age group 60 and above. CFR is <1%.

36.2 Epidemiology

The geographic range of anaplasmosis appears to be increasing, which is consistent with the expanding range of *I. scapularis*. In the USA anaplasmosis can occur during any month of the year, but most cases are reported beginning with the summer months and a peak is observed in June and July. This coincides with hyperactivity of nymphs of *I. scapularis*. The second, smaller peak occurs in October and November when adult blacklegged ticks are most active.

© Springer Nature Singapore Pte Ltd. 2024
K. G. Narayan et al., *Handbook of Management of Zoonoses*,
https://doi.org/10.1007/978-981-99-9885-2_36

36.2.1 Transmission

The primary tick vectors are *Ixodes ricinus* and *I. persulcatus* in the temperate regions of the USA, Europe and Asia and *I. scapularis* and *I. pacificus* in the eastern and western regions of the USA. *Dermacentor variabilis* is another tick vector. The nymphal and adult stages are mostly involved. Deer, elk and wild rodents are thought to be reservoirs. In the eastern states of the USA, *I. scapularis* is the vector and the white-footed mouse (*Peromyscus leucopus*) the major mammalian reservoir host. In Poland wild boars seem to be the natural reservoir. Experimental studies (de la Fuente and Gortazar 2012) in naturally and experimentally infected boars showed that they are susceptible to *A. phagocytophilum* but may not act as reservoir hosts.

In general, there is a potential risk of transmission through blood transfusion of anaplasmosis and other tick-borne diseases, including human ehrlichiosis, Rocky Mountain spotted fever and babesiosis, caused by *Ehrlichia chaffeensis* or *Ehrlichia ewingii, Rickettsia rickettsii* and *Babesia* spp., respectively. If the recipient of blood develops acute thrombocytopenia accompanied with fever, it should be considered that the donor had asymptomatic anaplasmosis. Blood is generally not tested for it before transfusion. Both *A. phagocytophilum* and *E. chaffeensis* can survive in refrigerated RBCs (CDC 2008). The same tick vector may transmit also other human pathogens; approximately 10% of patients with HGA exhibit serologic evidence of co-infection with Lyme disease, babesiosis or tick-borne meningoencephalitis.

36.3 Symptoms

The incubation period is usually 3 weeks (5–21 days post tick bite). The infection may be symptomless or too mild to seek any medical help. Majority, however, suffer from sudden onset of fever, chills, severe headache and myalgia—all non-specific symptoms confounded with influenza, human monocytic ehrlichiosis (HME), caused by *Ehrlichia chaffeensis* and other tick-borne illnesses such as Lyme disease. The immunocompromised and aged suffer from a severe form of the disease. There are prolonged fever, shock, confusion, seizures, pneumonitis, renal failure, haemorrhage, opportunistic infections and death. Infection is thought to induce long-term immunity but rarely re-infection occurs.

According to Chapman and the tick-borne rickettsial disease (TBRD) working group (Chapman 2006), TBRD continue to cause severe illness and death in adults and children in spite of the availability and low cost of the effective antibiotics. Delay in the early diagnosis when the therapy is most effective is the most challenging. The signs and symptoms are dangerously confounding.

36.4   Diagnosis

- History of exposure to ticks or tick bites and also the symptoms leads to initial diagnosis.
- Haemogram shows low white blood cells and platelets and elevated liver-specific enzymes (transaminases).
- A peripheral blood smear stained with Wright-Giemsa stain demonstrates inclusions compatible with *A. phagocytophilum* morulae in infected neutrophils. Negative finding does not rule out the infection.
- Specific antibodies (indirect IFA, ELISA, immunohistochemical staining) and PCR are confirmatory tests.

36.5   Treatment

It is an easily treatable disease with antibiotics like tetracycline and doxycycline administered for 10–14 days. However, delay in treatment may lead to serious consequence.

Biggs et al (2016) developed guidelines for assisting clinicians and other health-care and public health professionals to (1) identify epidemiological features and clinical manifestations, (2) develop a differential diagnosis which includes and ranks TBRD, (3) understand the recommendations for doxycycline as treatment of choice for adults and children, (4) understand that early empiric antibiotic therapy can prevent severe morbidity and death and (5) report the cases of suspect or confirmed of TBRD to local public health authorities to assist them with control measures and public health education efforts.

References

Biggs HM, Behravesh C, Bradley KK, Dahlgren FS et al (2016) Diagnosis and management of tick borne rickettsial diseases: rocky mountain spotted fever, Ehrlichioses, and Anaplasmosis-United States: a practical guide for physicians and other health-care and public health professionals. MMWR Recomm Rep 65(2):1–44

CDC (2008) *Anaplasma phagocytophilum* transmitted through blood transfusion—Minnesota, 2007. MMWR 57(42):1145–1148

Chapman AS, S in collaboration with the Tick-Borne Rickettsial Diseases Working Group (2006). http://www.cdc.gov/mmwr/preview/mmwrhtml/rr5504a1.htm

de la Fuente J, Gortazar C (2012) Wild boars as hosts of human pathogenic Anaplasma phagocytophilum variants. Emerg Infect Dis 18(12):2094

Chapter 37
Anthrax

Synonyms

Anthrax (anthrax = coal in Greek because of black eschar), also known as Siberian plague/fever, Splenic fever, Malignant oedema, Woolsorters' disease, Cumberland disease, Maladi Charbon, Malignant pustule, Malignant Carbuncle, Milzbrand.

Anthrax is an acute infectious disease of almost all warm-blooded animals and humans caused by a spore-forming bacterium *Bacillus anthracis* that affects the skin, intestine, lymphatics, respiratory tissues, kidneys and meninges, resulting into sudden deaths of animals. Distribution is worldwide. The name anthrax was derived from the Greek word 'anthrakis' which means coal because coal black skin lesions are formed in the cutaneous form of anthrax (Goel 2015).

37.1 Aetiology

Bacillus anthracis is a rod-shaped, encapsulated, Gram-positive aerobic bacterium, growing in chains. It is a member of *Bacillus cereus* sensu lato consisting of nine species of Gram-positive, endospore-forming bacteria including *B. cereus* and *B. thuringiensis,* family *Bacillaceae* (Carroll et al. 2017). The infectious endospores are resistant to heat (<135 °C 5–10 min dry heat; <100–105 °C 4–5 min moist heat), cold (4–5 cycles of freeze-thaw), drought (years in soil in sun and light and in dried blood), UV and gamma radiations. Endospores are more resistant than other pathogens to commonly used disinfectants (e.g. liquor cresolis, carbolic acid, mercuric chloride, formaldehyde) at the respective recommended concentrations, and therefore, it is advisable to allow a contact time of 24 h. Being a relatively new species, having diverged only very recently from *B. cereus*, *B. anthracis* has little genetic variation and is genetically and phenotypically extremely homogeneous (Okutani et al. 2019). Virulent *B. anthracis* isolates have two plasmids: pX01, which codes

© Springer Nature Singapore Pte Ltd. 2024   379
K. G. Narayan et al., *Handbook of Management of Zoonoses*,
https://doi.org/10.1007/978-981-99-9885-2_37

for a tripartite protein exotoxin complex, and pX02, which encodes the antiphago-cytic polyglutamic capsule genes. Additionally, a few *B. cereus* isolates that have plasmids closely related to pX01 have caused anthrax-like diseases. Isolates of *B. cereus* biovar *anthracis* carry both pX01 and pX02 like plasmids and may be virulent like *B. anthracis* (Baldwin 2020; www.cfsph.iastate.edu).

37.2 Virulence Factors

It is believed that endospores (a) start germinating after entering the human or ani-mal body in situ or (b) are phagocytosed and transported to the lymphatics and regional lymph glands where they germinate or both (a and b). Poly-D-glutamic acid (gamma-DGA) capsule protects the bacterium from phagocytosis.

The bicarbonate-responsive transcriptional regulator AtxA controls the expres-sion of pX01 and pX02.

The toxin PA binds to the cellular receptor to translocate toxins, EF and ET into cells. The signalling pathways in the host cells is so altered as to interfere with the innate immune response in the early part of infection and vascular collapse later (Moayeri et al. 2015).

B. anthracis toxin consists of two components, A and B. A component consists of two LF and EF. B component is binding and translocating the protective antigen (PA) which self-assembles at the cell surface to form two 'classic' binary toxins, LT (LF + PA) and oedema toxin ET (EF + PA). Neither LF nor ET alone (without PA) is toxic. The LF is a Zn-metalloprotease which interferes with signalling pathways, finally damaging the cells. EF is a calmodulin-dependent adenylate cyclase that increases intracellular cAMP level and helps *B. anthracis* to spread in the host, evading the immune system. PA or protective antigen (used for making vaccine) is the central component responsible for binding and delivery of ET and LT into the cytosol (Liu and Nestorovich 2021). Interestingly PA is considered to be a channel that can be used to transport anthrax toxin molecules to tumours for therapeutic use.

The master virulence regulator AtxA of *B. anthracis* regulates the expression of three toxins and genes for capsule formation required for pathogenicity. AtxA appears to function as a global regulator because it affects a large number of genes on the chromosome and plasmids. Furuta et al. (2021) detected eight direct regulons of AtxA, five protein-coding gene including 2/3 toxin genes and three genes encod-ing small RNAs XrrA, XrrB and XrrC. These three genes, XrrA, XrrB and XrrC controlled the cell physiology. These appear to be the first layer of the gene regula-tory network for the pathogenicity of *B. anthracis*.

HitRS and HssRS are two component systems (TCS) in *B. anthracis* to sense host-induced stresses and respond to alterations in the environment. The cross-regulating TCS, HitRS responds to cell envelope disruption and HssRS to high level of *heme*. Studies revealed the protein homeostasis regulators, DnaJ and ClpX, main-tained *B. anthracis* signal transduction activities through TCS regulation (Laut et al. 2022). PA is responsible for stabilization.

B. anthracis succeeds in evading natural defence, invades macrophages, multiplies and bursts macrophages to release a large number of bacilli and concomitantly toxins. LF caused macrophages to form 'TNF-alpha' and 'interleukin 1 beta (IL1B)'—both are cytokines regulating inflammation and apoptosis (programmed cell death)—over production of which leads to septic shock and death. The endothelial cells are also targeted by the bacilli, resulting into vascular leakage and ultimately hypovolemic shock (low blood volume) and septic shock. Observed sudden death in animals is thus explained. Sweeney et al. (2010) studied the effects of ET and LT (read as EF and LF) toxins in a dog model. Both reduced vascular resistance and were associated with renal and hepatic dysfunction. LT might also cause depressed myocardial function in addition to causing progressive hypotension while ET caused rapid hypotension.

37.3 Epidemiology

Anthrax is common in parts of Africa, Asia, the Middle East and South and Central America where control measures in animals are inadequate. It has been infrequently reported from parts of Europe, North America and Canada. In the tropical forests of sub-Saharan Africa *B. cereus* var. *anthracis* seems to be widespread. *B. cereus* with pX01-like plasmids has been reported from human cases from Florida, Texas and Louisiana and anthrax-like cutaneous lesions in India.

The estimated annual number of human cases worldwide range from 2000 to 20,000. Forgotten in western countries, anthrax is still endemic in some parts of the world such as the Middle East, Central Asia and African countries (Doganay et al. 2010). The disease is most prevalent in those countries of tropical or subtropical latitudes where pastoral agriculture is prevalent and veterinary infrastructure is poor.

Carlson et al. (2019) estimated 1.83 billion people live in the regions of anthrax risk but with little occupational exposure risk; precisely a global total of 63.8 million poor livestock keepers and 1.1 billion livestock live within such regions. The rural rainfed systems throughout arid and temperate land across Eurasia, Africa and North America present risk to both human and livestock.

The disease is one of the oldest and deadliest diseases known to impact both economy and human health. Anthrax cases are increasingly reported; partly it is real because of the recurrent outbreaks and partly because of better and multi-disease tracking agencies, e.g. the FAO Global Animal Disease Information System (EMPRES-i), the Program for Monitoring Emerging Diseases (ProMED-mail), the Center for Infectious Disease Research and Policy (CIDRAP) and others. Recurrent outbreaks are attributed to (a) poor-quality vaccine, (b) bioterrorism and (c) penicillin-resistant virulent strain in medical practice.

It causes significant losses in domestic and wild animals and consequential human health problems worldwide. It is underreported in countries with poor/inadequate veterinary services. Endemic areas are sub-Saharan Africa, Latin America, Eastern Europe, Russia and Asia. Sporadic cases occur in southern European countries, regions of North America and Australia. Soil in certain specific areas of some countries allows for survival of spores of *B. anthracis* and hence recurrent of outbreaks is predictable.

Poor countries have weak veterinary services and public health services. Sustenance of vaccination and implementation of control programmes is difficult. Other contributory factors may be political unrest, civil unrest and natural disaster. Poverty may compel slaughter of moribund cattle and selling meat—a process that exposes human to zoonotic anthrax, as seen in some African and Asian countries.

37.3.1 Source of Infection and Transmission

Anthrax is a soil-borne infection. Spores of *B. anthracis* can survive for many years in soil.

That the spores are characterized by a high floating capacity suggest that water plays an important role in the ecology and distribution through flowing water (rain water) away and to concentrate in the low areas. Heavy rains and flood followed by hot and dry environmental conditions bring the spores on the surface. Livestock ingest the spores and get infected while grazing on contaminated pastures or eating contaminated feed.

Nature favours replicative cycle. Better opportunity is offered by wild and domestic ruminants' bodies where the development of pathogenicity overcomes body's defence and rapid and intense multiplication by the vegetative cells leads to the death of the host quickly. Dark non-clotting blood oozing from the natural body openings—nose, mouth and anus—of anthrax-dead animals is considered diagnostic and a warning. These contaminate soil. Opening the carcass contaminates soil heavily as the bacillus forms spores as soon as it comes in contact with air/oxygen. When anthrax carcass is not opened, the bacterium dies in the body of the carcass.

Use of contaminated bone meal as fertilizer may add spores. Certain environmental conditions favour long survival, resulting into 'defined anthrax areas' where spore concentration per unit of soil is high. Soil rich in organic matter and humid warm conditions are favourable for spore germination and multiplication of bacilli. Outbreaks are more common in areas where soil is rich in alkaline, calcium and other minerals, e.g. endemic anthrax in Zimbabwe, usually in the Gonarezhou. In the driest months of September and October, ruminants ingest the spores while browsing the remnants of vegetation and are infected. The spores naturally occur in soil of Canadian prairies and affect cattle, sheep, goats, horses and bison and generally surface during hot and dry summer months when heavy rains and flood precede.

Pigs get infection after eating flesh, bone meal and meat meal concentrates made from carcasses contaminated with anthrax spores. Insects like blow flies and scavenging wild carnivores and vultures devouring anthrax carcass can spread the spores of *B. anthracis* from the body fluids/discharges and contaminated meat, respectively. Contaminated vegetation eaten by browsing animals (non-carnivores) may lead to infection. Contaminated shoes and clothing also spread spores. Contaminated animal products like infected wool, hairs, hide, leather, etc. spread it to users distantly located. With modernization such items are replaced with safer ones. At the same time, newer sources of human infection are emerging. Human-to-human transmission has not been reported (Cross et al. 2019).

Fasanella et al. (2013) brought evidence of suspected vector transmission. The DNA from the scab of cutaneous anthrax and dead sheep matched. The patient and owner of the outbreak affected flock in Basilicata, Italy, reported that he had no contact with infected or dead sheep but was stung by gadflies.

37.3.2 Species Affected

The susceptibility to *B. anthracis* differs with species of animals. Domesticated and wild herbivores are susceptible and often rapidly die. Anthrax in unvaccinated ruminants can be a serious economic problem in endemic regions. The carnivores and omnivores are less susceptible, develop clinical disease and may even recover from illness.

Domestic animals—such as cattle, sheep, goats, horses, donkeys, pigs and dogs—as well as wild ruminants, such as antelopes, gazelles and impalas, elephants and hippopotami (in some parts of Africa) and wild carnivores, such as lions, hyenas and jackals, are susceptible. Birds seem to be resistant.

According to Spickler (2017), *B. cereus* biovar *anthracis* has been reported in nonhuman primates, chimpanzees (*Pan troglodytes*), duikers (*Cephalophus* spp.), mongooses (family *Herpestidae*) and porcupines (family *Hystricidae*).

Anthrax endemicity in wildlife has been reported in Africa and North America. Epizootics in wildlife cause concern; ungulates die in large number.

Anthrax is known to occur in an enzootic form in many national parks and wildlife reserves.

Some ecologists consider that anthrax enzootic is a part of the natural ecological system to keep a 'check on population of herbivores'. However, the infection may spill over to livestock and human beings. Control of anthrax in wildlife is challenging as vaccination of free-living wild animals is very difficult.

37.3.3 Outbreaks

In developed nations, human anthrax has all but disappeared (Thappa and Karthikeyan 2001). However, recent reports (OIE 2016; Sidwa et al. 2020) suggest otherwise.

37.3.3.1 Russia (https://outbreaknewstoday.com/ anthrax-kills-2349-reindeer-in-siberia-oie-data-34491/)

Six clusters of anthrax outbreaks were reported in July 2016 in reindeer in the Yamalo-Nenets Autonomous Okrug of the Russian Federation where no anthrax outbreaks had occurred since 1941. Grazing reindeer herds is a livelihood for a pastoralist population there. There were approximately 111,000 susceptible animals. A total of 2657 cases were reported (2.39%), with a fatality of 88.67%. Human cases, including hospitalized and fatal, were reported among those who had contacts with the animals. The cases included gastrointestinal anthrax in those who consumed meat or blood from the reindeer.

37.3.3.2   Texas, USA (Sidwa et al. 2020)

As compared to 63 culture-positive cases in 18 years (2000–2018), 25 culture-positive animals and a human case were recorded in 1 year (up to August 2019). These were cattle, horses, white-tailed deer, antelope and a goat. Unconfirmed numbers reported to DSHS staff suggest that >1000 animal losses might be attributed to the 2019 outbreak. The human case had removed a deer carcass from his porch and was bitten by a fly.

37.3.3.3   Bangladesh (Ahmed et al. 2010)

Anthrax is endemic in Bangladesh, commonly reported from Pabna, Sirajganj and Tangail areas where cattle population is dense. Twenty seven human cases were reported during 1980–1984. In 1997, 19 cases were detected from 624 tannery workers examined in Dhaka City. Outbreaks were reported during 2009–2010. There were 55 cases in animals and 99 human cases during Oct 2009–June 2010. During August–October 2010, there were 140 cases in animals and 607 human cases. All human cases were cutaneous anthrax.

Outbreaks occur every year in African countries. Eastern Europe and Central Asia report animal and human anthrax. Most human cases in Central Asia during May to November, with a peak during July to August, believed to be related with animal movement for grazing.

New outbreaks suggest a re-emergence potentially linked with climate change. There are multiple new or continuing anthrax outbreaks in endemic countries worldwide. These warrant more attention for heightened awareness and effective control measures to prevent anthrax infection in animals and limit its transmission to humans.

37.4   Symptoms

37.4.1   Animals

The incubation period of animal anthrax may be as short as 1 day or as long as 14 days. Characteristically animals in good conditions die suddenly without manifesting any signs. Overt signs of acute anthrax in cattle, sheep and wild herbivores are fever, depression, difficulty in breathing and convulsions followed by death if not treated in 2–3 days. Death may occur 2–30 days, most frequently 8 days, after exposure. Few animals suffer from mild form showing general malaise. Pigs, dogs, cats and wild carnivores have swelling in throat that causes breathing problem. Anthrax is rare in dogs and cats.

37.4.2 Human

The following classification approximately defines 'persons at risk':

1. Agricultural anthrax—contact with sick or dying animal, such as ranchers, vets, butchers and slaughterhouse workers while handling sick animals and skinning, shearing, butchering and handling dead animal bodies in 'carcass utilization centres' or 'rendering plants' and also lab workers while handling specimen in lab (occupational anthrax).
2. Industrial anthrax—spores are generated during cleaning and industrial processing—rocessors of hides, leathers, tanners, hairs, wool, bone, tusk and meat—handlers in 'industries' (occupational anthrax). The agent possibly does not withstand dyeing of yarn as most infections occur prior to making yarn and weaving.
3. Outside the above two—contact with products from anthrax-infected animals, e.g. anthrax-contaminated bristle shaving brushes, animal skins, animal hair or yarn (users' anthrax).
4. Injection anthrax (drug addicts' anthrax).
5. Bioterrorism-related anthrax (target groups, mainly army).

Transmission from animal to human and human to human is not so easy. Outbreak of animal anthrax does not necessarily mean that human infection will occur. Transmission occurs if proper precautions while handling affected animals and carcasses are not taken. Abraded/cut skin provides entry of the bacillus.

In endemic areas, it is occupationally acquired. Occupationally exposed ones are advised vaccination, though mass vaccination is not recommended.

Further sub-classification of human anthrax is largely based on the portal of entry of the anthrax bacilli and tissues affected.

The three forms are cutaneous, pulmonary and gastrointestinal forms, depending upon the routes of entry (percutaneous, inhalation, ingestion) of spores of *B. anthracis.* Spores are reactivated, and the vegetative form rapidly multiplies. Pulmonary form is the most dangerous and fatal. Gastrointestinal form is less so but may be fatal. Cutaneous form is the most common, accounting for >90% of all natural infections. Generally, it is non-fatal.

Infective dose may range between 2500 and 760,000 endospores (Wright et al. 2010). Incubation periods vary depending upon the route of entry of the bacilli. According to Oregon Public Health Department April 2013 report, IP for the cutaneous, gastrointestinal and inhalational forms are 1–12, 1–7 and 2–60 days, respectively.

In Romania, all exposed in an outbreak associated with slaughter, handling and eating of undercooked meat from a cow had to be observed for a period of 30 days from the date of exposure (Popescu et al. 2011). Illness begins with rise in body temperature, 100 °F and above, accompanied with chills, cough, shortness of breath, muscle ache, headache, anorexia, nausea, vomiting, abdominal discomfort and diarrhoea. The disease occurs primarily in three forms: cutaneous, respiratory and gastrointestinal.

37.4.2.1   Cutaneous Form (*Pustula maligna*)

A sore resembling one that appears following an insect bite progresses into a vesicle in 1–2 days that might be pruritic, red, indurated and raised erythematous lesion with small ulcers oozing serosanguineous fluid, surrounded by a blanched halo. It develops into a painless ulcer of 1–3 cm diameter, the centre of which is black and necrotic (eschar/carbon).

Cutaneous anthrax can be self-limiting; the lesions resolve without any complications or scarring in 80–90% of cases with treatment. It accounts for 95% of human cases globally, and <1% cases are fatal, if not treated properly (Dixon et al. 1999). The draining lymph nodes in the adjacent area of cutaneous lesion are inflamed. The cutaneous forms can disseminate, become systemic and prove fatal if not treated in about 20% cases. It is estimated that there are approximately 2000 cases annually worldwide (Sweeney et al. 2011).

37.4.2.2   Inhalation/Pulmonary Form

In the pulmonary form such as 'woolsorters' disease' or 'ragpickers' disease', endospores (a) may be taken up by nasal-associated lymphoid tissues in <24 h and spread to the mandibular lymph nodes or, (b) when in particles ≤5 μm, reach the alveoli, engulfed by macrophages and transported to the mediastinal and peribronchial lymph glands. These may remain dormant there for weeks or months. The incubation period is thus variable. Endospores germinate and multiply in the lymph nodes and release toxins, causing haemorrhagic mediastinitis and necrosis. Although initial symptoms are confounded with upper respiratory tract infection, severe dyspnoea develop in 2–3 days. The disease may progress to worsening dyspnoea, shock, cyanosis and death. X-rays show the characteristic widened mediastinum. Spores may germinate also in the pulmonary epithelia and proliferate in systemic fulminant forms, usually ending fatally. Meningitis may be another complication. The fatality is high, may be 75%, even after possible care is taken.

B. anthracis dispersed in particle size <5 μm pose risk over large areas.

Bush et al. (2001) reported a fatal case of inhalation anthrax, the index case in the US Bioterrorism. The prodromal symptoms included fever, myalgia and malaise that continue for several days. Fulminant course followed; seizures and respiratory failure without clinical and at autopsy pneumonia were observed. Chest radiography suggested haemorrhagic mediastinitis, confirmed at autopsy, possibly resulted in respiratory failure. Death occurred in 6 days at onset of symptoms. Earlier in a biological weapon facility of Russia, an accidental release of endospores caused human anthrax as far as 4 km from the site and in animals as far as 50 km. This index case probably got infected while handling a suspicious letter containing powder on 19 September, 8 days before the onset of symptoms. In the Russian outbreak the incubation period was 10 days. Examination of haemorrhagic spinal fluid showed Gram-positive bacilli.

37.4.2.3   Gastrointestinal

It may be subclinical or clinical.

After per os infection, the disease may present in two forms: (a) oropharyngeal form—cervical lymphadenitis, oedema, swelling, pharyngitis, sore throat, fever and dysphagia—and (b) gastrointestinal form. The primary site of infection is the epithelia of the stomach and intestine and intestinal Peyer's patches in mice. Clinical form manifests into vomiting, fever, anorexia and abdominal pain. Severe forms show haematemesis and bloody diarrhoea, progressing to septicaemia, toxaemia, shock and death. The intestine and mesentery show extensive oedema. Fatality rate may be 20–65%.

Lay Mayo et al. (2010) reported an investigation of gastrointestinal anthrax in New Hampshire.

A 24-year-old woman from New Hampshire was diagnosed with gastrointestinal anthrax. The clinical findings strongly suggested and *B. anthracis* was isolated. She had participated in a drumming event a day before in a building where drums of multiple ages and origins were played.

Drums were set up, vegetarian meal prepared and participants ate the dinner in the main drumming room. The lady was in good health and participated in the drumming event. The next day, 05 December 2009, she was down with influenza-like symptoms, which continued for the following several days with increasing pain in the head, neck and back. On 12 Dec, she complained worsening, vomiting, abdominal cramp and dizziness. She was admitted to an emergency department of a hospital on 14 Dec. Abdominal computed tomography showed massive ascites, oedema of small bowel and multiple retroperitoneal lymph nodes. On 24 December she was diagnosed as a case of gastrointestinal anthrax.

The investigation included 84 potentially exposed persons. Three environmental sites, two from drumheads and one composite sample of three electrical outlets in the main drumming room were positive for *B. anthracis*. Additionally, two samples from one drum and four from environmental locations in the building were also positive. These suggested aerosolization of anthrax spores from drumheads. All isolates were identical based on multiple-locus variable-number tandem repeat analysis using eight loci (MLVA-8). Animal-hide drums should be considered as potential source of anthrax spores.

37.4.2.4 Meningitis

Meningitis may occur in any of the three forms: cutaneous, gastrointestinal and pulmonary when septicaemia (10^7–10^8/mL) occurs and haematogenous spread takes place. Commonly about 5% of cutaneous form cases get this complication. There are increased vascular permeability and disseminated intravascular coagulation. The patient feels restless, headache and pain in lower back and legs. CSF contains pus and/or blood. The course is rapid, ending fatally.

37.4.2.5 Injection Anthrax

The term 'injection anthrax' has been proposed by Ringertz et al. (2000), when the first case of heroin-related anthrax was described. 'Injection anthrax' occurs when a contaminated drug is introduced through subcutaneous, intramuscular or intravenous route. The case fatality rate is 34%–47% among its infected patients despite antibiotic treatment (Tan et al. 2019). It is difficult to diagnose when the symptoms differ from the classical cutaneous anthrax and a case is inadequately treated. According to Grunow et al. (2013), there were three outbreaks with 69 laboratory confirmed cases in Europe between 2000 and 31/12/2012; the fatality rate was >30% despite therapeutic intervention. Massive oedema or necrotizing fasciitis, and NOT the papule or vesicle with central eschar, occurs. Septic and cardiovascular shock, meningitis and death, absent in the classical cutaneous form, occur despite antibiotic therapy. The 'injecting drug users (IDU)' show non-specific soft tissue infections at the site of injection. They take anthrax-contaminated heroin through injection.

Injection anthrax was identified in 2000 in Norway in a drug user. A molecular study of the first isolate and the isolates from cases in 2009–2010 and 2012 in the UK, Germany, France and Denmark failed to detect any difference, suggesting a single source contamination of heroin (Grunow et al. 2013).

Genotyping of strains of 2009–2010 outbreaks revealed that these were related to a single *B. anthracis* strain type that belonged to Trans-European *B. anthracis* group Ba4599. Strains associated with the European drug use originated in Turkey (Hanczaruk 2014). Molecular epidemiological studies (whole genome sequence) on 60 *B. anthracis* isolates associated with injection anthrax cases in an outbreak and a closely related reference strain were made by Keim et al. (2015). Two clusters were identified: one associated with the 2009–2010 outbreak located primarily in Scotland and the other with the 2012–2013 outbreak cases and a single case in Norway. Most likely, separate events of contamination originated from the same geographic region and possibly the same site of drug manufacturing or processing.

37.4.2.6 Bioterrorism-Related Anthrax

The fact that anthrax affected livestock and draft animals prompted Germany to use it during World War I and II. Defence research continued in some countries for its use as a weapon. A leakage from a lab in Russia caused 64 deaths of 96 affected.

In 2001 spores mixed with powder were delivered in envelopes through mails result-ing into 22 cases in the eastern USA—11 each of cutaneous and inhalation anthrax. Five of the inhalation cases died. Twenty cases occurred among mail handlers in the place where these were received and processed—possible modes of infection were inhalation and contact. In the remaining two, cross-contamination might have led to infection (Wright et al. 2010).

Both the 'attacker' and the target population' may be benefitted with the out-come of research in this area. For example, if 50 kg of anthrax spores were dis-persed aerially over 5.0 million persons, 95,000 are likely to die and 125,000 need hospitalization. The 'attacked country' needs to prepare for the 'dead' and 'victims'—the quantum and areas are defined. The army needs protection. Preparation includes procurement, stocking, availability of protective drugs and vaccine and administration on time. The Department of Home Security intro-duced in 2003 'BioWatch and Public Health Surveillance Evaluating Systems for the Early Detection of Biological Threats for quick detection of specific biologi-cal agents that could be released in aerosolized form during a biological attack'. A signal is generated if a sample is positive. A review suggested to 'establish better testing and collaboration with public health system' to improve its effectiveness.

What to do if suspicious parcel/envelope is received? Every country has devel-oped some guidelines. In general, suspicion arises if the sender is unknown, spelling incorrect, senders' address absent, letter is 'personal'/confidential' and the envelope has unusual weight/shape, powdery substance and strange odour. Things to do: do not handle/damage, isolate, put into a plastic pouch, seal and hand over to the authority. All who have touched it should wash and take a shower with soap and water. The surface should be disinfected (WHO Global Alert Response). Killing of spores and thus decontamination of mail may be attained if domestic electrical iron set at 204 °C is applied for 5 min.

37.5   Diagnosis

Sudden deaths and bleeding from natural openings—nose, mouth and anus—raise strong suspicion. The blood sample is collected in a sealed container for laboratory diagnosis. Other specimens useful for examination are hides, skin, wool, soil, etc.

Safety requirement for diagnostic laboratory is Biohazard level 3.

Chains of encapsulated bacilli are seen in characteristic McFadyean's reaction. The sample is cultured for bacilli.

Bacteriological culture is the gold standard. In the case of contaminated speci-mens, PLET (polymyxin-lysozyme-EDTA-thallous acetate) may be added to the medium to make it selective. *B. anthracis* grows well on 5% sheep blood agar at 35 °C or ambient room temperature. Colonies are flat, irregular with swirling pro-jections, referred to as 'medusa head', and non-haemolytic. It is lecithinase positive on egg yolk agar. Confirmation is made by observing sensitivity to gamma bacteriophage. A smear from 6-h-grown colonies on defibrinated sheep blood agar shows chains of encapsulated bacilli.

Immunohistochemical staining demonstrates *B. anthracis* antigens in tissues using both *B. anthracis* cell wall and capsule monoclonal antibodies.

Serological tests applied are indirect haemagglutination, precipitin (ASCOLI's—on slaughtered/autopsied) and enzyme-linked immunosorbent assay to detect antibodies. A fourfold rise in serum antibodies to PA between acute and convalescent sera specimens using the Centers for Disease Control and Prevention (CDC) quantitative anti-PA IgG ELISA testing is diagnostic.

Animal inoculation test—mice is inoculated with suspected bacterial suspension in saline isotonic solution of opalescent corresponding to McFarland standard 0.5 in volume 0.2–0.3 mL subcutaneously. Gram-positive encapsulated bacilli in chains are observed in the impression smear from the liver, spleen and heart.

Genomic—PCR (directed against the virulence plasmid marker) is a rapid and most dependable method.

Multiple-locus variable-number tandem repeat analysis using eight loci (MLVA-8).

37.6 Treatment

Ciprofloxacin, doxycycline and penicillin—oral or intravenous—and antimicrobial PEP (post-exposure prophylaxis) for 7–14 days may be considered in cases of gastrointestinal exposure from eating undercooked carcass of anthrax-infected animal.

Raxibacumab is a human IgG1 monoclonal antibody against the *B. anthracis* protective antigen for use in the prevention and treatment of inhalation anthrax.

The US FDA has approved its use for treatment in injection form in combination with appropriate antibacterial drugs for treatment. It can be used prophylactically when alternative therapy is unavailable.

Review of guidelines for anthrax post-exposure prophylaxis and treatment and update was done by a panel of experts of CDC (Hendricks et al. 2014). Salient recommendations are (1) a 60-day antimicrobial therapy, particularly for those exposed to aerosolized endospores for two reasons: (a) acquired immune response might be blunted because of antimicrobial therapy and (b) endospores lying dormant for long in the lungs, (2) manage shock and (3) antitoxins (raxibacumab or anthrax immunoglobulin intravenous) may be combined with antimicrobial drugs in cases of systemic anthrax.

37.7 Prevention

37.7.1 Vaccines

Anthrax was the first disease for which the principle of a bacterial vaccination was found to be effective. The Sterne strain, isolated in 1937 (Sterne 1937), is toxinogenic and non-capsulated. A live vaccine is still used and provides satisfactory protection. The worldwide use of this vaccine has played its role in controlling the incidence of anthrax in livestock and wild animals. Because of its residual virulence, the live vaccine is not considered suitable for human use (Mock and Fouet 2001).

1. Anthrax Vaccine Adsorbed (AVA)/MDPH-PA/MDPH-AVA; trade name *BioThrax*
   V770-NP1-R *B. anthracis* Vollum strain, a non-encapsulated mutant, is used. The vaccine is an inactivated cell-free product that contains mainly protective antigen, small amounts of oedema and lethal factors. It is also available as a post-exposure prophylaxis (PEP) under an Emergency Use Authorization. The *Advisory Committee on Immunization Practices* (ACIP) updated the following recommendations (Wright et al. 2010): (a) the pre-event and pre-exposure series reduced from 6 to 5 doses (omit vaccination 2 weeks), administered intramuscular (not s/c), (b) may be administered to aerosol-exposed pregnant women under post-exposure prophylaxis and (c) 60 days antimicrobial prophylaxis in conjunction with three doses of AVA for optimal protection of previously unvaccinated persons after exposure to aerosolized spores.
2. Anthrax Vaccine Precipitated (AVP)—A British anthrax vaccine—three doses for 3 weeks apart with a booster after 6 months, to repeat once a year. The Sterne strain is used.
3. Russian Anthrax Vaccine—A live attenuated, non-encapsulated spore vaccine widely used for humans; aerosol/scarification/subcutaneously administered; used in Russia and China.

The Sterne (veterinary) vaccine—34F2 strain—protects for 9 months. Livestock are vaccinated every year and they should not be receiving any antibiotics.

37.7.2 Surveillance, Control and Prevention

Soil samples are useful in surveillance. *B. anthracis*-positive soil samples delineate the risk area. Targeted intervention measures follow (Fasanella et al. 2011).

Surveillance marks the 'areas where anthrax cases are most likely to occur'. Veterinary services (VS) should ensure 'effective mandatory reporting'. Diagnosis on-site or in laboratory but without delay enables 'rapid action'.

The approach to control and prevention needs to cover four areas: (a) preventing infection of livestock and vaccination, (b) improving industrial hygiene, (c) decreasing the use of contaminated raw imported materials, and (d) additional measures are required in case of human death. These are avoid contact with dead body, exuded body fluids from natural openings, beddings, clothing etc. quarantine. Use disposable personal protective for collection of sample/handling dead body- rubber gloves, gum boots. Autoclave non-disposable, bury/burn disposable after use.

Preventing infection of livestock and vaccination:

- Proper disposal of carcass.
- Vaccination is strategically planned in the endemic areas and implemented at least 1 month prior to the established period of outbreak. This practice should not be interrupted.
- Avoid feeding fodder, hay cut close to soil, particularly to non-vaccinated animals.

In the face of outbreak:
- All susceptible animals on the affected premises and surrounding households should be vaccinated; more than one booster shot may be given depending upon the severity of the outbreak and potency of vaccine.
- Quarantine—movement of animals and animal by-products from the affected premises is stopped/restricted and traced.
- Anthrax responds to antibiotic therapy and so treat the affected and animals under incubation period. Antibiotics administered after the development of toxaemic phase are ineffective.
- Safe disposal of carcasses—burning is preferred than burial as the former destroys even spores and eliminates chances of exhuming. Carcass may be soaked with formaldehyde and buried.
- Control of scavengers.
- Decontamination and disinfection of premises and all contaminated surfaces, footwear, instruments, etc.; wash clothes worn when attending to sick animals separately.

Oxidizing agents such as peroxide, ethylene oxide, chlorine dioxide and sodium hypochlorite in liquid bleach products slowly destroy spores. When combined with certain catalytic agents, spore destruction is speeded up and is completed in <30 min. These are iron and tetra-amido macrocyclic ligands. These are combined with sodium carbonate and bicarbonate to convert into spray. This is applied to the infested area followed by another spray of tert-butyl hydroperoxide.

- Epidemiological investigation to trace the source and extent of the affected area and intensive surveillance and monitoring in the surrounding area for early detection of cases.

37.7.2.1 Industrial Hygiene

Animal products from endemic areas should preferably be decontaminated. Spores may be inactivated by boiling, steam/dry heat sterilization, ethylene oxide gas, formaldehyde and hypochlorite as follows:

- Bales and fleece should be treated first with warm alkali and detergent followed by 2.0% formaldehyde and dried in hot air.
- Hair and bristle should be autoclaved or treated with warm vapour of formaldehyde.
- Hides may be freed of spores in 7–16 days by H_2S, in 24 h by 1 in 5000 mercury chloride and 1% formic acid and in 2 days by 2% hydrochloric acid and 10% sodium chloride following 14 days of storage.

37.7.2.2 Awareness Programme About the Process of Transmission, Spread and Protection

As soon as anthrax is recognized in an animal population, public health and animal health agencies must come together, to heighten awareness among medical and animal health communities, as well as among ranchers and other inhabitants of at-risk areas.

- Use 'personal protective equipment' while handling a carcass and slaughter and meat by-products
- Consequences of eating uncooked/partially cooked meat from moribund animals—anthrax suspects
- Protective mask as a safety measure against inhalation anthrax—while shearing sheep
- Encourage reporting of suspected cases, clandestine slaughter and sale/consumption of carcass meat of affected animals through incentives
- Local vets and public health services to act on such reports

37.7.3 One Health Approach

Anthrax provides a suitable platform for development of 'One Health approach for control' (Shadomy et al. 2016). Rapid detection of anthrax-related illness for expeditious treatment and source identification including intentional (bio-terror) requires laboratory and healthcare providers reporting suspected anthrax. Chain of transmission is broken and environmental load of contaminant is reduced with accrued benefits of poverty alleviation and human health. Personnel in provincial, district and local health centres, the Ministry of Health and Veterinary Services and Ministry of Agriculture and Animal Husbandry are activated.

'Synergistic efforts of stakeholders' are required for achieving success. These are:

- Communities—their attitude changed through awareness; citizens committee constituted.
- Veterinary service to identify laboratory or create a 'lab response network' for diagnosis and investigate, monitor and implement vaccination programmes.
- Wildlife parks, reserve organizations—monitoring, reporting and organizing rapid vet service actions like quarantine, carcass disposal, disinfection of premises, etc.
- Public health efforts to treat zoonotic anthrax

The programme is monitored, information shared and reviewed and the programme is amended if needed.

Anthrax is a notifiable disease in most countries. Even a single 'clinically suspected case' is considered 'alert threshold' as in Romania. A case is a 'clinically compatible and laboratory confirmed'. It has to be reported to the local public health authority within 5 days in a standardized form. The National Centre for Communicable Diseases Surveillance and Control maintains the register for communicable diseases. The European Early Warning and Response System notifies laboratory-confirmed cases to the WHO. Germany follows this system. Anthrax is a 'federally' reportable disease in Canada. Animal producers, veterinarians and laboratories are required to report suspect cases to the Canadian Food Inspection Agency (CFIA) which in turn is required to comply with its international reporting obligations to trading partners and the World Organisation for Animal Health (OIE).

References

Ahmed B-N, Sultana Y, Fatema D, Ara K, Begum N et al (2010) Anthrax: an emerging zoonotic disease in Bangladesh. Bangladesh J Med Microbiol 4(1):46–50

Baldwin VM (2020) *B. cereus* – A review of Bacillus cereus strains that cause Anthrax-Like Disease. Front Microbiol 11:1731. https://10.3389/fmicb.2020.01731

Bush LM, Abrams BH, Beall A, Johnson CC (2001) Index case of fatal inhalation anthrax due to bioterrorism in the United States. N Engl J Med 345:1607–1610

Carlson CJ, Kracalik IT, Ross N, Alexander KA, Hugh-Jones ME et al (2019) The global distribution of *Bacillus anthracis* and associated anthrax risk to humans, livestock and wildlife. Nat Microbiol 4(8):1337–1343

Carroll LM, Kovac J, Miller RA, Wiedmann M (2017) Rapid, high-throughput identification of anthrax-causing and emetic *Bacillus cereus* group genome assemblies using BTyper, a computational tool for virulence-based classification of *Bacillus cereus* group isolates using nucleotide sequencing data. Appl Environ Microbiol 17:e01096–e01017

Cross AR, Baldwin VM, Roy S, Essex-Lopresti AE, Prior JL, Harmer NJ (2019) Zoonoses under our noses. Microbes Infect 21:10–19

Dixon TC, Messelson M, Guillemin J, Hanna PC (1999) Anthrax. New Eng J Med 11:815–826

Doganay M, Metan G, Alp E (2010) A review of cutaneous anthrax and its outcome. J Infect Public Health 3:98–105

Fasanella A, Di T, Battisti A, Longobardi C, Panerai F et al (2011) Old animal anthrax outbreaks discovered through the analysis of soil. Giornale Italiano Di Medicina Tropicale 16(3–4):1–4

Fasanella A, Garofolo G, Galella M, Troiano P et al (2013) Suspected vector transmission of human cutaneous anthrax during an animal outbreak in southern Italy. Vector Borne Zoonotic Dis 13(10):769–771

Furuta Y, Cheng C, Zorigt et al (2021) Direct regulons of AtxA, the master virulence regulator of *Bacillus anthracis*. mSystems 6:e0029121

Goel AK (2015) Anthrax: a disease of biowarfare and public health importance. World J Clin Cases 3:20–33

Grunow R, Klee SR, Beyer W, George M, Grunow D et al (2013) Anthrax among heroin users in Europe possibly caused by same *Bacillus anthracis* strain since 2000. Euro Surveill 18(13):20437

Hanczaruk M (2014) European injectional anthrax cases linked to strain from 2009 outbreak. Emerg Infect Dis 20:322–323

Hendricks KA, Wright ME, Shadomy SV, Bradley JS et al (2014) Centers for Disease Control and Prevention expert panel meetings on prevention and treatment of anthrax in adults. Emerg Infect Dis 20(2):e130687

Keim P, Grunow R, Vipond R, Grass G, Hoffmaster A et al (2015) Whole genome analysis of Injectional anthrax identifies two disease clusters spanning more than 13 years. EBioMedicine 2(11):1613

Laut CL, Leasure CS, PiH et al (2022) Dnaj and CIpX are required for HitRS and HssRS two-component system signalling in Bacillus anthracis. Infect Immun 90(1):e0056021

Liu W, Nestorovich EM (2021) Anthrax toxin channel: what we know based on over 30 years of research. Biochim Biophys Acta Biomembr 1863(11):183715

Mayo L et al (2010) Gastrointestinal anthrax after an animal-hide drumming event—New Hampshire and Massachusetts, 2009. MMWR 59(28):872–877

Moayeri M, Lappla SH, Vrentas C et al (2015) Anthrax pathogenesis. Ann Rev Microbiol 69:185

Mock A, Fouet A (2001) Anthrax. Ann Rev Microbiol 55:647–671

OIE (2016) Anthrax, Russia. http://www.oie.int/wahis_2/public/wahid.php/Reviewreport/Review?page_refer=MapFullEventReport&reportid=20689. Accessed 10 Sept 2016

Okutani A, Inoue S, Morikawa S (2019) Comparative genomics and phylogenetic analysis of *Bacillus anthracis* strains isolated from domestic animals in Japan. Infect Genet Evol 71:128–139

Popescu R, Pistol A, Miltaru L, Caplan D, Cucuiu R, Popovici F (2011) Two cases of infection with *Bacillus anthracis*, Romania, October 2011. Euro Surveill 16(45):20008

Ringertz SH, Hoiby EA, Jensenius M, Mahler J et al (2000) Injectional anthrax in a heroin skin-popper. Lancet 356:1574–1575

Shadomy S, Idrissi AE, Riazman E, Brini M, Palamara E et al (2016) Anthrax outbreaks: a warning for improved prevention, control and heightened awareness. Empress Watch 37:1–8

Sidwa T, Salzer JS, Traxler R, Swaney E et al (2020) Control and prevention of anthrax, Texas, USA, 2019. Emerg Infect Dis 26(12):2815–2824

Sterne M (1937) Avirulent anthrax vaccine. Onderstepoort J Vet Sci Animal Ind 21:41–43

Sweeney DA, Cui X, Solomon SB, Vitberg DA et al (2010) Anthrax lethal and edema toxins produce different patterns of cardiovascular and renal dysfunction and synergistically decrease survival of canines. J Infect Dis 202:1885–1896

Sweeney DA, Hicks CW, Cui X, Li Y, Eichacker PQ (2011) Anthrax infection. Am J Respir Crit Care Med 184:1333–1341

Tan LM, Ha HTT, Thai PQ, Tuan LA, Hung TTM et al (2019) Injectional anthrax among people who inject drugs and implications for research in Vietnam: a literature review. Vietnam J Prev Med 29:7–19

Thappa DM, Karthikeyan K (2001) Anthrax: an overview within the Indian subcontinent. Int J Dermatol 40:216–222

Wright JG, Quinn CP, Shadomy S, Messonnier N (2010) Use of anthrax vaccine in the United States recommendations of the Advisory Committee on Immunization Practices (ACIP), 2009. MMWR 59(RR-6):1–36

Chapter 38
Bartonellosis

Bartonellae are emerging zoonotic agents causing a clinically complex disease, bartonellosis. These are Carrion's disease, cat scratch disease, chronic lymphadenopathy, trench fever, chronic bacteraemia, culture-negative endocarditis, bacillary angiomatosis, bacillary peliosis, vasculitis and uveitis. Bartonellae are also linked to loss of weight, hallucination, fatigue, partial paralysis, paediatric acute-onset neuropsychiatric syndrome (PANS) and vasoproliferative tumours (Cheslock and Embers 2019).

These are often classified as:

Pathologies: Endocarditis, blood culture-negative endocarditis (BCNE), myocarditis, bacillary angiomatosis (*B. henselae* and *B. quintana*), peliosis hepatis (*B. henselae*).

Diseases: Cat scratch disease, Oroya fever, Carrion's disease, verruga peruana (*B. bacilliformis*), trench fever (*B. quintana*).

Zoonotic transmission occurs through sandflies, cat fleas and human body louse and suggested insects like ticks, red ants and spider have been suggested to transmit them. *B. quintana* survive in bed bug faeces for 18 days and enter the host through scratch (Cheslock and Embers 2019).

38.1 Aetiology

Bartonella are facultative intracellular in erythrocytes and endothelial cells, but can be cultivated on blood-enriched media and are pleomorphic, coccobacillary flagellate (e.g. *B. bacilliformis*, *B. clarridgeiae* and *B. schoenbuchii*) and non-flagellated (*B. henselae*) bacteria.

Bartonellae are fastidious, microaerophilic, pleomorphic, non-capsulated, non-sporing, Gram-negative bacteria belonging to alpha-2 subgroup of the class Proteobacteria. Primary isolation requires special medium and trypticase soy agar

© Springer Nature Singapore Pte Ltd. 2024
K. G. Narayan et al., *Handbook of Management of Zoonoses*,
https://doi.org/10.1007/978-981-99-9885-2_38

supplemented with 5% rabbit blood/haemoglobin. The incubation period is extended, 21 days, and requires 5% CO_2 and temperature of 35–37 °C. *B. bacilliformis* prefers ambient CO_2 and temperatures of 26–28 °C.

Presently there are 45 species, 13 associated with human diseases (Table 38.1). *Bartonella* species are increasing with expanding range of new animal reservoirs including marine mammals.

38.2   Epidemiology

Bartonella spp. are haemoparasites. Mammals are reservoir hosts. Some species of *Bartonella* are pathogenic to humans and animals. Most are zoonotic.

The bacteria are maintained in animal-arthropod vector cycle. Vectors may be ticks, mites, sandfly, flea and lice. There is persistent asymptomatic intraerythrocytic bacteraemia in a diverse array of mammalian reservoir hosts, cats, dogs, rabbits, rodents, horses, cattle and other wild animals. Man gets infected directly and indirectly through vectors.

B. quintana and *B. recurrentis* are human diseases transmitted directly from human reservoir to susceptible human through lice.

Oroya fever (Carrion's disease), cat scratch fever and trench fever are emerging human diseases caused respectively by *B. bacilliformis*, *B. henselae* and *B. quintana*. Humans are the hosts and reservoirs for *B. bacilliformis* and *B. quintana*.

38.2.1   Distribution

Bartonelloses in human, domestic and pet, wild animals and fishes occur in forms of sporadic to epidemic worldwide.

Cat scratch fever and trench fever are distributed worldwide. *B. bacilliformis* is limited to South America and *B. henselae* and *B. quintana* to Asia and Australia. *B. koehlerae* was reported from Israel, whereas *B. tamiae* from a febrile patient in Thailand. Bartonellae are reportedly the cause of endocarditis, cat scratch fever, prolonged fever, uveitis and other less frequent manifestations in Asia and Australia.

38.2.2   Reservoir

Large numbers of animals are potential reservoirs: cats, rats, mice and other rodents, wild rabbits, dogs, coyote, mammals, birds, bats and fishes. More than one *Bartonella* species may simultaneously infect cats and rodents.

Bartonella species have been isolated or detected in rodents, bats and marine animals such as beluga whales and sea turtles, in most cases without any serious

Table 38.1 Human bartonelloses (based on Saisongkorh et al. 2009; Okaro et al. 2017; Cheslock and Embers 2019)

Bartonella species	Disease in man	Reservoir	Vector
B. henselae	Cat scratch fever, bacteraemia; endocarditis, angiomatosis, peliosis; oculoglandular, neuroretinitis; osteomyelitis, arthropathy	Cats (domestic and feral—*Felis catus*), dogs horse[b]	Ticks, *Ctenocephalides* spp. lice, spider[b]
B. bacilliformis	Carrion's disease—Oroya fever (acute haemolytic anaemia); (chronic verruga peruana)	Human	Sandfly *Lutzomyia* spp.
B. clarridgeiae	Cat scratch fever lymphadenopathy, fever, papule	Cat, dog saliva agents' DNA+	Cat flea, ticks[b]
B. koehlerae	Cat scratch fever, endocarditis	Cats, dogs	Fleas[b]
B. rochalimae	Bacteraemia, fever, splenomegaly	Rats, *foxes, raccoons, coyotes, dogs*[b]	Flea, ticks[b]
B. grahamii	Neuroretinitis	Mice, voles Europe	*Ctenophthalmus nobilis*
B. elizabethae	Bacteraemia, endocarditis, retinitis	Rats, human[b], dogs, small mammals	*Xenopsylla cheopis*
B. vinsonii ssp. *auropensis*	Fever, bacteraemia in cattle rancher; endocarditis	Dog, rodent, cats, coyotes	Ticks
B. vinsonii ssp. *berkoffi*	Endocarditis	Cat. dog, rodents, wild canines	Vector (suspected) for wild canines, dogs, flea[b], ticks[b]
B. washoensis	Myocarditis	Ground squirrel	Vector (suspected) for wild canines, dogs flea[b], ticks[b]
B. quintana[a]	Endocarditis, angiomatosis, bacteraemia, trench fever	Human, cats, macaques,[b] dogs[b]	Human body lice, fleas, bed bugs[b]
B. alsatica[a]	Endocarditis	Rabbit, human[b]	Flea,[b] ticks[b]
B. ancashensis[a]	*Verruga Peruana*		
B. mayotimonensis[a]	Endocarditis	Bat[b], human[b]; patients had exposure to mouse faeces and earlier owned a cat. Bats and their ectoparasites	Human body lice, fleas, bed bugs[b]
B. tamiae[a]	Fever	Rodents, human[b]	Chigger mites and ticks
Following from Cheslock and Embers (2019)			
B. bovis		Cattle, cat, dog, human	Biting flies, ticks
B. schoenbuchensis		Cattle	Biting flies, ticks
B. chomelii		Cattle	Biting flies, ticks

(continued)

Table 38.1 (continued)

Bartonella species	Disease in man	Reservoir	Vector
B. melophagi		Sheep, human	Sheep keds
B. rattimassiliensis		Rats	Fleas
B. tribocorum		Rats	Fleas
B. doshiae		Rats, human	Fleas
B. birtlesii		Mice	Fleas
B. grahamii		Mice, human	Fleas
B. myotimonensis		Bats, human	Bat flies, fleas, ticks
B. rousetii		Bats	Bat flies

Bold face—vast majority of human cases causing species
[a]Okaro et al. (2017)
[b]Cheslock and Embers (2019)

disease. Bacteria and reservoirs seem to have co-evolved, e.g. *B. bacilliformis* and *B. quintana* with human, *B. henselae* with cats, *B. vinsonii* subsp. *berkhoffii* with dogs, *B. bovis* with cows, *B. melophagi* with sheep and *B. australis* with kangaroos.

Rodent-adapted *Bartonella* species are growing (Okaro et al. 2017), e.g. ground squirrels (*B. washoensis*), grey squirrels (*Candidatus B. durdenii*), flying squirrels (*Candidatus B. volans*), and even groundhogs (*Candidatus B. monaxi*).

Bats have been identified as the reservoirs of diverse and novel species of *Bartonella* in eastern Africa (Kenya) and Guatemala and Peru. High prevalence may possibly be due to (a) bats' long life of 10–20 years, (b) direct inter- and intra-species transmission (*Carollia* and *Glossophaga* bats share roosts) and (c) vector transmission, being hosts to a wide variety of ectoparasites such as fleas, bat flies, soft ticks and mites.

38.2.3 Vector

Bartonella spp. live in the gut of blood-sucking arthropod vectors (fleas, lice, ticks and sandflies). Transmission of *Bartonella* spp. is influenced by vector preference, e.g. sandfly transmission for *B. bacilliformis*, louse transmission for *B. quintana* and *B. recurrentis*, flea transmission for *Bartonella* species and permissive mammalian host such as rodents influence transmission. Natural infections occur mostly from rodent communities worldwide and a few other mammalian species like cats. *B. henselae* infects cats through *Ctenocephalides felis*. Infected pet and stray cats show no symptoms but are common cause of 'cat scratch fever'. Infection is high in hot and humid climate. *B. clarridgeiae* can be a co-infecting bacterium. Two species *B. koehlerae* and *B. weissii* (now termed *B. bovis*) are reported worldwide in domestic cats but are relatively uncommon.

38.2.4   Transmission

Generally, Bartonellae are transmitted to human from cattle and pets like cats and dogs. *B. henselae* and *B. koehlerae* causing cat scratch fever have been isolated from owners' cats and dogs.

The transmission cycle involves reservoir mammals—blood-sucking arthropods. *Bartonella* spp. invade erythrocytes and remain intra-erythrocyte for a prolonged period in asymptomatic hosts, e.g. in 1% of erythrocytes *B. quintana* persisted for months to years with no or subclinical symptoms.

Transmission by blood-sucking arthropods facilitates survival and dispersal while avoiding the host immune system. The endothelial cells in the mammalian host are the primary niche. It is suggested that some bacteria are released periodically from these and infect erythrocytes. There is intraerythrocytic multiplication and the blood-sucking arthropods pick up these to continue transmission.

38.3   Virulence Factors and Pathogenesis

Okaro et al. (2017) described the virulence factors and pathogenesis.

38.3.1   Virulence Factors

Of the many virulence factors of *Bartonella*, TAAs and T4SSs are the two major factors facilitating infection.

TAAs of Gram-negative bacteria are a family of proteins. All *Bartonella* have at least one TAA gene. TAA protein in *B. henselae* is termed BadA, in *B. quintana* Vomps and in *B. vinsonii* Brps (*Bartonella* repeat proteins).

BadA facilitates *Bartonella* infection through adherence to extracellular matrix proteins or target endothelial cells, evading phagocytosis, stimulating endothelial cell proliferation by inducing a proangiogenic host cell response.

There are four Vomps, A–D, found in *B. quintana*. These function like adhesin, mediate host cell adhesion, autoaggregation and suppressor of host immune response.

VirB/VirD4 T4SS (best characterized in *B. henselae*) is a multi-protein system (VirB2 to VirB11) which translocates Beps (Bartonella effector proteins) to target cells. Bartonellae gain entry into human endothelial cells through an invasome-mediated uptake mechanism that requires VirB/VirD4 T4SS. The VirB/VirD4 T4SS delivers (1) BepG for invasome-mediated uptake and/or (2) BepC and BepF to rearrange the actin cytoskeleton. Aggregation of bacteria, engulfment by host cell membranes and entry into endothelial cells via the invasome occur. VirB/VirD4 T4SS is also crucial for inhibition of endothelial cell apoptosis and intraerythrocytic infection.

Hbps—Bartonellae use hemin binding proteins (Hbp) for survival in vectors' gut. *B. henselae* replicates in the cat flea gut and is excreted in the flea's faeces. *Bartonella* uses HbpA probably for iron acquisition and to bind hemin required for bacterial growth.

Hbps serve also as adhesins, bind fibronectin and facilitate entry into endothelial cells. It protects Bartonellae from toxic concentration of hemin present in mammalian bloodstream.

Biofilm—Biofilm formation by Bartonellae possibly enhances transmission. Replication of *B. henselae* in cat flea gut and excretion in faeces occur and carried to the cat's claws. It is possible that the bacteria form biofilm in the gut of flea and also faeces of flea and persist there before transmission to the cat's claws.

Bartonellae have unique invasion mechanism driving angiogenesis.

38.3.2   Pathogenesis

First Bartonellae must cross/evade the innate immune system. The TLR (Toll-like receptor) fails to identify lipopolysaccharide on the surface of *Bartonellae* because of reduced endotoxic activity. The invading *B. quintana* causes overproduction of anti-inflammatory interleukin-10 and antagonizes pro-inflammatory factors like Toll-like receptor-4, thus reducing the host's inflammatory response. *B. bacillifor-mis* uses 'primary amino acid sequence changes in flagellin' to evade TLR.

Bartonellae reach and invade the primary niche 'endothelial cells' and multiply, reinfect blood and cause bacteraemia. Invasion of endothelial cells by *B. henselae* results into large aggregate of bacteria termed as 'invasomes' following VirB/VirD4 T4SS-dependent and VirB/VirD4 T4SS-independent mechanism.

B. henselae caused the proliferation of endothelial cells by inducing the production of the vascular endothelial growth factor (VEGF) and suppressing apoptosis of vascular endothelial cells. VEGF stimulates angiogenesis increasing microvascular endothelial cells. VEGF production required BadA. The suppression of apoptosis is caused by the delivery of Bartonella effector proteins (Beps), viz. BepA by the VirB/VirD T4SS of *B. henselae*.

Bartonellae infection causes angiogenesis, i.e. formation of new blood vessels. This involves migration, growth and differentiation of endothelial cells forming the inner lining of blood vessels. Bartonellae target endothelial cells. The three major pathogenic species, *B. bacilliformis*, *B. henselae* and *B. quintana*, invade the endothelium, resulting in the angiogenic response by the hosts.

Angiogenesis is achieved by the following suggested pathway (paracrine angiogenic loop) by *B. henselae*:

BadA facilitates adherence to or phagocytosis by macrophages. VEGF production causes endothelial cell proliferation and angiogenesis. Another path adopted by B. henselae involves VirB-enabled adherence/infection of endothelial cells. Beps induced increased interleukin 8 plus the increased VEGF from the macrophages caused angiogenesis.

The human progenitor endothelial cells can be reprogramed by *B. henselae*. *B. bacilliformis* stimulates endothelial cell proliferation and induces angiogenesis.

Chronic and asymptomatic carrier state is created through attenuation of host immune response.

Example is *B. quintana* asymptomatic infection and carrier state in homeless patients.

38.4   Pathologies

Clinical response to *Bartonellae* infection in human is mainly dependent upon the immune status. The response is granulomatous and suppurative in immunocompetent individuals vasoproliferative in immunocompromised.

The long-recognized diseases such as Carrion's disease, trench fever and cat scratch disease are dealt with separately. The newer clinical manifestations such as bacillary angiomatosis (BA) and peliosis hepatitis, endocarditis and Parinaud oculoglandular syndrome are described here under.

38.4.1   Bacillary Angiomatosis (BA)

BA has been reported from the USA, Africa, Southeast Asia, Middle East, Australia and South America, mostly in men (Akram et al. 2022).

The causative agents are *B. henselae* and *B. quintana*. Both cause cutaneous lesion. The latter is associated more frequently with subcutaneous and osseous lesions. The former (*B. henselae* genotype I) is more frequently linked to splenic and hepatic peliosis. *B. henselae* genotype II is more frequently linked to lesions in the skin or lymph nodes or both. Genotypic difference between types 1 and II is based on 16S rDNA sequences and multi-locus variable number tandem repeat analysis (MLVA).

B. henselae is maintained in cats by episodes of asymptomatic bacteraemia. Cats acquire infection from infected cat flea, *Ctenocephalides felis*, vector for also *B. quintana*. *Pediculus humanus* transmits *B. quintana*.

Cat flea-human transmission has been hypothesized, not documented. Tick-human transmission has been observed.

Human and Japanese macaques (*Macaca fuscata*) are considered reservoir of *B. quintana*.

BA is a proliferative disease of vascular epithelium wherein abnormal vascular endothelial cell proliferation and neovascularization occur. It is also known as epitheloid angiomatosis.

The condition is manifested as a solitary or multiple papulonodular cutaneous lesions originally observed in HIV. BA occurs among the non-HIV patients, e.g. leukaemia, chronic hepatitis B, transplant cases and those on immunosuppressant therapy.

The cutaneous lesions are highly vascular, bruising or bleed easily with regional lymphadenopathy. These could be superficial to deep sub-dermal even involving bones.

BA may also affect mucous membranes of the mouth, conjunctivae and the gastrointestinal tract, including the perianal area. Visceral organs affected include the liver, spleen, lymph nodes and bone marrow.

Diagnosis should be attempted regardless of the immune status of patients as BA occurs also among immunocompetent patients at sites of burn or cat scratch masquerading as a pyogenic granuloma.

38.4.2 *Peliosis Hepatis:* B. henselae

Peliosis is a Greek word means blue/black or discoloured extravasated blood. Such a condition may involve spleen, bone marrow, lungs, lymph nodes and other abdominal organs but most commonly liver, hence Peliosis hepatis.

Peliosis hepatis was originally described in association with tuberculosis. A disseminated bartonella infection has been found associated with other pathological conditions, e.g. immunodeficient/immunocompromised, HIV and other infectious and non-infectious conditions like neoplasia, exposure to toxins and anabolic steroids.

Patients report abdominal pain, fever and weight loss. Peliosis hepatis is characterized by hepatomegaly, multiple vascular, haemorrhagic parenchymatous and cystic lesions ranging from a few mm to 3 cm distributed throughout the liver. Histological examination shows dilated capillaries, proliferation of the sinusoidal hepatic capillaries, vascular hyperplasia, inflammatory cells and cystic blood-filled cavities.

Ahsan et al. (1998) described it in a case of kidney transplant. There was severe anaemia, persistent thrombocytopenia and hepatorenal syndrome. PCR detected *B. henselae* and *B. quintana* DNA in peripheral blood and liver. A 3-month erythromycin treatment resulted in clinical recovery.

Peliosis hepatis in a 6-year-old spayed Golden retriever was described by Kitchell et al. (2000). The bitch suffered from general weakness and abdominal distension. Ultrasound showed large fluid accumulated in peritoneum and multiple small, nodular masses and cyst-like structure in enlarged liver. Diagnosis was based on PCR detection of *B. henselae* DNA and gross and histopathological changes in liver.

38.4.3 Blood Culture-Negative Endocarditis (BCNE)

It is generally defined as endocarditis where the microbial aetiology cannot be established after at least three different blood samples in a standard blood culture system fail to grow an organism after at least 5 days of incubation. In France it accounts for 20–30% of all documented *Bartonella* endocarditis which is next to *Coxiella burnetii*—endocarditis (Edouard et al. 2015). Incidence of BCNE varied between 2.5% and 76% of all infective endocarditis cases and in different geographic regions mostly by *B. quintana* and *B. henselae*. Culture negativity varied from 50% in Africa, Algeria and Pakistan against 12–20% in Japan, the UK and France, probably because of differences in availability of diagnostic facility. Present estimate is around 5% of all endocarditis (Okaro et al. 2017). Culture negativity may be due to antimicrobial pre-treatment, right-side endocarditis, implanted device like pacemaker or defibrillator and fastidious nature of bacteria.

García-Álvarez et al. (2022) presented epidemiologic, clinical characteristics, management and outcomes of infective endocarditis cases from GAMES (Grupo de Apoyo al Manejo de la Endocarditis infecciosa en España) cohort. Twenty-one cases of Bartonella infective endocarditis (IE) represented 0.3% of cases and 2% of BCNE of the cohort. Diagnosis was based on PCR and serology. Only one case was culture positive. Endocarditis was caused by *B. henselae* (62%) and *B. quintana* (38%). IE presented as cardiac failure (87.5% in *B. quintana* and 61.5% in *B. henselae*). In 85% of cases aortic valve was affected (100% in *B. quintana* IE and 76% in *B. henselae* IE). Echocardiograph showed vegetations. Less than 40% cases had fever.

Pathogenesis: Vomps of *Bartonellae* are essential for infection and evasion of host's immune system. After entry, *Bartonellae* adhere to and infect erythrocyte and endothelial cells causing prolonged bacteraemia (may last for years).

1. *B. quintana* induces intracellular signals for decreased apoptosis and increased proliferation of vascular endothelial cells. This leads to chronic infection and intracellular aggregation (colonization) in endothelial cells, including vascular and valvular endothelial cells.

   These pathogenic mechanisms underlie the insidious clinical presentation and subtle variations in clinical findings of endocarditis caused by *B. quintana*.
2. *B. henselae* endocarditis: accounts for about one-fourth of *Bartonella* endocarditis cases. The majority of cases have a history of contact or interaction with a cat. *Bartonella* adhesin A (BadA) and the TAA are expressed in *B. henselae* as well as in *B. quintana*. *B. henselae* shows similar tropism for endothelial cells, replicates and persists in the endothelium.

Symptoms: Nonspecific, fatigue, fever and weight loss; 50–70% showed exertional dyspnoea, a symptom of heart failure; examination revealed heart murmur. Aortic valve alone or with others are commonly affected. Majority of the valves affected were native valves. Prosthetic valves are also affected and may be aggressively leading to perforation and heart failure.

Additional pathological changes include splenomegaly, thromboembolism, hepatomegaly, digital clubbing, anaemia, thrombocytopenia, leucocytosis, increased ESR, positive rheumatoid factor, elevated liver enzymes and evidence of renal failure.

Advocated diagnosis: B. henselae or *B. quintana* positive PCR, IgG serology at ≥1:800 by IFA or a positive Western blot assay should be considered Major Duke Criteria for *Bartonella* endocarditis. Valvular specimen was better than blood. Edouard et al. (2015) suggested that any patient with a *Bartonella* IgG titre of less than 800 and a medical history evocative of endocarditis should be tested by Western blotting and RT-PCR following cardiac valve removal.

The number of reported *Bartonella* endocarditis increased from 2005 to 2013 and is increasing rapidly, probably because of better understanding, interest and improvement of diagnostic tools (Edouard et al. 2015). *Bartonella* endocarditis death rate is reducing, earlier ranging between 7 and 30%. *B. quintana* accounts for about three-fourths and *B. henselae* for one-fourth.

38.5   Diagnosis

The lysis centrifugation method for sample preparation increases isolate recovery.

Blood culture and tissue culture (of surgically excised valve) have 20–30% sensitivity. There is no *Bartonella*-specific strain.

Bartonella endocarditis relies heavily on serology and/or molecular testing of blood or valvular tissue specimens.

ELISA and IFA are not species-specific.

- The VirB5 17-kDa antigen recombinant protein expressed in *Escherichia coli* reacted with sera from cat scratch disease (CSD) and *B. henselae* IgG antibody by ELISA and for IgM capture assay with high specificity and sensitivity.
- Use of subcellular fractions as an antigen in an ELISA to detect IgG for the diagnosis of CSD.
- Cross-adsorption (other bacterial species, especially *Chlamydia* spp. causing endocarditis) and Western immunoblotting techniques also have been reported with high specificity and sensitivity in detecting *Bartonella* endocarditis.

38.5.1 Molecular Tools

38.5.1.1 PCR Using 16SRNA

PCR detection of (a) *Bartonella* 16S rRNA gene sequences in the lesions of patients with bacillary angiomatosis and (b) of *B. henselae* 16S rRNA gene sequences in skin test antigens to diagnose CSD. It is useful with other specimens like whole blood, plasma and serum also.

Laboratory diagnosis is important for management of cases. Specific diagnosis helps in specific treatment.

38.6 Treatment

The mild form with lymphadenopathy and fever needs no treatment because of the self-limiting nature of the disease (Bass et al. 1998). However, use of a single anti-microbial regimen (azithromycin, ciprofloxacin, gentamicin, trimethoprim-sulfamethoxazole and rifampin) will reduce the duration of the symptoms significantly. Combinations of antimicrobial drugs worked.

References

Ahsan N, Holman MJ, Riley TR, Abendroth CS et al (1998) Peloisis hepatis due to *Bartonella henselae* in transplantation: a hemato-hepato-renal syndrome. Transplantation 65(7):1000–1003

Akram SM, Anwar MY, Thandra KC et al (2022) Bacillary angiomatosis. In: StatPearls. StatPearls Publishing, Treasure Island, FL. https://www.ncbi.nlm.nih.gov/books/NBK448092/

Bass JW, Freitas BC, Freitas AD, Sisler CL et al (1998) Prospective randomized double blind placebo-controlled evaluation of azithromycin for treatment of cat-scratch disease. Pediatr Infect Dis J 17(6):447–452

Cheslock MA, Embers ME (2019) Human Bartonellosis: an underappreciated public health problem? Trop Med Infect Dis 4(2):69

Edouard S, Nabet C, Lepidi H, Fournier P-E, Raoult D (2015) *Bartonella*, a common cause of endocarditis: a report on 106 cases and review. J Clin Microbiol 53:824–829

García-Álvarez L, García-García C, Muñoz P, Fariñas-Álvarez MDC et al (2022) On Behalf of Grupo de Apoyo Al Manejo de la Endocarditis Infecciosa En España Games. Pathogens 11(5):561

Kitchell BE, Fan TM, Kordick D, Breitschwerdt EB et al (2000) Peliosis hepatis in a dog infected with Bartonella henselae. J Am Vet Med Assoc 216(4):519–523

Okaro U, Addisu A, Casanas B, Anderson B (2017) *Bartonella* species, an emerging cause of blood-culture-negative endocarditis. Clin Microbiol Rev 30:709–746

Saisongkorh W, Rolain JM, Suputtamongkol Y, Raoult D (2009) Emerging Bartonella in humans and animals in Asia and Australia. J Med Assoc Thail 92(5):707–731

Chapter 39
Cat Scratch Fever/Disease (CSF/CSD)

Cat scratch fever/disease (CSF/CSD) is characterized by non-painful bump or blister at the site of injury and painful lymph gland draining the area, fever and malaise. The incubation period is 3–14 days. The clinical syndrome of CSD was described in 1950 for the first time (Debre et al. 1950) and organism could not be observed until 1983 when a small, pleomorphic Gram-negative bacillus in infected lymph nodes of patients was described (Wear et al. 1983). It was successfully isolated and cultured in 1988 (English et al. 1988). Initially, it was named *Afipia felis*, after the Armed Forces Institute of Pathology, where this organism was discovered (Brenner et al. 1991), but later it was designated as *Bartonella*.

39.1 Aetiology

B. henselae and *B. clarridgeiae.*

39.2 Epidemiology

Cat scratch fever/disease is distributed worldwide with cases reported from the USA, Europe, Japan, New Zealand and Australia (Florin et al. 2008). Seroprevalence (antibodies to *B. henselae)* in humans and bacteraemia was found to be highest in regions with warm and humid climates. Specific location is dependent upon the population of kitten in which *B. henselae* is more prevalent. In turn, breeding of cat is responsible for turn over population of kitten, means cat breeding season, which is warm months. About 20% cats are carriers in the USA and cats remain so for long even for life. Cats show no symptoms and may act as sentinel. Veterinarians may examine the mouth, eyes, heart (laboured breathing) and urinary system of cats.

© Springer Nature Singapore Pte Ltd. 2024   409
K. G. Narayan et al., *Handbook of Management of Zoonoses*,
https://doi.org/10.1007/978-981-99-9885-2_39

Twenty percent of cats are carriers in the USA and cats remain so for long even for life.

Asymptomatic cats (>50%) are bacteraemic and may harbour cat flea (explain for persistence in flea). *B. henselae* has also been isolated from fleas recovered from infected cats. The bacterium multiplies in the gut of fleas, is shed in faeces and survives in it for 3 days post exposure, as seen experimentally. Cat-to-cat transmission may be flea bite, ingestion of flea and flea faeces. Flea-to-human transmission is not known. Cat scratch transmission of *B. henselae* to human is indirect, through flea faeces carrying the bacterium.

CSD is common in age group 5–9 years, in southern USA, with 22,000 diagnoses and 2000 hospitalization per year. More than 90% of cases reported some contact with cats. Most cases occur during fall and early winter (September through January) attributed to the breeding pattern of cats, adoption and temporal presence of fleas on cats (Okaro et al. 2017). Human illness from other cats *Bartonella*, *B. clarridgeiae* and *B. koehlerae* is uncommon.

Zoonotic bacillary angiomatosis and CSD in man is associated with contact with cats. Cats' oral swab and claws carry *B. henselae*. Zangwill et al. (1993) presented findings of an epidemiological study over 60 patients. A significant number of cases were seropositive compared to control (*P* < 0.001). The positive predictive value of the serologic test was 91%. A significant number of serum samples from cats of patients were positive for *R. henselae* as compared to cats from control patients (*P* < 0.001). The odd ratio for kitten-owning households to contract CSD or bitten was 12.4 (95% confidence interval).

39.2.1   Transmission

Cat is a natural reservoir. *B. henselae* has been isolated from fleas and recovered from infected cats. Kittens are more likely transmitter. Fleas (*Ctenocephalides felis*) are vectors. They excrete viable bacteria in faeces that enter intradermally in cats. Transmission between cats is mainly by the cat flea; *Ixodes* ticks have been proposed.

In man *B. henselae* enter through a scratch wound and cat saliva as the bacterium is found in the kittens' mouth and their claw. Scratch by or, less likely, the bite or lick of cats transmits infection to man. Tick can also occasionally transmit.

39.3   Symptoms

Cat scratch disease primarily affects children and young adults; 80% of those affected are under 21. Most patients develop regional lymphadenopathy, preceded by an erythematous papule at the site of inoculation. Most common sites were the axillae and neck.

Scratch by a cat is followed by local inflammation; a bump/blister at the site 10–14 days later and a significant enlargement of regional lymph nodes, fever, sore throat, malaise, loss of appetite and body weight develop and could last for several weeks. Majority of cases are benign and recover. Severe form is rare and manifests as chills, prolonged fever, rash and pain in joint and back. Serious complications reported such as meningitis, encephalitis, osteomyelitis and endocarditis are known. Oculoglandular syndrome (Parinaud's oculoglandular syndrome) is a granulomatous conjunctivitis with pre- and post-auricular lymphadenopathy and may be expanding ocular involvement presenting as an optic nerve granuloma.

39.4   Diagnosis

Confounding conditions are brucellosis, lymphadenitis and Lyme disease.

Laboratory diagnosis is based on growing *Bartonella* from clinical specimen and/or genome analysis. Growing *Bartonella* on artificial medium is difficult and time-taking because (a) it is intracellular, (b) slow growing and (c) antibiotic administered to patients. Recently developed medium is *Bartonella* alpha-Proteobacteria growth medium (BAPGM) for isolation of seven species of *Bartonella*.

Whole cell fatty acid/cellular fatty acid analysis is also useful for identification of *Bartonella* species.

PCR is a rapid, sensitive and specific test for detecting bacteria in clinical specimen.

Studying *B. henselae,* Diddi et al. (2013) observed that growing *Bartonella* on BAPGM followed by PCR provide a complimentary diagnostic approach Restriction fragment length polymorphism (RFLP) analysis of PCR-amplified genes (boiling method of DNA extraction was the easiest, less time-taking and cost-effective and gave a good yield of DNA)—followed by PCR might differentiate between species of *Bartonella* genus.

39.5   Treatment

Azithromycin and doxycycline are drugs of choice.

39.6   Prevention

Primarily control of fleas (minimal contact and washing hands after handling a cat or cat faeces); keeping cats inside to protect from likely infestation outside.

1. Avoid rough play with cats, particularly strays and kittens, to prevent scratches. Wash hands promptly after handling cats.
2. Treat cats for fleas.
3. Use flea collar or similar topical preventive on dogs.

References

Brenner DJ, Hollis DG, Moss CW et al (1991) Proposal of *Afipia* gen. nov., with *Afipia felis* sp. Nov. (formerly Cat-scratch disease bacillus), *Afipia clevelandensis* sp. Nov. (formerly the Cleveland Clinic Foundation strain), *Afipia broomeae* sp. Nov., and three unnamed genospecies. J Clin Microbiol 29(11):2450–2460

Debre R, Lamy M, Jammet M, Costil L, Mozzicona P (1950) La maladie des griffes de chat. Bull Mem Soc Med Hop Paris 66:76–79

Diddi K, Chaudhury R, Sharma N, Dhawan B (2013) Strategy for identification and characterization of *B. henselae*. Indian J Med Res 137:380–387

English CK, Wear DJ, Margileth AM, Lissner CR, Walsh GP (1988) Cat-scratch disease: isolation and culture of the bacterial agent. JAMA 259(9):1347–1352

Florin TA, Zaoutis TE, Zaoutis LB (2008) Beyond cat scratch disease: widening spectrum of *Bartonella henselae* infection. Pediatrics 121(5):e1413–e1425

Okaro U, Addisu A, Casanas B, Anderson B (2017) *Bartonella* species, an emerging cause of blood-culture-negative endocarditis. Clin Microbiol Rev 30:709–746

Wear DJ, Margileth AM, Hadfield TL, Fischer GW et al (1983) Cat-scratch disease: a bacterial infection. Science 221(4618):1403–1405

Zangwill KM, Hamilton DH, Perkins BA, Regnery RL et al (1993) Cat scratch disease in Connecticut—epidemiology, risk factors, and evaluation of a new diagnostic test. N Engl J Med 329:8–13

Chapter 40
Oroya Fever

Synonyms

Carrion's disease, Peruvian warts or commonly known verruga peruana are various names of the conditions caused by *Bartonella bacilliformis*.

Carrion's disease is a biphasic illness. Oroya fever is the acute phase of life-threatening disease of immunologically naïve population such as children. Oroya fever is characterized by acute haemolytic anaemia. Peruvian warts or verruga peruana is a chronic phase characterized by chronic vascular proliferative cutaneous lesions.

40.1 Aetiology

It is caused by *Bartonella bacilliformis*. Humans are the only established reservoir. Once infected, a man acts as a reservoir for infecting sandflies. Man-sandfly-man transmission maintains the bacterium in nature. The disease is reproducible in rhesus macaques, chimpanzees and orangutans, suggesting possibility of alternate reservoir and their use as sentinels.

40.2 Epidemiology

Carrion's disease is endemic in high-altitude valleys of South American Andes and in low income group and is linked with poverty. The distribution of Carrion's disease correlates with the presence of vector in the endemic areas. Appearance of Carrion's disease in other areas suggests extension/expansion of vector activity. Over the last two decades numerous outbreaks have occurred and areas seem to be expanding. According to Garcia Quintanilla et al. (2019), a total of 1389 cases of bartonellosis were reported during 2009–2013, and 16% were Carrion's disease (~3% Oroya fever and ~13% verruga peruana) in Colombia. South Americans (ca 1.7 million) are estimated to be at risk in an area covering roughly 145,000 km^2 of Ecuador, Colombia and Peru (Minnick et al. 2014). The prevalence matches geographic boundaries of vector *L. verrucarum*, 1–3 km of altitude in the Andes Mountains in Peru. Other phlebotomine sandflies, *L. maranonensis* and *L. robusta*, may serve as vectors in areas devoid of *L. verrucarum*. It is sporadically reported among travellers returning from visits to areas of endemicity.

Sandflies are weak fliers and breed in close proximity to their blood-meal source. Transmission mechanism of *B. bacilliformis* by sandflies is still unclear. It has been demonstrated experimentally that 'bacterium massively multiplied, invaded red blood cells during the first three days, infection persisted in the gut of *L. verrucarum* for seven days'. Transmission during the second blood meal was not attempted. Faecal droplets were not examined for bacterium (Minnick et al. 2014). Epidemiological observations in Peru are supportive.

L. verrucarum is anthropophilic but multiple host feeders—feeds on animals and human and vice versa—rests inside human dwellings and feeds readily indoors, preferentially on humans. The population density and activity are influenced by atmospheric temperature and humidity. The density of their population is low during dry winter (June–July) and highest in November when temperature and humidity increased (before summer and onset of rains in Dec.). Feeding time also appears to be so regulated, e.g. 18.00–20.00 h during March to July (coldest winter in Peru) and throughout the night in August through November. Epidemics of bartonellosis in Peru (Caraz and Cusco) were coincident with abundance of vectors because of El Niño in 1997–1998 as the rainy season was extended, humidity and minimum monthly temperature rose. Evidences suggest that ticks might be potential vectors.

40.3   Pathogenesis

GroEL of *B. bacilliformis* increases apoptosis and regulates the growth of endothelial cells. Invasion-associated locus proteins A and B (IalA, IalB) are important for invasion into erythrocytes, facilitated by flagella. Flagellin is not recognized by Toll-like receptor 5 (TLR5), as a result the host's inflammatory response is not activated. Erythrocyte invasion model revealed substantial and long-lasting deformations in erythrocyte membranes where bacteria are localized. Invasion of endothelial cells and proliferation (similar to angiogenesis) cause the formation of verruga peruana. Endothelial cell model studies of *B. bacilliformis* dissemination through the blood stream led to rapid (1 h) invasion of endothelial cells, activation of release of tissue plasminogen activator (t-PA) involved in angiogenesis, rapid proliferation due to bacteria-derived proteinaceous mitogen and large vacuolic inclusions after 12 h. There is a strong induction of angiopoietin-2 in endothelial cells and vascular endothelial growth factor (Garcia Quintanilla et al. 2019). The study by Hicks and Minnick (2020) demonstrated that infected vascular endothelial cells (VECs) cause overproduction of epidermal growth factor (EGF) and cells multiply more rapidly. VECs migrate towards the bacterium and form capillary-like tubes—processes that occur during an actual infection.

40.4 Transmission

According to Pons et al. (2017) sandfly-human transmission is the most relevant route of transmission. *Lutzomyia verrucosum and L. peruensis* are known vectors. Some other species have also been proposed.

Other routes of transmission should not be ignored. These are blood transfusion, direct contact or inoculation of infected human blood, tissue and fluids, mother to child (vertical transmission) and probably organ transplant.

About 52% of humans are seropositive, asymptomatic and carriers in endemic areas and appear to be the main reservoir (Garcia Quintanilla et al. 2019).

40.5 Symptoms

Infection with *B. bacilliformis* may be asymptomatic. Symptoms depend upon the cells invaded. The disease is biphasic, with both an acute haemolytic anaemia (Oroya fever) and a chronic form with vascular proliferative lesions (verruga peruana), occurring independently or sequentially. The acute phase (Oroya fever) is serious and life-threatening, causing deaths if not treated. It occurs mainly in immunologically naïve population such as children. High mortality, miscarriages, preterm birth and foetal deaths occur in pregnant women (Pons et al. 2017).

Oroya fever occurs approximately 60 days following the bite of an infected sandfly. Young children (>60%) are mainly affected. The bacterium invades erythrocytes and endothelial cells. There is an intraerythrocytic replication, resulting in erythrocyte rupture.

The first phase is erythrocytic acute febrile illness (sometimes known as Oroya fever) characterized by fever (ca. 102 °F), generalized lymphadenopathy, myalgia, headache, hepatosplenomegaly, jaundice, transient immunosuppression and severe haemolytic anaemia with fatality rates of as high as 88% in untreated as against 10% in treated (Garcia Quintanilla et al. 2019). Some cases may show heart murmur, probably related with affection of the circulatory system. Complications occur due to secondary infections and may increase fatality. Meningeal and cerebral involvement up to 20% of patients with Carrion's disease and manifestations like delirium, paralysis and seizures may occur.

The second or subsequent chronic phase is cutaneous eruptive phase (Peruvian warts or verruga peruana) of the disease. Cases report fever, malaise, myalgia, anorexia, bone pain, joint pain, arthralgia, lymphadenopathy and hepatosplenomegaly. There is a characteristic development of verrucous dermal eruptions that result from proliferation of vascular endothelial cells. Invaded endothelial cells proliferate to produce eruptions of varied sizes, military (most common), nodular or subdermic and mular (Carrion's disease). These skin lesions ulcerate and bleed. There may be dermal infection and necrosis.

The chronic verruga peruana phase can occur presenting as blood-filled nodular haemangioma-like lesions in the skin.

B. bacilliformis infection results in a lifelong humoral immunity which confers partial immunological protection. Convalescent serum is protective. An analysis of immune response among carriers revealed that infection induces immunosuppression (IL10 overproduction) in the acute phase that is maintained in the later phase with low levels of bacteraemia (up to 3 years), a mechanism for establishment and persistence of infection. A RT-PCR study estimated 37% and 52% carriers in post outbreak and endemic areas, respectively. This study by Pons et al. (2017) also identifies serum biomarkers useful for surveillance.

40.6   Diagnosis

It can be diagnosed by examining Giemsa-stained blood smear, IF and PCR.

Rhesus monkeys are the ideal model for a study of *B. bacilliformis*. Disease manifestation mimics disease in human. A prolonged irregular intermittent fever is induced. The erythrocyte invaded by the bacterium can be seen by microspore and can be cultivated from peripheral blood for as long as 58 days. Chimpanzees and orangutans are the only other animals in which Carrion's disease can be reproduced.

40.7   Treatment

It is treatable with antibiotics like azithromycin, erythromycin and others considering combined infections.

40.8   Prevention

Conventional protection methods against fly bites are bed nets and vaseline-citronella ointments as a means of warding off sandflies. Peak biting activity occurs shortly after sundown.

40.8.1 Control of Sandfly Population

Sandfly population control experiments have been cited (Minnick et al. 2014). Adult *Lutzomyia* flies dwell/rest in deep crevices and deep cracks during daylight. Rodent burrows are suspected habitats for adult and immature stages. Larvae feed upon rodent faeces. Vegetation was sprayed with sugar solution containing *Bacillus sphaericus* and a dye. The number of marked flies entering significantly exceeded the number coming out, suggesting that toxic bait was effective. This method could be used for targeted population. Systemic insecticide-incorporated baits, like ivermectin or spinosad, in rodent burrow have shown cent percent mortality of blood-feeding sandflies with the effect lasting for a week. Another medicine, 'fipronil' in rodent baits produced rodent faeces toxic for coprophagous insects for 21 days.

References

Garcia Quintanilla M, Dichter AA, Guerra H, Kempf VAJ (2019) Review Carrion's disease: more than a neglected disease. Parasit Vectors 12(1):141

Hicks LD, Minnick MF (2020) Human vascular endothelial cells express epithelial growth factor in response to infection by *Bartonella bacilliformis*. PLoS Negl Trop Dis 14(4):e0008236

Minnick MF, Anderson BE, Lima A, Battisti JM et al (2014) Oroya fever and verruga peruana: Bartonelloses unique to South America. PLoSNegl Trop Dis. 8(7):e2919

Pons MJ, Gomes C, Aguilar R, Barrios D et al (2017) Immunosuppressive and angiogenic cytokine profile associated with *Bartonella bacilliformis* infection in post-outbreak and endemic areas of Carrion's disease in Peru. PLoSNegl Trop Dis 11(6):e0005684

Chapter 41
Trench Fever

Synonyms

Five-day fever, Quintan fever (*febris quintana* in Latin), Urban trench fever, Wolhynia fever, Shin bone fever, Meuse fever, His disease and His-Werner disease (after Wilhelm His, Jr. and Heinrich Werner).

Trench fever (occurred among armies' troops in trenches during World War I, hence the name) is a re-emerging disease affecting homeless population in cities in the USA and Europe (Foucault et al. 2006), characterized by chronic bacteraemia, endocarditis, bacillary angiomatosis and lymphadenopathy.

41.1 Aetiology

Bartonella quintana belongs to family *Bartonellaceae*. Old names are *Rochalimaea quintana and Rickettsia quintana*.

    B. quintana is closely related to *Bartonella henselae*, the agent of cat scratch fever, and is transmitted person to person by the body louse, *Pediculus humanus*.

41.2 Epidemiology

B. quintana and *B. bacilliformis* are specifically human pathogens. *B. quintana* infection persists as long as 8 years in infected humans. Huang et al. (2011) brought out evidences that *B. quintana* has other reservoir hosts also and these are rhesus macaques. *B. quintana* was isolated from 2/36 captive rhesus macaques.

© Springer Nature Singapore Pte Ltd. 2024
K. G. Narayan et al., *Handbook of Management of Zoonoses*,
https://doi.org/10.1007/978-981-99-9885-2_41

Further, 12/33 had antibodies. These monkeys had contact with human only and
no ectoparasite was recovered. Detection of *B. quintana* in cat fleas and dental
pulp of cat suggested bacteraemia, and simultaneous isolation from cat and its
owner patient of chronic adenopathy suggested that the mode of transmission was
similar to those of cat scratch fever caused by *B. henselae* (Foucault et al. 2006).
It appears that more studies are required to understand the natural history of
this agent.

Trench fever is prevalent in every continent except Antarctica. The vector is
Pediculus humanus corporis. Its stomach wall carries the bacterium. It is distributed
in Asia, North Africa and Europe. The incidence dropped after World War I, reappeared during World War II and is re-emerging among homeless population in cities
of Europe and America.

Trench fever in Europe affected over 1.0 million soldiers during World War
I. Frequent epidemics of louse-borne relapsing fever (LBRF) occurred in Europe
during the early twentieth century, causing 13 million cases and five million deaths
between 1919 and 1923 in the social upheaval in Russia and Eastern Europe. LBRF
occurs sporadically or as outbreaks in sub-Saharan Africa, particularly in regions
affected by war and in refugee camps. It appears to be endemic in Ethiopia, Sudan,
Eritrea and Somalia. The illness can be severe, with mortality of 1% in treated and
30–70% untreated cases in outbreaks. Epidemic typhus outbreak occurred during
civil war in Burundi. *B. quintana* was isolated from three countries, Congo,
Zimbabwe and Burundi (Roux and Raoult 1999).

The increasing prevalence in the recent years is attributed to a possible emergence of a more virulent strain due to horizontal transfer of gene. Poor living conditions of socially disadvantaged people, especially related to bedding and clothing,
favour the lice. The disease is re-emerging because of the changing social and economic order and unrest. Makeshift arrangement for continuously coming refugees
to European cities in 2015 was associated with the re-emergence. Recrudescence of
body lice is considered to be another factor. Changing living conditions such as
sharing the same accommodation by many who work in shift in factories or call
centre are ascribed.

41.2.1   Vector

Lice are relatively least known pathogens. These are tiny blood suckers. Detection
of a number of bacteria in *Pediculus humanus humanus*, e.g. *B. quintana, Borrelia
recurrentis, R. prowazekii, Serratia marcescens, Acinetobacter baumannii, A. lwoffii,
C. burnetii, R. conorii, R. rickettsii, R. typhi* and *Yersinia pestis,* confirms its role as
vector and role of lice as main vectors of the first three pathogens is significant.

Three types of sucking lice parasitize human: head lice, body lice and carb
(pubic) lice, depending upon specific regions of the body. *Pediculus humanus*
appears in two ecotypes *P. h. capitis* (head louse) and *P. h. humanus* (the body or

clothing louse). *P. h. capitis* live exclusively in the scalp region, lay eggs at the base of hair shaft and are prevalent worldwide among school children causing irritating pruritus.

P. h. humanus are more potent vector than *P. h. capitis*, probably due to larger blood meal. These feed on body regions, females lay and secure eggs to clothing, were common in the past but almost vanishing in the modern times, with exception to poor hygienic conditions of camps under forced conditions of life like camps and jails. *P. h. capitis* also has been increasingly recognized as vectors in poor African countries, the USA and France (Amanzougaghene et al. 2017).

Amanzougaghene et al. (2017) detected in head lice *B. quintana, Coxiella burnetii* and *Rickettsia aeschlimannii* as well as DNA of potential new species of *Anaplasma* and *Ehrlichia* in Mali.

41.2.2   Mode of Infection

There are three mitochondrial clades in genus *Pediculus*, A, B and C. Drali et al. (2015) described the fourth clade, D. This comprised both head lice and body lice. It is considered that clade D may be a vector of *B. quintana* and *Yersinia pestis*. This clade is prevalent in a highly plague-endemic area near Rethy Health District, Orientale Province, Democratic Republic of the Congo.

Pediculus humanus humanus are blood-sucking ectoparasites. It is believed that the body louse is the only recognized vector of louse-borne diseases. The two divergent mitochondrial clades, A and B, exhibit different geographic locations. Louni et al. (2018) studied genetic diversity of body lice collected from homeless individuals in Algeria. *Bartonella quintana, Coxiella burnetii, Anaplasma phagocytophilum* and several species of *Acinetobacter* were detected in human body lice from Algeria.

According to Hou Hamdi et al. (2005), the human louse *Pediculus humanus humanus* is the vector. It lives and multiplies in human clothes. Cold weather and poor hygiene are favourable conditions. The body louse transmits three human pathogens, viz. *Rickettsia prowazekii* (epidemic typhus), *Borrelia recurrentis and Bartonella quintana*. Epidemic typhus invaded Burundi during the civil war after the world war. Relapsing fever occurs in Ethiopia and neighbouring regions after it caused massive outbreaks in Eurasia and Africa. The aetiology of trench fever, bacillary angiomatosis, chronic bacteraemia, endocarditis and lymphadenopathy is re-emerging. *Acinetobacter baumannii* is the fourth pathogen found associated with louse.

The epidemic typhus in Burundi occurred among displaced population living in appalling conditions in camps following the civil war in 1993. The epidemiological study (Raoult et al. 1998) revealed *R. prowazekii* in 75% patients. *B. quintana* infection was established serologically among 13/102 original patients and 19/232 suspected cases. The study concluded that a gigantic outbreak of *R. prowazekii*-caused typhus and *B. quintana*-caused trench fever was continuing.

Sangaré et al. (2014) tested 616 head lice and 424 body lice from nine African countries. *B. quintana* DNA was found in 54% of body lice and in 2% of head lice. *B. quintana*-positive body lice and head lice were more common in poor countries than in wealthy areas. It was suggested that head lice in Africa may be infected by *B. quintana* when patients lived in poor conditions and are also exposed to body lice.

It appears head lice and body lice influence human infection differently. According to Boutellis et al. (2013) body lice have been known to be the vector of *Borrelia recurrentis* since the 1800s and in 2011 they found 23% of head lice from patients with louse-borne relapsing fever were positive for *B. recurrentis* and *B. quintana*. Whether this transmitted infection was yet to be determined.

The human body louse is responsible for person-to-person transmission. The bacteria multiply in the gut of lice that have sucked blood of an infected man. *B. quintana* is present in lice faeces. Infection occurs through the abrasion in the skin caused by scratches in the pruritic area and crushing of lice or at the site of bite.

B. quintana is intra-erythrocytic in a state of prolonged bacteraemia. Non-haemolytic colonization protects against host defences and drugs and is a potential risk of transmission through blood transfusion.

Other potential modes of transmission suggested are cat fleas, monkey fleas and cat dental pulp wherein *B. quintana* has been detected.

Transmission from person to person by head lice is not yet known. Head lice from patients with louse-borne relapsing fever are infected with *B. recurrentis* and *B. quintana*. DNA fragments of *B. quintana* were detected in head lice, *Pediculus humanus capitis* De Geer, and body lice *Pediculus humanus humanus* L in 2006. Both head lice (7%) and body lice (18%) from persons in Ethiopia were positive for *B. quintana* (Sasaki et al. 2006). The study of lice collected from nine African countries detected *B. quintana* DNA in 54% of body lice and 2% of head lice, and it was suggested that head lice may also infect when patients live in poor economic conditions and are also exposed to body lice (Sangaré et al. 2014). Further, *B. quintana* DNA was found in (a) nits and adult head lice, (b) in head lice from homeless children from Nepal where head lice genotype C exists, (c) in lice pools from 138 homeless persons in the San Francisco area and (d) from Ethiopia at altitudes >2121 m only in patients infected with head lice without infected body lice (Angelakis et al. 2011).

41.3   Pathology

The bacterium prefers (tropism) and infects endothelial cells. It is located in red cells during asymptomatic bacteraemia and also in erythroblasts in the bone marrow. It proliferates in cells. Intra-erythrocytic *B. quintana* colonization suppresses apoptosis, releases pro-inflammatory cytokines, increases vascular proliferation and causes lesions protruding in the vascular lumina (bacillary angiomatosis), causing obstruction or even occlusion of blood flow. Lymphadenitis and bacteraemia are the results. Monocytes produce excess of interleukin-10 that weakens the immune response, enabling *B. quintana* to persist. Bacillary angiomatosis is seen commonly among immunocompromised and HIV cases, characterized by the proliferation of blood vessels, resulting in the appearance of tumour-like masses in the skin and other organs (liver, spleen, bone marrow). Chronic lymphadenopathy (e.g. intraparotid granulomatous abscess and lymphadenitis) in both immune-depressed and immunocompetent individuals may also be the case seen with the pathological features of a granulomatous reaction and without fever and/or other symptom/signs (Vitale et al. 2009).

41.4   Symptoms

The incubation period ranges between 5 and 20 days. The onset is sudden acute fever, chill, severe headache, pain in moving eyeball (retro-orbital headache), pain and hyperaesthesia of shins, bone pain, splenomegaly and diaphoresis. Fever is typically '5 days fever', may be relapsing at 5 days interval (so-called quintan fever) and is rarely continuous. It takes long, a month, for recovery. Chronic course lasts several weeks, during which bacteraemia is common; cardiac involvement may complicate the course with insidious onset of endocarditis.

Rashes are less common. Patients die if untreated or develop endocarditis. The disease may end into neurasthenia, myalgia and cardiac disturbance. 'Culture-negative endocarditis' cases are most likely due to this infection.

Trench fever manifests in three forms: (a) *classical relapsing* associated with peritibial (shin) pain, headache and dizziness; (b) *typhoidal showing prolonged fever*, splenomegaly and rash often persistent for months; and (c) *transient maculo-papular rash*, the abortive form of a brief and less intense course (Foucault et al. 2006).

41.5   Diagnosis

- Blood culture
- Serology—IF, immunohistochemical on biopsied tissues like cardiac valve in the cases of endocarditis and skin
- DNA hybridization, restriction fragment length polymorphism, Western blot and PCR

41.6   Treatment

Erythromycin, doxycycline and azithromycin may be useful.

41.7   Prevention

Alleviation of poverty, social and personal hygiene and home hygiene.

References

Amanzougaghene N, Fenollar F, SangareÂ AK, Sissoko MS et al (2017) Detection of bacterial pathogens including potential new species in human head lice from Mali. PLoS One 12(9):e0184621

Angelakis A, Diatta G, Abdissa A, Trape JF, Mediannikov O et al (2011) Altitude-dependent Bartonella quintana genotype C in Head lice, Ethiopia. Emerg Infect Dis 17(12):2357–2359

Boutellis A, Mediannikov O, Bilcha KD, Ali J et al (2013) *Borrelia recurrentis* in head lice, Ethiopia. Emerg Infect Dis 19(5):796–798

Drali R, Shako JC, Davoust B, Diatta G, Raoult D (2015) A new clade of African body and head lice infected by *Bartonella quintana* and *Yersinia pestis*—Democratic Republic of the Congo. Am J Trop Med Hyg 2015(93):990–993

Foucault C, Brouqui P, Raoult D (2006) *Bartonella quintana* characteristics and clinical management. Emerg Infect Dis 12(2):217–223

Hou Hamdi L, Parola P, Raoult D (2005) Lice and lice-borne diseases in humans. Med Trop (Mars) 55(1):13–23

Huang R, Liu Q, Li G, Li D, Song X, Birtles RJ et al (2011) *Bartonella quintana* infections in captive monkeys, China. Emerg Infect Dis 17(9):1707–1709

Louni M, Mana N, Bitam I, Dahmani M, Parola P, Fenollar F et al (2018) Body lice of homeless people reveal the presence of several emerging bacterial pathogens in northern Algeria. PLoS Negl Trop Dis 12(4):e0006397

Raoult D, Ndihkubwayo JB, Tissot-Dupont H, Roux V et al (1998) Outbreak of epidemic typhus associated with trench fever in Burundi. Lancet 352(9125):353–358

Roux V, Raoult D (1999) Body lice as tools for diagnosis and surveillance of reemerging diseases. J Clin Microbiol 37(3):596–599

Sangaré AK, Boutellis A, Drali R, Socolovschi C, Barker SC et al (2014) Detection of *Bartonella quintana* in African body and head lice. Am J Trop Med Hyg. 91(2):294–301

Sasaki T, Poudel SK, Isawa H, Hayashi T, Seki N et al (2006) First molecular evidence of *Bartonella quintana* in *Pediculus humanus capitis* (Phthiraptera: Pediculidae), collected from Nepalese children. J Medl Entomol 43(1):110–112

Vitale G, Incandela S, Incandela C, Micalizzi A, Mansueto P (2009) Isolation and characterization of *Bartonella quintana* from the parotid gland of an immunocompetent man. J Clin Microbiol 47(3):862–864

Chapter 42
Brucellosis

Synonyms

Remitting fever, Undulant fever, Mediterranean fever, Maltese fever, Gibraltar fever, Crimean fever, Goat fever, and Bang disease.

Brucellosis is a direct occupational anthropozoonosis characterized by insidious onset of bouts of irregular fever over a period of weeks and months which are not pathognomonic (Maxwell and Bill 2008). It is a chronic disease, considered as pyrexia of unknown aetiology. Remissions are common and hence it is also known as *undulant fever*.

Brucellosis is one of the most ancient and widespread bacterial zoonoses with global, economic and public health significance (Akpınar 2016; Sayer 2016). It is one of the world's major zoonoses, a threat to livestock economy due to abortion, loss of offspring, infertility and reduced milk yield, leading to cause a serious reduction in the availability of quality food, especially the animal proteins.

Human and animal brucellosis remains endemic in many parts of the world, including Spain, the Middle East, Latin America and Asia (Pappas et al. 2006). It is endemic with high prevalence rates in the Middle East, the Mediterranean Basin (Portugal, Spain, Italy, Greece, Turkey, the Near East, North Africa), South and Central America, Southeastern Europe, Asia, Africa and the Caribbean (Godfroid et al. 2005).

While a number of industrialized countries have successfully controlled *B. abortus* infection in domestic animals, *B. melitensis* infection in bovines has emerged as a threat to public health.

42.1 Aetiology

The causative agent was first isolated from the spleen of soldiers inflicted with relapsing fever in 1887 by Sir David Bruce, who named it *Micrococcus melitensis*. It was later renamed as *Brucella melitensis* in his honour. But the zoonotic nature

© Springer Nature Singapore Pte Ltd. 2024
K. G. Narayan et al., *Handbook of Management of Zoonoses*,
https://doi.org/10.1007/978-981-99-9885-2_42

was demonstrated in 1905 by Zammit by isolating *B. melitensis* from milk of goat in Malta (Zammit 1905).

Brucella are Gram-negative coccobacilli belonging to the family *Brucellaceae* together with *Ochrobactrum* spp., their closest phylogenetic relatives. This family belongs to the order *Rhizobiales*, which contain several genera of plant-associated alpha Proteobacteria (Whatmore 2009).

At present, the genus *Brucella* has 12 species divided into six classical species with 15 biovars based on host preference and phenotypic differences and six recently discovered species (Table 42.1). The species are *Brucella abortus* (cattle; biovars: 1–6, 9), *B. melitensis* (sheep, goat; biovars: 1–3), *B. suis* (pig, hare; biovars: 1–5), *B. canis* (dog), *B. ovis* (sheep, goat) and *B. neotomae* (desert rat). Interestingly, *B. ovis* and *B. neotomae* have never been associated with human infection.

The concept of host restriction of different *Brucella* species is gradually eluding as reports from Brazil and Columbia show that *B. suis* biovar 1 has become established in cattle, thus becoming a more important reservoir than pigs. Congruently *B. melitensis* infection in cattle is emerging as an impending threat in some southern European countries, Israel, Kuwait and Saudi Arabia. *B. melitensis* infection is particularly problematic as *B. abortus* vaccines do not protect effectively against *B. melitensis* infection and *B. melitensis* Rev. 1 vaccine has not been fully evaluated

Table 42.1 Year of isolation of different species of *Brucella*

S. no.	Species	Host	Year of isolation	Reference
1.	*B. abortus*	Cattle	1897	Bang (1897)
2.	*B. melitensis*	Sheep/goat	1887	
3.	*B. suis*	Swine	1914	Traum (1914)
4.	*B. ovis*	Sheep	1953	Buddle and Boyes (1953); Simmons and Hall (1953)
5.	*B. canis*	Canine	1968	Carmichael and Bruner (1968)
6.	*B. neotomae*	Desert wood rat	1957	Stoenner and Lackman (1957)
7.	*B. ceti*	Cetacea	2007	Foster et al. (2007)
8.	*B. pinnipedialis*	Pinnipeds	2007	Foster et al. (2007)
9.	*B. microti*	Voles	2009	Audic et al. (2009)
10.	*B. inopinata*	Human breast implant	2010	Scholz et al. (2010)
11.	*B. papionis*	Stillbirth in baboons		Whatmore et al. (2014)
12.	*B. vulpis*	Red foxes	2016	Scholz et al. (2016)
Atypical isolates				
13.	*B. inopinata*-like strain BO2	Chronic pneumonia in a human patient	2010	Tiller et al. (2010a)
14.	Strains isolated from wild rodents	Rodents	2010	Tiller et al. (2010b)
Atypical isolates from non-mammalian host				
1.	Big-eyed tree frog	*Leptopelis vermiculatus*		Fischer et al. (2012)
2.	African bullfrogs	*Pyxicephalus edulis*		Eisenberg et al. (2012)
3.	White's tree frog	*Litoria caerulea*	2015	Whatmore et al. (2015)

for use in cattle. Seropositivity is intermittently expressed by infected animals with huge individual and seasonal variations on incubation period and seroconversion. Infected individuals can spontaneously recover, develop a chronic form or relapse. Although vertical transmission is known to exist, only a small proportion ($\approx$5% in cattle) of the infected offspring remains infected until the first delivery.

42.2   Sources

Traditionally said to be associated with domestic (cattle, sheep, goat, dog, camel, horse, etc.) and wild animals, it has recently been reported to be associated with marine mammals with zoonotic implications (Olsen and Palmer 2014). Presence of brucellae in soil, foxes and bats has been recently indicated.

42.3   Transmission

Primarily a disease of animals, brucellosis is transmitted to humans accidentally by contact with vaginal discharges and foetal fluids or by ingestion of infected animals' products such as unpasteurized milk and their products with protean symptoms. Careless handling of *Brucella* culture in the laboratory may lead to infection. The bacteria may enter through the conjunctival mucosa and even intact skin. Human-to-human infection does not occur.

42.4   Infection: Pathology

Brucella do not express classical virulence factors/markers, such as exotoxins, endotoxic lipopolysaccharide (LPS), cytolysins, capsules, fimbria, plasmids, lysogenic phages, drug-resistant forms and antigenic variation (Moreno and Moriyón 2002; Seleem et al. 2008).

Brucellae have been shown to replicate within the professional as well as non-professional phagocytes (Atluri et al. 2011) with pronounced tropism for genital organs of sexually mature animals causing orchitis, epididymitis and infertility in males besides abortion and infertility in females (Moreno and Moriyón 2006). Such genital tropism is also seen in man, where they cause epididymo-orchitis and infect the placenta even though rarely implicated in abortion (Anderson et al. 1986). Sexual secretions and abortion materials do contain a huge number of *Brucella* organisms to contaminate the environment causing transmission directly or indirectly, emphasizing importance of their localization and fierce multiplication inside the reproductive tract in their biology (Letteson et al. 2017). Though genital tropism is known since long, the exact reasons for the underlying genital tropism and multiplication are still elusive. Considering their nature, *Brucella* has better been described as intracellular facultative extra-cellular bacteria (Moreno and Moriyón 2002) instead of facultative intracellular bacteria. True to its nature, *Brucella* has also been referred to as a stealthy bacterium (Barquero-Calvo et al. 2007; Martirosyan et al. 2011; Waqas et al. 2016).

42.5 Infection in Human

Most cases in humans are caused by contact with infected animals or ingestion of animal products, such as unpasteurized milk and cheese prepared from infected unpasteurized milk (Pappas et al. 2005).

An occupational direct zoonosis, incidence of human brucellosis is much higher among rural population living in close association of animals. Humans get infection accidentally (Corbel 2006) and brucellosis in man is not considered contagious, rather man is supposed to be a dead-end-host (Ducrotoy et al. 2017; Mandal et al. 2017). Less than 10% of human cases of brucellosis may be recognized and reported (Wise 1980), primarily because of misleading clinical symptoms (Young 1983; Corbel 1997). The incidence/prevalence among humans has a direct correlation with the incidence and prevalence of infection in animals. A single case of human brucellosis is indicative of endemicity of disease in the region—man acts as sentinel for brucellosis in livestock. For every case in human, 15 cases in small ruminants and 150 cases in cattle are estimated (Zinsstag et al. 2005).

42.5.1 Human Brucellosis

Brucellosis is a multisystem disease. Brucellae can get distributed to almost any organ of the body with osteoarticular symptoms, the most common complication. Brucellosis in man has low mortality even in non-treated cases with majority of deaths due to endocarditis (Alici et al. 2014). Resistance to rifampicin and co-trimoxazole in both human and animal isolates of *Brucella* is a cause for concern, necessitating the use of antibiotic sensitivity tests for *Brucella* isolates in endemic areas (Lalsangzuala et al. 2020).

The incubation period for brucellosis is highly variable, usually 5–60 days, but it can be as long as several months or more. It causes systemic febrile illness in humans which runs an acute or chronic course. The onset is gradual. There are weakness, malaise and moderate rise in temperature. Although the patient is ill enough to be bedfast, he does not appear critically ill and often feels well on arising but worsens as the day progresses.

Brucellosis presents an extensive trail of symptoms: indigestion, diarrhoea and constipation and headache. There are insomnia, profuse sweating (sweat of peculiar and disagreeable odour) especially at night, loss of weight, generalized body ache, etc. often confused with typhoid and influenza. Gums are spongy and bleed easily during acute and chronic phase. Joints are sore and painful, and the most affected joints are hip, knee, ankle and shoulder.

Pulmonary symptoms like bronchitis and pneumonia may be seen in some, bronchitis persisting for long. Complications include epistaxis, pleurisy with effusion, hepatosplenomegaly, endocarditis, spondylitis and orchitis.

Swelling of testes and burning micturition due to orchitis and urethritis, respectively, are also peculiar symptoms of the disease in man (Smits and Kadri 2005). The presence of neurological symptoms, subcutaneous nodules, headache, stiff neck and photophobia were also reported. Brucellosis in man may be classified into three different phases: acute (initial, 2 months), sub-acute (2–12 months) and chronic (more than 12 months) (González-Espinoza et al. 2021).

Worldwide millions of individuals are at risk, especially in countries where infection in animals is endemic and has not been brought under control, pasteurization of milk is not practised and hygiene in animal husbandry is poor.

42.5.2   Brucellosis in Animals

In animals, the disease is characterized by abortion in the last trimester, stillbirth and reproductive problems.

In cattle, *B. abortus* causes abortion, stillbirth and weak calves with abortions usually occurring during the third trimester of gestation. In 75%–90% of cases, infected cows abort only once. Few of the heifers born to *Brucella*-infected dams become latent carriers and are serologically detected only at their first calving (Plommet et al. 1973). The exact mechanism enabling *Brucella* to cause latent infection is unknown (Blasco and Molina-Flores 2011). Infection persists for long, often lifelong. Brucellae multiply and localize intracellularly in monocytes and reticuloendothelial cells, causing little harm to the hosts. Such animals remain a serious threat to control and eradication programme.

Clinical forms are placentitis and abortion, urogenital infection and mastitis and *Brucella* exit in massive number, transmission occurs. Large numbers of brucellae are shed in uterine discharges starting 1 week before abortion or during parturition and continue for a month. Subsequent shedding is intermittent for weeks. Brucellae are shed in milk continuously or intermittently throughout lactation.

Testicular abscesses are sometimes seen in bulls. Arthritis can develop after long-term infections. In sheep and goats, *B. melitensis* can cause abortion, retained placenta, orchitis and epididymitis. Abortions usually occur late in gestation in sheep and during the fourth month of gestation in goats. There is no evidence that the clinical features of *B. melitensis* infection in sheep and goats vary according to the biovar involved (Fensterbank 1987). In pigs, the most common symptom is abortion (any time during gestation) and weak or stillborn piglets. Temporary or permanent orchitis may be seen in boars. Boars can also excrete *B. suis* asymptomatically in the semen and sterility may be the only sign of infection. Swollen joints and tendon sheaths or lameness can occur in both sexes. In horses, *B. abortus* and occasionally *B. suis* can cause inflammation of the supra-spinous or supra-atlantal bursa, respectively, known as 'fistulous withers' or 'poll evil'. The bursal sac becomes distended by a clear, viscous, straw-coloured exudate and develops a thickened wall. *Brucella*-associated abortions are rare in horses. *B. canis* causes abortions, stillbirths and infertility in bitches. Most infections are seen in kennels.

Among wild animals, hare and rodents are infected by *B. suis* biotype 2 and *B. suis* biotype 3, respectively. *B. suis* biotype 4 from caribou can infect human and sled dogs. Mink and silver foxes get infected while feeding on infected viscera and foetus and are likely to transmit it to humans.

42.6 Epidemiology

The epidemiology of brucellosis has undergone sea change over the past decades globally. Brucellosis is a major health problem in the Mediterranean, Middle East, India, Latin America, Africa, parts of Mexico and parts of Asia. Syria has the highest annual incidence worldwide, reaching an alarming 1603 cases per million per year (Godfroid et al. 2013). It is prevalent mostly in low- and middle-income countries in the Mediterranean Basin, the Middle East and Central Asian countries (Dean et al. 2012a). Brucellosis continues to be an important public health concern in developed countries as well (Rubach et al. 2013).

The disease remains a serious concern in low-income under-developed countries where most human cases are seen besides huge economic loss to the livestock industry (Dean et al. 2012a, b; Rubach et al. 2013). Brucellosis has an adverse impact on livelihood of poor people in endemic regions due to chronic disability in man and lowered productivity of livestock. New cases result from direct contact with membranes and secretions, when other animals contact with expelled birth tissues from infected animals (Refai 2002).

Incidence of brucellosis varies widely between countries as well as within countries, which is influenced by demographic, occupational and socioeconomic factors (Dean et al. 2012b). An estimated 500,000 human infections per year occur worldwide. Brucellosis has been reported by 93 countries with incidence varying from <1/100,000 population in the UK, USA and Australia to >20–30/100,000 in southern European countries such as Greece and Spain and up to >70/100,000 in Middle Eastern countries like Kuwait and Saudi Arabia (Godfroid et al. 2013; Pappas et al. 2006; Pappas 2010).

Brucellosis causes huge economic losses in countries where it is endemic and is grossly underestimated. However, a conservative estimate of the economic impact of bovine brucellosis has been estimated at US$ 32 million, 23.5 million and 60 million in Brazil (Poester et al. 2002), Paraguay (Veirano 2001) and Argentina (Samartino 2002), respectively. In India, brucellosis costs around Rs. 350 million in the form of food, animal and labour losses (Kunen 1994) and about three million man-days annually (Patel et al. 1986). Earlier, Schwabe (1984) reported its impact on the national economy of India to the tune of Rs. 240 million annually due to cattle and buffalo brucellosis. Most recently, brucellosis in livestock has been shown to be responsible for a median loss of US$ 3.4 billion ≈ Rs. 22,000 crores (Singh et al. 2015).

Only 17 countries claim to be free of brucellosis. Brucellosis-free status has been granted by the European Union (EU) to Sweden, Denmark, Finland, Germany, the UK (excluding Northern Ireland), Austria, Netherlands, Belgium and Luxembourg. Norway and Switzerland are also considered brucellosis-free (Godfroid et al. 2002). Brucellosis has been re-emerging in many parts of the world like in Israel, Kuwait, Saudi Arabia, Brazil and Columbia (Seleem et al. 2010).

42.6.1   Role of Animals

Four possibilities of epizootics and spread of brucellosis are:

- Epizootic confined to wildlife as *B. neotomae* in desert wood rats in Utah.
- Wildlife may be infected from domestic animals, but infection is not sustained.
- Domestic animals ⇌ wildlife, e.g. *B. abortus* biotype 1 to and from American bison and elk.
- Wildlife may be the primary source—spreading to domestic animals like *B. suis* biotype 2 from European hare to domestic swine in Central and Western Europe.

Epidemiology of brucellosis in domestic animals is particularly influenced by a variety of *host factors, such as unvaccinated animals, herd size, population density, age, sexual maturity and use of maternity pens*. Replacement animals in large dairy herd are often a particular risk of getting infection if an infected animal is purchased.

Brucellae are sensitive to direct sunlight, disinfectant and pasteurization. However, aborted foetuses are left within reach of livestock, carnivores and humans. Scavenging animals like dogs and jackals may mechanically spread infection to distant location. Expansion of livestock industries with poor adoption of scientific methods of animal husbandry coupled with continued traditional practices contributes to brucellosis in domestic animals (Nicoletti 1980). Congregations and movement of animals such as animal fare, local, national and international trade contribute to infection and spread.

Co-husbandry of two species of domestic animals presents a possibility of interspecies transmission or even contamination of animal produce, e.g. cow's milk may get contaminated with *B. suis*.

Occupational—Veterinarians, farmers and laboratory workers are at risk.

Habit/faith/custom—Raw (unboiled or pasteurized) milk is considered healthier and having medicinal value by some. Malta fever occurred due to ingestion of infected raw milk.

Standards of hygiene—Personal and environmental, processing of milk and its products.

Season—Incidence rates are influenced with birthing season of cows, she-goats and ewes.

In India, the disease has been reported to be endemic (Smits and Kadri 2005) particularly in areas with high rainfall and humidity (Mathur 1968) with varying prevalence among animals and man in different states of the country (Boral et al. 2009).

42.7   Diagnosis

Diagnosis of brucellosis has never been easy. It is impossible to determine which species of *Brucella* has induced antibodies against sLPS (smooth LPS) in the host, and, thus, *the gold standard in brucellosis diagnosis is the isolation of the bacteria.*

Isolation and identification of *Brucella* is tedious with highly varying success (Ray 1979). A sound strategy is first to estimate the apparent prevalence of brucellosis by serology and then attempt to isolate the bacteria from a selected subset of samples.

The available serological tests are not able to effectively detect infected animals in all phases of the infection or are not suitable for use under different epidemiological settings (Kittelberger et al. 1997). The most used serological tests are the serum agglutination test (SAT), Rose Bengal test (RBT), complement fixation test (CFT) and enzyme-linked immunosorbent assay (ELISA) (Al Dahouk et al. 2003). All tests have limitations concerning specificity and sensitivity, especially when testing individual animals. RBPT has been recommended as a screening test with CFT and ELISA as confirmatory tests (OIE 2016). In the case of dairy herds, milk ring test (MRT) has been successfully used to detect the *Brucella*-infected herd. Alternative diagnostic approaches include DNA amplification and detection methods, but the effectiveness of such approaches on readily available material such as blood, serum, swabs and milk has yet to be fully evaluated and existing information is conflicting.

42.8   Treatment

Treatment of brucellosis in animals is not recommended by the OIE. In the cases of human brucellosis, a combination of two drugs should be used for the treatment since use of antibiotic singly results in more cases of relapse. The recommended treatment of uncomplicated brucellosis in adults is doxycycline 100 mg twice daily with rifampin 600–900 mg daily orally for 6 weeks. Rifampicin can be replaced with streptomycin 1 g daily intramuscularly for 2–3 weeks or gentamicin (5 mg/kg) daily parenterally in 1 dose for 7–14 days (Ariza et al. 2007).

Alternatively, fluoroquinolones (ciprofloxacin and ofloxacin) can be used to treat acute uncomplicated cases of brucellosis along with rifampin or doxycycline in place of doxycycline-rifampin combination. The children and pregnant women are treated with trimethoprim-sulfamethoxazole in combination with rifampin as drug of choice. Cases of relapse are treated successfully with the same regimens.

42.9   Prevention and Control

Human brucellosis is acquired from domestic animals, mainly cattle, sheep and goats, and their produce, milk and milk products. Protecting human from *Brucella* infection lies in eliminating infection from animals (Olsen 2013; Pappas et al. 2006). Vaccines are effective.

42.9.1   Vaccines

Live attenuated brucellosis vaccines have been available for protecting domestic livestock against *B. melitensis* and *B. abortus* for decades. Current vaccines are effective in preventing abortion and transmission of brucellosis, but poor at preventing infection or seroconversion. In addition, they can induce abortions in pregnant animals and are infectious to humans.

Although they have been a valuable tool for reducing the prevalence of brucellosis in natural hosts and eradicating the disease, the available vaccines have many shortcomings, which include:

- Production of antibodies which is difficult to be distinguished from natural infection
- Have potential to induce human infection
- Can induce abortions in pregnant animals
- A limited ability to prevent infection and seroconversion after continued exposure

Over the years, a wide variety of killed vaccines have been developed for protection against brucellosis. They have had limited acceptance and success. None have approached the protection levels afforded by the live attenuated vaccines. Killed vaccines developed are *B. abortus* strain 45/20 and *B. melitensis* H38. *B. abortus* strain 45/20 was used in cattle and sheep, while *B. melitensis* H38 was tested in mice and cows. In addition to the lack of desired protection, killed vaccines such as strains 45/20 and H38 induced persistent antibody titres.

Many antigenic fractions of *Brucella* have been examined as vaccine candidates, with or without adjuvant(s), but none have seen the light of day to replace the conventional live attenuated vaccines.

42.9.2   Current Vaccines Against Brucellosis

In endemic areas, vaccination has been found to be the most economic measure for control of brucellosis. When sanitary and animal movement control is also put in place, the effect is increased many folds. It also minimizes economic losses due to the abortion, infertility and weak offspring and decreased milk production.

Brucellosis vaccines are highly effective in decreasing transmission and production losses, but less effective at preventing infection by field strains (Olsen and Stoffregen 2005). Young (4–8 months) female calves are vaccinated by a single intramuscular or subcutaneous injection. However, in areas of high prevalence of brucellosis with no or little movement control, mass vaccination, including adult cows, is required. Males are not vaccinated since it can cause tissue damage in male genital tract.

Currently, there are two live attenuated vaccines for the control of *B. abortus* infection in cattle: *B. abortus* strain 19 (S19) and *B. abortus* RB51 (OIE 2009). *B. abortus* strain 45/20—a rough strain—was used as a heat-killed vaccine with an adjuvant in some European countries; however, because of variability in protection, unpredictable serological response and occurrence of reactions at the site of vaccine injection in some animals led to discontinuation of this vaccine (Dorneles et al. 2015).

The strain *B. abortus* S19, isolated in the early twentieth century and attenuated naturally after virulent culture was left at room temperature for 1 year (Thomas et al. 1981), has been effective in the control of brucellosis in adult bovines. It prevents abortion and decrease prevalence in herds. A low rate of abortion in livestock and reduction in milk production has been reported with *B. abortus* S19 vaccination.

In calves (3–6 months), S19 vaccination can be performed with full dose $(5–8 \times 10^{10}$ viable organisms). Vaccination of adult cattle with low dosage S19 $(3 \times 10^8$ to 3×10^9 organisms) can be done in infected herds (OIE 2016). However, vaccination of pregnant animals can cause abortion (Dorneles et al. 2015).

The live vaccine *B. abortus* RB51 is a laboratory-derived rough mutant obtained by serial passage of the virulent *B. abortus* 2308 in the presence of rifampicin and penicillin (Schurig et al. 1991). RB51 does not induce a positive response in typical serological diagnostic test. Effectiveness of RB51 and absence of side effects remain controversial especially under situations of high endemicity (Moriyon et al. 2004; Blasco and Moriyon 2010).

In small ruminants, live attenuated *B. melitensis* Rev. 1—developed by Herzberg and Elberg in the mid-1950s—is used to control brucellosis (OIE 2016). It is given by subcutaneous or conjunctival route. Like *B. abortus* S19, *B. melitensis* Rev. 1 also induces a positive antibody response in vaccinated animals and can infect humans. The vaccination is recommended prior to the first gestation between 3 and 7 months of age to avoid abortion in pregnant animals (OIE 2016).

A live attenuated *B. suis* strain 2 vaccine has been extensively used in several animal species in China (Xie 1986) with no persistent antibodies. An orally administrable brucellosis vaccine, *B. suis* strain 2 vaccine is claimed to produce effective immunity in sheep, goats, cattle and pigs.

42.10   Control and Eradication

In animals, brucellosis control or eradication programmes are generally based on combinations of sanitation, isolation, vaccination and test and removal programmes, depending on economic resources. In general, vaccination is the most economical approach for preventing brucellosis in domestic livestock. A prevalence level of ≤2% achieved by vaccination is considered 'brucellosis has been controlled'.

The basic principles for eradication are (a) checking the introduction of infected animals into healthy flocks/herds, (b) vaccination of young replacement stock and (c) test and slaughter of seropositive animals. Continued for at least one generation usually leads to attaining a '*Brucella*-free' status.

Although expensive, control and eradication programmes have a highly positive cost-benefit ratio with benefit to both public health and livestock sectors. In Mongolia, with high prevalence of brucellosis, the cost-benefit ratio for mass vaccination against brucellosis was estimated to be 3.2 (Roth et al. 2003). Similarly, in the Czech Republic, it was estimated that the cumulative benefit/eradication cost ratio was 7:1 (Kouba 2003). The major benefits are financial due to improved productivity of livestock and savings in health costs for human treatment and hospitalization.

A sustained vaccination of animals is required with proper permanent identification for the control of movement particularly before sale or purchase. The vaccination should cover at least ≥80% of the population.

Calf-hood vaccination is not very useful in areas where the prevalence of brucellosis is high and animal movement not controlled. Development of herd immunity takes a long time. Mass vaccination of livestock should be the first option.

References

Akpınar O (2016) Historical perspective of brucellosis: a microbiological and epidemiological overview. Infez Med 24(1):77–86

Al Dahouk S, Tomaso H, Nockler K, Neubauer H, Frangoulidis D (2003) Laboratory-based diagnosis of brucellosis—a review of the literature. Part II: Serological tests for brucellosis. Clin Lab 49:577–589

Alici H, Ercan S, Davutoglu V (2014) *Brucella* infective endocarditis. Cor et Vasa 56(5):e433–e435

Anderson TD, Cheville NF, Meador VP (1986) Pathogenesis of placentitis in the goat inoculated with *Brucella abortus*. II. Ultrastructural studies. Vet Pathol 23(3):227–239

Ariza J, Bosilkovski M, Cascio A, Colmenero JD, Corbel MJ et al (2007) Perspectives for the treatment of brucellosis in the 21st century: the Ioannina recommendations. PLoS Med 4:e317

Atluri VL, Xavier MN, de Jong MF, den Hartigh AB, Tsolis RM (2011) Interactions of the human pathogenic *Brucella* species with their hosts. Ann Rev Microbiol 65:523–541

Audic S, Lescot M, Claverie JM, Scholz HC (2009) *Brucella microti*: the genome sequence of an emerging pathogen. BMC Genomics 10:352

Bang B (1897) The etiology of epizootic abortion. J Comp Pathol 10:125–149

Barquero-Calvo E, Chaves-Olarte E, Weiss DS, Guzma'n-Verri C, Chaco'n-Dı'az C et al (2007) *Brucella abortus* uses a stealthy strategy to avoid activation of the innate immune system during the onset of infection. PLoS ONE 2(7):e631

Blasco JM, Molina-Flores B (2011) Control and eradication of *Brucella melitensis* infection in sheep and goats. Vet Clin N Am Food Anim Pract 27:95–104

Blasco JM, Moriyon I (2010) Eradication of bovine brucellosis in the Azores, Portugal-outcome of a 5-year programme (2002–2007) based on test-and-slaughter and RB51 vaccination. Prev Vet Med 94:154–157

Boral R, Singh M, Singh DK (2009) Status and strategies for control of brucellosis—a review. Indian J Anim Sci 79(12):1191–1199

Buddle MB, Boyes BW (1953) A *Brucella* mutant causing genital disease of sheep in New Zealand. Aust Vet J 29:145–153

Carmichael LE, Bruner DW (1968) Characteristics of a newly recognized species of *Brucella* responsible for infectious canine abortions. Cornell Vet 48(4):579–592

Corbel MJ (1997) Brucellosis: an overview. Emerg Infect Dis 3:213–221

Corbel MJ (2006) Brucellosis in humans and animals. WHO Press, World Health Organization, Geneva

Dean AS, Crump L, Greter H, Schelling E, Zinsstag J (2012a) Global burden of human brucellosis: a systematic review of disease frequency. PLoS Negl Trop Dis 6(10):e1865

Dean AS, Crump L, Greter H, Hattendorf J, Schelling E, Zinsstag J (2012b) Clinical manifestations of human brucellosis: a systematic review and meta-analysis. PLoS Negl Trop Dis 6(12):e1929

Dorneles EM, Sriranganathan N, Lage AP (2015) Recent advances in *Brucella abortus* vaccines. Vet Res 46(1):76

Ducrotoy M, Bertu WJ, Matope G, Cadmus S, Conde-Álvarez R et al (2017) Brucellosis in sub-Saharan Africa: current challenges for management, diagnosis, and control. Acta Trop 165:179–193

Eisenberg T, Hamann HP, Kaim U, Schlez K, Seeger H et al (2012) Isolation of potentially novel *Brucella* spp. from frogs. Appl Environ Microbiol 78(10):3753–3755

Fensterbank R (1987) Some aspects of experimental bovine brucellosis. Ann Res Vet 18:421–428

Fischer D, Lorenz N, Heuser W, Kämpfer P, Scholz HC, Lierz M (2012) Abscesses associated with a *Brucella inopinata*-like bacterium in a big-eyed tree frog (*Leptopelis vermiculatus*). J Zoo Wildl Med 43(3):625–628

Foster G, Osterman BS, Godfroid J, Jacques I, Cloeckaert A (2007) *Brucella ceti* sp. nov. and *Brucella pinnipedialis* sp. nov. for *Brucella* strains with cetaceans and seals as their preferred hosts. Int J Syst Evol Microbiol 57(Pt 11):2688–2693

Godfroid J, Saegerman C, Wellemans V, Walravens K, Letesson JJ et al (2002) How to substantiate eradication of bovine brucellosis when a specific serological reactions occur in the course of brucellosis testing. Vet Microbiol 90(1–4):461–477

Godfroid J, Cloeckaert A, Liautard JP, Kohler S, Fretin D et al (2005) From the discovery of the Malta fever's agent to the discovery of a marine mammal reservoir, brucellosis has continuously been a re-emerging zoonosis. Vet Res 36(3):313–326

Godfroid J, Garin-Bastuji B, Saegerman C, Blasco JM (2013) Brucellosis in terrestrial wildlife. Rev Sci Tech 32:27–42

González-Espinoza G, Arce-Gorvel V, Mémet S, Gorvel JP (2021) *Brucella*: reservoirs and niches in animals and humans. Pathogens 10:186

Kittelberger R, Reichel MP, Joyce MA, Staak C (1997) Serological cross reactivity between *Brucella abortus* and *Yersinia enterocolitica* 0:9 III. Specificity of the in vitro antigen-specific gamma interferon test for bovine brucellosis diagnosis in experimentally *Yersinia enterocolitica* 0:9-infected cattle. Vet Microbiol 57(4):361–371

Kouba V (2003) A method of accelerated eradication of bovine brucellosis in The Czech Republic. Rev Sci Tech 22(3):1003–1012

Kunen AV (1994) Brucellosis. In: Kunen A (ed) Infectious diseases, diagnosis and management in clinical practice. CBS Publishers, New Delhi, pp 448–449

Lalsangzuala C, Sinha DK, Kuma MS, Singh DK et al (2020) Antimicrobial susceptibility testing of *Brucella* spp. isolated from livestock and human in India. J Vet Pub Hlth 18(1):10–14

Letteson JJ, Barbier T, Zúñiga-Ripa A, Godfroid J et al (2017) *Brucella* genital tropism: what's on the menu. Front Microbiol 8:506

Mandal SS, Duncombe L, Ganesh NV, Sarkar S et al (2017) Novel solutions for vaccines and diagnostics to combat brucellosis. ACS Cent Sci 3(3):224–231

Martirosyan A, Moreno E, Gorvel JP (2011) An evolutionary strategy for a stealthy intracellular *Brucella* pathogen. Immunol Rev 240(1):211–234

Mathur TN (1968) The epidemiology of human brucellosis in Haryana with regard to 215 strains of *Brucella* isolated from man and animals. Indian J Pathol Bacteriol 11(4):244–248

Maxwell JR, Bill DE (2008) Developing a brucellosis public health information and awareness campaign in Iraq. Mil Med 173(1):79–84

Moreno E, Moriyón I (2002) *Brucella melitensis*: a nasty bug with hidden credentials for virulence. Proc Natl Acad Sci USA 99:1–3

Moreno E, Moriyón I (2006) The genus *Brucella*. In: Dworkin M, Falkow S, Rosenberg E, Schleifer K-H, Stackebrant E (eds) The prokaryotes, vol 5 Part 1, Section 31. Springer-Verlag, New York, pp 315–456

Moriyon I, Grillo JM, Monreal D, Gonzalez D, Marin C et al (2004) Rough vaccines in animal brucellosis: structural and genetic basis and present status. Vet Res 35:1–38

Nicoletti P (1980) The epidemiology of bovine brucellosis. Adv Vet Sci Comp Med 24:69–98

OIE (2009) Bovine brucellosis. Manual of diagnostic tests and vaccines for terrestrial animals. World Organisation for Animal Health

OIE (2016) Infection with Brucella abortus, *B. melitensis* and *B. suis*. Chapter 2.1.4—OIE. In: Manual of diagnostic tests and vaccines for terrestrial animals. OIE, Paris, France

Olsen SC (2013) Recent developments in livestock and wildlife brucellosis vaccination. Rev Sci Tech 32(1):207–217

Olsen SC, Palmer MV (2014) Advancement of knowledge of *Brucella* over the past 50 years. Vet Pathol 51(6):1076–1089

Olsen SC, Stoffregen WS (2005) Essential role of vaccines in brucellosis control and eradication programs for livestock. Expert Rev Vaccines 4:915–928

Pappas G (2010) The changing Brucella ecology: novel reservoirs, new threats. Int J Antimicro Agents 36(Suppl 1):S8–S11

Pappas G, Aknitidis N, Bosilkovski M, Tsianos E (2005) Brucellosis. N Engl J Med 352:2325–2336

Pappas G, Papadimitriou P, Akritidis N, Christou L, Tsianos EV (2006) The new global map of human brucellosis. Lancet Infect Dis 6:91–99

Patel PR, Anjaria JM, Dave MR, Desai H (1986) Serological evidence of brucellosis in human beings in Kaira district of Gujarat. Indian J Public Hlth 30:197–200

Plommet M, Fensterbank R, Renoux G, Gestin J, Philippon A, Experimental bovine brucellosis. XII. (1973) Persistence to adult age of congenital infection in the heifer. Ann Rech Vet 4:419–435

Poester F P, Gonc‚ Alves VSP, Lage AP. Brucellosis in Brazil. Vet Microbiol 2002; 90 (1–4): 55–62

Ray WC (1979) Brucellosis (due to *Brucella abortus* and *B. suis*). In: Steel JH (ed) Handbook series in zoonosis, vol 1. CRC Press, Baca Raton, FL, pp 99–185

Refai M (2002) Incidence and control of brucellosis in the near east region. Vet Microbiol 90:81–110

Roth F, Zinsstag J, Orkhon D, Chimed-Ochir G, Hutton G et al (2003) Human health benefits from livestock vaccination for brucellosis: case study. Bull World Health Organ 2003(81):867–876

Rubach MP, Halliday JE, Cleaveland S, Crump JA (2013) Brucellosis in low-income and middle-income countries. Curr Opin Infect Dis 26(5):404–412

Samartino LE (2002) Brucellosis in Argentina. Vet Microbiol 90(1–4):71–80

Sayer K (2016) Brucellosis in fact and fiction: the story of a zoonosis. Vet History 18(2):165–183

Scholz HC, Nöckler K, Göllner C, Bahn P, Vergnaud G et al (2010) *Brucella inopinata* sp. nov., isolated from a breast implant infection. Int J Syst Evol Microbiol 60(Pt 4):801–808

Scholz HC, Revilla-Fernández S, Dahouk SA, Hammerl JA, Zygmunt MS et al (2016) *Brucella vulpis* sp. nov., isolated from mandibular lymph nodes of red foxes (*Vulpes vulpes*). Int J Syst Evol Microbiol 66(5):2090–2098

Schurig GG, Roop RM, Bagchi T, Boyle S et al (1991) Biological properties of RB51; a stable rough strain of Brucella abortus. Vet Microbiol 28(2):171–188

Schwabe CW (1984) Veterinary medicine and human health. Waverly Press Inc. Mount Royal Guilford Avenues, Baltimore, M. D. 21202. US. pp 16–39

Seleem MN, Boyle SM, Sriranganathan N (2008) *Brucella*: a pathogen without classic virulence genes. Vet Microbiol 129:1–14

Seleem MN, Boyle SM, Sriranganathan N (2010) Brucellosis: a re-emerging zoonosis. Vet Microbiol 140(3–4):392–398

Simmons GC, Hall WTK (1953) Epididymitis of rams. Aust Vet J 29(2):33–40

Singh BB, Dhand NK, Gill JPS (2015) 2015. Economic losses occurring due to brucellosis in Indian livestock populations. Prev Vet Med 119(3–4):211–215

Smits HL, Kadri SM (2005) Brucellosis in India: a deceptive infectious disease. Indian J Med Res 122(5):375–384

Stoenner HG, Lackman DB (1957) A new species of Brucella isolated from the desert woodrat, Neotoma lepida Thomas. Am J Vet Res 18(69):947–951

Thomas EL, Bracewell CD, Corbel MJ (1981) Characterisation of Brucella abortus strain 19 cultures isolated from vaccinated cattle. Vet Rec 108(5):90–93

Tiller RV, Gee JE, Frace MA, Taylor TK, Setubal JC et al (2010a) Characterization of novel Brucella strains originating from wild native rodent species in North Queensland, Australia. Appl Environ Microbiol 76(17):5837–5845

Tiller RV, Gee JE, Lonsway DR, Gribble S, Bell SC et al (2010b) Identification of an unusual Brucella strain (BO2) from a lung biopsy in a 52-year-old patient with chronic destructive pneumonia. BMC Microbiol 10:23

Traum J (1914) Report to the chief of the Bureau of Animal Industry. US Department of Agriculture, Washington, p 30

Veirano FR (2001) Livestock from the past and the future. Study Series production and environment. Foundation for Socio-Economic Development, Asuncion, Paraguay

Waqas A, Zheng K, Liu Z-F (2016) Establishment of chronic infection: Brucella's stealth strategy. Front Cell Infect Microbiol 6:30

Whatmore AM (2009) Current understanding of the genetic diversity of Brucella, an expanding genus of zoonotic pathogens. Infect Genet Evol 9(6):1168–1184

Whatmore AM, Davison N, Cloeckaert A, Al Dahouk S, Zygmunt MS et al (2014) Brucella papionis sp. nov., isolated from baboons (Papio spp.). Int J Syst Evol Microbiol 64(Pt 12):4120–4128

Whatmore AM, Dale E, Stubberfield E, Muchowski J et al (2015) Isolation of Brucella from a White's tree frog (Litoria caerulea). JMM Case Rep 2(1). https://doi.org/10.1099/jmmcr.0.000017

Wise RI (1980) Brucellosis in the United States: past, present, and future. JAMA 244:2318–2322

Xie X (1986) Orally administrable brucellosis vaccine: Brucella suis strain 2 vaccine. Vaccine 4:212–216

Young EJ (1983) Human brucellosis. Rev Infect Dis 5(5):821–842

Zammit T (1905) A preliminary note on the susceptibility of goats to Malta fever. Proc R Soc 76B:377–378

Zinsstag J, Roth F, Orkhon D, Chimed-Ochir G, Nansalmaa M et al (2005) A model of animal human brucellosis transmission in Mongolia. Prev Vet Med 69:77–95

Chapter 43
Ehrlichiosis

Ehrlichiosis is a disease caused by invasion of white blood cells and affects various mammalian species, cattle, horse, sheep, goat, dogs, deer, mice and human beings. It occurs worldwide. It is transmitted through tick-bite and rarely by blood transfusion.

The type of white cells infected vary with infecting species; *E. chaffeensis* infects monocytes or macrophages and so disease is named as HME (human monocytic ehrlichiosis); *Anaplasma phagocytophilum* and *E. ewingii* infect granulocytes and so the condition is known as HGE/HGA (human granulocytic ehrlichiosis/anaplasmosis). The clinical manifestations of both are almost the same and so the term ehrlichiosis is used for both.

43.1 Aetiology

Ehrlichiosis comprises a group of diseases caused by various species of *Ehrlichia*. These are HME (human monocytic ehrlichiosis) caused by *E. chaffeensis*; human ewingii ehrlichiosis caused by *E. ewingii* and also *E. canis, Neorickettsia sennetsu* and recently described Panola Mountain *Ehrlichia* species (Reeves et al. 2008). The Panola Mountain *Ehrlichia* species is genetically closely related to *E. ruminantium* and more distantly related to *E. chaffeensis.* The first two are well known.

A 31-year-old man from Atlanta, Georgia (GA), in the United States of America (USA) hiking in Panola Mountain State Park in Georgia presented with a persistent sore neck of 3 weeks duration following a tick bite. DNA from the Panola Mountain species, which was recently discovered in a goat in Georgia, was detected in a blood sample (Reeves et al. 2008).

E. muris eauclairensis, carried by blacklegged tick *(I. scapularis)* has been found in Wisconsin and Minnesota (https://www.cdc.gov/ehrlichiosis/index.htmlPage last reviewed: May 9, 2022)

© Springer Nature Singapore Pte Ltd. 2024
K. G. Narayan et al., *Handbook of Management of Zoonoses*,
https://doi.org/10.1007/978-981-99-9885-2_43

These are obligate intracytoplasmic tiny Gram-negative bacteria (0.2–2.0 microns). These multiply in the vacuoles of cytoplasm of infected white blood cells to form clusters, large mulberry-shaped aggregate, called morulae. Wright-Giemsa stains these inclusion bodies in mononuclear phagocytic cells, detected 5–7 days after infection. The infected white blood cells burst after intracellular multiplication of *Ehrlichia*, releasing new crop into circulation to infect other white blood cells.

The surface membrane protein antigens are complex and consist of thermolabile and thermostable components. The key antigens associated with HME have molecular weight of 27, 29 and 44 kD, whereas those associated with HGE have 40, 44 and 65 kD. This may be useful in differential diagnosis.

43.2   Vector and Natural Hosts

Amblyomma americanum (the lone star tick) is the primary vector of both *Ehrlichia chaffeensis* and *Ehrlichia ewingii* in the southern, eastern and south central USA, coincident with the tick habitat. Cases outside this known area have generally a history of travel to the endemic areas about a fortnight earlier to the date of reporting illness. The natural reservoir host of *E. chaffeensis* is white-tailed deer and act as host for all stages of the lone star tick. Coyotes, dogs and goats also suffer naturally.

43.3   Symptoms

The incubation period (tick bite to illness) is generally 5–14 days. All infections do not result into clinical illness. It ranges from asymptomatic to mild. The clinical manifestations are fever, fatigue, headache and myalgia. Other signs and symptoms that may be observed are nausea, vomiting, diarrhoea, cough, arthralgia and occasional rash. Associated blood picture shows increased white cells, low platelets and elevated liver enzymes. In severe cases, thrombocytopenia with disseminated intravascular coagulation (DIC) resulting into haemorrhages in the skin may occur.

The average reported annual incidence is 0.7 cases per million. It affects all age group, mainly young adults (Cunha 2009). Incidence of ehrlichiosis increases with age, with the highest incidence reported among persons aged 60+ years. Male:female ratio is 4:1, suggesting more opportunities of exposure and infection. The estimated mortality rate is 1–5%, much greater in the immunocompromised (Cunha 2009).

43.4   Diagnosis

• History of exposure to ticks or tick bites and also the symptoms leads to initial diagnosis.

- Haemogram shows low white blood cells and platelets and elevated liver-specific enzymes (transaminases).
- A peripheral blood smear stained with Wright-Giemsa stain demonstrates inclusions compatible with *Ehrlichia* morulae in infected neutrophils. Negative finding does not rule out the infection.
- Specific antibodies (indirect IFA, ELISA, immunohistochemical staining) and PCR are confirmatory tests.
- A positive PCR reaction, with confirmation of the amplicon identity, is sufficient for laboratory confirmation of a case of human ehrlichiosis.

43.5   Treatment

It is treatable with tetracycline, usually doxycycline. However, diagnosis is difficult and delays proper treatment, leading to possible serious complications. Ehrlichiosis and RMSF have almost the same geographical distribution as the same ticks (*Amblyomma* and *Dermacentor*) transmit. Helpful clues to consider cases as ehrlichiosis are:

Absence of (a) petechial rash and (b) bilateral periorbital oedema, oedema of the dorsum of hands and feet and conjunctival suffusion and commonly observed neutropenia in ehrlichiosis help to differentiate the case from RMSF. Absence of nuchal rigidity and normal CSF profile in ehrlichiosis differentiate it from other bacterial meningitis.

43.6   Prevention

Use dogs and ticks on body as sentinels. Dogs do not transmit but ticks do. Detection of disease in dogs is possible with diagnostic tests like ELISA and IF. Symptoms are suggestive—anaemia, lameness, neurological, swollen limbs and vision problem.

References

Cunha BA (2009) Ehrlichiosis: overview, http://emedicinemedscapecom/article/235839-overview Updated: Feb 5, 2009
Reeves WK, Loftis AD, Nicholson WL, Czarkowski AG (2008) The first report of human illness associated with the Panola Mountain Ehrlichia species: a case report. J Med Case Rep 2:139

Chapter 44
Glanders

Synonyms

Equina, Farcy, Malleus, Droe.

Glanders is infectious life-threatening disease of horses, mules and donkeys, transmissible to dogs, cats, goats, camels and felines living in the wild, bears, wolves and human. The acute form is characterized by fever, cough, infectious nasal discharge, pneumonia, septicaemia and death within days. Chronic form presents nodules that ulcerate eventually in the upper respiratory and nasal mucosa, lungs and subcutaneous tissues. Death occurs within months. Survivors act as carriers.

It was described by Aristotle in the third century that it is highly contagious and was recognized as far back as in 1664. By the beginning of nineteenth century, it was found to be zoonotic. It is OIE-listed and occurrence must be notified.

44.1 Aetiology

Burkholderia mallei (also known as *Pseudomonas pseudomallei*) is Gram-negative, coccobacillary, aerobic, non-motile, facultative intracellular human and animal pathogen, measuring 1.5–3.0 × 0.5–1.0 microns. It belongs to the order *Burkholderiales*, family *Burkholderiaceae*, genus *Burkholderia*.

© Springer Nature Singapore Pte Ltd. 2024   443
K. G. Narayan et al., *Handbook of Management of Zoonoses*,
https://doi.org/10.1007/978-981-99-9885-2_44

44.2   Pathogenesis, Pathology

B. mallei penetrates the mucosa and spreads through lymphatics to regional lymph glands, multiplies and enters the bloodstream for further dissemination to different tissues and organs including bones. Bacterial capsule and lipopolysaccharide and intracellular localization enable the bacteria to escape phagocytosis.

Pathological lesions are nodules under pleura, diffuse miliary granulomatous nodules with caseous centre, oedema in lungs and serosanguineous fluid accumulated in paranasal sinuses and nasal cavity. Histopathology suggests granulomatous or pyogranulomatous inflammation with haemorrhagic foci.

44.3   Epidemiology

44.3.1   Reservoir

B. mallei does not persist outside a host. Solipeds (single-hooved), particularly horses, are the only reservoirs. Donkeys are more likely to suffer from acute form, horses with chronic and latent form, and mules from all the three forms of disease. Mules are susceptible and infection may be latent, and disease acute and chronic.

B. mallei does not penetrate intact skin. Entry and invasion occur through abraded or lacerated skin, inhalation and invasion of nasal, oral and conjunctival mucous membrane.

44.3.2   Source

Pre-symptomatic and carrier animals constitute the potential source. Chronically infected non-symptomatic horses remain highly infectious. Shedding of bacteria from nose or skin may be intermittent or continuous. Sneezing, coughing and contaminated aerosol from grooming equipment spread infection through air.

44.3.3   Distribution

It has worldwide prevalence but has been considerably reduced through veterinary services over the past 100 years. It has been eradicated from America, Australia, Japan and Europe. It is reported only sporadically in equines, camels and zoo animals in United Arab Emirates, Bahrain, Iran, Iraq, Kuwait, Lebanon, Mongolia, India, Myanmar, Afghanistan, Pakistan and Philippines, Brazil in South America and in few countries such as Eritrea and Ethiopia in Africa. No glanders epidemic in human has been recorded; sporadic outbreaks and deliberate use as bioweapon are on records.

According to the status report (Singha et al. 2020a), high prevalence of glanders in the past century led to the adoption of 'Glanders and Farcy Act 1899' in India. Resurgence of glanders took place during 1960–1970s. In 1990 and 1998 outbreaks occurred in Punjab and Haryana. Glanders emerged in 2006 and after alleged unrestricted movement of equines. Sero-surveillance was conducted for the period 2006–2018 after capacity building.

Glanders is endemic in India. Malik et al. (2012) reviewed major outbreaks reported from different parts between 1976 and 1982. Sporadic cases appeared in 1988, 1990 and 1998. For nearly 8 years no case was reported. In 2006–2007 outbreaks occurred in eight different states. Repeated outbreaks occurred in Himachal Pradesh and Uttar Pradesh. Fresh outbreaks reported from Chhattisgarh in 2009–2010. The distribution of most of 164 cases was: Uttar Pradesh, 77; Maharashtra, 23; Uttarakhand, 21; and Andhra Pradesh, 16. Euthanasia of infected and biosecurity measures controlled glanders.

Sero-surveillance was carried out during Jan 2015–Dec 2018 in 299 districts of 21 states and one Union Territory. The method used was Hcp1 indirect ELISA followed by confirmatory CFT. A total of 932 glanders cases were detected. These were distributed in over 120 districts in 12 states. Increasing trend of cases since 2016 was observed with maximum cases from northern India. Seasonal shifting from March to June (winter to summer) was observed. Re-emergence was noted after a gap of 10 years in Maharashtra, Haryana and Punjab. Glanders appeared, making ingress into states like Jammu and Kashmir, Gujarat, Rajasthan, Madhya Pradesh, Delhi and Tamil Nadu (Singha et al. 2020b).

International trading of horses might cause re-emergence in countries from where it stands eradicated.

44.4 Glanders in Human

Humans are accidental hosts. Human-to-human transmission is rare. Occupational exposure in medical practice and work like conducting autopsies pose a risk in hospital setting. In home setting too it is possible that care givers of glanders-affected individual got infected (Van Zandt et al. 2013).

44.4.1 Zoonotic Transmission

Zoonotic transmission occurs from the infected solipeds. Although zoonotic infection is relatively uncommon and restricted to areas/regions where horses continue to be used for transport and farming and with inadequate veterinary care, the possibility of frequent and close contact with infected animals and contact with latent/subclinical infected horses and mules exists. Occupational exposure makes veterinarians, veterinary students, farriers, flayers, transport workers, soldiers, equine slaughterhouse workers, farmers and stable hands high-risk groups. Transmission is through aerosolised fomites, direct and indirect contacts. *B. mallei* enters through nasal, oral, and conjunctival mucosa and less likely per os—through contaminated food and water and abraded skin of hands, arms, face and neck in particular. Inhalation leads to deposition of bacteria deep in the lungs. Aerosolized *B. mallei* is highly infectious.

44.4.2   Laboratory Infection

In a *laboratory*, seven persons working with the bacterium got infected in the 1940s in the USA before the advent of the modern laboratory containment practices. Six of them performed normal laboratory procedures that could generate aerosols such as washing, centrifugation and aerating. The seventh case had collected a blood sample via a finger-stick from a person for monitoring diabetes before entering the laboratory (Van Zandt et al. 2013).

In 2000, one case occurred in a research laboratory worker in the USA after accidental exposure (https://www.cdc.gov/glanders/index.html). An authentic zoonotic case of glanders was a pathologist in Punjab Veterinary College, Lahore, erstwhile India, reported in 1913. Two Japanese laboratory workers were accidentally exposed at the Ping Fan Institute in 1937 and died (CD Alert GLANDERS427247804.pdf).

ELISA and CFT tests on serum samples collected from 538 humans including equine handlers and veterinarians exposed to glanderous equids failed to detect any one positive (Singha et al. 2020c).

44.4.3   Biological War

Van Zandt et al. (2013) presented an overview on human glanders. High infectivity, small infective dose, degree of incapacitation and high case fatality caused in human beings make *B. mallei* a useful and easily available bioweapon. Clinical symptoms are nonspecific and thus diagnosis and treatment are very likely delayed. Infection in horses and mules caused deadly disease and incapacitation.

B. mallei was used as bioweapon in the twentieth century, in World War I against animals in WWI in Europe, Russia and the USA affecting supply convoys and artillery. It is alleged that the Soviet Union used it against opposition forces in Afghanistan between 1982 and 1984. In Russia, human cases increased during and after the war. During WWII also it was used by Japan to deliberately infect horses, prisoners of wars and also civilians in China.

44.4.4 Symptoms

According to Van Zandt et al. (2013) an exposure may cause localized infection, acute pulmonary and chronic disease. In general, incubation period varies between 1 and 14 days. There is a swelling and weeping discharge in the affected area observed within 5 days of entry of bacteria. It may progress to septicaemia in nearly 2 weeks' time. Septicaemia may also develop immediately after infection.

Acute pulmonary symptoms may appear within 10–14 days of airborne exposure. There is rapid onset almost always ending in death between 10 and 30 days. Chronic form may take 12 weeks for symptoms to appear.

The localised form is characterized by a local lesion with regional swelling with foci of suppuration. Abscess ulcerates and drains for long time. The accompanied symptoms include low grade fever, malaise, fatigue, chills, headache, myalgia, headache and backache. There is lymphadenopathy. Cases may complain of sore throat and chest pain. The patients feel better and recovered for a few days to 2 months. Some patients suffer a second wave of illness. Localized lesions can disseminate to cause pulmonary, septicaemic of multi-tissue infection.

The laboratory-acquired infection seven cases were closely followed. The description of glanders in human by Van Zandt et al. (2013) is mostly based on this. Most cases reported afternoon to evening low-grade fever, malaise, fatigue, headache, myalgias including backache, lymphadenopathy and chest pain. They showed signs of recovery over a period of time. About half of the observed cases had a second wave of symptoms appearing after few days to 2 months. This temporary improvement is thus deceptive and may lead to discontinued therapy which should not be.

Depending upon routes of infection glanders cases may be described as *skin (cutaneous), mucosal, pulmonary and disseminated septicaemic forms.*

44.4.4.1 Skin (Cutaneous) Form

Entering through abraded skin, *B. mallei* produces a painful inflammatory swelling. A single blister appears and slowly develops into haemorrhagic ulcer. The lesion may extend along the regional lymphatics as lymphangitis with a number of suppurating foci. It has chronic indolent course.

44.4.4.2 Mucosal Form

Contact infection of eye causes conjunctivitis, lacrimation, and photophobia. Nasal entry causes inflammation and swelling of nose, copious nasal discharge, invasion of nasal septum and bony tissues causing destruction of tissues and fistulae, swelling of face and regional lymph glands. Infection may extend further, causing bronchitis accompanied with cough, and mucopurulent sputum may appear.

Patient may present constitutional signs and symptoms such as low-grade fever, chill with or without rigor and severe headache within the first few days of infection.

44.4.4.3 Pulmonary Form

Airborne infection results in pneumonia, pulmonary abscess, pleuritic chest pain and pleural effusion. The patients complain of sore throat, cough, pleuritic chest pain, fatigue, chills and headache. There is fever >102 °F, dyspnoea, tachypnoea, mucopurulent nasal discharge and sputum. Signs and symptoms may develop over 2–3 weeks.

Mortality rate in untreated cases may be as high as 90–95% against 40% in treated patients.

44.4.4.4 Disseminated Form

Local, cutaneous or mucosal form may disseminate, resulting into septicaemia and infection of internal organs developing into abscess in spleen, liver and lungs. This may end into septic shock and death. Septicaemic and cutaneous forms becoming septicaemic cause 90–95% without treatment against 50% despite treatment.

44.5 Glanders in Animals

Glanders is a contagious fatal disease of horses, donkeys and mules, characterized by farcy (skin form) and development of nodules and ulceration in the respiratory tract and lungs (respiratory form) caused by *Burkholderia mallei*. It is a zoonosis. *B. mallei* evolved from *B. pseudomallei* cause of melioidosis in human and animals (OIE 2018). Both are potentially fatal.

Generally, glanders in donkeys and mules is acute and in horses a chronic form of disease. Chronic and subclinical cases are permanent and intermittent shedders and potential sources of infection and spread of disease.

44.5.1 Symptom

Incubation period may be days to months, commonly 2–6 weeks. *B. mallei* may invade through mucous membranes of nose and gastrointestinal tract. Glanders could be acute, chronic or latent.

44.5.1.1 Acute Form

Mules and donkeys usually suffer from acute glanders. There is moderate to high fever, depression, malaise, anorexia, cough, thick yellow nasal discharge. Septicaemia or pneumonia/respiratory failure cause death within a few days.

44.5.1.2 Chronic Form

Chronic form of glanders in horse manifests in intermittent fever, loss of weight and cough. Nodules ulcerate eventually in upper respiratory and nasal mucosa, lungs and subcutaneous tissues. The nasal discharge is yellowish green and bloody. Horse is lame because of swelling of joints in the hind quarters. Glanders can persist for years interspersed with episodes of illness and recovery and progressive debilitation and eventual death.

Glanders cases present any combination of the following forms:

44.5.1.3 Nasal Form

There is thick yellow (bloody) discharge from deep nodules and ulcers in nasal passage. Healing ulcers leave a characteristic star-shaped scar. Infection spreading under the jaw causes enlargement and rupture of submaxillary lymph nodes. Infection extending further may affect the lower respiratory tract.

44.5.1.4 Pulmonary Form

Pulmonary form causes cough and breathing difficulty. Reddish nodules and abscess with central grey necrotic zone form in the lungs. There is progressive debility, febrile episodes, coughing and dyspnoea.

44.5.1.5 Skin Form

Skin form is known as Farcy and presents characteristic crater-shaped ulcers around muzzle and limbs. Farcy manifests as enlarged lymph vessels and nodular abscesses (buds) along their course which ulcerate discharging thick yellow pus. Common sites are hock and thigh. There is oedematous swelling. Pyogranulomatous nodules are found also in the liver and spleen. Animals lose weight and ultimately die within months, and survivors become carriers.

44.5.1.6 Latent Form

The clinical signs of disease are minimum. There are fever, nasal discharge and breathing difficulty with visible lesions.

Survivors, latently infected and discharges from the respiratory tract and skin lesions constitute source of infection. Close contact, inoculation, inhalation and ingestion of contaminated feed and water trough spread infection.

Erdemsurakh et al. (2020) described four equine glanders cases in Mongolia. These presented nasal discharge and multiple cutaneous nodules or papules in hind limbs and abdomen. Diagnosis was based on Rose Bengal agglutinin, complement fixation and Mallein tests. Monoclonal antibody to *B. mallei* BpaB was used for histochemistry. Bacterial antigen was detected in the cytoplasm of neutrophils, macrophages, epithelioid cells and multinucleated giant cells in the pyogranulomas and abscesses in target organs including alveolar type II cells and bronchiolar epithelial cells.

44.5.2 Prognosis

Glanders-positive case is usually euthanized in non-endemic areas. Acute and chronic cases ultimately usually die.

44.5.3 Glanders in Animals Other Than Equines

Camels are naturally infected. The disease manifests as fever, lethargy, emaciation with severe mucopurulent nasal discharge because of nodules and ulcers in the nasal passage.

Carnivores, like dogs, cats and wolves and tiger, get infected per os after eating infected meat or by contact. In the beginning enlarged lymph nodes are noticed, which later ulcerate. Lesion is detected in nostrils. The pets cough and manifest respiratory distress. Nodules may be found in bronchioles and lungs in the respiratory or pneumonic form. Cutaneous lesions or Farcy are pus-filled ulcers found on the limbs and body. Irregular-shaped ulcers may appear along the enlarged lymph nodes. Internal organs like the spleen and liver may also show ulcers.

Infection may be contracted by small ruminants if kept in close contact with a horse suffering from glanders (OIE 2018).

44.6 Diagnosis

Clinical signs and symptoms are suggestive. Laboratory confirmation can be done by culture and isolation of *B. mallei* from secretions, sputum, blood, urine or by PCR even when antibodies have appeared. Bacteriological culture—inoculated on chocolate agar characteristic colonies of *Burkholderia mallei*—develop in 72 h at 37 °C.

Tests to detect immune response are:

- Complement fixation test (CFT) is the OIE (World Organization for Animal Health)-recommended diagnostic test.
- Enzyme-linked immunosorbent assay (ELISA) may be used for human glanders diagnosis.

Elschner et al. (2019) found the WB and all ELISAs, except BimA, were significantly more specific than the CFT (the intracellular motility A protein [BimA]).

- Indirect haemagglutination test (IHA) has been used for melioidosis. Sheep RBC coated with *Burkholderia* antigen agglutinate when the test serum from suspected animal is positive. Test is not specific.
- Western blot.
- Mallein test is used in animals. Purified protein derivatives of *B. mallei* are intradermally injected and delayed-type hypersensitive reaction is observed.

It is also known as intra-dermo-palpebral test. It has replaced the earlier s/c or ophthalmic tests. 0.1 mL of mallein is injected i/d in the lower eyelid with a tuberculin syringe. After 48 h there is marked oedema of the eyelid with blepharospasm and a severe purulent conjunctivitis in positive animals. Some infected animals may show a general hypersensitivity reaction.

These tests are useful in detecting infection in individual and also in population.

- Animal inoculation test—Guinea pig and hamster are highly susceptible.

Strauss test—Male guinea pig inoculated intra-peritoneally develops lesions in the scrotum in case the specimen contains *B. mallei*. Cultivation of the bacterium from the lesions is confirmatory. The test is named after Strauss who developed it as early as in 1886 (Arms 1910).

Marmoset inoculation test—Nelson et al. (2014) reproduced disease in marmoset. They suggested it as animal model for specific and differential diagnosis. Marmoset (*Callithrix jacchus*) inoculation—subcutaneous inoculation of 1.0×10^2 cfu of *B. mallei* caused a lethal disease in 93% of experimental marmosets in 5–10.5 days manifesting lymphatic spread of the bacterium and non-necrotic multifocal solid lesions with severe necrosis and pneumonia. Additional advantage was differentiation from melioidosis. Subcutaneous inoculation of 1.0×10^2 cfu *Burkholderia pseudomallei* caused lethal disease within 22–85 h post-inoculation, characterized by a high level of bacteraemia, focal microgranuloma progressing to non-necrotic multifocal solid lesions in the liver and spleen and multiorgan failure.

Marmosets (*Callithrix jacchus*) offer a model to study *B. mallei* infection. Jelesijevic et al. (2015) observed intranasal inoculation of 2.5×10^4–10^5 strain ATCC23344 caused acute lethal infection in 83% within 3–4 days. Signs and symptoms observed were lethargy, off-feed, conjunctivitis, mucopurulent and haemorrhagic nasal discharge, increased respiratory problem. Lesions, characteristics of glanders and recovery of *B. mallei* from the lungs, spleen and liver confirmed the experimental infection.

44.7 Treatment

Human glanders has been successfully treated with sulphadiazine and antibiotics. Most deaths were reported earlier to 1940 when antibiotics were not available. *B. mallei* is sensitive to antibiotics. However, it is intracellular pathogen and only antibiotics that can penetrate inside cells are effective. Glanders requires long treatment. Suitable supportive and antibiotics therapy with patience result into recovery.

NCDC, Delhi, India, recommended sulphonamides (trimethoprim-sulfamethoxazole, TMPSMX) and piperacillin/tazobactam as an alternative for ceftazidime (NCDC 2017, CD Alert GLANDERS427247804.pdf). Another drug found effective in hamster model is doxycycline. Tetracycline derivatives, aureomycin; imipenem and doxycycline i/v for 1 month followed by oral azithromycin and doxycycline for 6 months; imipenem, meropenem and ceftazidime with or without trimethoprim-sulfamethoxazole have been useful.

44.8   Prevention

There is no vaccine for human.

44.8.1   Other Measures

Countries free from glanders must quarantine new arrival stringently; animal must prove negative to tests that detect glanders. Quarantine of pet dog is problematic unlike horse. Glanders is zoonotic. Euthanasia may have to be considered.

Screening of apparently normal, early detection in susceptible animals, humane elimination of positives, safe disposal of carcass and contaminated material, strict quarantine and disinfection of premises are necessary. Awareness among susceptible animal owners and compensation in case euthanized are required.

The OIE Animal Health Code for Terrestrial Animals (2018) enunciates detailed instructions for import of equines and equine products such as semen or serum from glanders-infected and glanders-free countries.

International animal trade requires certificate attesting that the animal(s) showed no symptoms of glanders and were kept in an exporting country free of the disease for at least 6 months prior to shipment.

Diagnosis is often difficult. Germany reports an interesting case of glanders after 1955. Apparently, healthy horse was readying for export. Blood sample tested positive for glanders. It was quarantined. Subsequent test results also were positive. It was euthanized for diagnosis. Organs were negative, and skin samples initially showed doubtful results. Scabs of skin samples fixed in formalin showed positive results using a different test. Source could not be traced (Horsetalk n.d., http://horsetalk.co.nz/2015/02/08/case-much-feared-glanders-confirmed-german).

44.8.2 Prevention and Control in India (CD Alert GLANDERS427247804.pdf)

Veterinary authorities in India test destroy affected horses and notify glanders outbreak under the Glanders and Farcy Act, 1899 (Act 13 of 1899). The act has been replaced by the 'Prevention and Control of Infectious and Contagious Diseases in Animals Act, 2009' in India.

Action plan for control and containment of glanders in equines (May 2016, GOI, Ministry of Agriculture, Department of Animal Husbandry, Dairying & Fisheries) has all the details spelled out and should be used.

References

Arms BL (1910) The Strauss reaction for the diagnosis of Glanders. JAMA 55(7):591–593

Elschner MC, Laroucau K, Singha H, Tripathi BN, Saqib M et al (2019) Evaluation of the comparative accuracy of the complement fixation test, Western blot and five enzyme-linked immunosorbent assays for serodiagnosis of glanders. PLoS One 14(4):e0214963

Erdemsurakh O, Purevdorj B, Ochirbat K, Adilbish A, Vanaabaatar B et al (2020) Pathological and immunohistochemical analyses of naturally occurring equine glanders using an anti-BpaB antibody. Vet Pathol 57(6):807–811

Horsetalk (n.d.). Horsetalk.co.nz | 8 February 2015 10:01 am; Case of much-feared glanders confirmed in German horse. HTTP://HORSETALK.CO.NZ/2015/02/08/CASE-MUCH-FEARED-GLANDERS-CONFIRMED-GERMAN-HORSE/#AXZZ3ISYUOLTJ. Read more: http://horsetalk.co.nz/2015/02/08/case-much-feared-glanders-confirmed-german-horse/#ixzz3isyw9h2k

Jelesijevic T, Zimmerman SM, Harvey SB, Mead DG et al (2015) Use of the common marmoset to study *Burkholderia mallei* infection. PLoS One 10(4):e0124181

Malik P, Singha H, Khurana SK, Kumar R, Kumar S et al (2012) Emergence and re-emergence of glanders in India: a description of outbreaks from 2006 to 2011. Vet Ital 48(2):167–178

NCDC (2017) CD alert Glanders: a public health concern. Directorate general health services. CD alert GLANDERS427247804.pdf: www.ncdc.gov.in

Nelson M, Salguero FJ, Dean RE, Ngugi SA, Smither SJ et al (2014) Comparative experimental subcutaneous glanders and melioidosis in the common marmoset (*Callithrix jacchus*). Int J Exp Pathol 95(6):378–391

OIE (2018) World organization for animal health (OIE). Glanders and Melioidosis in OIE Terrestrial Manual. pp. 1–13. https://www.oie.int/fileadmin/Home/eng/Health_standards/tahm/3.05.11_GLANDERS.pdf

Singha H, Shanmugasundaram K, Malik P, Khurana SK, Virmani N, Gulati BR et al (2020a) Glanders status report in India: beginning of eradicating the dreaded ancient disease. Ind J Comp Microbiol Immunol Infect Dis 41:66–74

Singha H, Shanmugasundaram K, Tripathi BN, Saini S, Khurana SK et al (2020b) Serological surveillance and clinical investigation of glanders among indigenous equines in India from 2015 to 2018. Transbound Emerg Dis 67(3):1336–1348

Singha H, Shanmugasundaram K, Saini S, Tripathi BN (2020c) Serological survey of humans exposed to *Burkholderia mallei*-infected equids: a public health approach. Asia Pac J Public Health 32(5):274–277

Van Zandt KE, Greer MT, Gelhaus HC (2013) Glanders: an overview of infection in humans. Orphanet J Rare Dis 3(8):131

Chapter 45
Melioidosis

Synonyms

Whitmore disease, Vietnamese time bomb, Nightcliff gardener's disease, Morphia injector's septicaemia, and Paddy-field disease

Melioidosis is a serious disease of horses closely resembling glanders but with more diverse presentation. *Burkholderia mallei* and *B. pseudomallei* cause serious, potentially fatal zoonotic diseases. These must be handled in a biosafety laboratory (level 3).

45.1 Aetiology

Burkholderia pseudomallei is a Gram-negative saprophytic bacterium classified as a Tier 1 biological select agent. It is a saprophyte, ubiquitous soil bacterium and stable in environment. It is resistant to various antibiotics and disinfectants. A variety of characters that contributed to its survival, pathogenicity and long-term persistence within the host have been identified by in vivo and in vitro experimental studies (Nathan et al. 2018).

45.2 Epidemiology

Melioidosis can be considered an emerging disease. It is endemic in Thailand and is the third most common cause of death. It is the most common cause of community-acquired septicaemic pneumonia in northern Australia. Melioidosis has been increasingly reported from many countries like China, India, Madagascar, Costa Rica, El Salvador, Kenya, Brazil and Venezuela (Limmathurotsakul et al. 2012) Multiple cases have been reported from Southeast Asia, India, the Middle East, Africa and South America.

© Springer Nature Singapore Pte Ltd. 2024
K. G. Narayan et al., *Handbook of Management of Zoonoses*,
https://doi.org/10.1007/978-981-99-9885-2_45

According to Arushothy et al. (2020) it accounted for about 20% of all community-acquired septicaemias in northeastern Thailand where 2000–3000 new cases are reported annually. In Malaysia, >2000 patients die every year. It caused an estimated 165,000 cases/year with a fatality of about 50%. There were about 1500 isolates of *B. pseudomallei* during 2017–2019 according to the National Surveillance for Antibiotic Resistance in Malaysia. Of these 60% were from cases of septicaemia.

45.2.1 Source of Infection

B. pseudomallei is naturally found in soil and water of endemic areas (Nathan et al. 2018). It prefers deeper layers of soil with high moisture and located close to the roots of plant.

B. pseudomallei affects a wide range of animals including wildlife, farm animals and humans. It is excreted in mastitic milk and diarrhoeic faeces and has been frequently isolated from abscesses in lymph glands and organs such as the spleen, liver and lungs. The environment and objects around them get contaminated and constitute the source of infection.

According to Musa et al. (2015), animals such as cattle, deer, dogs, cats and poultry act as risk factors significantly associated with high *B. pseudomallei* infection.

45.2.2 Modes of Infection and Spread

Infection may occur through inoculation, inhalation and ingestion of the bacteria. Infected animals or contaminated materials in the environment, especially of infected animals, spread the infection. Infection may also be inapparent.

45.2.3 Season

In a study in Australia, Currie et al. (2010) observed seasonal association with infection, 81% infection occurred during the monsoon wet season. There was a high proportion of inhalation pneumonic cases during December to February with severe weather conditions.

Wet weather and seasonal association with occurrence of infection has also been reported by Nathan et al. (2018) in Malaysia. There was the highest frequency of hospitalization during the rainy season, November to February. Heavy rains and flood churn out *B. pseudomallei* from the soil habitat.

45.2.4   Occupation

Those who have regular contact with/exposure to soil or water by occupation stand at risk of getting infection through abraded skin or pre-existing wound (inoculation) or inhalation. These are agricultural, forestry and fishery workers, construction workers, those engaged in rescue operations, military personnel and ecotourists. Incidence of melioidosis is generally high in those states of Malaysia that are active in agriculture (Nathan et al. 2018). In Australia, occupational exposure accounted for 18% of infection. Another 22% had recreational or occupational exposure (Currie et al. 2010).

Bush clearance releases *B. pseudomallei* located in the deeper layers of soil in air and causes inhalation pneumonia or contact-borne infection among bush-cleaning workers (Musa et al. 2015).

Musa et al. (2015) studied the risk factors for human melioidosis. Animals like livestock, dogs and wallabies were found to be significantly associated. The average body temperature of chicken and optimum growth temperature of *B. pseudomallei* match and so these may be considered as amplifying hosts. It has been speculated that the bacteria may be dispersed from Australia to outside.

45.3   Symptoms

45.3.1   Human

Although there is no age susceptibility, most cases in Malaysia fell between 40 and 60 years.

Nathan et al. (2018) classified the clinical cases reported in Malaysia into four: acute pulmonary (33–63%), (b) acute blood stream infection (19–61%), (c) disseminated infection (16–37%) and (d) acute localized infection (10%).

Currie et al. (2010) described the clinical spectrum and epidemiology of human melioidosis in Australia. Pneumonia was the principal presentation accounting for 51% of the cases. Genitourinary, skin, bacteraemia without evidence of any foci, septic arthritis/osteomyelitis and neurological melioidosis followed. Prognosis of bacteraemia cases is grave. Such cases end up into septic shock. Fatality is three times more than in non-bacteraemia cases. A sizeable number of cases, 55% developed bacteraemia and 21% septic shock even ending fatally. Abscesses in the internal organs and secondary foci in the lungs and joints were common. Inadequate or poor adherence to therapy led to recurrence. Diabetes, alcohol intake and chronic disease of the lungs and kidneys were identified as risk factors. According to Limmathurotsakul et al. (2012) melioidosis is the most common cause of fatal community-acquired septicaemic pneumonia in northern Australia. Acute phase cases required prompt treatment and most cases could be saved from ending fatally. Survivors from acute phase are likely to have recurrence.

Infection may also be dormant for a prolonged period, possibly because *B. pseudomallei* lie protected in phagocytic cells, in enclosed abscess or in a protective covering impermeable to the drugs.

Important causes of relapses include incomplete course of therapy, immunocompromised state of patient and delayed diagnosis.

Factors contributing to mortality included age of >40 years and comorbid condition, though independent. Comorbidity may be diabetes mellitus (Nathan et al. 2018).

45.3.2   Animals

Animal melioidosis in Malaysia has been recorded since 1921. It has been reported in local goats, sheep, cattle, pigs, horses, cats, dogs, rabbits, deer and monkeys (pig-tailed macaques, spider monkey, including fatal infection among orangutans) (Nathan et al. 2018).

The incubation period in animals is not known.

Inoculation expectedly involves the skin. Initially the lesions resemble fungal eczema which develop into papules and abscess over time. Cutaneous and subcutaneous nodules and ulcers in limbs are confounded with farcy. Infection of the conjunctiva leads to conjunctivitis and keratitis.

Inhalation involves the respiratory tract, in which the lungs are always affected. There is acute bronchopneumonia. There are abscesses and ulcers on the mucosa of the upper respiratory tract, nasal septum and epiglottis.

Severe enteritis is common. Autopsy may show multiple microabscesses on the internal organs like the kidneys, liver and spleen.

45.4   Diagnosis

Diagnosis is challenging because of the absence of pathognomonic clinical presentation of melioidosis. The attending physicians and laboratories especially in rural settings are not familiar with it.

Bacterial culture of specimens and identification of isolates that are non-motile, Gram negative and oxidase positive is done manually or by automated biochemical systems. It takes 3–5 days for most laboratories in Malaysia. Antibiotic susceptibility tests for amoxicillin-clavulanate, colistin and gentamicin and the *B. pseudomallei*-specific latex agglutination assay were recommended by Melioidosis Diagnostic Workshop 2013 (Nathan et al. 2018).

Serological tests for detecting anti-*B. pseudomallei* antibody—indirect haemagglutination and ELISA—are commonly used. In acute cases, IgM-antibody-ELISA detection may be useful.

Detection of *B. pseudomallei* in soil samples may be done by simplified bacterial culture method (Limmathurotsakul et al. 2012) or by lateral flow immunoassay (Rongkard et al. 2016).

PCR is the least time-taking method.

45.5 Treatment

There is no approved antibiotic regimen for infection of horses (OIE 2018).

45.6 Control and Prevention

Screening of apparently healthy-looking equids, testing of suspected clinical cases and elimination of reactors are recommended. Stable hygiene using minimum of water, frequent removal of faeces, disinfection of hooves and lower limbs and soil hygiene are useful. Soil may be freed of *B. pseudomallei* after all infected animals are removed. Culling of infected equids in non-endemic countries is proposed to maintain non-endemic status.

Personal protective equipment while handling suspected infected animals or fomites are required to prevent self-infection of animal handlers and veterinarians (OIE 2018).

References

Arushothy R, Amran F, Samsuddin N, Ahmad N, Nathan S (2020) Multi locus sequence typing of clinical *Burkholderia pseudomallei* isolates from Malaysia. PLoS Negl Trop Dis 14(12):e0008979

Currie BJ, Ward L, Cheng AC (2010) The epidemiology and clinical spectrum of melioidosis: 540 cases from the 20 year Darwin prospective study. PLoS Negl Trop Dis 4(11):e900

Limmathurotsakul D, Wuthiekanun V, Amornchai P, Wongsuwan G et al (2012) Effectiveness of a simplified method for isolation of *Burkholderia pseudomallei* from soil. Appl Environ Microbiol 78(3):876–877

Musa HI, Hassan L, Shamsuddin ZH, Panchadcharam C, Zakaria Z et al (2015) Case-control investigation on the risk factors of melioidosis in small ruminant farms in peninsular Malaysia. J Appl Microbiol 119(2):331–341

Nathan S, Chieng S, Kingsley PV, Mohan A et al (2018) Melioidosis in Malaysia: incidence, clinical challenges, and advances in understanding pathogenesis. Trop Med Infect Dis 3(1):25

OIE (2018) World Organization for Animal Health (OIE). Glanders and melioidosis in OIE terrestrial manual. pp 1–13. https://www.oie.int/fileadmin/Home/eng/Health_standards/tahm/3.05.11_GLANDERS.pdf

Rongkard P, Hantrakun V, Dittrich S, Srilohasin P et al (2016) Utility of a lateral flow immunoassay (LFI) to detect *Burkholderia pseudomallei* in soil samples. PLoS Negl Trop Dis 10(12):e0005204

Chapter 46
Leptospirosis

Synonyms

Rat-urine fever, Rat catcher's yellow, Weil's disease, Stuttgart disease, Mud fever, Swineherd' disease, Severe Pulmonary Haemorrhagic Syndrome, Haemorrhagic jaundice, Harvest fever, Cane field/cutter's fever, Rice-Field fever, Swamp fever, Fort Bragg fever, Red water of calves, and Canicola fever of dogs.

Leptospirosis is emerging and re-emerging zoonotic infection affecting primarily the liver and kidney but may affect lungs and other organs also. It has serious economic and social impact on agrarian communities. The distribution is worldwide. South and Southeast Asia, Oceania and parts of Latin America and the Caribbean report the highest morbidity. Hawaii, Florida and Puerto Rico in the USA have experienced outbreaks following floods.

The estimated annual number of cases is 1.03 million and number of deaths is 58,900. Leptospirosis is thus the leading zoonotic cause of morbidity and mortality. It is endemic in the poorest regions of the world where routine surveillance is not done (Costa et al. 2015). According to Torgerson et al. (2015), the estimated disability-adjusted life years was 2.90 million mostly because of premature deaths and suffering of disproportionately young male adults in resource-poor tropical countries.

Human leptospirosis is a neglected disease with an estimated median global annual incidence in endemic regions, excluding outbreaks, of 5 cases per 100,000 population (WHO 2011). During outbreaks and in high exposure groups, the incidence may be high, >50/100,000. Endemic human leptospirosis rates varied by region from 0.5/100,000 population in Europe to 95/100,000 population in Africa (Haake and Levett 2015). A recent report estimates an annual worldwide incidence of >1 million cases including 59,000 deaths (www.cdc.gov/leptospirosis).

© Springer Nature Singapore Pte Ltd. 2024
K. G. Narayan et al., *Handbook of Management of Zoonoses*,
https://doi.org/10.1007/978-981-99-9885-2_46

46.1 Aetiology

Leptospires are spirochetes, about 0.1 mm in diameter by 6–20 mm in length. These belong to order Spirochaetales, family Leptospiraceae and various species of *Leptospira* that are saprophytes and pathogens. Lipopolysaccharide antigens of *Leptospira* differ. Related ones are identified as serovars, further grouped into 24 serogroups. There are more than 250/300 pathogenic serovars. *L. interrogans* and *L. biflexa* represented pathogenic and saprophytic leptospires, respectively, till 1989. Genotyping reclassified the genus *Leptospira* into 21 species. However, correlation between genotyping and serotyping is poor. Same serotypes may be genetically different. Reverse is also true. Therefore, the older serovar/serogroup method is still commonly used in clinical practice, although serogroups are no longer considered valid in formal taxonomy.

L. interrogans, L. borgpetersenii, L. alexanderi, L. alstonii, L. inadai, L. fainei, L. kirschneri, L. licerasiae, L. noguchi, L. santarosai, L. terpstra, L. weilii and *L. wolffii* have been isolated from clinical cases.

Icterohaemorrhagiae, Canicola, Pomona, Grippotyphosa and Bratislava infect both dogs and human. These are commonly associated with leptospirosis in Canada and the USA.

Six *Leptospira* species were identified (*L. borgpetersenii, L. kirschneri, L. santarosai, L. interrogans, L. noguchii* and an intermediate species within the *L. licerasiae* and *L. wolffii* clade) in two low-income rural communities near the coast of Ecuador. Genotyping of human clinical samples showed multiple species of *Leptospira*, and these were also detected from a variety of animals. In absence of evidence of transmission, no potential reservoir could be identified (Barragan et al. 2016).

46.2 Epidemiology

Leptospirosis occurs worldwide and causes high morbidity especially in tropical and subtropical areas with high rainfall. It has been commonly reported in low-income countries, particularly from urine-polluted environment and where situation offers opportunity for contact with urine of infected animals. Leptospirosis is reported from several Southeast Asian countries, namely, India, Indonesia, Thailand and Sri Lanka, during rainy season and floods. The incidence has been high in Thailand, Cambodia, Laos, the Philippines and Vietnam, considered endemic countries.

Leptospirosis is an underreported and neglected disease partly because it is often not diagnosed. The symptoms are 'flu' like and often confounded with other liver diseases. Pulmonary haemorrhage often develops in early stage of leptospirosis. Jaundice is often absent in leptospirosis. Rapid detection test reports are not always reliable. Laboratory detection is scarce.

Epidemiology of leptospirosis is complex. A man gets infected while carrying out normal daily activities. Poor sanitation and climatic conditions are the only two commonly identified factors. Rodents and livestock are considered reservoirs. Molecular reverse tracing to source and infectious dose of *Leptospira* bacteria necessary for understanding epidemiology revealed multiple gaps in knowledge. Genetic mechanism of reproduction, survival and persistence in environment needs to be understood.

46.2.1 Maintenance Cycle

Leptospira maintain itself widely in nature through a cycle in environment-host combination. Its relationship with the maintenance hosts is like that of a commensal (without significant ill effect). The leptospiral cycle involves persistence in environment, acquisition by a new host, hematogenous spread in the host, colonizing the brush border of the proximal renal tubular epithelium and persistent shedding in urine.

46.2.2 Reservoir

Important reservoirs/primary hosts are small mammals, rodents including rats, mice and moles. Added to the list is banded mongoose from Botswana (Jobbins et al. 2013). Pets and domestic animals such as dogs, cats, cattle, buffalo, sheep and pigs; besides deer, hedgehogs, raccoons, opossums, skunks and rabbits and certain marine mammals act as carriers, transmit infection and act as secondary hosts. *Leptospira* has been isolated from a large number of mammalian species like bats and pinnipeds and also from poikilothermic animals such as frogs, toads and amphibians (Haake and Levett 2015). According to Kakita et al. (2021), cats may be an important source of infection and also used as sentinel animal. Cats shed pathogenic *Leptospira* in urine for a long period (eight months) after infection. Cats are the most common companion animal in Japan, estimated to be 9,778,000 in 2019, higher than that of dogs. The worldwide prevalence ranged from 4% to 33% and 0% to 67.8%, respectively, for *Leptospira* antibodies and DNA. They observed that *cats (including stary)* may be maintenance host of *L. borgpetersenii* serogroup *Javanica* and the source for human infection. MLST (multi-locus sequence typing) revealed that *L. borgpetersenii* detected in urine samples and isolated from cats, black rats, a mongoose and humans (all) belonged to ST143, suggesting an infection cycle between cats and rats in Okinawa Island.

Certain serovars generally tend to adapt to one or more hosts, and these may or may not show clinical signs of infection, for example, serovar Canicola to dogs, Bratislava and Pomana to pigs, Bratislava to horse and Hardjo to cattle, sheep and farmed red deer.

The urine is infective and can transmit so long the soil is moist. Animals, such as dogs, are infected by licking infective urine off the soil or grass or by drinking from contaminated accumulated water, for example, muddy banks of river and canals, gullies, ditches and animal farms. *Leptospira* bacteria may be distributed in tissues of infected animals—vaginal discharges, reproductive organs and aborted or stillborn foetuses. Serovar Hardjo may be detected in reproductive tract of both cows and bulls for more than a year (Spickler and Larson 2013). Semen of infected animals can also transmit *Leptospira* bacteria.

Humans are accidental hosts. Infection may result into potentially fatal disease with rare human-to-human transmission. Rodents serve as natural reservoir hosts and are resistant to fatal outcome.

46.2.3   Source of Infection

Leptospira bacteria are shed in urine, placenta and vaginal fluids. Direct and indirect contact with the infected bodily fluids causes infection. Leptospira penetrates the skin through small abrasions or mucosal membrane, such as of eyes and the mouth.

The survival in environment, pathogenicity, virulence of *Leptospira* bacteria and the outcome of interaction with human hosts determine infection and disease causation.

Environmental source: A maximum of 10^4 *Leptospira* bacteria/ml has been generally found. Infected and reservoir animals seed environment with leptospires shed in their urine. Based on available information, estimated number of *Leptospira* bacteria shed by rats is 5.7×10^6 and by others like cows, deer, dogs, mice and humans have been reported to shed an average of 3.7×10^4, 1.7×10^5, 1.4×10^2, 3.1×10^3 and 7.9×10^2 Leptospira bacteria/ml of urine, respectively. Pathogenic *Leptospira* bacteria metabolize urea, survive for 6–18 h in pure urine (pH 7–8) longer in diluted urine, resist changes in osmolality and remain infectious for 43 days in wet soil and 20 months in freshwater.

The build-up of environmental source is likely determined by factors such as volume of urine excreted and period of shedding. Infected animals and humans shed leptospires in urine for months and years. Humans excrete for 60 days or so. Heavy black rats have higher leptospiral load in urine. Density of infected animals and prevalence has direct effect upon the build-up of environmental source. This in turn would be deciding the epidemiological settings, rural, peri-urban or urban; for example, *Leptospira* bacteria have been isolated from samples of water and soil from rural and peri-urban settings where standing water gets contaminated by urine from wild or domesticated animals. South Andaman Island showed higher positivity in urban sewage water and household drainage water than in ponds or civic toilet drainage. Higher positivity was found in rural paddy field water than in streams, ponds and other water sources (Barragan et al. 2017).

46.2.4   Agent

Human febrile illness is caused by multiple species of *Leptospira* detected from a variety of animals. Apparently environmental conditions determine the survival and persistence of *Leptospira* outside the hosts' body, and this has important bearing on direct infection. However, the rate of survival differs among species and strains. Leptospires can remain viable for weeks to months outside host and in warm and humid conditions, at temperatures between 28 °C and 32 °C under neutral to slightly alkaline pH. *L. interrogans* has been shown to survive and retain virulence in water for up to 344 days. Environmental bacterial biofilm provides shelter. Leptospira co-aggregate and live within environmental bacterial biofilms from paddy field water, sewers and stagnant rainwater. *Leptospira* bacteria move on viscous matrices (around 15 m/s) and liquid surfaces (5 m/s)—that is, they can move to host in aquatic environment and in blood (Barragan et al. 2017).

46.2.5   Host

The status of human skin (abrasion/covered), genetic susceptibility (HLA DQ6 allele) and age of the host determine infection, disease and fatal outcome (increase with age).

In Thailand, during 2003–2012, the incidence rate was 6.6/100.000, case fatality rate was 1.5% and 72.3% of cases worked in agriculture lived in northeastern region, and since 2015, the occurrence of leptospirosis has shifted to southern region that has different ecology, housing and lifestyle. Both parts taken together account for 85% of all cases in Thailand every year since 2010 (Narkkul et al. 2021).

Leptospirosis is associated with poverty, income level and poor sanitation. Inadequate sanitation (absence of indoor toilets, inadequate drainage facilities and open drains, inefficient solid waste disposal) and poor housing both in urban and rural overcrowded slum communities and proximity to rodent-infested uncollected trash are by far the most important exposures, affecting millions of people living, many walking barefoot in tropical regions (Haake and Levett 2015).

Exposure to leptospire-contaminated soil and animal urine is high with certain occupational groups; agricultural workers, for example, rice field workers, banana farmers and sugar cane and pineapple field harvesters; sewers, miners, cable layers, inland fishermen, dairy farmers and workers, veterinarians and abattoir workers; hunters and trappers; animal shelter workers; soldiers; scientists; and technologists handling animals in laboratories or during fieldwork (Spickler and Larson 2013).

Leptospirosis may occur in high income groups due to *avocational exposures* as they afford to travel (endemic areas) and participate in recreational activities and adventure sports, for example, water sports including caving, canoeing, kayaking, rafting and triathlons can be associated with leptospirosis. This type of exposure has increased over the past 20 years. Studies by Chaiwattanarungruengpaisan et al. (2020) suggested that environments of an elephant camp can be a potential source of infection. The elephant camp setting presented an environment shared by inter-acting animal-environment-human. Leptospira were isolated from pond mud and river water samples, and 89% belonged to pathogenic clade and 61% to saprophytes. Two isolates from riverbank had DNA highly similar to pathogenic *L. interrogans* and *L. santarosai*.

46.2.6   Season and Environment

It has seasonal occurrence in the temperate and round the year in tropical countries. Leptospirosis outbreaks are more likely during heavy rainfall and flood. It is endemic in many of the 11 countries in south-eastern region, like India, Indonesia and Thailand where about 60% of the workforce is engaged in agriculture and has to wade through contaminated water and wells and work outdoor in warm and wet areas. Water sports are likely sources of infection.

Rainfall and flood have direct relationship with outbreaks as experienced in Mumbai and Maharashtra in India and northeast of Thailand. Heavy rains, flood, hurricane, typhoon and other climate change that are related to flowing water spreading the contaminated urine and also stagnation contribute.

However, exception suggests that leptospirosis can occur at any site and in any season. Maroun et al. (2011) described a fulminant case that developed haemoptysis, bilateral infiltrates on radiography and MAT + (microscopic agglutination test) and multiorgan failure in the middle of January in New York City.

In a cross-sectional study, Narkkul et al. (2021) identified (a) risk associated with human -animal-environment-water interface and human-animal-environment contact. The odd ratios were 4.31 for occupations related to animals or environmental water and 10.74 those who consumed water from more than two sources. Summarizing, the risk factors include (1) increased rainfall and flooding; (2) inadequate drainage for flood water; (3) poor housing, hygiene and sanitation; (4) slum dwelling and overcrowding; (5) proximity to sewers; and (6) contact with animals and workplace exposure.

Della Rossa et al. (2016) studied the role of rodent and environmental habitat in the epidemiology of *Leptospirosis* in Thailand. High incidence of human leptospirosis was observed in non-patchy habitat close to river and dominated by agricultural land, steep slopes, low altitudes and high population. Rodents positive for *Leptospira* were trapped from forest and patches of forests located on hills. Predominant crops cultivated were rice and maize. The latter was cultivated on the slopes of hill, and this practice was found associated with significant increase in rodent population. However, the location of human leptospirosis did not relate with the rodent-infested areas. There was an overall decrease in population of livestock. The authors observed that the proximity to water (river) was related to human leptospirosis.

Detection of *Leptospira* bacteria or their DNA in environmental samples is a valuable epidemiological information. The observed strong correlation between host species and pathogen type seems to be changing due to observed genetic diversity of a pathogen in a single reservoir species.

Knowledge of eco-epidemiology of *Leptospirosis* seems to be important. Gamage et al. (2020) used eDNA (environmental DNA) barcoding to understand the eco-epidemiology of leptospirosis by examining samples of irrigation water from two agro-ecological regions of Sri Lanka, namely, Kandy (wet zone mid-country region 2) and Girandurukotte, Badulla (intermediate zone low-country region 2). Analysis of eDNA showed (a) different microbiomes in both regions, (b) higher biodiversity of circulating *Leptospira*, (c) higher number of sequence reads of pathogenic *Leptospira* spp. associated with clinical cases such as *L. interrogans* in Kandy than in Girandurukotte and (d) several pathogenic abortion-causing bacterial species including *Arcobacter cryaerophilus* associated with pathogenic *Leptospira*.

46.3 Transmission

Humans are infected percutaneously or permucosally with *Leptospira* spp. by direct contact with the urine of maintenance hosts or by indirect contact with soil or water contaminated with infected urine. Human-to-human infection may occur during sexual intercourse and transplacental and breastfeeding.

Portals of entry include cuts and abrasions in skin or mucous membranes such as the conjunctival, oral or genital surfaces. Human gets infected by contact with water or soil and/or by eating/drinking water contaminated with urine from infected animals. Bush meat (including banded mongoose) is consumed and may be a means of transmission. *Leptospira* can enter also through the eyes, nose and vagina.

46.4 Leptospirosis in Animals

Infection in animals may not be noticed as the symptoms may be nil or mild. However, leptospirosis in animals may also be acute and chronic. The incubation period varies between 2 and 20 days. Leptospirosis occurs also in cattle, sheep, goats, horse, pigs, South American camelids and farmed cervids and zoo animals and wildlife (sea lions, seals).

Sudden onset of agalactia (in adult milking cattle and sheep); icterus and haemoglobinuria, especially in young animals; meningitis; and acute renal failure or jaundice in dogs are indicative of acute leptospirosis. Abortion, stillbirth, birth of weak offspring (may be premature), infertility, chronic renal failure or chronic active hepatitis in dogs and cases of periodic ophthalmia in horses are observed in chronic form of disease (OIE 2014).

Reproductive loss is caused by *Leptospira* bacteria in pigs, cattle, horse and camels. Sows abort after 1–4 weeks and cows after 2–12 weeks of infection. Prominent post-mortem lesions include inflamed kidney and liver.

Dogs suffer most often with pathology of the liver, kidney and also lungs (pulmonary form with severe lung haemorrhage). Polydipsia, polyuria, oliguria and haematuria occur when kidneys are involved. The hepatic form is manifested as vomiting, diarrhoea, abdominal pain, grey stools, weight loss, jaundice, conjunctivitis and abortions. Leptospiral pulmonary haemorrhage syndrome is manifested as coughing, tachypnoea or dyspnoea.

Infected animals are potential source of human infection for several months to year. The infection is passed on to human by direct contact with animals and indirectly via animal products. The seroprevalence in humans, buffaloes and cattle and pigs were 23.7%, 24.8%, 28.1% and 11.3%, respectively, in Thailand during the period 2010–2015 as observed by Chadsuthi et al. (2017). The serovar Shermani was the most common across humans, buffaloes, cattle, pigs and regions suggesting transmission between humans and livestock. Bratislava, Panama and Sejroe in human; Shermani, Ranarum and Tarassovi in buffaloes; and Shermani and Ranarum in cattle and pigs were also prevalent.

46.5   Leptospirosis in Human

46.5.1   Pathogenesis

Haake and Levett (2015) have described *Leptospira*-human interaction progressing to disease and death. Leptospires enter through abraded skin or through mucous membrane to reach bloodstream, persist during leptospiraemic phase and use flagella to move between cell layers. Detection in blood for the first eight days by quantitative PCR is possible, as high as 10^6/ml. Organs like the liver, lungs, heart and kidney are rapidly invaded. Peri-sinusoidal spaces and liver sinusoids appear congested. Apoptosis of hepatocytes and leakage of bile into bloodstream cause jaundice.

Leptospires can move between epithelial cells and adhere to adhesion molecules of cells to colonize. Leptospires bind to cells such as endothelial cells of blood vessels and kidneys, macrophages and fibroblasts. Leptospires passing between and adhering to epithelial cells lining renal tubules colonize the lumen and the proximal tubules. The leptospiral surface immunoglobulin-like (Lig) proteins-LigB and LipL32 controlled by genes found in pathogenic species are used to bind to a number of proteins like thrombin, fibrinogen, plasminogen, complement proteins and extracellular matrix (a mesh consisting of protein and carbohydrate located between cells). Inflammatory response is triggered. Damage of endothelial cells may be a key factor in pulmonary pathology.

The hosts' defence is evaded. Leptospires escape opsonization because the extracellular matrix is broken. Complement proteins (C3) are degraded by proteases. Binding thrombin blocks or reduced formation of fibrin and degradation of fibrin clot increased the risk of bleeding. Petechiae to frank bleeding occur in interalveolar spaces and alveolar septum in lungs occur. Leptospires produce sphingomyelinase and haemolysin to attack red cells and secrete toxin to cause interstitial nephritis, atrophy, fibrosis and kidney failure.

Most infections are asymptomatic to mild in endemic areas. Human innate immune system responds. Capillary endothelial cells are activated; cytokines and antimicrobial peptides are produced which mobilize white blood cells; macrophages engulf leptospires. Agglutinating antibodies IgM and IgG are produced and are directed mainly against LPS. Leptospires that escape proliferate.

The Toll-like receptor 2 (TLR2) in monocytes recognizes the LPS of leptospires and is activated. TRL4 is not able to recognize. TRL4 of mice recognizes leptospiral LPS, suggesting that the murine innate response is adapted to leptospiral infection and is reflected in nature—'mice are resistant to fatal infection and serve as natural reservoir'. Humans are accidental hosts, which rarely transmit infection which is potentially fatal. The brush border of proximal renal tubular epithelium is colonized in the reservoir hosts, detected by immunohistochemistry, and there is persistent shedding of leptospires in urine.

Severe disease depends possibly upon epidemiological condition, host susceptibility and virulence of the pathogen. Patients with the HLA DQ6 allele are at higher risk, and leptospiral superantigen stimulates lymphocytes, damaging organs. Cytokine flush occurs in case of severe leptospirosis—high levels of interleukin 6, tumour necrosis factor alpha (TNF-alpha) and interleukin 10; sepsis-like life-threatening symptoms appear.

Mortality increases with age, >60 years. Prognosis is grave with high levels of bacteraemia.

Kidney pathology and Weil's syndrome result because of the inflammatory response of infection seen on tubular epithelium, intensity increasing during the first two weeks of illness. Interstitial nephritis sets in, characterized by infiltration with lymphocytes, monocytes and plasma cells and occasionally neutrophils. There is thinning and/or necrosis, oedema, distension of lumen, hyaline casts and cellular debris.

Renal function is restored after acute renal failure in most of the cases but in some tubular atrophy or interstitial fibrosis causes persistent dysfunction.

46.5.2 Symptoms

Leptospirosis may be asymptomatic and mild to fulminant life threatening. The signs and symptoms are protean; diagnosis becomes difficult. Mild cases recover spontaneously, with proper supportive care.

After 7–21 days (range 2–30 days) of exposure, a mild flu-like illness may appear not necessarily seeking medical attention. Resolution without treatment is possible. Illness begins with non-specific symptoms: sudden onset of fever, chills, myalgia and headache.

Other symptoms are fever, vomiting, abdominal pain, headache, retro-orbital pain, aseptic meningitis, rashes, purpura, petechiae, epistaxis and haemoptysis.

About 10% of cases are severe, potentially fatal with multiorgan dysfunction. Leptospirosis is a biphasic fever with temporary reduced fever in between. The acute febrile illness may have an approximate seven-day septicaemic phase. Severe headache may be bitemporal or frontal throbbing. Some patients may complain of retro-orbital pain and photophobia. Chills, myalgia of calves and lower back and conjunctival suffusion are characteristics of leptospirosis. Other symptoms may be abdominal pain, nausea, vomiting, diarrhoea, cough and skin rash. The second phase is the immune phase when antibodies appear and the examination of urine may show leptospires.

Leptospirosis progresses through pre-icteric and non-icteric to icteric stages. In the pre-icteric stage, conjunctivital suffusion and sub-conjunctival haemorrhage may be seen. Jaundice appears in 5–9 days, is most intense in 4–5 days later and may continue for a month.

Severe leptospirosis is a more advanced stage but may develop suddenly also. There is dysfunction of multiple organs, for example, liver, kidneys, lungs and brain. Patients present signs of bleeding, petechiae, ecchymoses, epistaxis and coagulation disorders (prothrombin time is prolonged), thrombocytopenia, melena or hematemesis, jaundice, renal failure, aseptic meningitis, cardiac arrhythmias, pulmonary insufficiency and haemodynamic collapse.

46.5.2.1   Hepatic Failure

In one of the severe forms of leptospirosis, there is progressive liver failure. Weil's disease presents a combination of hepatomegaly (jaundice) and (nephropathy) renal failure. Nearly 70% cases show pulmonary symptoms like respiratory distress and massive pulmonary haemorrhage. The overall case fatality rate is 1–5%, 5–15% in icteric and 30–60% in pulmonary cases.

46.5.2.2   Renal Failure/Interstitial Nephritis

Leptospires appear to be renal-tropic in the reservoir hosts. Kidney is the common target organ. Symptoms include pyuria, haematuria and elevated levels of proteins in urine. Serum blood urea nitrogen and creatinine levels are high. Leptospirosis causes 'non-oliguric potassium wasting nephropathy' in which sodium reabsorption is impaired and potassium is wasted.

46.5.2.3   Severe Pulmonary Haemorrhage Syndrome (SHPS)

In leptospirosis, acute respiratory distress syndrome may occur either sporadic or as a part of outbreak. Patients present cough and massive haemoptysis and need mechanical ventilation. Lung injury is diffuse (diffuse alveolar infiltrates seen on X-ray). Case fatality is >50%. This is often confounded with viral pneumonia. Silver staining and immunohistochemistry of post-mortem lung tissue reveal leptospires.

Ludwig et al. (2017) presented a case of fatal leptospirosis (*L. interrogans* serovar *icterohaemorrhagiae* strain 17) diagnosed after death by PCR. Infection was traced back to his pet rat bought about four weeks before his hospitalization. Abdominal symptoms and haematemesis were the leading symptoms. A 34-year-old case presented with dyspnoea and haemoptysis after a week of influenza-like symptoms. He was initially diagnosed as a case of severe sepsis, acute kidney failure and severe haemolysis. Multi-organ failure developed within 29 h and this could not be reversed.

Seventy-four percent of cases of severe pulmonary haemorrhagic leptospirosis treated without extracorporeal membrane oxygenation (ECMO) die. This patient could not be saved even after ECMO, plasmapheresis (beneficial in Weil's disease), cortisone and beta-lactum antimicrobial and extracorporeal cytokine absorbent therapy.

46.5.2.4 CNS Involvement

Leptospirosis may involve CNS (central nervous system). Anicteric meningitis, meningoencephalitis and neurological complications like Guillain-Barre syndrome, hemiplegia and myelitis may be caused.

Fort Bragg fever in soldiers in North Carolina presented pretibial erythematous rash on both legs on the fourth day of illness besides headache, malaise and splenomegaly and later diagnosed to be caused by *L. interrogans* serovar Autumnalis.

Some patients reported 'persistent complaints after acute leptospirosis'. Complains included fatigue, myalgia, malaise, headache and weakness, lasting for >24 months in some.

46.6 Prognosis

Severe leptospirosis presents grave prognosis. Haake and Levett (2015) have compiled such factors and associated odd ratios. Predictors of death could be age of patient and clinical presentations such as pulmonary form, mental status, acute renal failure, etc.

Age: The risk of a fatal outcome increases with increased age; the odd ratios are 3, 7 and 7.3 for the age group of patients 40–49 and 60 years or older compared to 19–29 years.

Clinical Presentation

Oliguria (5.28), age over 36 years (4.38), respiratory insufficiency (2.56), dyspnoea (11.7) or alveolar infiltrates on chest X-ray (7.3) and altered mental status (9.12).

46.7 Management of Leptospirosis

Leptospirosis present non-specific symptoms necessitating laboratory diagnosis which is complex. Recognition and management of leptospirosis increase dramatically if clinical expertise is combined with laboratory diagnosis, epidemiologic information and awareness (Shivakumar 2013).

46.7.1   Recognition

46.7.1.1   Faine's Criteria (WHO Guidelines, 1982)

Clinical data (Part A), epidemiological factors (Part B) and bacteriological and lab findings (Part C) are combined (Table 46.1). A score of A + B + C = 25 or more is diagnostic of leptospirosis. The sensitivity, specificity, positive predictive value and negative predictive value were to be 81.8%, 72.9%, 40.9% and 94.5%, respectively.

Guidelines of the Regional Medical Research Centre (ICMR) and WHO Regional Office for Southeast Asia have defined leptospirosis as the following:

Suspect consists of only clinical features. *Probable* consists of clinical features + rapid diagnostic tests. *Confirmed* consists of clinical features + positive MAT/PCR/culture. Suspect/probable/confirmed cases have been defined for the primary, secondary and tertiary health-care levels.

The symptoms of a 'suspect' case: fever ≥38.5 °C, with or without headache, myalgia, prostration and/or conjunctival suffusion with a history of exposure. 'Probable' presented additionally any two of the following—tenderness of calf muscles, cough with or without haemoptysis, jaundice, haemorrhages, meningeal irritation, anuria/oliguria and/or proteinuria, breathlessness, cardiac arrhythmia and rashes on skin.

Based on *laboratory diagnosis* (available, as in the cases of secondary and tertiary health-care levels) a 'probable case' is a 'suspect case' found positive to rapid IgM test and/or MAT (titre 200 in a single sample) and/or any three of the following—(1) urine positive for proteins, blood and pus cells, (2) neutrophilia >80% with

Table 46.1 Process of preparing score card

Clinical data (Part A)	Epidemiological factors (Part B)	Lab diagnosis (Part C)
Headache 2 Fever 2 Temperature >39 °C 2 Conjunctival suffusion 4 Meningism 4, muscle pain 4 Conjunctival suffusion + Meningism + muscle pain 10 Jaundice 1 Albuminuria/nitrogen retention 2	Contact with animals or contact with known contaminated water 10	Isolation of *Leptospira* in culture—diagnosis certain—25 **Positive serology (MAT)** *Leptospirosis endemic*: Single positive low titre 2 Single positive high titre 10 *Leptospirosis nonendemic:* Single positive low titre 5 Single positive high titre 15 Rising titre (paired sera) 25

Total score: Presumptive diagnosis of leptospirosis is made as follows: Part A and Part B score, 26 or more, and Parts A, B and C score (total), 25 or more
A score between 20 and 25 suggests leptospirosis as a possible diagnosis

Modification (2004): ELISA IgM positive –15; SAT positive –15 were added. Any of the three tests, MAT, ELISA and SAT result, is considered for the score

Modification (2012): PCR –25 was added to isolation in culture; score of either of the two considered. Rapid tests –25, for example, Latex agglutination test/Lepto dipstick/Lepto Tek lateral flow/Lepto Tek Dri-Dot test –25, are added. Epidemiological –10 was subdivided as Rainfall 5, Exposure to contaminated environment 4 and Animal contact 1.

lymphopenia, (3) platelets <100,000/cu mm and (4) serum bilurubin >2 mg%, liver enzymes (serum alkaline phosphatise, S amylase, CPK) raised moderately.

A 'confirmed' case is defined as a 'suspect'/'probable' case with any of the following—clinical specimens positive for leptospires—by (1) isolation, (2) PCR and (3) sero-conversion from negative to positive or a fourfold rise in titre by MAT or MAT of ≥400 in a single sample. In places with limited laboratory capacity, positive by any two different 'rapid diagnostic tests' is also considered a confirmed case.

Some may categorize a case as 'suspect' and 'confirmed' and define a 'confirmed' case as a 'suspect case with positive laboratory test report'.

46.7.2   Management

Acute febrile illnesses may be due to malaria, leptospirosis, dengue, scrub typhus and viral respiratory diseases. Leptospirosis co-infection is possible, with malaria, scrub typhus, viral hepatitis and dengue. Laboratory diagnosis is needed. Mild cases of acute febrile illness have no complications and can take oral drugs. Doxycycline and chloroquine can treat all febrile illness. Right way would be to depend upon and begin treatment on the basis of symptoms and epidemiological criteria in the first week based on clinical presentation without waiting for laboratory confirmation.

A patient of acute febrile illness with complications should be suspected for severe leptospirosis and hospitalized. Complications could be organ dysfunction and/or persistent fever. Dialysis for acute kidney injury and ventilatory support for respiratory failure would definitely reduce mortality.

46.8   Diagnosis

Patients' history of possible exposure and liver and kidney function tests are strong guidelines.

Specimens for demonstration of *Leptospires* in laboratory examination include blood, cerebrospinal fluid for the first seven days and urine and kidneys after that to ten days.

Specimens need to be transported in medium that preserves leptospires. Recommended options are Ellinghausen-McCullough-Johnson-Harris (EMJH) or Fletcher's medium, Ringer lactate solution or un-chlorinated sterile tap/well water containing 10% of serum.

Following are laboratory tests:

- Microscopic agglutination test (MAT) is the gold test and should be available in referral laboratories. Most laboratories maintain 24 live serogroup cultures. Antibodies titre peak in second–third week and persist for 5–10 years.
- Dark field microscopy, silver staining—not to be used as the *only* test.

- ELISA-IgM is a suitable alternative to MAT. IFT and immunohistochemical staining are also used.
- Other rapid tests are MSAT, latex agglutination test/Lepto dipstick/Lepto Tek lateral flow/Lepto Tek Dri-Dot test

Confirmatory tests are the following:

- PCR is useful in early stage of illness.
- Culture in EMJH medium. Incubation temperature is 28–30 °C. Growth is time taking −3 weeks to 3 months and this test is of only academic value.

PCR results are available in the first week of leptospirosis but serovars cannot be identified. The latter takes weeks to months.

Serological tests are conducted on a panel of different strains. Serotyping of isolates is epidemiologically important.

46.8.1 In Order to Detect/Establish Endemicity, Animals Are Often Examined as Sentinel

According to OIE (2014), the isolation or demonstration of leptospires in (a) several of the internal organs (such as the liver, lung, brain and kidney) and body fluids (blood, milk, cerebrospinal, thoracic and peritoneal fluids) of clinically infected animals gives a definitive diagnosis of acute clinical disease or, in the case of a foetus, chronic infection of its mother; (b) the kidney, urine or genital tract of animals without clinical signs is diagnostic only of a chronic carrier state.

46.9 Treatment

Early treatment of suspected cases reduces case fatality rate. Penicillin G, ampicillin, amoxicillin and ceftriaxone are effective. Glucose and salt solution transfusion is helpful. Care should be taken for the specific organ/system such as renal/hepatic/pulmonary /haemorrhagic/neurological depending upon the case.

46.10 Prevention

Leptospirosis risk reduction is multidimensional and requires multisectoral, multidisciplinary cooperation and coordination, for example, One Health approach.

Environmental and climatic conditions, particularly rainfall, influence dynamics of rodent population, size and behaviour, agriculture and animal farming and put pressure on drainage of water and sanitation. Input from the Intergovernmental

Panel on Climate Change seems important. Data on livestock leptospirosis collected from veterinary services, slaughter houses and post-mortem and microbiome studies should help in locating hot spots empowering the public health services for pre-emptive/preventing action plans.

Leptospirosis Burden Epidemiology Reference Group of WHO estimates *Leptospira*—disease burden—coordinates and directs global research and action against human leptospirosis.

Mass chemoprophylaxis—Doxycycline 100 mg twice daily or amoxicillin/ampicillin 2 mg twice daily for seven days should be used in case of laboratory accidents. Likewise, high-risk group in endemic area may be protected with antibiotics, for example, doxycycline given once a week.

Avoiding contact with rat urine-contaminated water is essential.

A study in Thailand supports this public health approach. Della Rossa et al. (2016) observed the sudden increased incidence in 2000 in Nan province of Thailand related to flooding. Regular awareness campaigns (encouraging farmers to wear boots and controlling rodent populations) and prophylaxis by allowing large distribution of antibiotics during flooding events reduced the incidence, in Tha Wang Pha and Pua districts. Public health awareness may have led to better diagnosis and reporting.

Vaccines—Suspension of killed leptospires constitutes vaccine. Protection is serovar-specific and vaccine must contain the serovars matching those circulating in the area. Dogs, pigs and cattle can be immunized similarly. Immunization prevents diseases but renal carriage is not always prevented. Polyvalent vaccine (icterohaemorrhagiae, canicola) is effective in dogs, protection lasting or one year. Vaccine for cattle contains serovar Hardjo and for swine Pomona.

References

Barragan V, Chiriboga J, Miller E, Olivas S, Birdsell D, Hepp C et al (2016) High *Leptospira* diversity in animals and humans complicates the search for common reservoirs of human disease in rural Ecuador. PLoS Negl Trop Dis 10:e0004990

Barragan V, Olivas S, Keim P, Pearson T (2017) Critical knowledge gaps in our understanding of environmental cycling and transmission of Leptospira spp. Appl Environ Microbiol 83(19):e01190–e01117

Chadsuthi S, Bicout DJ, Wiratsudakul A, Suwancharoen D et al (2017) Investigation on predominant *Leptospira* serovars and its distribution in humans and livestock in Thailand, 2010-2015. PLoS Negl Trop Dis 11(2):e0005228

Chaiwattanarungruengpaisan S, Thepapichaikul W, Paungpin W, Ketchim K et al (2020) Potentially pathogenic *Leptospira* in the environment of an elephant camp in Thailand. Trop Med Infect Dis 5(4):183

Costa F, Hagan JE, Calcagno J, Kane M, Torgerson P, Martinez-Silveira MS et al (2015) Global morbidity and mortality of leptospirosis: a systematic review. PLoS Negl Trop Dis 9(9):e0003898

Della Rossa P, Tantrakarnapa K, Sutdan D, Kasetsinsombat K et al (2016) Environmental factors and public health policy associated with human and rodent infection by leptospirosis: a land cover-based study in Nan province, Thailand. Epidemiol Infect 144(7):1550–1562

Gamage CD, Sato Y, Kimura R, Yamashiro T, Toma C (2020) Understanding leptospirosis eco-epidemiology by environmental DNA metabarcoding of irrigation water from two agro-ecological regions of Sri Lanka. PLoS Negl Trop Dis 14(7):e0008437

Haake DA, Levett PN (2015) Leptospirosis in humans. Curr Top Microbiol Immunol 387:65–97

Jobbins SE, Sanderson CE, Alexander KA (2013) *Leptospira interrogans* at the human-wildlife interface in Northern Botswana: a newly identified Public Health threat. Zoonoses Public Health 61(2):113–123

Kakita T, Kuba Y, Kyan H, Okano S, Morita M, Koizumi N (2021) Molecular and serological epidemiology of Leptospira infection in cats in Okinawa Island, Japan. Sci Rep 11(1):10365

Ludwig B, Zotzmann V, Bode C, Staudacher DL, Zschiedrich S (2017) Lethal pulmonary hemorrhage syndrome due to Leptospira infection transmitted by pet rat. IDCases 8:84–86

Maroun E, Kushawaha A, El-Charabaty E, Mobarakai N, El-Sayegh S (2011) Fulminant Leptospirosis (Weil's disease) in an urban setting as an overlooked cause of multiorgan failure: a case report. J Med Case Rep 5:7

Narkkul U, Thaipadungpanit J, Srisawat N, Rudge JW, Thongdee M et al (2021) Human, animal, water source interactions and leptospirosis in Thailand. Sci Rep 11(1):3215

OIE (2014) OIE Terrestrial Manual 2021, ch. 3.1.12-Leptospirosis. https://www.woah.org/fileadmin/Home/fr/Health_standards/tahm/3.01.12_LEPTO.pdf

Shivakumar S (2013) Indian guidelines for the diagnosis and management of human leptospirosis. API Medicine Update ed 23 Chapter 7:23–29. file:///C:/Users/kgnar/Downloads/GuidelinesforDiagnosisofHumanLeptospirosisveterinarycollegeIJVASR.pdf

Spickler AR, Larson KL (2013) Leptospirosis. Retrieved from http://www.cfsph.iastate.edu/DiseaseInfo/factsheets.php

Torgerson PR, Hagan JE, Costa F, Calcagno J et al (2015) Global burden of leptospirosis: estimated in terms of disability adjusted life years. PLoS Negl Trop Dis 9(10):e0004122

WHO (2011) Report of the Second Meeting of the Leptospirosis Burden Epidemiology Reference Group

Chapter 47
Louse-Borne Relapsing Fever (LBRF)

Louse-borne relapsing fever are caused by *Bartonella quintana* and *Borrelia recurrentis*. *B. recurrentis* enters a susceptible man via mucous membranes and then invades the blood stream. There is no animal reservoir. *Bartonella quintana* caused angiostoma, endocarditis and lymphadenopathy. *Acinetobacter baumannii* has been added to the list of LBRF.

Characterized by remissions of symptoms that increase in intensity over five days (average 2–7 days) coincident with bacteraemia and then subside with disappearance of spirochaete from blood, first remission is accompanied with reappearance of spirochaete in blood. In untreated patients, less than ten relapses occur usually.

47.1 Aetiology

B. recurrentis are helical, 8–30 µm long and 0.2–0.5 µm in diameter, are motile and have 8–30 flagella. *Borrelia recurrentis* is closely related to *Borrelia duttonii*, the causative agent of tick-borne relapsing fever. It is a human-restricted pathogen.

47.2 Epidemiology

Body lice are the principal vectors of *B. recurrentis*. Viable *B. recurrentis* is found in lice excrement. Authentic relationship between *B. recurrentis* and body lice was found experimentally. Body lice were fed on experimentally spirochaetemic rabbit.

© Springer Nature Singapore Pte Ltd. 2024
K. G. Narayan et al., *Handbook of Management of Zoonoses*,
https://doi.org/10.1007/978-981-99-9885-2_47

Lice remained infected for life but did not transmit borreliae to their progeny. *B. recurrentis* spread to haemolymph on day 5 of infection and formed clumps. *B. recurrentis* was excreted beginning 14 days after infection (Houhamdi et al. 2005). Prolonged excretion enhances transmission. Head lice can also carry this borreliae, as was reported in Ethiopia in 2013. *B. recurrentis* DNA was found in 23% of head lice from patients with louse-borne relapsing fever (Boutellis et al. 2013). Four pathogenic bacteria are transmitted by Pediculus humanus humanus. These are Rickettsia prowazekii ,Borrelia recurrentis, Bartonella quintana and Acinetobacter baumannii (Houhamdi et al. 2005)

Infection spread from person to person most commonly slum dwellers, prisoners and among those living in impoverished overcrowded unhygienic conditions.

In the first half of twentieth century, major outbreaks occurred in Eastern Europe, Balkans, former Soviet Union and Africa linked with war and famine. According to Houhamdi et al. (2005), there was a massive outbreak of relapsing fever (*Borrelia recurrentis*) in Eurasia and Africa earlier and is prevalent in Ethiopia and neighbouring countries.

LBRF has declined with improvement of living conditions. It is endemic foci in Ethiopia, Somalia and Sudan and also recorded in rural Andean community in Peru and in Northern China.

47.3   Symptoms

There were twenty-seven confirmed cases of louse-borne relapsing fever (LBRF) in European Union countries and Switzerland between July and October 2015. These cases, diagnosed among refugees from countries of the Horn of Africa. An increase of refugees from LBRF-endemic areas was observed in the EU since 2014. Body lice infestation is linked to low socioeconomic status, over-crowding and poor personal transmission of LBRF among migrants within the EU. Most likely overcrowding in temporary shelters facilitated secondary spread and cases (ECDC 2015). Incubation period is 2–15 days, bacteraemia, sudden onset, high fever, malaise, chills, sweat, myalgia/arthralgia, nausea and vomiting meningism; injected conjunctiva, petechiae and erythematous rash, cardi-respiratory affection—tachycardia, tachypnea and non-productive cough; hepatomegaly and splenomegaly; neuropathy, cranial nerve palsy, iritis, ophthalmitis; meningitis, meningoencephalitis; common complications—haemorrhage such as epistaxis, blood-tinged sputum and gastrointestinal haemorrhage.

Antigenic variation being common, immunity is only partial. Mortality is 10–40% among untreated and 2–5% among treated

Confounding diseases are malaria, typhoid, viral haemorrhagic fever, leptospirosis, tick-borne relapsing fever, typhus, non-typhoidal salmonellosis and meningitis.

47.4   Diagnosis

- Thrombocytopenia
- Spirochaete demonstration in blood smear, sampled during febrile stage—Giemsa stain/dark-field/phase contrast microscopy
- Culture
- Nucleic acid detection

47.5   Treatment

Tetracyclin, penicillin G, erythromycin and chloramphenicol are useful antibiotics. Antibiotic treatment of LBRF may cause potentially severe to fatal Jarisch-Herxheimer reaction often observed a few hours after the first antibiotic treatment. Two successive phases appear: (a) the chill phase manifests as rigours, high fever, anxiety or confusion, increasing metabolic rate, and (b) the flush phase manifests into decrease in temperature, drenching sweat and significant decrease in arterial pressure and myocardial dysfunction requiring supportive care for monitoring fluid balance and arterial/venous pressure.

47.6   Risk and Management

Migrants from endemic countries are likely to bring LBRF with them and secondary transmission could spread. Most of the 27 confirmed cases of LBRF diagnosed between July and October 2015—Germany (15), Finland (1), Italy (8), the Netherlands (2) and Switzerland (1)—are likely to have got LBRF in country of their origin during their journey to Europe. Migrants increased since 2014. Relief workers caring refugees are at risk, which could be minimized, if they wear gloves. Differential diagnosis in clinical cases to arrive at correct diagnosis will minimize suffering.

Lice are transferred from person to person by direct contact, sharing clothes and bedding. Lice multiply rapidly—increasing by 11% per day. These are susceptible to cold, freezing and desiccation.

- Washing clothes at 60 °C or above
- Dusting powder with insecticide

References

Boutellis A, Mediannikov O, Bilcha KD, Ali J et al (2013) *Borrelia recurrentis* in Head Lice, Ethiopia. Emerg Infect Dis 19(5):796–798

European Centre for Disease Prevention and Control (2015) Louse-borne relapsing fever in the EU – 17 November 2015. Stockholm: ECDC; 2015. © European Centre for Disease Prevention and Control, Stockholm, 2015

Houhamdi L, Parola P, Raoult D (2005) Lice and lice-borne diseases in human. Med Trop (Mars) 65(1):13–23

https://www.ecdc.europa.eu/en/louse-borne-relapsing-fever/facts

Chapter 48
Borreliosis

Synonyms

Lyme disease.

Borreliosis is characterized by affection of multiple systems. During the long course of the disease, skin are affected including vital organs such as brain, heart and joints.

48.1 Aetiology

The causative agent is a Gram-negative spirochaete, in the family Spirochaetaceae, genus *Borrelia*. It is spiral shaped, 20–30 × 0.2–0.3 microns, and moves in a corkscrew-like motion using endoflagella in periplasmic space. The outer surface proteins play a role in virulence. *B. burgdorferi sensu lato* or *B. burgdorferi s. l.* is a bacteria species complex that includes aetiological agents of Lyme borreliosis (Lyme disease) in the Northern hemisphere. It consists of >20 named and proposed genospecies that use vertebrate hosts and tick vectors for transmission in Americas and Eurasia (Wolcott et al. 2021).

Genetic variability within and between each species has a considerable impact on pathogenicity, clinical picture, diagnostic methods, transmission mechanisms and its ecology. The distribution of distinct genospecies varies with the different geographic area and over a time (Derdáková and Lencáková 2005).

There are three closely related species. *B. burgdorferi sensu lato* occurring predominantly in America, extending into Canada, is also present in Europe. *B. garinii* and *B. afzelii* occur predominantly in Europe and Asia. In North America, *Borrelia mayonii* also causes Lyme disease. *B. mayonii* was identified in 2013 collaboratively by the Mayo Clinic, state public health agencies and CDC (Centers for Disease and Control). It has been found in black-legged ticks in north-western

© Springer Nature Singapore Pte Ltd. 2024
K. G. Narayan et al., *Handbook of Management of Zoonoses*,
https://doi.org/10.1007/978-981-99-9885-2_48

Wisconsin and Minnesota (Borrelia mayonii | Ticks | CDC. www.cdc.gov.). Rudenko et al. (2023) reported the isolation of *B. garinii* from cotton mouse (*Peromyscus gossypinus*) in South Carolina, USA. It is closely related to group of isolates from Europe. Their study indicated that the Canadian isolates might have been introduced from Europe or Iceland by seabirds and ticks associated with them. The isolates from the USA formed a part of ancestral lineage from East Asia and might have arrived from Europe.

48.2   Epidemiology

Lyme borreliosis is an important emerging tick-borne zoonosis in Europe, North America and Far Eastern countries. The geographic distribution is influenced by the association of host vector and species of *B. burgdorferi s. l.*

48.2.1   Distribution

Lyme disease is the most common tick-borne disease in North America and Europe and one of the fastest-growing infectious diseases in the USA. The annual incidence in Germany is estimated at 100–150 cases/lakh (Nau et al. 2009). Leighton et al. (2012) predicted that the range of *I. scapularis* tick was expanding. There was an increase of 17% (42,743 confirmed and probable cases) in 2017 (https://www.fda. gov/news-events/press-announcements/fda-clears-new-indications-existing-lyme-disease-tests-may-help-streamline-diagnoses) from 2016 according to CDC, USA (also Content current as of 07-29-2019). According to Ogden et al. (2009), the range of *I. scapularis* is expanding and the number of endemic areas of Lyme disease increasing in Canada. The surveillance data for the period 2010–2016 in Eastern Ontario, Canada, demonstrated that *I. scapularis* and *B. burgdorferi* rapidly spread northwards followed by increasing incidence of Lyme disease; most spread occurred during 2011–2013 (Kulkarni et al. 2019).

A meta-analysis estimated the seropositivity for *B. burgdorferi* for the period 2005–2020 in China (Stark et al. 2022). The point prevalence with a fixed-effects model was 9.1%. The positivity rate with a two-tier testing approach using EIA (Enzyme Immunoassay) plus a confirmatory Western immunoblot was 1.8%. The seropositivity rates in high- and low-risk groups were 10.0% and 4.5%, respectively. The north-eastern and western provinces had the highest seropositivity. Russia, China, Japan, Thailand and Nepal are other countries where *B. burgdorferi sensu lato*-infested ticks are being found more frequently. Li et al. (1998) characterized 59 isolates of *B. burgdorferi s.l* collected from *Ixodes persulcatus* ticks and *Apodemus peninsulae* rodents in Northeastern China. Fifty-eight percent were *B. garinii*, and 28.8% *B. afzelii*; findings were resembling those isolated from Eastern Russia and Japan. According to Masuzawa (2004), *I. persulcatus* carries Eurasian-type

B. garinii (20047 type), *B. afzelii*, and *Asian-type B. garinii* (variant NT29) in Northern Asian countries where *B. burgdorferi sensu stricto* has not been isolated. The Asian-type *B. garinii* has not been found in the European vector tick *Ixodes ricinus*. These *Borrelia* spp. cause Lyme borreliosis in their respective countries.

  B. burgdorferi sensu lato seems to be widely distributed, reported from Morocco, Algeria, Egypt, Tunisia and Kenya in Northern Africa, Central Europe particularly Slovenia and Austria and Italy, Portugal and other countries in this continent. In South America, ticks carrying *B. burgdorferi sensu lato*, as well as canine and human tick-borne disease, are reported widely in Brazil.

48.2.2 Disease Burden

Economic burden of Lyme disease for the period 2014–2016 in the USA was estimated by Hook et al. (2022). The diagnosed cases were approximately 476,000 cases/year. The aggregate cost of these could be $345–968 million (2016 US dollars) to the US society. Patients with confirmed disseminated disease or probable disease had approximately doubled the societal cost of those with confirmed localized disease.

48.2.3 Biocoenosis *and* Natural Nidii

Lyme disease causing *Borrelia* is maintained in nature in reservoir rodents and feeding hard ticks. The infection in these and several other mammals and birds is latent constituting multiple foci. Most common reservoir hosts are white-tailed deer (*Odocoileus virginianus*) and white-footed mice (*Peromyscus leucopus*) for *B. burgdorferi*, rodents for *B. afzelii*, birds for *B. garinii* and *B. valaisiana* and both rodents and birds for *B. burdorferi sensu stricto* and dormouse and hedgehog for *B. spielmanii*.

48.2.4 Life Cycle of Ticks and Seasonality of Disease (Fig. 48.1)

The vector tick species are different in different locales: *I ricinus* (sheep tick or castor bean tick) in Europe; *I. persulcatus* (taiga tick) in China, Asia; *I. scapularis* (black-legged or deer tick) on the east coast and *I. pacificus* (Western black-legged tick) on the west coast; and *I. dammini* in the north-eastern and midwestern parts are the vectors in America.

  Black-legged ticks can feed from mammals, birds, reptiles and amphibians. The ticks need to have a new host at each stage of their life. These (e.g. *I. dammini*,

Life cycle (2 years -span) of the vector tick *I. dammini*
(Transovarial & transstadial transmission of *B. burgdorferi*)

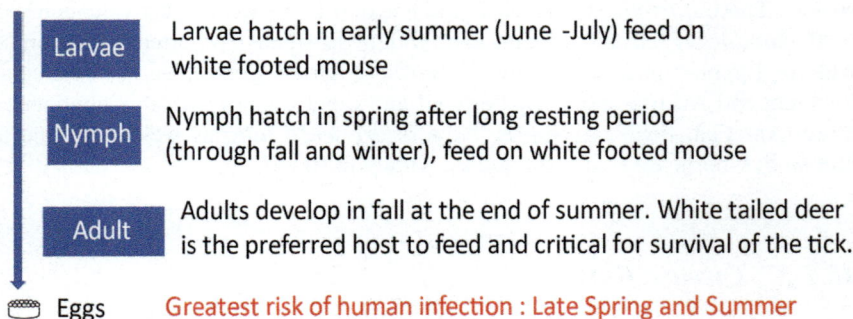

Larvae	Larvae hatch in early summer (June -July) feed on white footed mouse
Nymph	Nymph hatch in spring after long resting period (through fall and winter), feed on white footed mouse
Adult	Adults develop in fall at the end of summer. White tailed deer is the preferred host to feed and critical for survival of the tick.

Eggs   **Greatest risk of human infection : Late Spring and Summer**

The infection is transmitted to humans by a <u>bridge tick</u>, *I. pacificus*. *I. neotomae* and Kangaro rat maintains enzootic cycle. *I. neotomae* does not feed on human.

Fig. 48.1 Transovarial and transstadial transmission of *Borrelia burgdorferi*

I. scapularis) take two years, from eggs and larvae in one calendar year to nymph and adult in the next (Fig. 48.1). Generally, these abound in deciduous forest, tall grasslands and shrubs bordering edge of forest, and distribution is related to the distribution of their reproductive host, white-tailed deer.

White-tailed deer is the preferred host for adult *I. dammini* and is critical to the survival of ticks. A critical population density of white-tailed deer may thus be controlling the ticks' density, and this may be exploited by ecologists to control Lyme disease.

The larval and the nymphal stages of *I. dammini* feed on the preferred host, white-footed mouse. The enzootic is maintained in North California in dusky-footed wood rat (*Neotoma fuscipes*) and California Kangaro rat (*Dipodomys californicus*) by *I. neotomae*, which does not feed on humans. The infection is transmitted to humans by a *bridge tick*, *I. pacificus* (Walker et al. 1996). The distribution of Lyme disease mirrors the distribution of the vector ticks.

Ixodes dammini mate on hosts' body and the male dies. Females oviposit during March and April (spring). It takes four weeks for larvae to emerge. They feed actively on the preferred hosts (white-footed mouse) for 2–3 days, generally once during June and July (early summer). Following spring, larvae moult and nymph appear and feed for 3–4 days on white-footed mouse. The life cycle of the spirochete depends upon horizontal transmission between immature ticks and mice. Adults emerge during end of summer and in September. Infection in ticks being trans-ovarial and trans-stadial, there is a build-up of infection in increased population of infected vectors which feed during spring and summer, and this is reflected in the seasonal occurrence of Lyme disease. Its seasonal occurrence coincides with ticks' activity; most cases occur during May through September. Studies in Canada indicate *I. scapularis* prefer warmer regions, and projected increases in temperature with climate change are expected to permit and accelerate the expansion of hotspots. Adult ticks abound in bush about a metre from the ground. This positioning helps them attach easily on grazing mammals and human. Seasonality of occurrence of the disease was related to life cycle of ticks. In Germany, most cases occurred between June and August, only 15% during November and April (Nau et al. 2009).

48.2.5 Transmission

Mostly nymph bites but also adult tick bites cause infection. The victim remains unaware of tick bite for two reasons: nymphal stage of tick is very small (<2 mm) and bite is painless, usually in armpit, groin and scalp. Ticks remain undetected. For the transmission of infection, the tick must remain attached to host for long, at least a day (24–36 h). The *Borrelia* in the gut of tick migrates to the salivary gland only after contact with blood (post attachment takes time) and then to the human host through the punctured wound.

Ticks are often found at the hairline in children. Careless manoeuvring to remove the ticks or covering with ointments or oil may lead to regurgitation of blood increasing the likelihood of transmission. It is advised to use tweezers.

Requirement of a bridge tick and long feeding on susceptible host may be the reason for delay in the detection of natural foci of infection. The recognition of Lyme disease was delayed possibly because of this. In 1975, first cluster of 15 cases was detected in Lyme, Connecticut, USA, and hence the name of the disease. In the next 10 years, 1500 more cases were added.

Other means of transmission and spread: Clinical disease occurs in horses, cattle, sheep, dogs and man. Spirochete is shed in semen, breast milk, cows' milk and urine. Congenital transmission from mother to foetus and transplacental in women and mares occurs during pregnancy. Infection during the first three months of pregnancy harms the foetus.

Oral infection in experimental white-footed mouse has been observed. Bite from asymptomatic infected horses may also transmit.

The same tick may be carrying more than one pathogen, and multiple co-infections are possible, complicating diagnosis, for example, *Theileria microti* and *Anaplasma phagocytophilum*.

48.2.6 Population at Risk and Activities

Persons at risk irrespective of age and sex are hunters, hikers, campers and foresters, dog owners and rural folk and farmers exposed to tick habitat. Deforestation and encroaching upon the forest regions due to urbanization bring the human closer to the forest and so the tick habitat. On the other hand, reforestation may present increasing opportunities of expansion of biotopes and enzootic area. Recreational activities such as hiking and camping in forest areas are likely to expose to the tick habitat and bite.

48.3   Symptoms

According to Nau et al. (2009), *Borrelia burgdorferi sensu stricto, B. afzelii, B. garinii* and *B. spielmanii* are the causative agents of human Borreliosis in Europe, and till date *B. spielmanii* caused erythema migrans only; *B. afzelii* acrodermatitis chronica atrophicans (ACA) only and *B. garinii* often caused neuroborreliosis. The other species apparently caused all the clinical symptoms.

48.3.1   Pathogenesis: Mechanism of Infection, Pathology and Persistence in Hosts' Body

Tick saliva disables the local immune system to allow *Borrelia* to establish infection at the site of tick bite. Erythema chronicum migrans (ECM) or Bull's eye appears. Neutrophils fail to appear in this area and clear infection. The spirochete survives, multiplies and spreads to multiple organs of the body evading antibodies. The mechanisms may be, decreasing expression of and changing structure (antigenic variation) of surface proteins of the spirochaete that are targeted by antibodies, inactivating complement, hiding in the extracellular matrix.

Lyme disease pathology may be a 'pathogen-induced autoimmune disease'. The spirochete's resemblance to hosts' body tissues (a) protects it from being killed by hosts' immune system and explains (b) some of the chronic symptoms that arise from autoimmune reaction and (c) persistence of symptoms (chronic arthritis) even after the body has been cleared of the spirochete. Ogrinc et al. (2022) demonstrated that borrelial meningoradiculoneuritis presented unique immune and genetic pathophysiology.

48.3.2   Clinical Presentation

Infected tick initiates infection in human. Silent infection is common. An expanding skin lesion, erythema migrans, appears within days to weeks at the site of tick bite. In untreated cases, infection may disseminate involving other organs. As reported by Nau et al. (2009), the rate of seroconversion ranged between 3% and 6% in Germany. Overt disease appears in 0.3–1.4% of tick bites. A study reveals 313 cases in Wurzburg (Bavaria, Germany), 89% cases manifested in ECM, 3% a stage II neuroborreliosis, 2% borrelial lymphocytoma, arthritis in 5%, ACA in 1% and carditis in <1% and none stage III (chronic) neuroborreliosis.

The spirochaete affects multiple body system and so produces a variety of symptoms, all may not be seen in every patient, and some may be non-specific, seen in other diseases also.

Lyme disease has a long duration and may be classified as early or late. The clinical manifestation may be classified as local or generalized and varies with age of the patient, species of pathogens and others. An untreated patient passes through three different stages—1, 2 and 3—each lasting for several weeks, two to several months and months to years, respectively. Most cases end with stage 1. Most cases recover in stages 1 and 2.

48.3.2.1 Stage 1. Early Localized (Days to Weeks After the Tick Bite)

Characteristic circular expanding skin lesion called ECM (erythema chronicum migrans or bull's eye, Fig. 48.2) appears at the site of bite about 3–32 days (may be longer) of infected tick bite (incubation period). Thigh, groin and axilla are the common sites. ECM begins as red macule and expands as annular bright red rings. There is diffuse erythema and urticaria. There may be two or more rings suggesting systemic bacterial dissemination. Some cases present flu-like symptoms, fever, severe headache, musculoskeletal pain, arthralgia, stiff neck, chill, depression and malaise. Patients continue to feel constant fatigue and lethargy for months. ECM resolves spontaneously in few days to weeks if left untreated.

Jairath et al. (2014) described a series of five cases recorded in a period of three months in a village of Haryana, India. Three cases got the exposure while farming (Fig. 48.3). Two recalled they had tick bite. A young boy of 17 years had a tick bite in the groin while he was playing football. The fifth case was a boy of seven years. He had visited a resort two weeks earlier. Erythematous patch measuring 15 cm × 10 cm was seen around the right ear extending onto the right side of the

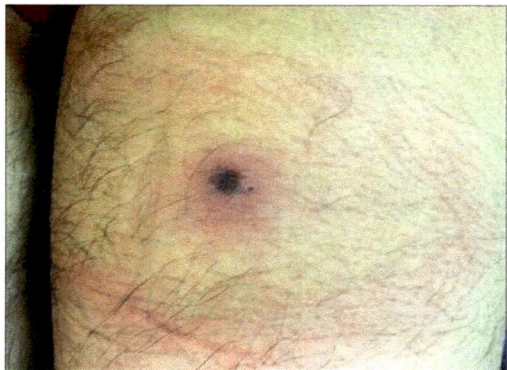

Fig. 48.2 Bull's eye lesion with a central necrotic ulcer with a 10 cm × 10 cm diameter ring of erythema on thigh of a 17-year-old villager (Jairath et al. 2014)

Fig. 48.3 Blister on an erythematous latch 6 × 7 cm patch over right arm of a 32-year-old farmer (Jairath et al. 2014)

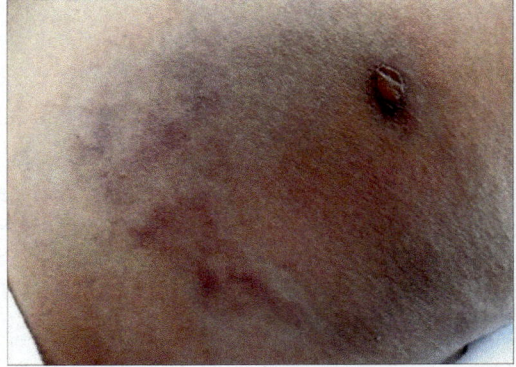

neck. All cases reported associated symptoms like fever, myalgia, fatigue, arthralgia and lymphadenopathy.

48.3.2.2   Stage 2. Early Disseminated (Weeks to Six Months After the Tick Bite)

Dissemination of *Borrelia* through blood stream begins within days to weeks after infection, and it spreads to the skin, heart, joint, peripheral nervous system and central nervous system during course of disease. ECM appears at sites other than tick bite.

Borrelial lymphocytoma or lymphadenosis is a cutaneous manifestation appearing within two months of tick bite. ECM often accompanies. It appears as a benign, purple-coloured lump in the ear lobe, nipple and scrotum of patients. Patients complain of migrating pain in the muscle, joints and tendons.

According to Ogrinc et al. (2022), Lyme neuroborreliosis (NLB) is common in Europe and the second most common in North America. In adults, it begins with painful meningoradiculoneuritis (also known as Garin-Bujadoux-Bannwarth syndrome or Bannwarth syndrome) or with cranial neuritis and is by peripheral facial palsy (PFP) or lymphocytic meningitis. It is the leading manifestation of stage 2. There is lymphomonocytic meningitis, radiculitis (inflammation of spinal nerve roots) and cranial nerve deficits (Nau et al. 2009). Neurological symptoms are seen in about 5% of cases, characterized by clear symptoms of meningitis (severe headache, nuchal rigidity, photophobia), encephalitis and cranial neuritis. There is facial palsy/Bell's palsy and radiculoneuropathy (shooting pain). Memory loss and sleep disturbance occur in mild neurological borreliosis. These may resolve within months. Later chronic neurological disorders may appear. Children usually suffer with peripheral facial palsy.

Borrelial carditis may appear after 4 days to 7 months of tick bite (usually after 21 days) and is a rare complication in Europe than in North America (Nau et al. 2009). Cardiac symptoms appear in some and last for few weeks. Erythema migrans or neurological deficits often accompany. There is atrioventricular block of variable severity which resolves in six weeks. Symptoms are dizziness, palpitations and syncope.

48.3.2.3   Stage 3. Late or Persistent (Longer Than Six Months After the Tick Bite, Perhaps Years After It)

Multiple body system may be affected in untreated or incompletely treated patients leading to severe and chronic myriads of disabling symptoms, like paraplegia. Organs such as the brain, heart, eyes, nerves and joints may be affected.

Borreliosis induced chronically progressive meningoencephalitis, cerebral vasculitis and extra pyramidal motor disease. Chronically progressive meningoencephalitis and multifocal cerebral encephalitis cause irreversible neurological damage. In a study in Germany, <5% of all neuroborreliosis cases suffered with it (Nau et al. 2009). Chronic neurological symptoms include shooting pain, numbness and tingling in the hand and feet, difficulty in concentration, short-term memory and profound fatigue. Chronic progressive encephalomyelitis manifests as cognitive impairment, leg weakness, back pain and facial palsy. Rarely psychosis may develop.

Oligoarticular arthritis of large joints, particularly of the knee, and symmetrical polyarthritis and ACA (acrodermatitis chronica atrophicans of Herxheimer) are the two typical manifestations of stage 3. The inflammatory skin lesions may appear as a transition to atrophic stage of ACA six months to several years after tick bite on the external surfaces of the limbs, face or trunk. The lesion looks like thin skin with altered pigmentation and prominent veins. There is pain, pruritus, hyperaesthesia or paresthesia.

Prognosis: Early cases are successfully treated. Delay in diagnosis and antibiotic therapy, co-infection with other tick-borne diseases and immune suppression or deficiency complicates the case. Neurocognitive symptoms, physical disability and fatigue and pain in the muscle and joints may persist for years. Rare cases end fatally.

48.3.2.4   Post-Treatment Lyme Disease Syndrome (PTLDS)

Some patients complain pain, fatigue and difficulty in thinking for six months after completion of course of treatment. The reason is unclear. Three possibilities may be (a) auto-immune response as seen in Campylobacter (Guillain-Barré syndrome), Chlamydia (Reiter's syndrome) and strep throat (rheumatic heart disease), (b) a persistent but difficult-to-detect infection and (c) other causes unrelated to the patient's *Borrelia burgdorferi* infection. There is no defined treatment. Patients feel better overtime, maybe months for complete recovery.

48.4 Diagnosis

* History of possible exposure to ticks and tick bite.
* Symptoms.
* Physical examination revealing ECM, facial paralysis and arthritis.
* Neuroborreliosis is diagnosed by observing in CSF pleocytosis—leucocytes <1000/ml predominately lymphocytes, high protein (1 g/L or higher), intrathecally formed specific antibody IgG and IgM (antibody index) [Nau et al. 2009].
* Serodiagnosis by IFA, ELISA, SDS-PAGE and Western blot. Sera samples taken in early and late stage of disease yield erroneous results. Western blot—IgM—may be used in diagnosis of early cases.
* Two-tier approach used EIA followed by Western blot to confirm a clinical diagnosis. The FDA reviewed data from clinical studies of the ZEUS ELISA *Borrelia*VlsE1/pepC10 IgG/IgM Test System, ZEUS ELISA *Borrelia burgdorferi* IgG/IgM Test System, ZEUS ELISA *Borrelia burgdorferi* IgM Test System and the ZEUS ELISA *Borrelia burgdorferi* IgG Test System that showed this alternative approach, referred to as a modified two-tier test and cleared, July 29, 2019 (https://www.fda.gov/news-events/press-announcements/fda-clears-new-indications-existing-lyme-disease-tests-may-help-streamline-diagnoses).
* Demonstration of spirochete by dark ground illumination, IFA in specimens from the skin, blood, affected tissue, synovial fluid and CSF.
* Culture.
* PCR for spirochete-DNA sample may be blood and CSF.
* CSF levels of B-cell chemoattractants CXCL12 and CXCL13, T-cell chemoattractants CXCL9 and CXCL10 and Th17 cytokine, IL-17, are markedly elevated in patients of meningoradiculoneuritis. These immune modulators may be used for diagnosis and markers of disease progress or resolution (Ogrinc et al. 2022).
* Nanotechnology-based test has been developed (Lerner et al. 2013). Single-walled carbon nanotube (SWNT) field-effect transistors (FETs) are a fast and accurate sensors of Lyme disease antigen. As little as 1 ng/mL of Lyme flagellar protein can be detected in 20 min.

48.5 Treatment

Depending upon the patients' condition and stage of disease—doxycycline, amoxicillin and erythromycin are useful, respectively, for adults, children and pregnant women. Ceftriaxone, cefuroxime and cefotaxime are also useful. The course of treatment is generally 14–28 days. Tetracycline should not be given to pregnant women. Spirochete crosses blood-brain barrier in neuroborreliosis, and minocycline also does so and is therefore useful.

48.6   Prevention

Prediction of Lyme disease or detection of host spots are useful in preventing the occurrence.

According to Tkadlec et al. (2019), data on rodent host densities and climate indices dynamics of Lyme disease and tick-borne encephalitis can predict the risk of these diseases one year in advance .

Ogden et al. (2009) advocated the use of risk maps and risk algorithms to identify the areas where *Ixodes scapularis* ticks are getting established. Active surveillance driven by risk maps identified expected additional emerging population in Southern Quebec in the absence of clear indications from passive surveillance.

Animal sentinel: Lyme disease can occur in dogs and deer. Dogs may suffer with joint disease or glomerulonephritis and may be fatal. Dog should be examined for ticks in the head, neck and ears.

Protection against exposure and infection:

- Protective measures against ticks' exposure and bites.
- Examination of shelter workers, foresters, campers and their pets and animal owners and their animals after they return from forest for ticks.
- Removal of ticks carefully.
- Outer Surface Protein A (OspA) of *B. burgdorferi*-based recombinant vaccine (LYMErix, Glaxo Smith Kline) protected 76% of adults and 100% of children with mild to moderate transient side effects. Newer vaccines are being developed with Osp C and glycoprotein. Valeneva's VLA5 (www.valneva.com) is a multivalent protein subunit vaccine, targets OspA of all serotypes of Borrelia and produces excellent anamnestic response to booster given 12–15 months after first injection. Antibodies prevent *Borrelia* migrating from tick to human after bite. The company announced (Saint-Herblain, France July 1, 2019) 'second phase testing' (Valneva. Valneva initiates second phase 2 study for its Lyme disease vaccine candidate VLA15 (https://valneva.com/press-release/valneva-initiates-second-phase-2-study-for-its-lyme-disease-vaccine-candidate-vla15).
- Dogs may be protected with available vaccines.
- Domesticated guinea fowl are voracious eaters of insects and like ticks in particular—maybe used as a biological control measure.

References

Derdáková M, Lencáková D (2005) Association of genetic variability within the *Borrelia burgdorferi sensu lato* with the ecology, epidemiology of Lyme borreliosis in Europe. Ann Agric Environ Med 12(2):165–172

Hook SA, Jeon S, Niesobecki SA, Hansen AP et al (2022) Economic burden of reported Lyme disease in high-incidence areas, United States, 2014–2016. Emerg Infect Dis 28(6):1170–1179

Jairath V, Sehrawat M, Jindal N, Jain VK, Aggarwal P (2014) Lyme disease in Haryana, India. Indian J Dermatol Venereol Leprol 80(4):320–323

Kulkarni MA, Narula I, Slatculescu AM, Russell C (2019) Lyme disease emergence after invasion of the blacklegged tick, Ixodes scapularis, Ontario, Canada, 2010–2016. Emerg Infect Dis 25(2):328–332

Leighton P, Koffi P, Lindsay O (2012) Predicting the speed of tick invasion: an empirical model of range expansion for the Lyme disease vector *Ixodes scapularis* in Canada. J Appl Ecol 49(2):457

Lerner MB, Dailey J, Goldsmith BR, Brisson D, Johnson ATC (2013) Detecting Lyme disease using antibody-functionalized single-walled carbon nanotube transistors. Biosens Bioelectron 45:163–167

Li M, Masuzawa T, Takada N, Ishiguro F et al (1998) Lyme disease *Borrelia* species in northeastern China resemble those isolated from far eastern Russia and Japan. Appl Environ Microbiol 64(7):2705–2709

Masuzawa T (2004) Terrestrial distribution of the Lyme borreliosis agent *Borrelia burgdorferi sensu lato* in East Asia. Jpn J Infect Dis 57(6):229–235

Nau R, Christen HJ, Eiffert H (2009) Lyme disease--current state of knowledge. Dtsch Arztebl Int 106(5):72–81

Ogden NH, Lindsay LR, Morshed M, Sockett PN, Artsob H (2009) The emergence of Lyme disease in Canada. CMAJ 180(12):1221–1224

Ogrinc K, Hernández SA, Korva M, Bogovič P et al (2022) Unique clinical, immune, and genetic signature in patients with borrelial meningoradiculoneuritis. Emerg Infect Dis 28(4):766–776

Rudenko N, Golovchenko M, Horak A, Grubhoffer L et al (2023) Genomic confirmation of *Borrelia garinii*, United States. Emerg Infect Dis 29(1):64–69

Stark J, Li X, Zhang J, Burn L, Valluri SR et al (2022) Systematic review and meta-analysis of Lyme disease data and seropositivity for *Borrelia burgdorferi*, China, 2005–2020. Emerg Infect Dis 28(12):2389–2397

Tkadlec E, Václavík T, Široký P (2019) Rodent host abundance and climate variability as predictors of tickborne disease risk 1 year in advance. Emerg Infect Dis 25(9):1738–1741

Walker DH, Barbour AG, Oliver JH, Lane RS, Dumier JS et al (1996) Emerging bacterial zoonotic and vector borne diseases. JAMA 275(6):463–469

Wolcott KA, Margos G, Fingerle V, Becker NS (2021) Host association of *Borrelia burgdorferi sensu lato*: a review. Ticks Tick-Borne Dis 12(5):101766

Chapter 49
Southern Tick-Associated Rash Illness (STARI)

Synonyms

Masters' disease.

Southern tick-associated rash illness (STARI) or Masters' disease is erythema migrans characterized by expanding annular erythema (3 inches or 8 cm or more), which tends to have lymphocytic infiltrate. *Borrelia lonestari* was considered to be a causative agent but further research did not support. The cause of STARI remains unknown (https://www.cdc.gov/stari/disease/index.html).

The natural history is not completely known. The adult female tick bears a white dot on its back, hence called lone star tick, *Amblyomma americanum*; all the three stages feed on the reservoir white-tailed deer and human and transmission takes place. The ticks are active in eastern south-eastern and south-central states. The range of the lone star tick has increased over the years. STARI occurs during spring summer coincident with tick activity. Lone star ticks have not been found transmitting Lyme disease (*Borrelia burgdorferi*).

Symptoms are very similar to Lyme disease but mild. The causative agent has not been cultivated from skin lesion biopsy, blood and tissues or ticks. But the bite of tick may cause redness and discomfort because saliva of tick is irritating. It may not indicate that transmission has taken place.

The incubation period is 7 days. Rash mild fever, generalized fatigue, headache, stiff neck, myalgia, arthralgia and swollen lymph nodes within 30 days of tick bite require consulting a physician.

Diagnosis is arrived at by observing (a) history of tick bite, (b) rash on the skin, (c) spring summer seasonality, (d) absence of antibodies to *B. burgdorferi* and (e) PCR. Doxycycline is effective.

© Springer Nature Singapore Pte Ltd. 2024
K. G. Narayan et al., *Handbook of Management of Zoonoses*,
https://doi.org/10.1007/978-981-99-9885-2_49

Chapter 50
Mycobacteriosis

One or the other species of *Mycobacterium* caused chronic inflammatory conditions in human beings. Classical tuberculosis is caused by *M. tuberculosis*, primarily transmissible between human beings. This and other species of *M. tuberculosis* complex infect both animals and human beings and are transmissible both ways and hence classed as zooanthropozoonosis and anthropozoonosis. The animals' and birds' mycobacterioses are also transmissible to human (direct anthropozoonosis) causing primarily extra-pulmonary TB (tuberculosis). There is a larger group of glandular and skin infections caused by environmental mycobacteria classed as nontuberculous mycobacteria (NTM). Many of these are classed as saprozoonosis.

50.1 Aetiology

Mycobacteriosis is caused by species of the genus *Mycobacterium*, family *Mycobacteriaceae* of phylum *Actinobacteria*. There are >190 members of the genus *Mycobacterium*.

Mycobacteria are Gram-positive, non-motile and non-sporing rod-shaped (0.2–0.6 × 1.0–10 microns). These grow into rough or smooth colonies of varying colours white to pink. Most are aerobic.

These are distributed widely, living in natural tap and chlorine treated water and foods except the obligate parasitic species which cause tuberculosis and leprosy. These are small rod-shaped, encapsulated, aerobic, acid fast non-motile (except *M. marinum*) bacteria. There is an outer membrane. The cell wall is thicker than most other bacteria and made up of layers of hydrophobic mycolate and peptidoglycan held together by polysaccharide.

Pathogenicity is determined by hosts' body, survivability in environment and ability to colonize. Mycobacterial infection in most is asymptomatic. One-fourth of the world's population has latent TB and cannot transmit.

© Springer Nature Singapore Pte Ltd. 2024
K. G. Narayan et al., *Handbook of Management of Zoonoses*,
https://doi.org/10.1007/978-981-99-9885-2_50

Mycobacterial cell wall is very thick. Of the four layers, the innermost consists of peptidoglycan and others of lipids. The cell wall is uniquely resistant enabling it to survive acids, alkalis, detergents, oxidative bursts and lysis by complement and impermeable to various dyes.

Infection is notoriously difficult to treat. Mycobacteria are naturally resistant to many antibiotics that disrupt cell walls, for example, penicillin. Mycobacteria, like other pathogenic bacteria, produce a number of secretory proteins that contribute to virulence.

50.1.1   Medical Classification

Medical classification: Mycobacteria fall in four groups:

1. *Mycobacterium tuberculosis* is a complex cause of tuberculosis in man and similar disease in animals.
2. *M. leprae* and *M. lepromatosis* are causes of Hansen's disease or leprosy.
3. *M. avium* complex (MAC) are agents causing disseminated infection (not lung), leading to deaths in individuals with AIDS and immunocompromised.
4. Non-tuberculous mycobacteria (NTM) are all the other Mycobacteria which can cause pulmonary disease resembling tuberculosis, lymphadenitis, skin disease or disseminated disease. These atypical, environmental Mycobacteria are classed as Mycobacteria other than tuberculosis (MOTT).

50.2   Forms of Tuberculosis

Following types of mycobacteriosis are described:

- Classical TB
- MDR and XDR
- TB-HIV
- Nosocomial
- Anthropozoonotic
- Zoonotic

  - Wildlife
  - Bovine – TB and others
  - NTM

50.2.1   Classical TB

A communicable disease TB is a major cause of ill health and one of the leading causes of death worldwide by a single infectious agent, except for the recent pandemic causing coronavirus COVID-19.

The manifestation of infection ranges from simple sensitivity to mild cough and common cold to serious pulmonary form. About 25% world's population get infected but most do not fall ill. An estimated 90% of cases are adults, more males than females, and 50% die if not treated.

Those sick with pulmonary form are infectious and spread infection through talk, sneeze and cough. Left untreated, each person with active TB will infect on an average between 10 and 15 persons every year. TB bacilli may remain dormant and are protected for years by a thick waxy coat and the hosts' immune system. Weakening of the hosts' immune system increases the chance of precipitation of sickness. TB affects development in any country. Poverty and undernourishment fuel TB. HIV, diabetes and smoking contribute to infection. Currently, recommended treatment regimen of 4–6 months cures 85%.

50.2.1.1   Global Picture/Status

TB is a global problem. WHO Global's report on TB in the year 2022 covers 99% of the world's population from 202 countries and territories. In 2021, Southeast Asian countries accounted for 46% of new cases followed by the WHO African region with 23% and the WHO Western Pacific with 18%. In 2020, 30 countries accounted for 87% of new cases. India, Indonesia, China, the Philippines, Pakistan, Nigeria, Bangladesh and South Africa accounted for two-thirds of cases (WHO 2022a).

COVID-19 pandemic has impacted. Progress made up to 2019 has slowed, stalled or reversed, achieving global targets delayed. Access to diagnosis, treatment and burden were affected.

Burden of reported newly diagnosed cases dropped. India, Indonesia and the Philippines accounted for 67% of global total, and reports from these led to the most reduction in 2020. They made partial recovery in 2021 yet accounted for 60% of the global reduction compared with 2019. Treatment of rifampicin-resistant tuberculosis (RR-TB) and multidrug-resistant tuberculosis (MDR-TB) dropped. Global spending on essential TB services declined. Estimated number of deaths increased between 2019 and 2021. There were 1.4 million deaths among HIV-negative (95% uncertainty interval [UI]: 1.3–1.5 million) and 187,000 deaths (95% UI : 158,000–218,000) among HIV-positive people, for a combined total of 1.6 million compared to 1.5 million in 2020 and 1.4 million in 2019. In 2021, 10.6 million (95% UI: 9.9–11 million) fell ill, an increase of 4.5% from 10.1 million (95% UI: 9.5–10.7 million) in 2020. Incidence per 100,000/year rose by 3.6% between 2020 and 2021. There were 450,000 (95% UI: 399 000–501 000) new cases of RR-TB. Burden of drug-resistant TB (DR-TB) increased between 2020 and 2021. The rate of success for people treated for TB was 86% in 2019 and the same was maintained in 2020.

Milestones of the End TB strategy for incidence and death have been achieved or passed by Kenya, United Republic of Tanzania and Zambia; Ethiopia is very close.

Yet COVID-19 affected badly. Against the WHO END TB Strategy milestones for 2025 (against 2015) of reduction in (a) incidence (50%), (b) deaths (75%) and percent of people with TB facing catastrophic cost to 0%, the achievements in 2021 were 10%, 5.9% and 48%, respectively.

People with TB-receiving treatment increased from about 6.0 million in 2015 to 7.0 million in 2018 and 7.1 million in 2019. TB-preventing treatment is recommended by WHO for people living with HIV, household contacts of those bacteriologically confirmed pulmonary TB and clinical risk groups such as receiving dialysis. The number of people receiving TB-preventive treatment increased from 1.0 million in 2015 to 2.2 million in 2018 and 4.1 million in 2019.

In most of European countries, the overall rate of TB has been declining during the past five years (ECDC-WHO 2021). In 2019, the rate of notification was 9.6/100,000 population in the EU/EEA. The target notification rate is 2.4 per 100,000 populations by 2030 under the United Nations Sustainable Development Goal 3. A total of 49,752 cases of TB were reported; 76.9% were new cases and 67.1% were confirmed by culture or smear or nucleic acid amplification tests. Most of new and relapse cases (65.3%) were in the age group of 25–64 years and 4.1% under 15 years. Male-to-female ratio was 1.8.

Between 2019 and 2020, there was a drop by 24% in notified new cases and relapse TB partly due to COVID-19 pandemic strain on the health system. Despite this, the 163,602 incident TB cases were reported in the European union. The EU and European Economic Area continued with less than 10 TB cases/100,000 population (ECDC 2022).

50.2.1.2 Modes of Transmission

Mycobacteria may enter a susceptible host either through respiratory, oral or skin routes. The transmission through inhalation is most common. Aerosolized respiratory excretion (droplets 0.5–5.0 micron)—cough, sneeze (40,000 droplets/sneeze), sputum and saliva (speech)—may carry *M. tuberculosis* in droplet and reach lung alveoli to precipitate infection. The infective dose may be as low as 1–3 Mycobacteria. Ingestion is a common route for infection with fresh milk from infected udder. Active TB case can infect 5–15 other people through close contact over the course of one year. Risk of falling ill after infection is 5–10% lifetime, and it is higher for those comorbidities like HIV, diabetes, malnutrition and smokers.

Mycobacteria enter tonsils or intestinal mucosa. Infection occurs with milk from infected cows or indirectly contaminated milk. Accidental cuts/injuries through butchers' knife, post-mortem implements and injection needle introduce Mycobacteria. More important is that transmission often occurs before detection of transmitter (diagnosis of a case).

50.2.1.3 Epidemiology

Open cases of tuberculosis shed Mycobacteria. Duration of infectious status-sputum positive, concentration of Mycobacteria in sputum, duration of contact and also density of persons around determine secondary attack rate. One infectious case is expected to shed one infectious *Mycobacterium* in air per 200 cubic feet. Estimation of incidence/prevalence is based on sputum analysis, tuberculin testing and chest X-ray. Infection is favoured by a number of factors.

Innate resistance is suggested. Incidence is high among Gurkhas compared to Marathas. TB incidence peaks during spring and summer. It seems that incidence is influenced by low temperature, low humidity, low rainfall and climate change.

High risk factors are poverty, malnutrition, drug addiction and certain ethnic minorities and exposure to those who have contact with high-risk category patients.

Crowding and confinement aid in transmission. Reporting of TB in prisons is poor. Prisoners had a relative risk of 15.8 compared to general population in the same country. There were 185 new and relapse cases reported from 13 EU/EEA countries (ECDC-WHO 2021).

Inadequate and poor health-care facilities, poverty, poor nutrition and low socio-economic condition contribute to infection. As per WHO (2022b), >80% cases and deaths were reported from low- and middle-income countries. Around 2.2 million new TB cases in 2019 were attributable to malnutrition (risk factor of 3). Similarly, alcohol and tobacco smoking increased risk of infection and death. People with HIV stood 16 times risk of developing active TB. Other comorbidities impairing immune system also increased the risk of active infection and death. Alcohol use disorder accounted for 0.74 million and tobacco smoking to 0.69 million new TB cases in 2021 worldwide.

Certain occupations and overcrowding reduce social distance. Semilan et al. (2021) determined the occupational exposure and incidence of TB in the Makkah region. TB incidence has been reported as highest (25.13/100,000 persons) in this region of Saudi Arabia through 2005–2012. In a planned cross-sectional study, incidence among workers was 9 compared to 31 per 100,000 non-workers in 2016. Among the workers, two occupational groups, namely, supporting basic engineering (car drivers, building construction labourers, mechanics, blacksmiths, carpenters) and agriculture, animal husbandry and fishing, had the highest incidence of TB, 13 and 12.11 per 100,000, respectively, attributable to close contact, long period of contact and low socioeconomic. Low income leads to more of treatment dropouts. Working hours was not but both medium educational level and low educational level, and the incidence rate of TB had an inverse association.

Study by Karande and Bavdekar (2002) in slum areas of Mumbai suggested that dense population; overcrowded slum, that is, poor housing and sanitary conditions; and the presence of children with HIV (mostly vertically infected) contributed to increased TB, MDR and TB-HIV. Most sputum-negative children went undiagnosed and were not covered by the Revised National Tuberculosis Control Programme and Directly Observed Treatment Short Course (DOTS).

Slum dwellings combine all such factors. Smoking and occupational exposure to metallic and stone dust (pneumoconiosis) prepare a favourable tissue for precipitating Mycobacterial infection. More males are occupied in such operations and higher incidence in males is thus observed. Health workers, nurses and young doctors attending patients with respiratory symptoms (undiagnosed) in outpatient wards stand at high risk of infection.

Similarly, prolonged period of exposure is posed by a number of open cases of tuberculosis (especially uncured/prechemotherapy period) to family members and health-care workers.

Availability of health-care facility—rapid diagnosis followed by chemotherapy and BCG vaccination and awareness—contributes to reduction in prevalence, transmission and incidence. Migrating labourers contribute to transmission and treatment—dropouts and increase in MDR-TB. Migratory labourers have no identity proof and often have no access (and often not sustained) to government diagnostic and treatment services. Guidelines and strategy to track migrants are missing in TB control programme. They constitute a large proportion of urban slum dwellers. Maharashtra has one-fifth of India's slum dwellers. They are deprived of these facilities. They constitute a large number of TB cases, both drug sensitive and MDR-TB.

50.2.1.4   Pathogenesis – Primary, Progressive

Infection depends upon species of *Mycobacterium*, virulence, dose of infection and host species, for example, *M tuberculosis* infects human, non-human primates and guinea pigs. Cattle, cats and rabbits are susceptible to *M. bovis* but resistant to *M. tuberculosis*. Dogs and swine are susceptible to both *M. tuberculosis* and *M. bovis*.

Incidence of TB has three components—(a) recurrent TB in patients who have had previously disease, (b) rapid progression to TB among individuals infected or re-infected within relatively short period (say, less than two years) of infection and (c) reactivation of TB contracted many years ago. Molecular and conventional epidemiological investigation methods identify each.

The host defence may thwart the infection. In weak and susceptible individual, primary infection sets in. *Mycobacterium* is naturally equipped with factors that enable it to overcome the body's natural defence mechanisms. These invade and multiply in endosome of alveolar macrophages. The structure of the cell wall (rich in lipid-mycolic acid) prevents fusion of the phagosome with lysosome and blocks bridging molecule early endosomal autoantigen 1 (EEA1) without affecting the fusion with vesicle filled with nutrients; thus bacterium continues to grow unchecked in the macrophages; the gene UreC prevents acidification of the phagosome; the neutralizing reactive nitrogen intermediates too are evaded. *M. tuberculosis* reproduces in macrophages and kills these.

Protective immunity is due to CMI (cell-mediated immunity) response. Granuloma form around the invading bacteria to arrest progress and localize the infection. This process is interfered, or the localized infection is reactivated with compromised immune status, stress, old age and HIV infection.

Primary Infection

It is symptomless. Infection converts a person from tuberculin insensitivity to sensitivity and this takes 3–8 weeks.

M. tuberculosis disseminating by blood forms tiny white tubercle, 'miliary TB'. It is common among children and those with HIV infection. Post-primary infection lesions may appear in meninges, bones, joints or kidneys in about one year. Fatality is about 30% even with treatment. Meningeal TB may occur in three months, pleural effusion and pneumonia to appear in 3–6 months. The invading Mycobacteria spread are engulfed by macrophages and brought to the regional draining lymph gland. Formation of 'tubercle'—the epithelioid granuloma—is initiated by a number of chemicals secreted by *M. tuberculosis*, such as peptidoglycan, glycolipid, wax D, phosphatides, cord factor (trehalose dimycolate), etc. In case body defence takes over, Ghon complex forms, that is, healed and calcified lesions, commonly in the upper part of the lower lobe or the lower part of the upper lobe of lungs. Simon focus occurs in apex of lungs as a result haematogenous infection.

Progressive Pulmonary Tuberculosis

It is the other alternative seen when the 'primary infection' proceeds further, spread by haematogenous route to invade any organ commonly lungs producing pulmonary lesions, granuloma, necrosis, caseation and cavitation.

Granulomatous inflammation and caseous necrosis: TB granuloma are aggregate of macrophages, B and T lymphocytes, epithelioid cell and fibroblasts in which lymphocytes surround infected macrophages. Healthy macrophages attacking the infected macrophages fuse together and form a giant multinucleated cell in alveoli.

Latent TB: Dissemination of *Mycobacterium* is prevented. Cells of immune system act locally. Mycobacteria are protected inside granuloma from destruction by hosts' immune system. Mycobacterial antigen is prevented from presentation to lymphocytes for immune response. Mycobacteria become dormant and infection is latent. Cells in the centre of granuloma die and necrosis sets—caseous necrosis. Alternatively, the lesions heal and calcify and a stage known as 'quiescent TB' results.

Investigation of an outbreak of pulmonary TB in a school (summarized in Table 50.1) demonstrates the spread from one sputum-positive student to three

Table 50.1 Outbreak (2016–2019) of pulmonary TB in a school (Fang et al. 2021)

Index case (one student sputum positive) attended before diagnosis approximately for three months; three isolates from class mates positive for identical TB (MIRU-VNTR alleles)			
Case definition	Test (s)	Students (*n*/%)	Teachers (*n*/%)
Latent	Tuberculin skin (TST)	30/405 or 7.4%	7/26 or 26.92%
Probable	TST+, chest X-ray+, productive cough for two weeks	3 from TST negative	
Confirmed	Two or more sputum test+/one sputum smear (SS) test+ and chest X-ray+ or culture+	1 from TST negative	
4/17 or 23.53% students with latent TB in 2016 refused prophylaxis and became probable/confirmed in 2019. All of six teachers who refused prophylaxis maintained status quo (latent TB).			
Summary of OB investigation (3 years): 52 cases (6 confirmed + 9 probable + 37 latent)			

students and one teacher and progress from latent to probable/confirmed state in absence of prophylaxis and treatment in a period of three years (2016–2019). Latent TB prevailed in 2016 (7.4%) in students and 26.92% among teachers. The ratio of rates of prevalence among teachers and students was 0.28 (odds ratio).

This investigation suggested the following:

Delayed detection of index case and long-term contact among students and teachers in classroom and dormitory led to this outbreak. Refusal of chemoprophylaxis led to conversion from latent to probable/confirmed TB. History revealed that the father of the index case had contracted TB two years before. This reverse tracing suggested TB transmission from community to school.

50.2.1.5 Symptoms

Latent TB does not present any symptom and does not spread.

Pulmonary TB constitutes almost 90% of active cases. The incubation period is uncertain and long. Signs of cold and cough and non-specific pneumonia are prominent in case of primary pulmonary TB. Fever is mild, often undetected, and occurs in the afternoon. As the disease progresses, chills, loss of weight, fatigue and night sweating are observed. Advanced stages of pulmonary TB show bad cough lasting for three weeks or longer, dyspnoea, chest pain, cough, phlegm from deep inside lungs, haemoptysis and cyanosis.

Extra-pulmonary TB (15–20%): Pleurisy and adenitis are most common of the extra-pulmonary TB. Enlarged hilar lymph node in children causes bronchial obstruction. Other forms may be pericarditis and peritonitis.

TB of the gastrointestine, urogenital system, adrenal glands, muscles and skin, bones and CNS (meningitis) may occur. Alimentary tract infection occurs through ingestion of contaminated milk, sputum and discharges from laryngeal ulcer. Relapse of TB may be the result of reactivation of 'quiescent TB' usually after five years of the primary infection. This is manifested as chronic wasting condition associated with night sweating and prominent respiratory symptoms. Relapse may also occur as a result of reinfection.

Scrofula denotes chronic lymph adenitis of cervical lymph nodes, commonly seen in children below five years of age and may be caused by *M. bovis*, *M. scrofulaceum* and *M. intracellulare*.

Miliary TB makes up about 10% of extra-pulmonary TB. It is a widespread, serious disseminated form of TB.

50.2.1.6 Diagnosis

The philosophy of TB diagnosis is unique because its control and eradication are 'infection and patient-centric'. Identifications of both (a) infection and (b) clinical cases are important. Diagnostic tools are selected accordingly. Identification of 'an infected individual' is essential to prevent the progress to a 'clinical disease' and thus becoming a source of infection to others. Identification of clinical case has to be rapid, and test results are expected to reveal more than mere presence of acid fast bacilli (AFB). Early detection enables rapid intervention, stops transmission and reduces mortality. Slow-growing nature of *Mycobacteria*, contamination of specimens, drug resistance, HIV-TB and immune status of host all need to be considered. Progress in the control of tuberculosis is greatly hampered because the diagnostic tests are slow and relatively insensitive.

Tests are listed below:

1. Radiography—chest X-ray. Result is suggestive.
2. Serological.

   - Tuberculin (Montoux test).
   - Lymphocyte proliferation.
   - Y-interferon.
   - ELISA.
   - The rapid test (RT) is a coloured latex-based lateral flow technology. A mix of selected *M. bovis* antigens is used including ESAT-6, CFP10 and MPB83. Tschopp et al. (2010) used to detect specific antibodies in animal serum. Results can be read in 20 min after adding buffer solution to the test serum. A coloured line appears in addition to the control-coloured line if the test serum is positive.

3. Microscopic examination of sputum and cerebrospinal fluid.

   - Acid fast *Bacilli* (sensitivity 5000–10,000 Mycobacteria/ml) not necessarily TB bacilli).
   - Fluorescent antibody test (specific test).

4. Mycolic acid profile determination by TLC or HPLC.
5. Isolation by bacteriological cultural method (sensitivity 10–100 Mycobacteria/ml).

   Tests are often complimentary. Montoux, microscopic and ELISA-IgG and IgM may be done to diagnose paediatric tuberculous meningitis.

6. Molecular methods such as Multiplex PCR, using primers specific for the genus *Mycobacterium*—further sequenced over the 16S rRNA locus s– and primer specific for *M. tuberculosis* complex.

   - Spoligotyping.
   - Mycobacterial interspersed repetitive unit (MIRU) analysis.
   - IS6110-based restriction fragment length polymorphism (RFLP) analysis.

Genotyping combined with epidemiological data helps identify a patient (s) involved in the chain of transmission.

Detection of a TB patient is the first step to extend care and stop transmission. The result should be dependable and reveals the sensitivity/resistance of *M. tuberculosis* to drugs. The WHO is making effort to improve the quality and expand the capacity of TB diagnostic laboratories through the WHO and the Stop TB Partnership

Global Laboratory Initiative (GLI) together with the GLI network of international collaborators (http://www.stoptb.org/wg/gli).

Boehme et al. (2010) developed a rapid molecular detection of tuberculosis and also rifampin resistance, *MTB/RIF* (rapid molecular detection of tuberculosis and rifampin resistance test). Result is available in less than 2 h. Single-step specimen processing is simple and reduces viable tubercle bacilli. Infectious aerosol is not generated, and so biosafety cabinet is not necessary and cuts the cost. DNA extraction, amplification and detection are automated and done in a sealed cartridge to ward off amplicon contamination. WHO launched this test as Xpert MTB RIF test (http://www.who.int/tb/laboratory/policy_statements/). The procedure is simple.

To each volume of the sample, two volumes of the 'sample reagent' are added. The mixture is shaken, incubated at room temperature for 15 min and shaken again. In a test cartridge, 2–3 ml of this is transferred. The cartridge is loaded into the instrument. The instrument carries out the subsequent steps, 'semi-nested real-time amplification and detection'. A printable test result, such as 'MTB detected; RIF resistance not detected', comes out.

Diriba et al. (2022) used the Xpert MTB/RIF assay on 13,772 presumptive TB patients in Addis Ababa, Ethiopia. *M. tuberculosis* was detected in 17%, of which nearly 9.9% were rifampicin resistant (RR-TB) and 1.0% RR-intermediate. Of all the RR-TB cases, more than half (53.6%) were males, and 105 were new TB cases. Rate of RR-TB was more (11.0%) among extra-pulmonary (EPTB) patients than pulmonary (PTB) patients (9.6%).

- **Nosocomial**

Pai et al. (2006) highlighted the problem of nosocomial tuberculosis and suggested implementation of control measures with the indigenously available resources. The authors studied the incidences of tuberculosis and TB infection in hospital settings, among interns, residents and nurses. The incidences of TB and TB infection were ten times higher than the national average among residents. Pleural TB was predominant among health workers, and it is thought to be progression of newly acquired primary infection. The authors hypothesized that in a hypothetical Indian hospital with 1000 workers, ≈500 (50%) will likely have latent infection, and ≈25 (5%) of uninfected workers will be newly infected each year. If this is not taken care of, it may seriously affect TB control programme.

Three essential components of control of TB in health-care settings are 'early detection, isolation of patient and rapid and effective treatment'. Implementation of the basic TB infection control programme is important. Recommendations from WHO and other agencies are available:

- Educating health-care workers, interns, residents and patients and their attendants and using simple surgical masks on infectious patients who are coughing.
- Improving sputum collection practices.
- Evaluation of suspected TB patients in outpatient settings.
- Separation or segregation of smear-positive TB patients in private or semiprivate rooms or wards with simple mechanical exhaust ventilation (e.g. window fans)/

natural ventilation through open windows and sunshine could be feasible in some settings, particularly in the private sector and well-funded public hospitals.

– Infectious TB must not be admitted to the same wards as patients with HIV infection.
– Periodic testing of health-care workers, junior staff, interns and residents to detect latent infection and suitably treating them.
– Evaluation of symptomatic health-care workers for active TB.

Ultimately, implementing adequate infection control measures is the responsibility of each health-care facility.

- **MDR, XDR (Emergence, Prevalence)**

Emergence

Most TB cases respond to a six-month DOTS. Some do not because the TB bacillus has developed resistance.

Multiple drug resistance tuberculosis (MDR-TB): It is a TB case that does not respond to at least isoniazid and rifampicin, the two most powerful anti-TB drugs. MDR-TB develops because of mismanaged treatment, inappropriate, incorrect, ineffective formulations and premature interruptions.

XDR-TB: During the course of treatment of MDR-TB, the patient does not respond because the bacterium has developed additional resistance (extensively drug resistance). Such cases are XDR-TB. This development is explained by interrupted treatment of MDR-TB. Treatment of MDR-TB is expensive; medicines are not always available and cause adverse effects. These lead to interruption and development of XDR, that is, additional resistance to more anti-TB drugs.

MDR-TB and XDR-TB develop during the course of treatment. Human-to-human transmission spreads such resistant bacteria and certain settings promote this. These are crowded settings, such as slum, prison and hospital.

Prevalence

According to the revised Global XDR TB task force definition, XDR-TB is MDR-TB with further resistance to ≥ 3 of the six classes of second-line drugs. Based on a study of 17,690 isolates reflecting 48 countries, 3520 (19.9%) were MDR-TB and 347 (9.95) XDR-TB (Shah et al. 2007).

XDR-TB isolates were extensively distributed. Percent of MDR-TB isolates recorded as XDR-TB from industrialized nations; Russia, Eastern Europe and Republic of Korea were 6.5, 13.6 and 15.4, respectively. In the Republic of Korea, this made 1.7% of all *M. tuberculosis* isolates tested for XDR-TB. Therefore, the authors (Shah et al. 2007) concluded that further investigation of population-based trends and expanded efforts to prevent drug resistance and effectively treat patients with MDR-TB are crucial for protection of public health and control of TB.

According to Raviglione (2007), XDR has been invading far and wide. Between 2006, March (first described) and June 2008, 49 countries recorded at least one case. Key to the emergence of XDR is failure of the ongoing treatment. Such cases are largely clustered in low-income areas. Logical reason is the inadequate infrastructure and commitment to tuberculosis control programmes. XDR is often considered untreatable and has short course and high fatality. Aggressive treatment supported with bacteriological and clinical monitoring that enables selection of and opportunity to make changes in the drug regimens succeed in reducing deaths. Cox et al. (2008) explained distribution of MDR/XDR-TB patients, their fate and the need for strain characterization by DNA fingerprinting.

The estimated number (WHO 2014) of MDR-TB cases in 2013 was 480,000 (3.5% of new and 20.5% of previously treated cases) and 9.0% of these had XTR-TB. More than half of the estimated MDR cases were clustered in India, China and Russian Federation. Since 2009, detection of MDR-TB has increased, and three times more patients (total of 97,000) were put on treatment. Average rate of success was 48%, and 5 (Ethiopia, Kazakhstan, Myanmar, Pakistan and Vietnam) of 27 countries with high MDR-TB burden showed a success rate of ≥70%.

As per WHO (2018), the estimated number of people who developed MDR-TB in 2016 was 490,000, and additional 110,000 had rifampicin-resistant TB. Around 6.2% of these were estimated to be XDR-TB. Forty-seven percent of global MDR/RR-TB cases clustered in China, India and Russian Federation.

During 2017 and 2019, the number of people enrolled for MDR/RR-TB treatment increased by 10% over 2018. In 2019, 3.3% of new TB cases and 17.7% of previously treated cases had MDR/RR-TB globally. The countries with biggest increase in enrolment include India, China the Russian Federation, Indonesia and Angola in descending order. In 2018–2019, the total number of people treated was 333, 304 (WHO 2020).

Of 24,812 tested in the EU/EEA, 834 or 3.4% revealed MDR-TB in the EU/EEA in 2019. XDR-TB cases were detected in 21.9% of 584 MDR-TB cases tested for second-line drug susceptibility. Romania and Lithuania accounted for 75% of XDR-TB (ECDC-WHO 2021). The region has 9/30 countries with highest MDR-TB burden in the world (ECDC-WHO 2022).

Only 57% of MDR-TB cases are successfully treated worldwide. In the EU/EEA, 63.7% were treated successfully and 0.8% unsuccessfully and 6.7% died in 2018. Of the 937 MDR-TB notified in 2017 (24 months), 15.2% died and 45.7% were treated successfully and 11.0% unsuccessfully. Of the XDR-TB reported in 2016 (36 months), 26.2% died and 34.9% were treated successfully and 18.0% unsuccessfully (ECDC-WHO 2021).

Longer regimens lasted for 20 months. Acceptability of recently recommended short regimen of 9–11 months is high. Resistance to fluoroquinolones should be excluded prior to the initiation of treatment with this regimen. Eighty-nine countries started by the end of 2019. One-hundred nine countries improved the effectiveness by using bedaquiline.

Detection of MDR-TB and drug resistance is required to be done by rapid molecular tests, culture methods and sequence technology.

- **HIV-TB (Prevention)**

TB and HIV are two independent lethal diseases. A person having infections of both, HIV and *M. tuberculosis*, latent or active, is a case of TB and HIV co-infection. Co-infection speeds up progression of each, latent to active TB, progression of HIV. HIV/TB co-infection leads acquired immunodeficiency syndrome (AIDS) to defining conditions. Co-infected individuals stand at a two times risk of death than HIV-infected individuals without TB. Untreated latent TB infection is more likely to develop clinical TB after HIV infection than a person without HIV because the latter weakens the immune system. HIV cases are 18 (15–21) times more likely to develop active TB disease than people without HIV. TB appears earlier, within weeks to months rather than years to decades. The risk of progressing from latent to active TB is 12–20 times. Extrapulmonary TB is more likely. TB occurs earlier in the course of HIV infection than many other opportunistic infections. A TB-infected HIV person becomes infectious to others and is a potentially faster spreader of TB; he becomes a potential annual spreader from a lifetime one.

TB is a leading cause of death among HIV-positive cases. HIV is one of the most significant contributing factors to increase the incidence of TB since 1990 in Africa. It also impedes the progress of tuberculosis control programme. Mycobacterial species that normally do not cause severe/disseminated infection do so in HIV patients. Examples are *Mycobacterium avium-intracellulare-scrofulaceum* complex and MOTT and saprophytic like *M. chelonae* and *M. fortuitum.*

A further complication may be the development of drug-resistant strain. Hong et al. (2013) described a BCG strain resistant to rifampicin from a HIV infant in Vietnam. BCG strain is naturally resistant to pyrazinamide. She happened to acquire HIV from her mother and was BCG-vaccinated at birth. She was hospitalized when a voluminous ipsilateral axillary mass appeared at the site of vaccination accompanied with fever, hepatomegaly and loss of weight. She was put on anti-*Mycobacterial* drugs without microbiological examination. After six months, recurrent fever, axillary lymphadenitis and fistula led to hospitalization and was confirmed by microbiological examination.

HIV/TB may have few and non-specific symptoms and normal chest X-ray, so-called sub-clinical TB and so often not recognized and treated. Those with pulmonary infection may manifest classic TB symptoms. Countries like South Africa where HIV is more common, HIVTB may be extra-pulmonary. Risk of death in co-infected is twice the one infected with HIV alone.

According to WHO (2020), 64% of TB patients tested HIV positive in 2018. It increased to 69% in 2019. Overall, 88% of TB patients known to be living with HIV were on antiretroviral therapy (ART). The burden is high in the WHO African region (86% of TB patients had HIV). The estimated TB deaths among HIV-negative people in 2019 were 1.2 million (range, 1.1–1.3 million). There was a reduction from 1.7 million in 2000. Death among HIV-positive people was 208 000 (range, 177 000–242 000) (a reduction from 678 000 in 2000). About 187 000 people died of HIV-associated TB in 2021.

In EU/EEA, TB-HIV co-infection showed a decline. Such cases peaked (23) in 2016, 21 in 2018 and 19 in 2019. An overall 3.1% of TB cases were HIV positive (ECDC-WHO 2021).

Prevention

Co-infected is tested for TB infection and disease and treatment initiated accordingly. Detection of TB in a co-infection is more difficult than to diagnose a TB individual. Sputum smear test yields false-negative result on many. However, diagnosis of HIV is straight. HIV-TB is detected by testing TB patients for HIV. This constitutes the first intervention for reducing HIV-associated TB.

Collaborative TB-HIV activities are the answer. Cases have to be put on antiretroviral therapy (ART). In order to prevent TB among HIV patients, isoniazid preventive therapy (IPT) is initiated. However, only 21% of countries globally and 41 high TB/HIV burden countries reported to have provided this in 2013. In 2018 and 2019, 5.3 million people living with HIV (88% of the five-year target of 6.0 million) were provided with TB preventive treatment.

In 2018, 64% of notified TB patients had HIV, an increase by 60% over the previous year (2017). In the WHO African region, 87% of TB patients were HIV-TB. Among HIV patients, 56% were TB positive and 86% were on antiretroviral therapy. Success rate of treatment was 85% for TB and 75% for HIV-associated TB (Kanabus 2020; https://tbfacts.org/tb-hiv).

50.2.1.7   Prevention and Control – Drugs, DOTS, International Recommendations - results

Tuberculosis is not currently a candidate for eradication efforts; eradication is defined as the achievement of a status whereby no further cases of a disease occur anywhere and control measures are unnecessary.

Tuberculosis elimination has been defined arbitrarily as no more than one new case per million populations per year or a prevalence of TB infection of below 1% in the general population. However, this leaves a chance of re-emergence through (a) migrants and (b) complacency because of likelihood of reduction of TB vigilance.

Patient-centric approach stops transmission of TB controls prevalence to an undetectable level. Successful treatment of a case stops transmission and ultimately controls tuberculosis. The principal steps are (a) detect, treat and cure cases of TB, the first time, and (b) ensure zero transmission from the patients.

Anti-Mycobacterial Drugs

The first-line drugs are isoniazid, rifampin, ethambutol and streptomycin. Curing a patient relieves him from the suffering. At the same time, it makes him non-infectious and stops transmission.

However, strains that are resistant to a single drug have been documented in every country surveyed. Not only this, strains resistant to all major anti-TB drugs have emerged. DOTS prevents emergence of resistant strain in patients infected with susceptible strains.

MDR-TB or the multidrug-resistant strain-caused TB is dangerous, which is defined as the disease caused by TB bacilli resistant to at least isoniazid and rifampicin, the two most powerful anti-TB drugs.

It is possible to treat drug-resistant TB. Extensive chemotherapy lasting up to two years or more with the second line of anti-TB drugs is required. The second-line drugs consist of six classes: (i) aminoglycosides other than streptomycin, like kanamycin and amikacin; (ii) cyclopeptides such as capreomycin; (iii) fluoroquinolones, for example, Cipro-, Oflo-, Levo and Max-floxacin; (iv) thioamides, for example, prothionamide and ethionamide; (v) serine analogues, for example, cycloserine and terizidone; and (vi) salicylic acid derivatives—para-amino salicylic acid (PAS). The second-line drugs included in the WHO Model List of Essential Medicines are amikacin, capreomycin, ciprofloxacin, cycloserine, ethionamide, kanamycin, levofloxacin, ofloxacin, p-aminosalicylic acid and prothionamide.

These drugs are more costly, toxic and less effective than first-line drugs used for routine treatment of TB. The toxic drug reactions may be severe but are manageable. Treating MDR-TB with second line of drugs may cure >65% of patients and thus stop further transmission. This latter is observed in high-income countries and additional efforts—DOTS plus—are required in low-income countries.

Quality-assured second-line anti-TB drugs are available at reduced prices for projects approved by the Green Light Committee, WHO.

Directly Observed Treatment Short (DOTS)

DOTS is a 6–8-month treatment course of a TB patient who is observed and administered with medicine by a health worker. Administration of quality medicines without break and also monitoring of the response are assured. Sputum is examined after two months and at the end of treatment for absence of TB bacilli. Expanding of high-quality DOTS; addressing TB-HIV and MDR-TB; strengthening health system, at the level of primary health; partnering all care providers; empowering people and communities; and promoting research are the components of strategy 'Global pal to stop TB, 2006-15'. It targets 50% reduction of global burden of TB by 2015 in line with the Millennium Development Goals with 1990 as baseline and elimination as public health problem by 2050 (Raviglione 2007).

International Recommendations and Results

Nathanson et al. (2006) list the international recommendations for the control of MDR-TB. These are (a) the monitoring, (b) access to/assured supply of quality-assured second-line drugs at reduced price, (c) a well-functioning DOTS programme, (d) long-term political commitment, (e) rational case finding strategies and (f) awareness on preventive measures

WHO recommendations for MDR/XTDR-TB (Tuberculosis: Multidrug-resistant tuberculosis (MDR-TB) (who.int).

- Speed up detection by rapid tests like Xpert MTB/RIF.
- 'Standardized shorter (9-12 months course) regimen' which is cheaper, $1000/patient.

It is less expensive than current regimens. Adherence to treatment is better and loss to follow-up is reduced.

Nathanson et al. (2006) designed this study in low-income countries—precisely in Estonia, Latvia, Lima (Peru), Manila (the Philippines) and Tomsk Oblast (Russian Federation). All projects used Drug Sensitivity Test (DST) results and previous treatment history to design the individualized regimen. The approach is patient-oriented and so the duration of treatment varied, usually 18–24 months. The median duration of follow-up after declaring completion of treatment or cure of a patient varied between 24 and 36 months. Success rate of treatment was 70%. Cost of treatment per patient averaged $3400 in the Philippines and $9000–10,000 in Estonia and Tomsk (the latter was due to considerable hospitalization).

A word of caution has come from Pietersen et al. (2014) who followed XDR-TB cases in South Africa. They observed that a substantial number of patients failed treatment, were sputum positive and discharged from hospital as facilities for long stay were scarce. They are likely to transmit infection into community.

The emergence of extensively drug-resistant (XDR) TB, particularly in settings where many TB patients are also infected with HIV, poses a serious threat to TB control and confirms the urgent need to strengthen basic TB control and to apply the new WHO guidelines for the programmatic management of drug-resistant TB.

In 2016, an estimated 490,000 people worldwide developed MDR-TB, and an additional 110, 000 people with rifampicin-resistant TB were also newly eligible for MDR-TB treatment. The countries with the largest numbers of MDR/RR-TB cases (47% of the global total) were China, India and the Russian Federation. It is estimated that about 6.2% of these cases were XDR-TB (Tuberculosis: Multidrug-resistant tuberculosis (MDR-TB) (who.int).

50.2.2 *Anthropozoonotic Mycobacteriosis* – **Mycobacterium leprae**

Mycobacterium leprae-caused leprosy affects skin, mucosa of eyes and upper respiratory tract and peripheral nerves and may cause progressive and permanent disabilities.

It is reported from all the six WHO regions that majority of annual new cases are from Southeast Asia. Over 120 countries report >200,000 new cases annually. Elimination (prevalence of <1 case/10,000) was achieved in 2010 in most countries. Data of 2019 show that 45 countries reported 0 and 99 <1000 cases. Brazil, India and Indonesia reported more than 10, 000 new cases, while 13 other countries each reported 1000–10,000 new cases (WHO 2023).

50.2.2.1 Infection and Symptoms

The incubation period may be several months or years. The exposed and infected can become carriers and infect others, only 5% develop leprosy; leprosy may be tuberculoid (paucibacillry) and lepromatous (multibacillary). The tuberculoid leprosy progresses slowly and easily treatable. The lepromatous is caused by strongly proliferative bacteria and progresses rapidly. It manifests as ulcers distributed over hands, feet, face and ears. If diagnosis and drug intervention are delayed, nerves may be irreversibly damaged. Leprosy patients face social problems, stigma and discrimination.

50.2.2.2 Diagnosis

Mycobacterium leprae cannot be cultivated. Animal model, like seven-banded armadillos, is used to grow it and carry out drug sensitivity. This takes a year time. The microscopic diagnostics of skin or nasal smears is often difficult as samples are false-negative. Molecular testing (PCR) of the samples from lesion is the best choice.

Leprosy can be diagnosed on the basis of clinical manifestation and with the help of laboratory tests. Finding at least one of the following cardinal signs diagnoses leprosy: (i) definite loss of sensation in a pale or reddish patch on skin, (ii) thickened or enlarged peripheral nerve with loss of sensation and/or weakness of the muscles supplied by that nerve and (iii) microscopic detection of bacilli in the slit-skin smear. The cases are then classified as 'paucibacillary' (PB), a case with 1–5 skin lesions with slit-skin smear negative, and 'multibacillary' (MB), a case with >5 skin lesions/pure neuritis or skin lesions with neuritis/slit-skin positive for bacteria irrespective of number of skin lesions.

50.2.2.3 Treatment

It is treatable. The multiple drug therapy (MDT) recommended includes dapsone, rifampicin and clofazimine. The duration of treatment is six months for PB and 12 months for MB cases. MDT kills the pathogen and cures the patient. WHO has been providing MDT free of cost.

50.2.2.4 Prevention

Reverse tracing and chemoprophylaxis: with the consent of index case, household contacts, neighbourhood and social contacts are reached. Single dose of rifampicin preventing chemotherapy is administered.

WHO released the strategy 'Towards zero leprosy: global leprosy (Hansen's disease) 2021-20230' which aims at zero—leprosy, infection and disease, disability, stigma and discrimination and finally elimination (interruption of transmission). The strategic pillars are (a) implementing integrated, country-owned zero leprosy roadmaps in all endemic countries, (b) scaling up leprosy prevention alongside integrated active case detection, (c) managing leprosy and its complications and prevent new disability and (d) combatting stigma and ensuring human rights are respected. Global and national investment in research is required.

50.2.3   Zoonotic Mycobacteriosis

50.2.3.1   *Mycobacterium tuberculosis* **Complex**

M. tuberculosis complex consists of *M. microti* from wild voles and wood mice, *M. africanum* from monkey and *M. caprae* from dromedary camel. *M. pinnipedii, a variant of M. bovis,* caused disease in fur seals, sea lions, cattle, gorilla, llama, tapirs and trainer of seals in New Zealand (Thoen et al. 2009).

M. tuberculosis

Most reported cases of TB in captive animals resulted from infection with *M. tuberculosis*, with only a few cases caused by *M. bovis because of high level of exposure through direct/indirect human interaction.* Infected human can transmit infection to in-contact animals, like cattle, dogs, cats and monkeys. This reverse zoonosis (Fig. 50.1) has been reported also recently in Ethiopia (Romha et al. 2018); *M. tuberculosis* has been reportedly isolated from domestic animals. Infection thus transferred to cattle may only sensitize it so that it becomes 'human tuberculin' positive. Animals too transmit the infection to humans.

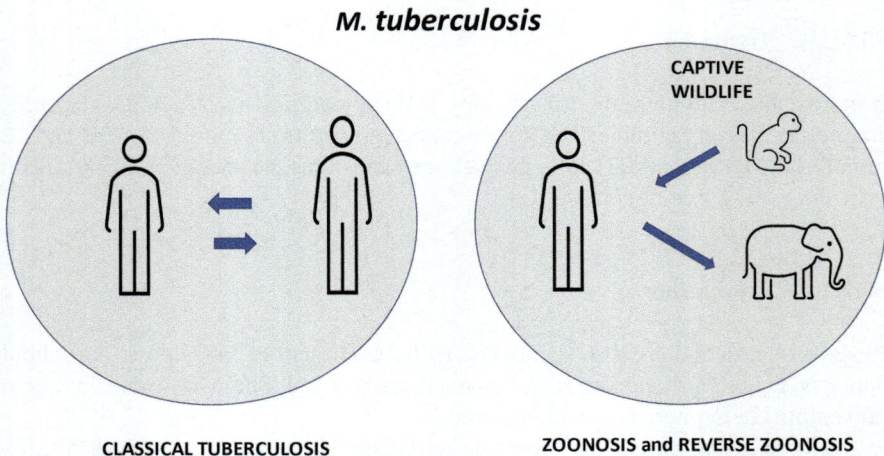

Fig. 50.1 Classical tuberculosis, zoonosis and reverse zoonosis

Ntivuguruzwa et al. (2022) demonstrated *M. tuberculosis* complex in 1.7% (5/300) and *M. bovis* from 1.3% (4/300) of sampled slaughtered cattle. Non-tuberculous mycobacteria were identified in 12.0% (36/300) of the sampled cattle. A possible zooanthroponotic transmission was indicated by isolation of one RR-*M. tuberculosis* from cattle.

Clinical TB may occur in dogs, monkeys and wild animals. Wildlife is uncultivated flora and fauna existing without human interference. Free ranging wildlife is expected to be free from tuberculosis. Most TB cases reported are in captive wildlife of various species—carnivores like leopards, bear, tigers, etc., non-human primates, deer, antelope, Indian bison, elephants, rodents, birds and amphibians.

Domestic animals are let loose in forest for grazing, even under a planned programme like social forestry; thus these share grazing areas and water sources with wild animals. Humans visit forest for activities related to livelihood—hunting, firewood, timber, leaves and grasses to feed their animals, adventure and enjoyment. Forest area is shrinking. Encroachments around zoo are common. Monkeys in cities are often captured and released into forest. Many of these suffer with tuberculosis. The distance between wildlife and human and his pets and domestic animals are thus reducing.

Transmission of mycobacteria involving human, domestic animals and wild animals is thus frequent. Wild animal-associated TB thus impacts health of domestic animals and humans and also threatens certain wildlife species.

Wildlife

Alexander et al. (2002) described transmission of *M. tuberculosis* from human to animals and also the epizootic affecting two wildlife species—suricates (*Suricata suricatta*) and free-ranging banded mongoose (*Mungos mungo*) in South Africa. Increased human visitors to forests, foraging by these animals in garbage pits or roadside possibly contaminated with human sputum and a known human case of TB lived near the suricate burrow, led to infection of mesenteric lymph glands from where *M. tuberculosis* was isolated. They suffered with progressive weakness, emaciation, cachexia and ataxia, separated themselves from the rest during foraging and exhibited no fear from human.

M. tuberculosis infection in elephants has been frequently reported (Chandranaik et al. 2017; Simpson et al. 2017; Miller et al. 2018). TB in elephants caused by *M. tuberculosis* and *M. bovis* and transmission to other mammals and veterinarians has been reported from Africa and Asia. Investigation by Michalak et al. (1998) suggested transmission between human and elephants. Between 1994 and 1996, three elephants from an exotic animal farm in Illinois died of pulmonary disease due to *M. tuberculosis*. In October 1996, a fourth living elephant was culture-positive. Twenty-two handlers at the farm were screened for tuberculosis (TB); eleven had positive reactions to intradermal injection with purified protein derivative. One had smear-negative, culture-positive active TB. DNA fingerprint comparison by IS6110 and TBN12 typing showed that the isolates from the four elephants and the handler with active TB were the same strain.

Oh et al. (2002) brought out evidence of transmission of TB from zoo animals to human beings. Investigation in the Los Angeles during 1997–2000 revealed *M. tuberculosis* in two Asian elephants (*Elephas maximus*), three Rocky Mountain goats (*Oreamnos americanus*) and one black rhinoceros (*Diceros bicornis*), no active case in human beings. DNA finger printing suggested recent transmission. Those associated with training of elephants and attending elephant necropsy showed tuberculin skin test conversion.

Angkawanish et al. (2010) studied TB in four elephants referred to the National Elephant Institute Hospital, Thailand, during 2005–2008. Elephants showed nasal discharge, lateral recumbency, anorexia, chronic weight loss and lesions at necropsy comparable to TB; specimens—standard—is trunk wash. Infection confirmed as *Mycobacterium tuberculosis* by bacterial culture, other diagnostic procedures and sequencing of 16S–23S rDNA internal transcribed spacer region, 16S rRNA and gyrase B gene sequences. Genotyping showed that the infectious agents originated from four sources in Thailand. To identify infections, a combination of diagnostic assays is essential.

Simpson et al. (2017) reported TB and treatment in Albuquerque Biopark, New Mexico. Two African elephants (31 and 8 years old) from a small travelling circus in poor condition were quarantined in 1997 for one year and then shifted to *Albuquerque Biopark*. One tested positive in 2000 for *M. tuberculosis* IS6110 and was treated. A third elephant proved positive for the same genotype of *M. tuberculosis*. Infection was acquired possibly through contact for more than ten years of cohabitation. None of the 178 workers of the park tested positive. Trunk washings were tested, either twice or once weekly. *M. tuberculosis* showed remarkable genome conservation. Drug (*isoniazid* and *pyrazinamide combination*) administration per os was not accepted by the elephants, and so administered per rectal, serum drug concentration was monitored. This $20,000 regimen (per elephant per year) was ultimately used for one year to successfully treat elephant.

Zachariah et al. (2017) reported 3.8% of 88 elephants undergoing post-mortem examination; these were confirmed cases of *M. tuberculosis* in the Muthanga range of the Wayanad Wildlife Sanctuary in Southern India. They believed that the infection spilled over from human (reverse zoonosis).

Three elephants in a Swiss zoo were weak, had weight loss and failed exercise and were euthanized. Post-mortem findings and isolation of *M. tuberculosis* from the trunk mucosa and tracheobronchial and pharyngeal swab in two out of three elephants confirmed TB. Whole-genome sequence (WGS) analysis of eight isolates confirmed a single source of infection the route of transmission between the three animals. The lineage detected is very common in humans; reverse zoonotic transmission from human to elephant most likely occurred (Ghielmetti et al. 2017).

M. bovis

M. bovis affects lymph glands, lungs and other parts of the body like *M. tuberculosis*. Symptoms depend upon the organs affected. When left untreated, they can be fatal. Zoonotic TB caused extra-pulmonary disease. It accounted for a significant proportion before the introduction of pasteurization of milk in the Western world. It stands greatly controlled or eliminated from high-income countries.

Burden

The WHO (2017) estimates of global zoonotic TB burden in 2016 were incidence 147,000 and deaths 12,500. These are distributed in Africa, the Americas, Eastern Mediterranean, Europe, Southeast Asia and Western Pacific. The respective incidences are 72,700, 822; 7660, 1160; and 46,700, 18,000. The number of deaths in the respective regions are 9300, 41; 654, 84; and 2080, 350.

Data on the global prevalence and distribution of human infection with bovine TB are scarce, yet it is suggested that it is prevalent in all major livestock-producing countries posing risk of exposure.

In a study (Müller et al. 2013) that is based on data collected from 61 countries, zoonotic TB or TB in humans are referred to as those caused by *M. bovis* or *M. caprae*. Most zoonotic TB is caused by *M. bovis* and cattle are the major reservoirs. Data for the WHO region of Southeast Asia including major cattle-producing countries like Bangladesh, India, Indonesia, Myanmar and Pakistan were not available. Ample data were available from low-risk and high-income countries. In contrast, nationwide surveys were lacking in potential high-risk settings. Estimation of global occurrence of zoonotic TB was difficult.

Incidence of zoonotic TB was low. Crude estimate was 7/100,000/year (base 2010 data) in African countries included in this study. This accounted for a median of 2.8% of all TB cases. Ethiopia, Nigeria and Tanzania had most cases. Outside Africa it was <1.4%. Pasteurization of milk and regular meat inspection is almost absent. Additional contributory factors are behaviour and prevalence of HIV.

Proportion of *M. bovis* infection among HIV-TB cases is high compared to HIV-negative patients and significantly higher in the USA. The relative risk for an infection with *M. bovis* among TB patients was 2.6–8.3 times higher in HIV co-infected patients than in HIV-negative patients. No significant association between *M. bovis* infection and HIV status was identified in surveys in Africa or other countries of the Americas.

In the Americas, zoonotic TB was of minor consequences. However, *M. bovis* can be a substantial cause of deaths in certain population group and settings. The median proportion was 0.3% mostly confined to specific areas of Mexico and the USA affecting mainly the Hispanic and attributed to consumption of unpasteurized contaminated cheese.

In the UK, bovine TB incidence was 40% in the 1930s and so was human TB >50,000 with around 2500 deaths every year (6% of total TB deaths) due to zoonotically acquired *M. bovis* infection before the introduction of animal disease control programme. In 2012, 35 of 5200 culture-positive cases of human TB (0.7%) were due to *M. bovis* and 97.1% due to *M. tuberculosis*. Since 2000, the UK has maintained a low number of B-TB cases (12–36, mean 23). Most cases (57%) occurred in the age group 65+ years and were born in the UK. This was followed by 15–44 years (26%), most born in the UK. It is important to note that majority of these cases (61%) were due to *M. tuberculosis*. *M. bovis* cases in age group 0–14 years were very low (2%). Most cases of *M. bovis* appear to have resulted from activation of latent infection acquired prior to the widespread milk pasteurization and compulsory TB control programme in cattle (tuberculin testing and slaughter of reactors) or infection acquired outside the UK. *M. bovis* has been found to infect deer, camelids (alpaca and llama), pigs, cats and sheep commonly in Great Britain. Infection of non-bovine animals was culture confirmed in 98 incidents in 2012. Two cases of transmission from infected alpacas and recent events involving infected cats have provided evidence that close contact with infected animals may result in latent and also active TB (Anonym 2014; ETS/ESMI 2014).

Studies in Europe showed 0.4% median proportion, most cases from Austria, Germany, Greece and Spain. Both *M. caprae* and *M. bovis* were responsible. MDR-*M. bovis*—caused two nosocomial outbreaks.

Zoonotic TB occurred also in Eastern Mediterranean – Egypt Suez Canal region and Djibouti.

Median proportions of *M. bovis* infection were 0.2% in western pacific region—Australia, New Zealand and parts of China; generally New Zealand showed a higher proportion and incidence and also increasing trend than Australia. Among other domesticated animals, pigs get infected with *M. bovis* and *M. avium* through eating garbage and milk. They may show clinical disease. The infection in cattle is proportionately related to infection in human and pigs, as control of *M. bovis* infection in cattle is reflected in the proportionate decline in prevalence in human and pigs.

Risk Factors

Butchers, veterinarians and sty attendants are the likely professionals at risk of infection through direct and indirect contact. Undercooked contaminated pork may cause infection among consumers.

Highest bovine TB incidence is observed in the region where intensive dairy production, such as milk sheds in large cities, is located, particularly if veterinary support is inadequate. Crowding as in markets, corrals, watering ponds, dips, etc. contribute to the spread of infection.

Zoonotic TB (*M. bovis*) and classical TB (*M. tuberculosis*) cases are indistinguishable. The former is extra-pulmonary in most cases. It is more likely to be misdiagnosed. Laboratory diagnosis cannot differentiate the two. The prevalence of zoonotic TB is underestimated. Treatment is challenging because *M. bovis* is resistant to one of the drugs, pyrazinamide listed as first line of treatment, and treatment begins in most cases without drug sensitivity test.

M. bovis continues to be a relevant zoonotic agent (Fig. 50.2). Infection in humans and domesticated and wild animals are reported. It occurs in industrialized countries and in immigrants from endemic countries. Laboratory facilities for culture and identification of *M. bovis* are inadequate. It is the main cause of underreporting. In Latin America, less than 1% of tuberculosis cases are reported as being due to *M. bovis* (Thoen et al. 2009).

The proportion of zoonotic TB caused by M. *bovis* out of the total human TB cases is unknown. Further consequences of *M. bovis* infection should be a matter of concern. HIV cases being more susceptible to *M. bovis* infection would be

Mycobacterium bovis

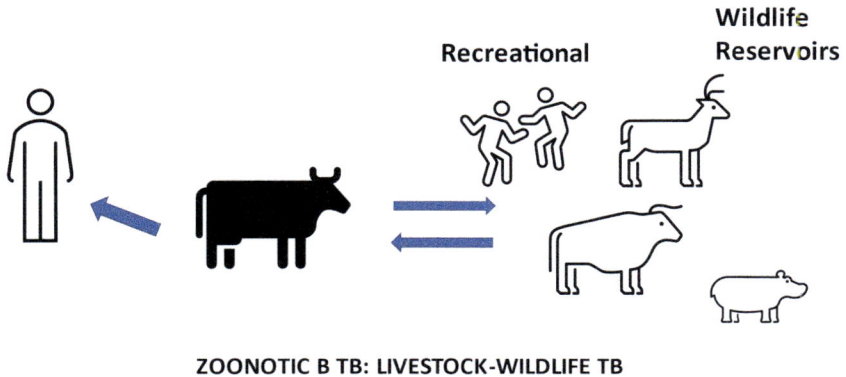

Fig. 50.2 Zoonotic bovine tuberculosis

potential source of continuous person-to-person spread. In hospital settings, outbreaks of MDR- *M. bovis* among HIV patients have been reported. This zoonotic TB is a potential threat in countries/regions/areas where bovine TB and HIV co-exist, sub-Saharan Africa, Asia and Latin America, for example (Silva et al. 2018).

Bovine TB continues to be endemic where its control and eradication have not been implemented or improperly carried out. People continue to consume unpasteurized milk. A cross-sectional study in an urban area of Brazil 1.6% or 3/189 TB patients were found co-infected with *M. tuberculosis* and *M. bovis*. Further study concluded that zoonotic exposures (endemic bovine TB, consumption of unpasteurized milk and its products) increased the risk of zoonotic TB especially among EPTB (extra-pulmonary TB) patients.

Routes of Infection

Ingestion of unpasteurized milk, inhalation and direct contact with infected excretions and secretions (sputum, urine, faeces and pus) are the common routes of infection.

Animal Reservoirs

M. bovis affects cattle, pigs, domestic cats, human and a number of wild animals, brush tail possum, mustelids, rodents, foxes, coyotes, ferret and deer. *M. bovis* disease has been reported from captive and non-human primates. *M. bovis* subtype *Almaty* (infection of bovine/wild animals and from these to human) is probably not known). Kubica et al. (2006) described eight isolates from eight patients living in Kazakhstan having molecular marker typical of *M. bovis* but growth and biochemical characteristics intermediate between *M. bovis* and *M. tuberculosis*.

The natural hosts of *M. bovis* are cattle, buffalo and bison. Almost all warm-blooded animals are susceptible to it, and this makes the control very difficult particularly when certain wild life species sustains the infection so much so as to become its reservoir. *M. bovis* may be silently maintained undetected in a geographic area in wildlife or domestic buffaloes/cattle. *M. bovis*—susceptible wildlife—may be grouped into reservoirs, potential reservoirs and others (Wilkins et al. 2008; Thoen et al. 2009; Miller and Sweeney 2013).

Wildlife Reservoirs

Cape buffalo (*Syncerus caffer*) and greater kudu (*Tragelaphus strepsiceros*) live in Southern Africa; *Brushtail possums* (*Trichosurus vulpecula*) in New Zealand; Elk (*Cervus canadensis*), white-tailed deer (*Odocoileus virginianus*) and American bison (*Bison bison*) in Canada; *Cervids*—white-tailed deer (*Odocoileus virginianus*) – mule deer (*Odocoileus hemionus*), red deer (*Cervus elaphus*), lechwe (*Kobus lechwe*) and wood bison (*Bison athabascae*) in the USA; badgers (*Meles meles*) in Europe; Feral swine (*Suis scrofa*) in Spain; red lechwe (*Kobus lechwe kafuencis*) in Zambia; and Feral water buffalo in Australia.

The geographical distribution may overlap in some.

Potential Wildlife Reservoirs

Free ranging axis deer (*Axis axis*), greater kudu (*Tragelaphus strepsiceros*), llama (*Lama glama*), fallow deer (*Dama dama*), roe deer (*Capreolus capreolus*), feral water buffalo (*Bubalis bubalis*), giraffe (*Giraffa camelopardalis*), European wild goat (*Capra aegagrus*) and impala (*Aepyceros melampus*).

Carnivores and scavengers can acquire bovine TB—fox, tiger, coyote, wolf, fox, lion, cheetah, leopard, weasel, bob cat raccoon, hyena, black bear and opossum.

Wildlife: Domestic Cattle Tuberculosis

Emerging *M. bovis* in North American wildlife poses a serious and emerging risk for the livestock and recreational hunting industry besides human health. Bovine TB (B-TB) has been detected in nine geographically distinct wildlife population of North America and Hawaii. It is endemic in at least three populations including species of *Bovidae*, *Cervidae* and *Suidae*. Transmission of B-TB from cattle to wildlife occurs. It was transmitted to deer in Michigan around 1955 and caused epizootic. A reduction in population density of deer by 50% and concurrent management actions reduced the prevalence from 4.9% to 1.7% in adult deer in five counties. Widespread culling and rigorous sampling led to decline to 1.2% in 2005 and undetectable level by 2010. An opposite experience was the reported outbreak in 11 cattle herds around the Riding Mountain National Park in Manitoba, Canada, where infected herd of elk was implicated. *M. bovis* is considered endemic in bison. Free-ranging bison population around the Wood Buffalo National Park, Canada, is the largest reservoir (Miller and Sweeny 2013).

Bovine TB restricted to livestock can be controlled but is impossible if it has spread to free-ranging maintenance hosts. Miller and Sweeney (2013) identified four common risk factors associated with establishment of *M. bovis* in uninfected wildlife populations in North America: (1) commingling of infected cattle with susceptible wildlife, (2) supplemental feeding of wildlife, (3) inadequate surveillance of at-risk wildlife and (4) unrecognized emergence of alternate wildlife species as successful maintenance hosts. Increasing game ranching (*combining exotic and native hoof stock*) in the US animal agriculture industry and *recreational hunting* added to the risk.

Enzootic infection is a danger to human beings exposed occupationally (hunters, taxidermists, trappers, venison processors) and eaters. Two cases however have been epidemiologically linked to the infected deer, and the isolates have been found to be genotypically identical with the strain enzootic in deer. One of the two cases got infected with the contaminated knife that pierced his finger while processing the carcass.

Bovine TB in wildlife (Fig. 50.2) has been detected in New Zealand, the USA and the Great Britain in llamas, alpacas (*camelids*), badger, wild boar and deer. Infection in camelids turns rapidly into progressive and extensive disease, and the 'spit' (a mixture of gastric content and saliva) is infectious. These appear to be 'spill-over host'. Endemic TB in badger mitigates efforts to control bovine TB in Great Britain. These animals generate aerosols in 'spits', and so the infected camelids are likely to transmit infection to human handlers, owners and keepers.

M. bovis survives for days, weeks and even years in environment such as stagnant water, pasture in dry state and faeces.

de Garine-Wichatitsky (2010) traced the spread of B-TB in Southern Africa since 1990 when African buffaloes (*Syncerus caffer*) in South Africa's Kruger Park were found positive. By 2008, B-TB were detected in African buff in the Gonarezhou National Park, Zimbabwe. The authors considered epidemiological links between the two positive Parks. Movement of infected livestock led to transboundary spread: cattle-buff-unidentified wild spp., for example, Kudu *(Tragelaphus strepsiceros)*—buff transmission.

Sharing same pasture or territory provides opportunity of transfer and spread of infection. Examples are badgers (*Meles meles*) in the UK and possums (*Trichosurus vulpecula*) in New Zealand. Matos et al. (2014) reported *M. bovis* from brain and mediastinal lymph nodes of red foxes in Portugal suggesting disseminated infection involving cerebral. The rural-urban barrier is porous.

Detection of TB-infected badger is extremely difficult, as the clinical signs manifested even in very late stages are non-specific. Soil or faeces around badger setts may be found positive for *M. bovis*, but to identify individual infected animal is not possible. Badgers avoid grazing cattle but forage in and contaminate grazing land, feed stores and cattle sheds and may also come in direct contact with cattle. Deer could pose a significant risk of cattle infection only if the prevalence of TB infection in deer is high. Domestic and feral pigs are infected directly or indirectly from natural host 'cattle' (when raised together) or wildlife, say badger or deer, and may sustain the agent when their density of population is high.

Bovine TB and Control

M. bovis can infect cattle of any age, but opportunities for exposure to the bacterium accumulate with time (i.e. age in itself may not be a factor of susceptibility). The infection may be acquired through inhalation, ingestion and congenital transmission.

Bovine TB affects livestock trade and productivity and causes zoonotic transmission through milk and meat. A significant proportion of infection in cattle is latent, a state comparable to *M. tuberculosis* infection in human. This partially explains why a large proportion of skin test reactors and gamma interferon positive from a herd that is culture-positive have no gross visible TB lesions and attempts to culture and isolate *M. bovis* fail. However, disease has the potential to re-emerge in many of such animals under stress at later stage. Such animals are therefore potential transmitters. However, immune responses in TB-infected cattle usually develop before visible signs of disease are evident to the veterinarian or meat inspector. Regular herd testing and speedy removal of all skin (and gamma interferon) test reactors are therefore required to control TB. Shedding of B-TB bacilli can take place at any stage of infection, though shedding is more frequent in early stage of infection. Cattle having lung lesions are akin to human 'open cases' and pose a risk to other cattle, wildlife and human beings. In majority of bovine TB cattle, lesions are located in lymph glands of the head and chest with or without affecting lung tissues, yet the latter is considered to pose a risk of transmission. Nasal excretion and transmission may occur in the early stages, observed in experimental infections 20–30 and 80–90 days post inoculation (Mc Corry et al., 2005 cited in Anonym (2009)).

Control

Battle against bovine TB has to be fought at two levels, cattle and wildlife. It worked in Australia, New Zealand, Ireland and England.

The bovine TB advisory group in England (Anonym 2009) recommended (a) review of TB control in non-bovine species; (b) development of effective diagnostic test and validation for use in camelids; (c) improved surveillance in wildlife including badger, wild boar and wild deer; and (d) development and deployment of vaccine for badger and cattle [which will require the development of a test to differentiate vaccinated from unvaccinated cattle (DIVA)]. Twenty-five thousand cattle were slaughtered because of bovine TB in 2009, especially in the West and Southwest England, costing 63 million British pounds in England alone.

Without controlling TB in badgers, bovine TB cannot be controlled. TB in badger can be controlled by culling only in high incidence area and vaccination in the rest. Vaccine is injectable and is thus of limited use.

Gloucestershire, Dorset and Somerset are the areas where B-TB is endemic in badger. The control efforts hit the targets for the area in 2015. Vaccination and culling of badger are two methods, but there is no vaccine for cattle. Culling of badger under a four-year license worked. A reduction in TB incidence in cattle due to culling persists for at least 6.5 years after the last cull. There are two culling procedures. 'Proactive', repeated culling across all accessible land, and 'reactive', in response to bovine TB outbreaks in cattle. The Badger Edge Vaccination Scheme proposes vaccination in the Edge Area. Study on naturally infected >800 wild badgers vaccinated with BCG injectable vaccine in Gloucestershire showed a 74% reduction in badgers.

Bovine TB control (The Bovine TB Science Advisory Body (Bovine TB Science Advisory Body (bTB SAB)and (Strategy for Achieving Officially Bovine Tuberculosis Free Status for England) salient features are the following:

- Testing of herds: Four yearly low-risk and annually – high risk and edge areas (surveillance); post-mortem inspection for signs of TB in slaughterhouses. Sheep and cattle in Taiwan are compulsorily and deer optionally tested under *M. bovis* surveillance but not humans (Jou et al. 2008) and prevalence was low.
- Compulsory testing of animals of >42 days moving out (except for slaughter) of annually tested herd; it must test negative for TB in a skin test 60 days before they are moved.
- Control and eliminate infection detected in a herd if any animal is found positive by rapidly removing it, imposing movement restriction and frequent testing of the remaining.
- Early detection of positive animal in herds in Edge area, with increasing incidence.
- Biosecurity.
- Penalty, if animal is not tested on time.
- Details of TB history on animals made available at the time of sale enabling buyer to take decision.

'Official Tuberculosis Free status' is withdrawn if evidence of TB is found in at least one of the animals at slaughter.

In New Zealand, *M. bovis* is endemic in possums in 38% (vector areas) of the area. Possums or ferret contribute to 70% of herd infections. Terminally ill possums turn effective transmitter: erratic behaviour leads them to venture out in day to feed and seek a place to keep warm like paddocks. Inquisitive cattle and deer are attracted (contact exposure).

The goal of the Animal Health Board is to eradicate *M. bovis* from possum from an identified area-at-risk that is nearly one-fourth of the country by 2026, eventually eradicating the disease.

Possum population was controlled by trapping, ground-baiting and aerial spray of sodium fluoroacetate (biodegradable) where ground operation is impractical. Sustained control programme in cattle, checking cross-infection and breaking disease transmission brought down the herd infection rates in cattle and deer reduced from >1700 in 1994 to <100 herds in 2011. During 1988–1994, TB-infected possum density was reduced by 87.5% at Hohota, reflected into reduction of TB by 83.4% in cattle herds.

WHO, OIE, FAO and the International Union Against Tuberculosis and Lung Disease – 'Roadmap on tackling zoonotic TB, October 2017' – is centred on one health approach and aims at controlling bovine TB in animals and improving food safety and suggested it as priority Global Health agenda (Global Tuberculosis Report WHO, 2017 https://www.who.int/tb/publications/global_report/gtbr2017_main_text.pdf).

Mycobacterium africanum

Mycobacterium africanum is a member of the *M. tuberculosis* complex. It has been isolated in Africa around equator from humans. Desmond et al. (2004) described five cases in California; three had lived in Africa. It has been reported also from Europe. The isolates were identified as *M. africanum* by spoligotyping, single nucleotide polymorphisms, a deletion mutation and phenotypic traits. The disease manifestation is very similar to those caused by *M. tuberculosis*. The California cases (25–34 years) suffered with productive cough, low-grade temperature, weight loss, anorexia and fatigue. X-ray of lungs revealed infiltration and cavities. The patients were treated successfully with drugs like rifampicin, INH, PZA, and ethambutol given for 6–10 months under DOTS. One case required treatment with capreomycin, ofloxacin, PAS, clofazimine and cycloserine for longer period.

Mycobacterium microti

Tuberculosis in wild rodents was first studied in 1937. Field voles, bank voles, wood mice, shrews and also cats and New World camelids domesticated in Europe are susceptible to *M. microti*, whereas guinea pigs, rabbits, mice and rats are resistant. Infection is widespread in wild small rodents and sporadic in others in the UK and Western Europe. *M. microti* seems to be less virulent as it has been extensively tried as candidate vaccine.

There have been only 6 published reports of human infections, comprising 13 patients in total. This underreporting may be due to (a) poor growth on conventional solid egg media and in the modern automatic liquid culture techniques and (b) generally not include in routine veterinary diagnostic and (c) poor formal reporting in literature.

Cats and pets are infected. Although infection of cats from infected wild rodents is suspected, the isolates from the two were not genotypically identical. Very little is known about the incidence and ecology of *M. microti* infection in farm and domestic animals. More recently, sporadic cases have been described in larger mammals. Xavier et al. (2007) isolated *M. microti* from 5 animals (2 cats, 1 each from llama, badger and ferret) and 4 humans in Scotland in a 12-year period (1994–2005) with no epidemiological linkage. Human-to-human transmission is uncertain. It affects apparently immunocompetent individuals, yet possibility of undetected specific immune defects needs investigation. This is so because inherited defects of interleukin receptor function are known to specifically predispose to intracellular infections—particularly mycobacterial.

Mycobacterium canettii

According to Miltgen et al. (2002), *M. canettii* was first isolated from a famer in 1969 by Gorge Canetti. In 1997, van Soolingen isolated So93, from TB lymph node from a child who had arrived in the Netherlands from Somalia in 1993. The strain

NZM 217/94 originated from abdominal lymphatic TB of a 56-year-old Swiss who had lived in Kenya. *M. canettii* was isolated from two cases of pulmonary TB who also had lived in East Africa. All cases originated from Horn of Africa. *M. canettii* is included in *M. tuberculosis* complex on the basis of genetic studies.

MAC is atypical *Mycobacterium*. Two main species are *M. avium* and *M. intracellulare*. It is difficult to differentiate and often collectively referred to as *M. avium-intracellulare* (MAI).

Mycobacterium avium (MAC)

Lung is primarily affected in MAC infection causing chronic obstructive pulmonary disease, chronic bronchitis and bronchiectasis. Other associated conditions are osteomyelitis, tenosynovitis and synovitis, and in the disseminated form, the lymph nodes, liver, spleen, bone marrow and CNS may be involved. Lung is rarely affected in immunocompetent hosts, and *M. intracellulare* is commonly responsible. Underlying lung disease is the risk. Lymphadenitis is common in children. Manglani et al. (2015) reported a case of pleural effusion in an immunocompetent middle-aged woman. She was admitted with right-side chest pain, productive cough and fever; examination revealed tachycardia, tachypnoea and right-side pleural effusion confirmed by X-ray. MAC is detected in pleural fluid. A six-month TB treatment became asymptomatic. Lady Windermere syndrome caused by MAC is a pulmonary infection or bronchiectasis without underlying lung disease in old ladies. Rao et al. (2016) described a case in a middle-aged immunocompetent non-smoker lady. She had a 10-year history of recurrent episodes of cough with expectoration, dyspnoea, fatiguability and pedal oedema caused by MAC.

Voluntary suppression of cough leads to stagnation of secretion that favours growth of MAC. Hot-tub lung is hypersensitivity pneumonitis (diffuse granulomatous lungs) caused by aerosolized MAC.

Mycobacterium avium (MAC)-*M. intracellulare*

Post-traumatic infection is also caused. Cutaneous *M. intracellulare* infection generally presents as abscesses, nodular lesions, erythematous plaques with yellow-crusted bases or ulcerations. Deeper infections are panniculitis, tenosynovitis and fasciitis. Pampaloni et al. (2020) described a post-traumatic skin infection (exogenous infection) with *M. intracellulare* (PCR diagnosed). It caused a cutaneous painful ulcer on the right foot of an immunocompetent person. It was chronic, deep-seated ulcer involving subcutaneous tissues up to metatarsal and accompanied hypoaesthesia.

MAC are distributed in water, dust, soil, bird-domestic fowl, crows, sparrows, water fowl, ducks, geese, turkeys, wild birds, starlings, pheasants and farm animals. Human infection occurs through inhalation and ingestion (unpasteurized milk).

Infection in Animals

Mycobacterium paratuberculosis (MAP) causes chronic inflammation of intestines and mesenteric lymph glands of animals (Johne's diseases). The herd prevalence ranged between 7% and 55% in Europe and 40% in US stocks of >300. It is endemic in India. Study of 28 years by Singh et al. (2014) suggested an increasing trend in India. Goats and cattle were more susceptible than sheep and buffaloes. The authors used multiple tests—microscopy, culture, ELISA and *IS900*PCR—for the study that revealed MAP was distributed widely, water, soil, human stool, blood, animal faeces, inflamed mesenteric lymph glands and tissues collected from slaughtered and post-mortem animals. Rabbits sharing water bodies with farm animals were positive. PCR positivity was found in blood samples from human with concurrent infection such as typhoid and dermatitis. The frequency of isolations from human beings classed on the basis of clinical laboratory diagnosis in decreasing order was liver>diabetes and anaemia> lipid profile. The MAP DNA from cattle, buffaloes, wild ruminants (blue bull, deer, bison) and rabbits were characterized as 'Bison type' using *IS1311*PCR-RE, further characterized as 'Indian Bison type'. It has wide distribution—milk, human, goats, sheep, rabbit, bison, deer, blue bull, primates, soil and water. However, role of animals in the epidemiology of human *M. avium* infection is unclear.

50.2.3.2   Non-tuberculous Mycobacteria (NTM; Fig. 50.3)

M. scrofulaceum

A retrospective chart review of patients with *M. scrofulaceum* culture positive over a period of 15 years identified that 10/17 had clinical infection. These were distributed as four pulmonary and pleural, two bone and joint infection with a foreign body, two skin and soft tissues, two brain abscess and one paediatric cervical adenitis. All patients, except for those who had joint and bone infection, had some or the other immunomodulatory and condition and/or structural lung disease (Wilson et al. 2019).

M. gordonae

It causes infection in immunocompromised cases and AIDS patients. Infection is disseminated affecting the skin, lungs, peritoneum, endocardium, liver, kidney, bone marrow and cornea. Patients respond to anti-mycobacterial drugs, except isoniazid. This agent is ubiquitous—common sources are soil and water.

Between January 2016 and December 2018, 7 cases of *M. gordonae* infection were diagnosed and treated at the National Taiwan University Hospital. One of the cases has comorbidity affecting immunity. Another had no underlying disease. The sites of infection were the lung (3), skin and soft tissue (3), and one had

NMT *Mycobacteria*

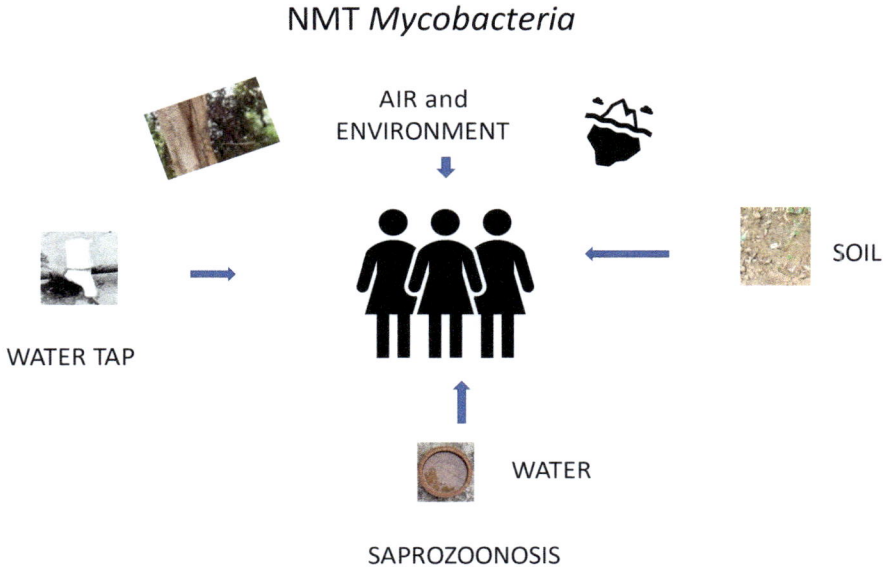

Fig. 50.3 Non-tuberculous mycobacteria

disseminated infection involving the lung and bone marrow. Six were treated successfully, the seventh succumbed due to refractory leukaemia (Chang et al. 2021).

M. kansasii

It is found in aquatic nidii and can infect cattle, pigs and human beings.

According to Akram and Rawla (2022), the prevalence of infection with NTM has been steadily increasing compared to tuberculosis. *M. kansasii* is a NTM readily recognizable by its characteristic yellow pigment when exposed to light. The major reservoir is tap water, city tap water, swimming pools, fish tanks, fish bites, brackish water and seawater.

Most infections are through aerosol route. No human-to-human transmission occurs. The symptoms are non-specific. The patients present fever, hepatosplenomegaly, pulmonary infiltrates and lymphadenopathy. The disseminated form commonly involves the bone such as vertebral osteomyelitis and sacroiliitis. Other pathologies reported include bone marrow granuloma, liver granuloma and abscesses.

Infection is common in males aged 45–62 years. There is a geographic cluster of cases, reported from the USA, Wales in the UK and Poland in Europe, and HIV-endemic areas due to increased susceptibility. During the 1960s and 1970s, *M. kansasii* was the most common NTM, increased during the 1980s due to HIV infections. The antiretroviral therapy led to reduction in infections.

M. kansasii infects both immunocompetent and immunosuppressed. The underlying conditions like chronic obstructive pulmonary disease, chronic kidney disease, malignancy, silicosis, pneumoconiosis, immunocompromised state and smoking are the risk factors.

About 90% of *M. kansasii* patients present chronic pulmonary cavitary disease (upper lobe commonly). The rest are nodular and bronchiectatic. There is progressive destruction of lung tissues. Cutaneous forms present nodules, pustules, erythematous plaques, abscess and ulcers.

Diagnosis is done by acid-fast bacteria (AFB) staining, bacterial culture and PCR. Once diagnosed, treatment is a must as colonization or environmental contamination is rare. Rifampin, ethambutol and isoniazid plus pyridoxine for 12 months is the recommended therapy and is effective.

M. simiae

According to Jabbour et al. (2020), *M. simiae* was isolated from Indian Rhesus monkeys in 1965. It is a slow-growing photochromogenic *Mycobacterium* found in water, municipal water sources, soil, salt, foodstuff and air. It has been detected in hospital drinking fountains, sinks and ice machines and can contaminate equipment which may be possible source of nosocomial outbreaks.

Transmission may be inhalation of aerosol and by inoculation. Man gets infected from environment source. Occupationally, those handling monkeys get infected and suffer with pulmonary infiltration, effusion and apical cavities. Human-to-human transmission does not occur. Only ten reported *M. simiae* strains have been genotyped.

The environment, temperature and humidity influence the physiology of *M. simiae*, and this is reflected in the restricted distribution in a geographic region. Regional prevalence has been reported from many countries/regions, Cuba, Middle East, South-western USA, western European countries, eastern Mediterranean countries and Asia-Pacific countries (South Korea). The frequency of isolation of *M. simiae* relative to potential pathogenic NTM ranged between 30% and 50% in Lebanon in the past two decades and 30% in Israel between 1975 and 1981 and 35% in Mumbai. Genetic predisposition of population also influenced the prevalence.

M. simiae infection may be asymptomatic to fatal disseminated disease, commonly pulmonary disease. The immunocompetent but with underlying conditions like chronic obstructive pulmonary disease, smoking or a history of pulmonary tuberculosis, cardiovascular disease, malignancy and diabetes mellitus develop respiratory infections. Symptoms ranged from non-specific to productive cough, haemoptysis, dyspnoea, fever, night sweats and weight loss.

Disseminated form occurs in immunocompromised and elderly. Osteomyelitis in the spine, pelvis and femur; lymphadenitis, meningitis and skin and soft tissue infections are observed as focal disease.

Most cases are environmental contamination than clinical disease. An estimated 9–21% of pulmonary isolates are of clinical significance. Of all the NTM, only

M. simiae is niacin-positive and can be confused with *M. tuberculosis*. Pulmonary (chest) imaging of *M. simiae* shows chronic lung disease in middle and lower lobes, whereas TB presents cavitary lesions usually in the upper lobe and bilateral lymphadenopathy. The distinction is not clear cut. Differentiation is important because the treatment regimens are different.

The recommended therapy is based on a combination of macrolides with moxifloxacin, clofazimine and streptomycin with reported success.

M. heidelbergense

M. heidelbergense has been found associated with cervical lymphadenitis and pulmonary infection in a child.

M. lentiflavum

This has been isolated from contaminated bronchioscope and cervical lymphadenitis and spondylodiscitis. Molteni et al. (2005) have reviewed past 14 cases mostly affecting young children with cervical lymphadenitis as the predominant lesion. Most of the reports are from Europe. A case of chronic pulmonary infection due to *M. lentiflavum* in an immunocompetent patient is described. Conventional bacteriological methods are inadequate for diagnosis. HPLC of cell wall mycolic acid and molecular techniques such as study of 16 S rRNA gene fragments—through nucleic acid probes, sequencing and amplification should be resorted to.

Treatment is difficult. In this case, the patient appeared to have recovered after three months of treatment with clarithromycin. Sputum was negative after one month of treatment. It came out to be positive again. New regimen with clarithromycin plus ethambutol, rifabutin and ciprofloxacin was started but stopped prematurely because of poor response. The patient continues to be radiographically + (reticulonodular) and sputum + and clinically manifests weakness, dyspnoea and intermittent haemoptysis.

M. genavense

It is an environmental *Mycobacterium*. *M. genavense* has been detected in tap water, healthy birds and gastrointestine of healthy individuals. It becomes difficult to distinguish between colonization and infection if this bacterium is detected in gastrointestinal or respiratory tract. It is considered as an opportunist pathogen, associated mostly with HIV-infected patients with CD4 counts less than 100/micro L. It can cause disease in birds and dogs also. It causes cervical lymphadenitis, Whipple-like syndrome, sclerosing cholangitis and skin lesions. It is often fatal if untreated.

Hoefsloot et al. (2013) made a retrospective observational study of medical charts in the Netherlands to identify 14 cases of *M. genavense* infection from

January 2002 to January 2010. Thirteen (93%) had clinically relevant disease. They were severely immunocompromised, for example, HIV, immunosuppressive therapy, chemotherapy for non-Hodgkin lymphoma and solid organ transplant recipients. Two patients had non-disseminated pulmonary disease. Eight of twelve patients treated recovered.

M. triplex

M. triplex is a slow-growing non-pigmented *Mycobacterium* described in 1996. Phylogenetically *M. triplex* and *M. lentiflavum* are closely related to *M. simiae* and *M. genavense*.

A presumptive identification may be made by observing—non-pigmentation, slow growth, reduction of nitrate, production of urease and semi-quantitation of catalase and three-clustered mycolic acid profile.

However, HPLC analysis of mycolic acids provides a triple-clustered profile that closely resembles but distinguishes it from *M. simiae*, *M. genavense* and *M. sherrisii* but not from that of *M. lentiflavum*. Conclusive identification is based on sequencing the 16S rRNA hypervariable region.

It has been isolated from lymph node, sputum and cerebrospinal fluid specimens and the pericardial and peritoneal fluid of a 13-year-old female liver transplant patient (Hoff et al. 2001).

M. triplex is known to cause infection in AIDS cases in immunosuppressed and also immunocompetent persons (Piersimoni et al. 2004). The pulmonary cases manifest in fever, cough, fatigue, haemoptysis, lung infiltration, nodules, multifocal bronchiectasis and cavitation. It is unresponsive to anti-Mycobacterial therapy. Ethambutol, rifampin, clarithromycin and ciprofloxacin in different combination led to clinical recovery in ten months in one of three cases, but cases were sputum and culture positive even after two years.

M. ulcerans

M. ulcerans (Buruli ulcer, other names—Bairnsdale ulcer, Daintree ulcer and Mossman ulcer in Australia).

M. ulcerans infection is considered as the third most frequent mycobacterial infection after *M. tuberculosis* and *M. leprae*. It is characterized by indolent skin ulcer, extensive tissue necrosis and absence of systemic symptoms. It is considered as one of the neglected tropical diseases with a poorly known global prevalence and mainly affects remote rural African communities.

van der Werf et al. (2005) have reviewed *M. ulcerans* infection-related literature. Accordingly, the disease is known since 1897 when Sir Albert Cook described chronic ulceration in Uganda. The name Buruli arises from the name of the county in Uganda where large number of cases clustered in a refugee camp at Kinyara. Many countries in sub- Saharan Africa are considered endemic. The increasing number of cases has been reported in the riverine areas of Benin, Côte d'Ivoire and Ghana. Other foci in tropical areas are Sri Lanka, Papua New Guinea, Malaysia (Asia) Mexico, Peru and Guyana (Latin America). The disease occurs also in temperate climate and riverine areas in Bairnsdale, Victoria and Melbourne in Australia. In addition to human beings, Koalas (*Phascolarctos cinereus*), ring-tailed possums (*Pseudocheirus peregrinus*), brushtail possums (*Trichosurus vulpecula*), an alpaca (*Llama alpaca*) and a potoroo (*Potorous longipes*) have been reported to develop natural infections in endemic areas.

The source is environmental. Aquatic insects, fish and molluscs in endemic areas are infected without any overt disease. Biofilm of water plant has been found infected. Molluscs feed on biofilm, and certain aquatic insects, *Naucoridae*, appear to concentrate *M. ulcerans* in its salivary gland which may also feed on molluscs. Experimentally infected water bugs transmitted the disease in tail of mice through bite.

Role of insects in human infection is not yet established. Johnson et al. (2007) observed that mosquitoes, *Ae. camptorhynchus* and *Ae. Notoscriptus*, were positive for *M. ulcerans*. Number of mosquitoes and PCR-positive mosquitoes increased during spring and summer followed by cluster of new cases in autumn and winter, and this matched with the period of exposure to reporting and diagnosis.

Penetrating skin injuries followed by infection seems to be route of infection as may occur during fishing and farming activities. Swamps and recycled water from sewage facility used for irrigation are potent sources. Wading in water is one of the risk factors. Aerosol transmission has been suggested. Rare but human-to-human infection may occur.

Guarner et al. (2003) reported the results of WHO's initiated study in Ghana. Phanzu et al. (2006) made an exhaustive study for 28 months (2002–2004) in the Democratic Republic of Congo. A cross-sectional survey for the period July–August 2008 was made by Mavinga Phanzu et al. (2013). A total of 775 patients (259 active and 516 inactive) were detected in a population of 237,418, an overall prevalence of 3.3/1000 inhabitants in Songololo Territory. There was gross underreporting. The Buruli Ulcer cases in the hospital-based reporting system reflected only the tip of the iceberg of the true active prevalence.

M. ulcerans is an environmental pathogen. It is common in swampy areas and water having pH 6.1–6.9. It has been isolated from river Kimu, near Angolan refugee camp. It invades through skin injury such as those caused by grass thorns. The ulcer is deep, chronic and metastatic, often reaching the bone. Osteomyelitis is important complication. Most common site is the lower limb followed by the upper limb. It is a disfiguring and disabling skin disease. The sequelae are often a deformity/crippling in about 25% or scarring. There may be mortality also in those who turn up for treatment in very advanced stage.

The first case was reported in 1950 in the Democratic Republic of Congo in an American boy. Since then, it has been detected/suspected in 31 countries. It is highly prevalent in West and Central Africa. Seventy eight of 124 skin-biopsy specimens suspected for buruli ulcer in Ghana were diagnosed as positive for acid fast bacilli on histopathological examination.

Johnson et al. (2007) suggested that incubation period in Australia was 3–7 months. Quek et al. (2007) observed that 67% of cases in south-eastern Australia were >60 years contrasting with most cases of <15 years observed in studies in Africa.

The lesions showed necrosis of subcutaneous tissues and more frequent dermal collagen fibres. *M. ulcerans* produced a lipid called mycolactone, chemically identified as ketolide. In experimental guinea pigs, this lipid produced cutaneous histopathological lesions similar to those seen in clinical case. Genes for mycolactone synthesis appear to be located on a giant plasmid. Strains of *M. ulcerans* from one locality show remarkable similarity. Isolates from different geographic locations differ in the type of mycolactone production and perhaps explains the regional difference in virulence of strains and the disease (van der Werf et al. 2005). Mycolactone is immunosuppressive, suppressing (a) production of interleukin 2 by T cells, (b) tumour necrosis factor by monocytes and (c) induction of macrophage apoptosis. Gooding et al. (2001) observed that T cell anergy and lack of interferon production (IFN-gamma) might account for *M. ulcerans* pathology—indolent ulcer and extracellular persistence of *M. ulcerans*. Buruli ulcer is a localized toxin (mycolactone)-mediated immunosuppression.

The median age of patient is 15–17 years. More males than females are affected—possibly related to males more frequently reporting to hospital.

Methods of diagnosis included acid fast staining, culture, histopathology and PCR. Ideally, the specimen should be processed on the day it is collected. In semi-solid transport medium held at 4⁰C for a week, recovery percentage is over 60.

The patients, both acute and healed lesions, showed antibodies (85% of Buruli ulcer patients tested IgM positive compared to 4.5% healthy control) to culture filtrate of *M. ulcerans*.

Diagnostic methods include microscopic detection, isolation and cultivation of the bacterium, histopathology, polymerase chain reaction (PCR) and serological test. *Antigens used for serologic and/or CMI-based test may be (a) pathogen-derived and (b) recombinant proteins. Using pathogen-derived antigens better differentiated patients from control group than the recombinant proteins* (Avumegah et al. 2020).

Surgical debridement and anti-mycobacterial drugs like streptomycin and rifampicin followed by physiotherapy are the possible approaches to treat.

There is often a delay in presentation of cases for treatment. Diagnosis too is delayed as laboratory confirmation is desired but time taking. The period of hospitalization is consequentially lengthened. Recurrence rates increase. Recovery is slow. It ends into disability. All these taken together caused bad socio-economic effect. Approaches to minimize the adverse consequences require a multidisciplinary action, education of population in endemic areas, counselling and training of the health workers and establishment of specific diagnostic and treatment facilities.

M. intermedium

M. intermedium was originally isolated from sputum of a patient of pulmonary disease. Edson et al. (2006) describe its association with chronic granulomatous dermatitis. The source of infection is traced to contaminated water used in hot tub bath.

In support, water-borne non-tuberculous mycobacterial infections have been cited. *M. kansasii*, *M. xenopi*, *M. avium*, *M. fortuitum*, *M. chelonae* and *M. gordonae* were isolated from domestic and environmental water sources and were resistant to chlorine contributing its persistence in even treated water. Public and private hot tubs, whirlpools and public spas are likely to be the source of infection. Infection acquired from such sources caused *M. avium*, complex pneumonitis; *M. fortuitum*, amputation stump infection and lower extremity furunculosis; and *M. abscessus*, soft tissue infection.

M. haemophilum

The natural distribution and reservoirs of *M. haemophilum* may be wide and several—most likely water. Cases from the USA, Brazil and Israel are known, mostly distributed around large water bodies.

   M. haemophilum was first detected as the cause of cutaneous lesion in a patient of Hodgkin disease. It has been identified as cause of lymphadenopathy (cervical, submandibular, perihilar) in children and pulmonary nodules in adults both immunocompetent and immunocompromised. There is fever and loss of weight. Common lesions in adults are seen in the skin, erythematous to plaques, and joints, effusion, tenosynovitis and pyomyositis. Isolations have been made less frequently from respiratory tract, blood, bone marrow, bone and central venous catheters in the USA, Canada, the UK, France, Israel and Australia. Sampaio et al. (2002) describe isolations in Brazil from three patients—(a) nasal ulcer of a HIV-sero-positive, (b) osteomyelitis in the elbow of HIV sero-positive and (c) blood of a kidney transplant patient receiving immunosuppressive drugs.

   The infection seems to be more common than actually diagnosed. *M. haemophilum* does not grow on routine media. The organism is slow growing. Optimal growth temperature varies from 30-32^{0}C. It requires iron—for primary isolation and so ferric ammonium citrate or hemin-enriched media, chocolate agar is useful. It induces Mantoux reaction similar to *M. tuberculosis*. Thus, Mantoux positive and culture negative could be lost. Bruijnesteijn van Coppenraet et al. (2005) considered that real-time PCR was sensitive and specific for detection and identification in clinical specimens like sputum, CSF and synovial fluid. It is alcohol-acid-fast, catalase negative. Final identification is based on polymerase chain reaction.

M. marinum

The source is salt water fish and the bacterium invades through abraded skin of human being when exposed to infected water of swimming pool or fish tank. Abrasion is often caused by fin of the fish and the man is unaware of both abrasion and invasion. *M. marinum* produces nodular or ulcerating skin lesions on extremities. Delayed diagnosis and immune suppression contribute to the pathogenesis. Delay in appropriate treatment may allow the lesions to spread deeper—synovia, bursae and bone. Lahey (2003) described a case. The patient had a nagging, chronic erythematous lesion on left ring finger persisting for the past five years not responding to surgical debridement and antimicrobial therapy. The left elbow developed swelling and tenderness lasting for about five months. *M. marinum* was isolated from the lesion aspirate. Treatment on the basis of drug sensitivity test was successful with rifampicin and ethambutol given for 11.4 months. The patient was doing well after nine months. According to Lahey (2003), the average age of cases was 43 years. More men suffered and most had tenosynovitis; some had septic arthritis and osteomyelitis. Skin lesions may be single or multiple. Systemic infection is rare and occurred in immunocompromised individuals. Delayed diagnosis was common.

M. xenopi

It was isolated from a tumour-like lesion on the leg of a toad by Schwabacher in 1959. It can grow at high temperature and thus fowls are infected, suffer and may even die.

Human beings residing in areas like sea coast and estuary probably acquire infection from seagulls. van Ingen et al. (2008) described the clinical relevance of this mycobacterium.

Sources—heated water systems and natural water; it is able to resist flowing water and common disinfectants and contaminate medical instruments like bronchoscope; cross- contamination occurs.

Modes of transmission—environment through aerosol inhalation and ingestion; human-human and from animal reservoir to human not confirmed.

Infection of respiratory system is most common, though extra-pulmonary infection occurs. Impaired immunity (medication or HIV); pre-existing pulmonary disease and systemic diseases like haematologic malignancy predispose.

Isolation is infrequent and clinical relevance is often uncertain. Treatment of *M. xenopi* infections is time-consuming and often complicated. van Ingen et al. (2008) retrospectively reviewed medical files of all patients in the Netherlands in whom *M. xenopi* was isolated from January 1999 through March 2005 and found 49 patients, mostly White men, with an average age of 60 years and pre-existing pulmonary disease; of these, 25 (51%) met the diagnostic criteria. Mycobacterial genotype, based on 16S rRNA gene sequencing, was associated with true infection. Most infections were pulmonary, but pleural and spinal infections (spinal in HIV-infected patients) were also noted. Treatment regimens varied in content and duration; some patients were over treated and some were under treated.

M. goodie

M. goodie is a rapidly growing NMT and belongs to *M. smegmatis* group. It has been found to cause sporadic cellulitis, bursitis, osteomyelitis, lipoid pneumonia and infection at the site of pacemaker. Ferguson et al. (2004) have described three cases of nosocomial postsurgical infection at a Colorado hospital leading to removal of prosthesis. There was painful swelling at the site, erythematous wound and septic requiring drainage, debridement and patch removal. Diagnosis was delayed as NMT was not suspected. Specimens from drainage, joint fluid and patches decontaminated with either Sputagest 50 mucolytic agent or N-acetyle-L-cysteine-NaOH yielded Mycobacterial growth in 3, 7 and 11 days. The three isolates had closely related PFGE (pulsed field gel electrophoresis) pattern. Attempts to locate the common source of infection were inconclusive.

In general, NTM are relatively resistant to disinfectants and antiseptics. *M. smegmatis* is sensitive to povidone iodine, chlorhexidine gluconate and alkaline glutaraldehyde, and these may be used in absence of information on suitable antiseptic for *M. goodii.*

M. goodii infection is amenable to therapy. Drugs of choice are amikacin, ethambutol and sulfamethoxazole, followed by ciprofloxacin, doxycycline and tobramycin. Oral administration of drug of choice given for 4–6 months is effective against mild infection. Severe wound infection requires surgical debridement and initial combination followed by oral therapy given for six months.

M. kyorinense

Mycobacterium kyorinense is a non-pigmented slow-growing *Mycobacterium* first isolated from a pneumonia patient in Japan in 2007 (Ohnishi et al. 2013). It is different from but related to *M. celatum* and *M. branderi.* The authors reviewed the characteristics of 11 patients, 10 from Japan and 1 from Brazil. Respiratory problem was the most common (9/11); one each had lymphadenitis and arthritis. Four of the nine respiratory patients died. All strains were relatively resistant to rifampin. The first line of TB drugs—mainly rifampin, isoniazid and ethambutol—were not effective in all cases. A combination of fluoroquinolones and macrolides and/or aminoglycosides is recommended.

M. celatum

M. celatum was first described in 1993. It caused cervical lymphadenitis and fatal pulmonary disease similar to TB and also a disseminated form in immunocompromised cases. Piersimoni et al. (2003) described serious pulmonary infection resembling pulmonary TB in an immunocompetent patient who appeared to respond to anti-mycobacterial therapy, clarithromycin.

M. celatum is indistinguishable from *M. avium* complex but can be distinguished from *M. xenopi* on the basis of biochemical tests. Its mycolic acid pattern closely resembles those of *M. xenopi*. Sequencing of 16S rRNA shows three different types of *M. celatum*. Accuprobe assay (Gen-Probe Inc., San Diego, CA) for *M. tuberculosis* complex showed cross reactivity. The types 1 and 2 differed from the probe used in the Accuprobe by one and four nucleotides as revealed by DNA sequencing.

M. szulgai

The source of *M. szulgai* is environment. It has been reported from snails, aquarium water, swimming pools, tropical fish and hospital water supplies. Human-to-human transmission does not occur.

M. szulgai infection is uncommon in humans. In a study of over 36,000 NTM samples from 14 countries throughout Europe and the Middle East, only 0.2% were *M. szulgai*. Pulmonary infection is common. Tenosynovitis of the hand, olecranon bursitis, osteomyelitis, keratitis, cervical lymphadenitis and renal or cutaneous infection are extra-pulmonary manifestations. Infection leads to disease indistinguishable from tuberculosis caused by *M. tuberculosis*. It has been isolated from nodules in lungs and osteomyelitis in HIV-positive patients.

Nunes et al. (2022) described a case of disseminated *M. szulgai* infection in a 25-year-old patient of systemic lupus erythematosus. He had recurrent fever and non-productive cough. He had lost weight. He reported asthenia. There were two violaceous plaques with superficial ulceration in the gluteal region. Bronchial lavage and skin biopsy were culture positive. It took ten months for recovery with isoniazid, rifampin, ethambutol and pyrazinamide. The authors claimed only 16 cases of disseminated *M. szulgai* which have so far been reported.

Gido et al. (2019) presented a case of *M. szulgai* pulmonary infection. A 42-year-old male with normal immunity had chronic obstructive pulmonary disease, asthma and polyneuropathy. He was a smoker, one-half-pack-per-day for 30 years. He was found to have pulmonary disease. He was successfully treated in Niagara Falls, NY, USA, with regimen of rifampin, isoniazid, pyrazinamide and ethambutol for two months, followed by rifampin, isoniazid and azithromycin for an additional eight months.

M. malmoense

Cowan et al. (2009) presented a case of pulmonary infection in a Canadian woman aged 53 years. She possibly picked up infection from environment as *M. malmoense* is commonly found in soil and water and there is no evidence of human-to-human transmission. They dealt with the history of this *Mycobacterium*. *M. malmoense* derived its name from the City of Malmo, Sweden, where four cases of pulmonary infection were investigated and the causative agent was described by Schröder and Juhlin in 1977. It is a slow-growing non-photochromogenic *Mycobacterium*.

It is relatively common in the UK and Northern Europe and rarely reported in North America and Canada.

Pulmonary form of disease is more common than cervical adenitis which is seen commonly in children. Often the pulmonary form is misdiagnosed as symptoms are variable and non-specific. Symptoms include cough, dyspnoea, haemoptysis, sputum production, malaise and weight loss. The infection is common with certain comorbidities of lungs like chronic obstructive bronchial disease, bronchiectasis, cystic fibrosis, previous tuberculosis and occupational exposure such as pneumoconiosis. The lesions in AIDS patients are pulmonary infiltration and mediastinal lymphadenopathy. A retrospective (January 2002–January 2006) medical file of patients in the Netherlands from whom *M. malmoense* was isolated pinned down 51 patients. Forty of 51 (78%) were from pulmonary lesions and 32 or 80% of these met the diagnostic criteria of the American Thoracic Society (ATS) for non-tuberculous mycobacterial (NTM) diseases. Cavitary disease was most common (88%). Most patients were males of average age 56 years suffering with pre-existing chronic obstructive pulmonary obstructive disease. Cervical lymphadenitis was the most common extra-pulmonary condition. The response to treatment was good (Hoefsloot et al. 2009).

Laboratory diagnosis may be done by staining for AFB and cultivation (up to 8–12 weeks may be required to grow the organism in the laboratory) of at least two sputum samples and/or at least one bronchial lavage, molecular tools and high-performance liquid chromatography.

Prompt treatment is recommended. Patients respond to anti-mycobacterial therapy—rifampicin, isoniazid and ethambutol administered for 18–24 months.

References

Akram SM, Rawla P (2022) Mycobacterium Kansasii. [Updated 2022 Oct 9]. In: StatPearls [Internet]. StatPearls Publishing, Treasure Island (FL). Jan-. Available from: https://www.ncbi.nlm.nih.gov/books/NBK430906/

Alexander KA, Pleydell E, Williams MC, Lane EP, Nyange JF, Michel AL (2002) *Mycobacterium tuberculosis*: an emerging disease of free-ranging wildlife. Emerg Infect Dis 8(6):598–601

Angkawanish T, Wajjwalku W, Sirimalaisuwan A, Mahasawangkul S et al (2010) *Mycobacterium tuberculosis* infection of domesticated Asian elephants, Thailand. Emerg Infect Dis 16(12):1949–1951. https://doi.org/10.3201/eid1612.100862. Erratum in: Emerg Infect Dis. 2011 Apr;17(4):758

Anonym (2009) Bovine tuberculosis in England: towards eradication. Final Report of the Bovine TB Advisory Group Presented to the Minister for Farming and the Environment, and the Chief Veterinary Officer for Defra. 8 April 2009

Anonym (2014) Bovine tuberculosis: guidance on management of the public health consequences of tuberculosis in cattle and other animals (England) Published September 2014 PHE publications gateway number: 2014324

Avumegah MS, Waidyatillake NT, Michalski WP, O'Brien DP et al (2020) Cell-mediated and serology-based tests for *Mycobacterium ulcerans* disease: a systematic review and meta-analysis. PLoS Negl Trop Dis 14(4):e0008172

Boehme CC, Nabeta P, Hillemann D, Nicol MP, Shenai S et al (2010) Rapid molecular detection of tuberculosis and rifampin resistance. N Engl J Med 363:1005–1015

Bruijnesteijn van Coppenraet LE, Kuijper EJ, Lindeboom JA, Prins JM, Claas EC (2005) *Mycobacterium haemophilum* and lymphadenitis in children. Emerg Infect Dis 11(1):62–68

Chandranaik BM, Shivashankar BP, Umashankar KS, Nandini P et al (2017) *Mycobacterium tuberculosis* infection in free-roaming wild Asian elephant. Emerg Infect Dis 23(3):555–557

Chang HY, Tsai WC, Lee TF, Sheng WH (2021) *Mycobacterium gordonae* infection in immunocompromised and immunocompetent hosts: a series of seven cases and literature review. J Formosan Med Assoc 120(1, Part 2):524–532

Cowan CD, Hawboldt JJ, Bader M (2009) Pulmonary infection due to *Mycobacterium malmoense* in a patient with Crohn disease. Can J Hosp Pharm 62(6):496–499

Cox HS, Sibilia K, Feuerriegel S, Kalon S et al (2008) Emergence of extensive drug resistance during treatment for multidrug-resistant tuberculosis. N Engl J Med 359(22):2398–2400. Erratum in: N Engl J Med. 2010 Oct 21;363(17):1682

de Garine-Wichatitsky M, Caron A, Gomo C, Foggin C, Dutlow K et al (2010) Bovine tuberculosis in buffaloes, Southern Africa. Emerg Infect Dis 16(5):884–885

Desmond E, Ahmed AT, Probert WS, Ely J et al (2004) *Mycobacterium africanum* cases, California. Emerg Infect Dis 10(5):921–923

Diriba G, Alemu A, Tola HH, Eshetu K et al (2022) Detection of *Mycobacterium tuberculosis* and rifampicin resistance by Xpert® MTB/RIF assay among presumptive tuberculosis patients in Addis Ababa, Ethiopia from 2014 to 2021. IJID Reg 5:97–103

ECDC (2022) Tuberculosis surveillance and monitoring in Europe 2020. 24 March 2022

ECDC-WHO (2021) European Centre for Disease Prevention and Control, WHO Regional Office for Europe. Tuberculosis surveillance and monitoring in Europe 2021 – 2019 data. Copenhagen: WHO Regional Office for Europe; 2021. Publication series: Tuberculosis surveillance in Europe; 22 Mar 2021

ECDC-WHO (2022) European Centre for Disease Prevention and Control, WHO Regional Office for Europe. Tuberculosis surveillance and monitoring in Europe 2022 – 2020 data. Copenhagen: WHO Regional Office for Europe and Stockholm: European Centre for Disease Prevention and Control; 2022. Licence: CC BY 3.0 IGO. 24 Mar 2022

Edson RS, Terrell CL, Brutinel WM, Wengenack NL (2006) *Mycobacterium intermedium* granulomatous dermatitis from hot tub exposure. Emerg Infect Dis 12(5):821–823

ETS/ESMI (2014) Enhanced Tuberculosis Surveillance (ETS), Enhanced Surveillance of *Mycobacterial* Infections (ESMI). May 2014. Prepared by: TB Section - Public Health England, Colindale

Fang Y, Ma Y, Lu Q, Sun J, Pei Y (2021) An outbreak of pulmonary tuberculosis and a follow-up investigation of latent tuberculosis in a high school in an eastern city in China, 2016–2019. PLoS ONE 16(2):e0247564

Ferguson DD, Gershman K, Jensen B, Arduino MJ et al (2004) *Mycobacterium goodii* infections associated with surgical implants at Colorado hospital. Emerg Infect Dis 10(10):1868–1871

Ghielmetti G, Coscolla M, Ruetten M, Friedel U, Loiseau C et al (2017) Tuberculosis in Swiss captive Asian elephants: microevolution of *Mycobacterium tuberculosis* characterized by multilocus variable-number tandem-repeat analysis and whole-genome sequencing. Sci Rep 7(1):14647

Gido RDS, Wojciechowski AL, Bajwa RP (2019) Pulmonary infection with *Mycobacterium szulgai*: (2019). A case report. SAGE Open Med Case Rep 7:2050313X18823448

Global tuberculosis report 2017. Geneva: World Health Organization; 2017. Licence: CC BY-NCSA 3.0 IGO

Gooding TM, Johnson PD, Campbell DE, Hayman JA et al (2001) Immune response to infection with *Mycobacterium ulcerans*. Infect Immun 69(3):1704–1707

Guarner J, Bartlett J, Whitney EA, Raghunathan PL, Stienstra Y et al (2003) Histopathologic features of *Mycobacterium ulcerans* infection. Emerg Infect Dis 9(6):651–656

Hoefsloot W, van Ingen J, de Lange WC, Dekhuijzen PN et al (2009) Clinical relevance of *Mycobacterium malmoense* isolation in the Netherlands. Eur Resp J 34:926–931

Hoefsloot W, van Ingen J, Peters EJG, Magis-Escurra C, Dekhuijzen PNR et al (2013) *Mycobacterium genavense* in the Netherlands: an opportunistic pathogen in HIV and non-HIV immunocompromised patients. An observational study in 14 cases. Clin Microbiol Infect 19:432–437

Hoff E, Sholtis M, Procop G, Sabella C, Goldfarb J et al (2001) *Mycobacterium triplex* infection in a liver transplant patient. J Clin Microbiol 39(5):2033–2034

Hong DN, Huyen MN, Lan NT, Duong NH, Ngo VV et al (2013) Rifampin-resistant *Mycobacterium bovis* BCG-induced disease in HIV-infected infant, Vietnam. Emerg Infect Dis 19(7):1168–1170

Jabbour JF, Hamieh A, Sharara SL, Kanj SS (2020) *Mycobacterium simiae*: harmless colonizer or deadly pathogen? PLoS Pathog 16(4):e1008418

Johnson PD, Azuolas J, Lavender CJ, Wishart E, Stinear TP et al (2007) *Mycobacterium ulcerans* in mosquitoes captured during outbreak of Buruli ulcer, southeastern Australia. Emerg Infect Dis 13(11):1653–1660

Jou R, Huang WL, Chiang CY (2008) Human tuberculosis caused by *Mycobacterium bovis*, Taiwan. Emerg Infect Dis 14(3):515–517

Kanabus A. Information about tuberculosis, GHE, 2020. TB & HIV - Co-infection, statistics, diagnosis, treatment. https://tbfacts.org/tb-hiv

Karande S, Bavdekar SB (2002) Children and multidrug-resistant tuberculosis in Mumbai (Bombay), India. Emerg Infect Dis 8(11):1360–1361

References													537

Kubica T, Agzamova R, Wright A, Rakishev G et al (2006) *Mycobacterium bovis* isolates with *M. tuberculosis* specific characteristics. Emerg Infect Dis 12(5):763–765
Lahey T (2003) Invasive *Mycobacterium marinum* infections. Emerg Infect Dis 9(11):1496–1498
Manglani RP, Khaja M, Hennessey K, Kennedy O (2015) Pleural *Mycobacterium avium* complex infection in an immunocompetent female with no risk factors. Case Rep Pulmonol 2015:760614
Matos AC, Figueira L, Martins MH, Matos M, Morais M et al (2014) Disseminated *Mycobacterium bovis* infection in red foxes (*Vulpes vulpes*) with cerebral involvement found in Portugal. Vector Borne Zoonotic Dis 14(7):531–533
Mavinga Phanzu D, Suykerbuyk P, Saunderson P, Ngwala Lukanu P et al (2013) Burden of *Mycobacterium ulcerans* disease (Buruli Ulcer) and the underreporting ratio in the territory of Songololo, Democratic Republic of Congo. PLoS Negl Trop Dis 7(12):e2563
Michalak K, Austin C, Diesel S, Bacon MJ, Zimmerman P, Maslow JN (1998) *Mycobacterium tuberculosis* infection as a zoonotic disease: transmission between humans and elephants. Emerg Infect Dis 4(2):283–287
Miller MA, Finnegan M, Storms T, Garner M, Lyashchenko KP (2018) Outbreak of *Mycobacterium tuberculosis* in a herd of captive Asian elephants (*Elephas maximus*): antemortem diagnosis, treatment, and lessons learned. J Zoo Wildl Med 49(3):748–754
Miller RS, Sweeney SJ (2013) Mycobacterium bovis (bovine tuberculosis) infection in North American wildlife: Current status and opportunities for mitigation of risks of further infection in wildlife populations. Epidemiol Infect 141:1357–1370. https:10.1017/S0950268813000976
Miltgen J, Morillon M, Koeck JL, Varnerot A, Briant JF et al (2002) Two cases of pulmonary tuberculosis caused by *Mycobacterium tuberculosis* subsp *canetti*. Emerg Infect Dis 8(11):1350–1352
Molteni C, Gazzola L, Cesari M, Lombardi A, Salerno F, Tortoli E et al (2005) *Mycobacterium lentiflavum* infection in immunocompetent patient. Emerg Infect Dis 11(1):119–122
Müller B, Dürr S, Alonso S, Hattendorf J, Laisse CJ et al (2013) Zoonotic *Mycobacterium bovis*-induced tuberculosis in humans. Emerg Infect Dis 19(6):899–908
Nathanson E, Lambregts-van Weezenbeek C, Rich ML, Gupta R, Bayona J et al (2006) Multidrug-resistant tuberculosis management in resource-limited settings. Emerg Infect Dis 12(9):1389–1397
Ntivuguruzwa JB, Michel AL, Kolo FB, Mwikarago IE et al (2022) Prevalence of bovine tuberculosis and characterization of the members of the *Mycobacterium tuberculosis* complex from slaughtered cattle in Rwanda. PLoS Negl Trop Dis 16(8):e0009964
Nunes A, Coimbra A, Carvalho R, Figueiredo C et al (2022) *Mycobacterium szulgai*: a rare cause of non-tuberculous mycobacteria disseminated infection. J Med Cases North Am. https://www.journalmc.org/index.php/JMC/article/view/3885/3205
Oh P, Granich R, Scott J, Sun B, Joseph M et al (2002) Human exposure following *Mycobacterium tuberculosis* infection of multiple animal species in a Metropolitan Zoo. Emerg Infect Dis 8(11):1290–1293
Ohnishi H, Yonetani S, Matsushima S, Wada H, Takeshita K et al (2013) *Mycobacterium kyorinense* infection. Emerg Infect Dis 19(3):508–510
Pai M, Kalantri S, Aggarwal AN, Menzies D, Blumberg HM (2006) Nosocomial tuberculosis in India. Emerg Infect Dis 12(9):1311–1318
Pampaloni A, Tosto S, Locatelli ME, Gentile A, Scuderi D et al (2020) Skin and soft tissue infection by *Mycobacterium intracellulare* in an immunocompetent patient. IDCases 19:e00720
Phanzu DM, Bafende EA, Dunda BK, Imposo DB, Kibadi AK et al (2006) *Mycobacterium ulcerans* disease (Buruli ulcer) in a rural hospital in Bas-Congo, Democratic Republic of Congo, 2002–2004. Am J Trop Med Hyg 75:311–314
Piersimoni C, Zitti PG, Nista D, Bornigia S (2003) *Mycobacterium celatum* pulmonary infection in the immunocompetent: case report and review. Emerg Infect Dis 9(3):399–402
Piersimoni C, Zitti P, Mazzarelli G, Mariottini A, Nista D, Zallocco D (2004) *Mycobacterium triplex* pulmonary disease in immunocompetent host. Emerg Infect Dis 10(10):1859–1862
Pietersen E, Ignatius E, Streicher EM, Mastrapa B, Padanilam X et al (2014) Long-term outcomes of patients with extensively drug-resistant tuberculosis in South Africa: a cohort study. Lancet 383(9924):1230–1239

Quek TY, Athan E, Henry MJ, Pasco JA, Redden-Hoare J, Hughes A, Johnson PD (2007) Risk factors for Mycobacterium ulcerans infection, southeastern Australia. Emerg Infect Dis 13(11):1661–1666. https://10.3201/eid1311.061206. PMID: 18217548; PMCID: PMC3375781

Rao R, Sheshadri S, Patil N, Rao K, Arivazhahan A (2016) Lady Windermere Syndrome: a very rare entity in Indian Medical Scenario. J Clin Diagn Res 10(1):OD01-2

Raviglione MC (2007) The new Stop TB Strategy and the Global Plan to Stop TB, 2006-2015. Bull World Health Organ 85(5):327

Romha G, Gebru G, Asefa A, Mamo G (2018) Epidemiology of Mycobacterium bovis and Mycobacterium tuberculosis in animals: transmission dynamics and control challenges of zoonotic TB in Ethiopia. Prev Vet Med 158:1–17

Sampaio JL, Alves VA, Leão SC, De Magalhães VD et al (2002) Mycobacterium haemophilum: emerging or underdiagnosed in Brazil? Emerg Infect Dis 8(11):1359–1360

Semilan HM, Abugad HA, Mashat HM, Abdel Wahab MM (2021) Epidemiology of tuberculosis among different occupational groups in Makkah region, Saudi Arabia. Sci Rep 11(1):12764

Shah NS, Wright A, Bai GH, Barrera L, Boulahbal F et al (2007) Worldwide emergence of extensively drug-resistant tuberculosis. Emerg Infect Dis 13(3):380–387

Silva MR, Rocha ADS, Araújo FR, Fonseca-Júnior AA, Alencar AP et al (2018) Risk factors for human Mycobacterium bovis infections in an urban area of Brazil. Mem Inst Oswaldo Cruz 113(8):e170445

Simpson G, Zimmerman R, Shashkina E, Chen L, Richard M et al (2017) Mycobacterium tuberculosis infection among Asian elephants in captivity. Emerg Infect Dis 23(3):513–516. Erratum in: Emerg Infect Dis. 2017; 23(4):724

Singh SV, Singh PK, Singh AV, Sohal JS, Kumar N et al (2014) 'Bio-load' and bio-type profiles of Mycobacterium avium subspecies paratuberculosis infection in the domestic livestock population endemic for Johne's disease: a survey of 28 years (1985-2013) in India. Transbound Emerg Dis 61(Suppl 1):43–55

Thoen C, LoBue P, Enarson D, Kaneene J, Kantor I (2009) Tuberculosisis a re-emerging disease in animals and humans. Vet Ital 45:35–181

Tschopp R, Aseffa A, Schelling E, Berg S, Hailu E, Gadisa E et al (2010) Bovine tuberculosis at the wildlife-livestock-human interface in Hamer Woreda, South Omo, Southern Ethiopia. PLoS ONE 5(8):e12205

van der Werf TS, Stienstra Y, Johnson RC, Phillips R, Adjei O, Fleischer B et al (2005) Mycobacterium ulcerans disease. Bull World Health Organ 83(10):785–791

van Ingen J, Boeree MJ, de Lange WC, Hoefsloot W, Bendien SA et al (2008) Mycobacterium xenopi clinical relevance and determinants, the Netherlands. Emerg Infect Dis 14(3):385–389

WHO (2014) Global Tuberculosis Report 2014 9789241564809_eng

WHO (2018) 16 January 2018 Tuberculosis: multidrug-resistant tuberculosis (MDR-TB) https://www.who.int/news-room/q-a-detail/tuberculosis-multidrug-resistant-tuberculosis-(mdr-tb)

WHO (2020) Global tuberculosis report 2020. Geneva: World Health Organization; 2020. Licence: CC BY-NC-SA 3.0 IGO. ISBN 978-92-4-001313-1 (electronic version)

WHO (2022a) Global tuberculosis report 2022. Geneva: World Health Organization; 2022. Licence: CC BY-NC-SA 3.0 IGO. (electronic version ISB N 978-92-4-006172-9)

WHO (2022b) Fact Sheet 27 October . Tuberculosis (who.int) COPIED IN WORKING FILE

WHO (2023) Leprosy 2023. https://www.who.int/news-room/fact-sheets/detail/leprosy

Wilkins MJ, Meyerson J, Bartlett PC, Spieldenner SL, Berry DE et al (2008) Human Mycobacterium bovis infection and bovine tuberculosis outbreak, Michigan, 1994-2007. Emerg Infect Dis 14(4):657–660

Wilson JW, Jagtiani AC, Wengenack NL (2019) Mycobacterium scrofulaceum disease: experience from a tertiary medical centre and review of the literature. Infect Dis (Lond) 51(8):602–609

Xavier EF, Seagar AL, Doig C, Rayner A, Claxton P, Laurenson I (2007) Human and animal infections with Mycobacterium microti, Scotland. Emerg Infect Dis 13(12):1924–1927. https://10.3201/eid1312.061536. PMID: 18258049; PMCID: PMC2876740.

Zachariah A, Pandiyan J, Madhavilatha GK, Mundayoor S, Chandramohan B, Sajesh PK et al (2017) Mycobacterium tuberculosis in wild Asian elephants, southern India. Emerg Infect Dis 23:504–506

Chapter 51
Plague

Plague is one of the oldest known diseases that caused devastating pandemics. The Plague pandemic of China and India spread all over the world and established new natural plague foci in Central, Eastern and Southern Africa, South America and the western part of North America and in large areas of Asia. Eradication seems impossible.

All continents except Oceania has the enzootic plague (*Y. pestis* in animal reservoir and a vector/natural foci). Risk of human plague exists wherever human population co-exists with these natural foci.

Geographical Distribution: It is endemic in 25 countries in tropics, subtropics and warmer areas of temperate regions between 55 degrees North and 40 degrees South, western USA, Central Asia, Kurdistan, Western Asia, Northern India and Uganda. The causative bacterium *Yersinia pestis* is enzootic in population of fleas carried by rodents in natural nidii from where it spills over occasionally to cause outbreaks.

Urban plague has been controlled. Ships one time blamed for spreading rats from one continent/country to other to cause outbreaks are better sanitized. Yet, potential for re-emergence of plague exists. According to WHO (2017), plague can be very severe with case-fatality rate of 30–60% for bubonic and always so in pneumonic if left untreated.

Plague outbreaks/cases have occurred on three main continents during 2000–2018: Asia, America and Africa. Africa reported the most (96.7%) of global cases during 2013–2018, 80.5% of them were located in Madagascar. Currently, plague is endemic in the Democratic Republic of the Congo, Madagascar and Peru (WHO 2022).

© Springer Nature Singapore Pte Ltd. 2024
K. G. Narayan et al., *Handbook of Management of Zoonoses*,
https://doi.org/10.1007/978-981-99-9885-2_51

51.1   Aetiology

There are 11 species in the genus *Yersinia*, family Yersiniaceae. Three are considered human pathogens, namely, *Y pestis*, *Y. pseudotuberculosis* and *Y. enterocolitica*. *Y. pestis* and *Y. pseudotuberculosis* are very close but genetically distinguishable by whole genome sequencing.

Y. pestis is a pleomorphic Gram-negative bacillus appearing as single bipolar cells (safety pin) or short chains in direct smears on staining with Giemsa, Wright's or Wayson stains. It grows at an optimal temperature of 28 °C as pin-point colonies in 24 h on sheep blood agar.

51.1.1   Y. pestis *Phylogeny*

Insights into *Y. pestis* phylogeny are emerging from ancient DNA (aDNA) paleo-genomic studies and *Y. pestis* DNA recovered from the teeth of prehistoric individuals (Demeure et al. 2019). Early divergence of *Y. pestis* occurred 5000–5700 years ago, and most basal lineages persist toady, for example, 0.PE4 (*microtus*) and the diverse lineages that led to all known plague pandemics. Whole genome-based phylogenies have defined a five-branch (0, 1–4) of *Y. pestis* biovars (1–5).

The *Biovars* are Antiqua (ANT), Medievalis (MED), Orientalis (ORI), Intermediate (IN) and Pestoides (PE) including Microtus isolates, as well as six novel Pestoides clusters.

The *branches* are 0, 1.2.3 and 4. There are lineages in each of the branches, for example, lineages: 0.ANT4 and 0.ANT5 caused Justinian plague and are extinct, branched between current 0.ANT1 and 0.ANT2 lineages.

Prehistoric plague pandemic: Evidence of the prevalence of virulent pathogen *Y. pestis* among Neolithic human remains support the existence of prehistoric plague pandemics. The exact birthplace of the successful *Y. pestis* lineage that led to the historically recorded pandemics remains unclear. Paleo-genomic studies also provided unambiguous evidence, the two recorded plague pandemics:

- The Justinian's Plague (6th–8th centuries) – lineages – Biovar Antiqa (ANT) – Branch 0, sub-branches – 0.ANT4 and 0.ANT5 (Africa, South-eastern Russia, Central Asia)
- The Black Death – Mediaevalis plague (14th–18th centuries) – lineages – Biovar Mediaevalis (MED) – Branches – 2.MED0,1,2,3 and 2ANT1,2,3 (Caspian Sea)
- The Third pandemic – Orientalis plague (1855=1959) – lineages – Biovar Orientalis (ORI), sub-branches ORI1, ORI2 and ORI3 (Asia, Western Hemisphere)

Kutyrev et al. (2018) had genotyped 359 modern *Y. pestis* strains from the natural foci in the former Soviet Union countries. They defined seven subspecies (ssp.) of *Y. pestis*. The ssp. *pestis* included the vast majority of virulent lineages associated with historically recorded pandemics (ANT, MED, ORI and possibly IN too). Six other clusters (new sub-species) included ssp. *Caucasica*, 0.PE2; ssp. *angolica*, 0.PE3; ssp. *central asiatica*, 0.PE4; spp. *Tibetica*, 0.PE7; ssp. *ulegeica*, 0.PE5; and *ssp. Qinghaica*, 0.PE10.

51.2   Pathogenesis

Y. pestis diverged from *Y. pseudotuberculosis* around 5700–6000 years ago and emerged as a pathogen with two virulence-associated plasmids *pFra/pMT1* (the gain of *Yersinia murine toxin, ymt)* and *pPla/pPCP1* and by the inactivation (promoter mutation) of the virulence-associated gene *pde3. Y. pestis* was equipped with ability to cause bubonic plague through flea-borne transmission 5000 years ago and fulminant lung infection through acquired I259T mutation in the plasminogen activator (Pla).

51.2.1   Virulence Factors

Virulence factors are encoded primarily on chromosome and three plasmids of *Y. pestis*: pPst, pMT1 (synonym pFra) and pPla. *pFra* codes for phospholipase D that enables transmission through fleas.

HPI Pathogenicity Island encodes for several proteins that help adhesion to and invasion of host's cells. Pla (plasminogen activator), Ail and F1 have been detected in outer membrane vesicles, which may contribute to pathogenesis by dispersion and delivery of virulence factors. *pPla* codes for protease Pla which is an outer membrane protein effecting virulence through its adhesive, invasive, fibrinolytic and coagulase properties. It activates plasminogen in human hosts that might degrade clots helping systemic infection and rapid replication in airways to cause primary pneumonia. F1 is antigenic, elicits humoral response and is antiphagocytic. The V and W antigens are produced at 37 °C and help escape from phagocytosis and survival in macrophages.

Antigens F1, V and W are not available in strains isolated from environment and fleas and are readily phagocytosed and killed by neutrophils but not by mononuclear cells. These antigens are developed by strains engulfed by mononuclear cells. As a result, bacteria released by mononuclear cells are able to evade phagocytosis and destruction by neutrophils.

Outer membrane protein A (Omp A) enhances intracellular survival. *Yersinia* outer proteins (Yops) have pleiotropic role *(Pleiotropy = disorders where multiple unrelated organ systems are affected)*. These induce cell death by multiple sophisticated mechanisms including inhibiting phagocytosis, platelet aggregation and preventing an effective inflammatory response. The type III secretion systems (T3SS) supplement leading to infection and pathogenesis.

All outer membrane protein contributes to cell attachment. T3SS enables *Y. pestis* to inject YOPs into macrophages and other immune cells. The *YOPs* cause pores in the host cell membrane and enter cytoplasm. These limit phagocytosis and innate immune system, prevent release of some cytokines and cause apoptosis of macrophages.

Sequestration of essential metals like iron and zinc is a mechanism to protect against plague.

Y. pestis carries *HPI Pathogenecity Island* which has genes to regulate uptake and storage of iron. *Y. pestis* secretes the siderophore yersinia bactin (Ybt) to acquire iron. Ybt is necessary for zinc uptake. Ybt, the ABC transporter ZnuABC and YbtX, Yfe and Feo metal transporters play a role in bubonic and pneumonic plague. Ybtx contributes to the development of pneumonic plague in mice. There are similar four other factors with undefined role (Demeure et al. 2019).

Y. pestis thus succeeds in invading and establishing infection.

51.2.2   Pathogenesis

Demeure et al. (2019) described pre-inflammatory phase *(transition from an absence of immune response and clinical symptoms)* when intervention is most likely to prevent progression of plague to severe and fatal form. Migration, multiplication and immune evasion happen during the pre-inflammatory phase. Intracellular replication continues evading phagosome, innate resistance and upregulating T3SS. The target organ, lymph nodes, is invaded by phagocytes (i.e. macrophages, dendritic cells or neutrophils) carrying the bacteria or by flowing lymph.

An intervention at the onset of disease to trigger a fast response of innate immunity, fostering neutrophils (the first line of defence) or macrophages, could possibly counteract and prevent the progress of illness. Early intervention is possible with early diagnosis. Inflammatory phase follows; if not checked by appropriate antibiotics, systemic dissemination and tissue destruction occur with consequential clinical signs.

Pestis minor: Despite opsonic antibodies against F1 and V antigens inducing phagocytosis by neutrophils, *Y. pestis* succeeds invading lymph nodes and proliferates to cause lymphadenopathy. Lymphadenitis and peri-glandular oedema develop. These are recognized as buboes. It is controllable.

Buboes: Flea bite injects *Y. pestis* into the skin. The optimal temperature of flea and human skin is almost similar, ~30 °C. *Y. pestis* is phagocytosed and eliminated effectively by neutrophiles but survives and replicates when phagocytosed by macrophages. A small papule, vesicle, papule and furuncle appear at the site of flea bite, noticed by <10% victims. *Y. pestis* move to the draining regional lymph gland through cutaneous lymphatics. Inflammation causes swollen painful buboes and surrounding oedema. Buboes contain proteinaceous exudate, bacteria, polymorphonuclear cells, lymphocytes and fewer macrophages. Unchecked it progresses into haemorrhagic necrosis.

Bacterium entering circulation invades other organs/system. Rapidly progressing multilobular pneumonia, consolidation and 'pneumonic plague' may develop into 'septicaemic form'.

Pneumonic plague characterized by marked intra-alveolar oedema and congestion could be primary or secondary.

Primary pneumonic plague is caused by direct inhalation of 100–500 *Y. pestis* droplets from infected human or cats, causing primary pneumonic plague. *Y. pestis* grown at 37 °C in infectious patient's lungs (than grown below 30 °C in fleas) have an upregulated T3SS. Neutrophils attracted to lungs during pre-inflammatory stage associated with clinical symptoms are responsible for the pneumonia and necrosis destroying the lungs. Haemorrhages in trachea, bronchi and pneumonic foci along medium and large bronchi and involvement of hilar lymph nodes are seen in primary pneumonia. Secondary pneumonic plague is a complication of Bubonic or Septicaemic plague caused by haematogenous spread. Lesions like central exudate with peripheral congestion are seen along the route/passage of infection.

Distinction between the two is difficult.

Septicaemic plague may be primary and secondary. Primary septicaemic plague is systemic toxicity. There is no apparent preceding lymph node involvement. Overwhelming sepsis causes death within days after onset of illness if suitable antibiotic is not administered within 24 h. Fatality is 100%. There is multiorgan involvement showing foci of necrosis and haemorrhage and fibrin thrombi in glomerular capillaries or purpuric skin lesions and shock. Secondary septicaemic plague occurs commonly with either bubonic or primary pneumonic plague.

51.3 Epidemiology

51.3.1 *Epizootic-Enzootic* Y. pestis

Human plague is an epiphenomenon of zoonotic plague, the incidence of which fluctuates in time and is modulated by numerous factors. Understanding enzootic is important.

The natural persistence of plague seems to follow two cycles. In the western North America, there is an alternate infrequent sylvatic plague epizootic and enzootic. *Y. pestis* maintains a continuous virulence. Epizootic is caused by efficient transmission. Rodent and flea population decimate. Enzootic phase follows. Threat to public health is low. Asian field studies suggest a long but benign relationship between *Y. pestis* and adapted rodent hosts. Reversion to efficient transmission results in epizootic. A five to six times increase in incidence was observed in Asia during Vietnam war, possibly because of disrupted local ecosystem and reduction in the distance to humans. Most exposure occurs in the peri-domestic environment. Infected rodent fleas can be brought in home by free roaming pets.

High population density, poverty, poor living conditions, namely, filth, household waste around, poor civic services and slums all contribute to favour rodents and increase their density. These were consistently observed through two pandemics, the second and third, and also the Surat plague of 1994 in India. For example, Stuart London was never free from plague but was worst affected in 1665 [most preferred site for plague: *The Plague of 1665 (http://historylearning-site.co.uk/plague_of_1665.htm)*. Bubonic Plague epidemic was declared in the city in September 1896. By the first few weeks of 1897,s mortality rate was 75–85%. Half of the population fled by January 1897 to the countryside. More than 70% of the immigrant workers lived in chawls (density 700/acre in some wards), primitive habits and poor sanitation (https://en.wikipedia.org/wiki/Bombay_plague_epidemic).

51.3.2 Rodent-Flea Cycle (Fig. 51.1)

The plague bacteria, *Y. pestis*, affect wild rodents primarily and are spirally transmitted by fleas (vectors). Rodents are reservoirs. The population of rodents presents a variable resistance and hence some act as carriers. *Y. pestis* is maintained in nature in a rat-flea spiral cycle.

Y. pestis is maintained by enzootic flea-wild rodent cycle (including rock to squirrels, ground squirrels, prairie dogs) in plague biotope. Humans and domestic animals that are bitten by fleas from dead animals are at risk for naturally contracting plague, especially during an epizootic. Cats usually become very ill from plague can directly infect humans when they cough infectious droplets into the air. Dogs are less likely to be ill, but they can still bring plague-infected fleas into the home (Fig. 51.2). In addition to flea bites, people and wood rats can be exposed while handling skins or flesh of infected animals.

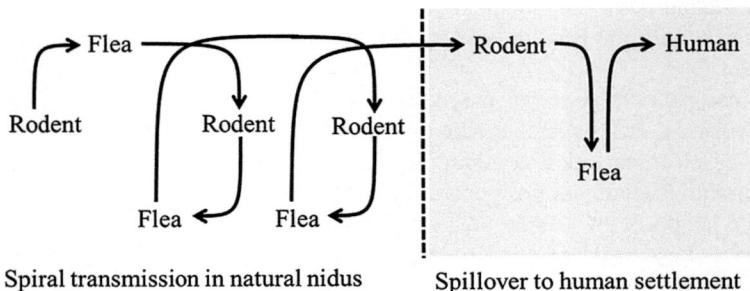

Spiral transmission in natural nidus   Spillover to human settlement

Fig. 51.1 Spiral transmission of *Y. pestis*

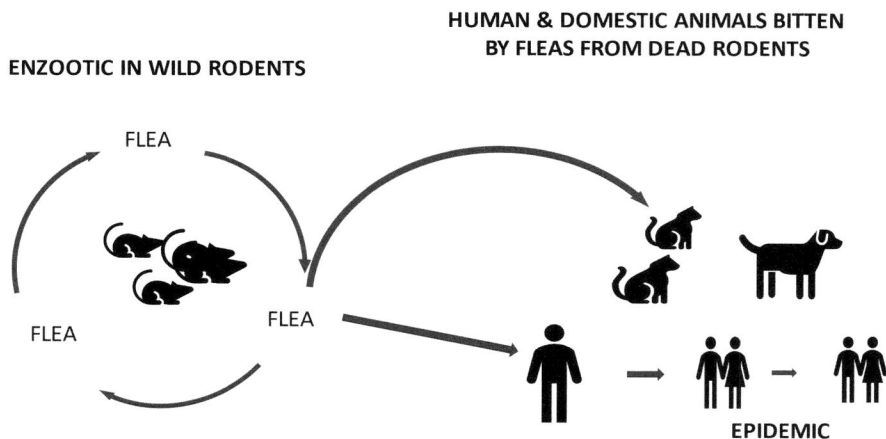

Fig. 51.2 Transmission of *Yersinia pestis*

51.3.3 Process of Infection

The population of susceptible rats increases following breeding. *Y. pestis* infects rats through flea bites. Those developing acute bacteraemia die, and the feeding flea leaves dead rat and attaches another live rat.

According to Hinnebusch (2005), mechanical transmission by flea (flea is not infected) requires that level of septicaemia is high and *Y. pestis* survived on the blood-tainted mouth parts of the flea between two consecutive feedings. Commonly *Y. pestis* is conveyed to the bite site by regurgitation when blocked fleas attempted to feed. Complete blockage is not necessary for pumping out (which is not a continuous process) *Y. pestis* by the infected flea. Partial blockage of the proventriculus actually made the flea better transmitters through an open channel.

In the proventriculus of flea, *Y. pestis* elaborates a coagulase that clots ingested blood to form a cohesive biofilm between the oesophagus and midgut blocking the incoming flow of blood; stage is 'occluded flea'. The optimum growth temperature of *Y. pestis* is 28 °C. *Y. pestis* multiplies in the fibrin matrix of coagulated blood. When the occluded flea feeds upon a host, blood regurgitates and returns to the body of the rat washing with it huge number (25,000–100,000) of plague bacilli. The hungry flea attempts feeding repeatedly and the plague bacilli are injected/introduced in the rats/human repeatedly. It takes 1–2 weeks or longer for a feeding flea to become infective (extrinsic incubation period), and flea can harbour the plague bacilli for 47 days. Infective flea (occluded flea) can become non-infective when the fibrin matrix of the coagulated blood occluding proventriculus dissolves by fibrinolytic factor and trypsin-like enzymes secreted by *Y. pestis* at 22 °C. Phagocytes and antibody in rats' blood help in this process.

F1 capsule, pla and the type III secretion system are known mammalian virulence factors. These are not required for infection of flea, *X. cheopis*. Ymt and Hms (product of genes *ymt* and *hms*) are flea-specific phenotype transmission factors, not required for virulence in mammals. The genes controlling virulence and transmission factors are different.

Mechanism of maintenance of the bacterium in the flea digestive tract involves several proteins. Phospholipase D (PLD) allows the bacilli to survive in the flea midgut. The hemin storage systems (Hms) and the Yersinia murine toxin (Ymt) are used for formation of biofilm in the proventriculus resulting into occluded flea and transmission of blood back to mammalian host (Hinnebusch et al. 1996, 2002).

Y. pestis transmitted by occluded fleas caused higher percentage of terminal disease in experimental mice. Early phase or mass transmission (three days of infectious meal on a host with high-level (10^8–10^9 CFU/ml) bacteraemia) led to survival and immune response. Transmission was non-productive in the sense bacteraemia did not develop (Bosio et al. 2020). In the early phase or mass transmission, infected fleas take one to few days to be able to transmit *Y. pestis* in their next blood meal on a naïve host. Simultaneous feeding by 5–10 infected fleas on a naive host results in transmission.

Plague is spread by migration and population reshuffle in rodents. Rodents in synanthropic domestic biotope are generally not infected. Ecological linkage with wild rodent biotope is likely to introduce zoonotic plague (*Y. pestis*) to synanthropic biotope. In the rat-flea-rat cycle, flea bites man in absence of a rat. Human-human transmission (demic plague) occurs in pneumonic plague and plague spreads like a wildfire.

The infective dose is small, 1–10 organisms to cause infection via the subcutaneous, intradermal, oral or intravenous routes.

51.3.4 Natural Nidus

Fleas and a large number of mammals maintain *Y. pestis* in nature.

Nearly 80 species of fleas and 200 species of wild rodents have been found to be infected or susceptible to experimental infection. The ability to transmit *Y. pestis* varied in different species (Hinnebusch 2005).

Vector fleas are *Xenopsylla cheopis*, oriental rat; *X. brasiliensis*, *X. astia* and *X. gerbilliminax*, gerbil; and *Pulex irritans*, uncommon human flea and *Ctenocephalides*.

Hosts: About 230 species serve as definitive hosts.

Rodents: Prairie dogs (*Cynomys* spp.), particularly the black-tailed prairie dog (*C. ludovicianus*), great gerbils (*Rhombomys opimus*), Mongolian gerbils (*Meriones unguiculatus*), ground squirrels (*Spermophilus* spp.), rats (*Neotoma* spp., *Rattus* spp.), mice (*Peromyscus* spp.) and chipmunks (*Tamias* spp.).

Wild and domestic felids: bobcats (*Lynx rufus*), mountain lions (*Puma concolor*), domestic cats (*Feliscatus domesticus*), wild and domestic canids, coyotes (*Canis latrans*), black-footed ferrets (*Mustela nigripes*), American badgers (*Taxidea taxus*), cervids, mule deer (*Odocoileus hemionus*), pronghorn antelope (*Antilocapra americana*), wild and domestic lagomorphs, domestic dogs (*Canis familiaris*), goats, camels, sheep, non-human primates and humans (*Homo sapiens*).

In India, the common rodents are *Tatera indica*, *Bandicota bengalensis*, *Mas. platythrix*, *Rattus* and *R. norvegicus*. Madon et al. (1997) identified *Y. pestis* in 28 species of wild or domestic mammals—wild rodents, predators/carnivores, fleas and bubonic, septicaemic and fatal human cases in the USA. Prairie dogs (*Cynomus luduvicianus*) are the commonest hosts. Other rodents susceptible to epizootic plague are wood rats (*Neotoma*) and some ground squirrels (*Spermophilus*). Voles, many mice, other ground squirrel species and rabbits are moderately susceptible while kangaroo rats (*Dipodomys*), certain mice populations and selected carnivores are resistant.

51.3.5 Pet-Associated Plague

Epizootics and increased deaths among susceptible animal hosts (viz. rodents) precede outbreaks in human. Cat-associated human plague cases (23 with 5 deaths) occurred in 8 Western states of America between 1977 and 1998 through bites, scratches and other contacts with infectious material while handling infected cats (Gage et al. 2000).

Exposure to dogs was found to be a significant risk factor for plague among infected patients in New Mexico. The odds ratios were 18.5 for contact and 5.7 for sleeping in same bed (Gould et al. 2008). *Pulex irritans*, the human flea, was the predominant flea species (72.4%) in houses of villages with high plague frequency and may be an indicator of plague potential in rural areas and may play a role in plague epidemiology in Tanzania (Laudisoit et al. 2007). Cats can be useful sentinel animals.

51.3.6 Plague Ecology and Disease in Animals

Livestock do not develop clinical signs. There may be reduced thriftiness (reduced milk and meat production) and sudden death. The incubation period is 2–6 days.

Infected rodents and wildlife may present fever, anorexia and enlarged lymph nodes and sometimes abscess and draining. Ulcers on the tongue and in the mouth may be seen. Acutely infected are found dead. Post-mortem examination reveals evidence of vascular oedema, mucohaemorrhagic diarrhoea, ulcerative gastroenterocolitis, mesenteric lymphadenopathy and necrotic lesions in the liver and spleen.

Y. pestis is a telluric bacterium. Soil could be a reservoir harbouring it in a free state, an L-form, or inside amoeba (Fig. 51.3). A bacterium with such a vast source—soil, mammals and ectoparasites, maintaining its virulence—is always a potential threat.

In a plague biotope, there may be assemblage of rodents of varying susceptibility. The grasshopper mouse (*Onychomys leucogaster*) is an alternate resistant host

Approximate Ecology of *Y. pestis* in a multi-host system

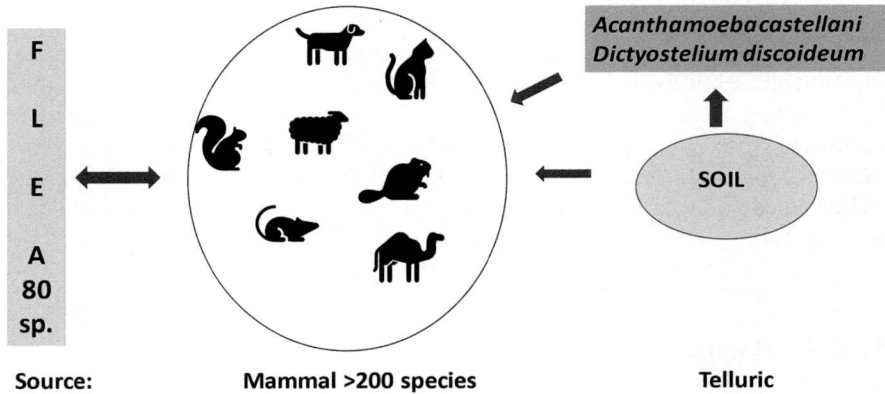

Fig. 51.3 Ecology of *Y. pestis* in a multi-host system

INTER - EPIZOOTIC PERSISTENCE

Y. pestis nearly ends with plague-decimated prairie dogs; **persists** by tissue sequestration in plague resistant grasshopper mouse

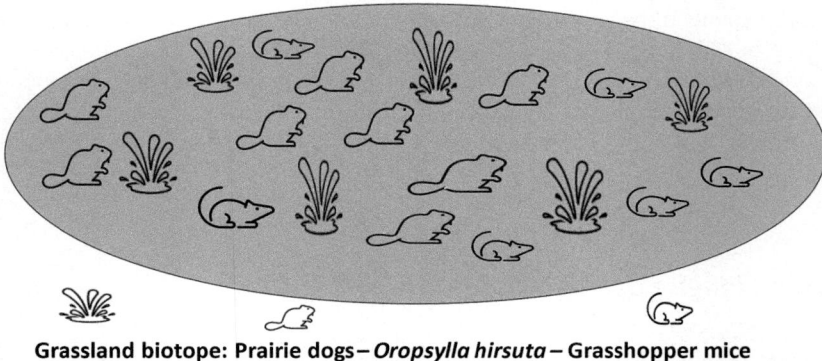

Grassland biotope: Prairie dogs – *Oropsylla hirsuta* – Grasshopper mice

Fig. 51.4 Inter-epizootic persistence of *Y. pestis*

(Fig. 51.4). Salkeld et al. (2010) explained it by percolation thresholds of alternate host (grasshopper mouse) abundance.

In sylvatic plague biotope, rodents with benign relationship with *Y. pestis* (because of resistance arising from selection pressure from epizootic) explain persistence (Fig. 51.5). According to Barbieri et al. (2021), the inter-epizootic persistence is a multi-factorial phenomenon. *Y. pestis* may be transported by flea/rodents/transporter species carrying infected fleas like coyotes (*Canis latrans*) and swift fox (*Vulpes velox*) or ungulates or by sequential host ferrying.

EPIZOOTIC – ENZOOTIC - EPIZOOTIC

Y. pestis maintains virulence

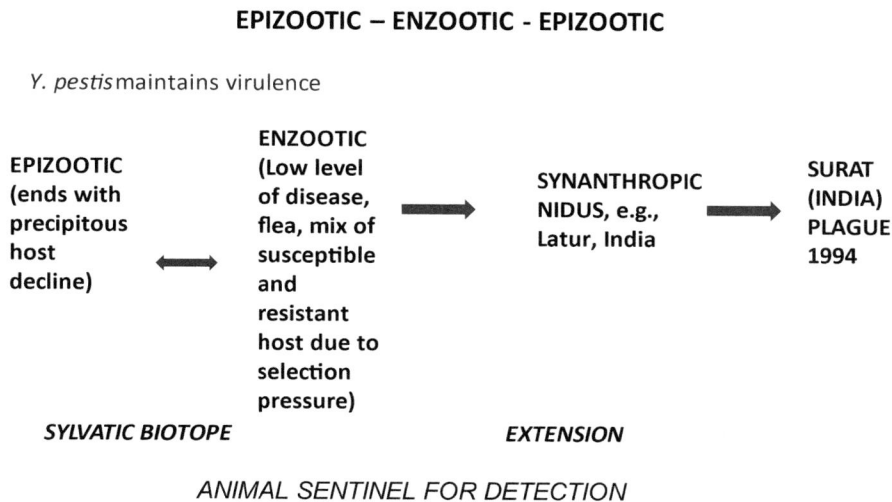

Fig. 51.5 Persistence of *Y. pestis*

51.3.7 *Prairie Dogs*

Plague is an important cause of morbidity and mortality in prairie dogs. Prairie dogs (*Cynomys ludovicianus)* are highly susceptible to plague; the CFR is 90%. They lack natural immunity. The endangered black-footed ferret and many others depended upon prairie dogs for food. Therefore, plague management has become a significant focus in wildlife conservation strategies.

Plague is non-native but enzootic to the western USA. Persistence of plague requires a stable biotope. Distribution of sylvatic plague is profoundly influenced by wild rodents and gradually shifted eastward into the mid-western USA, ~102° west longitude. Explanation for persistence of plague in the USA, in absence of clear evidence of carrier rodents, probably lies in the fleas playing a potential role and therefore needed detail study (Wimsatt and Biggins 2009). Plague persists in the American grasslands in quiescent outbreak pattern and erupts as sporadic epizootics in prairie dogs (*Cynomys ludovicianus*) decimating colonies. Daniel et al. (2010) observed that plague can persist in prairie-dog colonies for prolonged periods, because host movement is highly spatially constrained. Plague bacilli persists in a multi-host system. In the American grasslands, the grasshopper mouse (*Onychomys leucogaster*) is another (alternate) host of *Y. pestis*. The study revealed a clear threshold phenomenon between abundance of grasshopper mouse and outbreak among prairie dogs; a few percent increase in mouse density resulted into dramatic increase of the total number of infected prairies dogs. Abundance thresholds of alternate hosts permit percolation of the disease throughout the primary host population.

Flea burden and burrow density are significant contributors to the rate of disease spread.

In the Democratic Republic of Congo, two major outbreaks occurred in the equatorial forest of the tropical regions in the Ituri highlands. Small and stable endemic focus of plague persisted in this tropical region with ≥ 1 zoonotic host circulating *Y. pestis*. The clusters of sporadic bubonic cases round the year and outbreaks of pneumonic plague with CFR 36% to 52% in five health zones of Ituri occurred as a result (Abedi et al. 2018). Plague transmission in rats in urban areas was favoured by low temperature and humidity and in wild rodents in semi-arid regions of Madagascar by the end of the dry season. During the dry season, fewer fleas were observed on rodents in Uganda. Plague in rodents was linked to agricultural practices in Tanzania. The risk for plague tends to increase in highlands covered by savannas or meadows with a relatively dry climate.

51.4   Transmission to Human

Plague bacilli spill over from the wild biotope to domestic biotope through population reshuffle and migrating rats. A synanthropic domestic rat biotope is generally free from *Y. pestis*. However, if direct linkage is established between infected wild rat biotope with synanthropic domestic rat biotope, an infected synanthropic nidus is created. Human beings can be infected by both—infected flea and rat. Every infected animal can transmit infection to human through contact with skin tissue.

Multiple ways of transmission are possible. These are the following:

- Air-borne and droplets (sneezing, coughing)
- Direct contact with infected person including sex, carcass of rodents (marmots), rabbit, hare, coyotes (wild cats) and goats
- Indirect contact (contaminated soil, surface, nosocomial)
- Ingestion of contaminated meat (camel meat and the liver, Leslie et al. 2011)
- The most important vector (flea) bite

Risk of infection among those in contact of plague patients varies with intensity of exposure and environmental factors. Droplet can spread infection at distance of 3.7 feet. Pneumonic plague spreads like wildfire through sneezing, coughing and direct contact with infected tissue.

51.5   Symptoms

A common nursery rhyme composed during Black Death describes best the symptoms.

Ring a ring of roses—Red circular blotches on the skin developing into large pus-filled sacs, primarily under the armpits and in the groin—called *buboes* that are very painful.

A pocket full of posies—refers to the belief that the plague was spread by a cloud of poisonous gas that was colourless (known as a miasma). This miasma could be stopped, if only you carried flowers with you. The smell of the flowers would overpower the germs carried by the miasma. Also, sweet smelling flowers would cover up the unpleasantness when a victim's breath started to go off as the disease got worse.

Attischo, Attischo, We, all fall down—the final symptom was a sneezing fit that was promptly followed by death.

The incubation period varies between one and seven days. Plague begins with non-specific systemic symptoms such as sudden onset of fever, chills, head and body aches, weakness, vomiting and nausea.

There are two main forms of plague, depending upon route of infection.

51.5.1 Bubonic Plague

Bubonic plague is the most common form of plague and is caused by the bite of an infected flea. Buboes are enlarged, tense, smooth, painful lymph nodes that swell in the groin or armpit or neck, draining the site of flea bite/scratch and resulting from replication of plague bacillus, *Y. pestis*. The inflamed lymph nodes can turn into open sores filled with pus.

Symptoms of bubonic plague may appear suddenly or 2–5 days after exposure. These are fever 38–41 °C (101–105 °F), malaise, headache, aching joints, nausea and vomiting; untreated cases die, with CFR (case fatality rate) of 80% in 8 days, averaging 30–75%.

Human-to-human transmission of bubonic plague is rare. Bubonic plague can advance and spread to the lungs, which is the more severe type of plague called pneumonic plague.

51.5.2 Pneumonic Plague

Pneumonic plague occurs as a progression of bubonic plague or via inhalation of *Y. pestis* in droplet from a patient of pneumonic plague (human-to-human transmission). Incubation can be as short as 24 h. If not diagnosed and treated early, it can be fatal (CFR 90–95%). Symptoms include fever, chest pain, cough and frothy sputum. Sputum is blood tinged and may become free-flowing bright red as the disease progresses. However, recovery rates are high if detected and treated in time (within 24 h of onset of symptoms).

51.5.3   Septicaemic

Septicaemic plague is manifested as high fever, nausea, vomiting, abdominal pain, diarrhoea and purple patches on the skin/purpura (subepidermal haemorrhages) due to intravascular coagulation of blood—and the extremities would darken with a form of gangrene, CFR 100%, but this form is least common.

The course of pneumonic and septicaemic forms is rapid.

51.5.4   Other Symptoms

Meningitis (meningismus, altered mental status) may occur as a complication; *Pharyngitis* is a result of inhalation/ingestion of *Y. pestis*; *Pestis minor*—Patients usually have a febrile illness with localized lymphadenopathy. The nodes drain and patients recover without therapy. *Gastroenteritis* after ingestion/handling of camel meat (odds ratio 4.4) manifested as vomiting, diarrhoea, pharyngitis and lymphadenitis fatality (17/83 or 20.5%) reported by Leslie et al. (2011) on the basis of PCR and sero-conversion in one patient.

51.5.5   Potential Biological War

Properties of *Y. pestis* that make it a potential bioweapon are ready availability, production in large quantity, aerosol delivery, human-to-human transmission, high fatality rate and possible genetic manipulation to enhance virulence or induce drug resistance.

Features that suggest bioweapon attack: illness of many cases of acute multilobar pneumonia with haemoptysis and fulminant clinical course over several days (IP 2–4 days) in urban area, with no history of plague exposure and absence of buboes.

51.6   Diagnosis

Y. pestis is classified under WHO risk group 4.

Objective should be to diagnose a plague-suspected patient before the onset of severe symptoms to start treatment without any delay.

- Symptoms and signs
- Detection of *Y. pestis* (bipolar/safety pin-shaped bacteria) by Gram's stain in sample of pus from a bubo, lymph node aspirate, blood and sputum
- Culture of the above specimen on blood agar at 28 °C
- Antigen detection—techniques

One of them is a laboratory-validated rapid dipstick (diagnostic) test (F1RDT) now widely used in Africa and South America, with the support of WHO. It is based on detection of F1 antigen of *Y. pestis*. It is a practical method that can be implemented by trained staff at local points of care, can provide results within 15 min and has been validated for diagnosis of bubonic plague.

- Antibody Detection

  Anti-F1 serology—paired sera samples (onset and convalescence), fourfold rise in antibody titre detected by HA, passive HA, CFT, counter-immune-electrophoresis, ELISA, dot ELISA and FAT

- Genome sequencing—PCR and real-time PCR. It takes 2–4 h for the result to be available. Same ribotype *Y. pestis* isolates were detected in specimens from fleas, domestic and sylvatic rodents and human patients in case of the Surat plague.

In the case of field studies, specimens from fleas and rodents are tested.

WHO (2021) revised the guidelines for defining a case of plague for initiating immediate response at the level of public health and point of care.

Use of F1RDT (alert tool) to detect bubonic plague in plague-endemic areas: Use F1RDT in people with suspected bubonic plague to rapidly detect plague and implement an immediate public health response. In the meantime, use a confirmatory test (such as culture or molecular testing) before declaring a confirmed plague outbreak. Use F1RDT in people *at the point of care*: it helps both the clinician and the patient with early diagnosis.

Laboratory-validated conventional PCR and RT-PCR: the latter is rapid, performed on clinical specimens and culture. A combination of at least two different targets (Table 51.1 for options) is necessary, and two of these must be positive to satisfy the conditions for laboratory confirmation. It is recommended that the following genes be targeted:

Table 51.1 *Y. pestis* genes targeted by PCR (Bertherat and Jullien 2021)

Gene	Gene location	Gene product
caf1	pFra/pMT1 plasmid	F1 antigen of the pseudocapsule
Pla	pPla/pPCP1 plasmid	Tissue plasminogen activator
ypo2088	Chromosome	Methyltransferase
ypo2486	Chromosome	Hypothetical protein
inv (pseudogene with insertion of IS200-type element)	Chromosome	Invasin of *Y. pseudotuberculosis*

NB: This new case definition can be considered as the reference standard for notification under the International Health Regulations and should be used to the extent possible in epidemiological surveillance and field investigations. But like all case definitions, it can be adapted to the epidemiological situation, local conditions and the resources available

51.7   Treatment and Chemoprophylaxis

When rapidly diagnosed and promptly treated, plague may be successfully managed reducing mortality from 60% to less than 15%. The antibiotics used for the treatment of the cases are doxycycline, ciprofloxacin and cotrimoxazole. For the pulmonary or septicaemic form case, gentamycin is administrated.

WHO (2021) guidelines for adding fluoroquinolones (ciprofloxacin, levofloxacin and moxifloxacin) to the first-line medicines recommended for treating bubonic, pneumonic or septicaemic plague.

Pre-exposure prophylaxis: the 2009 recommendations to continue, namely, tetracycline, doxycycline, sulfamethoxazole + trimethoprim and ciprofloxacin lasting until seven days after the end of the exposure.

51.8   Plague Pandemics and Outbreaks

51.8.1   Past Plague Pandemics

Three major pandemics were the following:

  (i) The Justinian pandemic
 (ii) The Black Death
(iii) The Plague pandemic of China and India (1855–1959).

 (i) The Justinian pandemic (572–767 AD, the sixth and seventh centuries) wiped
      out an estimated 40% of the population of Constantinople and 50% of Europe.

Quantum of information related to the pandemics gradually increased with developments in the areas of public health, reporting, recording and communication. Least information about prehistoric and Justinian plague is available. Justinian plague pandemic began in 541–544 and continued for 200 years. It affected the Eastern Roman Empire, the Sasanian Empire and port cities around the Mediterranean Sea. Studies on *Y. pestis* DNA recovered from the prehistoric individual's teeth offer evidence of epidemic, its location, etc. Justinian plague reportedly started in the region of the eastern Mediterranean basin. Keller et al. (2019) studied microevolution of the bacterium with eight reconstructed genomes of *Y. pestis* DNA from human remains from 21 sites of Austria, Britain, Germany, France and Spain from the period of Justinian Plague. The study provides evidence that these countries including the British Isles were visited by the pandemic, and the genome diversification in *Y. pestis* occurred during the epidemic period 541–750.

 (ii) The Black Death (in the fourteenth century) caused death of 50 million
       Europeans between 1347 and 1351 only.

Description of the Black Death is available and supplemented further with current studies on ancient DNA of *Y. pestis* recovered from human remains. The

Black Death of fourteenth century (syn. Great plague, Great pestilence) occurred in the 1330s in China and caused deaths estimated at 25 million Chinese in 15 years. It entered Constantinople in 1347 [The Black Death: Bubonic Plague (http://www.themiddleages.net/plague.html). Black sea-China ship trade link brought several dead and ill to Sicily in October 1347. Black rats infested with Oriental fleas were common passengers on the ships. Plague spread rapidly. The disease seemed to disappear in winter but only because fleas were dormant then. Plague visited each spring, killing new victims. After five years, 25 million people were dead, one-third of Europe's people. Plague was established and caused major outbreaks in Italy, London and Vienna in 1629, 1665 and 1679, respectively (Konstantinidou et al. 2009). Haensch et al. (2010) confirmed that *Y. pestis* caused the Black Death and later epidemics on the entire continent of Europe over four centuries on the basis of DNA—specific to *Y. pestis* extracted from human skeletons from the medieval mass graves. Several others (Bos et al. 2011; Schuenemann et al. 2011) also studied ancient genome from victims of Black Death buried in East Smithfield Mass Burial site (1348–1350) and confirmed this.

Plague persisted in Europe until the eighteenth century. Was it due to repeated introduction from Asia through several waves and trade routes for persistence? It is not settled. In the first case, genetically diverse *Y. pestis* should be detected in different plague victims. Persistence in an unknown reservoir or host of identical or similar *Y. pestis* from different periods of time needs to be proven. *Y. pestis* genome from rat skeletal remains found in a Polish ossuary suggested possible source of plague distribution in medieval Europe. Study of genomes of *Y. pestis* from victims of plague from varying points of times during almost five centuries (fourteenth–eighteenth) suggested genetic continuity in Western and Central Europe (Morozova et al. 2020).

(iii) The Plague pandemic of China and India (1855–1959) devastated population in China and India.

Central/Eastern Asia is the suggested plague foci for the Black Death. It was introduced to Western Europe, spread via commercial trade route and human migration and persisted in natural rodent-based foci until the eighteenth century. This became the source for contemporary pandemics in Central and East Asia.

The natural nidus of plague existed in Central Asia and caused death among migrants and also the established population in the region. In the Yunnan province of China, the third pandemic of plague originated from nidus that continues as risk. ORI arose in 1855 and was caused by the biovar Orientalis strains, of the 1.ORI branch. In a span of 1855–1959, it spread worldwide, Asia, Africa and America through the steamships that carried infected rats also. In India only, ten million died. Epidemic was characterized as a single event of introduction, rapid expansion and settling down in local rodent population as reservoirs in rodent-flea-rodent cycle of transmission, which seems essential for establishment in a newly colonized country.

51.8.2   Current Epidemics/Outbreaks

51.8.2.1   Plague in India

(a) *The Surat (India) Plague 1994*

A review by Dutta et al. (2006) reported that pneumonic plague patients over-crowded hospitals in Surat (Gujarat, India) on September 23, 1994. The suspected cases swelled to 1061 by the September 25. One-fourth (0.7 million) fled the city. Laboratory confirmation came on September 25. The isolates were genetically more heterogenous compared to others in the world. The episode lasted for a little over two weeks. It created unprecedented panic that had international implications. Reportedly, there were 5150 suspected cases of pneumonic and bubonic plague and 53 deaths (92.5% from Surat) during August 26–October 5. The plague spread from the City of Surat to the surrounding 40 km areas during first phase following the process of 'expansion diffusion (infection often intensifies in the originating region diffuses to contiguous areas following rules of distance decay at each step while new areas are added'. The process of 'relocation diffusion' followed. The infected but in incubation phase spread plague to Delhi, Mumbai, Kolkata and Nasik in Maharashtra (Nasik is located between Surat and Mumbai). The 'hierarchic diffusion' led to spread from Delhi to (i) Faridabad, Bhiwani and Amritsar and (ii) to Ambala, Ludhiana and Amritsar.

During the period August 26 through October 1994, there were a total of 693 suspected or pneumonic plague-positive cases and 56 deaths. No deaths occurred after October 11. As on October 19, no imported plague was detected in persons in other countries; WHO considered the outbreak was 'under control' (https://www.cdc.gov/mmwr/preview/mmwrhtml/00032992.htm).

Epidemiological investigation in Mamla, District Beed, Maharashtra, linked this epidemic with the 1993 earthquake in Latur. The rodent and flea population grew exponentially; the intensity of flea infestation was 1.8 between October 1993 and July 1994 (Saxena and Verghese 1996). Mamla village had the first warning, 'rat fall' in the middle of August 1994. By the middle of September, 10% of the village population had bubonic plague.

Diamond cutting and silk industry in Surat attract many people for jobs from villages. Most of them lived on the outskirts of city in slum and most unhygienic condition. Flood in early August made the conditions still worst but favourable for rats. It is highly probable that some infected villagers from Maharashtra travelled to Surat. They could not afford treatment and bubonic plague progressed systemically into pneumonic, and subsequently person-to-person spread occurred rapidly.

The survivors of earthquake in September 1993 had converted/used the old, damaged homes into granaries. The rat population had boomed uninhibited/uninterrupted in the abandoned damaged houses. A nidus of *Y. pestis* had emerged.

The Orientalis strains of *Y. pestis* isolated from patients and rodents from the 1994 plague outbreaks had similar MLVA, ERIC-PCR and ERIC-BOX-PCR profiles. These were closely related with Orientalis strains recovered from the rodents trapped on the Deccan plateau suggesting these were resident of the endemic region (Kingston et al. 2009).

Possibly it was beyond imagination that, despite an admirable relief and rehabilitation operation during and after earthquake, this site would become a natural nidus of *Y. pestis*, and epidemic would be caused after a year.

This might explain the 'unpreparedness' by the public health authorities.

Lessons learnt are the following:

- Environmental health in the earthquake-affected areas—disposal of dead bodies is not enough. The demolished houses and debris also need to be sanitized.
- The disaster management does not end with relief and rehabilitation operation.
- The disaster management need more holistic planning and inclusive

(b) *The Outbreak 2002, India*

A small outbreak of primary pneumonic plague occurred in the Shimla District, India, during February 2002. There were 16 cases, 4 died (CFR 25%). It was confirmed by PCR and gene sequencing. An unconfirmed previous outbreak suggestive of pneumonic plague in this region occurred in 1983. There were 22 cases and 17 deaths.

On January 28, 2022, the index case of the 2002 outbreak went for hunting. He hunted a wild cat, skinned and returned home on February 2. He reported headache, chill and fever and sought treatment. On February 4, he developed breathlessness, chest pain and haemoptysis. X-ray suggested that lobar pneumonia was put on augmentin, but he died on February 5. Thirteen of his relatives reported similar symptoms and two acquired infection in hospital within 4–5 days, consistent with the incubation period of 1–4 days for plague. This indicates that cats may transmit infection through bites, scratches and contact with their infected tissues. This might have happened with the index case. Primary pneumonic plague is acquired by inhalation of infective droplets from persons, animals and rarely accidental aerosol exposure. Face-to-face exposure within 2 m of a coughing patient (not necessarily airborne) may result in transmission. Secondary cases might have resulted like this. Wife and sister of the index case also died. Investigation did not find evidence of contact with rats and flea.

Mediaevalis and Antiqua biovars were recovered from the environmental reservoir on the Deccan Plateau and from the pneumonic patients of 2002 plague outbreak (Kingston et al. 2009).

51.8.2.2 The Outbreaks in Algeria

According to Bitam et al. (2010), plague foci have been known for decades in Algiers, Aumale, Kahelia, Philippeville and Oran, where in 2003 plague re-emerged after its absence for >50 years. In the 2003 outbreak, 9/95 *Xenopsylla cheopis* fleas were found infected with *Y. pestis* biovar Orientalis (Bitam et al. 2006). In the Laghouat region, it emerged. Patients got infected by bites of fleas. *Y. pestis* was detected in a native rodent species *M. shawii* jirds, living in close contact with human. It is a plague-resistant species and thus is an efficient *Y. pestis* reservoir, a new rural zoonotic focus of plague. An Orientalis biotype sharing the same Yp8 and Yp9 spacer sequences was found in Oran and Laghouat. The emergence is unexplained.

Y. pestis biotype Orientalis has been found to survive for 40 weeks in soil (Ayyadurai et al. 2008).

51.8.2.3   Outbreaks in Uganda

In West Nile region of Uganda, a total of 1092 plague suspect cases were recorded during January 2004—December 2012, maximum of 321 in 2007. Majority (84%) were bubonic plague. Overall mortality was 34%. Most culture-confirmed plague cases (88%) occurred during the months of October through December. Most patients (61%) were female and median age was 13 years. All 61 isolates belonged to 1.ANT lineage which evolved 628–6914 years ago and earlier known to be prevalent in East and Central Africa (Respicio-Kingry et al. 2016).

51.8.2.4   Outbreaks in Madagascar

Plague appeared in 1898 in Madagascar. It is endemic particularly in rural areas of middle-west (including Ambohidratrimo, Miarinarivo and Tsiroanomandidy) and the central highland regions situated at an altitude of 800 m. The first three districts have long been considered plague hotspots. Strong agricultural practices engaged individuals under 19 years old and more males.

Plague is dependent on environmental and climatic factors bringing infected rats and their fleas into contact with humans. The global climate change such as the El Niño Southern Oscillation and Indian Ocean Dipole possibly influenced. The cases increased in the three hotspot districts in the middle-west in the Central Madagascar. Difference in climate, vegetation, surface area and density of population, spatial control campaigns and diagnosis and patient management influenced the difference in the number of cases reported in different regions. For example, higher proportion of pneumonic cases in the Ambositra District than in the Tsiroanomandidy District was probably due to delayed diagnosis and patient management.

The Plague National Control Program was established in 1993 and includes human surveillance. Andrianaivoarimanana et al. (2019) presented the trends during 1998–2016. A total of 13,234 suspected cases were recorded, mainly from central highlands. Of these, 27% were confirmed and 17% presumptive. The proportion of bubonic plague and of pneumonic was 93% and 7% of the total of presumptive and confirmed cases. The median age of patients of bubonic plague was 13 years and of pneumonic 29 years. Fatality rate was 18% for confirmed plus presumptive case patients. It was higher for the pneumonic plague (25%) than for the bubonic plague (15%). Factors/risk (odds ratio) associated with deaths identified were delayed consultation, pneumonic plague and contact with another plague case, not reporting dead rats. For example, delayed consultation had OR 3.2 at days 2–5.0 at day 4.

The distribution of cases showed peaks, in September and November with progressive decrease until April and then few cases until August. This pattern is associated with temperature effects on flea abundance. Annual cases peaked during 2003 and 2004 and decreased to the lowest incidence in 2016.

Aborode et al. (2021) reported plague epidemic amid COVID-19. The problem was of misdiagnosis because of overlapping respiratory symptoms. From January 1 to March 11, there were 37 suspect and 21 confirmed cases and 9 deaths in Ambositra and Mandarina.

Rakotosamimanana et al. (2021) studied the dynamics of plague in the two districts, Ambositra and Tsiroanomandidy, of the central highland region using data of 2006–2015. Clinical forms were significantly different. Plague occurred every year in Tsiroanomandidy. Cases were absent in a year in Ambositra when they were reported in Tsiroanomandidy. These suggested that several factors other than biogeographical were operating.

51.8.2.5 Outbreaks in the Democratic Republic of Congo

According to Abedi et al. (2018), >95% of 15,396 cases reported globally during 2004–2014 occurred in Africa, 54% in the Democratic Republic of Congo (DRC), 36% in Madagascar, 3% in Uganda and 1% in Tanzania. The first cases reported in 1928 were in Ituri (Orientale Province) and DRC near Lake Alberta. Plague is persistent here. Ten years later in 1938, another focus of plague near Lake Edward (presently North Kivu) appeared but is silent since 1967. Control programmes brought the incidence low. Progressive collapse of control programme resulted in reappearance and rise of cases with peaks during 2000–2006 in Ituri. Study of plague in DRC during the decade 2004–2014 throws light on ecology of plague in attempt to explain 'persistence of plague focus'. Armed conflicts led to collapse of health care and population impoverishment living in unsanitary conditions. Approximately, 60% of inhabitants slept on the floor and were subject to flea bites. Over 75% had >1 burrow on the ground; 90% of houses had 1 or 2 rooms; and 23 of 30 live rodents captured were caught inside the houses.

According to WHO (2020), a 12-year-old girl reported on June 12, 2020, to local health centre in the health zone of Rethy in Ituri Province of the Democratic Republic of Congo. She had fever, headache, cough and an enlarged lymph gland and died the same day. By July 15, 45 cases with same signs and symptoms including 9 deaths (fatality rate of 20%) were reported form 11 villages within the health zone. Four of the nine dead had cough (progressing to pneumonic) and two had septicaemia. Fifty-eight percent (26/45) were male and 93% (42/45) of >5 years old. Since beginning of 2020, there were 64 cases including 14 deaths (CFR 21.8%) in Ituri Province as against 10 cases and 5 deaths (CFR 50%) during the same period in 2019 in a single zone. Lockdown due to COVID-191 may have interrupted the response activities.

Plague is endemic in Rethy health zone; cases of enzootic variants of *Y. pestis* are seen across the wild rodent population. First outbreak was reported in February 2020 with cases imported from Linga health zone. Rethy health zone received 112,714 internally displaced persons (due to atrocities and violence), most of whom have come from the Jiba and Linga health zones. The quality of water, hygiene and sanitation deteriorated in the reception areas and internally displaced person sites.

51.9 Control

Human faced plague pandemics when the present science of Public Health did not exist with human ingenuity. Two important ancient Public Health measures are valuable, useful and valid even today and are part of evolving of epidemic/pandemic management. These are 'quarantine' and 'practices under Venetian rule'.

51.9.1 Managing Black Death

51.9.1.1 Quarantine (Mackowiak and Sehdev 2002)

Principle of isolating diseased persons from unaffected ones has been in practice from ancient times—cases of Leprosy, skin disease or body discharges must live in camps away from others [Old Testament. In Leviticus, chapter 13, [1, Lev. 13.46]. Numbers, Chapter 5, prescribes a duty to expel from camp everyone with a dreaded skin disease or bodily discharge [1, Num. 5.2].

In 1374, Viscount Bernabo of Reggio, Italy, declared that every person with plague be taken out of the city into the fields, there to die or to recover. Jacob Padua, the chief physician of the City Ragusa (Dubrovnik of Croatia), advised establishing a place outside the city walls for treatment of ill townspeople and outsiders who came to town seeking a cure.

In 1377, the Great Council passed a law establishing a trentino or a 30-day isolation period (Stuard 1992). The four tenets of this law were as follows: (1) that citizens or visitors from plague-endemic areas would not be admitted into Ragusa until they had first remained in isolation for 1 month; (2) that no person from Ragusa was permitted to go to the isolation area, under penalty of remaining there for 30 days; (3) that persons not assigned by the Great Council to care for those being quarantined were not permitted to bring food to isolated persons, under penalty of remaining with them for 1 month; and (4) that whoever did not observe these regulations would be fined and subjected to isolation for 1 month. During the next 80 years, similar laws were introduced in Marseilles, Venice, Pisa and Genoa (Stuard 1992).

How 30 days (trentino) changed to 40 (quarantine) is not known. There are guesses—(a) ancient Greek doctrine of 'critical days'—contagious disease develops within 40 days of exposure, (b) lent—40-day period of spiritual purification and (c) others.

'Quarantine' became part of the modern lexicon during the Black Death in Europe.

51.9.1.2   The Venetian Rule

The Venetian state is considered pioneer in organization of public health. It established regulations and practices in the late middle ages including quarantine (isolation from 14 to >40 days depending upon the health of the port of origin), lazarettos (institutions where those with plague or other similar diseases were isolated), public health offices and 'cordoni di sanita'. The first *lazzarettos* were established in Corfu and Zante in 1588 and in Cephalonia and Leukada at the beginning of the eighteenth century.

The Venetians activated a system of inspection and interrogation of sailors arriving on ports and established garrisons along the coasts to isolate suspected case or to isolate plague-infested areas and control all local movements till the end of emergency. Plague affected was kept in *lazarettos*, and large numbers of infected persons were kept in hospitals and houses on the assumption that they remained isolated. Isolation and movement controlled were ensured by military personnel.

Plague was last observed in Venice in 1630, in Southeastern Europe until the nineteenth century (Konstantinidou et al. 2009).

Third pandemic: Three important developments shaped the management of plague. Swiss-born French bacteriologist Alexandre Yersin isolated the bacterium in 1894 in Hong Kong. He is credited for determining mode of transmission and contributing to developments of methods of modern treatment including antibiotics and insecticides, eventually plague vaccines. The French scientist Paul-Louis Simond demonstrated vector—role of fleas.

Plague can be successfully treated by modern regimen. Prevention and isolation can stop the spread. Management of the Surat plague 1994 in India followed the procedure very much similar to the one used during Venetian rule (Dutt et al. 2006).

51.9.2   The Principles of Management of Outbreak

It is based on WHO (2022).

Plague outbreak management includes (1) detection of source of infection and stopping (which includes collection of specimens despatch/examination); (2) protecting health workers and nosocomial infection; (3) ensuring correct treatment; (4) isolation of patients of pneumonic plague; (5) surveillance, identifying contacts of pneumonic plague patients and house members of bubonic plague patients and a seven-day chemoprophylaxis; (6) disinfection, soap water hand wash or alcohol hand rub and freshly made household bleach for larger areas; (7) safe burial, using disinfectant-soaked cloth/absorbent material instead of conventional spray of face and chest area; and (8) rodent and flea control.

A patient is considered infectious for the first 48–72 h after initiation of appropriate antibiotic therapy and evidence of clinical improvement. Mask, eye and face shield, gloves and gowns are personal protective with hand washings as standard precautions. Isolation of pneumonic cases is preferably in rooms or at distance of 2 m in shared rooms to protect spread by drops and droplets. Aerosol of *Y. pestis* is infectious for about an hour. On surface, it can survive for days, longer in dried blood and secretions. Chemicals like 0.5–1% sodium hypochlorite, 70% ethanol, 2% glutaraldehyde, formaldehyde and iodine-based and phenolic disinfectants can be used. Heating at 56 °C or exposure to sunlight for 4 h should kill.

Autopsy guidelines should be followed, such as scrub suit, surgical cap, impervious gown, goggles, double surgical gloves, shoe covers, N-95 mask, etc. (WHO 2021).

For reactive surveillance system, biological confirmation of cases is required for early detection and control of outbreaks. The National Institute of Communicable Diseases (NICD) has a Plague surveillance unit at Bangalore and the Central Plague Laboratory at Delhi. The Haffkine Institute established for this purpose in Mumbai is possibly the oldest one working on plague.

51.9.2.1   Sentinel

Statistically significant temporal association between human plague cases and seroprevalence rates in coyotes was found—suggesting the use of coyote as sentinel animal (Brown et al. 2011).

51.9.2.2   Vaccines

Killed whole cell vaccine produced in the USA and Australia is now stopped because of low efficiency and short-lasting (six months) protection. The live *Y. pestis* EV vaccine is used in Asia and Russia. It was previously used with benefit in Madagascar. It has not been licensed in occidental countries. Candidate vaccines are molecular vaccines combining *Y. pestis* F1 and V antigens. The USA's, the UK's and China's governmental agencies have developed rF1-V, RypVax and SV1 vaccines, respectively. rF1-V and SV1 have completed phase I and II trials. These are patented but not yet licensed. These protect 100% of experimental mice when two doses are administered against bubonic and pneumonic plague. Cynomolgus macaques were protected against aerosolized *Y. pestis* but not African green monkeys. Several other vaccine candidates have been proposed but have not progressed to clinical trials (Demeure et al. 2019).

Bhattacharya et al. (2010) developed a vaccine and claim that it would interrupt transmission among wild animals. A single dose administered orally protected them against challenge with ten times the lethal dose of *Y. pestis*. Protection lasted for 45 weeks.

References

Abedi AA, Shako JC, Gaudart J, Sudre B, Ilunga BK et al (2018) Ecologic features of plague outbreak areas, Democratic Republic of the Congo, 2004-2014. Emerg Infect Dis 24(2):210–220

Aborode AT, dos Santos Costa AC, Mohan A et al (2021) Epidemic of plague amidst COVID-19 in Madagascar: efforts, challenges, and recommendations. Trop Med Health 49:56

Andrianaivoarimanana V, Piola P, Wagner DM, Rakotomanana F, Maheriniaina V et al (2019) Trends of human plague, Madagascar, 1998-2016. Emerg Infect Dis 25(2):220–228

Ayyadurai S, Houhamdi L, Lepidi H, Nappez C, Raoult D, Drancourt M (2008) Long-term persistence of virulent *Yersinia pestis* in soil. Microbiology (Reading) 154(Pt 9):2865–2871

Barbieri R, Signoli M, Chevé D, Costedoat C, Tzortzis S et al (2021) *Yersinia pestis*: the natural history of plague. Clin Microbiol Rev 34:e00044–e00019

Bertherat E, Jullien S (2021) Revision of the international definition of plague cases. Wkly Epidemiol Rec 24:238–240

Bhattacharya D, Mecsas J, Hu LT (2010) Development of a vaccinia virus based reservoir-targeted vaccine against *Yersinia pestis*. Vaccine 28(48):7683–7689

Bitam I, Baziz B, Rolain JM, Belkaid M, Raoult D (2006) Zoonotic focus of plague, Algeria. Emerg Infect Dis 12(12):1975–1977

Bitam I, Ayyadurai S, Kernif T, Chetta M, Boulaghman N et al (2010) New rural focus of plague, Algeria. Emerg Infect Dis 16(10):1639–1640

Bos K, Schuenemann V, Golding G et al (2011) A draft genome of *Yersinia pestis* from victims of the Black Death. Nature 478:506–510

Bosio CF, Jarrett CO, Scott DP, Fintzi J, Hinnebusch BJ (2020) Comparison of the transmission efficiency and plague progression dynamics associated with two mechanisms by which fleas transmit *Yersinia pestis*. PLoS Pathog 16(12):e1009092

Brown HE, Levy CE, Enscore RE, Schriefer ME, DeLiberto TJ et al (2011) Annual seroprevalence of *Yersinia pestis* in coyotes as predictors of interannual variation in reports of human plague cases in Arizona, United States. Vector Borne Zoonotic Dis 11(11):1439–1446

Demeure CE, Dussurget O, Mas Fiol G et al (2019) *Yersinia pestis* and plague: an updated view on evolution, virulence determinants, immune subversion, vaccination, and diagnostics. Genes Immun 20:357–370

Dutt AK, Akhtar R, McVeigh M (2006) Surat plague of 1994 re-examined. Southeast Asian J Trop Med Public Health 37(4):755–760. PMID: 17121302

Gage KL, Dennis DT, Orloski KA, Ettestad P, Brown TL et al (2000) Cases of cat-associated human plague in the Western US, 1977-1998. Clin Infect Dis 30(6):893–900

Gould LH, Pape J, Ettestad P, Griffith KS, Mead PS (2008) Dog-associated risk factors for human plague. Zoonoses Public Health 55(8–10):448–454

Haensch S, Bianucci R, Signoli M, Rajerison M, Schultz M, Kacki S et al (2010) Distinct clones of *Yersinia pestis* caused the Black Death. PLoS Pathog 6(10):e1001134

Hinnebusch BJ (2005) The evolution of flea-borne transmission in *Yersinia pestis*. Curr Issues Mol Biol 7(2):197–212

Hinnebusch BJ, Perry RD, Schwan TG (1996) Role of the Yersinia pestis hemin storage (hms) locus in the transmission of plague by fleas. Science 273(5273):367–370

Hinnebusch BJ, Rudolph AE, Cherepanov P, Dixon JE et al (2002) Role of *Yersinia murine* toxin in survival of *Yersinia pestis* in the midgut of the flea vector. Science 296(5568):733–735

Keller M, Spyrou MA, Scheib CL et al (2019) Ancient *Yersinia pestis* genomes from across Western Europe reveal early diversification during the First Pandemic (541-750). Proc Natl Acad Sci U S A 116(25):12363–12372

Kingston JJ, Tuteja U, Kapil M et al (2009) Genotyping of Indian *Yersinia pestis* strains by MLVA and repetitive DNA sequence based PCRs. Antonie van Leeuwenhoek 96:303–312

Konstantinidou K, Mantadakis E, Falagas ME, Sardi T, Samonis G (2009) Venetian rule and control of plague epidemics on the Ionian Islands during 17th and 18th centuries. Emerg Infect Dis 15(1):39–43

Kutyrev VV, Eroshenko GA, Motin VL, Nosov NY, Krasnov JM et al (2018) Phylogeny and clas-
    sification of *Yersinia pestis* through the lens of strains from the plague foci of commonwealth
    of independent states. Front Microbiol 9:1106
Laudisoit A, Leirs H, Makundi RH, Van Dongen S, Davis S et al (2007) Plague and the human flea,
    Tanzania. Emerg Infect Dis 13(5):687–693
Leslie T, Whitehouse CA, Yingst S, Baldwin C, Kakar F et al (2011) Outbreak of gastroenteritis
    caused by *Yersinia pestis* in Afghanistan. Epidemiol Infect 139(5):728–735
Mackowiak PA, Sehdev PS (2002) The origin of quarantine. Clin Infect Dis 35(9):1071–1072
Madon MB, Hitchcock JC, Davis RM, Myers CM, Smith CR et al (1997) An overview of plague in
    the United States and a report of investigations of two human cases in Kern county, California,
    1995. J Vector Ecol 22(1):77–82
Morozova I, Kasianov A, Bruskin S, Neukamm J, Molak M et al (2020) New ancient Eastern
    European *Yersinia pestis* genomes illuminate the dispersal of plague in Europe. Phil Trans R
    Soc B 375:20190569
Rakotosamimanana S, Kassie D, Taglioni F et al (2021) A decade of plague in Madagascar: a
    description of two hotspot districts. BMC Public Health 21:1112
Respicio-Kingry LB, Yockey BM, Acayo S, Kaggwa J, Apangu T et al (2016) Two distinct *Yersinia
    pestis* populations causing plague among humans in the West Nile Region of Uganda. PLoS
    Negl Trop Dis 10(2):e0004360
Salkeld DJ, Salathé M, Stapp P, Jones JH (2010) Plague outbreaks in prairie dog populations
    explained by percolation thresholds of alternate host abundance. Proc Natl Acad Sci U S A
    107(32):14247–14250
Saxena VK, Verghese T (1996) Ecology of flea transmitted zoonotic infection in village Mamla,
    district Beed. Curr Sci 71(10):800–802
Schuenemann VJ, Bos K, DeWitte S, Schmedes S, Jamieson J et al (2011) Targeted enrichment
    of ancient pathogens yielding the pPCP1 plasmid of *Yersinia pestis* from victims of the Black
    Death. Proc Natl Acad Sci U S A 108(38):E746–E752
Stuard SM (1992) A state of deference: Ragusa/Dubrovnik in the medieval centuries. University
    of Pennsylvania Press, Philadelphia
WHO (31 October 2017). https://www.who.int/news-room/fact-sheets/detail/plague
WHO (23 July 2020) Plague - Democratic Republic of the Congo. https://www.who.int/
    emergencies/disease-outbreak-news/item/plague-democratic-republic-of-the-congo
WHO (2021) WHO guidelines for plague management: revised recommendations for the use of
    rapid diagnostic tests, fluoroquinolones for case management and personal protective equip-
    ment for prevention of post-mortem transmission. Web annex B: evidence-to-decision tables.
    World Health Organization. https://apps.who.int/iris/handle/10665/341496
WHO (2022) Plague (who.int) 7 July 2022
Wimsatt J, Biggins DE (2009) A review of plague persistence with special emphasis on fleas. J
    Vector Borne Dis 46(2):85–99

Chapter 52
Q Fever

Synonyms

Coxiellosis, Query fever, Nine-mile fever, and Quadrilateral fever.

Q (Query) fever is characterized by sudden onset of fever, sweat, severe retro-orbital headache, loss of appetite, weakness and pneumonia. An intracellular anthropozoonotic agent *Coxiella burnetii* is spread by domestic animals, goats, sheep and cattle through their placenta, amniotic fluid, urine, faeces and milk. It has worldwide distribution. It is a potential bioterrorism agent under category B because of its characters, contagious and stable in aerosol in a wide range of temperatures, survives for 60 days on surfaces and has the lowest infective dose (ID_{50} is 1).

It affects animal farming, causes economic loss and is a serious public health problem. Q fever epidemic occurred in the Netherlands during 2007–2010. It was linked to epizootic in goat farms. Thousands of humans suffered with large hospitalization. There were 95 deaths. The epizootic was controlled after culling 50,000 dairy goats from 55 farms. Severe disease has been reported in pregnant women, foetuses, new-born babies and infants. In 2019, 33 European countries reported 958/1069 (90%) confirmed cases of Q fever. Spain, France and Germany reported the highest number. Most cases were acquired locally (EFSA and ECDC 2021).

52.1 Aetiology

Coxiella burnetii is Gram negative and appears as small bipolar rods. It belongs to the order Legionellales. Earlier named as *Rickettsia burnetii* is identical with *R. diaphorica* isolated from *Dermacentor andersoni* ticks from Nine Mile Creek, Montana. Rolla Dyer, the director of NIH visiting the Rocky Mountain Laboratories, Montana, acquired this infection from laboratory within ten days and was down with fever, sweats, chills and a severe retro-orbital headache, which are classical

© Springer Nature Singapore Pte Ltd. 2024

K. G. Narayan et al., *Handbook of Management of Zoonoses*,

https://doi.org/10.1007/978-981-99-9885-2_52

symptoms of Q fever. This Nine Mile strain is used in laboratories. *C. burnetii* is obligately intracellular and filterable and differs from other *Rickettsiae* in G+C content.

C. burnetii belongs to the family Coxiellaceae and can replicate intracellularly. *Coxiella* occur in three forms, (a) small cell variant (SCV, highly infectious), (b) large cell variant (LCV, developed also in cell culture) and (c) spore -like particle (SLP). In mammalian cells, *C. burnetii* grow in large cell and spore-like forms.

SLP is infectious and resistant and can survive in environment for long, 7–10 months on sheep wool at 15–20 °C and for more than a month in meat stored in cold (4 °C) and >40 months in dry milk powder at room temperature. Infection-competent *C. burnetii* could be extracted after 4–5 months from formalin-fixed tissue or even paraffin-treated tissue. Gaseous formaldehyde sterilization is ineffective.

Effective inactivation of *Coxiella* is achieved by 1% phenol, 5% hydrogen peroxide, 5% chloroform and 0.5% hypochlorite and exposure to heat at 65 °C for >1 h, irradiation with 10 kGy gamma rays, 70% ethanol for 20 min, autoclaving at 131 °C for 15 min and 5% formaldehyde for 5 min.

It is biphasic and does not produce agglutinin to react in Weil Felix test. Recent isolates from vertebrate animals, ticks/arthropods or laboratory animals are usually phase I. Phase II antigen develops after a variable number of passages through immunologically incompetent hosts such as embryonated eggs or cell cultures. Reversion to phase I occurs even with a single passage through a susceptible host like guinea pigs. The phase I antigen is a lipopolysaccharide (LPS), resistant to heat at 121 °C for 15 min. Trichloroacetic acid treatment of the phase I antigen converts it to phase II antigen. Antigens of phases I and II have diagnostic value. The predominant antibody in acute Q fever in man is against phase II and in chronic against phase I antigen.

52.1.1   Genotypes and Plasmids

The 30 multi-spacer sequence typing (MST) grouping (Glazunova et al. 2005) was extended by single nucleotide polymorphism (SNP) analysis by means of real-time polymerase chain reaction (PCR) and melting point analysis considering insertions and deletions by bi-allelic and tri-allelic SNP by Hornstra et al. (2011) to construct a phylogenetic tree of *Coxiella* isolates. This tree consists of I–VI genogroups and 35 MST genotypes with individual groups containing between 1 and 15 MST. Most MST genotypes have worldwide distribution. MST 8 causes chronic infections and endocarditis frequently in humans, and goats act as the reservoir. According to Arbeitskreis Blut (2014), several authors suggested genotypes/genogroups based on nucleic acid sequence analysis including plasmids. Individual genotypes displayed only partial agreement but are sufficient to characterize outbreaks.

Four plasmids identified are QpH1, QpRS, QpDG and QpDV. Plasmidless strains may contain plasmid-related sequences integrated into their chromosomes. The absolute conservation of plasmid or integrated plasmid-like sequences in all isolates suggests an adaptive role. Plasmids QpRS, QpH1 and QpDV may be associated with differences in pathogenicity of genotypes. Plasmid genes encode Dot/Icm T4SS substrates that can modify host cell milieu to favour *C. burnetii* survival and growth. Each bacterial cell has one of the four plasmids and accounts for 2% of genetic information (Arbeitskreis Blut 2014).

52.1.2   Virulence Determinants

Phase I *C. burnetii* is highly infectious and virulent for humans. The human infective dose is just 1–10 *Coxiella*. BSL3 containment is required. Phase II bacteria can be safely handled in BSL2 labs.

The LPS determines virulence. Phase I LPS has full-length O side chains in the outer membrane. The bacterial surface antigens are masked. Passive phagocytosis occurs. The dendritic cells fail to recognize antigenic pattern and are infected without activation. The inflammatory response is delayed. Lysis (phagolysosome) of *Coxiella* is delayed or prevented because the components of complement are not activated or activation is delayed by the LPS. The infection persists.

Phase II LPS has truncated O side chains. Cell wall proteins are accessible to immune system. Phase II *Coxiella* is readily inactivated by complement system and is thus less infectious and virulent.

The type IV secretion system is considered another potential virulence determinant.

52.1.3   Host Cell Invasion and Replication

C. burnetii replicates intracellular and not extracellular in cells of both poikilothermic and homeothermic animals. It can survive in amoeba for several weeks. The doubling time in mammalian cells varies between 20 and 45 h.

The target cells include macrophages (e.g. in the lymph nodes, spleen, lungs and liver) and monocytes circulating in blood.

Martinez et al. (2014) identified *Coxiella*—invasion, precisely CBU_1260 (OmpA), as the first step in the host cell invasion. Three key steps of infection are (1) internalization within host cells, (2) vacuole biogenesis/intracellular replication and (3) protection of infected cells from apoptosis. Production of oxygen derivatives and NO, synthesis of interferon gamma and the formation of suppressor T-lymphocytes are suppressed.

Generally, intracellular bacteria reside in a vacuolar compartment after invasion. This compartment (PV) is modified by *C. burnetii* into an acidified lysosome-derived compartment referred to as *C. burnetii*-containing vacuole (CCV) that occupies most of the host cell cytoplasm.

C. *burnetii* encodes a Dot/Icm-type IV (defect in organelle trafficking/intracellular multiplication) secretion system (van Schaik et al. 2013). The type IV secretion system called Dot/Icm delivers bacterial effector proteins CBU0077, CBU1823 and CBU1524 into the host cytosol during infection and are detectable after 8 h (Newton et al. 2013). This required acidification of CCV and its maturation to a late endocytic compartment (a two-stage process). During the first two days of infection, CCV expands. The pH is 4.8. Metabolism is activated and replication initiated. Further expansion and replication continue for following several days.

52.1.4   SCV-LCV Cycle

The extracellular 'small cell variant (SCV)' is a spore-like small dense subpopulation that is infectious. It is quite resistant to drying and desiccation, long storage at room temperature, high temperature 60 °C, UV light and also some disinfectants, for example, phenolic and antibiotics. It can survive long in nature and also in vertebrate hosts without involving invertebrates.

The SCV passively enters hosts' cells, initially alveolar macrophages and monocytes, and localizes and multiplies into parasitophorous vacuoles (PV). There is phagosome pause. *Coxiella* produces a Type 4B Secretion System (T4BSS) that secrets effector proteins into the host cell to control a number of infection events including creation of low pH that prevents decomposition. Survival is enhanced, and transformation into metabolically active and fragile 'large cell variant (LCV)' is facilitated. Intracellular replication occurs over 5–6 days. A mixture of SCV and LCV accumulate in a vacuole created by PV. Eventually, all transform into SCV population ready to be released upon lysis.

52.2   Epidemiology

52.2.1   Prevalence

C. *burnetii* is commonly prevalent in nature because of (a) a wide range of hosts and (b) innate resistance to environmental conditions. It maintains in nature without involving human beings who are accidental hosts. Q fever zoonosis occurs all over the world but is under diagnosed and underreported.

52.2.2   Reservoirs

Lagomorphs, rodents and marsupials are reservoirs besides a big list of seropositive birds and animals suggestive of susceptibility. Indian studies identified shrews, household rats and mice, bandicoots and also poikilotherms such as snakes, pythons, king cobra, Indian monitor, tortoise, toads and frogs as reservoirs—possibly maintaining feral cycle of *C. burnetii* and also spilling and spreading it to domestic animals and human beings. Rats, bandicoots, shrews and house mice may act linking between domestic and feral cycles and also transmit infection to human beings.

A number of species of ticks (approximately 40) are natural reservoirs for life. These are *Ornithodorus*, *Dermacentor*, *Hyalomma*, *Haemaphysalis*, *Otobius*, *Aponomma gervaisi*, *Boophilus* and *Rhipicephalus* also *Argasidae*. Transovarial and trans-stadial infection occurs in ticks. Dried faeces of ticks infect domestic animals through inhalation.

Domestic animal reservoirs are cattle, buffalo, sheep, goats and pigs and game birds (pigeons and sparrows). Others include multiple vertebrate species, including wildlife, marine mammals, domestic mammals, birds and reptiles.

Any infected animal has the potential to transmit the infection through excretion and secretions. Human outbreaks and cases have been epidemiologically linked to exposure to multiple species including pigeons, dogs, cats and rabbits. *C. burnetii* is shed in large number in the birth products. The viable organisms might be shed also in urine, milk and faeces of infected animals. PCR is used to detect. These are resistant to heat and desiccation and can survive in the environment for months to years and get aerosolized and driven with wind infecting a man as far as 10 miles. In the Netherlands epidemic, 2 miles was a significant factor.

52.2.3   Q Fever in Animals

C. burnetii causes placentitis, abortion, stillbirth, premature delivery of weak offspring and infertility in ruminants. Pregnant animals seem to be more susceptible. *Coxiella* infection may be reactivated during pregnancy. Goats may also suffer with pneumonia, but most common symptoms are abortions, stillbirths and weak kids. Cows suffer with subclinical infection to mastitis, metritis and infertility. Chronic infection in cows and goats is more frequent than in sheep. Mammary glands and the uterus are the sites of localization. Consequently, cows' milk has been found positive for long, 32 months post-partum. Shedding in faeces, urine and vaginal secretion contribute to environmental contamination. It is discontinuous in goats, limited to kidding season. In experimental goats, shedding in vaginal mucus and milk has been observed in two successive kidding seasons. Shedding in milk lasts long.

C. burnetii-caused abortions are especially high in goats (up to 70–90%) and lower in sheep (usually below 6%). Epizootics in goats and sheep are commonly linked to human Q fever outbreaks. Rearing of goats, kidding/lambing season and spread of goat or sheep manure and close contact are attributed. According to Kilicoglu et al. (2020), *C. burnetii* has spread among sheep herds in Black Sea region. Infection in sheep and aborted foetuses was detected. A cross-sectional study in Chhattisgarh and Odisha, India, detected an overall prevalence of 14.2% in goats (11.93% PCR and 9.63% ELISA). Seropositivity among farmers and farm workers was 46.24% (Sahu et al. 2018). ELISA testing of sera and milk detected 29.91% and 26.73% *C. burnetii* infection among cattle. 84.21% of cattle and farm workers were sero-positive. The trans-PCR detected the pathogen in 12.94% sera, 14.73% vaginal swabs and 5.53% milk samples of cattle and in one soil sample. The sera of the farm workers and tick were tested negative (Dhaka et al. 2019).

According to Bellabidi et al. (2020), camels and their ticks in Algeria may play an important role as a reservoir for *C. burnetii* and can be considered as a significant source of Q fever transmission to other animal species and humans.

Dogs, cats and rabbits can be infected and contribute to human infection, but clinical presentation in these species is not well understood.

Álvarez-Alonso et al. (2020) selected four naturally infected flocks of sheep on the basis of *C. burnetii* DNA in bulk tank milk (BTM) and a high seroprevalence in yearlings during previous milking period for a longitudinal study for four consecutive lambings. *C. burnetii* faecal shedding and the bacterial burden detected in dust were significantly related. Vaginal shedding contributed to indoor aerosols. *C. burnetii* survived during the four lambing seasons and infection remained active for five years. A real-time PCR analysis was used in the study. Genotypes identified were SNP8 (three flocks, 52.9% of the samples), SNP1 (two flocks, 44.8% samples) and SNP5 (one flock, two environmental samples).

These results suggest that environmental contamination on the premises and surrounding areas of farms persists.

52.2.4   *Q Fever in Human*

Humans get infection through air, contact, ingestion (of contaminated milk and milk products), 'fresh cell therapy', xenotransplant and bite of infected ticks.

Generally, Q fever is considered as an occupationally acquired zoonosis. This includes livestock farmers and those helping in animal births, veterinarians, and those involved in farm hygiene, especially in removing and spreading manure. However, urban outbreaks have no known exposure to livestock and person of any occupation may be victims. The size of inoculum and route of infection determine the clinical outcome.

Although traditionally Q fever in Atlantic Canada is acquired from infected parturient cats or new-born kittens, Webster et al. (2009) described first case linked to ovine.

It is a notifiable disease in the USA. In the USA, acute Q fever cases were reported in any month but peaked in spring, most likely related to birthing time of livestock and manure spreading. Persons aged ≥40 years constituted more cases than young ones, and those aged 60–64 years had the highest risk. Probably occupation led to more cases in males than in females. Another explanation could be the protective effects of 17β-estradiol (Anderson et al. 2013). Another study from the USA reported the occurrence of cluster of cases of Q fever coincident with breeding season of domestic animals and related increased human activities. A ten-year study (Harris et al. 2013) in the Townsville region of Queensland showed that the incidence peaked in May. The increase in wildlife population and drier conditions immediately following the wet season possibly led to this increase in incidence.

The notification rate of Q fever in the EU/EEA was 0.19/100,000 in 2019 with no significant change during past five years. The case fatality rate was 0.63%. Spain reported all the four deaths. Q fever cases occur round the year; however, seasonality is observed. Cases appear during April–September with peaks in June and August and a fall in July, with some variations in countries. The maximum numbers of cases are recorded in June in Spain, April–July in France and August in Germany. Q fever appears to affect working age group, rate of notification increasing with age up to 64 years and highest in the age group 45–64 in both sexes. The male-to-female ratio was 2.4:1. Q fever-positive animals in the EU included sheep (8.9%), goats (10.8%), cattle (5.3%) and 1% other domestic animals and wild animals. Good hygiene practices in animal premises, particularly sheep and goats, help to prevent transmission of Q fever (ECDC 2021).

Q fever was described first in Brisbane, Queensland, Australia, among abattoir workers (occupationally acquired). Study of serologically confirmed acute cases during 2000–2010 revealed that the incidence was higher in the Townsville region of Queensland, Australia. The incidence peaked in May, following the peak rainfall in February. Drier conditions following the wet season and increased wildlife population possibly led to the increased incidence (Harris et al. 2013).

Mahamat et al. (2013) reported a unique clone of *C. burnetii*—genotype 17—and considered it as the most virulent described to date. It caused highest incidence in the world in Cayenne, the capital of French Guiana. It is related to the genotypes that harbour plasmid—QpH1-strains known to cause most severe clinical form of disease in experimental animal models. It was responsible for 24% of community-acquired pneumonia (CAP) and caused severe pneumonia and endocarditis. Seroprevalence is high among farmers in Thailand where it presents as CAP and later developing chronic form endocarditis.

52.2.5 Q Fever in the Netherlands

It has been endemic for decades in the Netherlands. The estimated seroprevalence was 2.4%, and independent risk factors identified were keeping ruminants, increasing age and being born in Turkey (Schimmer et al. 2012). Epidemic emerged since spring 2007. Roest et al. (2011) and van der Hoek et al. (2012) described the epidemic of 2007–2010. Disease (abortion) was diagnosed on two dairy goat farms in

2005. Thirty dairy goat and sheep farms recorded abortions during 2005–2009. In Southern Netherlands, where intensive dairy goat farms were located, human cases were detected in 2007. Proximity to aborting animals' farms (<5 km) and susceptibility led to 3523 human cases between 2007 and 2009 and >4000 by 2010. In most affected area, 15% of population was affected. The rate of hospitalization was 20%. Annual summer seasonal peak was observed. The isolate of *C. burnetii* was identified as genotype 1. The epidemic peaked in 2009.

C. burnetii genotype 1 DNA was detected in the placenta from horses and dogs (Roest et al. 2013). A study (Rijks et al. 2011) in roe deer (*Capreolus capreolus*) found no evidence of spillover of the most predominant epidemic strain. Infection in roe deer occurred round the year, but *C. burnetii* DNA load was highest in March, April and June. Study of an outbreak in rural area of the Netherlands (Karagiannis et al. 2009) showed that living in the area in which positive goat farms, cattle and small ruminants were located, smoking and contact with agricultural products like manure were associated with the epidemic. As observed in Europe (Marrie 2003), cases clustered among those who lived along the road over which farm vehicles travelled and animals moved, probably farm vehicles, caused aerosol from contaminated manure, straw and dust. The experience of the 2007–2010 epidemics in the Netherlands suggested that 20–55% of those living near (about 1–1.5 km radius) goat farms were at high risk of getting infected. Inhalation of the contaminated aerosols by susceptible human results in Q fever. This explains why, in many areas, annual outbreaks of Q fever occur around the time of livestock kidding.

52.2.6   Source

Most human infections are acquired from animals and their produce or excretions and environment contaminated by these. Density of infected animals determines environmental load and in turn influences the rate of human infection.

C. burnetii is excreted by an infected host in faeces, urine, milk and foetal membranes, particularly with aborted foetus. The concentration per gram is high in foetal membranes—say 10^9 in case of ewes and 10^5 in milk. Isolation of *C. burnetii* from water of ponds and frogs and toads is suggestive either aquatic nidus or contamination of water from the discharges of these and other animals. The bacteria can survive for long in dried tissues/faeces (nearly six months in soil) of reservoir hosts and ticks.

Tick faeces may contain 10^9 *Coxiella*/g and is a source for direct/indirect contact and get aerosolized for air-borne infection.

52.2.7 Modes of Infection

C. burnetii can enter through abraded skin, inhalation, conjunctival mucous membrane, ingestion and infected tick bite.

Ingestion of contaminated milk and milk products, for example, cheese, causes infection.

Inhalation of contaminated aerosol or dust is the main transmission pathway. *Coxiella* may be air-borne from dried excretions, secretions and discharges from infected hosts and man and animals. Risk persists for years after infected sheep herd has left the region.

Contact: Direct domestic and pet animal-human, human-human contact or indirect contact with infected tissues such as placenta or manure from goat and sheep or farm implement and bedding.

Vector—tick bite. Transcutaneous/percutaneous: Tick bites transmit infection between animals and rarely humans.

52.2.8 Human-to-Human Transmission

Human-to-human transmission is possible but uncommon. Contact with dead during post-mortem examination and during sex and parturient woman (intra-uterine infection) and transplacental have resulted into sporadic cases. *C. burnetii* has been isolated from human breast milk.

Sexual and transplacental Transmission: *C. burnetii* persist in genitalia of man and animals. Human-human transmission through sex is possible.

There is a risk of blood transfusion and bone marrow transplantation from infected donors.

Nosocomial infection is possible during autopsies and obstetrical procedures.

High-risk and occupational groups: Susceptibility to infection is high in debilitated and weak, comorbidities and reduced immune status because of drug of HIV infection. Human infections are mostly occupationally acquired. Examples of such risky occupations and exposures are animal farmers engaged in raising animals like cattle, buffalo, sheep, goats, camel, horse, dog, poultry, etc.; veterinarians; abattoir workers, particularly engaged in bone-grinding and animal waste (placenta, foetus, viscera) collecting units; pathologists and laboratory workers handling infected tissues and cultures; and scientists and experimental animals' (rodents, rabbits, guinea pigs, cats besides others) attendants. Infection among veterinary teachers and students has been traced to using infected sheep for teaching purpose. Cases clustered in a veterinary facility attending to infected cat and its litter. Mioni et al. (2020) demonstrated widespread distribution of *C. burnetii* in the State of São Paulo, Brazil, and observed that abattoir workers were exposed to contaminated aerosols generated during slaughter. Infection follows the route of transport of infected ewes. Infection may be trans-located with contaminated straw.

52.3   Clinical/Disease

Diagnosis of acute Q fever (AQF) is challenging because most infections (50%) are asymptomatic or present non-specific symptoms. It is a common cause of fever of unknown origin (FUO). Simple cases present unexplained malaise and fever only.

Matsui et al. (2019) reported two cases of AQF contracted during travel to Malawi. AQF epidemiology is not known in Malawi; however, seroprevalence of Q fever among cattle was reported as 6.5%. AQF among hospital admissions of febrile cases ranged from 2% to 9% in Africa. In Tanzania, 3% of children and 8% of adults admitted as febrile patients were diagnosed as AQF and may be linked to livestock parturition during dry season. Aerosolized *Coxiella* might have infected the two travellers from Japan to Malawi. The mother (40 years) and child (4 years) were hospitalized, child with high- and mother with a mild-grade fever. Mother had dry cough and child had no symptoms. The child had abnormal liver function and was diagnosed as viral fever. He spontaneously recovered after seven days. Mother was admitted two days later with dry cough. She had a history of Kawasaki disease without cardiac complications. Examinations revealed that she had bradycardia, bicytopenia and mildly elevated liver transferase and was negative for malaria and blood culture. She was suspected of having AQF because of her relative bradycardia and her indirect livestock contact in Malawi. Paired serum antiphase II IgM and IgG was significantly elevated in the convalescent phase in both cases. *C. burnetii* gene (IS1111) was detected from the mother's blood sample.

In hospitalized cases, fatality up to 2.4% has been observed in France (Arbeitskreis Blut 2014). Human do not have innate resistance. Immunity is built up after recovery from acute infection.

*Q fever can be acute and chronic. D*uration of illness may run in weeks or months if untreated. It occurs in two forms, acute and chronic. Acute Q fever cases have predominant *C. burnetii* phase II antibodies and are higher than the phase I antibodies. Chronic infection is associated with a rising phase I immunoglobulin G (IgG) titre.

52.3.1   Acute Q Fever

After an incubation period of 2–4 weeks/3–30 days, there is rapid onset of fever, 101–104 °F that runs for several days and lasts for 1–2 weeks. There is bacteraemia. Other symptoms include headache (at times not responding to analgesics), extreme fatigue, myalgia, retro-orbital pain, anorexia, general malaise, headache, myalgia, sweats, nausea and sometimes vomiting, diarrhoea, cough, chest pain and atypical pneumonia, diarrhoea and skin rash. Recurrent fever, headache and retro-orbital pain predominate. Transplacental infection may occur. Infection in pregnant women leads to spontaneous abortion and intrauterine growth retardation, foetal deaths, neonatal morbidity and mortality.

It is self-limiting except when serious complications follow in some cases. Digestive, respiratory, cardiovascular or central nervous system may be affected. Cases may show pneumonia, haemorrhagic gastroenteritis, granulomatous hepatitis and icterus, myocarditis, nervous signs and symptoms and miscarriages among pregnant. Less than 2% hospitalized may die. Timely diagnosis and correct treatment shorten the period of suffering. In the Netherlands epidemic, approximately 4000 cases were reported, and up to 50% of acute cases were hospitalized (Anderson et al. 2013).

Pregnant women are at risk of getting Q fever most likely without symptoms but might have the risk of recrudescent infection during subsequent pregnancies. Q fever causes miscarriage, stillbirth, premature birth or birth of retarded or underweight infant. Infection in the first trimester is likely to result into miscarriage. Premature delivery is more likely if infection occurred later in pregnancy. Chances of chronic Q fever are high when acute infection occurs during first trimester. It is evidenced by an increased phase I IgG titres that do not decrease after pregnancy.

In children, Q fever is less likely to be symptomatic. It is milder and self-limiting if symptomatic. Pneumonia is mild to moderate. Rash is more common in children than in adult. In 50–80% paediatric cases, gastrointestinal symptoms like anorexia, abdominal pain, vomiting and diarrhoea appear.

Q fever pneumonia in adults could be mild to severe. About 1–2% suffers with lobar pneumonia with high fever. It manifests as rapidly progressing atypical pneumonia, infiltration and consolidation. X-rays may show atelectasis, swelling of hilar lymph nodes and granulomas. Cough is often present and is non-productive in 50% of patients. Upper respiratory signs are less likely.

Some patients (1–5%) may progress into chronic pneumonia. Serious forms that most commonly (60–70%) manifest are endocarditis and vascular infections, as has been observed in France and the Netherlands. The fatality rate in such cases is high (25–60%) if not diagnosed early and treated.

52.3.2 Chronic Q Fever

Chronic form manifests after six months of primary Q fever in majority (75%) of cases although it may also appear after years. Chronic form may affect a number of tissues and accordingly appear as endocarditis, vasculitis, osteomyelitis, hepatitis, interstitial lung fibrosis and long-lasting or recurring fever. Immune defence cells migrate to the replication sites during the acute phase to cause granulomas that are typical for the chronic disease. Over years, granulomas may form in other tissues also and *Coxiella* survive in these. The clinical manifestation of chronic Q fever initially is nonspecific and highly variable, such as fever, fatigue, weight loss, night sweats, pain in the abdomen or chest or enlarged liver.

Kampschreur et al. (2012) made a case control study to elucidate the 'risk factors' as chronic form of Q fever was rising after the epidemic of acute fever subsided. Proven/probable/suspected chronic Q fever cases in the study were those who were diagnosed/suspected/without known risk factor, respectively, but manifested specific signs of chronic infection and were laboratory-diagnosed Q fever by phase I–IgG titre of >1024 and/or PCR + blood/tissues. Some earlier known risk factors and others identified in this study included pre-existing cardiac and valvular disease, valvular surgery, vascular prostheses, aneurysms, immunosuppression due to therapy or HIV or old age, pregnancy, renal inefficiency and >60 years age. Patient may present chronic hepatitis, interstitial pneumonia, septic arthritis and osteomyelitis. Following may be observed rarely—lymphadenopathy, Guillain-Barre syndrome, meningitis, encephalitis, peripheral neuropathy, paralysis of oculomotor nerve, confusion and epileptic fits. Arbeitskreis Blut (2014) has described chronic forms like endocarditis, hepatitis and neurologic manifestations.

Endocarditis: It is one of the major forms of chronic Q fever and accounts for about 10% of all endocarditis cases in England and Wales. It is rare in children. *C. burnetii* may be detected in blood in more than 50% cases. The whole of vascular system may be affected. The bacteria adhere as biofilm on the artificial valves and walls of aneurysms. Associated manifestation includes haematuria, anaemia, embolism and splenomegaly. Patients respond to antibiotics (doxycycline and chloroquine). Interrupted/incomplete therapy leads to development of resistance in three years and resistant form relapses.

Hepatitis: It is another manifestation of chronic Q fever frequently observed in France and Spain in the region where intensive sheep breeding is common. Consumption of raw milk and cheese seems associated with the disease. Hepatitis may occur in Q fever pneumonia cases also. Granuloma has a dense fibrin ring and forms in the liver.

Neurological infection: Chronic Q fever may cause aseptic meningitis and encephalitis. There is severe headache, paraesthesia, reduced vision and impaired sensory abilities. Examination of CSF reveals mononuclear cells and elevated protein.

52.3.3   Post-Q Fever Fatigue Syndrome

After symptomatic acute Q fever, healthy persons with no underlying medical or psychological problem report *debilitating fatigue* prominent among a complex of symptoms, such as nausea, pain in muscles and joints, severe headache, night sweat, sleeping difficulty and irrational irritability without involvement of any organ. It is observed in 10–25% of patients. This form was observed in 52% of the patients in the Netherlands epidemic six months after and in 26% one year after the acute illness. The possible explanation is dysregulation of cytokine production, induced by persistent antigens including LPS and proteins, rather than persistent latent *Coxiella* (Porter et al. 2011). The condition lasts for beyond a year and in many for several years. This and elevated antibody titres against *C. burnetii* antigen are diagnostic.

52.4 Diagnosis

Rapid diagnosis is important as treatment started within three days of onset of illness is effective. Detectable antibodies appear in about 7–10 days. Therefore, history of exposure or earlier infection (in case of chronic Q fever) helps the physician in making a near-correct judgement. It is advisable to start treatment and not wait for the availability of reports of laboratory diagnosis.

Demonstration of C. burnetii or its genetic material in blood, serum, sputum, milk, foetal stomach content, placenta or amniotic fluid by direct staining, immunohistological staining and biological and molecular methods summed up as follows:

- Giemsa or Gimenez or Stamp-Macchiavello stain to observe purple or pink or red rickettsia (non-specific)
- *C. burnetii* DNA

Cerebrospinal fluid, pleural fluid, blood, serum, bone marrow, bone biopsies, liver biopsies, milk, placenta and foetal tissue can be tested by PCR to provide rapid results and diagnose acute Q fever in approximately first two weeks after onset of symptoms and before administration of antibiotics.

1. Nucleic acid amplification test (NAT): Conventional PCR, nested PCR and real-time PCR are used.
2. TaqMan-based real-time PCR assay—targeting gene *icd* and transporase of the *IS1111a* element—test was specific and sensitive (detecting <10 genome equivalents per reaction). The *icd* as marker too was highly sensitive (Klee et al. 2006).
3. Molecular characterization could be done using multispacer sequence typing (Glazunova et al. 2005).

Coxiella DNA can be detected in paraffin-embedded tissue, in the blood by PCR two weeks after transmission.

- Immunohistochemistry on biopsy, for example, avidin-biotin-peroxidase complex
- IFA
- Inoculation in cell culture, chicken embryo egg sac, intra-peritoneal in mice, guinea pig and hamster. Inoculated animals show a rise in temperature of 40 °C. Rickettsiae are detected in blood/tissues like the liver. Examine serum before inoculation and 4–6 weeks post-inoculation for rising antibodies titre.

52.4.1 Serology

IFA: A fourfold increase in phase II IgG titre by IFA on paired acute and convalescent serum specimens is a gold standard to confirm acute Q fever, which has higher sensitivity and specificity than a single convalescent serum. A negative acute titre does not rule out Q fever because most cases seroconvert by third week.

- Rising antibody titre in paired serum samples taken 2–4 weeks apart may be demonstrated by micro- and capillary agglutination, CFT, neutralization test, IFT, ELISA and radio-immunoassay. During epizootics, haematoxylin stained phase I antigen is used to test samples of milk and serum (Luoto's capillary agglutination test). The first serum sample should be taken as early in infection as is possible. The indirect IFA IgG phase II is usually negative or has low titre, and the second sample shows a fourfold or higher titre in acute infections.
- In chronic infection, >1:800 phase I–IgG or higher than phase II–IgG antibodies plus a focus infection such as endocarditis is considered positive.

In acute infection, antibodies to phase II antigen are predominant, so titre is higher than the phase I antibodies. The titre barely decreases over 600 days and points to chronic infection. It is reverse in chronic infection.

IgM antibodies also appear nearly simultaneously with IgG and remain elevated for months or longer but has poor diagnostic value.

Seropositivity may be observed in otherwise healthy population, particularly those who are professionally exposed.

- Serology may also be used in epidemiological studies to search for the status of *C. burnetii* infection in animals (sentinel study).
- Skin test: An intradermal injection of extremely diluted inactivated vaccine (Coxevac) induces antigenic reaction in infected animals in a form of nodule of varying size. Test is easy and useful for application in rural areas (Porter et al. 2011).

52.5   Herd Screening

- Bulk tank milk-bulk tank milk sero-testing (e.g. ELISA) is useful for detecting infected herd and also the sanitary status of farms (Ruiz-Fons et al. 2011).

52.6   Checking Blood Donors

Blood donors are generally checked for the absence of any disease (no symptoms), acute or chronic. Q fever is asymptomatic in many adults during acute and chronic phase and they may have bacteraemia.

Seroprevalence of *C. burnetii* infection among blood donors has been reported from Germany, Spain, Turkey, Newfound land, France and the Netherlands. Detection of antibody indicates immunity and not infectivity. Increased titres of IgM and IgG titres in 38/942 donors tested in South France and 2/38 donors developed acute Q fever which was not diagnosed at the time of donation (Arbeitskreis Blut 2014). The exclusion criteria need to be made stringent.

52.7   Q Fever Management and Treatment

Q fever management based upon clinical evaluation and laboratory diagnosis has been recommended by CDC, USA (Anderson et al. 2013). Acute case is further evaluated for risk of chronic (endocarditis, vascular defects). Clinical and serological re-evaluation is recommended 'after six months in absence of risk'. Those classed as possible chronic cases should be re-evaluated after 3, 6, 12, 18 and 24 months. Those with clinical evidence of chronic Q fever, involvement of organ and laboratory evidence are treated for 18 months if native valve and 24 months if prosthetic valve is involved. The cases are monitored throughout the course of treatment. The treatment is discontinued after clinical recovery, and serological test demonstrates a decrease by fourfold phase I IgG antibody titre and negative phase II IgM. Serological monitoring every six months for a period of five years should be done for possible relapse.

Treatment should not be delayed waiting for serological report because seroconversion takes time. Treatment should not be discontinued on the basis of a negative acute specimen. Treatment for chronic Q fever should be started after confirmation. Drug of choice is doxycycline. A combination of doxycycline and hydroxychloroquine is preferred. Chloroquine is a lysosomotropic agent that raises phagolysosomal pH thus stopping replication of *C. burnetii*. Interferon IFNy has been successful in treating cases not responding to antibiotics. Alternate antibiotics that may be used are rifampin, erythromycin, clarithromycin and roxithromycin.

52.8   Control

It was experienced in the Netherlands that good monitoring and surveillance were important for assessing the magnitude of epidemic. Early diagnosis and treatment cut the transmission. Pasteurization of milk prevents per os infection in human.

A number of veterinary control measures were taken.

Vaccination of animals with Coxevac, culling of all pregnant sheep and goats and banning movement and breeding on infected farms and spreading of manure for at least 90 days controlled the epizootics in the Netherlands and consequently the epidemic in human beings. These measures were mandatory in farms with >50 animals.

Smaller herds may initiate action by detecting infection applying herd testing followed by detecting individual infected by skin testing. Culling of identified cases, vaccination of the rest, selective breeding, lime or calcium cyanide treatment of manure and restriction on the movement would be economical. Monitoring of the herd for elimination of infection and maintenance of 'infection-free' status should follow.

References

Álvarez-Alonso R, Zendoia II, Barandika JF, Jado I, Hurtado A et al (2020) Monitoring Coxiella burnetii infection in naturally infected dairy sheep flocks throughout four lambing seasons and investigation of viable bacteria. Front Vet Sci 7:352

Anderson A, Bijlmer H, Fournier PE, Graves S, Hartzell J et al (2013) Diagnosis and management of Q fever--United States, 2013: recommendations from CDC and the Q Fever Working Group. MMWR Recomm Rep 62(RR-03):1–30. Erratum in: MMWR Recomm Rep. 2013 Sep 6;62(35):730

Arbeitskreis Blut (2014) *Coxiella burnetii* – pathogenic agent of Q (Query) fever. Transfus Med Hemother 41:60–72

Bellabidi M, Benaissa MH, Bissati-Bouafia S, Harrat Z et al (2020) *Coxiella burnetii* in camels (*Camelus dromedarius*) from Algeria: seroprevalence, molecular characterization, and ticks (Acari: Ixodidae) vectors. Acta Trop 206:105443

Dhaka P, Malik SS, Yadav JP, Kumar M, Baranwal A et al (2019) Seroprevalence and molecular detection of coxiellosis among cattle and their human contacts in an organized dairy farm. J Infect Public Health 12(2):190–194

ECDC (2021) European Centre for Disease Prevention and Control. Q fever. In: ECDC (ed) Annual epidemiological report for 2019. ECDC, Stockholm

EFSA and ECDC (European Food Safety Authority and European Centre for Disease Prevention and Control) (2021) The European Union One Health 2019 Zoonoses Report. EFSA J 19(2):6406, 286 pp

Glazunova O, Roux V, Freylikman O, Sekeyova Z, Fournous G et al (2005) *Coxiella burnetii* genotyping. Emerg Infect Dis 11(8):1211–1217

Harris P, Eales KM, Squires R, Govan B, Norton R (2013) Acute Q fever in northern Queensland: variation in incidence related to rainfall and geographical location. Epidemiol Infect 141(5):1034–1038

Hornstra HM, Priestley RA, Georgia SM, Kachur S et al (2011) Rapid typing of *Coxiella burnetii*. PLoS ONE 6(11):e26201

Kampschreur LM, Dekker S, Hagenaars JC, Lestrade PJ, Renders NH et al (2012) Identification of risk factors for chronic Q fever, the Netherlands. Emerg Infect Dis 18(4):563–570

Karagiannis I, Schimmer B, Van Lier A, Timen A et al (2009) Investigation of a Q fever outbreak in a rural area of The Netherlands. Epidemiol Infect 137(9):1283–1294

Kilicoglu Y, Cagirgan AA, Serdar G, Kaya S, Durmaz Y, Gur Y (2020) Molecular investigation, isolation and phylogenetic analysis of *Coxiella burnetii* from aborted fetus and ticks. Comp Immunol Microbiol Infect Dis 73:101571

Klee SR, Tyczka J, Ellerbrok H, Franz T, Link S, Baljer G, Appel B (2006) Highly sensitive realtime PCR for specific detection and quantification of Coxiella burnetii. BMC Microbiol 6:2

Mahamat A, Edouard S, Demar M, Abboud P, Patrice JY et al (2013) Unique clone of Coxiella burnetii causing severe Q fever, French Guiana. Emerg Infect Dis 19(7):1102–1104

Marrie TJ (2003) *Coxiella burnetii* pneumonia. Eur Respir J 21:713–719

Martinez E, Cantet F, Fava L, Norville I, Bonazzi M (2014) Identification of OmpA, a *Coxiella burnetii* protein involved in host cell invasion, by multi-phenotypic high-content screening. PLoS Pathog 10(3):e1004013

Matsui T, Nakamoto T, Hayakawa K, Yamamoto K, Nakamura K et al (2019) Case report: two cases of acute Q fever from the same family who returned from Malawi to Japan. Am J Trop Med Hyg 101(6):1263–1264

Mioni MSR, Costa FB, Ribeiro BLD, Teixeira WSR et al (2020) *Coxiella burnetii* in slaughterhouses in Brazil: a public health concern. PLoS ONE 15(10):e0241246

Newton HJ, McDonough JA, Roy CR (2013) Effector protein translocation by the *Coxiella burnetii* Dot/Icm Type IV secretion system requires endocytic maturation of the pathogen-occupied vacuole. PLoS ONE 8(1):e54566

Porter SR, Czaplicki G, Mainil J, Guattéo R, Saegerman C (2011) Q Fever: current state of knowledge and perspectives of research of a neglected zoonosis. Int J Microbiol 2011:248418

Rijks JM, Roest HI, van Tulden PW, Kik MJ, IJzer J, Gröne A (2011) *Coxiella burnetii* infection in roe deer during Q fever epidemic, the Netherlands. Emerg Infect Dis 17(12):2369–2371

Roest HI, Tilburg JJ, van der Hoek W, Vellema P et al (2011) The Q fever epidemic in The Netherlands: history, onset, response and reflection. Epidemiol Infect 139(1):1–12

Roest HI, van Solt CB, Tilburg JJ, Klaassen CH, Hovius EK et al (2013) Search for possible additional reservoirs for human Q fever, The Netherlands. Emerg Infect Dis 19(5):834–835

Ruiz-Fons F, Astobiza I, Barandika JF, Juste RA, Hurtado A, García-Pérez AL (2011) Measuring antibody levels in bulk-tank milk as an epidemiological tool to search for the status of Coxiella burnetii in dairy sheep. Epidemiol Infect 139(10):1631–1636

Sahu R, Kale SB, Vergis J, Dhaka P, Kumar M, Choudhary M, Jain L et al (2018) Apparent prevalence and risk factors associated with occurrence of Coxiella burnetii infection in goats and humans in Chhattisgarh and Odisha, India. Comp Immunol Microbiol Infect Dis 60:46–51

Schimmer B, Notermans DW, Harms MG, Reimerink JH, Bakker J et al (2012) Low seroprevalence of Q fever in The Netherlands prior to a series of large outbreaks. Epidemiol Infect 140(1):27–35

van der Hoek W, Morroy G, Renders NH, Wever PC et al (2012) Epidemic Q fever in humans in the Netherlands. Adv Exp Med Biol 984:329–364

van Schaik EJ, Chen C, Mertens K, Weber MM, Samuel JE (2013) Molecular pathogenesis of the obligate intracellular bacterium *Coxiella burnetii*. Nat Rev Microbiol 11(8):561–573

Webster D, Haase D, Marrie TJ, Campbell N, Pettipas J, Davidson R, Hatchette TF (2009) Ovine-associated Q fever. Epidemiol Infect 137(5):744–751

Chapter 53
Tularemia

Synonyms

Pahvant Valley plague or deerfly fever (USA), Yato-byo or Ohara's disease (Japan), Lemming fever (Norway), Francis' disease, Market men's disease, Rabbit fever.

Tularemia

Tularemia is a bacterial disease of human and wild and domestic animals. It is a potentially fatal zoonotic disease if untreated. In man, it is characterized by sudden onset of high undulating fever, chills, fatigue, headache, pharyngitis and joint pain, dry cough and chest discomfort sometimes fatal pneumonia (if untreated), vomiting, abdominal pain, and diarrhoea and long course and longer convalescence.

53.1 Aetiology

Tularemia is caused by *Francisella tularensis*, which was first isolated from Tulare county of California in 1991 by Edward Fancis. It is a pleomorphic, bipolar, facultative intracellular, aerobic, small Gram-negative coccobacillus. The cell wall is rich in fatty acids and besieged by a semi-virulent capsule (Yeni et al. 2021). Low infective dose, high virulence, aerosol spread, long survival at low temperature in animal carcass, soil and water make it a select Tier 1 potential agent for bioterrorism and potential severe threat to public health and safety.

There are four subtypes of *F. tularensis*: *F. tularensis* subsp. *tularensis* (type A), *F. tularensis* subsp. *holarctica* (type B), *F. tularensis* subsp. *novicida* and *F. tularensis* subsp. *mediasiatica*. *F. tularensis* subsp. *tularensis* (type A) and *F. tularensis* subsp.

holarctica (type B) cause human tularaemia. *F. tularensis var novicida* is relatively non-virulent and may infect severely immunocompromised host. *F. tularensis var mediasiatica* is found primarily in Central Asian Republics in the former Union of Soviet Socialist Republics (Larson et al. 2020) has never been documented (Yeni et al. 2021).

The most virulent subspecies are *F. tularensis* subsp. *tularensis* and *F. tularensis* subsp. *holarctica.* There is an average nucleotide identity of 98–99% among the virulent species and subspecies including *F. tularensis* subsp. *novicida*, an opportunistic microbe. But the chromosomal disparities and the resultant differences in the genetic organization of the virulent subspecies contribute to differences in virulence (Larson et al. 2020).

Francisella tularensis uses type IV pili for binding to the host cells, breaks phagosomal compartment, evades phagocytosis, replicates intracellular and has type VI secretion system. It downregulates immune response.

53.2   Epidemiology

53.2.1   Distribution

Tularemia has been reported from most countries in the northern hemisphere, such as Nordic and Scandinavia countries, North America, Japan and Russia. Turkey, Yugoslavia, Spain, Kosovo and Switzerland have also reported. According to Larson et al. (2020), *F. tularensis* subsp. *tularensis* and *F. tularensis* subsp. *holarctica* have been reported from North America and the whole Northern hemisphere, respectively. *F. tularensis* subsp. *holarctica*, also known as type B, is found throughout the Northern Hemisphere (holarctic region), North America, Europe and Asia and is the leading cause of tularemia in Europe.

Tularemia has been reported from China and Japan (East Asia); Iran, Turkey (West Asia) and Kazakhstan, Uzbekistan and Turkmenistan (Central Asia); and Armenia and Azerbaijan (Caucasus nation).

53.2.2   Reservoirs

The range of hosts of *F. tularensis* is very wide covering more than 100 wildlife species and domestic animals and over 100 species of invertebrates (Yeni et al. 2021). The most important are Lagomorpha, Rodentia and Sciuromorph, Lagomorphs (cottontail rabbits), hares, jackrabbits, muskrats, beavers and a variety of rodents such as voles, field, mice, squirrels and lemmings, mink and fox. Sheep, cats, rabbits, dogs, pigs and horses are among the domesticated animals.

Infection in animals may be mild that recover without signs. Animal tularemia manifests in swollen glands, sudden onset of high fever, anorexia, lethargy, stiffness, reduced mobility, cough, increased rate of respiration, diarrhoea and frequent micturition. Severe cases end up in prostration and death within few hours to days. Recovery is associated with long-lasting immunity. Rapid diagnosis and treatment are effective. Reducing ticks may control.

The invertebrate reservoirs are ticks, mosquitoes, horseflies and fleas. It has been isolated from contaminated water and mud.

53.2.3   Modes of Transmission

It has a very wide host range and infects more than 100 species of wild and domestic vertebrates and over 100 species of invertebrates (Yeni et al. 2021). The infection is transmitted to susceptible host by a variety of arthropod vectors. The bacteria can survive for weeks outside mammalian hosts and have been recovered from grassland, haystack and water.

Tularensis is both direct zoonosis and also metazoonosis. Following modes of transmission have been observed:

- Direct or indirect contact with animals is most common, (a) handling/processing of carcass of infected hares and (b) bites by cats and squirrel.
- Arthropod vectors: Important tick vectors are *Dermacentor variabilis*, *D. andersoni*, *D. nuttalli*, *D. marginatus*, *D. reticulatus*, *Ixodes ricinus*, *Haemaphysalis concinna* and *Amblyomma americana* ticks. Other insect vectors are mosquitoes (*Aedes*, *Culex* and *Anopheles*), flea, lice, horseflies and deerflies.
- Aquatic environment and water: Ingestion of contaminated food or water/contact with aquatic environment.
- Inhalation of infectious aerosol, environmental (landscapers, lawn mowers, bush cutters).

Laboratory-acquired (Staples et al. 2006) infections require relatively higher dose. The route of entry often decides the clinical manifestation; *F. tularensis* entering through skin or oral route causes lymphadenitis and through inhalation causes pneumonia. Transmission from person to person is not known.

53.2.4   International Animal Trade Spread Tularemia

Avashia et al. (2004) brought out evidence for prairie-dog-to-human transmission associated with exotic pet trade. An outbreak of fatal oropharyngeal tularemia occurred among wild caught and commercially reared prairie dogs for wild pet trade. The agent was *F. tularensis* type B. Petersen et al. (2004) traced the infection originating from this source to pet shops in the Czech Republic and Texas through the infected pet trade. Isolates were identified as *F. tularensis* subsp. *holarctica* (type B).

53.2.5   Tularemia in the USA

Tularemia occurred mostly in hunters of rabbits and hares and so known as rabbit fever. Rabbits and hares are carriers/reservoirs. Tularemia emerged in the USA with the import of rabbits (*Sylvilagus floridanus*) in the late 1950s. Beginning with few cases, it became much more common in the early part of twentieth century with almost 1000 cases/year reduced down to 250. Tularemia became endemic (Yeni et al. 2021).

F. tularensis subspecies *tularensis* (type A) and *F. tularensis* subspecies *holarctica* (type B) account for almost all human cases of tularemia. *F. tularensis* subsp. *tularensis* has two distinct subpopulations—A. I (A-east; prevalent in the east and central) and A. II (A-west, prevalent in the west) in the USA. *F. tularensis* subsp. *tularensis* (type A) and *F. tularensis* subsp. *holarctica* (type B) are the main causes of tularemia in the USA. *F. tularensis* subsp. *holarctica*, also known as type B or biovar *palaearctica*, is generally less virulent than *F. tularensis* subsp. *tularensis* (*nearctica*, biovar type A). It causes severe and fatal illness in humans and rabbits in *North America*. It is able to produce acid from glycerol. The type B does not produce acid from glycerol and rarely causes death in humans. Type A-east and type B isolates were more likely than type A-west isolates to be recovered from the blood and lung. Type A-west isolates were more likely to be recovered from lymph nodes. Type B is most frequently isolated from rodent species, including muskrats (*Ondatra zibethicus*), mice (*Mus musculus*), beaver (*Castor canadensis*), voles (*Microtus* spp.) and water voles (*Arvicola terrestris*). Most type A infections were associated with lagomorphs. Both types A and B infections were associated with exposure to cats in the USA. Both type A-east and type B human infection were tick-transmitted. Biting flies transmitted type A-west (Staples et al. 2006).

Most cases of tularemia occur during summer and fall and are associated with arthropod bite transmission. Infections acquired by handling of animals/hunting/other exposure-related activities do not follow seasonality.

Tularemia is endemic in Martha's Vineyard, an island off the coast of Cape Cod, Massachusetts. Two outbreaks of tularemia occurred, 1978 and 2000. The 2000 outbreak occurred in summer 2000 and had 11/15 pneumonia cases. A case control epidemiological study demonstrated that lawn-mowing and bush-cutting were the risk factors (odds ratio 6.7). They pent spent more hours per week (exposure period) in the activity. A case control serological study was conducted. More landscapers (12% or 9.1%) were seropositive compared to single from the control group, and the number of lawns mowed was the factor most robustly associated. Increased participation in potential aerosol-generating activities and absence of evidence of exposure to arthropod and animal reservoirs suggested persistence of *F. tularensis* in aerosol created during mowing activities (Feldman et al. 2003).

Tularemia is endemic also in Canada.

53.2.6 Tularemia in Europe

Tularemia is widely distributed throughout Europe, including Russia and east European countries. Some Nordic countries, such as Sweden and Finland, are endemic. Countries known to be free are Albania, Greece, Iceland, the UK, Ireland and Liechtenstein.

53.2.6.1 Germany

In North Rhine-Westphalia, Germany, tularemia among hunters of hare was reported by Otto et al. (2015). The isolates from human and hares were identified as *F. tularensis* subsp. *holarctica*, FTN002–00 genetic subclade confirming hare-to-human transmission. Those infected through aerosol had respiratory symptoms, and others who skinned and processed the hunted hare had lesions of the skin and lymphadenitis.

53.2.6.2 Sweden

Tularemia has been known in Sweden since 1931 and is a notifiable disease since 1968. A case control epidemiological study by Eliasson et al. (2002) in endemic and non-endemic areas of Sweden identified three risk factors. The odds ratio for mosquito bites was 8.8, for farming in the endemic areas 3.2 and owning cats 2.5. Tularemia is endemic in central part of Sweden with only sporadic cases in other areas. The outbreak in the year 2000 reported large number (40%) of cases from south of tularemia-endemic areas. Farming and time spent in it appeared as a risk factor only in the disease-endemic area where small plots of arable land were interspersed in heavy forest. The reservoirs seem not to have come into contact with human settlement. The outbreak in 2003 in Sweden was investigated by Payne et al. (2005). It involved 698 cases with increased number from non-endemic areas, considered as an emerging zoonosis. The number of cases appeared ascending in July, peaking in August and September and tapering in November–December. The spatial distribution suggested insect bites as a route of infection. The highest number of cases was in the working age groups 45–64, followed by 25–44, 65–79 and 7–17 years reflecting exposure during outdoor activities/works in farms and gardens in rural areas. Epidemic may be traced to concurrent epizootic in rodents and lagomorphs. Population bloom of rodents and lagomorphs may be precipitating factor (Payne et al. 2005). In 2019, Sweden experienced its largest outbreak of tularemia in over 50 years. The number of cases exceeded in any single year since the 1960s and from the whole of Europe during a normal year. Dryselius et al. (2019) reported that the Public Health Agency of Sweden received a report of increasing number of tularemia cases in Gävleborg, a county in Central Sweden. The increasing cases/week peaked at 150, and by October 6, total number reached 979; 98% were registered since 24 July with 734 lab-confirmed cases—53% male and 47% female with a median age of males 52 years and females 55 years. The 52–55 years of age corresponds to the working age group engaged in farm/garden/outdoor activities. It appears that women were attracted to 'mushroom-picking' in the tularemia-risk areas and got infected (2019 was a good mushroom year). Mosquito-transmitted ulceroglandular tularemia cases begin reporting by the end of July or August, peak at the end of August or in September and then decline in December. The outbreak followed this pattern. The weather conditions in 2019, relatively wet spring and a mild summer and autumn, favoured mosquitoes and longer mosquitoes-host animal transmission. *Francisella tularensis* was detected in the mosquito species *Aedes cinereus* near the golf course in Ljusdal. These strongly suggested that the outbreak was caused predominantly by mosquitoe transmission.

53.2.6.3   Kosovo

Epidemiological investigation of an outbreak of tularemia in Kosovo suggested that the source of infection was rodents, whose population had exploded in fields, gardens, homes and outbuildings. The food and water in the area were contaminated with rodents' excreta. Cluster of patients reported fever, pharyngitis and pronounced cervical lymphadenitis confirmed by laboratory (Reintjes et al. 2002).

53.2.6.4   Turkey

Waterborne human tularemia (*F. tularensis* subsp. *holarctica*) spreads through contact with contaminated water. The bacteria survive and remain infectious in water through amoeba and reservoir hosts, beavers, muskrats, lemmings and water vole. The reservoirs shed bacteria in urine and faeces and contaminate water. The period of survival and infectivity in water may be over a month. An outbreak and sporadic cases were recorded around Bursa, Turkey, since November 1988. Helvaci et al. (2000) reported the observation based on 205 cases of tularemia. Most cases of both sexes were young and suffered with oropharyngeal form. Tularemia is waterborne in this region. Breakdown of health services during war affecting quality of drinking water led to an outbreak. It is a major public health problem as both sporadic and outbreaks have been reported worldwide in the last decades in countries such as Turkey, Kosovo, Bulgaria, Georgia, Norway, Sweden, Italy and Germany involving even >100 people. Ingestion and also various usages of water or aquatic activities like swimming, canyoning and fishing pose risk of waterborne tularemia (Yeni et al. 2021).

53.2.6.5 Spain

Contamination of river water with sewage, infection of fishes, its transfer to fishermen and fish processors (occupational) and to consumers in Spain was revealed in an interesting study carried out by Anda et al. (2001). Cray fish-associated outbreak of ulcero-glandular tularemia is caused by *F. tularensis* biovar *palaearctica*. Odds ratio (OR) of 39.7 for injury while handling of crayfish, 29.1 for catching or emptying net and 38.8 for cleaning were recorded. Washing hands with soap after cleaning reduced it to 0.3. *F. tularensis* was detected in the crayfish stomach and pancreas. Crayfish is known for bioaccumulation of toxins. Samples of river water, liver and crayfish four weeks after the outbreak were negative. Authors alerted on two accounts: (a) commercialization of crayfish farming and (b) *F. tularensis* is listed as an agent for bioterrorism.

53.2.6.6 Bulgaria

In the 1997–2005 tularemia outbreak in Bulgaria, 285 people were affected. Amplified fragment-length polymorphism typing of the ten isolates from humans, a tick, a hare and water and the strain Srebarna 19 of *F. tularensis* suggested that a new genetic variant was the cause. Patients suffered with oculoglandular, ulceroglandular and oropharyngeal (96.5%) forms. Isolates from the oropharyngeal patient and well water suggested the outbreak was waterborne. Rodents and/or their excreta could be the source contaminating water (Kantardjiev et al. 2006).

53.3 Symptoms

F. tularensis is a highly infectious agent, capable of infecting both man and animals via respiratory route. As few as ten organisms are enough to cause severe disease and death in human and one organism in experimental guinea pig (Hood 2009). Tularemia used to be fatal during the pre-antibiotic era. Its diagnosis is difficult as the clinical presentation is confounding. This is particular so with typhoidal and pneumonic form. Advancements in laboratory diagnosis have eased the situation. Serological diagnosis is resorted, but the appearance of antibody takes 3–4 weeks. Blood culture is possible but is not frequently used. Blood cultures may be positive after the incubation period.

Incubation period usually ranges between three and five days, may be as long as 10–21 days. Depending upon the portal of entry of *Francisella tularensis*, the tissue and organs are affected. The clinical forms are dependent upon the site and the mode of infection and are as follows: (a) primary pulmonary, (b) typhoid (systemic), (c) oropharyngeal, (d) ulceroglandular and (e) oculoglandular. Aerosol infection in farm and laboratory workers causes bronchopneumonia and pneumonia. Systemic infection is also known as typhoidal. Oropharyngeal form results from ingestion of meat of infected animals or contaminated water. It is characterized by fever, pharyngitis, ulcer in the mouth and pharynx, cervical lymphadenitis and suppuration and gastroenteritis. The ulceroglandular form occurs when the bacterium enters skin through insect bites/cuts/scratches and necrotic ulcers at the site of entry of pathogen develop. This may be accompanied by swelling of regional lymph nodes which may ulcerate. Lower eyelid is affected in the oculoglandular form.

The disease may be acute and fulminant if not specifically treated. The course of disease may be protracted and debilitating. Convalescence period runs in weeks to months with intermittent bouts of fever. Han et al. (2004) described a case of tularemia with peritonitis developing in a 50-year-old man soon after diagnosis of stomach cancer with metastasis. *Francisella tularensis* subsp. *holarctica* was isolated from ascitic fluid and identified by sequencing analysis of the 16S rDNA. The authors consider that most cases of tularemia occur in old age, alcoholic, diabetic, immunocompromised, transplant or deficient (AIDS) cases.

53.4 Diagnosis

The diagnosis of tularemia mostly made on basis of positive serology in combination with clinical and epidemiological correlates. History, signs and symptoms are helpful guides.

- Bacteriological culture and identification
- Biological test in guinea pig
- Direct examination of smears from exudates by IFT
- Skin test with ether-extracted antigen
- Serologic tests like agglutination and haemagglutination with patients' sera pre-adsorbed with *Brucella* antigen

53.5 Treatment

Aminoglycosides, tetracycline, quinolones and chloramphenicol are frequently used in the treatment of tularemia (Caspar and Maurin 2017).

Streptomycin, gentamicin, doxycycline and ciprofloxacin can be used for treatment usually for 10–21 days.

53.6 Prevention

- Prevention requires vector control, which can be done at individual level (protective clothing, repellents, etc.) and/or population level (fogging, sprays of insecticides).
- Environmental measures to prevent contamination of water.

- Occupational tularemia cases have been reported among laboratory workers, farmers, veterinarians, sheep workers, hunters or trappers, cooks or meat handlers and landscapers. They need to be made aware of the protective measures, for example, use of mask for landscapers, mowers and others and personal protective measures for handlers of fish, animal carcass, excreta, etc.
- Immunization of high-risk groups like laboratory workers and hunters.

53.6.1 Sentinel Survey

Raccoons (*Procyon lotor*) and skunks (*Mephitis mephitis*) have been suggested as sentinel animals for tularemia even though their reservoir capacity was unclear (Berrada et al. 2006).

References

Anda P, Segura del Pozo J, Díaz García JM, Escudero R, García Peña FJ et al (2001) Waterborne outbreak of tularemia associated with crayfish fishing. Emerg Infect Dis 7(3 Suppl):575–582

Avashia SB, Petersen JM, Lindley CM, Schriefer ME, Gage KL, Cetron M et al (2004) First reported prairie dog–to-human tularemia transmission, Texas, 2002. Emerg Infect Dis 10(3):483–486

Berrada ZL, Goethert HK, Telford SR III (2006) Raccoons and skunks as sentinels for enzootic tularemia. Emerg Infect Dis 12(6):1019–1021

Caspar Y, Maurin M (2017) *Francisella tularensis* susceptibility to antibiotics: a comprehensive review of the data obtained *in vitro* and in animal models. Front Cell Infect Microbiol 7:122

Dryselius R, Hjertqvist M, Mäkitalo S, Lindblom A, Lilja T, Eklöf D, Lindström A (2019) Large outbreak of tularaemia, central Sweden, July to September 2019. Euro Surveill 24(42):1900603

Eliasson H, Lindbäck J, Nuorti JP, Arneborn M, Giesecke J, Tegnell A (2002) The 2000 tularemia outbreak: a case-control study of risk factors in disease-endemic and emergent areas, Sweden. Emerg Infect Dis 8(9):956–960

Feldman KA, Stiles-Enos D, Julian K, Matyas BT, Telford SR 3rd, Chu MC et al (2003) Tularemia on Martha's Vineyard: seroprevalence and occupational risk. Emerg Infect Dis 9(3):350–354

Han XY, Ho LX, Safdar A (2004) *Francisella tularensis* peritonitis in stomach cancer patient. Emerg Infect Dis 10(12):2238–2240

Helvaci S, Gedikoğlu S, Akalin H, Oral HB (2000) Tularemia in Bursa, Turkey: 205 cases in ten years. Eur J Epidemiol 16(3):271–276

Hood AM (2009) The effect of open-air factors on the virulence and viability of airborne *Francisella tularensis*. Epidemiol Infect 137(6):753–761

Kantardjiev T, Ivanov I, Velinov T, Padeshki P, Popov B, Nenova R et al (2006) Tularemia outbreak, Bulgaria, 1997–2005. Emerg Infect Dis 12(4):678–680

Larson MA, Sayood K, Bartling AM, Meyer JR, Starr C et al (2020) Differentiation of *Francisella tularensis* subspecies and subtypes. J Clin Microbiol 58(4):e01495–e01419

Otto P, Kohlmann R, Müller W, Julich S, Geis G et al (2015) Hare-to-human transmission of Francisella tularensis subsp. holarctica, Germany. Emerg Infect Dis 21(1):153–155

Payne L, Arneborn M, Tegnell A, Giesecke J (2005) Endemic tularemia, Sweden, 2003. Emerg Infect Dis 11(9):1440–1442

Petersen JM, Schriefer ME, Carter LG, Zhou Y, Sealy T, Bawiec D et al (2004) Laboratory analysis of tularemia in wild-trapped, commercially traded prairie dogs, Texas, 2002. Emerg Infect Dis 10(3):419–425

Reintjes R, Dedushaj I, Gjini A et al (2002) Tularemia outbreak investigation in Kosovo: case control and environmental studies. Emerg Infect Dis 8(1):69–73

Staples JE, Kubota KA, Chalcraft LG, Mead PS, Petersen JM (2006) Epidemiologic and molecular analysis of human tularemia, United States, 1964-2004. Emerg Infect Dis 12(7):1113–1118

Yeni DK, Büyük F, Ashraf A, Shah MSUD (2021) Tularemia: a re-emerging tick-borne infectious disease. Folia Microbiol (Praha) 66(1):1–14

Chapter 54
Psittacosis

Synonyms

Ornithosis, Parrot fever, Chlamydiosis.

Psittacosis is an infectious zoonotic disease manifesting as mild, non-specific flu-like symptoms. It is caused by *Chlamydia psittaci* and is transmitted from infected birds. *C. psittaci* affects animal health and is economically relevant. Psittacosis is referred to infection transmitted from birds of the family Psittacidae. Ornithosis refers to infection acquired from other birds, domestic and wild. Both are considered the same. *C. psittaci* is listed as a potential bioweapon.

54.1 Aetiology

Chlamydiaceae family, genus *Chlamydia*, are Gram-negative obligatory intracellular coccoid bacteria with a wide range of hosts. The growth cycle and hosts of different genotypes have been summarized by Radomski et al. (2016).

54.1.1 Growth (EB-RB) Cycle

Chlamydia spp. are biphasic and have a metabolically inactive, infectious form, the elementary body (EB), and a metabolically active, non-infectious form, the reticulate body (RB). Prior to activation of the type III secretory system (T3SS), the EBs attach the surface of hosts' cells. Effector bacterial proteins, such as TARP, are injected into the cytoplasm triggering a process for active endocytosis of *C. psittaci*. Preloaded effectors are further injected that protect *Chlamydia* from lysosomal

© Springer Nature Singapore Pte Ltd. 2024
K. G. Narayan et al., *Handbook of Management of Zoonoses*,
https://doi.org/10.1007/978-981-99-9885-2_54

Table 54.1 Genotypes of *C. psittaci* and respective hosts

Genotype	Hosts
A	Endemic in psittacine birds and causes respiratory disease in humans
B	Pigeons, chickens, passerines and wild birds
C and D	Waterfowls and poultry (chicken, turkeys)
E	Pigeons, waterfowl, turkeys and human
F	Parakeets
G	Red-tailed hawk
WC	Cattle
M56	Rodents
E/B	Ducks

fusion. The chlamydial vacuole (inclusion) interacts with the Golgi and actively recruits lipids for the inclusion membrane. EBs differentiate into RBs (the metabolically active form of *Chlamydia*). RBs replicate actively by binary fission in inclusion growth. The T3SS is active in RBs. Chlamydial effectors are secreted in the host cytoplasm. The Inc proteins are inserted into the inclusion membrane. RBs re-differentiate into infectious EBs at the end of the cycle.

54.1.2   Hosts

Avian chlamydiosis is caused by *C. psittaci*. *C. gallinacean*, *C. avium*, *C. ibidis* and *C. buteonis* are new avian chlamydial species. Pigeons and psittacines commonly harbour *C. avium*. A flock and also the same bird may harbour more than one species of *Chlamydia*. *C. gallinacean* has been reported in asymptomatic poultry flocks and linked to chlamydiosis in workers.

   C. psittaci possesses several such properties that make it an efficient zoonotic pathogen. These are a wide range of avian and non-avian hosts, rapid and efficient invasion of target cells and efficient distribution within the host, all combined leading to a systemic infection and even fulminant psittacosis (Table 54.1). The bacterium is able to manage immune response and may be associated with cancer.

54.2   Epidemiology

54.2.1   Prevalence

Psittacosis is reportable in most countries. It occurs locally as sporadic outbreaks. Most cases of psittacosis are sporadic occupational infections. Young- and middle-aged adults are commonly affected.

Psittacosis goes undiagnosed and unreported under all of pneumonia cases. The real disease burden is largely underestimated. During 2003–2014, 112 human cases of psittacosis were reported to the Centres for Disease Control (Balsamo et al. 2017). According to Vande Weygaerde et al. (2018), only ten cases/year are reported in Belgium despite a very high prevalence in poultry. There is a rapid growth of psittacine bird population in Egypt. Available information on chlamydial infection in birds and human are few (Abd El-Ghany 2020).

54.2.2 Common Source and Risk Groups

C. psittaci infections occur in 30 different bird orders. *Psittacidae* (which include parakeets, parrots, cockatoos and lories) and Columbiformes (pigeons) seem to be most commonly affected. Exposure to infected pet birds like cockatiels, parakeets and macaws generally accounts for most of human cases.

Psittacosis in humans contracted from turkeys and ducks is often as severe as at contracted from psittacine birds. High-risk groups include bird owners, pet shop employees handling wild birds, bird's fanciers, pigeon fanciers, zookeepers, veterinarians and those working in poultry-processing plants, landscapers and diagnostic laboratory workers.

54.2.3 Non-avian Source

Chan et al. (2017) made an epidemiological study of a cluster of cases in a veterinary school and a case in the local stud after the New South Wales Health notified it in November 2014. Five of the nine people exposed to foetal membrane of the mare fell sick with psittacosis. Two had to be hospitalized. In contrast to the RR = 0.5 for contact with birds, RR = 11.77 was observed for direct contact with mare's foetal membrane. The odd value for manipulation of foetal membrane was 2.33. The risk of exposure was higher with direct contact with foetal membrane than with manipulation. Other risk factors were ruled out. The clinical presentation of cases was consistent with those reported for psittacosis.

This outbreak linked to mares (non-avian host) questions the speculation that 'passages of *C. psittaci* through non-avian hosts might result in a striking reduction in or loss of virulence (non-avian *C. psittaci* strains belong to risk group 2, whereas avian strains are classified in risk group 3)'.

54.2.4 Avian Chlamydiosis

Chlamydia psittaci infection or avian chlamydiosis in birds constitutes the source of human infection. The bacteria are shed in faeces and nasal discharge and remain infectious for several months. Infection in birds may be latent. The bacteria remain quiescent. When such birds are exposed to stress, the bacteria are activated. The latent infection turns patent and bacteria are shed. Birds are highly mobile, fly to long distance and hence can spread *C. psittaci* widely.

According to Abd El-Ghany (2020), most chlamydial infection is recorded in Psittaciformes, Passeriformes, Galliformes, Columbiformes and Anseriformes. Over 465 avian species including companion, domestic and wild birds as well as 30 different orders of birds, are susceptible. *C. psittaci* infects pet birds, domestic poultry species and wild birds, particularly *Psittacidae* (parrots, parakeets, cockatoos, cockatiels, amazon parrots and macaws) and *Columbiformes* (pigeons and doves). Zoo, fancy or pet birds are very susceptible and can transmit the infection to human and other domestic birds. Captive parrots are the main global reservoir of *C. psittaci*. Wild and domestic, pet birds and poultry are affected. These may get infected from parrots, cockatiels, parakeets, macaws, canaries, pigeons, chickens, ducks and turkeys.

C. psittaci infection in birds is systemic. The incubation period may be 3 days to several weeks. Infection can be inapparent, severe, acute or chronic. The infected birds may show signs of poor appetite, loss of weight and inflammation of eyes (runny eyes). The breathing is difficult. The droppings are watery and green urates. The shedding of bacteria is intermittent or sometimes continuous for weeks to months. Th rate of shedding increases with stress like transport, high temperature, overcrowding and reproductive activities.

The bacteria can remain infective for several months if protected by organic debris like litter and faeces. Infection in birds is transmitted either by inhalation or ingestion through soiled feathers, vertically through eggs and contact mostly from parents to young. Insects, mites and lice may help in mechanical transmission/spread.

The avian strains of *C. psittaci* infect mammals (such as sheep, goats, pigs, dogs and rabbits) including humans.

54.3 Mode of Infection

Birds to human through mouth-to-beak contact, bites from infected birds, handling plumage or tissues of dead birds, aerosol from feather dust, faeces, respiratory discharges of infected birds and rarely and human-to-human transmission may occur.

Recent reports suggest that the exposure to infected animals (not only birds) can cause psittacosis (Abd El-Ghany 2020). Exposure to foetal membranes of a mare caused a cluster of cases among veterinarians (Chan et al. 2017). The odd values for

direct contact with foetal membrane were 11.77 (95% CI 1.02–∞) and for manipulation of foetal membrane 2.33 (95% CI 0.99–5.49).

After entry into human host, the bacterium spreads via the bloodstream to the
reticuloendothelial system. *C. psittaci* is able to invade virtually any type of cell
(e.g. macrophages, epithelial cells, fibroblasts).

54.4 Symptoms

The incubation period ranges between 5 and 19 days. The infection ranges from
more common asymptomatic through a brief self-limiting flu-like symptoms to less
common severe mainly atypical pneumonia. Before the advent of antimicrobial
agents, 15–20% human respiratory infections with *Chlamydia* spp. ended fatally
(Balsamo et al. 2017). The duration of illness may be 3 weeks.

The onset of high fever is abrupt and accompanied with chills, arthralgia, myalgia, fatigue and diarrhoea. Initial symptoms mimic typhoid. A pulse-temperature
dissociation (fever without increased pulse rate) may be observed. There is splenomegaly towards the end of the week. Other symptoms may be bleeding from the
nose, conjunctivitis and appearance of skin lesions—rose spots/Horder's spot.
Pneumonia suggestive of severe lung infection appear. Severe psittacosis cases
complain of headache (suggesting meningitis) and nuchal rigidity and may develop
stupor and coma.

In the second week of illness, there is continuous high fever, headache, sore
throat, pharyngitis, cough and dyspnoea. Severe cases may require intensive care in
hospital. Fatality is <1% of cases.

Clinical diagnosis is based on respiratory symptoms, splenomegaly with or without epistaxis and patchy infiltration (seen on chest X-ray).

Likely serious complications are inflammation of the heart (endocarditis, myocarditis), liver, joints, brain and keratoconjunctivitis.

Vande Weygaerde et al. (2018) presented a case as an 82-year-old lady suffering
with fever (up to 39 °C) for a week, myalgia, generalized skin rash, oedema of
hands and feet and general weakness. She had bronchitis and non-productive cough.

She had been keeping a small parakeet (*Pyrrhura molinae molinae*) as a pet for
over 10 years. The bird did not show any signs of illness nor had he been ill in the
past. C-reactive protein, ESR and liver enzymes were elevated/increased with limited leukocytosis. Imaging showed diffuse patchy infiltrates on both lungs.

Imaging was compatible with an atypical infectious pneumonia. Aetiologies for
atypical pneumonia were ruled out. She had a history of contact with psittacine
birds. The nasopharyngeal swab and faeces of her pet bird tested *C. psittaci*-PCR
positive. The presence of *C. psittaci* genotype A in both the patient and the pet bird
confirmed the zoonotic infection.

An emerging pathology *C. psittaci* triggered lymphoma recorded in the
Netherlands, the East Coast of the USA and Germany. *C. psittaci* has been reported

as a potential trigger for ocular adnexal MALT (mucosa-associated lymphoid tissue) lymphoma.

54.5   Diagnosis

Clinical laboratory investigation shows normal to marked leucocytosis, elevated aspartate transaminase, ESR and C-protein.

Epidemiological—history of exposure to bird—is an important clue. However, Chan et al. (2017) observed equine-linked psittacosis and cited other reports where chlamydial species causing community-acquired pneumonia had no evidence of contact with birds.

Specific diagnosis is based on the following:

- Microbiological culture of patient's respiratory excretions/secretions/bronchial lavage. Biosafety level 3 facility is required. Specimens may be patient's sputum, pleural fluid or clotted blood during acute illness and before treatment with antimicrobial agent.
- Serological tests (e.g. CFT, IFT, ELISA) increase in specific (*C. psittaci*) antibody titres or fourfold increase in antibodies in paired sera samples collected 2–4 weeks apart, ideally 21 days apart.
- Histological—for typical inclusions called 'Leventhal-Cole-Lillie bodies' seen in the macrophages in bronchial lavage fluid.
- PCR on respiratory swab specimen.

Psittacosis is a notifiable disease in most countries because of a zoonoses of public health significance. Specific and rapid diagnostic test is required for tracing the source and preventing further spread. *C. psittaci*-PCR has been developed for this. Specific real-time PCR on a human respiratory sample enables correct diagnosis, the correct treatment modality and the source of infection (Vande Weygaerde et al. 2018). It helps in understanding of the epidemiology and clinical impact of this bacterium in animals and humans particularly in outbreaks.

54.6   Treatment

Chlamydia psittaci are sensitive to both macrolides and tetracyclines. However, tetracyclines are the drugs of choice, unless contraindicated. Macrolides are the drug of choice for children aged <8 years; however, tetracyclines could be considered when the benefits outweigh the risks, such as in life-threatening conditions or when macrolide failure is suspected (CDC 2022).

54.7   Control

The infection in pet birds and domestic poultry can be controlled by isolating infected birds, taking help of veterinary services for testing, treatment and other control measures that prevent spread of chlamydiosis.

There is no vaccine. Treatment or extermination of avian reservoir is recommended to prevent further spreading.

Isolation in a clean cage, proper husbandry and doxycycline for 21–30 days is recommended in relation to potential outbreak. PCR testing of samples should monitor the progress. The effective treatment period has not been scientifically established.

54.8   Prevention

Do not aerosolize while sweeping, brushing and cleaning bird cages. Burn or double-bag waste for disposal. Disinfectants with active ingredients like quaternary ammonium compounds, 3% hydrogen peroxide, isopropyl alcohol, alcoholic iodine solutions, 70% ethanol and household bleach (diluted to 1% sodium hypochlorite) may be used.

Use biosecurity measures to prevent infection in birds. Education and awareness programmes for those at risk should emphasize wearing protective clothing including gloves, eyewear, a disposable surgical cap and a properly fitted respirator with N95 or higher rating, washing hands with water and soap after being in contact with birds or their droppings.

Quarantine and testing of imported birds are critical to prevent introduction of the disease.

In the cohort study on outbreak of psittacosis, Chan et al. (2017) observed that none of the cohort had used mask or protective eyewear although had put on gloves, and 5/9 suffered; two were hospitalized. *The US Compendium of Measures to Control Chlamydophila psittaci Infection recommends the donning of PPE when handling potentially infected birds and using a biological safety cabinet and other strategies to prevent aerosolization of infectious particles, when performing necropsies of potentially infected birds.*

The same should be followed in veterinary practices, especially while examining foetal membranes.

Psittacosis is a public health problem. The vast number of bird reservoirs and the reports of non-avian animal exposures causing psittacosis makes it a serious veterinary public problem requiring an expanded health programme, such as one health.

The US Compendium of Measures to Control Chlamydophila psittaci Infection offers information and guidance regarding human illness, including diagnosis and treatment with the purpose of guiding public health officials, physicians, veterinarians, the pet bird industry and others concerned with the control of *C. psittaci* infection and the protection of public health.

References

Abd El-Ghany WA (2020) Avian chlamydiosis: a world-wide emerging and public health threat. Adv Anim Vet Sci 8(s2):82–97

Balsamo G, Maxted AM, Midla JW, Murphy JM, Wohrle R et al (2017) Compendium of measures to control *Chlamydia psittaci* infection among humans (psittacosis) and pet birds (avian chlamydiosis). J Avian Med Surg 31(3):262–282

CDC   (2022).   https://www.cdc.gov/pneumonia/atypical/psittacosis/hcp/diagnosis-treatment-prevention.html

Chan J, Doyle B, Branley J, Sheppeard V, Gabor M et al (2017) An outbreak of psittacosis at a veterinary school demonstrating a novel source of infection. One Health 3:29–33

Radomski N, Einenkel R, Müller A, Knittler MR (2016) Chlamydia–host cell interaction not only from a bird's eye view: some lessons from *Chlamydia psittaci*. FEBS Lett 590:3920–3940

Vande Weygaerde Y, Versteele C, Thijs E, De Spiegeleer A et al (2018) An unusual presentation of a case of human psittacosis. Respir Med Case Rep 23:138–142

Chapter 55
African Tick Bite Fever

Synonyms
African Tick typhus.

African tick bite fever (ATBF) is a disease characterized by an acute febrile illness accompanied frequently by headache, myalgia of prominent neck muscle, inoculation eschars and regional lymphadenitis.

Tick bite fever (TBF) was reported in Southern Africa in 1911. This differed from Boutonneuse fever (BF) discovered in Tunisia, North Africa, in 1910 in severity and epidemiology. The latter is more severe. The causative agent of TBF was identified as *R. africae*. Boutonneuse fever is caused by *R. conorii*. While TBF was associated with travel to grasslands and game parks, BF occurred in peri-urban or peri-domestic settings and association with dog ticks, *Rhipicephalus sanguineus*, *Rhipicephalus simus* and *Haemaphysalis leachi*.

In the 1990s, TBF cases had history of bites of the tick *Amblyomma hebraeum* that was predominant in Zimbabwe. In 1992, DNA extract from blood sample from a 36-year-old women resident of a small town in south-east Zimbabwe who was hospitalized with symptoms now described as characteristic of ATBF was positive for rickettsia now named as *R. africae*. This isolate was same as those collected from *A. hebraeum* (Mazhetese et al. 2021).

55.1 Aetiology

The causative agent *Rickettsia africae* is an obligate intracellular Gram-negative, coccobacillus. It has an outer slime layer and a trilaminar cell wall. The latter contains lipopolysaccharide antigens that are immunogenic and responsible for cross-reaction with other rickettsia. The outer membrane protein A (rOmpA) and B (rOmpB) are species-specific protein antigens.

55.2   Epidemiology

55.2.1   Distribution

R. africae was first reported from a patient in Guadeloupe in the West Indies in 1998. Since then, it has been detected in *A. variegatum* in eight additional territories and countries in the Caribbean including Martinique, Dominica, Montserrat, Nevis, St. Kitts, St. Lucia, Antigua and the US Virgin Islands. The rate of infection of ticks by *R. africae* on these islands is high (7–62%) posing a potential threat of acquisition of *R. africae* infection by travellers, hunters and military persons deployed to the endemic sub-Saharan areas (Parola et al. 2013). ATBF remains the most common tickborne rickettsiosis in sub-Saharan Africa. Out of 34 French tourists returning from South Africa, 10 suffered with ABTF (Consigny et al. 2005).

55.2.2   Vector

According to Parola et al. (2013), *Amblyomma* (4 spp.), *Rhipicephalus* (5 spp.) and *Hyalomma impeltatum* are the tick vectors. *A. variegatum* (the tropical bont tick) and *A. hebraeum* (the southern African bont tick) are principal vectors. Generally, they live in tall grass or bush. These are three-host ticks, and all stages (larvae, nymphs and adults) have been proved to be potential vectors of *Rickettsiae. These maintain R. africae* through transovarial and trans-stadial transmission through two generations. In Southern Africa, *A. hebraeum* is primarily distributed. In West, Central and Eastern Africa and the eastern Caribbean, *A. variegatum* is predominantly distributed. It is widely distributed, found in Zambia, north-eastern Botswana, the Caprivi Strip of Namibia, Angola, north-western Zimbabwe and Central and Northern Mozambique, Madagascar and several Indian Ocean islands (Mazhetese et al. 2021).

A. *variegatum* ticks collected from cattle, sheep and goats in Guadeloupe were found positive for *R. africae.* Animal and birds trade and migration led to expansion of the geographic region invaded by the tick *A. variegatum* over more than 15 islands in the Caribbean. It is likely that *R. africae* was brought to West Indies from Senegal to Guadeloupe through the cattle (Parola et al. 2005). If not controlled, *R. africae* and its vector *A. variegatum* may become established on the mainland America.

Most cases of ATBF are seen between November and April.

Its incidence in indigenous populations is low, but the number of reported cases among travellers from Europe and other areas to sub-Saharan Africa has increased. The incidence of ATBF has been estimated to be up to 5.3% in travellers to endemic regions, and risk factors include game hunting, safari tourism, travel in the rainy season (November through April) and travel to Southern Africa (Owen et al. 2006).

55.3 Symptoms

The incubation period is 4–10 days. The symptoms appear approximately 5–7 days after the infected tick bite. Onset of fever, fatigue, headache and myalgia is abrupt. Nearly 50–100% have eschar, frequently multiple. Regional lymphadenopathy accompanies. There is generalized maculopapular or maculovesicular rash and occasionally aphthous stomatitis. Severe cases report neurological and cardiac symptoms. Neurological complications are generally observed in elderly patients unusual symptoms (collected from a review of cases reported period 2004–2019) are: myocarditis, pericarditis, conjunctivitis, decreased vision, floaters, panuveitis and neurological signs such as faecal incontinence, urinary retention, hyperesthesia and depressed and significant irritability (Mazhetese et al. 2021).

55.4 Diagnosis

The disease can be diagnosed on the basis of symptoms and confirmed by culture. *R. africae* can be grown in the yolk sacs of developing chicken embryos and in cell cultures. The PCR and immunofluorescence are used for specific identification.

55.5 Treatment

No vaccine is available but can be treated with antibiotic doxycycline, chloramphenicol and azithromycin. Protection against exposure and bite of tick is recommended.

References

Consigny PH, Rolain JM, Mizzi D, Raoult D (2005) African tick-bite fever in French travelers. Emerg Infect Dis 11(11):1804–1806

Mazhetese E, Magaia V, Taviani E, Neves L, Morar-Leather D (2021) Review: *Rickettsia africae*: identifying gaps in the current knowledge on vector-pathogen-host interactions. J Infect Dev Ctries 15(8):1039–1047

Owen CE, Bahrami S, Malone JC, Callen JP, Kulp-Shorten C (2006) African tick bite fever: a not-so-uncommon illness in international travelers. Arch Dermatol 142:1312–1314

Parola P, Paddock CD, Raoult D (2005) Tick-borne rickettsioses around the world: emerging diseases challenging old concepts. Clin Microbiol Rev 18(4):719–756

Parola P, Paddock CD, Socolovschi C, Labruna MB, Mediannikov O et al (2013) Update on tick-borne rickettsioses around the world: a geographic approach. Clin Microbiol Rev 26(4):657–702

Chapter 56
Epidemic Typhus

Synonyms

Louse-borne typhus fever, Typhus fever, Epidemic typhus, Exanthematic typhus, *Historical typhus*, Classic typhus, Sylvatic typhus, European typhus, *Red louse disease*, Jail fever, and Brill-Zinsser disease.

Henrique da Rocha Lima discovered this bacterium in 1916. He along with his friend Stanislaus von Prowazek was studying the cause of 'jail fever' in a prison in Hamburg, Germany, and got infected. Prowazek died in 1915. Rocha Lima named the causative agent after his deceased friend.

Typhus is a Greek word meaning smoke and refers to the patients' common delirium state. It was confused with typhoid until eighteenth century. It was named 'exanthematous typhus' because the patients exhibited 'skin rash' and on postmortem the Peyer's patches did not show ulceration.

Epidemic typhus is one of the six quarantinable diseases and rare but potentially fatal. Characteristic features are sudden onset of high fever, myalgia, severe headache with skin rashes and neurological and vascular disturbance.

Infection leads to long immunity. In some cases, the immunity may wane sufficiently low to allow a latent infection reactivated months and (10–20) years later. The recrudescent form or Brill-Zinsser is mild and of short duration. This may be a mechanism of survival of *Rickettsia prowazekii*. It is a potential bioterrorism agent B (CDC classification) because of its ability to cause severe disease, aerosol infection and efficient arthropod transmission. Body lice are re-emergent worldwide and therefore also lice-borne diseases caused by *R. prowazekii*, *Borrelia recurrentis*, *Bartonella quintana* and recently added *Acinetobacter baumannii* (Houhamdi et al. 2005).

© Springer Nature Singapore Pte Ltd. 2024
K. G. Narayan et al., *Handbook of Management of Zoonoses*,
https://doi.org/10.1007/978-981-99-9885-2_56

56.1   Aetiology

R. prowazekii is a Gram-negative obligately intracellular alpha Proteobacteria. It is
often surrounded by a protein microcapsular and slime layer. It grows in cytoplasm
of infected host cells, preferentially endothelial cells. Lipopolysaccharide group
antigen and some biological characters differentiate it from spotted fever group of
rickettsia. It is resistant and can survive and replicate for days after the death of the
host cell. It survives for 100 days in died faeces of the lice and retains aerosol infectivity. This makes it a useful bioweapon.

   Strains of *R. prowazekii* may differ in virulence; however, a genetic analysis suggested that the strains found in squirrels are similar to other *R. prowazekii* and do
not belong to a different subsp. typhus.

56.2   Epidemiology

The term epidemic typhus comes from the old experience when extensive outbreaks
killing thousands and even million people occurred. *R. prowazekii* is carried/main-
tained in human for years without clinical signs and lice. In most parts of the world,
humans are the only reservoirs.

56.2.1   Epidemic Typhus

Epidemics During World War: According to Bechah et al. (2008), epidemic typhus
is said to have killed 20% of troops during Napoleonic Wars. Recent studies estimated that one-third of Napolean's soldiers were affected by this during the French
retreat from Russia. Epidemic typhus emerged again during World War I and continued causing heavy morbidity and mortality in World War II on almost all war
scenes—the USA, Eastern Europe and Russia (WWI), Northern Africa, Southern
Italy, Central and eastern Europe (terrible outbreak in concentration camp) and
China (WWII).

   Post-World War: Sporadic cases were reported after WWII in Guatemala and the
USA. Most were Brill-Zinsser cases among survivors of concentration camp or
immigrants from epidemic typhus foci. Epidemic typhus continues in certain areas,
including Burundi and Ethiopia in Central and Eastern Africa, Algeria, South Africa,
Uganda and Rwanda and in mountainous tropical areas like Tibet, Nepal and Peru.
During 1981–1997, it has been sporadic in Ethiopia. It has re-emerged since then.
Rural highlands of Africa and Central and South America report most cases. Massive
outbreak in Burundi during civil war in 1997 had 100, 000 infected and 15% death.
Outbreaks were recorded in Russia and in 1998 in Peru. It has been reported from
Afghanistan and Northern India also.

Disruption of social, economic or political system, natural catastrophes, famine force large number of people to share a crowded shelter often with poor sanitation. This leads to louse infestation among refugees and possible transmission of infection. Disease occurs in cold weather when heavy clothing and poor sanitation, both conducive for proliferation of lice, prevail.

Infestation is associated mainly with poor hygienic and living conditions and overcrowding; hence, refugees, prisoners and homeless people are more likely to be infested.

Recrudescent (Brill-Zinsser) epidemic typhus occurs in absence of vector body louse. It is reactivation of the old infection due to reduced immunity caused by stress or other factors. Persisting human infection and simultaneous infestation with *Pediculus humanus corporis* leads to emergence of epidemic foci.

56.2.2   Sylvatic Typhus

Human illness or outbreak linked to exposure to flying squirrel is also termed as sylvatic typhus. The southern flying squirrels (*Glaucomys volans*) maintains it in North America. These may cause sporadic zoonotic cases.

The rickettsiae are maintained essentially by human-lice-human cycle. Southern flying squirrel (*Glaucomys volans*) is a non-human potential reservoir of *R. prowazekii*. Livestock and donkeys are known to have antibodies. Flying squirrel-vector lice-man cycle of infection is not operative because infected lice from flying squirrel, *Neohaematopinus scuiropteri*, is host specific and does not feed on human. *Rickettsiae* strain from flying squirrel can multiply in human body lice. It appears therefore that lice faeces remain the source of infection and rickettsiae seem to be aerosolized by activities of flying squirrel. Study on the cluster of sylvatic epidemic typhus by Chapman et al. (2009) suggested that repeated and prolonged close exposure to flying squirrels and their nests had great potential for transmission. All patients had shared the same cabin with flying squirrel inside the wall adjacent to the bed. Flying squirrels around the cabin were trapped and 71% were infected with *R. prowazekii*. Occupational association and stepping into sylvatic nidus may lead to exposure and zoonosis.

56.2.3   Geographic Distribution

Some endemic foci continue in Asia, sub-Saharan Africa and Latin America. North Africa seems to be free, except Algeria. The southern flying squirrel are found in Eastern USA and Southern Canada. Zoonotic cases have appeared only in the USA (Spickler 2017).

56.2.4   Lice, the Vector

Lice belong to order of Psocodea, suborder of Anoplura and parvorder of Phthiraptera. These are referred to as sucking lice. Lice are host specific. Human lice are *P. humanus corporis (body lice)*, *P. humanus capitis* (head lice) and *Pthirus pubis* (crab lice).

These are ecotypes of *Pediculus humanus*. These cause pediculosis. The head lice commonly infest school children, cause body pediculosis (pruritis or irritating itching) and are transmitted by direct contact. The vector role is unclear. *Pthirus pubis* (crab lice) is sexually transmitted and is not vector of any pathogen.

P. humanus corporis is a known vector of serious three re-emerging infections, epidemic typhus, relapsing fever and trench fever. According to Ouarti et al. (2023), lice-borne diseases such as lice-borne-relapsing fever in East Africa and epidemic typhus represent regular threats and remain endemic in some regions. They identified 20 species of bacteria in human lice, all in *P. humanus capitis*.

56.2.5   Transmission

Human-to-human transmission does not occur.

The lice are haematophagous, feed five times a day and have a life span of about 4–12 weeks. These are susceptible to rapid dehydration and high temperature. Feeding blood and leaving a febrile (high body temperature) patient are means of survival. Otherwise, these are resistant to harsh conditions, for example, they can live for 3 days without nutrition. Lice live in clothing. They feed on human blood and lay eggs in clothes.

Transmission occurs through infected *Pediculus humanus corporis*.

The ingested Rickettsiae multiply in gut and are excreted in faeces which is dry (2% moisture) and rich in ammonia that attracts more and more lice. Rickettsiae are viable for 100 days in the faeces. Poor hygienic habit and humid weather help proliferation. Density of lice increases and is important for transmission which is facilitated by body contact and promiscuity. The rate of louse infestation during epidemic reaches 90–100%. Rickettsiae ingested with blood multiply in the gut epithelium, rupture the epithelial cells and reach body cavity. The lice look red. Lice are killed. Dead lice carry *R. prowazekii*. Lice defecate while feeding. *R. prowazekii* is excreted in faeces of the infected lice.

They remain infectious through their life. *R. prowazekii* is transmitted transstadially but not transovarially in lice. Infected lice die within 2 weeks.

56.2.6   Modes of Infection

• The bacterium enters through conjunctivae, mucous membrane and abraded skin- scratch after louse bite and crushed louse tissue.
• Inhalation of rickettsia in dried faeces of body louse.
• Accidental parenteral inoculation or inhalation such as in laboratory.

Sources could be faeces and tissues of infected lice and the infected flying squirrel.

Entry into human host: Bite wound breaks in skin and mucous membrane offer entry to *R. prowazekii* present in faeces and dead and crushed lice.

R. prowazekii surviving in faeces of lice and dead lice may be aerosolized and inhaled. Inhalation is considered as means of transmission of zoonotic rickettsiosis also. Infections acquired from squirrels can become latent in humans and may re-emerge later. In presence of lice, it may spread between people.

Theoretically, blood transfusion and organ transplant may be a possibility of transmission.

P. humanus capitis feed on human blood every 4–6 h and lay nits (eggs) at the base of the hair shaft. Human head lice (*Pediculus humanus capitis*) have been infected in the laboratory and can shed this organism, but role as vector is not clear. Role of other insect vectors in transmission is thought to be minimal.

56.3   Pathology

The median infective dose is estimated as <10 rickettsial particles (Anonym 2010*). Rickettsiae are intracellular parasite. The spread in human's body after entry is through lymphatic and bloodstream. *R. prowazekii* affects endothelial cells of small blood vessels and induce inflammatory, proliferative and degenerative changes leading to cellular infiltration and thrombosis. The pathology may be seen in lungs (interstitial infiltration), heart and CNS as endothelial cells of small capillaries in these organs are invaded and rickettsiae proliferate and accumulate till cells lyse. Infection results into vasculitis with increased vascular permeability.

56.4   Symptoms

The duration of acute febrile stage is of about 2 weeks in untreated patients. Recovery is slow and may take 2–3 months. It may be fatal if untreated.

The incubation period is about 7–14 days. The onset after an initial malaise of 1–3 days is abrupt with severe headache, body ache, cough, nausea, vomiting and pyrexia (39–41 °C). Severe myalgia forces patient to a crouching posture. By fifth day, skin rashes appear initially localized, as well as macules, petechiae or purpura. These may be non-confluent erythematous and blanching or non-blanching. There is no eschar. The skin lesions appear first on upper part of the trunk and move on the trunk, axilla and buttock, spreading to almost entire body-sparing face, palms and soles. In some patients, rash may be transient only. Rash can become dark, maculo-papular, petechial or even purpuric. Other signs may be arthralgia, splenomegaly, abdominal pain, nausea, vomiting and mild thrombocytopenia. One or more system is affected in most of the patients.

Cerebral thrombosis as a consequence of vasculitis and multiple organ failure may occur in severe cases. When CNS is involved, delirium, seizure and coma in second-third week may occur. When infection affects chest, cough, infiltration and pneumonia due to secondary bacterial infection are observed. Vascular disturbance includes tachycardia, hypotension and cyanosis. Ischaemia may lead to gangrene and necrosis of distal toes and fingers. Case fatality rate used to be high (even 60%) in pre-antibiotic era. Presently it is around 4%.

56.5   Diagnosis

Outbreak of fever of unknown origin in unhygienic settings generally observed in jails, during disaster, civil, social political collapse and in chronically poor and cold countries is suggestive. Confirmation by laboratory tests with specimens such as blood (human patient/lice), skin biopsy and serum is necessary.

- Guinea pig/mice inoculation for isolation
- Culture on L929 fibroblast monolayer to isolate followed by staining by Gimenez or specific IF staining
- Serological tests—Weil Felix (Brill-Zinsser not detected), more sensitive tests are indirect immunofluorescence and microagglutination. A fourfold increased increase in titre in convalescent compared to acute stage
- Molecular diagnostics—Westernblot (La Scola et al. 2000)—differentiates between endemic and epidemic typhus. A real-time PCR and a rapid version, quantitative real-time PCR, are specific and sensitive.

56.6   Treatment

Chloramphenicol and tetracycline are effective. Patients become afebrile in 2 days.

56.7   Prevention

Surveillance and prevention of lice-borne infections requires identification of lice. Head lice and body lice can be differentiated. Head lice can transform into body lice ecotype under certain conditions. Mitochondrial DNA analysis differentiated human lice into six clades, A–F. The clades B, C, E and F include head lice. The clades A and D include genetically indistinguishable head and body lice (Amanzougaghene et al. 2016).

Morphological identification has limitations: lack of differentiating criteria and documents and collecting damage-free samples.

Insects (mosquitoes, ticks, fleas and lice) could be identified quickly and correctly by matrix-assisted laser desorption/ionization time-of-flight mass spectrometry (MALDI-TOF MS). Huynh et al. (2022) identified mosquitoes in Vietnam using this technique. Benyahia et al. (2021) used this technique and recommended to identify lice stored in alcohol for any length of time.

Surveillance in human population may be made with diagnostics like PCR and serologic methods.

Environmental measures involve keeping out flying squirrels and vectors from recreation parks and rental cabins,

Ensure good keeping using the following:

• Delousing methods—like cleaning clothing with hot water
• Pesticides to kill lice such as 10% DDT, lindane, 1.0% malathion, 1.0% permethrin and carbaryl

Educate clinicians to evaluate patients with characteristic signs and symptoms for possible exposures.

Vaccines that have been used are the following:

• Formalin-treated vaccine is an effective immunizing agent.
• The attenuated Madrid E strain of *R. prowazekii*.
• The Cox vaccine (egg embryo type) is produced by cultivating *R. prowazekii* in chicken egg.
• The Durand vaccine (inactivated rat lung type).

References

Amanzougaghene N, Akiana J, Mongo Ndombe G, Davoust B, Nsana NS, Parra H-J et al (2016) Head lice of pygmies reveal the presence of relapsing fever Borreliae in the Republic of Congo. PLoS Negl Trop Dis 10(12):e0005142

Bechah Y, Capo C, Mege JL, Raoult D (2008) Epidemic typhus. Lancet Infect Dis 8(7):417–426

Benyahia H, Ouarti B, Diarra AZ et al (2021) Identification of lice stored in alcohol using MALDI-TOF MS. J Med Entomol 58(3):1126–1133

Chapman AS, Swerdlow DL, Dato VM, Anderson AD, Moodie CE et al (2009) Cluster of syl-
    vatic epidemic typhus cases associated with flying squirrels, 2004–2006. Emerg Infect Dis
    15(7):1005–1011
Houhamdi L, Parola P, Raoult D (2005) Lice and lice-borne diseases in humans. Med Trop (Mars)
    65(1):13–23
Huynh LN, Diarra AZ, Nguyen HS, Tran LB, Do VN, Ly TDA et al (2022) MALDI-TOF mass
    spectrometry identification of mosquitoes collected in Vietnam. Parasit Vectors 15(1):39
La Scola B, Rydkina L, Ndihokubwayo JB, Vene S, Raoult D (2000) Serological differentiation of
    murine typhus and epidemic typhus using cross-adsorption and Western blotting. Clin Diagn
    Lab Immunol 7(4):612–616
Ouarti B, Mbogning Fonkou DM, Houhamdi L, Mediannikov O, Parola P (2023) Lice and lice-
    borne diseases in humans in Africa: a narrative review. Acta Trop 237:106709
Spickler AR (2017) Typhus fever—Rickettsia prowazekii. http://www.cfsph.iastate.edu/
    DiseaseInfo/factsheets.php

Chapter 57
Indian Tick Typhus

Synonyms

East and South African tick fever, Marseilles fever, Boutonneuse fever, Mediterranean spotted fever.

Indian tick typhus (ITT) is caused by *Rickettsia conorii* characterized by fever, headache, vertigo, malaise and disturbance of vision, followed by arthromyalgia and a rash. The tick typhus occurs in Asia including India, East and South Africa and in Mediterranean region.

57.1   Aetiology

Rickettsia conorii subsp. *conorii* and Mediterranean spotted fever (MSF) were described in 1932. Subsequently, other subspecies were added. The subspecies, respective tick vector species and name of the disease are summarized in Table 57.1.

The causative agent is *R. conorii*, which are small, non-flagellate, Gram-negative, obligate intracellular organism.

R. conorii belongs to spotted fever group of *Rickettsia* and shares soluble antigens. Complement fixation test with washed rickettsial antigen separates it. Microscopic examination reveals these as minute rickettsiae in pair, purple with Giemsa stain and red when stained with Macchiavello's stain. It is intracellular and can grow both in cytoplasm and nucleus of cells of ticks, mammals and embryonated eggs.

© Springer Nature Singapore Pte Ltd. 2024   613
K. G. Narayan et al., *Handbook of Management of Zoonoses*,
https://doi.org/10.1007/978-981-99-9885-2_57

Table 57.1 Rickettsia, respective vectors, endemic areas and disease (Piotrowski and Rymaszewska 2020; Parola et al. 2013)

Rickettsia	Vector tick	Endemic region	Disease
Rickettsia conorii subsp. indica	Rhipicephalus sanguineus and R. turanicus	India	Indian tick typhus (ITT)
Rickettsia conorii subsp. conorii	R. sanguineus,	Europe and North Africa	Mediterranean spotted fever (MSF)
	R. sanguineus and R. bursa	Asia-Asiatic part of Turkey	MSF
	R. sanguineus, R. evertsi, R. simus, R. mushamae, Haemaphysalis punctaleachi and H. leachi	Sub-Saharan Africa	MSF
Rickettsia conorii subsp. israelensis	R. sanguineus	Europe, Asia and North Africa	Israeli spotted fever (ISF)
Rickettsia conorii subsp. caspia	R. pumilio and R. sanguineus	Astrakhan region of Caspian sea	Astrakhan fever

57.2 Epidemiology

The natural reservoir hosts are rodents (*Rattus* spp., *Otomys irroratus*, *Rhabdomys pumilio*) or striped mouse, rabbits and dogs and are latently infected. Seroprevalence in dogs is high in endemic areas.

Rhipicephalus sanguineus is the vector and reservoir also. Transmission in ticks is both transovarial and trans-stadial. Ticks once infected remain infected throughout their life or at least for 18 months. The larvae feed on rats, nymph on human and adult on dogs. A number of other ticks also transmit and maintain the rickettsia (Table 55.1). The distribution of ticks varies, *Dermacentor andersoni* in the west, *D. variabilis* in the east and *Haemaphysalis leachileachi* in South Africa, and determines the distribution of disease.

Piotrowski and Rymaszewska (2020) suggested the importance of understanding biology of tick in the prevention of disease. The habitats of people, animals and ticks overlap. Humid environment is required by *Ixodes* sp. *R. sanguineus* ticks are able to survive high temperature and low humidity. Meadows covered with forest are preferred by *Dermacentor*. *Amblyomma americanum* can live in dry forests. Ticks' access to host is interesting. Some ticks share habitat with human, for example, *R. sanguineus* are commonly found in homes and surroundings. Some ticks wait in grass in deciduous forest to climb to hosts; others are found in forest litter and fallen needles. Avoiding tick infestation is difficult.

Sharma and Mishra (2020) reviewed papers on the occurrence of rickettsial diseases in India. *R. sanguineus*, *Haemaphysalis leachi* var. *indica* and *Ixodes ricinus* have been found infected with *R. conorii* in Shrinagar, Imphal and Almora in India. In Pune, Maharashtra *R. conorii* was detected in *Boophilus microplus* and *Rhipicephalus haemaphysalis*. Sera from various species of rodents and gerbils (*Rattus blanfordi*, *R. rufescens* and *Suncus murinus*) and dog, cow, horse and sheep were detected (Padbidri et al. 1984). Other states in India from where Indian tick typhus has been reported are Karnataka, Kashmir, Kerala, Madhya Pradesh, Punjab, Uttar Pradesh and Tamil Nadu.

The geographic location and seasonality (April–September) of prevalence coincide with activity of ticks. Persons at high risk of getting infected are those who visit forest/or exposed natural nidii, such as foresters, eco-tourists, campers and hunters. Accompanying dogs may get infected or even bring infected ticks and then become a source of infection to other humans or create a synanthropic nidus. Proximity to sero-reactive dogs is a risk factor to human. Dog practitioners and attendants or kennel workers are thus likely to get infection.

In a study in Israel, Cohen et al. (2021) observed most cases reported during the summer and peaked in August. Only two patients remembered of exposure by tick bite. On the other hand, exposure to animals was common, and 80% of dogs was found exposed to *Rh. sanguineus* (the principal reservoir of *R. conorii*).

Solano-Gallego et al. (2006) reported acute illness in dogs caused by *R. conorii* spp. *conorii*. The diagnosis was based on PCR, DNA sequencing and sero-conversion. Important clinical manifestations are pain, erythema and oedema on experimental infection. The authors observed acute onset of fever, lethargy, thrombocytopenia, anaemia, mildly increased liver enzyme activities and hypo-albuminemia in the natural cases.

Travelers to endemic areas are likely to get infected (Parola et al. 2001).

57.2.1 Mode of Infection

The commonest mode of infection is tick bite. *R. conorii* may enter through abraded skin contaminated with faeces or tissue fluid of infected ticks (as may happen while removing ticks). Infection may occur through blood transfusion and inhalation (aerosol in laboratory).

57.3 Symptoms

The incubation period is seven (3–12) days. In most cases, there is sudden onset of fever (102–104 °F), severe headache, chill, arthromyalgia, extreme exhaustion, vertigo, photophobia and exanthema on extremities and trunk.

Fever may continue for 10–15 days. In severe cases, there may be delirium, renal failure, shock and death. Unlike other SFG rickettsiosis, IIT presents maculopapular rash turning into purpuric and absence of or presence of a single eschar.

Boutonneuse fever refers to the eschar that appears at the site of tick bite on 3–5 days of illness. Eschar is a maculopapular (ecchymotic in some), raised rash with black necrotic centre. The rash spreads on hands and soles. Multiple scars appear in some, most often in children. The regional lymph gland is enlarged. Fever is remittent lasting for 10–12 days. The skin lesions last for 10–20 days after symptoms disappear.

Illness may take serious course. Those at risk are old, with reduced immunity, alcoholic and treated with inappropriate antibiotics or treated late (Piotrowski and Rymaszewska 2020). Life-threatening course of illness is characterized by (a) cardiac symptoms, myocarditis, atrial fibrillation and coronary artery ectasia; (b) ocular symptoms, retinopathy, retinal vasculitis and uveitis; (c) neurological symptoms, meningitis, ischaemic strokes and loss of hearing; (d) acute respiratory distress syndrome; (e) haemophagocytic syndrome; and (f) acute renal failure, pancreatitis and splenic rupture. Fatality rates are reported at 13% in Portugal, an estimated 3.6% in African continent, and 54.5% in patients with neurological and multiorgan syndrome.

Tirumala et al. (2014) described a case of ITT from Nanded, Maharashtra, India, presenting life-threatening Purpura fulminans (retiform purpura all over the body), bullous eruptions and multiorgan failure. The Weil-Felix test confirmed the diagnosis. The case responded to doxycycline treatment.

About 30% of patients show enlarged liver and increased alkaline phosphatase (http://www.wrongdiagnosis.com/i/india_tick_typhus/intro.htm Indian tick typhus).

Cohen et al. (2021) reported a study of a series of hospitalized patients diagnosed SFGR over a decade in Israel of which *R. conorii* ITTS was the principal cause of severe disease with multiple organ failure and high mortality. They presented features typical of SFGR and eschar (rare in ISF) was seen in 12%. ISF caused purpura fulminans in 9% and meningoencephalitis in 24%. Fifty percent showed involvement of multiorgan including the liver, kidney, jaundice, rhabdomyolysis/myositis and coagulopathy. Severe illness requiring intensive care was common and 30% of ISF died in hospital.

57.4   Diagnosis

- History of tick bite/exposure and associated skin lesions and other symptoms.
- Weil Felix test is positive with OX 19 and OX 2.
- Staining of skin lesion biopsy with Giemsa or Macchiavellos' stain.
- Serological tests, CFT, IFT, IPT and Western Blot. These are useful after appearance of detectable antibodies, 10 days after onset of illness. IgM may appear earlier.
- Molecular methods include (a) nucleotide sequence analyses of the 16SrRNA and the rOmpA genes of the isolate, (b) Sequence comparison of gene coding for citrate synthase (*gltA*) and (c) polymerase chain reaction (PCR) amplification and sequence determination (Rydkina et al. 1999).

57.5 Treatment

Doxycycline is the most commonly used antibiotic but tetracycline, chloramphenicol and ciprofloxacin are also used.

57.6 Prevention

Dogs are considered to be the sentinels and serology constitutes a useful epidemiological marker.

- Avoid visit to tick infested area
- Protective clothing while visiting forests
- Tick repellents- N, N-diethyl-m-toluamide and dimethylphthalate
- Removal of tick from body carefully
- Insecticides like dieldrine, lindane, chlordane, DDT, diazinon and benzene hexachloride applied on selected areas

References

Cohen R, Finn T, Babushkin F, Paran Y, Ben Ami R et al (2021) Spotted fever group rickettsioses in Israel, 2010-2019. Emerg Infect Dis 27(8):2117–2126

Padbidri VS, Rodrigues JJ, Shetty PS, Joshi MV, Rao BL, Shukla RN (1984) Tick-borne rickettsioses in Pune district, Maharashtra, India. Int J Zoonoses 11(1):45–52

Parola P, Fenollar F, Badiaga S, Brouqui P, Raoult D (2001) First documentation of *Rickettsia conorii* infection (strain Indian tick typhus) in a traveler. Emerg Infect Dis 7(5):909–910

Parola P, Paddock CD, Socolovschi C, Labruna MB, Mediannikov O et al (2013) Update on tick-borne rickettsioses around the world: a geographic approach. Clin Microbiol Rev 26(4):657–702

Piotrowski M, Rymaszewska A (2020) Expansion of tick-borne rickettsioses in the world. Microorganisms 8(12):1906

Rydkina E, Roux V, Rudakov N, Gafarova M, Tarasevich I, Raoult D (1999) New Rickettsiae in ticks collected in territories of the former Soviet Union. Emerg Infect Dis 5(6):811–814

Sharma A, Mishra B (2020) Rickettsial disease existence in India: resurgence in outbreaks with the advent of 20th century. Indian J Health Sci Biomed Res KLEU 13(1):5–10

Solano-Gallego L, Kidd L, Trotta M, Di Marco M, Caldin M et al (2006) Febrile illness associated with *Rickettsia conorii* infection in dogs from Sicily. Emerg Infect Dis 12(12):1985–1988

Tirumala S, Behera B, Jawalkar S, Mishra PK, Patalay PV et al (2014) Indian tick typhus presenting as Purpura fulminans. Indian J Crit Care Med 18(7):476–478

Chapter 58
Murine Typhus

Synonyms

Endemic typhus, Flea-borne typhus (FBT).

Murine or endemic typhus/flea-borne typhus is an acute febrile self-limiting illness. Most cases fail to know or realize that they have had flea bite. Therefore, cases are either under recognized or not recognized and confused with viral diseases and epidemic typhus.

58.1 Aetiology

Murine typhus is caused by *Rickettsia typhi*, less often by *R. felis*. *Rickettsia typhi (mooseri)* is a member of typhus group. Spotted fever group (SFG) and typhus group (TG) are members of rickettsial species. *R. typhi* is a small (0.4 × 1.3 μm), Gram-negative, obligate, intracellular bacterium. Rickettsiae have evolved in such close association with arthropod hosts that they are adapted to survive within the host cells.

R. typhi is maintained by mammals and haematophagus insects, fleas and ticks. *R. felis* shares antigenic and genetic components of both TG and SFG Rickettsiae. The two species affecting human are serologically indistinguishable, and PCR analysis is required for differentiation.

© Springer Nature Singapore Pte Ltd. 2024   619
K. G. Narayan et al., *Handbook of Management of Zoonoses*,
https://doi.org/10.1007/978-981-99-9885-2_58

58.2   Epidemiology

Murine typhus has been documented worldwide in diverse geographic areas like Mediterranean, Africa, Southeast Asia and the USA. During the last decades, rickettsial diseases have shown re-emergence in the Americas with economic and public health implications. Murine typhus is prevalent mostly in tropical and subtropical coastal regions of the world. It has re-emerged in the southwestern USA.

The enzootic cycles involving small mammals and ectoparasites maintain *R. typhi*.

58.2.1   Natural History/Maintenance of R. typhi

R. typhi requires a combination of flea vector and mammalian hosts for its maintenance in nature. Human is an accidental host.

58.2.2   Vectors

The principal vectors are the oriental rat flea, *Xenopsylla cheopis*, and the flea *Nosopsyllus fasciatus*. These fleas naturally colonize the mouse *Mus musculus*. The cat fleas, *Ctenocephalides felis* (as well as seven other species of fleas), have also been implicated in the spread of the disease. The cat fleas have worldwide distribution. These feed indiscriminately, parasitizing cats, dogs, opossums and many other small mammals, and also readily bite human.

R. felis was detected in cat fleas *(Ctenocephalides felis)*, and opossums (*Didelphis marsupialis*) in the southern regions of California and Texas have been reported from Mexico, France and Brazil.

R. typhi multiplies in the epithelial cells of the flea's midgut and is shed in the faeces, which are deposited while the flea is feeding. Laboratory-infected *Xenopsylla cheopis* transovarially transmitted *R. typhi*, and the F1 fleas transmitted infection to >18% of rats they infested (Farhang-Azad et al. 1985). Fleas find hot and dry environment favourable for propagation.

58.2.3   Hosts

Rickettsia typhi (mooseri) is maintained in nature by rat-rat flea transmission cycle. Infection in rats is non-fatal. House mice are highly susceptible to experimental infection with *R. typhi*, which may establish a persistent intracerebral infection lasting for up to 5 months and is excreted in the urine. Rats serve as host for fleas. Infected rats carry rickettsia and make these available in blood for the vector fleas and help multiply the number of infected fleas that can then infect humans.

Rats, mice, cats and opossums are naturally infected. Opossums are peridomestic animals widely distributed in the USA. They have little natural fear of people and share habitat with domestic pets. Fleas can easily transfer between them.

Fleas feeding upon diseased rats ingest blood and get infected. Rickettsia are excreted in faeces and are not available in saliva. Bite is thus not infective.

R. felis was discovered in 1990. FBT persists primarily in South and Central Texas, the Los Angeles area and Hawaii. The prevalence of *Rickettsia typhi* (1.9%) and *R. felis* (24.8%) based on detection of DNA rat fleas (*Xenopsylla cheopis*) collected from mice on Oahu Island, Hawaii, suggested that *R. felis* may be a more common cause of rickettsiosis than *R. typhi* in Hawaii (Eremeeva et al. 2008).

Survey of fleas on dogs, cats and opossums in California, Texas and Georgia also confirmed that fleas were infected with *R. typhi* or *R. felis*, helping explain the spread of murine typhus into rural areas in the USA. Opossum (*Didelphis virginiana*) and cats have replaced rats as the primary reservoirs and the cat flea (*Ctenocephalides felis*) now as the most important vector in the former two areas. Maui County in Hawaii report 73% cases and has lower rainfall than other areas.

Cases of FBT are increasing in Texas and California. In 2018–2019, Los Angeles County experienced a resurgence of FBT, with rats as the reservoir.

58.2.4   Distribution

It is distributed worldwide in tropical, subtropical and temperate zone occurring in varying environments (generally warm and coastal region) in Southeast Asia, North America, the Mediterranean and Northern Africa. The worldwide seroprevalence of murine typhus has been estimated to range from 3 to 36%, with low mortality of 0–1% (Peniche et al. 2012).

58.2.5   Season and Other Contributing Factors

Murine typhus occurs in summer and autumn that favours rat-flea-rat cycle. Rats seek warm areas during winter to live near farmhouses or may share human dwelling (synanthropic nidus).

Most cases in Texas are reported from April through June, in California throughout summer and fall. Hawaii, particularly Maui, is exceptional. Infectious flea faeces in dust and unique round the year food supplies are possible explanation (Civen and Ngo 2008).

Rats, cats, opossums and their fleas can be found co-existing in suburban settings. Man gets infection while working, especially with earth (digging, farming) in high-density wild rat colonies and rodent-infested areas such as ports, granaries, farms and rat-infested buildings.

According to Eurosurveillance report (1998), malnutrition, poverty, overcrowding, disaster war and dirt are associated with infection. It is said that murine typhus can always be found everywhere if it is looked for. In Portugal, murine typhus is re-emerging. It was fairly common until the 1940s and was included in the list of notifiable diseases after 1955. Serum samples received and examined by the Centre for Vectors and Infectious Disease Research detected a case of *R. typhi* infection in a woman. Several other patients were also seropositive. Cases clustered on an island. High rainfall, increased vegetation and food and shelter led to increase rat population. Three of the five patients lived in Porto Santo Island but other had visited the island. All 26 users of the Health Centre at Porto Santo had history of contact with rat and flea and one described signs and symptoms of murine typhus.

Dzul-Rosado et al. (2022) studied seroprevalence of *R. typhi* and *R. rickettsia* in Teabo, Yucatan, Mexico. *R. typhi* was more prevalent. The presence of dogs in the peri-domestic area was correlated with rickettsial IgG seropositivity. The median height peri-domestic vegetation was also positively related to IgG seropositivity. More females than males were found seropositive, possibly because their confinement in houses caused exposure to multiple dogs, domestic animals and medium-height vegetations in the peridomestic area. *Rhipicephalus* and *Amblyomma* tick species were also found in the peri-domestic area.

According to Anstead (2020), history of flea-borne typhus (FBT) in the USA describes following three stages related to the rise and decline of primary reservoir *Rattus norvegicus* and *Xenopsylla cheopis*, the vector flea.

The rise (1930–1946): There were 42,000 cases during 1931–1946 with a peak of 5401 in 1944. It is associated with conditions favouring both the rats and flea. This situation is related to the depression, and World War II and post-war increased production, storage of food crops often in dilapidated houses, overcrowding, poor environmental sanitation and the difficulty of importing insecticides and rodenticides.

A vigorous intervention (1945–1952): The programme for the control of FBT was implemented vigorously by the US Public Health Service. Diagnosis and treatment improved. The incidence was brought down to 98 in 1956.

Persistence: FBT persists and is ascribed to population of companion animals, stray pets, opossums and the cat flea, an abundant and non-selective vector.

58.3   Modes of Infection

Fleas defecate while biting. *R. typhi* is present in faeces (poop/dirt) of fleas; *Rickettsia typhi* are resistant to drying and remain infectious for up to 100 days in rat faeces.

- *Inoculation (through cut, abrasion, wound)—R. typhi* enters through abrasion in the skin caused by bite by infected flea, *Xenopsylla cheopis*. The irritation of bite is felt by victim and the scratches. Entry of rickettsiae is facilitated.
- *Inhalation* of dried faeces of flea or dust laden with rickettsia from rodent urine. People can rub it (infected flea dirt) into eyes and get infected. Most common transmitters are rat fleas; less are cat and opossums-fleas.

- Laboratory personnel have been infected with this agent when inoculating rodents and handling infected animal; other occupational risk groups include farmers, cable layers, rat trappers, etc.

Human-to-human transmission does not occur.

58.4 Symptoms

Endemic/murine typhus may be acute, mild and rarely severe fatal. Sometimes, most cases recover even without treatment. Disease complications in 25% of patients and prolonged duration of fever in untreated have been reported (Doppler and Newton 2020). Cases left without treatment can turn into severe illness with damage of one or more organs.

Sable and Maayuf (2009) reported a case in adult Libyan of 18 years. He had fever, frontal headache, body ache, malaise, abdominal pain, nausea and vomiting, followed by a macular to maculopapular rash. Rash started on the arms and legs and then spread to the rest of the body, including the palms and soles. Eschar and lymphadenopathy were absent. He lived in a rat-infested house in peri-urban area.

R. typhi causes vasculitis and resulting rash and bleeding. The signs and symptoms resemble that of louse-borne typhus but are milder and shorter in duration. The incubation period varies between 6 and 14 days (average 10 days). Fever lasts generally for 12 days. The temperature may be 101–102 °F, even 105 °F. Blood pressure may be low and pulse rapid. The acute febrile disease is usually characterized by general malaise, headache, pain, nausea, vomiting, discrete rash (in 40–50% appearing 6 days after onset of signs) and chills, with signs ranging from mild to severe. Skin rashes appear under axilla and on arm, spreading to the shoulder, chest, abdomen and thigh, and last for 4–8 days.

Ocular manifestation of murine typhus has been reported (Hudson et al. 1997). Two patients (38-year-old male and 49-year-old female) reported fever, headache, rash, night sweats and pulmonary symptoms. They had noted the recent onset of diminished visual acuity and floaters. Examination revealed mild optic nerve head oedema (in one patient), intraretinal haemorrhages and small localized areas of retinal whitening. Both had history of exposure to flea. They serologically proved cases of acute murine typhus.

Rarely, *R. typhi* causes mild vitritis, retinal lesions and retinal vascular leakage. Post-infectious optic neuropathy is even less common (Zhang et al. 2011).

In Yucatan State of Mexico, Zavala-Castro et al. (2009) identified several cases of rickettsiosis caused by *R. felis* and *R. rickettsii*, some with fatal outcome, highlighted misdiagnosis and inappropriate treatment. Opossums, rats and mice often inhabit backyards and houses in rural and suburban areas. A 3-year-old girl was brought to the emergency room of the public hospital with a fever of a 3-day duration. As reported by mother, the child had flea bites on her legs and arms 2 days before the onset of fever. The child had close contact with mice, cat and dog as were present in the house. Symptoms of illness like high fever and abdominal, muscular and head pain led to diagnosis as viral pharyngitis and otitis media. She did not respond to treatment with nimesulide, amoxicillin and trimethoprim and had to be hospitalized after 10 days with high fever (39.8 °C), arthralgia in the hands and ankles and a petechial maculopapular rash on the thorax and extremities. She was diagnosed with typhoid and treated with sulfonamide, cephalosporin and acetaminophen but without remission of the symptoms. FA showed serum IgM and IgG antibody reactivity with *R. typhi* and IgG antibody reactivity with *R. rickettsii* and *R. akari*. PCR finally established *R. typhi* infection. Another case reported from Southeastern Mexico was a 23-year-old man who had a low-grade fever (37.6 °C) and maculopapular rash on the thorax and upper and lower extremities. He had a cat but without flea or tick infestation. He was diagnosed by PCR and treated with doxycycline (Zavala-Castro et al. 2014).

Respiratory involvement manifests in pulmonary congestion, irritating cough and even haemoptysis. Splenomegaly may be observed. An encephalitic syndrome appears in almost 45% cases (Mushatt and Hyslop 1991). Severe cases report persistent frontal headache even in the second week. There may be stupor, prostration, delirium, imbalance, meningitis, nuchal rigidity, seizures, coma and death, generally among old, debilitated and immunocompromised.

The symptoms resolve with lowering of the febrile response. Fatality rate for all ages is about 2% but increases with age. Proper antibiotic therapy is the most effective measure to prevent morbidity or mortality due to rickettsial infections.

Reviewing published reports, Doppler and Newton (2020) found duration of illness as 15 days and fatality rate of 3.6% in a patient series and 0.4% overall fatality rate if untreated. The rate of hospitalization was >50% with varied complications, 6–30% pulmonary, renal, gastrointestinal, muscular and CNS involvement. Age of patients ranged between 15 and 60 (mean 30.6) years most were males. The course of illness was mild to moderate in children. High rate of hospitalization and complications in untreated patients and duration of illness causes significant morbidity and disease burden highlighting importance of early diagnosis.

Risk of severe illness and complications stand with male sex, old age, delayed diagnosis, those with hepatic and renal dysfunction and glucose 6-phosphate dehydrogenase deficiency. Complications observed include culture-negative endocarditis, rupture of the spleen and CNS involvement like severe headache, stiff neck, papilledema and focal neurological deficits, such as hemiparesis or facial nerve palsy (Civen and Ngo 2008).

58.5   Diagnosis

Methods of diagnosis are the following:

1. Staining by (a) Gimenez and (b) immunohistology on skin biopsy during acute phase.

2. Serologic tests include (a) Weil-Felix test: Proteus OX 19 antigen is used. A titre of 1:50 or higher is considered positive. This is reached on the eighth day, peaked by the end of the second week and declined rapidly during convalescence. (b) CFT and HA with group-specific antigen. (c) IFA, EIA, micro-agglutination, CFT and neutralization with species-specific antigens. These are rarely diagnostic with blood serum collected at the onset of symptoms. A convalescent-phase specimen of blood serum is generally required to confirm diagnosis. A fourfold increase in titre between acute and convalescent phase is diagnostic.
3. Biological test: Guinea pig, cotton rat or white rat inoculation tests.
4. Molecular test: PCR.

58.6 Treatment

Treatment should be started without waiting for results from laboratory as lab diagnosis may take time. Clinical diagnosis is important.

Antibiotics like tetracycline, doxycycline and chloramphenicol are useful. Supplement with supportive therapy.

58.7 Control and Prevention

The approach includes (a) raticides for rat population control, (b) insecticides (DDT spray) for vector control and (c) personal protection.

Protect yourself:

- Personal protective measures—insecticide (dibutyl phthalate as repellent)—impregnated clothes while working; do not feed or pet stray and wild animals
- Inactivated rickettsial vaccine for nurses, doctors, laboratory workers and other high-risk group are recommended.
- Vector control—Insecticides (organochlorines, as well as others) as residual powders or sprays in areas where rats nest or traverse to control fleas.
- Rodent control—Rodenticides to control rat
- Note: Insecticides should be applied prior to using rodenticides. This will prevent fleas from leaving the dead rodents and feeding on human hosts.
- Maintain house, workplace and recreational areas free from rodents and opossums
- Keep a vigil of pets; maintain freedom from fleas.

Sentinel—presence of fleas on random-source dogs, cats and opossums raises the risk of transmission of murine typhus.

References

Anstead GM (2020) History, rats, fleas, and opossums. II. The decline and resurgence of flea-borne typhus in the United States, 1945-2019. Trop Med Infect Dis 6(1):2

Civen R, Ngo V (2008) Murine typhus: an unrecognised suburban vector borne disease. Clin Infect Dis 46:913–980

Doppler JF, Newton PN (2020) A systematic review of the untreated mortality of murine typhus. PLoS Negl Trop Dis 14(9):e0008641

Dzul-Rosado K, Cámara Herrera R, Miranda-Schaeubinger M, Arias-León J et al (2022) Socio-ecological determinants of rickettsial seroprevalence in a rural community of Yucatán, Mexico. Infect Genet Evol 102:105291

Eremeeva ME, Warashina WR, Sturgeon MM, Buchholz AE et al (2008) *Rickettsia typhi* and *R. felis* in rat fleas (*Xenopsylla cheopis*), Oahu, Hawaii. Emerg Infect Dis 14(10):1613–1615

Eurosurveillance report (1998) Is murine typhus re-emerging in Portugal? Eurosurveillance. 3(2). Surveillance report. http://www.eurosurveillance.org/ViewArticle.aspx?ArticleId=124

Farhang-Azad A, Traub R, Baqar S (1985) Transovarial transmission of murine typhus rickettsiae in Xenopsylla cheopis fleas. Science 227(4686):543–545

Hudson HL, Thach AB, Lopez PF (1997) Retinal manifestations of acute murine typhus. Int Ophthalmol 21(3):121–126

Mushatt DM, Hyslop NE (1991) Neurologic aspects of North American Zoonoses. Infect Dis North America 5:703–731. https://doi.org/10.1016/S0891-5520(20)30415-3

Peniche Lara G, Dzul-Rosado KR, Zavala Velázquez JE, Zavala-Castro J (2012) Murine typhus: Clinical and epidemiological aspects. Colomb Med (Cali) 43:175–80

Sable P, Maayuf M (2009) Case report. Endemic typhus (murine typhus) in an 18 year old Libyan adult. Southeast Asian J Trop Med Public Health 40(4):785–788

Zavala-Castro JE, Zavala-Velázquez J, Sulú-Uicab J (2009) Murine typhus in child, Yucatan, Mexico. Emerg Infect Dis 15(6):972–974

Zavala-Castro JE, Dzul-Rosado KR, Peniche-Lara G, Tello-Martín R, Zavala-Velázquez JE (2014) Isolation of *Rickettsia typhi* from human, Mexico. Emerg Infect Dis 20(8):1411–1412

Zhang J, Pau D, Lee AG (2011) Post infectious optic neuropathy in endemic typhus. J Neuroophthalmol 31(4):342–343

Chapter 59
Rickettsial Pox

Rickettsial pox has been first diagnosed in New York City in 1946 (Huebner et al. 1946). Cases have been reported from all continents including Europe (Croatia), Asia (Korea), Africa (South Africa) and South America (Akram et al. 2023). *Mus musculus* and wild rodents are the natural host of *R. akari*. This organism is also isolated from *Rattus rattus* and *R. norvegicus*, and the rat under certain circumstances may transmit the disease to humans. The vector is a mite, *Liponyssoides (Allodermanyssus) sanguineus.*

Clinical manifestation of disease caused by *R. akari* resembles murine typhus. The incubation period varies between 10 and 24 days. Patients complain of fever, headache and stiff neck. Rash of rickettsial pox commences as discrete maculopapular becoming vesicular on palm and soles. Eschar develops in most (90%) of cases as shallow ulcer with brown scab cover.

Diagnosis, treatment and control are similar to those described for murine typhus.

References

Akram SM, Jamil RT, Gossman W (2023) Rickettsia akari (Rickettsialpox) [Updated 2023 May 8]. In: StatPearls [Internet]. StatPearls Publishing, Treasure Island. https://www.ncbi.nlm.nih.gov/books/NBK448081/

Huebner RJ, Jellison WL, Pomerantz C (1946) Rickettsialpox, a newly recognized rickettsial disease; isolation of a Rickettsia apparently identical with the causative agent of rickettsialpox from Allodermanyssus sanguineus, a rodent mite. Public Health Rep (1896) 61(47):1677–1682

© Springer Nature Singapore Pte Ltd. 2024
K. G. Narayan et al., *Handbook of Management of Zoonoses*,
https://doi.org/10.1007/978-981-99-9885-2_59

627

Chapter 60
Rickettsiosis

Rickettsiosis is a disease complex. There are 26 known pathogenic species of the genus *Rickettsia*. Parola et al. (2005) reviewed species described/known prior to 1984, those emerging in 1984–2004 and newer ones in process of recognition.

The agents of the order Rickettsiales (both of known and unknown pathogenicities) are potentially transmitted to humans via the biting and/or contamination of mucous membranes/lesions by ectoparasites/arthropods such as hard or soft ticks, fleas, mosquitoes, mites, lice and fleas.

According to Piotrowski and Rymaszewska (2020), many species are distributed all over the world (Table 60.1). The vectors are species of ticks, principally of the genus *Ixodes*. The geographical distribution of Rickettsiae is related to their vectors. New location and new cases of rickettsiosis continue to be identified due to the variety and rapidly expanding and increasing density. Rickettsiae considered non-pathogenic are now known to cause disease. Novel Rickettsial species are detected in ticks around the world. The pathogenicity is unknown. Newer technologies, such as molecular recognition and swabbing of eschars followed by PCR, have enabled describing emerging tick-borne rickettsioses.

The order Rickettsiales, family *Rickettsiaceae*, diverged into three major phylogenetic groups with arthropod hosts (Gillespie et al. 2007):

- Ancestral group (AG) containing *R. bellii* and *R. canadensis*
- SFG (spotted fever group) associated with ticks, fleas and mites
- The TG (typhus group) including *R. prowazekii* and *R. typhi* associated with body lice and rat fleas, respectively

Recently, SFG has been divided into phylogenetic subgroups (El Karkouri et al. 2017):

© Springer Nature Singapore Pte Ltd. 2024
K. G. Narayan et al., *Handbook of Management of Zoonoses*,
https://doi.org/10.1007/978-981-99-9885-2_60

Table 60.1 Global distribution of Rickettsiae (Parola et al. 2013)

Geographic region	Tick-borne Rickettsiae spp.
Sub-Saharan Africa	*Rickettsia aeschlimannii, R. africae, R. conorii* subsp. *caspia, R. conorii* subsp. *conorii, R. massiliae* and *R. sibirica* subsp. *mongolitimonae (6)*
North Africa	*R. aeschlimannii, R. africae, R. conorii* subsp. *conorii, R. conorii* subsp. *indica, R. conorii* subsp. *israelensis, R. helvetica, R. massiliae, R. monacensis, R. raoultii, R. rickettsia, R. sibirica* subsp. *Mongolitimonae* and *R. slovaca (12)*
Europe	*R. aeschlimannii, R. conorii* subsp. *caspia, R. conorii* subsp. *conorii, R. conorii* subsp. *indica, R. conorii* subsp. *indica, R. conorii* subsp. *israelensis, R. helvetica, R. massiliae, R. monacensis, R. raoultii, R. sibirica* subsp. *Mongolitimonae* and *R. slovaca (12)*
Asia	*R. aeschlimannii, R. africae, R. conorii* subsp. *conorii, R. conorii* subsp. *indica, R. conorii* subsp. *Indica, R. conorii* subsp. *israelensis, R. heilongjiangensis, R. helvetica, R. honei, R. japonica, R. massiliae, R. raoulti, R. sibirica* subsp. *mongolitimonae, R. sibirica* subsp. *sibirica, R. slovaca* and *R. tamurae (16)*
North and Central America	*R. africae, R. massiliae, R. parkeri, R. philipii* (364D) and *R. rickettsii*
Pacific Islands	*R. africae*
Australia	*R. australis, R. honei* and *R. honei* strain marmionii
Pacific	*R. honei*
South America	*R. massiliae, R. parkeri* and *R. rickettsia*

- *Rickettsia slovaca* and *R. raoultii*, which are mainly associated with *Dermacentor* ticks, cause scalp eschar and neck lymphadenopathy (SENLAT) in humans
- *Rickettsia conorii* and *Rickettsia massiliae*, which are most often associated with *Rhipicephalus* ticks, cause Mediterranean spotted fever (MSF) in humans.

Genetic studies are contributing to understand the fitness and evolution of SFG rickettsia.

Rickettsial infections are caused by bacteria belonging to genera *Rickettsia, Anaplasma, Ehrlichia, Neorickettsia, Neoehrlichia* and *Orientia* (Nicholson and Paddock 2020).

Tick-borne Rickettsiosis are Anaplasmosis, Ehrlichiosis and Neoehrlichiosis. Anaplasmosis and Ehrlichiosis occur primarily in the USA, reported also throughout the world. Neoehrlichiosis are reported from Asia and Europe.

- *Anaplasma*—*A. phagocytophilum* with small mammals, rodents and deer as reservoir hosts causes human anaplasmosis.
- *Ehrlichia*—*E. chaffeensis, E. muris muris* with white-tailed deer, domestic ruminants, rodents and dogs as reservoir hosts. *E. ewingii, E. canis* and *E. muris eauclairensis* with dogs as the reservoir host. These cause human ehrlichiosis.
- *Neoehrlichia*—*N. mikurensis* with rodents as reservoir hosts causes neoehrlichiosis.

Other Rickettsiosis are described as follows:

* The Spotted Fever Group
* Typhus group of Rickettsiosis
* Scrub Typhus of Rickettsiosis

60.1   The Spotted Fever Group of Tick-Borne Rickettsioses

Rodents as Reservoir

* *Rickettsia rickettsia*—Rocky mountain spotted fever and Brazilian spotted fever
* *R. parkeri*—Maculatum infection
* *R. australis*—Queensland tick typhus
* *R. heilongjiangensis*—Far Eastern spotted fever
* *R. japonica*—Japanese spotted fever
* *R. sibirica mongolotimonae*—Lymphangitis-associated rickettsiosis
* *R. helvetica*—Aneruptive fever

Rodents and Dogs as Reservoir

* *R. conorii*—Mediterranean spotted fever or Boutonneuse fever

  Rodents and Reptiles as Reservoir

* *R. honei*, including strain 'marmionii'—Flinders Island spotted fever, Thai tick typhus

  Rodent and Lagomorph as Reservoir

* *R. slovaca*—Tick-borne lymphadenopathy (TIBOLA), *Dermacentor*-borne necrosis and lymphadenopathy (DEBONEL)

  Ruminant as R*eservoir*

* R. *africae*—African tick bite fever

  Unknown Reservoir, Possibly d=Dogs

* *R. massiliae*—Mediterranean spotted fever-like disease

  Lizards, Possibly Birds as Reservoir

* *R. monacensis*—Mediterranean spotted fever-like disease

  Unknown Reservoir

* *R. raoultii*—Tick-borne lymphadenopathy (TIBOLA), *Dermacentor*-borne necrosis and lymphadenopathy (DEBONEL)
* *Rickettsia aeschlimannii*—*Rickettsiosis*

  Domestic C*ats,* R*odents and* O*possums as* R*eservoirs*

* *R. felis*—Cat flea rickettsiosis

60.2   Typhus Group

R. prowazekii (body louse)—Epidemic typhus, sylvatic typhus—human body louse, flying squirrel ecto-parasites
  R. typhi (flea)—*Murine typhus*—*rodents*
  R. sibirica (Tick)—North Asian tick typhus, Siberian tick typhus—rodents

60.3   Scrub Typhus

Orientia tsutsugamushi (mite-larva/chigger)—*scrub typhus*—*rodents*
  Orientia chuto
Rickettsiosis are reported globally (table from Parola et al. 2013). Rickettsial zoonoses are among the oldest known zoonoses. Tick-borne rickettsiosis are complex, emerging and re-emerging, as many considered as non-pathogenic have been found causing human infections. There is geographic expansion of rickettsiosis.

Scrub typhus cases occurred in both the regions of China, Jiangsu and Jiangxi. Patients infected with *Anaplasma bovis*, *R. monacensis* and *Orientia tsutsugamushi* were detected. Multiple species of Rickettsiales were circulating in small mammals and ticks in both the provinces (Lu et al. 2019). A meta-analysis reported *R. aeschlimannii*, *R. africae*, *R. massiliae*, *R. monacensis*, *R. slovaca*, *R. conorii*, *R. conorii* subsp. *israelensis*, *R. conorii* subsp. *indica* and *A. phagocytophR. monacensisilum* from Italy. MSF and TIBOLA and HGA were the most frequent clinical manifestations (Guccione et al. 2021).

Neoehrlichia mikurensis is a tick-borne pathogen. Generally immunocompromised are infected. Cases occur in parts of Asia and Europe. *Neorickettsia sennetsu* cases have been reported from Japan, Malaysia and other parts of Asia after eating raw neorickettsiae- infected fish.

Ectoparasites, ticks, mites, fleas and lice transmit most rickettsia by bites and infectious fluids (faeces) through inoculation. Rickettsia may enter hosts also through conjunctiva and inhalation. Blood-borne rickettsia may be transmitted through transfusion and organ transplant.

Rodents are the reservoirs for most of the rickettsia. Other reservoirs like ruminants, dogs, etc., and the vectors share the environment with human. Areas where rodents abound, such as port cities and coastal regions and exposure to flea infested cats and dogs, travel to and stay/sleep in rodent infested areas are risky. Outdoor activities, such as hunting, hiking, eco-tourism and travel, spread rickettsiosis.

60.4   The Pathogen: Rickettsia

According to Parola et al. (2013), there are 26 *Rickettsia* species. Subspecies are being added, for example, *R. conorii* subsp. and *R. sibirica* subsp. Rickettsia genome is small sized, 1.11 Mb for *R. typhi (flea-borne)* to 2.1 Mb for *R. scapularis* (endosymbiont of *Ixodes scapularis*). Genome degradation, especially genome loss, drives rickettsia for adaptation to intracellular life within eukaryotic cells and possibly associated with increased virulence. The reductive evolution leaves noncoding sequences that function in biosynthetic pathways. Rickettsial genomes contain a variety of duplicated or repeated genes or fragments of DNA also. These are responsible for encoding substances related to pathogenicity and virulence, for example, type IV secretion system. There are multiple plasmids in several species of *Rickettsia*, suggesting possibility of lateral transfer of genes.

Rickettsiae use a variety of mechanisms to adapt to environment, ticks and other vectors, vertebrate hosts and environment. Many *Rickettsia* species multiply in arthropod vectors (amplify) and pass through the entire life of vectors, eggs to adult female (reservoir) and a mechanism of survival in symbiont invertebrate.

Transovarial transmission (TOT) is measured as 'the percentage of infected females that pass microorganisms to their progeny'. Filial infection rate (FIR) is measured as 'the per cent of infected progeny derived from infected female'.

Parola et al. (2013) cite examples of 100% FIR of *R. rickettsii* in naturally infected *Rhipicephalus sanguineus* ticks. The variations are likely, attributed to reproductive performance and survival of female tick

60.5   Rocky Mountain Spotted Fever (RMSF)

Synonyms: Rocky mountain spotted fever, Tick typhus, Tobia fever in Colombia, Sao Paulo fever or Febre maculosa in Brazil, Febre manchada in Mexico.

RMSF is an important tick-borne rickettsial zoonosis appearing as clinical disease in man and dogs. It is characterized by fever and headache followed by rash on the wrists, arms, ankle and feet. Vomiting and myalgia may also appear. RMSF was recognized first in man during the 1930s in western parts of the USA and later in dogs in the 1970s. Originally, it was known as 'black measles' because of the characteristic rash. Black measles was first recognized in 1896 in the Snake valley of Idaho and was a dreaded and frequently fatal disease in this area.

RMSF is recognized as one of the serious illnesses in the USA.

60.5.1   Aetiology

Spotted fever group of *Rickketsiae* are mainly *R. rickettsii* (the cause of RMSF), *R. parkeri* and *Rickettsia* species 364D. These are closely related genetically and antigenically. The rate of incidence and fatality of RMSF (*R. rickettsia)* in the USA is highest.

R. parkeri—rickettsiosis was described in 2004 and *Rickettsia* species 364D rickettsiosis in 2010. The former is ascribed to at least 40 cases till 2015 occurring during April–October in Kansas, Maryland, Oklahoma and Virginia (Biggs et al. 2016).

Rickettsia species 364D-caused rickettsiosis were reported from California during July-September. *Dermacentor occidentalis* is found in the coastal ranges of Oregon and California. Principal hosts of adult ticks are horses, cattle and black-tailed deer, whereas immature ticks feed on rodents and rabbits.

60.5.2 Epidemiology

The natural maintenance cycle of tick-borne rickettsial pathogens involve domestic or wild vertebrates and hard-bodied ticks (Akari: *Ixodidae*). The seasonal activities of vector tick and vertebrate hosts involved in transmission of these pathogens determine the geographic distribution. Human behaviours position persons at risk for tick attachment, bites and infection. Most cases occur during spring and summer months although cases appear all through the year in warm regions.

RMSF is endemic throughout the USA, Canada and several countries in Central and South America, including Argentina, Brazil, Columbia, Costa Rica, Mexico, and Panama.

Annual incidence determined by passive surveillance during 1997–2002 in the USA was 2.2/million reported from 48 states (Chapman 2006). More recently, Biggs et al. (2016) reported the figure for the period 2008–2012. The passive surveillance estimates for SFG was 8.9 cases/million/year in the USA (RMSF and SFG might not be differentiated), a substantial increase.

Highest rate of incidence was in the age group of 60–69 years and highest case fatality among children of <10 years of age.

The five states, Arkansas, Missouri, North Carolina, Oklahoma and Tennessee, continue to report the highest incidence and an increase from 56% (1997–2002) to 63% (2008–2012).

R. parkeri rickettsiosis cases are common along the Gulf Coast and the eastern seaboard. *Rickettsia* species 364D rickettsiosis cases occur in California.

Severe or fatal RMSF is associated with certain host factors: children and advanced age, male, race (American Indians, African Americans), chronic alcoholism, a sex-linked genetic condition and glucose-6-phosphate dehydrogenase deficiency (Amitai and Sinert 2009).

The disease is caused by *Ricketsia rickettsii* and spread to humans by ticks, *Dermacentor variabilis* in eastern, central and Pacific coastal states of the USA, *Dermacentor andersoni* in western USA and *Rhipicephalus sanguineus* in Central and South America, extending to Texas in the USA and Mexico (Chapman 2006).

According to Biggs et al. (2016), RMSF has emerged in parts of Arizona along the US-Mexico border. The incidence and case fatality rates are unusually high, particularly among children. The period of seasonal exposure to ticks, *Rhipicephalus sanguineus*, is prolonged and domestic and peridomestic exposures increased. Mexico has high incidence of RMSF and some cases acquiring infection there seek health care across the US-Mexico border. Several species of *Amblyomma* are also vectors of *R. rickettsii* from Mexico to Argentina. Their role in the USA has not been established.

D. variabilis are found commonly along the walkways and trails in wooded, shrubby and grassy areas, also in city parks and residential areas. Maximum activity of adult ticks is observed during late spring through early summer; these are active from spring through autumn. Adult *D. variabilis* and *D. andersoni* bite human, but larvae and nymph do not. The principal hosts tend to be deer, dogs and livestock.

Rh. sanguineus (the brown dog tick) is a recognized vector of *R. rickettsii* in Mexico. Canids, especially domestic dogs, are the preferred hosts for all stages. Dogs may be heavily infested and spread infected ticks among households. Humans are incidental hosts and may be bitten by all stages of ticks through contact with infested dogs or due to exposure to tick-infested environment. High incidence of RMSF among children <10 years of age may be because of their increased interaction with dogs and their habitat. *Rh. sanguineus* remain active round the year in the warm climate of Arizona and cases appear every month; however most RMSF cases occur during July–October after seasonal monsoon.

The incidence is seasonal, coincident with tick activity. In the USA, it occurs during April through September.

60.5.3   Transmission

Small mammals like chipmunks and squirrel act as reservoirs. Dogs and human are also reservoirs but are incidental hosts and are the only ones that manifest clinical disease. Ticks feeding on these get infected and are able to transmit/spread infection. The larvae and nymph of *Dermacentor* spp. feed on small mammals and adults prefer large mammals. *Dermacentor andersoni* (Fig. 60.1) takes 2–3 years for completion of its life cycle. *Rickettsia rickettsii* does not reach a high titre in blood of infected large mammals so as to infect ticks feeding on them.

RMSF rickettsia propagate in nature by infected ticks. Infected ticks pass rickettsia transovarially and transstadially. This way ticks remain infected throughout their life.

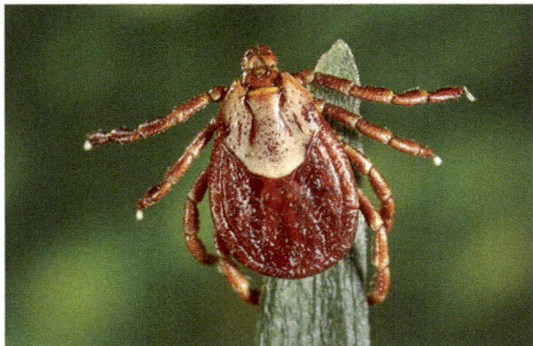

Fig. 60.1 Adult female *Dermacentor andersoni* [Source: Biggs et al. 2016, MMWR. 65(2):1–44]

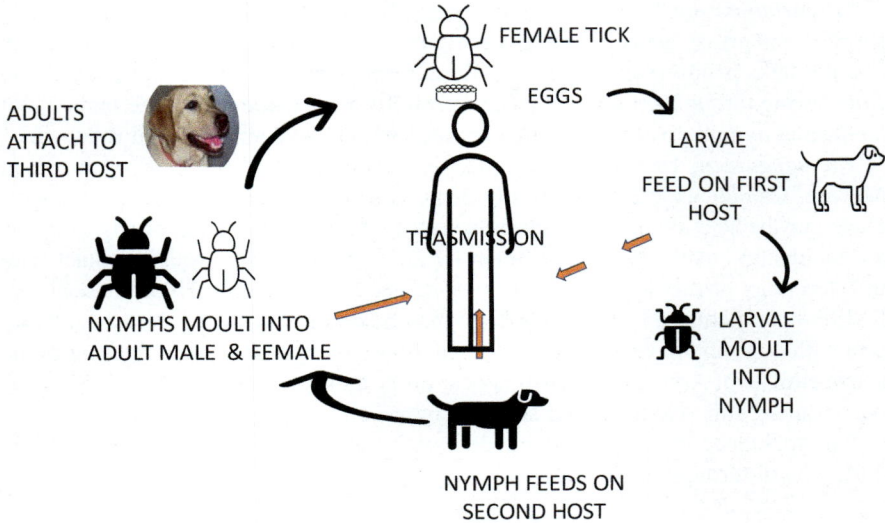

Fig. 60.2 Life cycle of *Rhipicephalus sanguineus* and transmission

The brown dog ticks, *Rhipicephalus sanguineus*, are found in parts of south-western USA and Mexico. The infected female ticks (feeding on the third host) lay eggs with *R. rickettsia*. The larvae hatch out, find the first dog host, feed upon and moult into nymph. Larvae may or may not transmit infection to human (broken arrow in Fig. 60.2). The nymphs attach the second dog host and can also to human, bite and transmit *R. rickettsia*. These falls from the body of dogs and moult into adult male and female. Adults find and attach the third dog host and human to transmit infection.

The larval and nymphal stages are therefore most often infected with *R. rickettsii*. Infected ticks transmit rickettsia through their saliva while biting for 5–20 h. Rickettsia may be present in haemolymph or excrement also. The remains of mouth parts of ticks while being pulled and also if crushed the infection can be transmitted through any cuts, abrasion and scratches and scrapes. The infected mammals do not transmit infection directly. Same infected ticks can pass infection to both dogs and human beings (pet and its owners while wandering in forests).

60.5.4   *Pathogenesis*

Tick bite is painless and often goes unnoticed, thus allowing time (5–20 h) for passing the rickettsia which enter skin and spread by lymphatics to bloodstream. This brings them to the target cells and vascular endothelium. In the endothelial cells of venules and capillaries, these multiply and spread. The pathological changes begin. There is vasculitis leading to oedema, haemorrhage, shock and vascular collapse. Most commonly, the end arterial organs—brain, skin, heart and kidneys—are most often affected. There is vascular hyperpermeability, hypovolemia, hypoalbumin-emia and mononuclear cell response.

RMSF is a multiple system disease and may affect blood vessels, tissues and organs throughout the body. Pulmonary form shows pulmonary oedema, interstitial pneumonia and adult respiratory distress syndrome. The latter is the most common cause of mortality. Microcirculatory vasculitis may cause myocarditis. When the kidney is affected, glomerular filtration rates decrease. Hepatic cell necrosis is focal and manifested as increased serum aminotransferase. Abdominal and gastrointesti-nal symptoms arise because of endothelial cell injury. There may be intestinal bleeding and anaemia. CNS involvement is manifested as encephalitis and menin-goencephalitis arising because of vascular injury. Ocular lesions tend to be bilateral, and these may be conjunctival hyperaemia, retinal haemorrhage and anterior uveitis.

60.5.5 Symptoms

Diagnosis of RMSF and initiating treatment in time is important. The disease pres-ents as with non-specific febrile illness and sepsis of unknown aetiology. Occurrence during spring and summer in the USA raises suspicion. RMSF progresses rapidly in absence of treatment. Delaying treatment is associated with increased hospitaliza-tion and requirement for intensive care and with fatality.

Infection may be asymptomatic in some. The incubation period (from bite of ticks to start of illness) is 5–10 days. The initial signs and symptoms are non-specific. These are fever (102 °F), nausea, vomiting, anorexia, severe headache and myalgia. These are followed by abdominal pain, joint pain, diarrhoea and petechial rash on the wrist, arms, trunk, ankles, palm and sole. The disease is severe and demands hospitalization.

The classical triad-tick bite, fever and rash characterize RMSF. There is a ten-dency of rash beginning from extremities and coursing towards trunk (centripetal). Rash appears (generally 2–5 days after onset of fever) as small, flat, pink non-itchy spots on the wrist, arms and ankles (Fig. 60.3a, b, c). The characteristic pink/red rashes appear on the sixth day of the onset of symptoms or later. Some patients do

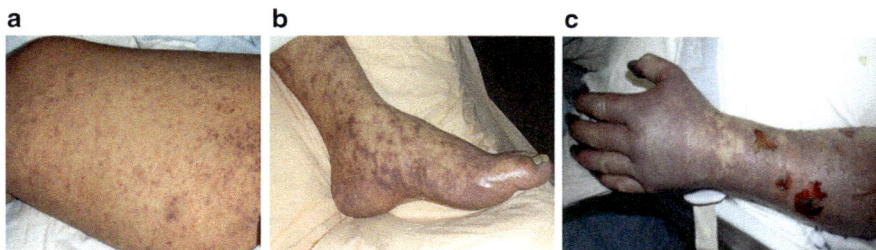

Fig. 60.3 (**a**) Maculopapular rash with central petechiae, (**b**) Late-stage petechial purpuric rash involving the sole of the foot in a patient (**c**) Gangrene of the digits in a patient with late-stage [Source: Biggs et al. 2016, MMWR. 65(2):1–44]

not show the classic distribution of rash on the palm and sole. Skin necrosis or gangrene, jaundice and CNS symptoms may be manifested by some patients. Death usually occurs eight days after the onset of symptoms. It may be as short as five days in fulminant cases. CFR used to be high (30%) before the advent of antibiotics. It has been reduced to 1.4% currently and mostly in cases of delayed diagnosis and treatment. The CFR in children <5 years and adults older than 70 years are 5% and 9%, respectively.

Among those who recover from severe, life-threatening disease requiring long hospitalization, most have long-term health effects persisting for >1 year after acute infection. These may be scarring—gangrene necessitating amputation of fingers, toes, arms or legs, cranial nerve damage leading to paralysis of the lower extremities, blindness or deafness, loss of bowel or bladder control and movement or speech disorder (Amitai and Sinert 2009).

It is considered that *R. rickettsii* infection leads to long-lasting immunity against reinfection. However, recovered cases are advised to take personal precaution against tick bites and report to physician in case of suspected illness following tick bite.

60.6   *R. parkeri* Rickettsiosis

Rickettsiosis caused by *R. parkeri* and *Rickettsia* species 364D have been described by Biggs et al. (2016).

IP 5 days (2–10 days), relatively less severe than RMSF and about one-third cases require hospitalization. There is an eschar formation at the site of infected tick bite. The eschar is a shallow ulcer of about 0.5–2 cm covered with a scabbed plaque surrounded by erythematous halo and few petechiae (Fig. 60.4).

Fever, myalgia and headache follow within a few days. In most cases, rash develops in a few (about 4) days on trunks and extremities like the palm and sole in some cases and faces in few. It is non-pruritic maculopapular or vesiculopapular. Draining/regional lymphadenopathy occurs. Rare cases show nausea, vomiting and

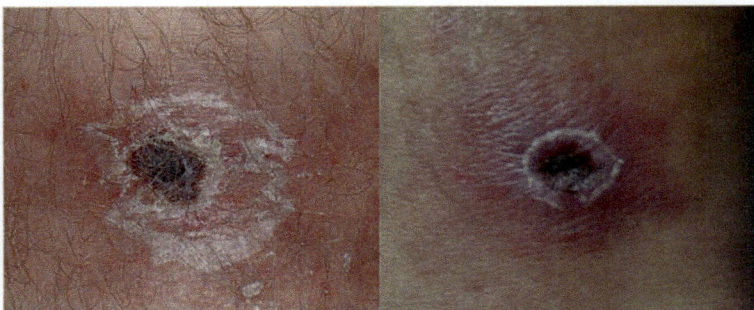

Fig. 60.4 Various appearances of eschars various appearances of eschars associated with *Rickettsia parkeririckettsiosis* [Source: Biggs et al. 2016, MMWR. 65(2):1–44].

gastrointestinal involvement. Laboratory investigation show mild thrombocytopenia, leukopenia and elevated hepatic transaminase.

R. parkeri is distributed throughout multiple tissues of the principal vector tick, *Ambylomma maculatum*, collected in the states along the Gulf Coast and the southern Atlantic region of the USA. *A. americanum* and *D. variabilis* are other vectors. A travel-related case in person returning from Honduras has been recorded. Dogs and cows have been found infected (Parola et al. 2013).

60.7   Rickettsia Species 364D Rickettsiosis

It is characterized by development fever, myalgia, fatigue, eschar or ulcerative skin lesion and lymphadenopathy. The disease is mild and easily treatable.

60.8   Diagnosis

- Classical triad—tick bite, fever and reddish rash.
- Thrombocytopenia (decreased blood platelets), hyponatremia (low sodium) and elevated liver enzymes.
- Serological—ELISA, CFT, and IFA microscopic and Latex agglutination; four-fold increase in IgG titre in case of paired serum samples or high (>1024) in case of single sample; IgM antibody (>8) indicates recent infection; titre declines after four weeks. Note—IgG titre increase 2–3 weeks post infection, lasting for 3–10 months.
- Histochemical staining (Fig. 60.5).
- Molecular—PCR of biopsy or samples from skin lesion to detect Rickettsia DNA through amplification of 16S rRNA.

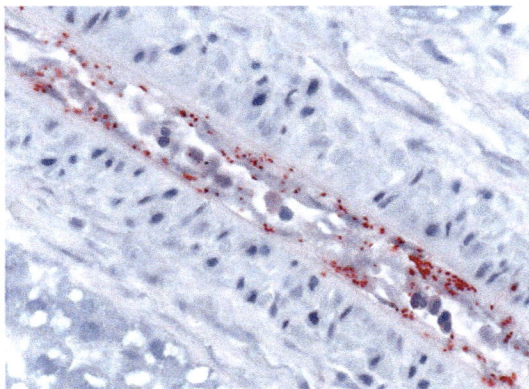

Fig. 60.5 Immunohistochemical stain demonstrating *Rickettsia rickettsii* [Source: Biggs et al. 2016, MMWR. 65(2):1–44].

60.9   Treatment

Tetracycline and doxycycline given at 100 mg every 12 h for adults and 4 mg/kg b. wt. in two divided doses per day for children <45 kg, continued for three days even after fever subsides and until clinical improvement. Generally, the course of treatment is 5–10 days.

60.10   Prevention

In absence of vaccine, personal protection against tick bite is the only method. Common sites where ticks reside are grassy, brushy or wooded areas or even on animals.

Sentinel: The presence of infected dogs is a valuable sentinel for human risk. These increase the risk of transmission to people where the vector is brown dog tick. Dogs and other infected animals do not pose a direct transmission risk in normal circumstances. Abundant and stray dogs can increase overall risk for other dogs and people.

RMSF is often seen in dogs and their owners. Associated cases frequently cluster in defined geographical area. How to detect?—Search ticks on dogs' body. If sick, look for suggestive symptoms: fever (up to 105 °F/40.5 °C), anorexia, lymphadenopathy, polyarthritis, dyspnoea, vomiting and diarrhoea, oedema on the face or extremities, evidence of haemorrhage in the retina, conjunctiva and oral mucosa. Carcass presents evidence of vascular endothelial damage, petechiae and ecchymoses and disseminated intravascular coagulation. Confirm with laboratory tests.

References

Amitai A, Sinert RH (2009) Rocky Mountain Spotted Fever: Overview. http://emedicine.medscape.com/article/785659-overview Updated: Mar 23, 2021, Author: Sunny Patel DO

Biggs HM, Behravesh CB, Bradley KK et al (2016) Diagnosis and Management of Tickborne Rickettsial Diseases: Rocky Mountain Spotted Fever and Other Spotted Fever Group Rickettsioses, Ehrlichioses, and Anaplasmosis — United States. A Practical Guide for Health Care and Public Health Professionals. Recommendations and Reports. MMWR Recomm Rep 65(2):1–44

Chapman AS (2006) Diagnosis and Management of Tickborne Rickettsial Diseases: Rocky Mountain Spotted Fever, Ehrlichioses, and Anaplasmosis — United States. A Practical Guide for Physicians and Other Health-Care and Public Health Professionals. https://www.cdc.gov/mmwr/preview/mmwrhtml/rr5504a1.htm

El Karkouri K, Kowalczewska M, Armstrong N, Azza S et al (2017) Multi-omics analysis sheds light on the evolution and the intracellular lifestyle strategies of Spotted Fever Group Rickettsia spp. Front Microbiol 8:1363

Gillespie JJ, Beier MS, Rahman MS, Ammerman NC et al (2007) Plasmids and Rickettsial evolution: insight from *Rickettsia felis*. PLoS ONE 2(3):e266

Guccione C, Colomba C, Tolomeo M, Trizzino M, Iaria C, Cascio A (2021) *Rickettsiales* in Italy. Pathogens 10(2):181

Lu M, Li F, Liao Y et al (2019) Epidemiology and diversity of Rickettsiales bacteria in humans and animals in Jiangsu and Jiangxi provinces, China. Sci Rep 9:13176

Nicholson WL, Paddock CD (2020) Rickettsial Diseases (including Spotted Fever & Typhus Fever Rickettsioses, Scrub Typhus, Anaplasmosis and Ehrlichioses). https://wwwnc.cdc.gov/travel/yellowbook/2020/travel-related-infectious-diseases/rickettsial-including-spotted-fever-and-typhus-fever-rickettsioses-scrub-typhus-anaplasmosis-and-ehr

Parola P, Paddock C D, Raoult D (2005) Tick-borne rickettsioses around the world: Emerging diseases challenging old concepts. Clin Microbiol Rev 18:719–756

Parola P, Paddock CD, Socolovschi C, Labruna MB, Mediannikov O et al (2013) Update on tick-borne rickettsioses around the world: a geographic approach. Clin Microbiol Rev 26(4):657–702. Erratum in: Clin Microbiol Rev 27(1):166

Piotrowski M, Rymaszewska A (2020) Expansion of Tick-Borne Rickettsioses in the World. Microorganisms 8(12):1906

Chapter 61
Scrub Typhus

Synonyms

Japanese fever, Tsutsugamushi disease, Tropical typhus, Bush typhus, Rural typhus, Chigger-borne rickettsiosis.

Scrub typhus is a mite larva (chigger) transmitted metazoonosis of life-threatening potential. Scrub typhus (ST) generates high annual disease burden. Yet, it remains neglected.

Orientia pathogenesis and immunity are less understood. Development of a cross protective vaccine is challenging.

The condition ranges from mild febrile illness to life-threatening severe illness. Lymphadenitis occurs in many cases. Rash is considered hallmark of rickettsiosis but not seen in all. Similarly, eschar formation is seen in 50–80% of Scrub typhus cases. Fatal multiple organ failure is reported in 7–15% with acute distress syndrome related to lung injury, hepatitis, renal failure, myocarditis, encephalitis and central nervous system involvement usually after two weeks and frequently among inappropriately treated cases.

Broad range of non-specific symptoms misleads and delays diagnosis. There is deficient acquired immunity. Detected serum IgG and IgM are from previous exposure. Delayed diagnosis and management may be fatal.

There is natural resistance of the pathogen to fluoroquinolones and beta-lactam drugs. Medical facilities are limited in rural endemic location.

Outbreaks are increasing within and outside of the *Tsutsugamushi* triangle and also the number of people at risk of contracting the disease. The resurgence may be due to awareness, increased surveillance and improvement of the diagnostic tests. Frequent outbreaks and re-infections occurring in the endemic regions may also be due to antigenic heterogeneity.

Luce-Fedrow et al. (2018) summarized 21 outbreaks of scrub typhus during 2000–2017 such as Soloman Island 1, Nepal 2, Thailand 1, India 14, Bhutan 1,

K. G. Narayan et al., *Handbook of Management of Zoonoses*,
https://doi.org/10.1007/978-981-99-9885-2_61

China 2 and Australia 1. According to Sharma and Mishra (2020), it was endemic in India in the 1960s and 1970s and was considered eradicated due to the use of insecticides and empirical use of chloromycetin and tetracyclines for treating PUO. It made a re-appearance in the 1990s in soldiers at the Indo-Pakistan border. There were nine outbreaks earlier to the year 2000, eight were mostly among soldiers and from Assam, Bengal. Indian tick typus, endemic typhus, Murine flea-borne typhus, spotted fever/malignant Mediterranean spotted fever and scrub typhus caused 23 outbreaks during 2000–2018; 11 were scrub typhus.

Fever of unknown origin involving multiple organs has increased over the past few years and scrub typhus in Asian countries coincident with urbanization of rural areas and widespread use of beta-lactum antibiotics. Possible contributory factors are deforestation, unplanned urbanization, movement/dispersal of reservoir rodents and vectors coincident with increasing travel and interest in investigation of causes of PUO.

61.1   Aetiology

Orientia tsutsugamushi belongs to the genus *Orientia*, family Rickettsiales, order Rickettsiaceae. The infectious particles of the genera *Orientia* and *Rickettsia* are located free in the cell cytoplasm.

Antigenic three prototypes of *O. tsutsugamushi* isolates were Karp, Kato and Gilliam initially determined by complement fixation, later by indirect and direct immunofluorescence assays. The 56-kDa protein was a major antigenic determinant. Sequencing and restriction-length polymorphism analyses determined high degree of genetic variability, multiple intragenic recombination events and a high rate of mutation. To date, only two fully assembled genomes, belonging to the Boryong (Korea) and Ikeda (Japan) isolates, exist for *O. tsutsugamushi* (Luce-Fedrow et al. 2018).

R. tsutsugamushi (R. orientalis, Orientia tsutsugamushi) is a natural and obligate intracellular parasite of mite, Gram's negative pleomorphic and stains well with Giemsa. It is alpha-proteobacterium, family Rickettsiaceae, genus *Orientia* (earlier *Rickettsia*). It has highly variable membrane protein and can have many antigenic strains. The classic antigenic strains are Karp, Gillam, Kato, Shimokoshi Kuroki and Kawasaki.

There are four major antigens (surface membrane proteins of 22 kDa, 47 kDa, 56 kDa and 110 kDa). The type specific antigen is 56 kDa and is useful in the serologic diagnostic tests. It enables the rickettsia to adhere, enter and invade host cells evading hosts' immune system. Isolates of *O. tsutsugamushi* from mites and rodents make great number of varying strains, differing in virulence.

61.2   Pathogenesis

Dermal dendritic cells and activated monocytes are the targets after intradermal entry by the pathogen which disseminates to lymph nodes. Scrub typhus is a disseminated endothelial infection with injury of organs (multi-organ failure) and death. Young white cells at the site of inoculation and then the endothelial cells lining vasculature are attacked. Phagocytes in circulating blood and macrophages in all organs are targeted. Attachment is mediated by membrane protein 56 kDa and surface cell antigens.

O. tsutsugamushi manipulates widely distributed cell receptor families and molecules for attachment to cells and active internalization—endocytic pathway for entering epithelial cells and fibroblast. The bacterium is transported into cytoplasm in a transportation bubble (vesicle) that is formed escaping phagosomal compartment. Exit (exocytosis) from the vesicle is facilitated by lysosome. It moves to perinuclear region, grows and multiplies in phagocytic, non-phagocytic cells, macrophages and dermal dendritic cells. Nitric oxide (NO), a potent free radical involved in the killing of engulfed microbes, enhances the cytosolic binary replication of *O. tsutsugamushi* in murine macrophages reaching a density of 10^3 bacteria in a single cell (Díaz et al. 2018). According to Luce-Fedrow et al. (2018), doubling time is approximately 8–9 h, until the host cell is filled in nearly 96–120 h post infection (strain dependent). The escape (exocytosis) is again in a vesicle using host cell membrane. The process is similar to the one used by some viruses. The released *Orientia* may employ different mechanisms to infect subsequent cells. Study on human autopsy and lethal and sub-lethal rodent infections suggest activation of endothelial cells and pathogenesis in severe scrub typhus. Activation of endothelial cells and immune cells play an important role in inflammatory response and immunopathology. Trent et al. (2019) explained the development of acute respiratory distress. Endothelial cells in damaged vasculature and lung alveoli are activated, proinflammatory cytokines are produced and neutrophils rushing to the site of inflammation also secrete chemokines. Protein-rich fluid (oedema) accumulates in the alveolar and interstitial space causing oedema.

61.3   Symptoms

High positivity is found in age group of 60–69 years.

The incubation period varies between 6 and 21 days. Erythematous, indurated multiple vesicles appear at the site of infective bite. The vesicles burst and ulcerate. Black crust form later. The pathognomonic features are eschar and lymphadenopathy. The lymph gland draining the area near the bite is first affected. Patients may present mental changes from confusion to coma.

Mahajan et al. (2006) isolated two new genotypes of *O. tsutsugamushi* from pyrexia of unknown origin in the Himalayan region and recommended more such studies to understand the epidemiology. They also observed that eschar formed in few secondary infections was rare in Southeast Asian patients, and indigenous persons of typhus-endemic had less severe illness often without rash or eschar. The study in Pondicherry (Vivekanandan et al. 2010) reported diverse clinical and laboratory manifestation. Untreated cases of scrub typhus (ST)- attributable acute febrile illness can progress to acute encephalitis syndrome (AES). ST accounted for two-thirds of acute encephalitis syndrome (AES) cases in Deoria and Gorakhpur, India. Generalized lymphadenitis and splenomegaly occur. Virulent strains may cause haemorrhage and intravascular coagulation. A haemophagocytosis syndrome is detected by cytologic findings of histiocytes containing phagocytosed blood cells in bone marrow aspirates. Prognosis is poor if untreated (Luce-Fedrow et al. 2018).

The onset is sudden presenting of acute febrile illness, high temperature 104–105 °F, chill, headache, myalgia, conjunctivitis and rapidly increasing rash on the trunk and extremities associated with gastrointestinal symptoms. Diseases progress to severe form with organ dysfunctions such as hepatorenal syndrome, coagulopathy or acute respiratory distress syndrome. Commonly scrub typhus patients develop mild interstitial pneumonia and resolve. Nearly 6–44% cases develop severe illness. Acute respiratory distress syndrome characterized by progressive dyspnoea, hypoxia and alveolar infiltrates (detected on X-ray) appear. Interstitial myocarditis occurs. Early stage of disease may present leucopoenia and abnormal liver function tests. Pneumonia, encephalitis and myocarditis are seen in the late stage. If untreated, patients may be die. Saifudheen et al. (2012) reported two cases of meningoencephalitis from Kerala, India. One died due to respiratory failure. Narvencar et al. (2012) evaluated all consecutive adult cases of fever of unknown origin between June 2009 and October 2010 at Goa Medical College. Thirty-four percent of the patients were identified at scrub typhus.

Fatality (about 1.4%) may occur even in untreated cases. It is high in neurological (14%) and multiorgan failure (24%) cases. Misdiagnosis/improper treatment of severe cases may lead to death in 30–70% cases.

Before the advent of antibiotic, case fatality rate was high (60%). One may thus infer that diagnosis and immediate start of antibiotic therapy are important.

There is no lasting immunity. Antigenic variation presents a problem for cross-protection.

61.4   Epidemiology

The endemic region covers the Russian Far East in the north, Japan in the east, northern Australia in the south and Afghanistan in the west—so-called Tsutsugamushi triangle, namely, Japan, Thailand, Korea, Myanmar, Australia, Papua New Guinea, India, Pakistan, Afghanistan and Russia. Scrub typhus is being reported from outside this endemic triangle, such as Africa, South America, the UAE and Maldives, and cases in endemic areas in Asia are increasing.

Scrub typhus is the most underdiagnosed disease. It accounts for about one-fifth of febrile cases in the hospital in some Southeast Asian countries. According to a recent review by Elliott et al. (2019), seroprevalence ranged between 9.3% and 27.9% (22.2% median). Rate of reported rise in incidence every decade is 4.6/100,000 (passive national surveillance systems). Fatality rate is 6% in untreated and 1.4% in treated cases. Calculated disability-adjusted life year estimated in Eastern China is 1.06/100,000. Nearly 1.0 million cases are recorded every year in the endemic area. Rodkvamtook et al. (2013) investigated ST in endemic region of Northern Thailand where every year >200 cases appeared. They demonstrated *O. tsutsugamushi* in children, rodent hosts and potential transmission between human and rodent reservoirs. Serologic and molecular laboratory test results showed that 65 of the children were positive for *O. tsutsugamushi*. Out of 55 rodents captured from grass, rice, banana fields, shrubs and woods, 81.8% were found infested with the chigger, *Leptotrombidium deliense*. *Bandicoot indica* and *B. savilei* had the highest chigger density.

Burden of diseases is huge in rural areas. Farmers are most affected. Infection is increasingly reported also in urban areas. Seroprevalence is high. South Korea, Japan, Thailand and China have the most cases and seropositive.

Scrub typhus is the most common rickettsial disease in India (8/9 earlier to 2000 and 11/23 outbreaks between 2000 and 2018) reported from sub-Himalayan belt from Jammu to Nagaland, Sikkim, Darjeeling, Himachal Pradesh, Bihar, Rajasthan, Maharashtra, South India-Puducherry, Tamil Nadu, Kerala and Karnataka (Sharma and Mishra 2020). Murhekar et al. (2021) reported high seroprevalence (IgG antibodies) of *O. tsutsugamushi* in rural Gorakhpur. Most infections were subclinical. Scrub typhus accounted for one-fifth of acute febrile illness reported during and post-monsoon to peripheral health facilities. Early administration of suitable antibiotic prevented progression of acute febrile illness to acute encephalitis syndrome. Nearly half of AES had serological or molecular evidence of ST. *L. deliense* was the predominant chigger with an index of 5.3/shrew (*Suncus murinus*) during July–November, peak in October. Natural infection with *O. tsutsugamushi* (PCR detected 5 kDa gene) was detected in the chigger during July–October; the peak coincided with peak of AES.

61.4.1   Vector

According to Elliott et al. (2019), free living trombiculid species of mites positive for *O. tsutsugamushi* were 23/31 and belonged to the genus *Leptotrombidium*. There is a good evidence about ten species transmitting *O. tsutsugamushi* to human. *L. deliense*, *L. akamushi*, *L. arenicola*, *L. imphalum*, *L. scutellare*, *L. pallidum*, *L. pavlovskyi* and *L. fetcheri* are the most important. The key vector in South and Southeast Asia was *L. delicense* and in South Korea and Japan were *L. pallidum* and *L. scutellare*.

In addition to *Rickettsia, Anaplasma, Borrelia* and *Hanataan virus* have been found in chiggers, but role in transmission is unclear. Arthropods feeding on rickett-siaemic hosts may be able to acquire *Orientia*, for example, ixodid ticks, flea and a non-chigger mite *Ornithonyssus bacoti*. Onward transmission is not documented; possibly the bacteria cannot cross the gut wall.

The mites live in moist soil (Fig. 61.1) covered in heavy scrub vegetation (bush, grasses). *The* female mites pass *O. tsutsugamushi* to its eggs transovarially, from eggs to larvae and then to adults transstadially. The chigger acts both as reservoir and a host.

Life cycle of trombiculid: There are at least two generations in tropical and one in temperate climate per year. One life cycle takes 2–3 months. Adults survive for 15 months or more. Egg deposition continues for 221 days at mean eggs of 2.4–21.7/day.

There are two six-legged stages, pre-larva and larva, and four eight-legged stages, protonymph, deutonymph, tritonymph and adult. The pre-larval, proto- and tritonymphal stages are inactive and nonfeeding, while the deuteronymph and adult stages are non-parasitic and generally feed on arthropod eggs or small arthropods.

Larval mites, often called chiggers, are the only parasitic stage. Six-legged larva emerge in 7–11 days (two stages: pre-larva and larva) for quiescent deutovum + 5–7 days manifest host-seeking behaviour, clustering on leaves, grass and twigs just above soil. Larva can survive for months waiting for opportunity to feed on verte-brate host. They gain entry into skin through hair follicles and pores of the host, inject salivary secretion using stylostome (feeding tube) that lyse host tissue and ingest digested tissue fluid sucking for 3–5 or more days, engorge and increase sev-eral folds in size and then detach to return to soil surface habitat. They remain attached for two days to several weeks and feed only once in its life. Adults over winter but several of the quiescent instars have the potential to persist in severe

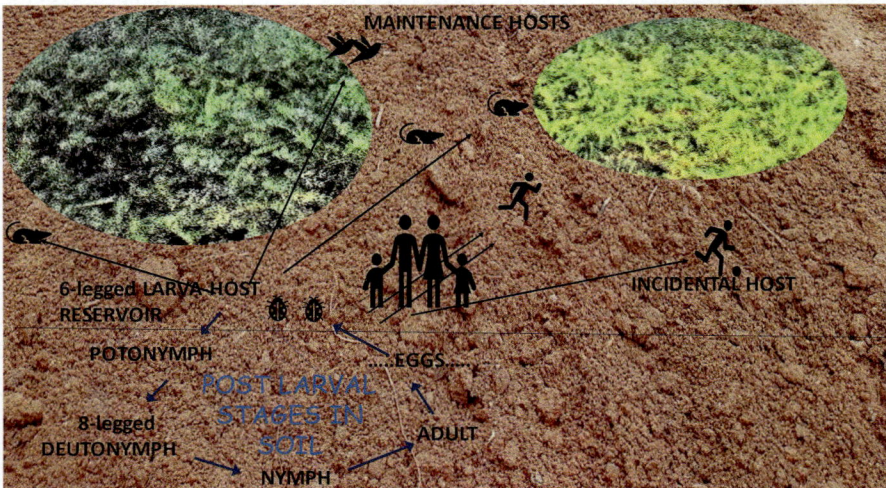

Fig. 61.1 Mite land

environmental conditions and overwinter. Successful transovarial and transstadial transmission is required for vectorial activity.

The chigger acts as a host, reservoir and an exceptional means of long survival for *O. tsutsugamushi*. Transovarial transmission of *Orientia* in lab-maintained chiggers is nearly 100% efficient for four generations in *L. akamushi*, *L. delicense* and *L arenicola*. This efficiency is 93–100% *L. chiangraiensis*, *L. fetcheri* and *L. Arenicola* in Malaysia and Thailand. Transovarial transmission continues through further generations, seen even after 17 generation but with marked decline. It is postulated that the lower rates of isolation of *O. tsutsugamushi* from eggs, deutova, nymphs and adults are because bacterium is in 'occult stage'. It is reactivated during feeding upon the host.

Chigger behaviour: CO_2 of exhaled air attracts. Larvae move <45 cm. Larvae become active at temperature >10 °C, crawl >12 °C at 10 cm /minute at 28 °C and survive for 60 days at 1–2 °C, one months at -20 °C and submerged water for two weeks.

Schoengastiella ligula, in the same superfamily Trombiculidae, but within the family Walchiidae, has also been implicated as a vector.

61.4.2   Hosts

A total 122 of 234 species of 'host' vertebrates (excluding humans) tested positive for *O. tsutsugamushi*. The *Muridae* had the highest proportion of positive tests at (25.5%). The rates of positivity for other groups of small mammals were 12.2%, 13.2% and 18%, respectively, for *Cricetidae*, *Soricidae* and *Canidae* (96% of *Canidae* tested positive using serological methods). Among the *Artiodactyla*, cows, goats and pigs tested 3.6% positive, by only serological methods. *Motacilla cinerea* (grey wagtail) and *Passer domesticus* (house sparrow)—10% birds—were positive in China. Chicken and pigeons could be experimentally infected rickettsia persisted for 42 days. *L. scutellare* and *L. pallidum* were found on chicken. *O. tsutsugamushi* was recovered from the liver and spleen of a chicken and *L. pallidum* in endemic area. Bipartite network analysis is becoming increasingly used to understand host-parasite interactions. The *Muridae* were both the most frequently tested and *O. tsutsugamushi*-positive (Elliott et al. 2019).

Suncus murinus, *Rattus blanfordi*, *R.r.rufescens* and *Mus booduga* are the rodent reservoirs in India.

Habitats are sandy beaches, mountain deserts and equatorial rain forests. Habitat is generally a damp area, classified as the following:

- Land use by man—scrub, fallow, fields, agricultural land, rice fields, grass, parks, riverside, orchards and plantations, settlements and urban and rural
- Crops—names (banana, tea, sugarcane and sweet potato) and general plant types (Miscanthus, lalang, palm, Pandanus and Lantana)
- Natural—mountainous, forest and forest edge

- Forest types—coniferous, deciduous, broadleaf, evergreen and bamboo

'Mite island' describes patchy distribution of human cases and chiggers. Small islands of mites may be 30 × 30 cm and patchy over few hundreds of metres. Large islands may be endemic areas of few to thousands of square miles bounded by ecological barriers.

Mite islands (intensity of vector chigger—host interaction) are determined by food, soil, microclimate and chigger predator. Rabbits or rats are used as bait to collect chigger and determine area of islands. Endemic areas in Japan showed 50% *L. pallidum* positive for *O. tsutsugamushi* compared to only 3.8% in a non-endemic area; 50.5% of rats collected from the site of outbreak in plantation workers were heavily infested with chiggers.

61.4.3   Natural nidii

The population of mites naturally and entirely maintains *Orientia tsutsugamushi*. Rodents and human are accidental hosts and are not required for maintenance of the rickettsia. *Leptotrombidium delicense* is the most common vector for rodents and human. The chigger, that is, larva, is the natural ectoparasites of reservoir small rodents and birds, feed, ingest lymph and tissue fluid to get infected. The reservoir hosts are small wild rodents (*Suncus murinus, Rattus blanfordi, R.r.rufescens* and *Mus booduga*) including rats, tree-shrews, field voles, bandicoots and mongoose, and migratory birds, and trombiculid mites (*Leptotrombidium akamushi, L. deliensi, L. pallidum, L. scutellare* and others) act as vectors. Carrier mites for countries may differ; *L. akamushi* is endemic in Japan, *L. imphalum* and *L. chiangraiensis* in Thailand and *L. Arenicola* in Malaysia and Indonesia.

Human activities and behaviours associated with risk are the following:

- Rural mass gathering of naïve human (arising from military action and training, civilian camping and orienteering, and refugee crises) in areas of high *O. tsutsugamushi*-infected chigger density (mite islands) cause outbreaks
- Human occupation, behaviour and activities promote exposure—farmers, plantation workers and the military and recreational exposure in suburban parks and gardens

Farmers and urban residents participate in agricultural activities, Chusok (Korean thanksgiving), chestnut harvest and mowing around graves. Outdoor leisure/recreational activities such as golf and climbing are increasing since 2004 and possibly add to risk of exposure.

The incidence is driven by human activities. In Japan, it is decreasing because of land development. More females in Korea and not in Japan are affected, possibly because of their active participation in gardening and tending plants (thus better chance of exposure to chiggers). Agricultural operations like plantation of oil palm and rubber, rice, etc. and recreational outings in the woods and mountains are associated with risk of exposure and infection. Kweon et al. (2009) reported the rapid increase in infected persons living in urban areas in South Korea. This was associated with the increase in population of mites and human activities and coincident with season. *Leptotrombidium pallidum* is a common mite in Korea. The mites increase beginning September and peak in October and November and another period April and May though to a lesser degree. Scrub typhus cases peak during October–November and secondary peak during April–May. This is associated with events and activities that increase exposure. Post-monsoon (August–November in India) is ideal for exposure because of increased agricultural activities. Rodents' habitat determines *nidii*, for example, agricultural fields, storing firewood indoors, animal feed fodder store, etc. Males engaged in farming and similar activities frequently get exposed and so more cases are males. Mites lay eggs which hatch to larva in humid condition, for example, moist soil covered with vegetation. Larval stage is infective.

During months following monsoon, there is also growth of secondary vegetation, the habitat of trombiculid mites. Clustering of most cases during July–November in India was possibly associated with farming operations exposing farmers to chigger bites. ST, caused by the bacterium *Orientia tsutsugamushi*, is transmitted by the bite of trombiculid mites, which live in moist soil covered with vegetation. Thangaraj et al. (2018) determined the odds ratios of possible factors associated with ST among children in Deoria and Gorakhpur, India. Important factors identified are playing in such area 5.2, agriculture feed/handling cattle fodder 2.05 and open defecation 2.0.

61.5   Diagnosis

Diagnostic methods are generally based on (a) serology, (b) isolation of pathogen and (c) molecular assay.

Sharma and Mishra (2020) presented useful comparison of the tests available.

61.5.1   Serologic Tests

IFA, indirect immuno-peroxidase and IgM capture ELISA are cent percent specific and 95–100 or 100% sensitive. Rapid immunochromatographic test for scrub typhus is a point of care test with 100% specificity but only 38% sensitivity. IgM capture ELISA is rapid and low cost requiring single acute serum and can be used at the district level hospitals. Weil-Felix test is cheap and easily available and has 77% sensitivity and 81.6% specificity.

61.5.2   Isolation of Organism (Shell Vial Assay)

Specimens include whole blood, serum and skin biopsy; cell lines required may be human, amphibian, avian and arthropod. Positive result is available in three days. It has cent percent sensitivity and specificity. Requirement of BSL-3 laboratory and invasive sampling are the limitations.

61.5.3   Molecular Assays

PCR, real-time PCR and LAMP detect rickettsial DNA. Specimens required include whole blood, buffy coat, eschar and biopsy. Result is available within 24 h.

61.6   Treatment

Chloramphenicol, tetracycline, doxycycline, macrolides, rifampicin and quinolones are effective.

61.7   Prevention

- Avoiding sitting or lying directly on the ground
- Use of insecticides on the skin and clothing
- Thorough washing of skin and clothing after outdoor activities
- Habitat clearing—rodent control

References

Díaz FE, Abarca K, Kalergis AM (2018) An update on host-pathogen interplay and modulation of immune responses during Orientia tsutsugamushi infection. Clin Microbiol Rev 31(2):e00076–e00017

Elliott I, Pearson I, Dahal P, Thomas NV, Roberts T et al (2019) Review Scrub typhus ecology: a systematic review of Orientia in vectors and hosts. Parasites Vectors 12:513

Kweon SS, Choi JS, Lim HS, Kim JR et al (2009) Rapid increase of scrub typhus, South Korea, 2001-2006. Emerg Infect Dis 15(7):1127–1129

Luce-Fedrow A, Lehman ML, Kelly DJ, Mullins K, Maina AN et al (2018) A review of Scrub typhus (Orientia tsutsugamushi and related organisms): then, now, and tomorrow. Trop Med Infect Dis 3(1):8.1-30

Mahajan SK, Rolain JM, Kashyap R, Bakshi D, Sharma V et al (2006) Scrub typhus in Himalayas. Emerg Infect Dis 12(10):1590–1592

Murhekar MV, Vivian Thangaraj JW, Sadanandane C, Mittal M, Gupta N et al (2021) Investigations of seasonal outbreaks of acute encephalitis syndrome due to *Orientia tsutsugamushi* in Gorakhpur region, India: a One Health case study. Indian J Med Res 153(3):375–381

Narvencar KPS, Rodrigues S, Nevrekar RP, Dias L et al (2012) Scrub typhus in patients reporting with acute febrile illness at a tertiary health care institution in Goa. Indian J Med Res 136(6):1020–1024

Rodkvamtook W, Gaywee J, Kanjanavanit S, Ruangareerate T, Richards AL et al (2013) Scrub typhus outbreak, northern Thailand, 2006-2007. Emerg Infect Dis 19(5):774–777

Saifudheen K, Kumar KG, Jose J, Veena V, Gafoor VA (2012) First case of scrub typhus with meningoencephalitis from Kerala: an emerging infectious threat. Ann Indian Acad Neurol 15(2):141–144

Sharma A, Mishra B (2020) Rickettsial disease existence in India: resurgence in outbreaks with the advent of 20th century. Indian J Health Sci Biomed Res 13:5–10

Thangaraj JWV, Vasanthapuram R, Machado L, Arunkumar G, Sodha SV, Zaman K et al (2018) Scrub Typhus Risk Factor Study Group. Risk factors for acquiring Scrub typhus among children in Deoria and Gorakhpur Districts, Uttar Pradesh, India, 2017. Emerg Infect Dis 24(12):2364–2367

Trent B, Fisher J, Soong L (2019) Scrub Typhus pathogenesis: innate immune response and lung injury during *Orientia tsutsugamushi* infection. Front Microbiol 10:2065

Vivekanandan M, Mani A, Priya YS, Singh AP et al (2010) Outbreak of scrub typhus in Pondicherry. J Assoc Physicians India 58:24–28

Part IV
Mycotic Zoonoses

Man is surrounded by fungi ubiquitously distributed in environment, plants and animals. Candidiasis is an important nosocomial infection in intensive care unit settings. These are saprophytes, live on organic matter, contribute to recycling of nutrients, for example, breaking down plant lignin. Zoonotic fungi are saprozoonoses. The infection often passes unnoticed. Viral and bacterial pathologies often overshadow these and when diagnosed the chronic condition has reached life-threatening stage. In several states of India, increased incidence of COVID-19-associated mucormycosis (Black fungus disease) was noticed, and it was declared as a notifiable disease. Black fungal disease (Mucormycoses) is angio-invasive infection with 46% global death.

Fungal infections are common and often serious in immunocompromised, immunodeficient and people with comorbidities, for example, cryptococcosis. The problem is challenging because drugs are limited and treatment is expensive, compounded by drug resistance, for example, *Candida auris* has been found resistant to azoles, polyenes and echinocandins.

Mycotoxins in foods cause serious diseases, for example, jaundice and liver cancer due to aflatoxins. Mycotoxic fungi may enter food chain right from the crop seeds, developing grains on plants or during postharvest storage and processing.

Altogether 11 mycotic diseases of zoonotic importance are discussed.

Chapter 62
Epidemiology of Mycotic Zoonoses

62.1 Classification of Mycotic Zoonoses

Fungi may appear in sexual or teleomorph and asexual or anamorph forms. The teleomorphic names are used in taxonomy. The teleomorphic groups are *Zygomycota* (form zygospores), *Ascomycota* (ascospores) and *Basidiomycota* (basidiospores). The fourth group of fungi is *Deuteromycota* (fungi imperfecta) for which the sexual state is either not known or nor described.

62.1.1 Zygomycota

Zygomycosis—(1) Mucormycosis caused by Mucorales (*Rhizopus* and *Mucor): Rhizopus microspores*, *R. oryzae*, *R. rhizopodiformis* and *Mucor circinelloides*, *M. racemosus* and *M. ramosissimus*. Others: *Rhizomucor pusillus*, *R. variabilis*, *Syncephalastrum racemosum*, *Cunninghamella bertholletiae*, *Apophysomyces elegans*, *Lichtheimia* (formerly *Absidia*), *Absidia corymbifera*, *Saksenaea vasiformis* and (2) Entomophthoramycosis is caused by Entomophthorales: *Basidiobolus ranarum*, *Cokeromyces recurvatus*, *Conidiobolus incongruous* and *Mortierella wolfii*.

62.1.2 Ascomycota

(1) *Dimorphic (yeast + mould)* **Onygenales** *causing* (a) **Coccidioidomycosis**—*Coccidioides immitis* and *C. posadasii*

(b) **Histoplasmosis**—*Histoplasma capsulatum*, **African histoplasmosis**—*H. duboisii*

Other conditions are Lobomycosis (*Lacazia loboi*); Paracoccidioidomycosis (*Paracoccidioidomycosis brasiliensis*); Blastomycosis (*Blastomyces dermatitidis*), Sporotrichosis (*Sporothrix schenckii*); Talaromycosis (*Talaromyces marneffei*).

(2) *Yeast like*—Candidiasis caused by *Candida albicans, C. auris, C. glabrata, C. lusitaniae* and *C. tropicalis*. Pneumocystosis caused by *Pneumocystis jirovecii*.

(3) *Mould like*—Aspergillosis caused by *Aspergillus*; others: Eumycetoma (*Exophiala jeanselmei*), Chromoblastomycosis (*Fonsecaea pedrosoi, F. compacta, Phialophora verrucose*), Geotrichosis (*Geotrichum candidum*), Allescheriasis (*Pseudallescheria boydii*)

(4) Dermatophyte—Dermatophytosis caused by *Tinea barbae/capitis, T. corporis, T. pedis, Epidermophyton floccosum, Microsporum audouinii, M. canis, Trichophyton verrucosum, T. tonsurans, T. rubrum* and *T. mentagrophytes/interdigitale*.

62.1.3   Basidiomycota

Cryptococcosis caused by *Cryptococcus neoformans* and *C. gattii*

Pragmatic classification of fungi (Table 62.1) into yeasts, moulds, dimorphic fungi and dermatophytes was suggested by Arendrup (2013).

Dimorphic fungi may become invasive with a fungaemic state. Most frequent invasive form is fungaemia; vast majority is Candidaemia. Others in decreasing order are *Cryptococcus, Rhodotorula* and *Trichosporon* (Arendrup 2013).

Kumudhavalli (2013) studied 200 suspected invasive fungal infection (IFI) cases in India. Most of them were males between ages 31 and 40 years. IFI occurred 1–10 years after immunosuppression in 77% cases. In about 40% of cases, aetiological agents were identified: *A. fumigatus, C. albicans, C. glabrata* and *Cryptococcus neoformans*. Diabetes mellitus was the most common risk factor followed by renal transplant. *A. fumigatus* and *C. albicans* were the common in diabetic cases. *C. neoformans* was the most common agent in AIDS patients. All isolates were

Table 62.1 Pragmatic classification of fungi (Arendrup 2013)

	Yeasts	Moulds	Dimorphic fungi	Dermatophytes
Genera	*Candida, Saccharomyces, Malassezia, Trichosporon* and *Cryptococcus*	*Aspergillus, Fusarium*, mucor and *Rhizopus*	*Histoplasma, Coccidioides, P. marneffei* and *Sporothrix*	Trichophyton, microsporum and epidermophyton
Normal habitat	Mucosa, skin (*Malassezia, Trichosporon*) and pigeon droppings (*Cryptococcus*)	Ubiquitous Inhalation/ inoculation	Endemic outside Denmark Inhalation/ inoculation	Ringworm of humans and animals
Disease entities	Mucositis, skin infections, haematogenous dissemination and meningitis (*Cryptococcus*)	Lung infections, sinusitis and haematogenous dissemination (*Fusarium*)	Lung infections, haematogenous dissemination and skin infections	Nail, inquina and body scalp

sensitive to Voriconazole. *C. glabrata* showed resistance to fluconazole. 5.2% of *C. albicans* was resistant to amphotericin B, itraconazole and fluconazole. Some isolates of *A. fumigatus* showed resistance to amphotericin B. *C. neoformans* isolates were sensitive to all antifungals. Mortality rate encountered was 2.5% and all the cases had proven IFI.

62.2 Specimens and Frequently Detected Fungi

- Blood—*Candida* spp., *Cryptococcus neoformans*, *Histoplasma capsulatum* and filamentous fungi are rarely isolated from blood with exception of *Fusarium* spp.
- Pus and other exudate—*Cryptococcus neoformans*, dimorphic fungi and *Fusarium* spp.
- Respiratory secretion—*Aspergillus* spp., *Candida* spp., *Cryptococcus neoformans*, dimorphic fungi, *Mucor* spp., *Scedosporium apiospermum* and *Rhizopus* spp.
- Cerebrospinal fluid—*Cryptococcus neoformans*, *Candida* spp., *Coccidioides immitis* and *Histoplasma capsulatum*
- Urine—*Candida* spp. and *Cryptococcus neoformans*
- Vitreous fluid—*Candida albicans* (most common)
- Synovial fluid—*Aspergillus* spp. and *Candida* spp.

Fungi are ubiquitous, found in environment, on plants, animals and human. These are saprophytes and natural recyclers of nutrients, for example, laccase enzyme breaks down plant lignin and helps wood rotting. However, some of the fungi are also opportunist pathogens and invade when a man offers an opportunity. When his innate immunity is weakened or compromised, these cause invasive infection. Some species of fungi are more aggressive, invade healthy human, but are intercepted and localized by the human defence system. Later in life, if immunity is compromised due to underlying infection/disease/comorbidity, the fungi get opportunity to disseminate and cause serious and life-threatening infection. The fungi invading seeds, developing grains on plants and harvested and even processed foods produce mycotoxins. Human is encircled within the web of harmful fungi and mycotoxins. These pathological conditions are beyond the listed acute viral and bacterial diseases and hence pass unnoticed. Extensive pathological damage has often been done before intervention. The antifungal drugs are expensive and toxic.

62.3 Diagnosis

It is difficult to diagnose disseminated fungal infection, such as histoplasmosis. Medical mycology laboratory is uncommon. Fungi take long time to grow. Serology is not sensitive for immunocompromised. Molecular diagnosis requires expensive laboratory, expertise and resources beyond reach of many. Staining, histopathology and antigen detection are useful.

62.4   Antifungal Compounds and Target Site

For fungal blood stream infections are the following:

- *Polyenes*—Amphotericin binds ergosterol in cell membrane and forms pores causing leakage of intracellular substances and eventual cell (fungal) death [side effect—nephrotoxic].
- *Azoles—The azoles* inhibit the enzyme P450 demethylase necessary for the ergosterol synthesis and arrest growth. Fluconazole is useful in cryptococcal meningitis. *Voriconazole* has anti-*Candida* activity but is reserved for resistant cases or situations where coverage of *Aspergillus* is also warranted [side effect—anaphylaxis Fluconazole—gastrointestinal discomfort, rash and hepatotoxic].
- The *echinocandins* inhibit formation of glucan in the fungal cell wall by inhibiting the enzyme 1.3-beta-glucan synthetase. These are less prone to cause cross reaction and interference with the human cell and are fungicidal against *Candida*.
- *Flucytosine*—It acts by inhibiting fungal DNA and RNA synthesis and is fungistatic in lower but fungicidal in higher dosages. It is used in combination with amphotericin, never as alone (which rapidly develops resistance), used for *Cryptococcus* and other rare yeast infections involving the CNS or other foci where drug penetration is a limiting factor [side effect—bone marrow suppression].
- *Terbinafine* is occasionally used for rare and very severe infections with resistant moulds like *Fusarium* in combination with other agents. It inhibits an earlier step in the ergosterol synthesis pathway.

Only the azole compounds can be given orally, are convenient and so are used extensively in the primary health-care sector. The other compounds are exclusively used in the hospital setting.

Outcome of treatment depends upon virulence of *Candida*, susceptibility (intrinsic and acquired resistance), severity of disease, timing of drug intervention and choice and dose of drug. Acquired resistance in *Candida* is a rather rare event. Resistant strains are rarely transferred from patient to patient. Mechanism of resistance cannot be transferred via plasmids among yeast. According to Ademe and Girma (2020), *C. auris* escapes from the microbicidal effect of all the classes of anti-fungal agents through different intrinsic mechanisms (Table 62.2).

Table 62.2 Resistance mechanism in *C. auris* (Ademe and Girma 2020)

Anti-fungal drugs	Resistance mechanism
Polyenes	Mutation 5 SNPs in different genome loci
Azoles	Point mutation in lanosterol 14-alpha demethylase (ERGII gene)
	ERGII upregulation due to mutation in Upc2 TF
	Upregulation efflux pump genes
Nucleoside analogues	Amino acid substitution (F2II) in FURI
Echinocandin	Mutation in FKSI/2 gene

C. albicans, *C. dubliniensis* and *C. tropicalis* are normally susceptible to all anti-fungals used for fungaemia; *C. glabrata* is less so; *C. krusei* is intrinsically resistant to fluconazole. *C. parapsilosis* is less susceptible to the echinocandins.

62.5   Antifungal Susceptibility Testing

Antifungal susceptibility testing of yeast and filamentous fungi is performed as per the Clinical Laboratory Standards Institute (CLSI) and US guidelines published in 1997. Non-species-specific breakpoints are provided for fluconazole, itraconazole and flucytosine and tentative ones also for amphotericin. This was revised subsequently leading to a harmonization of breakpoints and more appropriate interpretation of susceptibility results in a global perspective.

The European Committee for Antimicrobial Susceptibility Testing (EUCAST) subcommittee on Antifungal susceptibility testing (AFST) develop and validate breakpoints and methods for susceptibility testing of yeasts, moulds and dermatophytes. EUCAST-AFST has released ten new documents summarizing existing and new breakpoints and MIC ranges for control strains (Arendrup et al. 2017, 2020). A failure to adopt the breakpoint changes may lead to misclassifications and suboptimal or inappropriate therapy of patients with fungal infections.

References

Ademe M, Girma F (2020) *Candida auris*: from multidrug resistance to pan-resistant strains. Infect Drug Resist 13:1287–1294

Arendrup MC (2013) Candida and candidaemia. Susceptibility and epidemiology. Dan Med J 60(11):B4698

Arendrup MC, Mouton JW, Lagrou K, Hamal P, Guinea J (2017) Method for the determination of broth dilution minimum inhibitory concentrations of antifungal agents for yeasts. Clin Microbiol Infect 9:1–8

Arendrup MC, Friberg N, Mares M, Kahlmeter G et al (2020) How to interpret MICs of antifungal compounds according to the revised clinical breakpoints v. 10.0 European committee on antimicrobial susceptibility testing (EUCAST). Clin Microbiol Infect 26(11):1464–1472

Kumudhavalli KS (2013) A study on invasive fungal infections among immunocompromised patients in a tertiary care hospital. Thesis for MD Microbiology. The Tamilnadu Dr. M.G.R. Medical University

Chapter 63
Aspergillosis

Aspergillosis is a common saprozoonosis caused by certain species of *Aspergillus*. Common conditions are aspergillus bronchitis, rhinosinusitis, otitis externa and onychomycosis. The chronic pulmonary is more prevalent than the invasive. *Aspergillus* spp. produces aflatoxins that cause common mycotoxicosis.

Aspergillosis affects an estimated over 14 million people around the world (https://en.wikipedia.org/wiki/Aspergillosisis). According to Denning et al. (2013), an estimated 4,837,000 patients (range 1,354,000–6,772,000) of 193 adult active patients of asthma worldwide develop allergic broncho-pulmonary aspergillosis (ABPA). They are distributed in the AHO region such as Europe (1,062,000), Americas (1,461,000), Eastern Mediterranean (351,000), Africa (389,900), Western Pacific (823,200) and Southeast Asia (720,400). The global case burden of chronic pulmonary aspergillosis (CPA) was 411,100 (range 206,300–589,400) at a 10% rate with a 15% annual attrition. The global burden of ABPA potentially exceeds 4.8 million people and of CPA complicating ABPA ~400,000, which is more common than previously appreciated.

63.1 Aetiology

63.1.1 *Family* Trichocomaceae, *Genus*—Aspergillus

A. fumigatus is the most important airborne fungus with potential life-threatening invasive pulmonary aspergillosis in immunocompromised and allergy-inducing infections in those with atopic allergy. *A. flavus* is the common cause of sinusitis, cutaneous infection, keratitis and non-invasive fungal pneumonia.

© Springer Nature Singapore Pte Ltd. 2024
K. G. Narayan et al., *Handbook of Management of Zoonoses*,
https://doi.org/10.1007/978-981-99-9885-2_63

A. flavus, *A. niger*, *A. nidulans* and *A. terreus* have also been reported.

These are ubiquitous and found on vegetation, decomposing organic matter, compost, hay, grains and soil. *A. flavus* overwinters in soil in decaying matter and grows in hot humid climates. Sclerotia germinate, produce hyphae and asexual spores called conidia and are dispersed by winds and insects. Conidia are the primary inoculum. From the surface of sclerotia, conidiophores and conidia are produced (on crops/grains during spring).

The conidia are found in large number, $>10^8$/g in compost. These are found suspended in air with varying concentrations, generally high in indoor air. It may be as high as $>10^9$ conidia/m^3 in air of hay barn in comparison to outdoor air at other places 200/m^3. Fungi may settle down on surface of any object to contaminate, for example, *A niger*, *A. fumigatus*, *A. flavus* and *A. nidulans* were isolated from surface of goat meat in India (Narayan 2004).

A. flavus survives temperatures that other fungi do not. Minimum and maximum growth temperatures are 12 °C and 48 °C, respectively, optimum 37 °C. Growth is rapid between 30 °C and 55 °C and slow between 12 °C and 15 °C and stops at 5–8 °C. Moisture requirement ranges between 11% and 14% depending upon crops. *A. fumigatus* grows well at 40 °C and is able to grow at temperatures <20–50 °C; conidia survive at 70 °C.

A. fumigatus is the number one followed by *A. flavus*, the two leading causes of human aspergillosis primarily by inhalation of spores. It seems that the size of spores determines the site of infection. Big size spores settle in the upper respiratory tract.

Dry weather of Saudi Arabia and most Africa are prone to aspergillosis.

63.2   Mode of Infection and Pathogenesis

Pathogenesis and pathology of aspergillosis are complex. The pathogen *Aspergillus* possesses a number of virulence factors and other proteins; allergens spread on the surface of conidia and hyphae. Further, these produce mycotoxins. The hosts are grouped as those with normal intact immune system, compromised immune system and have previous other diseases like tuberculosis, fibrosis, etc. (a sort of susceptible host's continuum).

63.3   Pulmonary *Aspergillus* Overlap Syndromes (Kousha et al. 2011)

Invasive and allergic aspergillosis may co-exist or overlap, that is, progress from one to another entity, Aspergilloma to ABPA and ABPA to IP or chronic necrotizing *aspergillosis* (CNA), Aspergilloma to IP or CNA and reverse, IPA/CNA and ABPA to aspergilloma (Fig. 63.1), for example, fungal balls in patients of ABPA or IPA in a patient of ABPA. Shah and Panjabi (2014) described a case with three entities ABPA, AAS and Aspergilloma. Severe haemoptysis caused by aspergilloma in bronchiectatic cavity was treated by lobectomy. She developed left pleural effusion and associated underlying collapse of the left lung because of ABPA and AAS. Concurrently, all the three conditions were diagnosed in another case. Aspergilloma was treated (disappeared) with repeated oral course of prednisolone administered as maintenance therapy.

An aspergilloma may invade the cavity wall, causing local parenchyma destruction, as seen in patients with CNA. A pre-existing cavity is not needed. There is an overlap. There may be a chance coincidence or due to following factors:

- Concomitant development of aspergilloma and fibro-cavitary disease.
- Delayed detection of fungal balls in patients with fibrosis and cavitation associated with long-standing or poorly treated ABPA.
- Severe underlying lung disease (e.g. a patient with aspergilloma who develops chronic necrotizing aspergillosis (CNA).
- Corticosteroid therapy (IPA in a patient with aspergilloma or ABPA).
- *Aspergillus* fungal load.
- Genetic predisposition, for example, CFTR gene mutation, may lead to ABPA, and mannose-binding lectin gene mutations may result in CNA or IPA.
- Secondary viral infection—SBPA or aspergilloma case down with a viral illness.

Invasive procedures to rule out malignancy or tuberculosis could be avoided if it was known that aspergilloma could develop in ABPA patients.

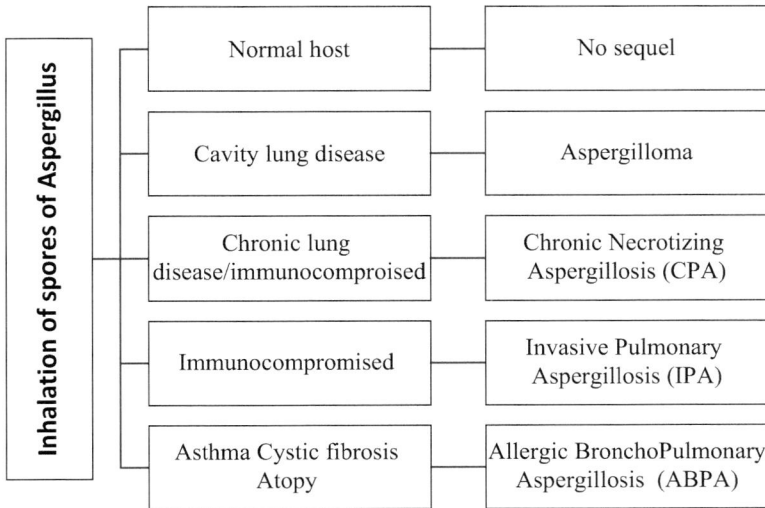

Fig. 63.1 Classification of inhalation Aspergillosis

63.3.1   Inhalation (Invasion)

Pathogenesis: Aspergillus spores suspended in air easily penetrate lung alveoli. Surface proteins of conidia and mycelium mediate interaction with host's cells.

Mucociliary clearance is initiated and neutrophils, alveolar macrophages and dendritic cells are drawn to the site and spores are phagocytosed. A large portion of inhaled conidia are cleared by cell-mediated immune response and antimicrobial peptides secreted by epithelium of airways.

Aspergillus use a number of factors to evade hosts' defence and invade and damage respiratory epithelium, for example, fibrinogen binding, proteases, elastase, gliotoxin, etc. Gliotoxin inhibits ciliary activity of cells, inhibits phagocytosis by macrophages, affects the spleen so that cytotoxic cell production is inhibited and inhibits complement pathways. According to Dasari et al. (2019), the conidia and hyphae of *A. fumigatus* activate all the three complement pathways, namely, alternate (AP), classical (CP) and lectin (LP). The resting conidia preferentially activate AP and the swollen conidia CP and LP. Complement orchestrates both the humoral and cellular responses of the human host. Studies identified Enolase and AfEno1 of *A. fumigatus* that is expressed on the surface of swollen (not resting) conidia and hyphae. It acts as immune-evasion and allergen. It binds four human complement regulator proteins factor H, FHL-1, C4BP and plasminogen (these four are present in the bronchoalveolar lavage fluids).

The invading fungus is able to survive in immunocompetent host. Additionally, it helps penetration, colonization and dissemination through damaging lung epithelial cells and degradation of ECM matrix proteins mediated through activated plasminogen. AfEno1 hijacks the human zymogen plasminogen and tPA (tissue-type plasminogen activator) to activate plasmin (Dasari et al. 2019). Increasing proteases and a number of other factors cause switching over the pro-inflammatory response to inhibitory response, resulting in the reduction of phagocytic clearance.

The conidia persisting in pulmonary tissues germinate; hyphae grow in the warm, moist nutrient-rich environment of pulmonary alveoli into mucus plugs. Growing filamentous hyphae penetrate epithelium and then vascular endothelium and inflict injury that induces pro-inflammatory response and related reactions causing thrombosis and infarction. Damage to pulmonary structure causes bronchiectasis and pulmonary fibrosis and aspergilloma usually in the upper lobe. Cases of bronchopulmonary aspergilloma have been reported from India.

In severely immunocompromised individuals, fragments of hyphae can spread through bloodstream. In already damaged lung tissues, due to previous disease such as tuberculosis, invading conidia finds it easier to colonize.

63.3.2 Clinical Disease

Aspergillosis can occur in any age, sex and everybody. Risk groups included are neutropenic, transplant recipient, children with chronic granulomatous disease, immunocompromised or immunodeficient. They usually suffer with acute invasive infection. Aspergillosis is fulminant and usually fatal. Human, animals and birds suffer with aspergillosis. It may occur as acute and chronic disease. Acute form affects those who are severely immunocompromised and bone marrow transplant stem cell recipient. Chronic form is a secondary infection causing complications, such as patients of asthma and chronic obstructive pulmonary disease.

63.4 Types/Classification and Symptoms

Aspergillosis may be broadly classed as (a) invasive (infection occurs) and (b) allergic (absence of infection).

63.4.1 Invasive Aspergillosis

Invasive aspergillosis usually occurs as an additional sickness in an already sick person, for example, cystic fibrosis, tuberculosis, asthma bronchiectasis, pneumonia, etc. generally suffer with aspergilloma. Pulmonary diseases and age were likely considered as highly associated risk factors for invasive aspergillosis (Wang et al. 2022).

Symptoms overlap and are difficult to delineate. When the lung is involved, common symptoms are shortness of breath, chest pain, cough (may be with blood) and fever. Infection may spread and other organs/system may get involved. Symptoms will vary accordingly.

Aspergillus grows unchecked in lungs and can spread to other parts because the victim is an immunocompromised (transplant case) or with weak immunity or impaired immunity (AIDS).

63.4.1.1 Aspergilloma

The fungus ball composed of the hyphae, inflammatory cells, fibrin, mucus and tissue debris. The most common cause is *A. fumigatus*. Other fungi likely to cause aspergilloma are *Zygomycetes* and *Fusarium*. Fungal infection (secondary infection) complicates many cavitary diseases. Of these, tuberculosis is the most common. Others may be pulmonary infections, bronchiectasis, bronchial cysts, sarcoidosis, neoplasm and other fungal infections. Fungus grows on the walls of pre-existing cavity usually due to inadequate drainage. The fungus ball generally does not invade (exceptions may be) the surrounding tissues or blood vessels, reduce in size or even resolve without treatment. The increase in size is rare.

Symptoms: Most may be asymptomatic. Severe haemoptysis, especially in tuberculosis patient, may be life-threatening. Haemoptysis is common as bronchial blood vessels bleed. The blood vessels lining the cavity are invaded and injured mechanically by the moving fungus ball or by the fungal endotoxin. Other symptoms may be because of the underlying disease or secondary bacterial infections and include fever, cough and dyspnoea.

Poor prognosis: recurrence of haemoptysis and/or increase in volume, underlying sarcoidosis, lung disease turning severe, increasing number and size of lesions in lungs, immunosuppression and increasing *Aspergillus*-specific IgG titres.

Diagnosis: Pulmonary aspergilloma is diagnosed by a combination of clinical, radiographic, serological or microbiological evidence of *Aspergillus* spp. Serum IgG is positive in many cases except those taking corticosteroid drugs. The fungus ball changing position with supine and prone position of the patient is visible in radiography.

In India, *A. fumigatus*, *A. niger* and *A. japonicus* have been isolated from patients (Narayan 2004).

Diagnosis – X-ray.

63.4.1.2   Acute Invasive Pulmonary Aspergillosis (Acute IPA)

A. fumigatus, *A. niger*, *A. terreus*, *A. nidulans* and *A. flavus* are associated with IPA. Pathogen entering lungs is recognized by Toll-like receptors, dectin-1 and mannose binding lectin (which identify fungal hyphae, produce cytokines and stimulate defence system).

Risk factors are as follows:

- Neutropenia (<500 cells/mm^3 for >10 days)—risk increases with duration.
- Transplantation (highest risk is with lung transplantation and haematopoetic stem cell transplant).
- Haematological malignancy (risk is higher with leukaemia).
- Prolonged (>3 weeks) and high-dose corticosteroid therapy.
- Chemotherapy-advanced AIDS.
- Chronic granulomatous disease.

Influenza infection is a risk factor for invasive pulmonary aspergillosis in both immunocompetent and immunocompromised hosts. The breaches in host defence occur during influenza infection allowing for the development of post-influenza fungal super-infection (Robinson 2022). Among immunocompetent persons, IPA is common in patients with severe chronic obstructive pulmonary disease (COPD) and critically ill patients. Susceptibility of COPD patients may be due to altered structural change in the lungs, mucosal lesions, impaired mucociliary clearance, invasive procedures, prolonged corticosteroid and antibiotic therapy and comorbidities.

Aspergillus spores enter commonly the human respiratory tract via inhalation reaching the lower respiratory tract and to sinuses. Spores may enter the gastrointestinal tract and skin. Pathology follows accordingly.

Acute IPA is the commonest and most severe with high case fatality. Manifestations vary. Fever does not respond to antibiotics. Patients report cough, sputum, dyspnoea and pleuritic chest pain. Haemoptysis associated with cavitation is most common in neutropenic patients and can be severe. The patients of febrile bronchopneumonic form report high fever, 103–104 °F chest pain, bronchopneumonia, lobar pneumonia, thrombosis, haemorrhagic pulmonary infarction and necrosis. Contiguous spread to mediastinum pleura (pleural friction) pericardium and oesophagus is possible. Spread to ribs, sternum and vertebrae may cause osteomyelitis. Osteomyelitis is often seen among children suffering from chronic granuloma. IPA can also complicate other viral infections such as SARS-CoV-2, respiratory syncytial virus, parainfluenza and adenovirus.

Diagnosis: Bronchoscopy with bronchoalveolar lavage is generally helpful in the diagnosis. Histopathology with demonstration and culture of fungus is the gold test. Neutropenic patients show scant inflammation, extensive coagulation necrosis with hyphal angio-invasion and high fungal burden. Transplant cases show the opposite.

Galactomannan and (13)-b-D-glucan are cellular wall constituents. Galactomannan is a polysaccharide released by *Aspergillus* during growth. It is species-specific. A double-sandwich ELISA was developed for the detection of galactomannan in serum (threshold of 0.5 ng/mL^{-1}), which can be detected several days before the presence of clinical signs, chest radiographic abnormalities or a positive culture. Galactomannan is detected in other body fluids such as bronchoalveolar lavage (BAL), urine and cerebrospinal fluid. PCR is another method (Kousha et al. 2011).

63.4.1.2.1 Aspergillus Tracheobronchitis (ATB)

Isolated invasion of tracheobronchial tree is a unique feature of IPA seen commonly among AIDS patients and lung transplant and cancer cases with mediastinal involvement. Three forms have been described:

- Obstructive—characterized by thick mucus plugs full of *Aspergillus* spp. Bronchial inflammation is absent.
- Pseudomembranous—characterized by extensive inflammation of the tracheobronchial tree. The fungus is located in the overlying membrane.
- Ulcerative involves the tracheobronchial tree, usually at the suture line in lung transplantation recipients.

Pseudomembranous ATB is the most severe with cough, dyspnoea and infrequent haemoptysis as symptoms.

Prognosis of obstructive and pseudomembranous ATB is poor. Mortality may be high. Ulcerative form responds to antifungal therapy favourably.

Diagnosis: Bronchoscopy combined with microscopic analysis of respiratory specimens obtained during the procedure.

63.4.1.2.2   Systemic Infection and Haematogenous Spread

Systemic Infection and Haematogenous spread to other organs occur in disseminated type of infection which is rare, fulminant and often fatal. It involved the lungs, heart, kidney, thyroid and brain.

63.4.1.2.2.1   *Acute Invasive Aspergillosis of Central Nervous System*

Haematogenous or non-haematogenous dissemination from the lung and sinus or acute fungaemia (infrequent) leads to invasion of CNS. Thrombosis or infarction with multiple lesions may be caused by hyphae. This can lead to ring-enhancing lesions, cerebral infarctions, intracranial haemorrhage, meningitis and epidural abscesses. Neural symptoms may include confusion, behavioural change, progressive depression, reduced consciousness, cranial nerve palsy and seizures. Cerebral aspergillosis has been recorded in India too.

63.4.1.2.2.2   *Acute Invasive Gastrointestinal Aspergillosis*

It is one of the disseminated forms of aspergillosis. Most common organ involved is oesophagus. Ulcers are the common lesion, which may perforate.

Other organs which may be affected by disseminated aspergillosis are the spleen, liver and heart (endocarditis, myocarditis). Fungal growth may occur on aortic and mitral valves. Growth may be the cause of embolism.

Affection of eyes may cause ocular pain, impaired vision, endophthalmitis, corneal ulceration and perforation.

63.4.1.2.2.3   *Aspergillus Otitis*

A. *niger* and A. *fumigatus* often invade and grow in auditory canal to cause otitis. There is pain, itching, reduced hearing and discharge. Fungal growth is fuzzy and greenish black.

3. Chronic Necrotizing Aspergillosis (CNA; Kousha et al. 2011)/Chronic Cavitary Pulmonary Aspergillosis.

It is semi-invasive or subacute invasive aspergillosis, relatively uncommon. There is local invasion of the lung tissue by the fungus causing destruction of lung parenchyma. An aspergilloma may invade the cavity wall, causing local parenchyma destruction, as seen in patients with CNA. A pre-existing cavity is not needed. There is an overlap.

It is an indolent, cavitary and infectious process of the lung parenchyma. It occurs commonly among middle- and old-aged persons, who have been receiving treatment for chronic lung disease. It has a slow progressive course. *Aspergillus* grows, over a period of ≥3 months; growing fungus causes cavities in lungs and one or more fungal balls in lungs. Dissemination is unusual. Chronic pulmonary aspergillosis manifested as fever, fatigue, malaise, weight loss of 1–6-month duration and productive cough which may include blood. The condition may range from mild to severe. Pathological changes include necrosis of lung tissue and acute or chronic inflammation of the cavity wall. Microscopic examination shows hyphae consistent with *Aspergillus* species. Chest X-ray and CT scan reveal the cavity in upper lobes, consolidation and thickening of pleura and aspergilloma.

Diagnosis: Serum IgG to *A. fumigatus*, not always positive, varies with time. Skin sensitivity test and culture of sputum or sample from bronchoscopy.

63.4.1.3   Cutaneous Aspergillosis

Aspergillus invades through the broken skin, for example, injury/burn or post-surgery or spread as in invasive aspergillosis. When it disseminates, the lesions appear in form of erythema, oedema, indurated plaque and necrotic ulcers with black eschar in the centre.

Azole-resistant *Aspergillus fumigatus* infection. If infection is not controlled, it may disseminate through circulation damaging organs. Fever, chills, shock, delirium, seizures and blood clots may appear. Patient may suffer with failure of the kidney or liver die soon.

63.4.2   Allergic Aspergillosis

Shah and Panjabi (2014) grouped allergic aspergillosis as (a) IgE-mediated *Aspergillus*-induced asthma (AIA), (b) allergic bronchopulmonary aspergillosis (ABPA), (c) allergic *Aspergillus* sinusitis (AAS) and (d) hypersensitivity pneumonitis.

63.4.2.1   IgE-mediated Aspergillus-induced asthma (AIA)

Is a classical immediate type I IgE-mediated hypersensitivity reaction to *Aspergillus* antigens. It is imperative to assess for sensitization to *Aspergillus* in patients with asthma. AIA patients have increased severity of airway obstruction, increased incidence of bronchiectasis, more severe form of asthma and higher mean duration of illness. Laboratory parameters such as mean eosinophil count and mean total IgE are increased. More usage of oral corticosteroids per year was observed in AIA.

63.4.2.2 Allergic bronchopulmonary aspergillosis (ABPA)

It is most recognized and occurring worldwide. It has a protracted course of illness characterized by repeated episodes of asthmatic exacerbation remissions eventually developing fibrosis. It occurs in 20–40 years of age, reported in children and also infants. ABPA patients are often misdiagnosed as having tuberculosis due to the radiological similarities in TB-endemic areas and are wrongly treated for a long duration while lung damage continues to progress silently.

Repeated inhalation of spores led to colonization and elicited allergic response. Exposure to municipal leaf compost, garbage collection site damp basements, barns and sewage treatment facilities is dangerous.

Pathogenesis: The conidia of *A. fumigatus* produce a number of proteins. These are immunoreactive and induce synthesis of both IgG and IgE. In a study, Singh et al. (2010) identified 66 immunoreactive proteins in the cytosol of germinating conidia of two strains of *A. fumigatus*. These included Asp f12 and Asp f22 (already known) and 4 predicted allergens (Hsp88, Hsp70, malate dehydrogenase and alcohol dehydrogenase). Recombinantly expressed proteins from this panel consistently reacted with IgE of individual sera of ABPA patients; thus they have diagnostic value and even may be used for desensitization.

Twenty-three allergens of *A. fumigatus* are known. The allergen Aspf2 is exposed on the surface of resting, and swollen conidia recruits human plasma regulators (factors H, FHL1) and plasminogen resulting into inhibition of opsonophagocytosis and killing of conidia by human neutrophils. The allergen Aspf22 also known as AfEno1 or enolase has immune -evasion potential. EfEno1-reacting IgE are seen in patients of allergic bronchopulmonary aspergillosis. Enolase binds human plasma proteins including plasminogen (Dasari et al. 2019). Common allergen of *A. flavus* are Asp fl 13 and Asp fl 18.

The immunopathology is probably because of the hypersensitivity reaction types I, III and IV. Conidia are trapped in sputum and colonize respiratory passage of susceptible patients. There may also be genetic predisposition suggested by personal/family history of atopic diseases. Germination and growth of hyphae are accompanied with secretion of proteolytic enzymes. Host responds in form of release of pro-inflammatory cytokines. The immunological response is primarily of the cellular T-helper cell (Th)-2 type, as evident by increased interleukin (IL)-4, IL-5, IL-10 and IL-13 production.

Immunocompetent patients respond with the strong humoral and cellular response.

Symptoms: ABPA manifests as wheezing, breathlessness, cough and in rare cases fever. Sputum contains typical plugs golden brown in colour. There may be recurrent pyrexia, eosinophilia and transient pulmonary infiltrations (non-homogenous or consolidation are common patterns) detected by X-ray. Permanent opacities reflect the irreversible fibrotic changes and tend to persist throughout life. Central bronchiectasis with normal peripheral bronchi is pathognomonic.

Staining and culture of plugs demonstrate the fungus. In about 10% cases, there is cystic fibrosis in later stages. Risk factors include conditions such as chronic asthma, cystic fibrosis, etc.

Diagnosis: A synthetic peptide epitope of Asp f 1, a major antigen of *A. fumigatus*, has been identified for its potential use in skin testing and development of immunodiagnostic test. A comparative study between total IgE and *A. fumigatus*-specific IgE revealed that the *A. fumigatus*-specific IgE increased in only five (38.5%) subjects during exacerbation. Thus, the total IgE is a useful test in monitoring treatment responses in ABPA while *A. fumigatus* specific IgE has limited utility (Agarwal et al. 2016). However, routine *A. fumigatus*-sIgE screening for asthma patients can significantly improve the diagnostic rate of ABPA (Lou et al. 2019).

Diagnostic criteria have been evolving. The International Society for Human and Animal Mycology criteria (Agarwal et al. 2013) suggested the following:

Predisposing conditions are bronchial asthma and cystic fibrosis.

Obligatory criteria: both should be present.

- Type I *Aspergillus* skin test positive (immediate cutaneous hypersensitivity to *Aspergillus* antigen) or elevated IgE levels against *A. fumigatus*
- Elevated total IgE levels (1000 IU/m^{-1}) [#]

Other criteria (at least two of three) include the following:

- Presence of precipitating or IgG antibodies against *A. fumigatus* in serum.
- Radiographic pulmonary opacities consistent with ABPA.
- Total eosinophil count .500 cells/mL^{-1} in steroid naıve patients (may be historical)

[#] : if the patient meets all other criteria an IgE value, 1000 IU/mL^{-1} may be acceptable.

63.4.2.2.1 Allergic Aspergillus sinusitis (AAS)

Conidia inhaled via sinusoidal route sets in immunopathology akin to in the bronchi in case of ABPA. About 25% of patients of perennial sinusitis are sensitized to *Aspergillus* antigens, that is, rhinitis is the risk factor. Rhinitis may be due to sensitization with antigens from *Aspergillus* (*Aspergillus*-sensitized) or other fungus (allergic fungal rhinitis), for example, *Alternaria*, *Curvularia*, *Bipolaris*, *Exserohilum*, *Drechslera* and *Cladosporium*.

There is a mucoid impaction in sinus in paranasal sinuses. Allergic sinusitis is common. It is estimated that 7% of sinusitis cases requiring surgical intervention are allergic. Maxillary, ethanoid, sphenoid and frontal sinus are affected in decreasing order. The polypoid antral lining is thickened and shows granulation tissue, gelatinous necrotic material and brownish or greenish cheese like mass. Allergic sinusitis cases experience headache, stuffiness, running nose and smell-loss/reduction. Characteristic nasal secretion is gelatinous and contains necrotic tissues. The nasal lavage is viscous and greasy.

Diagnosis (Shah and Panjabi 2014): Radiography—sinusitis of one or more paranasal sinus; histopathology of tissue from sinus—necrosed amorphous tissue along with oedematous polyps infiltrated with eosinophils.

Stain and culture—nasal discharge; eosinophilia; elevated total, as well as *Aspergillus*-specific IgE levels; type I and type III cutaneous hypersensitivity to *Aspergillus*; precipitating antibodies to *Aspergillus* antigens; characteristic computed tomography appearances.

63.4.2.2.2   Aspergilloma

A ball of *Aspergillus* grows in lungs or sinus (fungus ball) and does not spread. It is often asymptomatic. A patient of aspergilloma (fungus ball) suffers with general malaise and loss of body weight, has shortness of breath, coughs and may cough up blood. Aspergilloma formed in ABPA cavity is more evident. Aspergillomas may appear either prior to or after the onset of ABPA. Corticosteroid therapy often hastens aspergilloma formation. ABPA may occur in aspergilloma patient, possibly aspergilloma function as a nidus for antigenic stimulation in a genetically predisposed person. ABPA patient with multiple aspergilloma, though rare, is case of chronic pulmonary aspergillosis.

The invading conidia of *A. fumigatus* find already damaged lung tissue for seeding and growth. The growing fungus forms a ball usually in the upper lobe. The site may also be different, for example, paranasal *Aspergillus* granuloma.

Otomycosis, onychomycosis and keratitis are non-invasive manifestations.

63.4.2.2.3   Others

Aspergillosis of para-nasal sinuses may be (a) fulminant or acute invasive, (b) non-invasive and (c) allergic .

a. Fulminant or Acute Invasive Sinusitis

It is generally a life-threatening severe invasive aspergillosis. Lesions are necrotic and appear on hard palate and turbinates. It may spread deep to affect the facial bone and skull. Contiguous spread may reach to the meninges and brain. It may disfigure face and cause facial nerve paralysis. Arteritis and rupture of carotid artery may be seen.

b. Non-invasive Sinusitis

The infection is benign. It affects the skin, nose, turbinate, palate and orbit. It is painful. Patient feels heaviness, blurred vision, nasal obstruction and rhinorrhea. Surgical intervention may be required for clearing obstruction and drainage.

b.1 Ingestion/Aflatoxicosis

Aflatoxins are ingested without the knowledge of consumer of contaminated foodstuff of plant and animal origin. The toxins are AFB1, AFB2, AFG1, AFG2, AFM1, AFM2 and also B2a and G2a. The aflatoxin-intoxicated mother may pass on the toxin to infants across the placenta and through breastmilk feeding. *A. flavus* and related species grow on the crops (e.g. maize) and grains during storage, processing and distribution like rice bran, wheat bran, soyabean flour, oil seed cakes, animal feed, etc. and produce aflatoxins. The domestic animals and birds ingest toxins with contaminated feeds. The animal produce and products like milk, eggs, poultry meat and meat carry aflatoxins.

Aflatoxicosis suppresses immune system. Suppression of immune system involves impaired reticuloendothelial system, phagocytosis, antigen processing, complement system, cell-mediated immune response and protein synthesis. Aflatoxins cause reduced efficiency of immunization in children that lead to enhanced risk of infections (Kumar et al. 2017). Growth retardation and cancer are caused.

It causes infantile and childhood cirrhosis and adult human hepatitis. Early symptoms are fever, malaise and anorexia followed with abdominal pain, vomiting and hepatitis. In a study on aflatoxicosis in Bihar, 28.7% of foetal cord blood and 21.42% of breast milk were found contaminated with AFB1. Quantitative assay revealed a level of 30–90 mcg/l in icteric cord blood and death of the infant born in comparison with 20 mcg/l in normal cord blood. The urine samples from normal human had a range between trace to 30 mcg/l of AFB1 compared to 78 mcg/l in icteric patient for the past six months (Sinha 1999).

According to Kumar et al. (2017), toxicity may be acute and chronic. Acute toxicity is rare. Symptoms include oedema, haemorrhagic necrosis of the liver and profound lethargy.

63.5 Diagnosis

Allergic aspergillosis is indicated with history of recurrent pyrexia, cough, asthma, pneumonia and laboratory investigation supplements. Observation of eosinophilia supports. X-ray detects damages like uni- or bilateral infiltration; enlargement of hilar, paratracheal lymph node and consolidation and lobar contraction. As stated above, IgE total and specific for *Aspergillus* spp. brings closer to specific diagnosis. Demonstrating the fungus with silver staining and culture from the specimens such as plug or nasal lavage is the confirmatory.

- Silver staining and microscopy and culture for the fungus, PCR
- Skin test (allergen, sensitivity), lymphocyte proliferation migration tests for allergy
- Detection of fungal antigen by serologic tests, ELISA, Latex agglutination and radioimmunoassay
- Demonstration of antibodies by tests like immunodiffusion, ELISA and counter-immuno-electrophoresis

63.6   Prevention

HEPA filters in ICUs to keep out airborne fungus.

63.7   Treatment

Azole is the choice for treatment.

References

Agarwal R, Chakrabarti A, Shah A et al (2013) Allergic bronchopulmonary aspergillosis: review of literature and proposal of new diagnostic and classification criteria. Clin Exp Allergy 43:850–873

Agarwal R, Aggarwal AN, Sehgal IS, Dhooria S, Behera D, Chakrabarti A (2016) Utility of IgE (total and *Aspergillus fumigatus* specific) in monitoring for response and exacerbations in allergic bronchopulmonary aspergillosis. Mycoses 59(1):1–6

Dasari P, Koleci N, Shopova IA, Wartenberg D, Beyersdorf N et al (2019) Enolase from Aspergillus fumigatus is a moonlighting protein that binds the human plasma complement proteins factor H, FHL-1, C4BP, and plasminogen. Front Immunol 10:2573

Denning DW, Pleuvry A, Cole DC (2013) Global burden of allergic bronchopulmonary aspergillosis with asthma and its complication chronic pulmonary aspergillosis in adults. Med Mycol 51(4):361–370

Kousha M, Tadi R, Soubani AO (2011) Review: Pulmonary aspergillosis: a clinical review. Eur Respir Rev 20(121):156–174

Kumar P, Mahato DK, Kamle M, Mohanta TK, Kang SG (2017) Aflatoxins: a global concern for food safety, human health and their management. Front Microbiol 7:2170

Lou B, Xu Z, Yang G, Guo C, Zheng S et al (2019) Role of Aspergillus fumigatus -specific IgE in the diagnosis of Allergic Brochopulmonary Aspergillosis. Int Arch Allergy Immunol 178:338–344

Narayan KG (2004) Epidemiology, Diagnosis and Management of Zoonoses. ICAR, New Delhi

Robinson KM (2022) Mechanistic basis of super-infection: influenza-associated invasive pulmonary Aspergillosis. J Fungi 8:428

Shah A, Panjabi C (2014) Allergic aspergillosis of the respiratory tract. Eur Respir Rev 23:8–29

Singh B, Sharma GL, Oellerich M, Kumar R et al (2010) Novel cytosolic allergens of *Aspergillus fumigatus* identified from germinating conidia. J Proteome Res 9(11):5530–5541

Sinha BK (1999) Final report of the ICAR sponsored scheme (1996-99) on "Epidemiological and immunobiological studies on aflatoxicosis in animals and men in Bihar including its tribal areas". Department of Veterinary Microbiology, Bihar Veterinary College, Patna, Rajendra Agricultural University

Wang Y, Zhang L, Zhou L, Zhang M, Xu Y (2022) Epidemiology, drug susceptibility, and clinical risk factors in patients with invasive Aspergillosis. Front Public Health 10:835092

Chapter 64
Blastomycosis

Thomas Casper Gilchrist described first blastomycosis in 1894, and hence it is also referred to as Gilchrist's disease. It is an uncommon but potentially serious infection.

Blastomyces dermatitidis conidia cause a systemic pyogranulomatous infection upon inhalation manifesting as acute or chronic pneumonia. It is a pathogen infecting upper lobes of lungs causing pneumonia. Blastomycosis presents a wide range of radiographic features such as military disease or cavitary lesions, intermediate-sized nodules, air-space consolidation, mass-like lesions and interstitial disease. These are misdiagnosed as bacterial pneumonia and lung malignancy. Skin is the most common extra-pulmonary site (40–80%); the skin lesions, verrucous or ulcerated dermatitis can be mistaken for skin cancer and squamous cell carcinoma. The disease progresses in absence of correct diagnosis.

Dissemination to the kidney, prostate and epididymis may cause genitourinary tract infection. Brain is affected in some cases. Persons with weak immune system are more likely to develop the disseminated form.

The case fatality rate in primary blastomycosis has been estimated as 4–6%, 18% when CNS is involved and 25–40% among AIDS patients and immunocompromised. It has been as high as 89% in the Tennessee study (https://en.wikipedia.org/wiki/Blastomycosis).

64.1 Aetiology

Blastomyces dermatitidis is a dimorphic microfunguss belonging to family Ajellomycetaceae, phylum Ascomycota. It grows in mycelial form at room temperature (25 °C) in 2–4 weeks in form of white cotton colonies. The mycelia have branching hyphae with right-angled conidiophores ending in single-round conidia.

© Springer Nature Singapore Pte Ltd. 2024
K. G. Narayan et al., *Handbook of Management of Zoonoses*,
https://doi.org/10.1007/978-981-99-9885-2_64

At 37 °C, yeasts develop in infected hosts' tissues and in culture. Colonies of yeast are cream or tan coloured with wrinkled surface. Microscopy shows round yeasts of 8–15 microns in diameter with thick double refractile cell walls.

A wide range of mammals are susceptible, dogs and cats in particular. Dogs accompanying hunters or foresters may get infected. Dogs may be used as sentinel. The infection in dogs is often diagnosed as early as six months before in human in their respective owner. These suffer with respiratory infection progressing rapidly to death.

A new species named as *Blastomyces helicus* which is also a dimorphic fungus first isolated from a man with fungal encephalitis in Alberta, Canada (Schwartz et al. 2019), causes fatal pulmonary and systemic disease in humans and companion animals. It differs from *B. dermatitidis* in morphological presentation in culture and in histopathology, by primarily affecting immunocompromised persons, and in a geographic range that includes western regions of North America.

64.2   Epidemiology

The natural habitat is soil (grows in moist acidic soil enriched with animal droppings, decaying leaves and rotting wood) around water bodies.

Most epidemiological studies are sporadic and endemic based on the detection and reporting of clinical disease. Blastomycosis is reported predominately from North America. Endemic areas in the USA are valleys of Ohio, Mississippi and St. Lawrence Rivers, the Great Lakes. Cases have been reported from Arkansas, Kentucky, Mississippi, North Carolina, Tennessee, Louisiana, Illinois and Wisconsin. Hyperendemic areas are north-central Wisconsin, with cases as high as 40/100,000 (Saccente and Woods 2010). In Canada, blastomycosis is endemic in parts of Quebec, Ontario and Manitoba. Blastomycosis has been reported also from a non-endemic area like Africa (Cheikh Rouhou et al. 2008), India (Chakrabarti and Slavin 2011), Israel and Saudi Arabia. Cases from Africa and India are considered as autochthonous because it is thought that *B. dermatitidis* does not exist here. However, this may be because the physicians are not familiar with this infection; the fungus might be translocated with fomites from endemic areas and endogenous reactivation of foci after the infected person moved from endemic area. Saccente and Woods (2010) discussed some epidemics associated with exposure to common outdoor source.

Blastomycosis may occur in all weather, climate and atmospheric conditions except freezing. The natural habitat should have moisture and weather moderately warm. Such conditions favour survival of *B. dermatitidis* and may be released during relatively dry conditions into air by activity like excavation. The incidence per 100,000 in endemic areas is estimated at 0.5, occasionally rising to 12 (https://en.wikipedia.org/wiki/Blastomycosis).

Those infected have been aboriginals exposed during extensive excavation, associated with forests and open watersheds, as well as healthy and middle-aged individuals acquiring infection during trapping, working with wood and plants in forest, gardening or recreation and hunting fishing on sites that are apparently clean and attractive in endemic areas. These factors influence the possibility of exposure.

64.3 Mode of Infection

Inhalation of dust laden with the yeast, entry through penetrating skin injury, laboratory accident or bite of infected dogs. It is a saprozoonosis, a common source infecting both animals and humans. Human and his companion dogs have had shared exposure and diseases detected much earlier in dogs than human. Blastomycosis is generally not contagious; human-to-human transmission does not occur, except rarely through sex and intrauterine. Activities like cleaning with brush, excavation and disturbing soil and outdoor activities, namely, hunting and camping in forests, have been associated with epidemic.

64.4 Pathogenesis

Hosts' macrophages and neutrophils engulf inhaled conidia of *B. dermatitidis*. Transformation of conidia to the pathogenic yeast form is inhibited by alveolar macrophages. Some escape and rapidly transform into yeast phase. These have thick protective walls which resist phagocytosis. *BAD-1* is a glycoprotein virulence factor and an epitope is expressed. Multiplication of yeast occurs in lung tissues and dissemination occurs through blood and lymphatic channel. The pulmonary focus may resolve. Endogenous reactivation of pulmonary or extrapulmonary lesion may occur.

There is a mixed inflammatory reaction. The lesion presents polymorphonuclear leucocytes and often non-caseating granulomas consisting of epithelioid histiocytes and giant cells. There is pseudoepitheliomatous hyperplasia in infected skin and mucosa.

The cell-mediated immunity is important to check the progress of disease.

64.5 Symptoms

B. dermatitidis infection results in a wide range of consequences, from subclinical to fatal disseminated disease. Less than 50% infected manifest symptoms.

Incubation period ranges between three weeks and three months (after inhalation of spores). Infection among immunocompromised disseminates beyond the lung, mainly to the skin and bones.

Pulmonary blastomycosis may present in various forms, flu-like, pneumonic, acute respiratory distress syndrome (ARDS) and chronic form resembling tuberculosis and asymptomatic radiographic abnormality.

Chronic form is more common than the acute. There is a low-grade fever, mild but persistent productive cough, chest pain and haemoptysis accompanied with general malaise, fatigue and weight loss. Duration may be 2–6 months.

The fulminant or acute form occurs in small percentage of cases. Patients complain of fever, chill, chest pain, shortness of breath, night sweat, myalgia and exhaustion progressing to acute respiratory distress and dissemination in a week often ending fatally.

Patients suffering with moderately severe-to-severe pulmonary and extrapulmonary blastomycosis, namely, extensive pneumonia and respiratory failure due to ARDS, multiorgan involvement and haemodynamic instability, require hospitalization. Ventilator may be required within few days of admission.

Hussaini et al. (2018) described a case of pulmonary blastomycosis in a 52-year-old male, a former smoker. The problem and need of differential diagnosis have been discussed. He had non-productive cough, night sweats and weight loss and was initially diagnosed with pulmonary malignancy.

The disseminated dermal form presents subcutaneous abscesses growing from deeper foci, warts-like or ulcers with small pustules on the margin involving reticulo-endothelium system and lymphadenopathy.

Involvement of the bone and joints is painful. Inflammation of the prostate gland may or not cause pain while urinating. Patients of CNS blastomycosis may suffer with meningitis or abscess in epidural and brain. Uncommon sites include the liver, spleen, eyes, middle ear and other tissues.

64.6   Diagnosis

Sputum or biopsied tissue specimens or fine needle aspirate are examined.

Cytology or histopathology is used for diagnosis. Histopathological examination revealing pyogranulomas should prompt blastomycosis.

Cytology and histopathology show *budding yeast, round to oval multinucleated yeast cell, 8–15 micron diameter with thick double refractile wall, located intracellularly or extracellularly.*

KOH preparation, tissues stained with haematoxylin-eosin stain and periodic acid Schiff stain demonstrate the fungus. Histology demonstrates granulomatous nodules.

Culture is the golden test. The specimen 'sputum' has culture positivity of 86%. If collected by bronchoscopy, positivity is increased to 92%.

Commercially available urine antigen is used in case of negative cytology. The sensitivity of antigenuria is 85–93% and specificity 99–100%, which may be used to measure the progress of recovery during therapy. Antibody enzyme assay for *B. dermatitidis* surface protein Bad-1 is promising (Hussaini et al. 2018).

Saccente and Woods (2010) mention another commonly used commercially available test *–chemiluminescent DNA probe* for confirmation of *B. dermatitidis*. PCR has been used for molecular epidemiological studies.

64.7   Treatment

Itraconazole, ketoconazole and amphotericin B are the drugs. Fluconazole is useful when CNS is involved. ARDS cases are treated with conventional amphotericin B. Treatment options have been dealt with by Saccente and Woods (2010). Animal model studies suggested that liposomal amphotericin B reaches higher concentration in the CNS than the conventional amphotericin B. It is useful in treating pregnant blastomycosis cases also. Additionally, surgical intervention like drainage may be occasionally required in case of abscess in the brain and epidural and debridement of the bone.

64.8   Prognosis

Based on mortality data among cases under treatment for blastomycosis (https://en.wikipedia.org/wiki/Blastomycosis), possibility of survival varies with the status of the patient. While it is highest among immunocompetent (98–100%), it is increasingly reduced for immunocompromised (71%), AIDS (60%) and acute respiratory distress patients (32%).

64.9   Prevention

Personal protective like mask covering the nose to protect against entry of fungus through inhalation should be practised while working.

References

Chakrabarti A, Slavin MA (2011) Endemic fungal infections in the Asia-Pacific region. Med Mycol 49(4):337–344

Cheikh Rouhou S, Racil H, Ismail O, Trabelsi S, Zarrouk M, Chaouch N et al (2008) Pulmonary blastomycosis: a case from Africa. Sci World J 8:1098–1103

Hussaini SMQ, Madut D, Tong BC et al (2018) Pulmonary blastomycosis presenting as primary lung cancer. BMC Infect Dis 18:336

Saccente M, Woods GL (2010) Clinical and laboratory update on blastomycosis. Clin Microbiol Rev 23(2):367–381

Schwartz IS, Wiederhold NP, Hanson KE, Patterson TF, Sigler L (2019) *Blastomyces helicus*, a new dimorphic fungus causing fatal pulmonary and systemic disease in humans and animals in Western Canada and the United States. Clin Infect Dis 68(2):188–195

Chapter 65
Candidiasis

Synonyms

Candidosis, Moniliasis, Thrush.

The microbiome on the human skin, mucous membranes, gastrointestinal tract and female genital tract includes *Candida* and other yeast species. Candidiasis is an opportunistic infection caused by *Candida*, a type of fungi, which are eukaryotic organisms found in the form of yeasts, moulds or dimorphic fungi (Arya and Rafiq 2023). Nearly 10% of *Candida* species are pathogenic and associated with mild to severe and localized to serious even life-threatening deep-seated invasive infections. The incidence of candidemia is increasing and being reported from all parts of the world.

Candida spp. is now recognized as the fourth most common cause of bloodstream/invasive infections. Most common settings are intensive care units in healthcare facilities where at least 50% episodes of candidemia occur. The attributable fatality rates of candidemia are 15–35% in adults and 10–15% in neonates.

The late-onset septicaemia in very-low-birth-weight neonates and infants is commonly caused by *Candida* spp.

Candida albicans is the most common causative agent of candidemia and invasive candidiasis. Non-*C. albicans* species are increasingly reported and account for >50%, attributed to selection of species with reduced susceptibility to antifungal drugs.

Among the *Candida* species, *C. albicans* was the most common species (42/95; 44.21%), followed by *C. lusitaniae* (18/95; 18.95%), *C. parapsilosis* (13/95; 13.69%), *C. glabrata* (8/95; 8.42%), *C. kefyr* (6/95; 6.31%), *C. famata* (5/95; 5.26%), *C. africana* (2/95; 2.11%) and *C. orthopsilosis* (1/95; 1.05%), respectively (Hashemi et al. 2019).

The emerging multidrug-resistant species associated with invasive candidiasis and candidemia are *C. glabrata*, *C. guilliermondii* complex members, *C. krusei*,

© Springer Nature Singapore Pte Ltd. 2024   683
K. G. Narayan et al., *Handbook of Management of Zoonoses*,
https://doi.org/10.1007/978-981-99-9885-2_65

C. lusitaniae, C. lipolytica, C. rugosa, C. kefyr, C. haemulonii complex members and *C. auris* (Ahmad and Alfouzan 2021).

Cernáková et al. (2021) attempted to compare *C. auris* and other pathogenic *Candida* species. *C. auris* had higher pathogenic potential. The tissue fungal burden of *C. auris* and *C. albicans* was similar, and pathogenic potential was comparable in disseminated infection in immunocompetent hosts. It seems that there was no significant difference between *C. auris, Candida albicans, Candida glabrata* and *Candida haemulonii* as observed by (a) fungal load in the kidney followed by the spleen, liver and lung and (b) in vivo survival rate.

65.1   *C. albicans*

Candidiasis is an infection caused by a fungus called *Candida*, most commonly the *Candida albicans*. Candidiasis is the fourth leading cause of nosocomial infections. The occurrence is infrequent and considered by many as benign, managed by removing the contaminated device. Candidaemia is an emerging infection, particularly in the immunocompromised population.

Systemic candidiasis caused deaths, which range from 15% to 35%. Candida pericarditis mainly caused by *C. albicans* is a rare clinical entity with a high fatality. Other species have rarely been reported, for example, *C. tropicalis, C. glabrata, C. guilliermondii* and *C. parapsilosis*. It occurs commonly in patients with recent cardiothoracic surgery or debilitating chronic diseases.

65.1.1   *Aetiology*

Some 20 species of *Candida*, mainly *Candida albicans, C. glabrata, C. krusei, C. parapsilosis* and *C. tropicalis* account for most (90%) of invasive infections (Pfaller and Diekema 2007). *Candida auris* is an emerging multidrug-resistant organism causing serious infections and is reported from over 20 nations of the world (Pal 2020a, b).

Candida requires moisture for growth.

65.1.2   *Virulence and Risk Factors*

A number of virulence factors are used by *Candida*, namely, adherence, biofilm formation, haemolysin, phospholipases and proteases to overcome hosts' natural defences.

Risk factors: <1-month-old infant, old people, malnutrition, stress, diabetes, metabolic dysfunction, taking medicines like antibiotics, cytotoxic drugs, steroids for long, using too many cleansing products, hormone replacement and infertility therapy, transplant and underlying ailments like HIV/AIDS, cancer, mononucleosis, neutropenia, catheterization, dialysis and denture.

65.1.3   Mode of Infection

Source of *Candida*: *Candida* is normal flora of the mouth, throat, rest of gastrointestinal tract and urogenital tract.

- Endogenous.
- Direct contact of mucous membrane or macerated, abraded skin—neonates/infants—may acquire infection from mothers with vaginal candidiasis.
- Nosocomial.

Most *Candida* infections are endogenous in origin. Neonates/infants may acquire infection from mothers with vaginal candidiasis. Infection can also occur by direct contact of mucous membrane and injured, abraded skin with *Candida*-contaminated objects. Nosocomial infections are commonly observed in hospital settings throughout the world.

65.1.4   Pathology

Candida species are well known for causing infections in our mouth, skin and vagina but are also a common cause of life-threatening bloodstream infections in hospitals. Most *Candida* infections in people are caused by *C. albicans*, which has very low levels of drug resistance. A vast variety of pathological conditions are caused, namely, thrush, cheilitis, glossitis, stomatitis, oesophagitis, gastritis, pneumonia, lung empyema, pericarditis, endocarditis, cystitis, peritonitis, arthritis, osteoarthritis, meningitis, septicemia, endophthalmitis, otitis, vulvovaginitis, balanitis, paronychia and onychomycosis and others. These have been grouped into four (https://en.wikipedia.org/wiki/Candidiasis) as follows:

(a) Mucosal—oral (pseudomembranous, erythematous, hyperplastic, denture-related stomatitis, angular cheilitis, median rhomboid glossitis), vulvovaginitis, balanitis, esophageal, gastrointestinal and respiratory candidiasis
(b) Cutaneous—folliculitis, intertrigo, paronychia, perianal, congenital cutaneous, diaper candidiasis, onychomycosis and chronic mucocutaneous
(c) Systemic—candidaemia/fungaemia, invasive (disseminated, organ infection) candidiasis and chronic systemic candidiasis (hepatosplenic, sometimes during recovery from neutropenia)
(d) Antibiotics—iatrogenic candidiasis

Systemic candidaemia/fungaemia: The fungi/yeast present in blood may lead to sepsis. These are *Candida*, *Saccharomyces*, *Aspergillus* and *Cryptococcus*. Risk factors are diabetes, HIV, chronic haemodialysis, liver failure, asplenia and transplants—solid organ, stem cell and glucocorticoid intake.

Invasive candidiasis: It is a disseminated organ infection. Invasive candidiasis can be a serious and potentially fatal condition when the blood, brain, heart and eye are affected. Gastrointestinal infection causes gastric ulcer, gas and intestinal cramp. Symptoms include belching, bloating, indigestion, nausea, vomiting, diarrhoea and anal itching. There are red, popular or ulcerative perianal lesions. Increasing *Candida* population in bowel leads to dysbiosis (dysbacteriosis or disrupted bowel microbiota).

Invasive candidiasis is a common hospital-acquired infection. Host-related factors may be associated with a higher incidence among Blacks/African-Americans and babies <one month old, especially underweight (<2.2 pounds/1.0 kg).

65.1.5   Symptoms

Candidiasis may cause (a) common, (b) rare (dissemination because of compromised immunity) and (c) severe ailments. A patient of candidiasis complains tiredness, fatigue, joint pain and digestive problems. Symptoms vary widely. The mildest and most common forms are oral thrush and vulvo-vagintis. Most rare and severe forms affect the heart (endocardium) or brain (meninges).

65.1.5.1   Oral Thrush

It begins as creamy white patches or sores on the tongue or mucous membranes of the mouth. Corners of the mouth are red inflamed, sore, eroded and cracked (Perleche); angular cheilitis (crackings at the corners of the mouth) appear and difficulty/painful swallowing. Infection can overgrow to affect the throat and oesophagus.

Uncommon in healthy adult, imbalanced oral environment allows the already present *Candida* in small number to multiply (small number present also on the skin).

65.1.5.2   Candidiasis in Male (Balanitis)

Candida lives on the skin and mucous membrane. Increased growth (in diabetics) causes itchy rash, irritation, red skin with glazed appearance, swelling around the head of the penis, small papules or white patches under the foreskin, lumpy white discharge possibly with unpleasant odour, pain and difficulty in pulling back the foreskin and pain during sex or urination. It is not sexually transmitted but sex can transfer infection to partner.

65.1.5.3   Candidiasis in Female (Moniliasis)

Vulvovaginitis is common and affects every three out of four women at some point of time; many experience more than one attack. It is common among diabetics or pregnant. It appears first as leucorrhoea-thick white or yellow vaginal discharge. Vaginal yeast infection causes irritation, discharge and intense itchiness of the vagina, the vulva and tissues around the vaginal opening. It is not considered a sexually transmitted infection but risk of infection at the time first regular sex is increased; also transmission is possible during oro-genital sex.

65.1.5.4   Cutaneous Candidiasis

Superficial skin is infected. Lesions appear are well-circumscribed red patches of varying size. Small red pustules form a rim of the itchy lesion. Infection sites are commonly located in the skin fold, for example, the underarms, under breasts, navel, buttocks (diaper rash), groin, around the anus (perianal) and between toes and fingers. Infection may appear as crusts on scalp extending to the face, trunk and tips of the finger.

65.1.5.5   Nails (Candidal paronychia)

It is a painful swelling under nails. Pus develops. The infection may end with loss of nails of the finger or toes.

65.1.5.6   Chronic Mucocutaneous Candidiasis (Candida granuloma)

It is severe, rare and chronic form of Candidiasis affecting the skin, nails, scalp and mucous membranes. Generally, infants are affected. Lesions appear as red, pustules and thick crust on the nose and forehead.

65.1.5.7   Systemic Candidiasis

It is the most serious form of Candidiasis causing endocarditis, meningitis and osteomyelitis. It affects the membrane lining the heart (endocardium) and skull (meninges).

65.1.5.8   Invasive

Invasive yeast infections typically enter the bloodstream causing fungaemia. *Candida* is by far the most common fungal bloodstream pathogen causing Candidaemia. Others in decreasing order are *Cryptococcus, Rhodotorula* and *Trichosporon. C. albicans* remains the predominant species; a variety of other *Candida* species are involved in human infections.

Species according to reducing pathogenic potential are *C. albicans* and *C. tropicalis*; (ii) *C. glabrata, C. lusitaniae* and *C. kefyr*; and *(iii) C. parapsilosis, C. krusei* and *C. guilliermondii.*

Arendrup (2013) found this consistent by i/v mice inoculation. *C. albicans* and *C. tropicalis* challenged mice lost body weight and exhibited high inflammation score in the kidney and metastatic lesions in eyes. Mice challenged with *C. krusei* did not manifest these symptoms; instead they gained body weight. Frequency of species associated with cases in Norway during 1991–1996 was *C. albicans, C. glabrata, C. parapsilosis* and *C. tropicalis* 66%, 12.5%, 7.6% and 6.4%, respectively. *C. tropicalis* ending last is explained—it is virulent once it entered bloodstream but less so in intact gastrointestinal mucosa for which it is a less frequent colonizer. *C. albicans* and *C. tropicalis* followed by *C. glabrata* and *C. krusei* were ranked as causing mortality and fungal burden in challenged mice.

Most candidaemia cases probably arise from a smaller amount of yeast cells entering the bloodstream following a barrier leakage during gastrointestinal (GI) surgery or impaired integrity of the gastrointestinal mucosa during chemotherapy. Overall, *C. albicans* is the dominating cause of invasive infections. *C. tropicalis* follows as the significant pathogen in haematological setting. However, outside the oncology/haematology setting, *C. tropicalis* is less frequent in the Northern hemisphere. *C. parapsilosis* and *C. krusei* are very low-virulent, consistent with low prevalence and mortality in *C. parapsilosis* candidaemia cases and oral and vaginitis animal models. *C. parapsilosis* is able to form biofilm on plastic and other artificial surfaces and colonize the human skin without harming. Associated with nosocomial infection via intravenous catheters, parenteral nutrition and transfer through contaminated hands to neonates by nursing staff are more common in the southern hemisphere and in Asia.

65.1.6   Epidemiology (Nordic Countries, Denmark in Particular)

The observed high fungaemia incidence rate of 11/100,000 inhabitants of Denmark during 2004–2011 was observed. This was based on 3982 unique isolates, from 3867 episodes of fungaemia in 3689 patients. There was an annual incidence rate from 7.7 to 10.1 episodes/100,000 inhabitants over these eight years and was remarkably high in a Nordic perspective. In the early 1990s, the incidence rate of bloodstream fungal isolates was around 2/100,000. It has increased remarkably since then in all the three countries, Norway, Denmark and Finland, especially in Denmark.

Earlier reported rate of incidence ranged between 1.2 and 25 cases per 100,000 inhabitants or 0.19–2.5 per 1000 admissions. Among the Nordic countries, Norway (NO), Finland (FI) and Sweden report incidences of candidaemia around 3/100,000 inhabitant. The studies were dominantly based on data of university hospitals and all centres performing solid organ or bone marrow transplantation (not based on population surveys covering either a nation or defined geographic region).

When the surveillance was extended to the entire country, the high incidence remained a consistent finding, and the incidence rate was still increasing. A changing epidemiology was observed. A high and increasing proportion of the cases involved fluconazole-resistant isolates, significantly higher proportion in Denmark than in other Nordic countries, related to a significantly higher and increasing fluconazole use. Incidence was remarkably higher in the elderly population and in male, when compared to past two decades; this suggested an association with host-specific factors including antifungal consumption. Two peaks of incidences, namely, in infants (<1 year) and elderly >65 years, were observed. In age <1-year age, specific incidence rates were 11.3, 10.3 and 6.9 isolates/100,000 for Denmark, Norway and Finland, respectively. The second peak per 100,000 in Denmark was 37.1 in the age group 70–79, in Norway 8.4 in 80+ and in Finland 8.8 in >65 years. The overall species distribution has changed over the past years. *C. albicans* was the dominating pathogen (even at the main tertiary hospital in Copenhagen) in the mid and late 80s with significantly higher mortality than *C. parapsilosis. It has been reduced to half. C. glabrata* and *C. krusei* mainly emerged in the post fluconazole era and in settings with azole selection pressure. *C. glabrata* accounts for every third bloodstream fungal infection today.

It was observed that two-thirds of patients with fungaemia received abdominal surgery or intensive care treatment prior to the development of the fungaemia. It strongly suggested that the underlying clinical conditions and fungemia must be investigated for *C. albicans* and also other species for most appropriate treatment.

65.1.7   Diagnosis

Mycological, immunological, histopathological and molecular techniques are used. Isolation in pure growth on mycological media is still considered the gold standard.

Sign—mouth for white patches and irritation may make the diagnosis:

- Specimen—a scraping or swab of the affected area; a 3–5 ml fluid from duodenum for culture in case of gastrointestinal candidiasis (>1000 colony-forming units/ml is diagnostic).
- Microscopy—A drop of 10% potassium hydroxide is placed on the glass slide. Specimen is added. Skin cells but not the yeasts are dissolved. Pseudohyphae and budding yeasts are visible and can be stained by Gram's and Narayan stains.

- Culture—a sterile swab is rubbed on the infected skin surface and then on Sabouraud dextrose agar, CHROM agar and Pal sunflower seed agar, and incubate for several days at 37 °C.
- Multilocus sequence typing (MLST).

Arendrup (2013) used for detection of Candidaemia:

- Growth characteristics and colony appearance on CHROM agar, micromorphology on Rice and Tween or Corn Meal Agar, growth at 35 °C and 42 °C and carbon assimilation profiling using ATB ID32C
- Later rapid identification by latex agglutination for the separation of *C. albicans* and *C. dubliniensis*
- Sequencing of the ITS region (ITS for Internal Transcribed Spacer which is a non-functional piece of ribosomal DNA)

Sequencing resulted in separation of *C. dubliniensis* from *C. albicans* and improved identification for *C. guilliermondii*, *C. famata*, *C. lusitaniae*, *C. fermentati* and *C. palmioleophila* isolates.

He suggested to use a fungal blood culture flask in addition to the conventional aerobic and anaerobic ones if all *C. glabrata* infections (BACTEC) and all polymicrobial infections (BacT/ALERT) are to be diagnosed.

65.1.8   Treatment

Fluconazole-resistant species *C. glabrata*, *C. krusei* and *Saccharomyces cerevisiae* were significantly more common in patients exposed to at least seven days of antifungal prophylaxis (mainly fluconazole).

Caspofungin as the first line of treatment significantly improved the condition of patients infected with *C. glabrata*.

Outcome of treatment depends upon virulence of *Candida*, susceptibility (intrinsic and acquired resistance), severity of disease, timing of drug intervention and choice and dose of drug. Study in mouse model covers these observations, with possible extrapolation for use in human.

65.1.9   Prevention

- Oral hygiene—chlorhexidine mouthwash; those who use steroid inhalation should wash the mouth after inhaling the drug; disinfect denture regularly.
- Cotton underwear help to reduce infection of the skin and the vagina; avoid wearing wet clothes.
- Oral/intravaginal probiotics as pills or yoghurt.
- Control diabetes.

65.2   *Candida auris*

Candida auris is an emerging multidrug-resistant yeast associated with outbreaks of invasive infections in health-care facilities worldwide. It successfully sustains for prolonged periods in the intensive care unit, adeptly colonizes skin and spreads among patients, primarily staying for long periods in health-care facility. It causes life-threatening disease among immunocompromised. It is considered a global public threat by the Centres for Disease Control and Prevention, USA.

   C. auris has propensity to spread rapidly in critically ill patients. The resistance to commonly used antifungal drugs is responsible of high fatality due to *C. auris* candidemia. The crude 'in-hospital' mortality rate varies from 30% to 72%. The reported rates of a 30-day mortality in Colombia and Spain were 35.2% and 41.4%, respectively. It was >50% in Asia, Far East and the USA (Ademe and Girma 2020).

   C. auris infection has been associated with the development of pericarditis and urinary tract and respiratory infections. Khillan et al. (2014) reported a rare case of fungal pericardial effusion caused by a multidrug-resistant species *C. auris*. It was cultured from pericardial fluid, blood, bronchoalveolar lavage and urine of a chronic liver disease patient while on empiric fluconazole therapy and identified as *C. haemulonii* by the VITEK2 commercial identification system. It was confirmed later as *C. auris* by internal transcribed spacer and large ribosomal subunit sequencing. Wang et al. (2018) reported its isolation from bronchial lavage fluid of a 76-year-old woman with hypertension and nephritic syndrome.

65.2.1   *Aetiology*

Clinical presentation of *C. auris* is non-specific, not diagnostic. It has been commonly reported to be associated with infections of the bloodstream, bone, ear, urinary tract, surgical and other wounds and inflammatory conditions like myocarditis and meningitis. Isolated from ear canal of a Japanese patient first in 2009, it has been reported as a cause of disseminated infection with fatality rate as high as 60%.

   C. auris has been isolated in numerous countries on five continents. Whole genome sequencing has identified five distinct clades that represent the following geographical regions: South Asia (India/Pakistan), South Africa, South America, East Asia and the Middle East. Clinical *C. auris* isolates belonging to all four major clades (except the Middle East) formed multiple (yeast, filamentous, aggregated and elongated forms) colony and cellular morphologies that differed in antifungal resistance and virulence properties.

65.2.2   Epidemiology

C. auris possesses qualities of pathogen, resilience to survive and antifungal drug resistance, asymptomatic colonization and easy mode and pace of transmission among health-care workers and patients in hospitals.

65.2.3   Virulence Factors

Morphologic and metabolic plasticity: Both morphologic (e.g. aggregate/non-aggregate, biofilm) and metabolic plasticity confer an edge for virulence. This versatility allows the pathogenic organisms to rapidly adapt to different environmental conditions. Metabolic plasticity in *C. auris* is least studied. The bonding of *C. auris* mannan to IgG (e.g. in blood and sweat glands) was found to be 12–20-fold stronger than mannan from *C. albicans* suggesting likely role in its increased colonization of humans (Ahmad and Alfouzan 2021).

Phenotypic switching: It is a mechanism for adaptation to survive in harsh environment. Factors that stimulate it may be UV light, abnormal pH/temperature, nutrient limitation and biological factors present in serum. Examples are yeast-hyphal transition and white-opaque switching (white-opaque regulator gene controlled). The yeast-hyphal switching was rare in *C. auris* but heritable and depended upon cooler environment. The filamentous forms of *C. auris* could exist in the cooler hospital environment and perhaps also on the skin of colonized patients and enter and invade the body of the susceptible patients with multiple comorbidities, particularly in ICU settings.

Thermotolerance: C. auris is capable of growing at higher temperature (>40 °C) and thus able to colonize and infect human. Most fungi do not survive at normal physiological temperatures (36.5–37.5 °C) or during conditions of pyrexia ~40 °C.

Osmotolerance: C. auris unlike *C. haemulonii* complex members is also able to tolerate high (>10% NaCl) salt concentrations.

Thermotolerance and osmotolerance may help in the persistence and survival on biotic and abiotic surfaces for long periods of time.

Colonization, niche: Studies on synthetic sweat medium and porcine skin confirmed that *C. auris* adeptly colonize skin niches and withstand environmental stress. Outbreak surveillance reports implicated skin colonization as risk factor (Uppuluri 2020).

Aggregate: As per Ahmad and Alfouzan (2021), *C. auris* is a budding yeast and release daughter cells (non-aggregating). Some strains (aggregating) do not release and form aggregates of pseudohyphal-like cells which are resistant to physical, chemical and detergent disruption that makes eradication difficult. This phenotypic trait is inducible, stimulated by pre-exposure to triazoles or echinocandins. Although mortality rates for aggregative and non-aggregative strains were similar, clinical isolates were more pathogenic, predominately isolated from colonized patients, and had higher capacity for biofilm formation.

Biofilm: It has natural tendency to form biofilm and grow in it. Biofilms can resist desiccation. A robust biofilm growth and survival on dry surface make *C. auris* a successful pathogen. Adhesin genes are upregulated during biofilm formation, suggesting role in colonization. The biofilm-forming capacity of *C. auris* likely has a role in pathogenicity. Biofilm is able to trigger antifungal resistance and appears to be a fundamental factor to antifungal resistance in *C. auris* and persistent infection. Biofilm is resistant to all classes of antifungal drugs but sensitive to echinocandins and polyenes. Minimal biofilm eradication concentration of antifungal drugs (MBEC) was higher than minimal inhibitory concentration (MIC). *C. auris* biofilm on the skin is likely to contaminate intravenous catheter while it is puncturing skin. Biofilm formation on the surface of medical implants is an important determinant of bloodstream infections and other infections likely acquired by these. *C. auris* biofilm cells persisting on the skin could serve as source of continuing outbreaks in health-care facilities, spreading likely through horizontal transmission rapidly between hospital rooms (via human contact).

Virulence factors: Hemolysin, secreted aspartyl proteinases (SAPs), secreted lipases, phospholipase, integrin and adhesins (ALS3, ALS4) enable adhesion and tissue invasion (Ahmad and Alfouzan 2021).

Antifungal drug resistance: Most of the clinical *C. auris* isolates are resistant to main classes of antifungals (azoles, polyenes or echinocandins), and there is multi (MDR)- or pan-drug resistance to more than two antifungal classes (Ademe and Girma 2020). The South Asia clade has exhibited increased antifungal resistance compared to other clades of *C. auris*.

65.2.4   Risk Factors

Host-related risk factors are comorbidities (diabetes, hypertension, chronic lung or kidney disease), primary or acquired altered immunity and therapeutic management cases such as transplantation, on broad-spectrum antibiotics or immunosuppressive drugs. *C. auris* has been isolated from patients of both sexes and of all age groups.

It colonizes biotic surfaces, such as the skin of groin/axilla and nares commonly. The burden is roughly 2-log higher in nares than for axilla/groin colonization. Moisture or components in nasal secretions may be a factor in site preference.

Other risk factors: Longer stays in certain types of health-care facilities, for example, post-acute care facilities, may be associated with recent surgery, gastrostomy and parenteral nutrition, urinary or central venous catheters, tracheostomy, ventilator support and ICUs. An average stay of 25 days in Spain was associated with *C. auris* infection. This is suggestive of transmission through contaminated facilities in health-care institutions.

Colonization can progress into invasive and/or superficial infections.

Reservoirs: Prolonged and persistent colonization of clinical and screening case patients, environmental contamination and persistent and lack of an accepted decolonization regimen generated a large number of reservoirs.

Transmission goes on among patients with extensive exposure at and during health-care evident from culture of *C. auris* from rooms and equipment in multiple facilities and close contacts of case patients, highlighting infection control lapses. There is extensive and frequent contact with affected patients with multiple health-care facilities.

Fomite transmission: *C. auris* can survive for weeks on moist and dry surfaces of abiotic surfaces (e.g. plastic and steel). It endures for 1–2 weeks on the surface of objects in patient's room such as mobile phone, bedding, doors of bathroom, walls, faucets floor, sink, bedside trolleys and medical equipment and devices, including blood pressure cuffs and axillary thermometers. Colonization can spread to other patients.

Candida auris is an emerging fungal pathogen rapidly spreading throughout the world, 39 countries, 13 states (in the USA) and on all continents except Antarctica (Wickes 2020). *C. auris* bloodstream infection has been reported in India, the UK, Colombia, South Africa and the USA (Chowdhary et al. 2020). Nearly 1000 confirmed cases have been reported in the USA, mostly from Illinois, New Jersy, California and New York. These states reported more than 100 clinical cases of *C. auris* between May 1, 2020, and April 30, 2021, according to *tracking by the CDC*. Blood infection (fungemia) has been high, 76% in Colombia, 61% in New York and 58% in India. *C. auris* is an aggressive naturally resistant fungus. Strains are generally resistant to one class of antifungal drug, some resistant to all three including recently reported three pan-resistant cases in New York.

Adams et al. (2018) observed that a large outbreak continued through interconnected web of multiple health-care facilities with epidemiologic links in New York City. The numbers of cases were increasing for unknown reasons, possibly from a combination of three factors, namely, multiple introductions, aggressive case finding and presence of large interconnected health-care facilities. They defined 'case patient' as a person for whom a culture was positive for *C. auris* and 'screening cases' as those for which the culture was obtained for surveillance purposes.

Cultures from patients' blood, bile, urine, respiratory specimens and wounds were 61%, 6%, 8%, 8% and 6% positive, respectively. Cases were followed and cultures collected from a variety of sites typically axilla and groin and often the nares, rectum, urine and wounds. The clinical and screening case patients were followed up, and the 30-day and 90-day mortality rates among those with initial isolates from blood were 39% and 58%, respectively.

In another outbreak (2016–2018) in the New York reported by Zhu et al. (2020), *C. auris* was isolated from clinical specimen; most common specimen was blood. Genotyping revealed predominance of a single clade, Clade I, South Asia. Clade II, East Asia, was a minor clade. *C. auris* was recovered in large numbers (10^5 cfu); nonporous substrates were more heavily colonized than porous substrates. Urine specimens collected from some patients showed echinocandin resistance, suggesting that these isolates can be selected as drug-resistant strains and pose potential threat.

Known to persist on surfaces, *C. auris* can cause outbreak in health-care facilities. In June 2020, outbreaks occurred in skilled nursing facilities in Southern

California. *A single case introduced to a health-care facility in Orange County led to spread to 180* patients in 9 facilities due to interfacility transfers with knowing the patients' colonization status. As of October 2019, 181 patients were identified including 5 developing candidaemia and 36 deaths (none directly attributable to *C. auris*).

Secondary infection in COVID-19 cases was high. Candidaemia affected 15 (2.5%) of 596 COVID-19 cases in the ICU during April–July 2020 in New Delhi, distributed as *C. auris* 10 (67%), *C. albicans* 3 and *C. tropicalis* and *C. krusei* one each (Chowdhary et al. 2020).

All 15 had indwelling central lines and urinary catheter and acquired infection 2–7 weeks after hospitalization. Case fatality due to candidaemia was 53%. The ten *C. auris* patients had a prolonged hospitalization (20–60 days) and one or the other comorbidities such as diabetes mellitus, hypertension and chronic liver/kidney disease. Eight were of 66–88 years; seven were male. They developed candidaemia 10–42 days post-admission. Five (50%) had received ventilation. Case fatality was 60%. Whether fatalities (53% and 60%) could be attributed to *Candida* and *C. auris* is unclear. The patients were COVID-19 cases with comorbidity, and *Candida* were nosocomial secondary invaders. The observed case fatality rates do not subscribe. Isolates of *C. auris* were resistant to fluconazole, and 40% were resistant to amphotericin B.

65.2.5   Diagnosis

- *Biochemical phenotyping* resulted into misdiagnosis. *C. auris* infections have frequently been misdiagnosed, most often as *C. haemulonii* and less often as *C. famata*, *C. guilliermondii*, *C. lusitaniae*, *C. parapsilosis*, *C. sake*, *R. glutinis*, *C. duobushaemulonii*, *C catenulate*, *C. tropicalis* or *Saccharomyces cerevisiae*.
- *Matrix-assisted laser desorption ionization and time-of-flight mass spectrometry (MALDI-TOF MS)* are FDA approved.
- *Identification based on ITS or D1/D2 sequence has arguably been established as gold standard.*
- *Real-time PCR assay* was used in a study with 98.36%, 93.32% and 98.38% accuracy, sensitivity and specificity, respectively.

65.2.6   Major Causes of Concern

- High mortality rate, ranging from 28% to 78% depending on country.
- The cost to treatment is highest among the highest of all mycoses.
- The tendency to infect already severely debilitated patients.

- High frequency of drug resistance, >*90% of its isolates tested in vitro have shown this resistance. C. auris* is characterized by reduced susceptibility to azoles, polyenes and echinocandins.
- Tenacious persistence (for year or longer) on skin and in patients' environment makes *C. auris* most dangerous and difficult to eradicate.

Elevated resistance to fluconazole, with multidrug resistance, has been frequent and pan-fungal resistance has been described.

65.2.7 Prevention

Infection preventionists at University of California, Los Angeles (UCLA), used their electronic medical recording (EMR) system to screen each incoming patient for COVID-19 and *C. auris*.

In-house PCR for *early detection of C. auris* supplemented with IT and IP are proactive surveillance and communication between and with facilities, nursing, environmental services, etc. Patients are identified, flagged and notified.

Hospital having screening programme for carbapenemase-producing organism identified *C. auris*-infected patient; the patient was isolated in hospital (for 47 days), and their room was cleaned and disinfected using 0.5% chlorine-based solution and ultraviolet light. Following six months, *C. auris* colonization or a case did not appear/was reported.

65.2.8 Intervention Measures

Interventions blocking *C. auris* biofilm growth on the skin will help control the spread of this pathogen. Screening and detection of a first case, standard precautions, cleaning and disinfection to eliminate environmental biofilms and end/prevent colonization, management of inpatient transfer and outbreak and treatment were agreed upon by the experts of infection prevention and mycologists at a meeting organized by the Infection Prevention and Control Working Group of the International Society of Antimicrobial Chemotherapy (Kenters et al. 2019).

Ahmad and Alfouzan (2021) outlined the intervention steps and recommended infection control steps. Following are some of the salient steps:

- *Identification of C. auris cases:* Identify all *Candida* isolates from SITES (a) sterile, (b) non-sterile and (c) any site of the health-care facilities depending upon the need. Notify concerned officials and alert clinician; isolate the patient; search cases, retrospectively.
- *Surveillance culture:* Screening of *contact* and other patients in the health-care facility by examining specimens from the axilla, groin, nose, throat, urine, fae-

ces, wound drain fluid, insertion sites of venous catheters and respiratory specimens. Repeat/assess periodically. Alert officials and clinicians. Isolate culture-positive patients.

- *Contact precaution:* single room occupancy, follow transmission-based precautions.
- *Environment cleaning:* assess procedures and amend, namely, single patient-use items, disinfection of shared items and terminal cleaning of rooms with sodium hypochlorite (1000 ppm).
- *Hand hygiene:* hand wash followed by alcohol-based sanitizer.
- *Patient decolonization:* chlorhexidine body washes and mouth gargles; chlorhexidine-impregnated pads for catheter exit sites may offer some help.
- *Education of health-care workers.*

References

Adams E, Quinn M, Tsay S, Poirot E, Chaturvedi S, Southwick K et al (2018) Workgroup, C. *Candida auris* in healthcare facilities, New York, USA, 2013–2017. Emerg Infect Dis 24(10):1816–1824

Ademe M, Girma F (2020) *Candida auris*: from multidrug resistance to pan-resistant strains. Infect Drug Resist 13:1287–1294

Ahmad S, Alfouzan W (2021) *Candida auris*: epidemiology, diagnosis, pathogenesis, antifungal susceptibility, and infection control measures to combat the spread of infections in healthcare facilities. Microorganisms 9:807

Arendrup MC (2013) Candida and candidaemia. Susceptibility and epidemiology. Dan Med J 60(11):B4698

Arya NR, Rafiq NB (2023) Candidiasis. In: StatPearls. StatPearls Publishing, Treasure Island (FL)

Cernáková L, Roudbary M, Brás S, Tafaj S, Rodrigues CF (2021) *Candida auris*: a quick review on identification, current treatments, and challenges. Int J Mol Sci 22:4470

Chowdhary A, Tarai B, Singh A, Sharma A (2020) Multidrug-resistant *Candida auris* infections in critically ill coronavirus disease patients, India, April–July 2020. Emerg Infect Dis 26(11):2694–2696

Hashemi SE, Shokohi T, Abastabar M, Aslani N, Ghadamzadeh M, Haghani I (2019) Species distribution and susceptibility profiles of *Candida* species isolated from vulvovaginal candidiasis, emergence of *C. lusitaniae*. Curr Med Mycol 5(4):26–34

Kenters N, Kiernan M, Chowdhary A, Denning DW, Pemán J et al (2019) Control of *Candida auris* in healthcare institutions: outcome of an International Society for Antimicrobial Chemotherapy expert meeting. Int J Antimicrob Agents 54(4):400–406

Khillan V, Rathore N, Kathuria S, Chowdhary A (2014) A rare case of breakthrough fungal pericarditis due to fluconazole-resistant *Candida auris* in a patient with chronic liver disease. JMM Case Reports:1–5

Pal M (2020a) Zygomycosis: a highly infectious emerging opportunistic fungal disease of public health concern. Open Access J Mycol Mycol Sci 3(2). https://doi.org/10.23880/oajmms-16000123

Pal M (2020b) Candidiasis: an important opportunistic mycosis of global public health concern. Res Infect Dis Trop Med 2(1):49–51

Pfaller MA, Diekema DJ (2007) Epidemiology of invasive candidiasis: a persistent public health problem. Clin Microbiol Rev 2007(20):133–163

Uppuluri P (2020) *Candida auris* biofilm colonization on skin niche conditions. mSphere 5(1):e00972–e00919

Wang X, Bing J, Zheng Q, Zhang F, Liu J et al (2018) The first isolate of Candida auris in China: clinical and biological aspects. Emerg Microbes Infect 7:1–9

Wickes BL (2020) Analysis of a Candida auris outbreak provides new insights into an emerging pathogen. J Clin Microbiol 58:e02083–e02019

Wikipedia.: https://en.wikipedia.org/wiki/Candidiasis: This page was last edited on 8 August 2021, at 11:09 (UTC)

Zhu Y, O'Brien B, Leach L, Clarke A, Bates M et al (2020) Laboratory analysis of an outbreak of *Candida auris* in New York from 2016 to 2018: impact and lessons learned. J Clin Microbiol 58:e01503–e01519

Chapter 66
Coccidioidomycosis

Synonyms

Desert (rheumatism) fever, San Joaquin Valley fever, Posada's disease, California fever.

Coccidioidomycosis is a saprozoonosis characterized by respiratory symptoms resembling influenza.

66.1   Aetiology

Coccidioides was first discovered by a medical intern in 1892 and was later named *Coccidioides immitis* (Akram and Koirala 2023). Two species within the genus *Coccidioides* are recognized, namely, *C. immitis* and *C. posadasii*, which are diphasic. These are saprophytes and exist in soil as mycelia and arthroconidia and are pathogen in tissues as spherule and endospore.

  Coccidioides are filamentous fungi living under soil and require moisture (rain) for growth. These are able to survive in hot, dry (not less than 20% relative humidity), dessert, and sandy alkaline soil. The filaments grow both horizontally and vertically. The filaments degenerate during prolonged dry spell into barrel-shaped cells (spores) called arthroconidia. The arthroconidia have inner and outer refractile walls. The outer wall is thin and disintegrates readily along with the degenerating adherent cells. The aerial dispersal of released arthroconidia becomes easy.

K. G. Narayan et al., *Handbook of Management of Zoonoses*,
https://doi.org/10.1007/978-981-99-9885-2_66

66.2   Infection and Development Cycle

Upon inhalation, these spores reach alveoli and increase in size, spherules. Internal septation and segmentation occur. This is followed by development of endospores within spherule. Endospores are released with rupture of spherule. Endospores invade adjacent tissues, and lesions spread. It is intracellular in multinucleated giant cells within granuloma. Host responses lead to the formation of nodules around spherules. Thin-walled cavities form when nodules rupture and empty the contents in bronchi. Hematogenous spread occurs in those with weak immunity or comorbidity.

Infection through the skin is rare and can happen through broken skin (e.g. cut wound, splinter).

Laboratory-acquired infection.

66.3   Epidemiology

Coccidioidomycosis is endemic in arid and semi-arid certain areas of Central and South America. The estimated incidence is greater than 150, 000 every year in California, Arizona, New Mexico, Nevada, Utah, Texas, and northern Mexico of North America (Aduroja et al. 2021).

The fungus is found in alkaline sandy soil 10–30 cm under the surface. Coccidioidomycosis is endemic in western hemisphere, between $40°N$ and $40°S$, where the weather is mainly hot summer, low rains (10–50 cm), and mild winter.

The fungus grows in wet weather (rainy season). During succeeding dry weather, spores are spread by wind causing increased incidence.

Activities that stir up soil like agricultural- and construction-related and military training activities and natural happenings such as earthquake and windstorm create airborne arthroconidia. The likely exposed population who will inhale the arthroconidia include workers/participants of training/residents (of affected areas of earthquake and windstorm). Susceptibility to disseminated form of diseases appears to be high in certain ethnic groups, e.g. 175x in Filipinos and 10x in African Americans than non-Hispanic whites (https://en.wikipedia.org/wiki/Coccidioidomycosis). Cases outside endemic region are, generally, contracting infection in endemic region and disease manifestation outside.

Coccidioidomycosis occurs more in males than in females and is expected because of their outdoor activities. Old-age susceptibility is evidenced as over one-third deaths occur in the age group of 60–84 years. Patients with weak immune system (e.g. HIV), comorbidity like diabetes, solid organ transplant, corticosteroid or TNF inhibitor therapy, and monogenic defects along the interleukin-12-interferon-Y axis are susceptible to severe and disseminated coccidioidomycosis. A robust interferon-Y-mediated type 1 immune response, which requires cytokine interleukin-12 for initiation, helps in the resolution of infection. Type 2 immune responses may be deleterious in disseminated coccidioidomycosis, since eosinophilia and high IgE levels are associated with a worse prognosis (Tsai et al. 2020).

Elevated hormonal levels during third quarter pregnancy in women appear to stimulate growth and maturation of spherules and subsequent release of endospores leading to disseminated form of diseases.

66.3.1   Infection in Animals

Inhalation of dust laden with fungus causes infection in both man and animal, though infected animals cannot transmit it to human like domestic dogs suffering with mild to severe form of disease. Cats suffer commonly with skin form showing cutaneous lesions, fever, and loss of appetite. Cattle, sheep, horses and pigs suffer with localized infections, e.g., of mediastinal lymph gland. Coccidioidomycosis may occur in wild animals like llamas, primates, monkeys and apes, kangaroos, tigers, etc. native to the geographic area where the fungus is found.

66.4   Symptoms

Most infections (60%) show minimum to no symptom. The infection/exposure is detected by skin test, i.e. coccidioidin. Patients manifest a range of symptoms. Most of the cases recover and immune to fresh exogenous infection.

- Initial acute form or primary pulmonary form may progress to either
- Chronic coccidioidomycosis or
- Disseminated form includes primary cutaneous coccidioidomycosis.

The *initial acute form* is generally respiratory, bronchitis or pneumonia resembling influenza. Dimorphism enables the fungus transform into spore-filled spherule with potential invasion. The pathology progresses. It takes few weeks to resolve. Nearly one-fifth of cases of community-acquired pneumonia in endemic region are coccidioidomycosis. The pulmonary form may be severe in HIV cases.

The incubation ranges between 7 and 28 (average 10–16) days. Patients complain of chest pain, often pleuritic. In about three-fourth cases, it may be severe. There is anorexia, weight loss, malaise, fatigue, myalgia, arthralgia, cough, fever, sore throat, headache, and rash on the upper part of the body or legs. Some may complain loss of smell and taste. Duration of Valley fever may be few weeks to few months. Healthy individuals recover in several weeks to several months. Fatigue may be persistent, lasting for months. Some patients may have to continue taking antifungal drug for the rest of life.

Desert rheumatism is characterized by the classic triad of "fever, joint pain, and erythema nodosum".

Chronic form: Some cases (3–5%) do not recover and enter into chronic or disseminated form of coccidioidomycosis and are responsible for most of the morbidities and mortality. The residual lung lesions like nodule, fibrocavitary or cavernous, may be detected months or years later. Symptoms include productive cough, night sweating, and weight loss.

Disseminated form: Nearly 1% of infections progress to disseminated form. Disseminated coccidioidomycosis affects soft tissues, joints, skin, bones, and lining of the brain. The course of illness is prolonged and fatality is high, 40%. Skin lesions, erythema nodosum, skin ulcers, and abscesses may be seen throughout the body. Lesions in the bone and joints are very painful. Dissemination may cause inflammation of the heart and urinary tract. It takes months to years for development of meningitis and osteomyelitis. It may be metapulmonary coccidioidal granuloma (multiple lesions).

Significant mortality occurs with disseminated forms of this disease; almost 100% in case "shock'" develops.

Those with compromised/weakened immunity suffer with disseminated and severe form and complications, such as severe pneumonia, bronchopleural fistula, lung nodules, and lesions spread throughout the body. The disseminated form shatters the body system and even causes death.

66.5 Case Studies

66.5.1 Case 1

Aduroja et al. (2021) presented an unusual and infrequent case of coccidioidomycosis.

The patient was 61-year-old male, Hispanic, who spent his life in Texas as a worker in a ceramic and tile factory where he was exposed to high intensity of dust during the last 5 years. He was admitted for acute illness, was alert, then developed multiorgan failure and shock, and died on day 3.

66.5.1.1 Symptoms and Investigation

He complained suffering for 1 month with symptoms of vague abdominal pain, occasional nausea, and diarrhoea, 20-pound weight loss, generalized weakness with malaise, some arthralgia, and occasional cough that worsened and became productive of clear sputum over the last week before he was admitted for treatment of acute illness. Salient observations in life and on autopsy plus reports of investigation include the following:

Large lymph nodes (some >3 cm) in the cervical, supraclavicular, inguinal, and axillary areas.

Chest film showed a diffuse micronodular pattern (COVID-19-negative). CT scan revealed extensive diffuse bilateral micronodules in a miliary pattern and mediastinal and axillary lymphadenopathy with pericardial thickening (lymphoma and tuberculosis ruled out).

Abdomen and pelvis CT revealed enlarged lymph nodes in the para-aortic, gastrohepatic, inguinal, external, and internal iliac chains.

He was positive for HIV-1 with viral load 309,000 and CD4 count 38.

He was investigated for miliary tuberculosis, histoplasmosis, coccidioidomycosis, and cryptococcosis. Sputum culture was positive for *Candida albicans*. The patient died in hospital on day 3.

66.5.1.2   Autopsy Findings

Gross bilateral pleural lung effusions, congestion with areas of consolidation, and extensive intra-alveolar oedema; innumerable diffuse tan nodules showing miliary spread in the upper and lower lung lobes with predominance in the upper lobes in the lungs bilaterally nodules.

Extensive cervical, supraclavicular, inguinal, and axillary lymphadenopathy grossly showed a cut tan surface.

Microscopic granulomatous inflammation, alveolar spaces filled with proteinaceous material and *Coccidioides* fungal microorganisms—empty spherules or filled with endospores.

Normal lymph node architecture was replaced with caseating granulomas with *Coccidioides* fungal microorganisms.

66.5.1.3   Death Report

Diffuse coccidioidomycosis with negative AFB stain and malignancy. The cause of death was acute respiratory distress syndrome (ARDS) secondary to disseminated coccidioidomycosis and secondary to HIV/AIDS infection.

66.5.2   Case 2

A previously healthy 4-year-old boy, with no history of infection, immune deficiency, or autoimmunity (Tsai et al. 2020).

Symptoms: Fever and enlarging subcutaneous nodules on the forehead for the past 3 weeks.

Examination: Three tender mass 3–5 cm in diameter on the forehead and scalp, plaque on the posterior neck, tender right wrist, and ankle.

Lived in coccidioidomycosis endemic region of California.

Imaging: Focal consolidation in the right lung, lymphadenopathy, and multiple osteolytic lesions in his skull, vertebral bodies, ribs, right radius, and right tibia.

Biopsy: Skull lesion had fungal spherule; PCR confirmed *Coccidioides*; serology, CFT of CSF negative for *Coccidioides* IgG and IgM; blood 1:32 suggestive of disseminated coccidioidomycosis.

Coccidioidomycosis in animals: Animal infection is often detected at slaughter house after finding lesions. Granulomatous lesions are found in bronchioles and mediastinal lymph glands. Rare lesions are also seen in the lungs, maxillary and retropharyngeal lymph nodes.

Domestic dogs suffer with mild to severe form of disease like human beings and manifest similar symptoms. It manifests as fever, loss of body weight, anorexia, lethargy, depression, and chronic cough (may be dry/moist). The disseminated form can affect any organ of the body, commonly osteomyelitis (osteoarticular tissue) causing lameness.

66.6   Diagnosis

Signs and symptoms supplemented with X-ray, imaging, and laboratory confirmation together should enable detection of coccidioidomycoses.

Specimens commonly used for diagnosis are sputum, body fluids (pleural, gastric), exudates, and biopsy:

- Direct microscopic examination for fungus.
- Culture on Sabouraud agar.
- Histopathological examination demonstrates spherules, surrounding inflammation.
- Serological tests—to detect fungal antigen (in blood and urine) or host's antibody.

Intradermal test with coccidioidin—read 24–48 h later. An increase in skin thickness by 5 mm or more is considered positive. Complement fixation, tube precipitin (antibody not found in CSF), immunodiffusion, ELISA, and latex agglutination tests.

- PCR.

66.7   Treatment

Of those infected, less than 5% develop significant disease because of reduced immunity. Mild and asymptomatic infection does not require treatment. Those with severe disease can be treated with antifungal drugs, fluconazole, amphotericin B, itraconazole, and ketoconazole.

A life-threatening disseminated coccidioidomycosis was treated by supplementing antifungal agents with interferon-Y, and this slowed the progress of disease. Adding interleukin-4 and interleukin-13 blockade with dupilumab resulted in rapid resolution of the patient's clinical symptoms. It demonstrated that blocking of type 2 immune responses can treat infection. The immunomodulatory approach could enhance clearance of a refractory fungal infection (Tsai et al. 2020).

66.8   Prevention and Control

- Type-of-exposure-based respirator protection for occupational exposures, e.g. agriculture, construction, and other outdoor works in endemic areas.
- Dust control measures: Planting grass, metal roads, and sprinkling of water to settle down the dust should be adopted.

References

Aduroja O, Okudo J, Padilla A, Adnan M (2021) Disseminated Coccidioidomycosis presenting as septic shock with multiorgan failure. Case Rep Infect Dis 2021:1–6

Akram SM, Koirala J (2023) Coccidioidomycosis. In: StatPearls [internet]. StatPearls Publishing, Treasure Island, FL

Tsai MD, Timothy J, Thauland P et al (2020) Disseminated Coccidioidomycosis treated with interferon-γ and Dupilumab. N Engl J Med 382:2337–2343

Chapter 67
Cryptococcosis

Synonyms

Busse-Buschke disease, Cryptococcic meningitis, Cryptococcosis lung, Cryptococcosis skin, Torular meningitis, Torulosis.

Cryptococcosis is an invasive fungal disease that most commonly affects immuno-compromised individuals, typically causing pulmonary and central nervous system (CNS) symptoms. It has global distribution and is often transmitted through bird droppings or soil.

67.1 Aetiology

Cryptococcus neoformans is an environmental saprophyte. *C. neoformans* evolved a number of characteristics that enable it to survive within human and other mammalian and avian hosts. Human infection is accidental and dead end. *C. neoformans* is found as budding yeast in environment and in clinical specimens. The yeasts are spherical to oval cells with polysaccharide capsule.

C. neoformans is unicellular—yeast replicates by budding, makes hyphae during mating, and produces basidiospores at the end of hyphae, finally producing spores. Most of the clinical and environmental strains are mating-type alpha. Filaments of mating-type alpha undergo diploidization to form blastospores which are able to undergo meiosis, including recombination. The haploid basidiospores formed are dispersed in environment; the process is called monokaryotic fruiting.

Two varieties (now species) and five serotypes (based on capsular polysaccharide antigens) of *C. neoformans* were recognized, var. *neoformans*, now *C. neoformans* (serotypes A, D, and AD), and var. *gattii*, now *C. gattii* (serotypes B and C). The sexual state of *C. gattii* is known as *Filobasidiella bacillispora*.

The var. *neoformans is* more common in immunocompromised individuals and has been isolated from bird faeces, soil, plants, and contaminated foods. The var. *gattii* is

© Springer Nature Singapore Pte Ltd. 2024
K. G. Narayan et al., *Handbook of Management of Zoonoses*,
https://doi.org/10.1007/978-981-99-9885-2_67

more common in immunocompetent individuals and is distributed in tropical and sub-tropical regions in association with eucalyptus trees.

Genetic typing established nine molecular types of cryptococci associated with distinct amplified fragment length polymorphism (AFLP) profiles.

C. neoformans may be classified into VNI/VNII genotypes corresponding to AFLP1/1A/1B (serotype A), VNIII/AFLP3 (serotype AD), and VNIV/AFLP2 (serotype D). *C. gattii* may be distinguished as VGI/AFLP4 (serotype B), VGII/AFLP6 (serotype B), VGIII/AFLP5 (serotype B or C), and VGIV/AFLP7 (serotype B or C). VGV has recently been identified in the Central miombo woodlands of Zambia, Africa.

67.2   Epidemiology

67.2.1   Source

C. neoformans—birds' droppings (mainly pigeons), soil contaminated with birds' faecal material; decaying wood found in hollow parts of living trees. Cogliati (2013) lists a number of environmental sources, both animals and plants. The distribution of *C. gattii* is associated with *Eucalyptus* and other trees, birds' excreta, soil, and interaction of human with animals and environment. Wild felines, cats, and dogs are affected. *C. neoformans* caused systemic mycosis in cats. Cats and dogs manifest skin lesions occasionally but did not cause direct zoonosis. Asymptomatic nasal colonization by *C. gattii* in dogs and cats suggests a carrier status of these pets.

Cryptococcosis is a systemic mycosis that occurs in humans caused by either *C. neoformans* or *C. gattii* species, which has a predilection for the central nervous system and is generally believed to be acquired through the inhalation of airborne fungal propagules.

C. neoformans causes disease in predominantly immunocompromised individuals. *C. neoformans* var. *grubii* has worldwide distribution affecting AIDS patients. *C. neoformans* var. *neoformans* is more prevalent in South America and Europe.

Cryptococcus neoformans has worldwide distribution and is found in soil contaminated with bird, particularly pigeon, excreta, and decaying wood found in hollow parts of living trees.

Cryptococcus gattii is found primarily in tropical and subtropical but also temperate regions. Its distribution has been associated with several species of eucalyptus trees in Australia and spread with exported trees.

It is more aggressive species and causes infection predominantly in apparently immunocompetent man and animals. It is relatively more resistant to antifungal drugs and requires more prolonged treatment.

In a review, Mesquita da Costa et al. (2013) described epidemiology. Cryptococcosis is sporadic in occurrence with distribution worldwide. The estimated global incidence of *C. neoformans* meningoencephalitis in AIDS patients was about one million/year, and the fatality was approximately 625,000. The prevalence was high in sub-Saharan Africa with estimated mortality of 50% to 70%. The incidence of cryptococcal infection (including meningitis) reported from India was

6–8%. It was 5–11% in the USA, 33% in Africa, and 28.5% in Thailand. The mortality rate of acute cryptococcal meningoencephalitis after 3 months of treatment was 20%, and it could be 100% within 2 weeks after onset of clinical symptoms without antifungal treatment in AIDS patients.

Combined epidemiological analysis by Cogliati (2013) based on the study of a total of 68,811 *C. neoformans* and *C. gattii* isolates, reported by hundreds of global research studies, provides a detailed analysis of the geographical distribution of the major molecular types in each continent. The distribution of molecular types is summarized in Table 67.1.

67.2.2   Mode of Infection

Inhalation is the mode of infection. Basidiospores (<2 micron) in the environment are most suitable for aerial dispersal and survival in soil and directly reach alveoli of lungs to cause pneumonia and subsequently CNS upon dissemination to cause meningoencephalitis.

Table 67.1   Distribution of molecular types in (%) taken from figures (Cogliati 2013)

Molecular types	Oceania[a]	Asia[b]	Africa[c]	Europe[4]	Central and South America[d]	North America[e]
VNI	27	81	68	59.1	71	33
VNII	07	0.8	11		02	01
VNIII	01	2.6	02	18.5	0.4	05
VNIV	01	0.3		18.3	01	05
VNB			13			
VGI	39	13,2	01	3.4	04	07
VGII	22	1.7	0.25	0.3	17	0.2 + VGIIa 39
VGIII	03	0.1		0.1	03	04
VGIV		0.3	05		01	01
VGV						

The genotypes of *C. gattii* causing endemic or sporadic infections are distributed widely: *VGI* and *VGII* in Australia and Papua New Guinea, *VGIV* in South America including French Guiana and also Southeast Asia, *VGIV* and *VGV* in Southern and Central Africa, and *VGI* and *VGIII* in the United States. Recently in an outbreak setting in North America, *VGIIa* and *VGIIb* were involved (Paccoud et al. 2021)

These lineages seem to differ in geographic range, host susceptibility, and antifungal susceptibility; hence, genotyping is necessary. The infecting genotype seems to contribute to the phenotype of the infection. The clinical presentation is governed by a more complex combination of factors

[a]Oceania: Australia, New Zealand and Papua New Guinea

[b]Asia: India, China, Thailand, Malaysia, Vietnam, Taiwan, Japan, and Republic of Korea

[c]Africa: Senegal, Democratic Republic of the Congo, Uganda, Rwanda, Tanzania, Malawi, Zimbabwe, Botswana, and South Africa

[d]Central and South America: Guatemala, Honduras, Cuba, Puerto Rico, Aruba, Venezuela, Colombia, Perù, Uruguay, Brazil, Argentina, and Chile

[e]North America: Mexico, Canada

[4]Denmark, Sweden, Russia, Germany, Poland, Austria, Hungary, France, Croatia, Bulgaria, Italy, Switzerland, Greece, Spain, Portugal, Belgium, and The Netherlands

The desiccated yeasts are also small ~3 microns (growing yeasts measure 4–10 microns) and play a role in infection despite their fragility.

67.2.3   Virulence Factors

A number of properties of *C. gattii* and *C. neoformans* make these virulent enabling their survival in environment and damaging tissues and organs against the host's defence system. The virulent factors and mechanism have been elaborated by Bicanic and Harrison (2004) and Dixit et al. (2009).

Their ability to grow at 37 °C helps survival and persistence in host. Tolerance to low pH and high salt enable survival in environment.

The main virulence factors identified in *C. gattii* are outer polysaccharide capsule, melanin, mannitol, extracellular proteinase, products of the laccase pathway, superoxide dismutase, phospholipases, urease, the STE12α transcription factor that is present only in the α mating type, and the ability to switch capsular phenotype.

The capsule and associated polysaccharides are antiphagocytic, downregulate cellular and humoral response of host, and inhibit leucocyte migration into inflammatory sites. The polysaccharide capsule is composed of glucuronoxylomannan and galactoxylomannan of mannoprotein and is weak antigens and mask cellular components that could be recognized by the receptors of innate immunity and Toll-like receptors. Cryptococci survive and replicate in macrophage phagolysosome vesicles following which capsular polysaccharide accumulates in vesicles, makes permeable, and kills.

Melanin protects against UV radiation, oxygen, and nitrogen free radicals (oxidative killing by phagocytes) and may contribute to central nervous system tropism and negative cellular charge.

Mannitol protects against stress and oxygen free radicals and causes suggested increase in intracranial pressure.

Extracellular proteinase may contribute to degradation of proteins involved in tissue integrity and host immunity.

Products of laccase pathways contribute to diphenol oxidation, synthesis of melanin, and degradation of wood lignin.

Superoxide dismutase protects against oxidative stress and oxidative burst produced by immune effector cells.

Phospholipases degrade mammalian membrane lipids and lung surfactant.

Urease enhances the ability of *C. neoformans* to invade CNS.

STE12α transcription factor (in cells of α mating type): Upregulation leads to the synthesis of diphenol oxidase (which is a laccase). *Meiosis* in *C. neoformans* promotes recombinational repair in the oxidative DNA damaging environment of the host's macrophages.

Phenotyping switching: It is an adaptive mechanism. The size of capsule and the composition of polysaccharide may change in *C. gattii* and *C. neoformans*. Smooth variants are able to cross blood-brain barrier while mucoid variants are more virulent.

67.3 Pathogenesis

It is a facultative intracellular pathogen, detected in phagocytes and epithelioid cells. Primary pulmonary infection by inhalation of yeast or basidiospores is mostly asymptomatic, eliminated or contained within granuloma. The intracellular surviving cryptococci cause latent/silent infection and evade antifungal treatment and form the basis for disseminated disease. Haematogenous spread can disseminate infection to extra-pulmonary organs, mainly the CNS, to cause meningitis or meningoencephalitis.

Dissemination to extra-pulmonary sites (predilection for the brain) depends upon host factors, inoculum, and possibly virulence of the isolate, which happen either acutely or after a period of latency. Autopsy studies demonstrating cryptococcal cells within pulmonary granulomata in individuals dying of unrelated causes provided direct evidence of latency.

Human host response to primary pulmonary infection is phagocytosis of *C. neoformans* by alveolar macrophages. Oxidative and nitrosative agents are produced by macrophages to kill the cryptococci by damaging DNA. However, meiosis (sexual reproduction) may enable to it to survive by promoting DNA repair.

Haematogenous dissemination of pulmonary cryptococcosis may cause systemic infection and meningitis and meningoencephalitis in diabetics, normal, immunocompetent, and immunocompromised hosts with a fatality rate of 10–30%. The presentation of CNS infection may be varied, cryptococcomas, ischaemic stroke, spinal cord lesion, subdural effusion, isolated cranial nerve lesion, and dementia.

67.3.1 Immune Response

The protective response is active granulomatous inflammatory and depends upon cell-mediated immunity involving CD4 and CD8 cells, Th1 pattern of cytokine release. Tumour necrosis factor-α (TNF-α), interleukins 12 and 18 (IL-12, IL-18), and interferon-γ (IFN-Y) play important roles. The trio of pro-inflammatory cytokines TNF-α, IFN-Y, and IL-6 were shown to be associated with survival of patients and the rate of clearance of infection in CSF.

Deficient cell-mediated immunity and altered microglial and macrophage function led to the damage of parenchyma of the brain and yeasts tending to be located outside brain cells in meningoencephalitis in AIDS patients.

Certain evidences distinguish the two species (Tan et al. 2021). *C. neoformans* infects commonly immunocompromised individuals, and *C. gattii* infects apparently immunocompetent individuals. *C. neoformans* (worldwide distribution) is known to cause death by dissemination through the central nervous system (CNS). *C. gattii* primarily causes severe pulmonary symptoms and death without dissemination, and prevalence is restricted to tropical and subtropical regions where the lowest temperatures reached in the winter still remained above freezing, with an unusually high prevalence in Southern California. *C. neoformans* grows quickly in the brain and commonly causes meningitis or meningoencephalitis, while *C. gattii* grows faster in the lungs and customarily causes pulmonary disease and mortality up to 20–42% in transplant patients.

67.3.2   Risk Factors and Groups

Bicanic and Harrison (2004) cite an unprecedented outbreak of *C. gattii* infections that occurred since 1999 in over 50 immunocompetent patients and animals as diverse as dogs, cats, llamas, and porpoises on Vancouver Island, Canada. Cryptococcosis emerged as an important opportunistic pathogen among AIDS patient in the 1980s. The incidence before AIDS epidemic was less than one case per million persons per year in the USA, and it increased to 5–10% of AIDS patients in the USA, Europe, and Australia. There has been a consequential increase in HIV-associated community-acquired meningitis, accounting for 20–45% of laboratory-confirmed cases of meningitis in Southern Africa.

In non-HIV-infected individuals, incidence rates of 0.2–0.9% have been reported in the USA, mainly in organ transplant recipients. The infection prevalence can reach 15% when considering patients with AIDS accessing antiretroviral therapy (Mesquita da Costa et al. 2013).

Other risk groups include those with sarcoidosis and lymphoproliferative disorders and those on immunosuppressive therapy, steroid, organ transplant, chronic organ failure, malignancy, rheumatoid disease, systemic lupus erythematosus, and diabetes mellitus.

Immunosuppressive therapy results to extracellular invasion and dissemination of extra-pulmonary infection. A significant cluster of isolation of cryptococci from Africa who lived in France for >9 years compared to European patients was observed suggesting that African patients had acquired infection long before the development of clinical disease, a proof of latent/silent infection.

67.4   Disease

Conditions commonly reported are pulmonary, meningoencephalitis, septicaemia ocular, and gastrointestinal.

67.4.1   Immunocompromised

Immunocompromised cases show evidence of dissemination and flare-up of quiescent lesions in alveoli and hilar lymph node. Clinical course is rapid. In immunocompromised cases, dissemination to the CNS tends to be rapid in *C. neoformans* infection, and patients report meningeal symptoms rather than pulmonary. The acute respiratory failure associated with cryptococcal infection in AIDS patients is suggestive of dissemination shortly after acquisition of primary pulmonary infection.

67.4.2   Pneumonia

Cryptococcal pneumonia may be either asymptomatic or symptomatic, with or without evidence of dissemination. Disease may be subacute or chronic occurring as secondary infection among high-risk group. Pulmonary cryptococcosis mimics lung cancer, pulmonary tuberculosis, bacterial pneumonia, and other pulmonary mycoses, so diagnosis is difficult.

Symptoms include fever, malaise, cough with scant sputum, shortness of breath, tachypnoea, and pleurisy pain. Investigation may reveal nodular lesions, cavities, patchy infiltration-interstitial or alveolar, pleural effusion, hilar masses, and thoracic lymphadenopathy.

67.4.3   Meningoencephalitis

An estimated 223,100 cases of cryptococcal meningitis occur globally each year, leading to 181,100 deaths (Rajasingham et al. 2017). Cryptococcal meningoencephalitis is mild to subacute with varied symptoms and long course in immunocompetent. Development of symptoms takes a long time.

Symptoms: Patients present headache, pain in the neck, fever, nausea, vomiting, lethargy, sensitivity to light, coma, personality and behavioural changes, confusion, and memory loss over 2 to 4 weeks. There is a severe loss of vision in most patients with cryptococcal CNS invasion due to cranial nerve palsies and papilledema.

Complications of CNS cryptococcosis may be diffuse atrophy, hydrocephalus, and diffuse oedema. Mass lesions include hydrocephalus, motor or sensory deficits, cerebellar dysfunction, seizures, and diffuse oedema.

Unusual sites: Dissemination to other tissues is unusual but occurs. Patients of cirrhosis, liver transplant, ascites, and bleeding in the gastrointestinal tract are at risk of developing spontaneous cryptococcal peritonitis.

67.4.4   Immunocompetent

Healthy immunocompetent individuals have been affected by *C. gattii*, and *C. neoformans* infect healthy/immunocompetent individuals, but the former does it more frequently.

The major risk factors are exposure (living there or visit) in endemic areas, >50 years age, smoking, use of corticosteroids, and comorbidities like chronic lung disease, cancer.

Pulmonary cryptococcosis caused by *C. gattii* pass undetected or as a regressive lesion or misdiagnosed as malignant tumour. Cerebral mass lesions and/or hydrocephalus, pulmonary mass lesions, increased neurological deficits, and a slower response to treatment are more common in infections caused by *C. gattii* than by *C. neoformans.*

Neurologic sequelae requiring aggressive neurosurgical intervention are more common with *C. gattii* infection.

67.5   Cutaneous, Disseminated, CNS Forms

Bauer et al. (2018) reported a fatal case of cryptococcosis in immunocompetent 49-year-old woman. She complained headache for the last 3 weeks and developed discrete ataxia and impaired vision. Investigation revealed contrast-enhancing mass in the cerebellum (cranial MRI), subpleural nodule in the right inferior lung lobe, and slight leucocytosis. The mass was surgically removed from the brain. She developed non-treatable cerebral oedema and died 10 days post-surgery. Examination of surgical specimen and autopsy demonstrated fungal elements that were investigated. Cryptococcosis caused by *C. gattii* sensu lato, genotype AFLP6/VGII, recently described as *Cryptococcus deuterogattii* was confirmed. This is known to be endemic in Canada and the USA. The patient had spent her holidays in Vancouver Island, Canada, 2 years before the onset of disease.

Cases of cryptococcoses in patients with haematological malignancy are caused by both *C. neoformans* and *C. gattii.* Paccoud et al. (2021) described a case of *meningitis* caused by *C. gattii* in a patient receiving ibrutinib for relapsed chronic lymphocytic leukaemia in a hospital in Paris. This case happened to be an 88-year-old woman.

She had history of 5 days fever and headache and relapsed chronic lymphocytic leukaemia for which she was treated. She had no history of travel but reported extensive exposure to eucalyptus trees around and inside her house. Psychomotor slowing and meningeal syndrome were noted at the time of admission and accordingly investigated. The CSF was positive for *Cryptococcus* by India ink test and culture, antigen (titre of 11), and serum antibody (titre of 19). It was *C. gattii* serotype B. An India ink test on CSF was positive. *Cryptococcus* antigen (CALAS, Meridian Bioscience) was positive in the CSF (titre of 11) and in the serum (titre of 19). Fungal cultures of the CSF were positive, and the MALDI-TOF method (Bruker Biotyper) allowed the identification of the species *C. gattii,* molecular clade VGI, genotype ST197. This genotype belongs to the European-Mediterranean cluster. After 3 months of antifungal treatment, there was marked reduction in titres (4 and 3.1 in the CSF and serum, respectively).

Tan et al. (2021) described a case of meningitis—a 54-year-old male with a history of renal transplant, on chronic immunosuppressants, and with type 2 diabetes mellitus.

History includes syncope, multiple falls, worsening headaches, tinnitus, diplopia, and ongoing weight loss. He had multiple lung masses within the right upper and right lower lobes.

Diagnosis: A percutaneous biopsy of one of the lung masses in addition to a lumbar puncture (LP), both of which revealed positive *Cryptococcus* antigen confirmed to be *C. gattii*.

Amphotericin B and flucytosine therapy to treat cryptococcal meningitis was initiated.

His condition continued to worsen. Therapeutic lumbar puncture (LP) and temporary drainage was done. He was discharged when he could manage as outpatient and have serial LPs while concurrently taking fluconazole to prevent reaccumulation of cerebrospinal fluid (CSF) and recurrence of symptoms.

Cryptococcus and its capsular polysaccharide at the arachnoid granulations, inflammation, interstitial oedema, and reduced CSF outflow may cause increased intracranial pressure.

67.6 Cutaneous Cryptococcosis

Cellulitis and skin lesions are often seen on the face and neck. The lesions appear as papules, pustules, plaques, ulcers, subcutaneous masses, cellulitis, or acneiform.

Cutaneous lesions may be one of the first manifestations of cryptococcosis caused by *C. gattii* especially in immunocompetent patients living and coming from endemic areas.

Dora et al. (2006) reported a case of disseminated cryptococcosis presenting as cutaneous lesions in an immunocompetent patient. A 46-year-old male was admitted to a hospital in Brazil with a complain of fever, weight loss, and a 2-month-old nodular lesion progressing in size along 5 months in preauricular and scalp area. One month after the cutaneous lesion was noted, progressive holocranial headache was very intense. Examination revealed stiff neck; positive Kernig, Brudzinski, and Lasegue's signs; and right homonymous hemianopsia. Chest X-ray showed a nodule in the left lung, confirmed by CT scan. CT scan of the head showed a 2.0-cm left occipital ring-enhancing lesion.

Direct microscopy and culture of cerebrospinal fluid and skin biopsy were positive for *C. gattii*. Histopathology of biopsy of skin lesion showed innumerable encapsulated silver positive yeast. Serum cryptococcal antigen test was positive at a dilution 1:100.

This patient used to sleep under eucalyptus trees. This is in confirmation with the exposure of indigenous ethnic group to eucalypt reservoirs (*Eucalyptus camaldulensis* and *Eucalyptus tereticornis*) in tropical and subtropical areas and in Australia.

To sum up, it appears *Cryptococcus* initiated pulmonary infection by inhalation (lung X-ray and CT scan) and infection disseminated to skin and CNS.

Disseminated *Cryptococcus* presenting as cellulitis in a patient with decompensated cirrhosis has been reported (Clarey et al. 2020). The reported case is as follows:

A 64-year-old male with past medical history of ulcerative colitis, decompensated cirrhosis, and hypertension was admitted with a history of 3 weeks painful and warm erythematous plaques on his bilateral medial thighs, which was expanding despite treatment and diagnosed as cellulitis. Dermatologist considered the bilateral nature of the plaques and induration, the immunosuppressed status, and the upper lung ground glass opacities and went for detailed investigation. *Cryptococcus neoformans* was confirmed on the basis of biopsy (histology, yeast), serology (1:320 titre), CSF positive for yeast (staining), antigen, and culture.

Diagnosis: Disseminated cryptococcal cellulitis and meningitis.

The patient responded to treatment but developed acute kidney injury likely secondary to amphotericin administration. He died of acute respiratory failure with hypoxia in the setting of pulmonary oedema due to acute kidney injury.

Cryptococcal cellulitis is a rare diagnosis secondary to primary or disseminated infection. The risk of cryptococcemia and cryptococcal meningitis increases by 24 times in decompensated liver disease, and it accounts for 21–36% of *Cryptococcus* cases among non-HIV patients. High mortality occurs in disseminated cryptococcosis despite defined treatment algorithms. In one case series of 30 HIV-uninfected patients with disseminated disease (mean survival 21 days), it was 63% (Clarey et al. 2020).

The pulmonary cryptococcosis is reactivated by immunosuppression as indicated by cryptococcal antibodies observed in the majority of liver transplant patients prior to transplant.

67.7   Diagnosis

Diagnosis requires taking medical history; observing symptoms; conducting examination, X-ray, or CT scan; and collection of specimens for investigation. Six months post-transplant surgery, cryptococcosis can be detected in the asymptomatic recipient in the form of a pulmonary nodule containing *Cryptococcus*. A patient presenting as unexplained headaches, decreased levels of consciousness, failure to thrive, or unexplained focal dermatologic disease and a pulmonary nodule more than 6 months after transplantation should be suspected for cryptococcosis.

Specimens for laboratory investigation are biopsied tissues or body fluids, blood, serum, CSF, and sputum.

Confirmation is arrived at, on observing increased titres of cryptococcal antigen in the CSF, and positive CSF culture. High CSF pleocytosis indicate high fungal burden and severe inflammation, and high antibody titre. Histopathology - staining for polysaccharide capsule by India ink or Mucicarmine.

Diagnosis of pulmonary cryptococcosis is difficult by clinical and radiological methods. The sensitivity of culture of respiratory samples for *Cryptococcus* is poor. Cryptococcal antigen (CrAg) with lateral flow device is a fast and sensitive test, widely used on serum and cerebrospinal fluid, but sera from patients with pulmonary cryptococcosis are rarely positive in the absence of disseminated disease. Detection of CrAg from respiratory specimens by molecular detection techniques such as multiplex reverse transcription polymerase chain reaction (RT-PCR) could also provide better sensitivity but it still require validation for respiratory specimens (Setianingrum et al. 2019).

67.8   Prevention

Autopsy studies demonstrating cryptococcal cells within pulmonary granulomata in individuals dying of unrelated causes provided direct evidence of latency.

Immunosuppressive therapy results into extracellular yeasts and dissemination of extra-pulmonary infection. A significant cluster of isolation of cryptococci from Africa who lived in France for >9 years compared to European patients was observed suggesting that African patients had acquired infection long before the development of clinical disease, a proof of latent/silent infection (Bicanic and Harrison 2004).

If the risk groups such as HIV-infected are targeted for screening, activation and dissemination of silent pulmonary infection to invasion of CNS and progression to deadly meningoencephalitis could be prevented. Screening is possible with simple blood test to detect cryptococcal antigen. Cryptococcal infection can be eliminated before starting antiretroviral therapy.

[https://www.cdc.gov/fungal/diseases/cryptococcosis-neoformans/risk-prevention.html].

67.9   Treatment

Recommended therapy is antifungal medication for at least 6 months, often longer usually depending on the severity of the infection and the parts of the body that are affected:

- Fluconazole—*asymptomatic infections (*e.g. *diagnosed* via *targeted screening) or mild-to-moderate pulmonary infections.*
- Amphotericin B in combination with flucytosine followed by A fluconazole for an extended time to clear the infection—*severe lung infections or infections in the central nervous system* (brain and spinal cord).

The type, dose, and duration of antifungal treatment may differ for pregnant women, children, and people in resource-limited settings. Surgical removal fungal growths (cryptococcomas) may be required [https://www.cdc.gov/fungal/diseases/cryptococcosis-neoformans/treatment.html].

References

Bauer M, Wickenhauser C, Haak A, Pazaitis N, Siebolts U et al (2018) Case report: a fatal case of cryptococcosis in immunocompetent patient due to *Cryptococcus deuterogattii* (AFLP6/VGII). JMM Case Rep 5(10):e005168

Bicanic T, Harrison TS (2004) Cryptococcal meningitis. British Med Bull 72(1):99–118

Clarey DD, Sutton AV, Trowbridge RM (2020) *Cryptococcal cellulitis* in a patient immunocompromised secondary to cirrhosis. J Dermatol & Skin Sci 2(1):1–4

Cogliati M (2013) Global molecular epidemiology of *Cryptococcus neoformans* and *Cryptococcus gattii*: an atlas of the molecular types. Hindawi Publishing Corporation Scientica 2013:675213. 23

Dixit A, Carroll SF, Qureshi ST (2009) Review article *Cryptococcus gattii*: an emerging cause of fungal disease in North America. Inter-discip Perspect Infect Dis 2009:840452. 13

Dora JM, Kelbert S, Deutschendorf C et al (2006) Cutaneous cryptococcosis due to *Cryptococcus gattii* in immunocompetent hosts: case report and review. Mycopathologia 161(4):235–238

Mesquita da Costa M, Teixeira FM, Schalcher TR, Magalhães de Brito MTF et al (2013) Cryptococcosis, a risk for immunocompromised and immunocompetent individuals. Open Epidemiol J 6:9–17

Paccoud O, Bougnoux M-E, Desnos-Ollivier M, Varet B et al (2021) *Cryptococcus gattii* in patients with lymphoid neoplasms: an illustration of evolutive host–fungus interactions. J Fungi 7:212

Rajasingham R et al (2017) Global burden of disease of HIV- associated cryptococcal meningitis: an updated analysis. Lancet Infect Dis 17:873–881

Setianingrum F, Rautemaa-Richardson R, Denning DW (2019) Pulmonary cryptococcosis: a review of pathobiology and clinical aspects. Med Mycol 57(2):133–150

Tan S, Nasr G, Harding C (2021) Lung masses as a presenting sign of disseminated Cryptococcus. Cureus 13(5):e15185

Chapter 68
Dermatomycosis

Dermatomycosis is a superficial fungal infection with varying presentations depending upon site such as the hair, skin, and nails. The fungi require keratin for growth. Dermatophytosis is excluded. Piedra is a superficial infection of the skin, hair, and nails. Dermatophytosis is mycotic saprozoonosis, commonly known as ringworm.

Predisposing conditions: Moist and warm areas/conditions favour fungal growth, for example, folds in the skin, swimming pool relaxing chairs, lockers, tanning beds, sharing towels, brushes, clothing, and footwear.

68.1 Ringworm

Single or multiple patches of raised red rings of rash, which are itchy, appear to be about 4–14 days after exposure mostly in adults. Common sites are groin in males and the scalp and other parts in both sexes (Table 68.1). Lesions may show microvesicles and suppurative lesions or scales. Hairs are brittle. The scalp is the common site in children and groin in elderly. Bald patches appear on the scalp. Affected nails may thicken, crack, and change colour.

Ringworm is a zoonotic disease. Dogs, cats, pigs, and cattle are affected.

© Springer Nature Singapore Pte Ltd. 2024
K. G. Narayan et al., *Handbook of Management of Zoonoses*,
https://doi.org/10.1007/978-981-99-9885-2_68

Table 68.1 Sites and fungi (CDC 2021)

Species of fungus	Site	Symptoms
Tinea pedis	Feet (athletes' feet)	Itchy, red, swollen, peeling, skin between the toes; sole and heel may also be affected. Blister on the skin of feet is severe
T. onyx or T. unguium	Finger and toe nails and nail beds	
T. corporis	Arms, legs, trunk	
T. cruris	Groin (Dhobi's itch/jock itch)	Scaly, itchy, red spots, usually on the inner sides of the skin folds of the thigh
T. manuum	Hands, palm	
T. capitis	Scalp (ringworm), hair	Scaly, itchy, red, circular bald—Single /multiple spots; common in children
T. faciei	Face	
T. barbae	Scalp, hair (Barber's itch)	Scaly, itchy, red spots on the cheeks, chin, and upper neck; spots might become crusted over or filled with pus; affected hair might fall out
T. Interdigitale/ intertrigo	Skin folds	

68.2   Aetiology

It is multi-aetiological disease.

68.2.1   *Ascomycota*

Dermatophytosis caused by *Tinea barbae, T.capitis, T. corporis, T. pedis, Epidermophyton floccosum, Microspoum audouinii, M. canis, Trichophyton verrucosum, T. tonsurans, T. rubrum, T. mentagrophytes, and T. interdigitale.*

68.2.2   *Basidiomycota*

(a) *Malassezia furfur*—tinea versicolor, pityrosporum folliculitis.
   (b) *Trichosporon*—white piedra.
   These fungi generally survive for long in the shed epithelia, and thus fomites from man and animals may infect. *Microsporum* attacks the skin, hair, and rarely nails. *M. persicolor* does not invade the hair. The skin, hair, and nails are infected by *Trichophyton. Epidermophyton* very rarely invades the hair but invades the skin and nail.

The species of these fungi represent different stages of evolution; originally, the progenitor seems to be geophilic living in soil where keratinous tissues such as hooves, horn, hair, nails, and feathers (as component of fertilizer or naturally dumped) are decomposing, e.g. *Microsporum gypseum*. The zoophilic species *M. nanum* appears to have evolved to parasitize animals, particularly pigs. The anthropophilic species *M. audouinii* evolved from zoophilic fungi. The severity of infection by these in human differs. *M. audouinii* (anthropophilic) causes mild, *M. canis* (zoophilic) severe, and *M. gypseum* still severe disease in man.

Narayan (2004) has cited examples of zoonotic dermatophytosis. These are

- *T. verrucosum* and *T. mentagrophytes* affecting human are zoophilic.
- *Epidermophyton floccosum*, *M. audouinii*, *T. rubrum*, and *T. violaceum* are anthropophilic and affect lower vertebrates.
- Zoophilic dermatophytes: *M. canis* of dogs, *M. nanum* of pigs, *M. gallinae* of poultry, and *M. persicolor* of field voles and *T. mentagrophytes* var. *quinckeanum* of mouse, *T. mentagrophytes* var. *erinacei* of hedgehogs, *T. simii* of monkeys, *T. equinum* of horse, and *T. verrucosum* of cattle infect human beings.
- Geophilic dermatophytes affecting man and animals (saprozoonosis) are *M. gypseum*, *M. cookei*, *T. verrucosum*, *T. ajelloi*, and *T. terrestre*.

68.3 Source and Mode of Spread

Direct and indirect contact is the mode of infection. Sources are soil, fomites, and infected man and animals. Mere contact with sources like fomite is not enough. Microtrauma and moisture on the skin are required.

Cats, dogs, and, to a lesser extent, large animals are affected by *Microsporum canis*. *Trichophyton mentagrophytes*, *T. verrucosum*, and *T. erinacei* affect hedgehogs. A farmer may get infected with *M. gypseum* while working in field enriched with fertilizer made of hoof and horn and spread secondarily to others. He may get infection from cattle suffering with *T. mentagrophytes* var. *mentagrophytes*. Occupational exposure to laboratory workers with *T. mentagrophytes* var. *mentagrophytes* while handling infected rodents may occur. Zoophilic fungus *M. canis* originating from fomites of infected kitten caused infection in a man, and he subsequently spread the infection to others.

Aerosolization of fomites laden with arthroconidia has been reported to cause outbreak of *M. audouinii* and *T. tonsurans*.

Tinea capitis and *T. tonsurans* subclinical infections result into a carrier state. Carriers shed propagules for decades. Such carriers have been responsible for outbreaks in school hostel and hospital. The agent was isolated from air, comb, bed, and curtain in the school setting. In the hospital setting, index cases were a hospital staff and a visitor, and the agent was isolated from air, soil, linen, and chair backs. The fungus had spread so wide that it took months to eliminate.

Narayan (2004) has cited similar institutional outbreaks also in India. In one case, *T. violaceum* was found infecting 26% of 69 students. *Tinea capitis* was the cause in another school.

Tinea intertrigo causes malodourous moist erythema, weeping pruritus in skin folds. It is the most common in old, debilitated bedridden, and infants because of immobility and minimal aeration of intertriginous areas. It occurs commonly in nursing homes among patients.

Dermatophytosis caused by *Tinea pedis* and *T. interdigitale* spreads in swimming pool setting through towel, shoes, socks, and lockers. Sharing clothes, beds, toilet seats, etc. spread *T. rubrum* and *E. floccosum*. Pustular folliculitis was caused by *Tinea barbae*, *T. mentagrophytes* (contact with cattle), and *T. rubrum*. Public razor contributed to infection.

68.4 Diagnosis

Clinical presentation is diagnostic. Detection of causative fungi requires direct microscopy and culture of scales and hair specimens. A drop of 20% KOH on the specimen are covered with cover-slip and examined under microscope for fungi. Wood's lamp emits long-wave ultraviolet light and can detect fluorescence in the skin and hair. Healthy skin does not glow while blue green or dull blue glow indicates *T. capitis* infection.

68.5 Treatment

Topical application of fungicidal allylamines for short duration is useful. *Tinea capitis, T. barbae, T. manuum*, and onychomycosis may require systemic treatment.

68.6 Prevention

Care of the skin requires keeping it dry, and sharing of personal items like brush, towel, etc. must be avoided. Disinfection of the swimming pool, relaxing chairs, lockers, tanning beds, sharing towels, etc. is recommended.

References

CDC (2021) https://www.cdc.gov/fungal/diseases/ringworm/symptoms.html. Accessed 14 Jan 2021
Narayan KG (2004) Epidemiology, diagnosis and management of zoonoses. ICAR publication

Chapter 69
Histoplasmosis

Synonyms

Darling disease.

Histoplasmosis is an acute pulmonary almost always self-limiting infection caused by a dimorphic saprophyte. It may cause obstructive bronchopulmonary disease and death due to severe respiratory insufficiency. As a common secondary invader, *Histoplasma capsulatum* causes fatal infection in HIV patients and other immuno-compromised people due to disseminated form that can affect any tissue, the skin, gastrointestinal and respiratory organs, bones, joints, and the CNS.

69.1 Public Health Burden

HIV is complicated by TB and fungal infections especially histoplasmosis, cryptococcal meningitis, and *Pneumocystis jirovecii* pneumonia are a major contributor to mortality in Latin America and the Caribbean. Compared to TB, histoplasmosis causes similar or even higher incidence and deaths among people living with HIV in Latin America.

According to Nacher et al. (2020), the burden of disseminated histoplasmosis relative to HIV-TB was 43% in Latin American countries. Incidence of symptomatic disseminated histoplasmosis was more than that of tuberculosis. The Case fatality was higher than tuberculosis in 67% of countries; therapeutic immunosuppression was associated with disseminated histoplasmosis in HIV-negative cases.

69.2 Aetiology

Family Ajellomycetaceae, genus *Histoplasma*: Ajellomycetaceae are vertebrate-associated Onygenales.

© Springer Nature Singapore Pte Ltd. 2024

K. G. Narayan et al., *Handbook of Management of Zoonoses*,

https://doi.org/10.1007/978-981-99-9885-2_69

Histoplasma capsulatum is a dimorphic fungus, i.e. at body temperature (37 °C), it exists as yeast but at ambient temperatures (25 °C) as a mould (Akram and Koirala 2023). According to Mahajan (2021), Samuel T. Darling serendipitously identified a protozoan-like microorganism in an autopsy specimen in an attempt to understand malaria then prevalent during the construction of the Panama Canal. He discovered round oval bodies in a large number of mononuclear cells and in tissues of the lungs, spleen, liver, and lymph glands studded with pseudotubercles in 1905 in a 27-year-old Martinique Negro in Panama. He named it *Histoplasma capsulatum* because it invaded the cytoplasm (plasma) of histiocyte-like cells (Histo) and had a refractive halo mimicking a capsule (*capsulatum*), a misnomer. He suspected that it existed as saprophyte (Darling 1906). The infection was mistaken for tuberculosis. Infected ones were admitted to TB sanitoria, where they would have contracted TB. De Monbreum in 1934 cultivated it *in vitro* and reproduced disease in monkeys. Reverse tracing led to recovery of *H. capsulatum* from soil and 7/43 trapped rats (Emmons 1949).

There are three varieties spread globally: *H. capsulatum* var. *capsulatum, H. capsulatum* var. *duboisii,* and *H. capsulatum* var. *farciminosum.* The first two cause zoonosis. *H. farciminosum* is the cause of epizootic lymphangitis, farcy of Naples and farcy of Africa in equines.

There is a considerable genetic and phenotypic variability in isolates in a given region. *H. capsulatum* may have seven to eight distinct clades varying in virulence and also phenotypic differences. Most isolates have both alpha- and beta-glucan in their cell wall. A high infectious inoculum of the alpha-glucan yeast causes severe disease in mouse model. Most alpha-glucan strains infect immunocompetent and alpha-glucan⁺ HIV patients in North America (Horwath et al. 2015).

69.3   Epidemiology

H. capsulatum has a worldwide distribution. Low altitudes, high rainfall, moderate temperature, and river basins offer suitable conditions. The prevalence is related with soil conditions like nutrients, acidity, humidity, and temperature. The growth of fungus in nature is promoted by droppings of bats and birds. Bats are naturally infected and the fungus can be detected in the intestine and guano. Birds appear resistant, innately, or because of high body temperature (40 °C). Both play an important role in epidemiology. Droppings of domestic pigeons (*Columba livia*), chicken, Brewer's blackbird (*Euphagus cyanocephalus*), grackles (*Quiscalus quiscula*), red-winged blackbirds (*Agelaius phoeniceus*), oil birds (*Steatornis caripensis*), seagulls (*Larus delawarensis*), and starlings (*Sturnus vulgaris*) contribute to enrich soil for the production of a large number of conidia (Narayan 2004). The fungus is found around old poultry houses, in caves and areas harbouring bats, and around roosts of starling and blackbirds. Spores become airborne when soil is disturbed and inhalation precipitates infection. Human-to-human and animal-to-human infection does not occur.

Histoplasmosis is endemic in certain areas of the United States along the valleys of rivers, Ohio and Mississippi, the St. Lawrence River Valley of Canada, Central and South America, Africa, Gangetic West Bengal, Southeast Asia, India, and Australia. About 60% to 90% of people in the endemic areas in the United States have been exposed. A calculated incidence in adults aged ≥65 years is 3.4/100,000 (https://www.cdc.gov/fungal/diseases/histoplasmosis/statistics.html). Histoplasmosis is endemic in small regions along the Gangetic Plains of West Bengal and Uttar Pradesh in India. Disseminated histoplasmosis is not uncommon. The disseminated histoplasmosis in India manifests more commonly fever, weight loss, and mucocutaneous involvement than involvement of the lymph nodes, spleen, and liver. Mohapatra (1969) reported a prevalence of 0–12.3% on the basis of histoplasmin skin sensitivity testing. Kathuria et al. (2013) reviewed reported 61 immunocompetent patients with histoplasmosis between 1995 and May 2011. They were negative for risk and other predisposing factors. Their age ranged between 3 and 83 years; common were middle aged and elderly. Most were males. Thirteen had possible exposure to birds, working in moist damp areas, and mining were observed in 13 patients. Adrenal was involved in most (34/61 or 55.7%) cases. This was followed by the liver, skin, mucosa, spleen, lymph nodes, lungs, pharynx, bone marrow, larynx, gastrointestinal tract, testes, kidney, and epididymis. Adrenal insufficiency was limited to 4/34 patients.

69.4   Histoplasma

The fungus is dimorphic ascomycete. It is naturally found in soil in mitosporic saprophytic (hyphal) form at 25 °C. Survival, growth, and metamorphosis are dependent upon soil and environmental conditions. Soil with good water-holding capacity and rich in phosphorus, nitrogen, and organic matter favours growth. Bats and birds' droppings enrich soil. Large numbers of conidia of increased viability grow in soil and droppings of bats and birds. The mycelial form in nature survives drying and heat. The period of survival depends upon temperature, at 25 °C for 306 days, 34 °C for 95 days, and 37 °C for 62 days. The yeasts remain viable in frozen tissues at -40 °C for 5 months and survive alternate freezing and thawing for 198 days and 100 days in running water. *H. capsulatum* replicates by budding of unicellular yeast at 37 °C in media and hosts' tissues.

69.4.1   Virulence

Infection in human is dead end. It appears *H. capsulatum* is adapted to mammalian host. The mycelial form transforms to yeast at 37 °C. The yeast evades killing by macrophages by (a) degrading reactive oxygen species, (b) regulating lysosomal pH, and (c) capturing essential nutrients (Horwath et al. 2015). Elastase, collagenase, siderophore, and endotoxin-like substances elaborated by the fungus help invasion.

Exposures in endemic areas result into resistance to subsequent infection. Infection elicits both cellular and humoral immune responses; the protection is largely due to the latter.

Observations in mice model and human led to the understanding the importance of CD + 4 cells in histoplasmosis. In response to invasion by *H. capsulatum*, T and B cells increased. It was not so in patients with progressive disseminated form. The HIV epidemic in the 1980s and consequential increase in histoplasmosis brought to light that the progressive disseminated histoplasmosis was related with low CD+ T cells (<100/mm^3). Most HIV-histoplasmosis cases occur among HIV patient not receiving antiretroviral therapy and end up with mortality approaching 50%. Suppression of CD + 4 by medication increases the risk of histoplasmosis, particularly the disseminated form. High dosage of glucocorticoids and immunosuppressants targeting T cells is associated with cases of histoplasmosis. TNF-alpha was required for optimal control of histoplasmosis, and drugs used for blocking/suppressing it were associated with histoplasmosis (Horwath et al. 2015).

69.4.2   Mode of Infection

Inhalation of microconidia suspended in aerosolized dust is the mode of infection. Microconidia are small (<5 micron) and reach terminal bronchi and alveoli upon inhalation. The inhaled spores are transformed to intracellular yeast form. Most infections are subclinical or mild and resolve spontaneously. Successful infection depends upon strains, infectious dose, comorbidity, and the state of hosts' immunity.

69.4.3   Process of Infection

Dust generated by sweeping, destruction/demolition of buildings, digging, and excavation may be laden with *H. capsulatum*. Sites like poultry sheds, chicken coops, roosts of pigeon, blackbirds, oil birds and starlings, and caves (e.g. southern and east Africa) may harbour the fungus. Dust of poultry sheds sampled at a height of 6 inches to 2 feet from the ground has been positive for *H. capsulatum*. Association of these sites and activity with *Histoplasma* infection has often been confirmed by histoplasmin skin test.

Professional/occupational exposure leading to histoplasmosis has been observed among farmers, labours, miners, and cavers, who spent time in caves, entering a confined crawl space. Risk is associated with dirt in shelters like school after vacation, church steeples, industrial plants, attics, abandoned houses, and demolishing and bulldozing of buildings.

Weakened immune system or HIV infection is the important risk factor world over. Histoplasmosis is one of the most common opportunistic infections among people living with HIV, especially the disseminated type. According to PAHO/WHO (2020), about 5–15% HIV deaths annually in the Americas may be attributed to histoplasmosis, and the burden of the disease is concentrated in this region. Nonspecific symptoms are confounding. Histoplasmosis is indistinguishable from other diseases, tuberculosis in particular. Nearly 30% of HIV patients infected with histoplasmosis die in Latin America (https://www.cdc.gov/fungal/diseases/histoplasmosis/statistics.html). Histoplasmosis is an important health problem in areas where antiretroviral therapy is limited because ART helps keep HIV-infected people from reaching the stage where they are most vulnerable to histoplasmosis and other opportunistic infections.

69.4.3.1   Infection

Invasion of *H. capsulatum* activates adaptive immunity, particularly Th1 response. Macrophages, lymphocytes, and natural killer cells are attracted. The activated macrophages engulf these within an hour. The killer cells, hydrogen peroxide, halides, and myeloperoxidase together kill the invading yeast. The infection may be cleared without development of any symptom in most (>90%). Alternatively, infection sets in. Conidia (spores) transform into pathogenic yeast and replicate in macrophages. Macrophages spread these from lungs to all organs. Flu-like pulmonary symptoms appear. The victim may develop a chronic cavitary lung disease, and it may progress to disseminated form of histoplasmosis in immunocompetent individuals with exposure to a large infectious dose. HIV pandemic led to a dramatic increase in lethal histoplasmosis.

A. Infection in Animals

H. capsulatum infects dogs, cats, cattle, horses, sheep, and wild and captive animals such as rodents, squirrel, skunks, foxes, opossums, and others. The lungs, gastrointestines, eyes, and CNS may be involved. Signs and symptoms are non-specific. Lethargy, anorexia, fever, and body weight loss may be observed. Histoplasmosis may be the second most important fungal systemic infection of cats in the Midwest and South of the United States. Cats and dogs may suffer with primary gastrointestinal histoplasmosis showing diarrhoea with hematochezia or melena (Bromel and Sykes 2005). Cats may be more susceptible than dogs. The mode of infection is inhalation of conidia from the mycelial phase which is converted to yeast. It is phagocytosed and harboured by cells of the mononuclear phagocyte system. Three forms of infections are subclinical, clinical pulmonary granulomatous, and disseminated. The disseminated form affects predominately the liver, spleen, gastrointestinal tract, bone, bone marrow, skin, and eyes. Cutaneous form presents weeping ulcerated and nodular lesions. Protracted course in dogs is accompanied with weight loss, emaciation, persistent diarrhoea, anaemia, splenomegaly, hepatomegaly, lymphadenopathy, and ulceration in the nasopharynx and gastrointestinal tract. Acute histoplasmosis may end fatally after 2–5 weeks.

Information on the prevalence of animal histoplasmosis and its distribution in a geographic region is helpful. Infection in badger (*Meles meles*) has been used to identify endemic foci in Switzerland, Germany, and Denmark.

B. Disease in Human

Histoplasmosis may present clinically as asymptomatic infection, as acute or chronic pulmonary infection, and as disseminated infection.

The acute pulmonary form is almost always self-limited, except a massive infection that is rare and ends in death. Chronic cavitary histoplasmosis may cause death due to severe respiratory insufficiency. Progressive disseminated form has a high fatality rate, may be >90%.

B.1 Acute

Acute pulmonary histoplasmosis is a respiratory infection. Pulmonary histoplasmosis also may present as mediastinal lymphadenopathy or lung nodules. It may appear in the form of an outbreak. Immunocompromised may suffer as a result of exposure to fungus or a comeback or aggravated form of disease. Most people do not show any symptom or only mild symptoms. Those manifesting symptoms may complain of chills, fever, cough, shortness of breath, chest pain, stiff and painful muscle and joint, and small sores on lower limbs. The duration of illness may range from days to several weeks. Recovery is slow. Few cases, mostly with risk factors (HIV/immunocompromised/old age/comorbidities, etc.), may end up with complications like arthritis, arthralgia, erythema, and pericarditis.

B.2 Chronic

This is a type of accelerated obstructive bronchopulmonary disease leading to progressive pulmonary insufficiency. Infection in people with lung disease like emphysema may develop chronic histoplasmosis characterized by blood-tinged cough and loss of body weight. Often, acute pulmonary form progresses into chronic form. The symptoms are similar to tuberculosis and often misdiagnosed. Patients feel malaise, fatigue, low-grade fever, mild cough, and chest pain lasting few days and ameliorated by rest. Rest is a recommended treatment and most of early lesions heal. In others, there is a low-grade chronic illness characterized by chronic bronchitis, cough, sputum, anorexia, weight loss, and fatiguability.

B.3 Disseminated

Impaired cell-mediated immune response is associated with development of progressive disseminated histoplasmosis, and patient manifests symptoms during the acute period of dissemination.

Chronic progressive disseminated form progresses slowly and occurs mostly among older adults who are not overtly immunosuppressed. Their macrophages fail to effectively kill *H. capsulatum.* The symptoms are fever, malaise, anorexia, and weight loss. There are hepatosplenomegaly, lymphadenopathy, pallor, and petechiae and may be skin nodules, papules, ulcers, and also ulcers in mucous membrane. The progress of disseminated histoplasmosis in immunocompetent is slow.

B.3.1 Disseminated Histoplasmosis in Immunocompetent Individuals

Mansoor et al. (2013) described a case of disseminated histoplasmosis in India.

This case was immunocompetent, earlier diagnosed, and treated for tuberculosis of bone and soft tissue for 2 years. This strongly suggests the need for investigation of cases of disseminated granulomatous infection in immunocompetent individuals for histoplasmosis.

Case Study

A 48-year-old rubber tapper had multiple subcutaneous swellings over upper and lower limbs for >11 months and fever for >2 months. He was immunocompetent, non-diabetic, and not hypertensive and had no pulmonary TB, no high-risk behaviour, no history of travel, no blood transfusion, and no i/v drug abuse. He was heavy smoker long standing.

He had a history of traumatic fracture of L2 vertebrae and recovery 13 years ago. He had a second fall 2 years earlier and spinal implant which failed and removed but screw left behind; MRI showed para-spinal collection which showed granulomatous infection (sinus) on fine needle aspiration cytology and so treated for tuberculosis for 11 months without response. He complained of weakness of both lower limbs and had non-healing sinus. Swellings associated with ulcer over his right foot and left hand appeared and had fever for the last 1 month. X-ray of the foot revealed multiple periarticular lytic lesions. Biopsy and curettage from the lesions and bone marrow showed granulomatous inflammation. Later review showed the fungus.

He complained of anorexia, weight loss for 2 years. Examination showed ulcers over left and right hands and right foot; generalized lymphadenopathy, firm, non-tender, mobile, painless with no matting or overlying sinuses; and multiple subcutaneous swellings on the right leg, forearm, and elbow, cystic, painless, and mobile with local rise in temperature.

Investigation revealed a non-homogenous opacity in the left upper lobe (X-ray), multiple enlarged intra-abdominal lymph nodes (abdomen ultrasonography). Blood culture was negative.

An excision biopsy of the cervical lymph node showed necrotizing granuloma and capsulated yeast cells with narrow-based budding suggestive of *Histoplasma.* Pus from subcutaneous swellings was culture positive.

The case was diagnosed for disseminated histoplasmosis and treatment with liposomal amphotericin B, and itraconazole was planned for 12 months; when reviewed after 8 months, marked improvement was visible.

Another case of disseminated cutaneous histoplasmosis from Haryana, a non-endemic area, was reported by Kathuria et al. (2013). The two cases have a commonality—both were smokers.

A 50-year-old man probably got infected in Thailand. He was immunocompetent, non-diabetic, but chronic smoker. He suffered with multiple erythematous plaques and firm nodules and nodules on his face, neck, upper arms, and trunk. Laryngoscopy revealed multiple nodules over the tonsils and posterior pharyngeal wall. Eight months back, he had fever, significant weight loss, and generalized weakness lasting for 5 months. His fever subsided, and after a fortnight, there appeared skin lesions and sudden hoarseness, and 2 months later, there was a rapidly progressing dysphagia.

Staining and culture of biopsy of laryngeal and skin lesions confirmed histoplasmosis. He responded to antifungal therapy.

Dang et al. (2019) reported a rare case of disseminated histoplasmosis encroaching upon the oesophagus, colon, liver, spleen, and bone marrow in an immunocompetent 44-year-old Chinese man.

He reported intermittent high-grade fever (39.5 °C) with chills and rigor. Ultrasonography revealed hepatosplenomegaly, gastroscopy consecutive sheets of white bean curd-like substance attached to the oesophageal mucosa (fungal oesophagitis), and colonoscopy protuberant lesions with central depression and erosion along the mucous membrane of the colon.

Biopsy specimens of the colon identified granulomatous inflammation showing numerous yeast-laden histiocytes. The bone marrow showed oval or round organisms with amaranth nuclei and capsule-like unstained halos around in the cytoplasm of phagocytes.

H. capsulatum infection was diagnosed. The patient responded to treatment with amphotericin B.

B.3.2 Disseminated Histoplasmosis in Immunocompromised Individuals

Case Study

Disseminated CNS histoplasmosis was developed in a 54-year-old male patient of neurosarcoidosis with evidence of systemic sarcoidosis. He got this secondary infection. It progressed into a disseminated form involving the central nervous system, lungs, and bloodstream. Treatment of sarcoidosis with methotrexate and infliximab predisposed him to disseminated histoplasmosis. Neurosarcoidosis is considered to make blood-brain barrier dysfunctional, and this contributed dissemination of *Histoplasma* to the CNS (Bui 2018).

Abrahamowicz et al. (2021) report a case of disseminated histoplasmosis in a patient with multiple sclerosis (MS) treated with fingolimod, a sphingosine-1-phosphate receptor agonist. A 46-year-old man patient of MS was admitted with a history of 3 weeks of fever, night sweat, and 20-pound loss of body weight. Examination demonstrated moderate right upper quadrant abdominal tenderness. Repeated blood cultures were negative; colonoscopy showed innumerable sessile lesions, biopsied; histopathology showed lamina propria histiocytosis, severe disruption of crypts, and yeast-laden histiocytes. Liver biopsy showed multiple caseating granulomas replete with yeast-laden histiocytes. Molecular testing diagnosed *H. capsulatum*.

The patient recalled he had been renovating barn and encountered dead bats and rats. Fingolimod causes have been associated with fungal infections including primary cutaneous histoplasmosis.

The patient was treated with liposomal amphotericin B at 4 mg/ kg daily.

B.3.3 Presumed Ocular Histoplasmosis (POHS)

It is a serious condition with a potential of vision loss. *H. capsulatum* is suspected to cause it. The spread of fungus from lungs to eyes is unclear. People suffering with POHS never had symptoms of histoplasmosis. Small white spots develop deep inside eyes, detected by eye surgeons only. Choroidal neovascularization (formation of new blood vessels) can cause vision loss. Frequency of POHS is not known. The CDC quotes 13/100, 000 among people with private health insurance had POHS, and 25% of those with POHS had choroidal neovascularization. POHS is common in the histoplasmosis endemic areas around the Ohio and Mississippi river valleys. *Treatment*: Anti-vascular endothelial growth factor intraocular and laser therapy (CDC 2020).

69.5   *H. duboisii* (African Histoplasmosis)

African histoplasmosis caused by *H. capsulatum* var. *duboisii* is exclusive to Africa, spread in the continental Africa and Madagascar. Disease has been reported from Uganda, Nigeria, Democratic Republic of the Congo, and Senegal (https://en.wikipedia.org/wiki/African_histoplasmosis   African   histoplasmosis   – Wikipedia, 2021b).

It has been detected in intestinal content of hairy split-faced bat (*Nycteris hispida*) and Tadarida (*Chaetophora*) pumila. The former is a common bat in most of Africa, south of Sahara. It differs from *H. capsulatum* morphologically; yeast is large-celled. It is less virulent and causes similar disease affecting the skin, subcutaneous tissues and bones predominately, and rarely lungs. It affects immunocompetent individuals, less so in HIV cases probably due to under-reporting. It affects human and non-human primates, baboons (*Papio papio* and *P. cynocephalus*). These suffer with small papules and ulcerative granulomas without involving lungs and internal organs. Cats, dogs, and rodents are also susceptible. Infection in guinea pigs, rabbits, and pigeons is cleared spontaneously (https://en.wikipedia.org/wiki/Histoplasma_duboisii Histoplasmaduboisii – Wikipedia, 2021a).

Osteoarticular, ganglionic, and pulmonary forms of African histoplasmosis are known. The localized form presents lesions on the skin and lymph nodes and in bones. Cutaneous lesions appear as nodules, papules, or ulcers. In the disseminated form, cutaneous lesions are multiple spread all over the body: subcutaneous abscess, enlarged lymph nodes, spleen, liver, and other internal organs. Subcutaneous lesions may be seen as swelling, abscess, fistula, and ulcer.

69.6   Diagnosis

It is difficult to diagnose disseminated histoplasmosis. Medical mycology laboratory is uncommon. Fungi take long time to grow. Serology is not sensitive for immunocompromised. Molecular diagnosis requires expensive laboratory, expertise, and resources beyond reach of many. Biosafety level 3 laboratory is required.

Azar and Hage (2017) reviewed the diagnostic methods. Staining, histopathology, and antigen detection are useful. The gold standards are demonstration of yeast in pathological specimens and isolation of the fungus in culture media. Detection of antigen has the advantages of rapid, non-invasive, and sensitive test useful for treatment. Serologic test is useful for chronic disease manifestation. Sensitivity of detection of antigen is suboptimal. Molecular methods are being developed.

69.6.1   Culture and Staining

Calcofluor white is a fluorescent stain that binds chitin in the cell wall of all fungi and is useful to identify *H. capsulatum*. In appropriate culture medium grown at 25–30 °C, mycelia appear in 2–3 weeks, up to 8 weeks. Colonies on solid media can be teased with lactophenol cotton blue (tease mount) to study the morphology of the fungus. Depending upon maturity, a septate hyphae appear first, followed by smooth microconidia of 2–5 micron and finally the characteristic tuberculate macroconidia of 7–15 micron.

Grown on plates incubated at 37 °C, mycelia transform to yeasts, and microscopy shows small round, narrow-budding yeasts. Tuberculate macroconidia are highly suggestive but not specific. The rate of conversion of mycelia to yeast is low, and hence this method is not practical.

Sensitivity of culture method varies with burden of disease, clinical manifestation, and state of host's immunity: 74% in disseminated form, 42% acute pulmonary, and HIV patients 90% of respiratory specimens and 50% of blood cultures.

69.6.2   Histopathology

H. capsulatum yeast cells are ovoid in shape, measuring 2 to 4 micron with thin non-refractile cell walls.

Staining of tissue and aspirate specimens like bronchial lavage, fine-needle aspirate with Gomori methenamine silver, and periodic acid-Schiff stains are most useful to visualize *H. capsulatum* in tissues, highlighting the cell wall. Mucicarmine stain allows differentiation from *Cryptococcus*.

69.6.3   Antigen

Enzyme immunoassay of antigen commonly in urine and serum is done and is applicable to other specimens like CSF. It measures the burden of infection, disseminated, chronic, and acute pulmonary histoplasmosis, 91.8%, 87.5%, and 83%, respectively: lowest (30%) in subacute and highest (95%) in HIV patients. Monitoring antigenemia and antigenuria among HIV patients monitors the effect of treatment. Levels of <2 ng/ml have been proposed as one of the requirements for cure and discontinuation of antifungal drug.

69.6.4   Antibody

It takes 4–8 weeks for detectable levels of antibody to appear and hence is useful in subacute and chronic form including mediastinal histoplasmosis, antigen level is low, and so detection is suboptimal. Methods commonly used are immunodiffusion, complement fixation, and enzyme immunoassay.

69.7   Treatment

PAHO/WHO (2020) prepared guidelines for diagnosis and management of histoplasmosis among people living with HIV. The recommendations are conditional with low-certainty evidence. After detecting circulating *Histoplasma* antigen, a case is categorized severe or moderately severe and accordingly put on therapy.

Defining Disseminated Mild to Moderate Histoplasmosis in HIV Patients.

Severe or moderately severe—At least one sign or symptom involving vital organs is present: respiratory or circulatory failure, neurological signs, renal failure, coagulation anomalies, and a general alteration of the WHO performance status greater than 2, in which the person is confined to a bed or chair more than half of the waking hours and only capable of limited self-care. Mild to moderate histoplasmosis is defined as signs and symptoms that do not include the above features.

69.7.1 Induction Therapy

Severe or moderately severe histoplasmosis: liposomal amphotericin B, 3.0 mg/kg, for 2 weeks is recommended. The second choice, i.e. deoxycholate amphotericin B, 0.7–1.0 mg/kg, is recommended for 2 weeks. Involvement of the central nervous system may require extending induction therapy or increasing dosage.

Mild to moderate histoplasmosis: Itraconazole 200 mg three times daily for 3 days and then 200 mg twice daily is recommended (conditional recommendation, very low-certainty evidence).

Maintenance therapy: Itraconazole 200 mg twice daily for 12 months is recommended.

Shorter therapy (<12 months) can be considered when the person is clinically stable, antiretroviral therapy, and has suppressed viral load and the immune status has improved.

ART and TB therapy: Initiate antiretroviral therapy as soon as possible among disseminated histoplasmosis without involvement of the CNS (proven or suspected). Proceed for treatment of TB as per WHO guidelines for people co-infected with TB, HIV, and histoplasmosis.

69.8 Prevention

- Detection of endemic foci (screening samples of soil and animal sentinel).
- Spray of 3% formalin.
- Use of mask or covering the nose and mouth while cleaning, brooming, and dusting particularly of an abandoned poultry shed or any building frequented by pigeons, bats, etc., exploring caves, digging soil, and chopping wood.
- Risk group should keep away from such sites and activities.

References

Abrahamowicz AA, Chow EJ, Child DD, Dao A, Morrison ED et al (2021) Disseminated histoplasmosis in a patient with multiple sclerosis treated with Fingolimod. Neurol Neuroimmunol Neuroinflammation 8(3):e966

Akram SM, Koirala J (2023) Histoplasmosis. In: StatPearls [internet]. StatPearls Publishing, Treasure Island, FL

Azar MM, Hage CA (2017) Laboratory diagnostics for histoplasmosis. J Clin Microbiol 55:1612–1620

Bromel C, Sykes JE (2005) Histoplasmosis in dogs and cats. Clin Tech Small Anim Pract 20(4):227–232

Bui PV (2018) Case report disseminated histoplasmosis with Miliary Histoplasmosis, Neurohistoplasmosis, and *Histoplasma capsulatum* Bacteremia in Probable Neurosarcoidosis. Hindawi Case Rep Med 2018:3162403. https://doi.org/10.1155/2018/3162403

CDC (2020). https://www.cdc.gov/fungal/diseases/histoplasmosis/statistics.html. Accessed 22 May 2020

Dang Y, Jiang L, Zhang J et al (2019) Disseminated histoplasmosis in an immunocompetent individual diagnosed with gastrointestinal endoscopy: a case report. BMC Infect Dis 19:992. https://doi.org/10.1186/s12879-019-4542-x

Darling ST (1906) A protozoan general infection producing pseudotubercles in the lungs and focal necrosis in the liver, spleen and lymph nodes. JAMA J Am Med Assoc 4(17):1283–1285

Emmons CW (1949) Isolation of *H. Capsulatum* from soil. Public Health Rep 64:892–896

Horwath MC, Fecher RA, Deepe GS Jr (2015) *Histoplasma capsulatum*, lung infection and immunity. Future Microbiol 10(6):967–975

Kathuria S, Capoor MR, Yadav S, Singh A, Ramesh V (2013) Disseminated histoplasmosis in an apparently immunocompetent individual from North India: a case report and review. Med Mycol 51(7):774–778

Mahajan M (2021) Etymologia: Histoplasma capsulatum. Emerg Infect Dis 27(3):969

Mansoor CA, Bhargavan PV, Rajanish R, Nair LR (2013) Disseminated histoplasmosis. Indian J Orthop 47(6):639–642

Mohapatra LN (1969) Systemic mycoses in India – a critical review of the literatures. Bull AIIMS 3:7–19

Nacher M, Couppie′ P, Epelboin L, Djossou F, Demar M, Adenis A (2020) Disseminated histoplasmosis: fighting a neglected killer of patients with advanced HIV disease in Latin America. PLoS Pathog 16(5):e1008449

Narayan KG (2004) Epidemiology, diagnosis and management of zoonoses. ICAR publication

PAHO/WHO (2020). Guide lines for diagnosis and managing disseminated Histoplasmosis among people living with HIV

Wikipedia.: Histoplasma duboisii – Wikipedia. This page was last edited on 25 February 2021a, at 00:18 (UTC)

Wikipedia.: African histoplasmosis – Wikipedia. This page was last edited on 29 July 2021b, at 21:23 (UTC)

Chapter 70
Mucormycosis

Mucormycosis/black fungus disease (earlier called zygomycosis) is a rare but serious angio-invasive infection by a group of fungi, mucormycetes. It is an aggressive, life-threatening infection requiring prompt diagnosis and early treatment that includes antifungal medications and surgery. The global incidence rate varies from 0.005 to 1.7 per million population; highest is in India with $140/10^6$. The global death rate is 46%, while the case fatality rate was maximum for disseminated and 31% for cutaneous forms. Increased incidence of COVID-19-associated mucormycosis in several states in India made it a notifiable disease in May 2021. The current trend indicating the surge was higher in people with pre-existing diabetes and those on systemic corticosteroids. Aspergillosis and invasive candidiasis were other fungal infections in severe and recovering COVID-19 patients (WHO 2021; https://www.who.int/india/emergencies/coronavirus-disease-(covid-19)/mucormycosis).

70.1   Aetiology

The types of fungi that cause mucormycosis are called mucormycetes and belong to the scientific order Mucorales. The most common are species of *Rhizopus* (*Rhizopus microsporus*, *R. oryzae*, *R. rhizopodiformis*) and *Mucor* (*Mucor circinelloides*, *M. racemosus*, *M. ramosissimus*).

Others include *Rhizomucor pusillus*, *R. variabilis*, *Syncephalastrum* racemosum, *Cunninghamella bertholletiae*, *Apophysomyces elegans*, *Lichtheimia* (formerly *Absidia*), *Absidia corymbifera*, *Saksenaea vasiformis*, *Basidiobolus ranarum*, *Cokeromyces recurvatus*, *Conidiobolus incongruus*, and *Mortierella wolfii* (Pal 2020).

© Springer Nature Singapore Pte Ltd. 2024
K. G. Narayan et al., *Handbook of Management of Zoonoses*,
https://doi.org/10.1007/978-981-99-9885-2_70

70.2 Source

The causative group of fungi are ubiquitous. Their spores are found in soil, fallen leaves, compost, animal dung, and air.

70.3 Mode of Infection

Inhalation, ingestion, or traumatic inoculation and contact are common mode of infection.

Most people are exposed to fungal spores every day and probably impossible to avoid contact. These fungi are not harmful to most people except the high-risk group. The inhaled sporangiospores germinate and form hyphae in the host tissues, established infection, and then invade blood vessels. Inhaled spores of fungi infect sinuses and lungs and may spread to infect the eyes and brain.

Cutaneous and subcutaneous forms occur through contact with contaminated soil and vegetation entry of fungus through cut, burn, or other types of skin injury.

70.4 Transmission

Mucormycosis is not contagious (no person-person transmission). Zoonotic transmission is unknown. The disease is sporadic except in healthcare settings where outbreaks may occur. Transmission is linked to adhesive bandages, wooden tongue depressors, hospital linens, negative pressure rooms, water leaks, poor air filtration, non-sterile medical devices, and building construction. Mucormycosis is more common in summer and fall than in winter.

70.5 Pathogenesis

Mucormycosis infections are characterized by extensive angio-invasion. The blood vessels are thrombosed leading to ischemia and necrosis of tissues following the site of thrombosis. Ischemia likely prevents delivery of leucocytes and antifungal agents to the foci of infection. The angio-invasion continues, and the invading fungi spread haematogenously penetrating through the endothelial cells and extracellular matrix proteins lining the blood vessels.

70.6 High-Risk Group

It rarely occurs in immunocompetent and affects immunocompromised, i.e. those with comorbidities like diabetes and diabetic ketoacidosis (DKA); solid organ transplant; neutropenia; long corticosteroid therapy; hemochromatosis (iron overload); immunomodulating drugs; antifungal drug like voriconazole; skin injury due to surgery, burn, or wound; and low birth weight (neonatal gastrointestinal mucormycosis).

Ibrahim et al. (2012) explained neutropenia, DKA, and hemochromatosis (iron overload) predisposition. The mononuclear and polymorphonuclear phagocytes of normal hosts kill Mucorales by the generation of oxidative metabolites and the cationic peptides, defensins. The phagocytes in patients of diabetic ketoacidosis (DKA)—hyperglycaemia and low pH—are dysfunctional and have impaired chemotaxis and defective intracellular killing by both oxidative and nonoxidative mechanisms. Corticosteroid-immunosuppressed or animals with DKA die of progressive pulmonary and haematogenously disseminated infection. Pulmonary alveolar macrophages of immunosuppressed mice are unable even to prevent germination of the sporangiospores *in vitro* or after intranasal infection. *R. oryzae* grows poorly in normal serum and grows profusely on adding exogenous iron at acidic conditions but not at pH $\geq$ 7.4. Serum of patients with DKA have elevated levels of free iron, and such serum supports growth of *R. oryzae* at pH 7.3–6.88 (acidic) but not at 7.78–8.38 (alkaline).

70.7 Symptoms

Clinical presentation is classified according to the organ involvement. These are

- Cutaneous, subcutaneous, pulmonary, rhino-cerebral, rhino-orbital cerebral, gastrointestinal, pulmonary, and systemic or disseminated zygomycosis.
- Unusual forms are endocarditis, pyelonephritis, and osteomyelitis.

The most common forms are infections of sinuses and lungs.

Sinusitis: The patients complain severe frontal headache, nasal discharge, fever, chills, chest pain, sinusitis, and sputum with specks of blood.

Pulmonary form can spread to other organs if untreated. Symptoms include fever, cough, shortness of breath, and haemoptysis.

Gastrointestinal form causes abdominal pain, nausea, vomiting, and gastrointestinal bleeding.

Rhino-orbital-cerebral form is common in patients with diabetes mellitus. Symptoms are headache, fever, lethargy, seizures, slurred speech, one-sided facial swelling, partial paralysis, nasal/sinus congestion, black lesions on the nasal bridge or upper inside of the mouth quickly becoming more severe, bulging or displacement of eyes, and blurred vision.

Cutaneous form appears as skin lesions commonly on arms and legs resemble blisters or ulcers. There are pain, warmth, excessive redness, or swelling around a wound. Lesions appear as flat, erythematous, papular, dark yellow, nodular, pustule, and ulcerate. The lesions turn black. The lesions may also be deep abscess, large, painless, firm mass.

Disseminated form is difficult to identify because of the underlying disease; symptoms depend upon the organ affected, e.g. if the brain is affected, patients show altered mental status or coma.

70.8   Diagnosis

• Fungal staining (KOH mount) and culture of biopsy, drug sensitivity test. Treatment must not wait for test results.
• Imaging such as CT scan of the affected organ, e.g. lungs, sinus, etc.

70.9   Management/Treatment

Early detection/diagnosis and prompt administration of appropriate treatment—antifungal drug and surgical debridement (if required)—are important. Prognosis is difficult and depends upon the site and extent of infection, immunosuppression. Overall case fatality rate is nearly 50%.

Liposomal amphotericin B is the drug of choice and needs to be initiated early. Other drugs are posaconazole or isavuconazole.

70.10   Prevention

Management (WHO 2021) requires:

1. Attention/review of the underlying risk factors in the face of co-infection (e.g. COVID-19-associated mucormycosis), e.g. control of glycaemia, corticosteroids and immunomodulators, antibiotics, and antifungal drugs.
2. To prevent infection and the environmental spread of this pathogen, sterilization, disinfection of equipment, wound management, health facility management, protecting skin infection by wearing gloves while working with soil, wearing mask to protect against aerial infection in dusty areas, and avoiding contact with water-damaged buildings.

References

Ibrahim AS, Spellberg B, Walsh TJ, Kontoyiannis DP (2012) Pathogenesis of mucormycosis. Clin Infect Dis: An Official Publication of the Infectious Diseases Society of America 54(Suppl 1):S16–S22
Pal M (2020) Zygomycosis: a highly infectious emerging opportunistic fungal disease of public health concern. J Mycol Mycological Sci 3(2):000123
WHO (2021) Key facts: https://www.who.int/india/emergencies/coronavirus-disease-(covid-19)/mucormycosis

Chapter 71
Mycotoxicosis

Mycotoxicosis in animal and human can occur via inhalation, ingestion, or contact with mycotoxins largely due to contamination of feeds and foodstuffs. Mycotoxins are toxic secondary fungal metabolites of diverse nature and emerging toxic pollutants causing increased economic burden of concern for agriculture, aquaculture, and animal farming industries. Over 500 mycotoxins have been reported and new mycotoxins are often discovered. Common mycotoxins are aflatoxins, ochratoxins, fumonisins, trichothecenes, deoxynivalenol (DON), zearalenone (ZEA), patulin, sterigmatocystins (STCs), citrinin, ergotamine, etc.

Fungi grow on and in crops. Growth and mycotoxin production is favoured by too much or too little water during the growing season, temperature variations, pests, and unhygienic conditions for drying and storage (Fig. 71.1). There is a risk of accumulation of mycotoxin in fields and after harvest, including in commercial and traditional storage facilities. Higher temperatures, severe droughts, and unseasonal rain (global warming) during harvest times enhance this risk. Calamities like floods, wars, and famine favour mycotoxicosis to assume proportion of outbreaks or epidemic.

Aspergillus, *Fusarium*, *Penicillium*, and *Claviceps* genera are major fungi found on food and feed. Agriculturally important mycotoxins are aflatoxins, ochratoxin A, fumonisins, deoxynivalenol, and zearalenone.

Aflatoxin is carcinogenic. The WHO has estimated the global burden associated with exposure to aflatoxin toxicity (AFT) to be 21,757 (8,967-56,776) hepatocellular carcinoma (HCC) cases, resulting in 19,455 (7,954-51,324) deaths and 636,869 (267,142-1,617,081) DALYs (Gibb et al., 2015). Global hepatocellular carcinoma cases/year are caused by co-exposure to aflatoxins, and hepatitis B virus infection is between 5% and 28% of cases. Incidence is high in countries with poor regulations with respect to aflatoxin. High exposure of aflatoxin in children in developing countries may cause micronutrient deficiency. *Fumonisins* and *aflatoxins* or a combination of both has been linked to stunting in children in low- and middle-income

© Springer Nature Singapore Pte Ltd. 2024
K. G. Narayan et al., *Handbook of Management of Zoonoses*,
https://doi.org/10.1007/978-981-99-9885-2_71

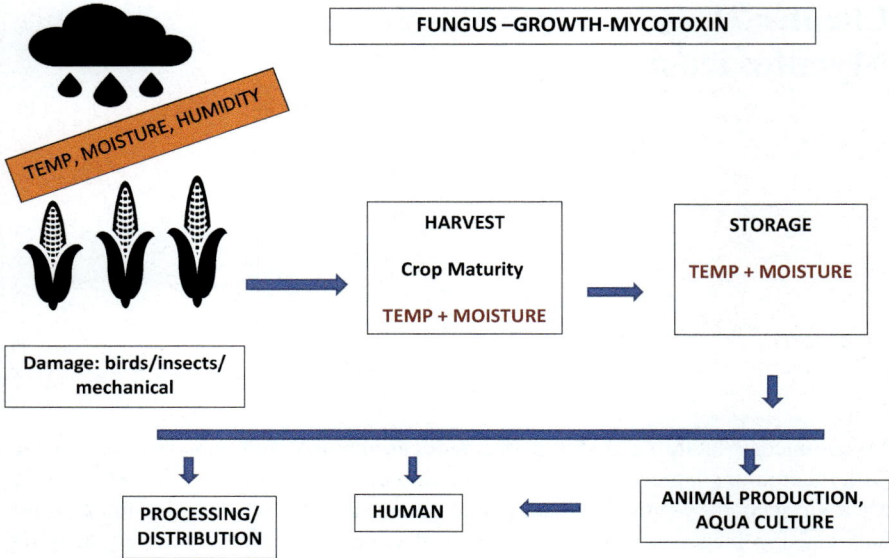

Fig. 71.1 Mycotoxin in food system

countries (Watson et al. 2018). *Other mycotoxins* affect the digestive, immune, reproductive, and excretory (kidneys) systems (Alshannaq and Yu 2017).

Modified mycotoxin: Parent mycotoxin may be modified structurally and have different physicochemical properties with varying biochemical mechanisms of action. Fungi other than the parent mycotoxin producer can bring about the modification. Modification can occur in the plant, during processing, or in human and animal's body, e.g. derivatives of mycotoxins such as *deoxynivalenol* and *zearalenone* can be deconjugated to their parent compound during digestion, thereby contributing to overall exposure to mycotoxins (Gratz et al. 2018; Vidal et al. 2018).

Occurrence and exposure with single mycotoxin or concurrently with others may occur, e.g. aflatoxins and fumonisins are common contaminants found in cereals and cereal-based foods. Interacting aflatoxin B1 and fumonisin B1 present in food posed a major concern for human's health (FAO and WHO 2016).

Combination may have synergistic, additive, or antagonistic effect.

Animal feed is often contaminated with more than one toxin, e.g. 64% of the samples, mainly from sub-Saharan Africa, Southeast Asia, and South Asia, were co-contaminated with two or more mycotoxins. Reduction in animal protein (reduced yield) and contaminated products such as milk results if mycotoxins in feed exceed the regulated or guideline concentration.

All taken together mycotoxins pose trade barrier. A harmonized control is required. Mycotoxins are not eliminated by processing and may be diluted. Several countries have established upper limit of mycotoxins in foods and regulate.

71.1 Mitigating Methods

- Good agricultural practices, a number of preharvest and postharvest measures.
- Biological and chemical processes.
- Appropriate packaging materials for storage.
- Non-toxigenic fungal strains of *Aspergillus flavus* outcompete toxigenic strains and are applied to commercial crops such as groundnuts, maize, pistachios, and cottonseed during preharvest.
- *Bacillus*, *Trichosporon*, *Sphingomonas*, *Pichia*, *Stenotrophomonas*, and lactic acid bacteria promote microbial degradation of mycotoxins—inoculate on susceptible crops preharvest or postharvest.
- Use of enzymes rather than microbes because of the lower safety concerns.
- Ease of use and higher specificity of enzymes.

71.2 Mycotoxins and Mycotoxicosis

Fungal metabolites when introduced in low concentration by a natural route in higher vertebrates and other animals evoke toxic response. These have low molecular weight (<1000 Da) and are termed mycotoxins.

Aflatoxins, ochratoxins, fumonisins, patulin, zearalenone, and trichothecenes including deoxynivalenol and T-2 toxin are commonly detected in foods and feed.

Mycotoxins may enter food chain directly from the plant-based foods (Fig. 71.1), right from the crop stage, such as maize cobs. The cobs on standing plant may be damaged by birds/insects/mechanically and get seeded by fungal spores. The infecting fungi grow under favourable weather moist and heat and produce toxin that accumulate while crop is maturing. Fungi make indirect entry on harvested crop during processing, packaging, distribution, and storage. Feverish temperature and humidity favour growth, mycotoxin production, and accumulation.

Mycotoxins are detected in maturing corn, cereals, soybeans, sorghum, peanuts, and other food and feed crops. Food crops differ in susceptibility, e.g. maize is susceptible, and rice is not. Mycotoxicosis in animals results from ingestion of mycotoxin -containing feed. Animal produce like milk, meat, and eggs are contaminated via feed. Generally, mycotoxins survive thermal processing such as pasteurization, frying, boiling, cooking, baking, and roasting, and thus a vast range of food are likely contaminated.

Toxicity can be acute or chronic. Mycotoxicosis is unavoidable and unpredictable world over causing public health problem and economic loss, even with good agricultural storage and processing. Most mycotoxins are resistant to heat and chemical and physical processing. Of the harvested crops in the world, 25% are reported as contaminated every year.

Aflatoxins pose most economic burden in the United States (US $52.1 million to $1.68 billion loss to corn industry) and European Union and hepatocellular carcinoma in Asia and Africa.

Dilution of mycotoxin to a limit considered harmless seems the only method to protect man and animals from toxicosis. This requires detection and regulatory permissible limits. The US Food and Drug Administration (FDA), World Health Organization (WHO), Food and Agriculture Organization (FAO), and European Food Safety Authority (EFSA) have developed and adopted such system, summarized in Table 71.1 by Alshannaq and Yu (2017).

Aflatoxins are regulated by established FDA action levels due to public health and economic impact; others are subject only to advisory levels.

Table 71.1 Major mycotoxins and US and EU limits on food and animal feed levels

Mycotoxin	Fungal spp.	Food commodity	US FDA (mcg/kg)	EU (E.C 2006) mcg/kg
Aflatoxins B1, B2, G1, G2	*Aspergillus flavus*, *Aspergillus parasiticus*	Maize, wheat, rice, peanut, sorghum, pistachio, almond, ground nuts, tree nuts, figs, cottonseed, spices	20 for total	2–12 for B1 4–15 for total
Aflatoxin M1	Metabolite of aflatoxin B1	Milk, milk products	0.5	0.05 in milk, 0.025 in infant formulae and infant milk
Ochratoxin A	*Aspergillus ochraceus* *Penicillium verrucosum* *Aspergillus carbonarius*	Cereals, dried vine fruit, wine, grapes, coffee, cocoa, cheese	Not set	2–10
Fumonisins B1, B2, B3	*Fusarium verticillioides* *Fusarium proliferatum*	Maize, maize products, sorghum, asparagus	2000–4000	200–1000
Zearalenone	*Fusarium graminearum* *Fusarium culmorum*	Cereals, cereal products, maize, wheat, barley	Not set	20–100
Deoxynivalenol	*Fusarium graminearum* *Fusarium culmorum*	Cereals, cereal products	1000	200–50
Patulin	*Penicillium expansum*	Apples, apple juice, and concentrate	50	10–50

Source: Alshannaq, A., and Yu, J.H. (2017)

71.2.1 Aflatoxins (AFs)

Aflatoxins are the most studied mycotoxin. AFs impact >5 billion individuals in regions of humid and warm climate, such as the tropical and subtropical areas. People in sub-Saharan Africa and southern China face regular exposure to AFs through polluted air and food beginning from intrauterine life to the entire lifespan.

Aflatoxins are a group of structurally related secondary metabolites produced by *A. flavus* and *A. parasiticus*. The fungi are naturally found in soil and organic matter. While *A. flavus* strains produce only aflatoxins B1 (AFB1) and B2 (AFB2), *A. parasiticus* strains produce AFB1, AFB2, and also G1 (AFG1) and G2 (AFG2). [In aflatoxin names, "2" shows that its structural isomer is missing a double bond in comparison with aflatoxins with a corresponding "1" (G) green or (B) blue fluorescence in ultraviolet light as well as their chromatographic mobilities.] In reducing the order of toxicity, AFs are in the order AFB1, AFB2, AFG1, and AFG2.

A number of cereals are infected and can be substrate wherein aflatoxin is produced; maize, rice, barley, oats, and sorghum. Other crops can be peanuts, ground nuts, pistachio nuts, almonds, walnuts, and cottonseeds.

Preharvest contamination can occur when plants in reproductive stage are stressed due to heat or drought. Inappropriate storage conditions, insect infestation, and excess moisture favour postharvest contamination. Stressors such as plant diseases, excess plant density, competition from weeds, plant oxidative stress, and insufficient plant nutrition augment production of AFs.

Cows eating feed contaminated with AFB1 metabolizes aflatoxin to excrete it in milk in the form of aflatoxin M1 (AFM1) within 12–24 h of consuming it. AFM1 is a hydroxylated AFB1.

Fungi of three genera, *Aspergillus*, *Fusarium*, and *Penicillium*, are commonly associated with mycotoxicosis. Growing crops of wheat, barley, and corn are generally infected with *Fusarium*. Stored foods and feeds are commonly infected with *Aspergillus* and *Penicillium*. AFs are produced primarily by *Aspergillus flavus*, *A. bombycis*, *A. pseudotamarii*, *A. nomius*, and *A. parasiticus*. *A. flavus* thrives as mycelia on plants and as sclerotia or conidia in soil. Warm climate between 16 and 35 °C is favourable, and it is uncommon beyond 45 °C. The preferred plants are oilseed crops, cotton, maize, peanut, and tree nuts. Lipids, especially triglycerides in cotton seeds, support the production of aflatoxin B1. *A. parasiticus* infects ground crops.

Aflatoxins' biosynthesis is complex and is influenced by several environmental conditions, including humidity and temperature. The range of temperature tolerated by *A. flavus* is wide, 19–35 °C: optimum for growth about 28 °C while for production of AFs 28–30 °C (up to 35 °C). Water activity (a_w) or free water in the substrate, e.g. host tissue, is an important determinant of growth and mycotoxin production. As low as a_w of 0.73 is required for growth by some strains of *A. flavus*, and optimal for AF production is a_w 0.85 (Valencia-Quintana et al. 2020). Changes in temperature and water availability related to actual climate changes (increased temperature, heavy rainfalls, and droughts) are modulating factors of mould growth and production of mycotoxins including AFs. Two or more aflatoxins may be produced by a fungus, e.g. *A. parasiticus* produces AFB1, AFB2, AFG1, and AFG2, and as a result, these aflatoxins are usually found as mixtures in foods.

Feed-Milk-Human: The AFB1 maximum residue level permitted in feeds of lactating cows is set at 5 μg AFB1/kg, 10 μg/kg, and 20 μg/kg of feeds in the EU, in China, and in the United States, respectively (Awuchi et al. 2021). AFM1 binds well with casein. It is stable to heat and carried in dairy products like cheese and may be in increased concentration. AFM1 contamination in milk is influenced by several factors, viz., seasons, farming systems' diversity, geographic location, and environmental conditions. Seasonal variation may be due to its influence on growth of fungi in feeds and storage period (circumstances necessitating storage). Human exposure to AFM1 occurs via milk. The maximum residue level of AFM1 permitted in milk has been set by the European Union and the United States at 50 ng/kg and 500 ng/kg of raw milk, respectively.

Toxicity: Aflatoxins are carcinogenic, teratogenic, hepatotoxic, mutagenic, and immunosuppressive. The International Agency for Research on Cancer has listed AFB1 as a Group 1 carcinogen, with high risks for hepatocellular carcinoma. AFM1 is listed in Group 2B (possibly carcinogenic to humans). The liver seems to be the target organ. The range of LD_{50} lies between 0.5 and 10 mg/kg body weight in different animal species.

AFs cause both acute and chronic toxicities. Chronic aflatoxicosis is a global problem. Acute toxicosis is common in developing countries and rare in developed countries.

71.2.1.1 Acute Toxicity

Acute toxicity can be fatal and has been reported in both humans and animals. Acute aflatoxicosis in human causes vomiting, abdominal pain, pulmonary and cerebral oedema, coma, convulsion, and death. Animals suffer with dysfunction of the digestive system resulting into reduced feed conversion and efficiency, low production (of eggs and milk), anaemia, and reduced reproduction.

Investigation into the cause of Turkey X disease killing 100,000 young turkeys in Great Britain in 1960 elucidated toxic groundnut meal imported from Brazil; further investigations led to the discovery of *A. flavus* and aflatoxin. An estimated exposure to between 2500 and 3500 μg of aflatoxins per kilogram in feed caused death of two-thirds of 600 feeder pigs. Draught-stressed *A. flavus*-contaminated maize had been stored in conditions that favoured the production of mycotoxins. Aflatoxin-contaminated commercial dog foods caused hepatic failure and death in dogs (Awuchi et al. 2021).

The first outbreak of human aflatoxicosis caused 100 deaths, which spread over 200 villages in western India (Krishnamachari et al. 1975). There were portal hypertension, rapidly developing ascites, and jaundice. They had consumed maize that was heavily contaminated with aflatoxin, an estimated daily intake of 2 to 6 mg of

AFB1 for up to a month. Aflatoxin B1 was detected in high concentration in the livers of those who died.

Ingestion of AF-contaminated Chinese noodles *loh see fun* caused 13 deaths among Chinese children in Perak, north western Malaysia, within hours of eating due to acute hepatic encephalopathy. The attack rate was significantly higher among those who had eaten the contaminated noodle than those who had not. Cases were scattered along the route of distribution of the contaminated noodles in six towns of two districts. Post-mortem confirmed aflatoxicosis (Lye et al. 1995).

Homegrown maize contaminated with aflatoxin caused one of the largest outbreaks in 2004 in Kenya with 317 cases and at least 125 deaths. Study revealed that 55% samples of maize products from the market had aflatoxin greater than the Kenyan regulatory level of 20 ppb; some had as high as >100 ppb and > 1000 ppb. Contaminated homegrown maize (odd ratio 2.71) entered the distribution system, resulting in widespread aflatoxin contamination of market maize (Lewis et al. 2005).

71.2.1.2 Chronic Toxicity

Chronic toxicity results into stunted growth, suppression of immunity, and hepatocellular carcinoma. Carcinogenesis may be brought about by the following mechanisms:

- The liver enzymes cytochromes P-450 3A4 and 1A2 are responsible for converting AFB1 to AFBO (bio-activated AFB1–8,9-epoxide). AFBO binds to cellular macromolecules particularly mitochondrial and nuclear nucleic acids and nucleoproteins resulting into general cytotoxicity. Protection of the liver from damage is provided by AFBO-glutathione conjugation, catalysed by glutathione S-transferase.
- AFB1 involves the p53 gene in humans for mutational effects. Nearly 50% of individuals with hepatocellular carcinoma residing in areas with a risk of exposure to aflatoxins harbour mutations in the p53 gene. Approximately 50% individuals that show hepatocellular carcinoma following exposure to aflatoxins are believed to have G–T transversions in p53 gene clusters (Awuchi et al. 2021).
- Synergistic action—AFB1 with hepatitis B virus, hepatitis C virus.

Around 25% of global cases of hepatocellular carcinoma can be associated with aflatoxin exposure, which commonly occurs in places with high hepatitis B prevalence, such as China, Southeast Asia, and sub-Saharan Africa. Lung carcinogenesis may also be due to exposure to aflatoxins (Awuchi et al. 2021).

71.2.2 Ochratoxins (OTs)

Ochratoxins (OTs) are ubiquitous and found in improperly stored food products. These are produced by *Aspergillus ochraceus*, *A. carbonarius*, *A. niger* industrial strains, *Penicillium verrucosum*, and other *Penicillium* species. It was discovered in 1965 in South Africa.

Ochratoxin A (OTA) is the most prevalent and important (B and C of less importance). *P. verrucosum* produces it generally under cool temperate conditions: 20 °C, pH 6–7, and a_w 0.86. *A. ochraceus* prefers hot tropical regions: 31 °C, pH 3–10, and a_w 0.8. Iron, zinc, and copper are required for optimal production (Awuchi et al. 2021).

Husks of grains have the most concentration of OTA, and removal of pericarp or outer layer is known to reduce almost half of OTA. Contamination of grains by ochratoxins largely depends on preharvest, periharvest, and postharvest conditions. Ochratoxins have been detected in a wide variety of agricultural commodities, corn, wheat, barley, flour, coffee, rice, oats, rye, beans, peas, and mixed feeds and also in wine, grape juice, and dried vine fruits. Ochratoxin A (OTA) get accumulated in animals and are found in produce such as meat and milk which also have been found to be contaminated with OTs. OTs can be found in human milk. Coffees and wines are a major source of human intake of OTA.

OTA is very stable in acidic environments. It can tolerate high thermal processing. It survives normal cooking and can be found in cereal products, beer, and roasted coffee.

The oral LD_{50} of OTA ranges from 3 to 20 mg/kg in different animals (Alshannaq and Yu 2017). Chronic exposure to OTA in low doses may have higher toxicity than acute exposures in high doses. Consuming 1.21 microgram every day combined with genetic predisposition and other toxins in the environment was found causing Balkan endemic nephropathy (BEN) in northwestern Bulgaria. Acute renal failure has been associated with inhalation of ochratoxin (Awuchi et al. 2021).

It is immunotoxic, teratogenic, neurotoxic, hepatotoxic, and nephrotoxic.

OTA has high affinity for protein, especially for albumin, and is fat-soluble. It explains its accumulation in organs of animals, especially pigs. It inhibits proper protein synthesis (*interferes phenylalanine hydroxylase activity in the kidney and liver*). In animals, it causes reduced feed conversion and loss of body weight and production. It circulates in blood; high level results in nephropathy. It is nephrotoxic. Acute toxicosis affects the pigs' kidneys the most.

According to Pfohl-Leszkowicz and Manderville (2007), OTA is suspected to be the main aetiology associated with chronic tubulo-interstitial disease (Balkan Endemic Nephropathy or BEN) which affects and causes high mortality in southeastern Europeans living near tributaries of the river Danube. There is a striking similarity between BEN and OTA-induced swine nephropathy. It has been associated with urothelial tumours, chronic interstitial nephropathy, and Balkan endemic nephropathy (BEN). Epidemiological associations of ochratoxin A in feeds/foods or its concentration in the blood with endemicity of BEN are reported.

Classed as group 2B carcinogen by the International Agency for Research on Cancer (IARC), OTA is genotoxic. OTA-mediated carcinogenesis may be (a) *direct, covalent DNA adduction* and (b) *indirect, oxidative DNA damage*. In human, epidemiological association with early-life OTA exposure to testicular cancer has been evidenced. Over 70 microgram/kg consumed daily may lead to renal tumour (Awuchi et al. 2021).

The upper limit of OTA is 5–50 parts per billion for several foodstuffs in EU. The permitted limits in some imported foods are 10.0 µg/kg for instant coffee, 5 µg/kg for roasted coffee, 2 µg/kg for grape juice, 2 µg/kg for wine, 3 µg/kg for processed cereal food products, and 5 µg/kg for unprocessed cereal grains.

71.2.3   Zearalenone (ZEA)

ZEA is produced by *Fusarium* species, mainly *F. graminearum* and *F. semitectum*. *Others are F. crookwellense*, *F. cerealis*, *F. equiseti*, and *F. culmorum*. Low temperature and high humidity favour fungi.

Corn, wheat, barley, sorghum and rye, maize, soybean, rice, rye, and oats (grain products) are known to be contaminated: commonly corn and wheat in the United States and Canada and wheat, rye, and oats in Europe. ZEA is stable under regular cooking temperatures. High temperature partially eliminates.

Structurally similar to oestrogen exerts estrogenic effects on human and animals causing lesions and alterations in female reproductive system, by binding with oestrogen receptors, Er alpha and Er beta. Contaminated feed may cause hyperoestrogenism, infertility, and reduced milk production. Pigs are more prone to its toxicities. Experimental lab animals, mice, guinea pigs, rats, and rabbits, have shown swelling of the vulva and uterus, ovarian atrophy, and embryo lethal resorption. Chronic administration can cause uterine fibroids, pituitary adenomas, testicular atrophy, cataracts, retinopathy, and nephropathy in rats (Awchi et al. 2021).

ZEA is classified as a Group 3 carcinogen by the IARC.

The tolerable daily intake (TDI) for zearalenone is set at 0.25 µg/kg bw/day (EFSA, Joint FAO/WHO Expert Committee on Food Additives). The European committee has regulated the maximum levels of zearalenone ranging between 20 and 100 ppb in various food commodities (EC No. 1126/2007).

71.2.4   Fumonisins

There are over 28 fumonisins grouped into 4 major groups, A, B, C, and P.

Fumonisins were isolated from cultures of *Fusarium moniliforme* (*F. verticillioides*) in 1988 in South Africa. The fungus contaminates maize in all regions, 80% of all harvested corn in the United States.

There are at least 14 other species of *Fusarium* including *F. nyagamai*, *F. oxysporum*, *F. globosum*, *F. fujikuroi*, and *F. proliferatum* which form fumonisins. *Aspergillus awamori* and *A. niger* have the biosynthetic gene cluster of fumonisins and produce fumonisin B2 (FB2) mostly.

Fumonisin B1 (FB1) is the most common (70–80%) of the family of fumonisins and frequently contaminates maize kernel.

Fumonisins are most significant in maize grown in warm and wet regions. These are produced in maize when the fungus is growing in the seed or plant, preharvest, or initial stage of drying/storage. Water activity of a_w 0.95 to 0.99 and temperature

20 °C–30 °C are optimum for production. Conditions for fumonisin production vary for different strains of fungi. *A. niger* require a_w 0.985–0.97 and temperature of 25 °C–30 °C. *Fusarium* prefers a_w exceeding 0.99 and temperature 20 °C to 25 °C.

Stability: stable at ≤150 °C; decomposition above this temperature; 90% decomposition at 175 °C after 60 min; least at pH 4, 10, and 7.

Levels of FB1 in dry milling of corn are highest in bran followed by germ fraction, used as animal feed. Fraction used for human food had the lowest.

FB1 is found in sorghum, wheat, barley, soybean, asparagus spears, figs, black tea, beer, rice, beans, medicinal plants, etc. besides corn and corn products. It is the most common contaminant of human food and also most toxic. In 2014, FB1, FB2, and FB3 were detected in 98.1% of corn product samples collected from Shandong Province, China.

Fumonisins are structurally similar to shingamine, inhibit sphingolipid synthesis to exert toxic effect, and target the liver and kidney mainly. These are hydrophilic, and so there are no carryovers into milk in cattle and accumulation in edible tissues. It is classified in Group 2B (probably carcinogenic) by the IARC. Fumonisins have been associated with pathological conditions such as cancer of the oesophagus and liver in human. High incidence of oesophageal cancer in area of Transkei, South Africa, was associated with detection of fumonisins in maize grown at a home. Maize and maize products are commonly consumed in China, Iran, the southeastern United States, northern Italy, and south-central Africa people stand at high risk of oesophageal cancer (Awchi et al. 2021).

Fumonisins are likely the cause of neural tube defect (NTD). Study by Missmer et al. (2006) observed that fumonisin exposure increases the risk of NTD, proportionate to dose, up to a threshold level, at which point foetal death may be more likely to occur. They made a case-control study because they had observed increased prevalence of NTD two times among Mexican-American women along the Texas-Mexico border during 1990–1991 coincident with epizootics attributed to exposure to fumonisin. The Mexican Americans in Texas consume large quantity of maize in the form of tortillas. The maternal exposure (eating known quantity of tortillas) during the first trimester was associated with increased odds ratios of 2.4 of having an NTD-affected pregnancy. Awchi et al. (2021) cite a study in Tanzania that demonstrated carryover of fumonisins from foods to maternal breast milk for infants' exposure; 44% of breast milk contained FB1, and 10% had >200 mcg/kg (EU limit for infants' food).

In animals, atherosclerosis in monkeys, leukoencephalomalacia in horses, pulmonary oedema and pulmonary artery hypertrophy in swine, and kidney and liver cancers in rodents are caused. It is hypothesized that pulmonary oedema in swine seemed to be the result of acute left-sided heart failure mediated by perturbation in the biosynthesis of sphingolipid.

Provisional maximum tolerable daily intake set at by WHO are 2 μg/kg body weights. The FDA recommended maximum levels are at 2–4 ppm in human foods such as corn and processed corn-based products and in animal feeds is at 5–100 ppm. The EU has put the maximum total fumonisin (fumonisins B1 and B2) limit at 1000 μg/kg for maize and maize products meant for direct consumption by humans and 800 μg/kg for snacks and breakfast cereals produced from maize.

71.2.5 Patulin (PAT)

PAT can be produced by at least 60 species of fungi; certain species of *Penicillium* [*P. expansum (P. leucopus), P. patulum (P.griseofulvum, P.urticae), P. crustosum, etc], Aspergillus (A. clavatus)*, and *Byssochlamys. P. expansum* is the most commonly PAT producing fungus.

The fungi thrives on fruits (apples, apple products, pears, peach and grapes), vegetables, cereals, legumes, seeds, nuts, etc.

Patulin is an organic compound classified as a polyketide and is mutagenic, teratogenic, carcinogenic, immunotoxic, and neurotoxic. Effects have been studied on cell cultures. It has neurotoxic and immunotoxic effects on animals. Reliable evidence of carcinogenic effect on human is wanting. Patulin causes toxicities, such as haemorrhages, ulcerations, vomiting, and nausea.

The upper limit of patulin set by the US, EU, and Chinese authorities are 50μg/L/kg in apple juices and fruit. The upper limit set by EU - 50 mcg/kg for concentrated fruit juices including cider, spirit drinks, fruit and reconstituted nectars, and other apple-derived fermented drinks or those with apple juice; 25 μg/kg maximum level for solid apple products, such as apple puree and apple compote, aimed at direct consumption by adults; and 10 μg/kg maximum level for solid apple products and apple juice, inclusive of apple puree and apple compote for young children and infants. The provisional maximum tolerable daily intake for patulin is set at 0.4 mg/kg body weight per day by the Joint FAO/WHO Expert Committee on Food Additives (Awuchi et al. 2021).

71.2.6 Trichothecenes (TCTC)

Trichothecenes (TCTC) were found to cause alimentary toxic aleukia (ATA) first reported in eastern Siberia in 1913. ATA reappeared in western Siberia in 1932. It is believed that overwintering and delayed harvesting of grains favoured the fungal infection, growth, and production of mycotoxin causing the outbreak. ATA manifested in fever; diarrhoea; abdominal pain; bleeding from the gum, mouth, and nose; necrotic angina, and agranulocytosis.

Of the three major types of mycotoxins, zearalenone, fumonisins, and trichothecenes produced by species of *Fusarium*, TCTC mycotoxins are the major group. Over 150 TCTC variants have been identified; few are of agriculture importance. These are chemically diverse compounds produced mainly by *Fusarium* species, such as *F. crookwellense, F. culmorum, F. graminearum*, and *F. poae*. Others may also produce, and these are *Acremonium (Cephalosporium), Cylindrocarpon, Dendrodochium, Myrothecium, Trichoderma, Trichothecium, Vertici monosporium, Spicellum*, and *Stachybotrys* species.

Deoxynivalenol (DON), also referred to as vomitoxin, is the most common trichothecene.

Plant-cereal disease: *F. graminearum* and *F. culmorum* infect and produce TCTC in crop plants and cause a disease of cereal grain crops, *Fusarium* head blight (FHB) which is of great economic importance world over. The cereals are mainly wheat, barley, oats, rye, maize, and rice. Others may also be infected, such as soybeans, potatoes, sunflower seeds, peanuts, and bananas. Processed cereal-derived foods that have been found infected are bread, breakfast cereals, noodles, and beer (Alshannaq and Yu 2017).

71.2.6.1 Deoxynivalenol (DON)

Deoxynivalenol (a trichothecene) is a very widely distributed *Fusarium* mycotoxin contaminating cereals in many countries like Japan, Korea, Europe, Southern Africa, and Australia. Though not most toxic, it impacts the economy seriously through contaminating corn, barley, oat, and wheat grains. *Fusarium* head blight intensity has a linear relationship with DON accumulation. Factors affecting FHB such as humidity, moisture, and temperature also affect its accumulation. The level of DON increases with increase in the number of damaged grains. With increase in the number of *Fusarium*-infested (damaged) kernel in a blend with non-infested, DON concentration increased. DON production can be controlled by maintaining storage moisture at <14% and controlling insects.

DON is heat-stable, between 170 and 350 °C; half an hour heating at 170 °C did not decrease its concentration. It is water-soluble and leaches out during cooking of contaminated noodles/pasta, but when contaminated, food is fried in oil.

Animal and Human Disease

DON is placed in carcinogenesis Group 3 by the IARC. It is highly toxic to human and animals. Human may suffer after exposure with DON-contaminated grain. DON may present in foods of animal origin like eggs, milk, the liver, and the kidney. Intoxication with DON results in fever, dizziness, headaches, diarrhoea, vomiting, nausea, and abdominal pain.

The oral LD_{50} for DON is 46–78 mg/kg. TCTC inhibits ribosomal protein synthesis followed by disruption of DNA and RNA synthesis. Experimental studies suggested that prolonged exposure in low doses impaired growth in children.

In animals, TCTC caused feed refusal, retarded growth, reduced milk production in cattle, drop in egg production, suppression of immune response, and intestinal haemorrhage. Sensitivity to DON varied with gender and age of animals; swines are most sensitive; dogs and cats are affected.

According to Awuchi et al. (2021), the advisory levels for finished wheat product (flour and bran) was 1 ppm DON that may be consumed by human and 5 ~ 10 ppm for all grains and grain by-products intended for animal consumption (US FDA).

71.3   Detection Methods and Challenges

Detection of low level of mycotoxin is required for proper regulation, consumers' health, international trade, and agriculture industry. Sensitivity of tests, i.e. detection of low level of mycotoxin, methods of extraction from complex food matrix, diverse chemical structure of mycotoxins, and occurrence of simultaneously more than one mycotoxin are problems (Alshannaq and Yu 2017).

Detection of exposure among consumers and sick and seeking epidemiological relationship are beset with a number of problems. Numerous food items usually contain mycotoxins, say aflatoxin. Estimating exact amount consumed or consumption pattern is challenging. Questionnaire and/or food diaries may be guiding but quantity consumed may not be estimated. Further, a foodstuff may be contaminated with more than one mycotoxin. The biomarkers are useful as the captured exposure of mycotoxin is reflected (Turner and Snyder 2021). Biomarkers are required for exposure assessment, bio-monitoring, and assessing the efficacy of interventions to mitigate exposure.

71.3.1   Aflatoxins

AFB1 is metabolized predominantly in the liver. Several hydroxy-metabolites, including AFM1, AFQ1, and AFP1, and two highly reactive epoxides, AFB1 exo-8, 9-epoxide and AFB1 endo-8,9-epoxide, are generated. The epoxides form covalent adducts with multiple macromolecules and proteins, e.g. with albumin AF-alb adduct, DNA AF-N7-Gua adduct, and AFB1-formamidopyrimidine adduct.

71.3.1.1   Testing of Urine and Serum

Urine: Aflatoxins AFB1, AFB2, AFG1, AFG2, and AFM1 have been observed in the urine, indicative of exposure. Study revealed a highly significant correlation between AF intake and total urinary AF. A non-specific AF enzyme-linked immunosorbent assay (ELISA) could capture multiple AF metabolites. Detailed urinary analysis revealed AFG1, AFP1, AFQ1, and AF-N7-Gua, and in refined regression analysis, AF ingestion was most strongly associated with AF-N7-Gua.

Serum: The AF-alb has a longer half-life and is a more useful biomarker. Result represents an integrated assessment of exposure over a period of 2–3 months. The concentration is 30x higher in chronically exposed than would be obtained from a single exposure. The AF-N7-Gua good marker for relatively recent exposure was predictive of a causal pathway to AF-induced hepatocellular carcinoma. It can alert and save one from developing hepatic carcinoma.

71.3.2   Fumonisins—FB1

FB1 has a sphingoid backbone and has the potential for ceramide synthase inhibition. The inhibition was demonstrated as a modulation of two physiologically important precursors in sphingolipid production, sphinganine (Sa) and sphingosine (So), leading to an increase in the ratio of Sa/So, appears to be the causal pathway for toxicity. This makes it (the ratio) a highly attractive biomarker for epidemiological purposes. It is suggested that serum sphinganine (Sa) and sphingosine (So)-phosphate adducts (Sa-Pi/So-Pi) be measured, as sphingoid bases were rapidly phosphorylated and accumulated in red blood cells. This biomarker should be used for population-based estimates for FB exposure in high-risk settings.

Summarizing, assessment of exposure can be made: for AFs, urinary AF-N7-Gua, AFM1, and serum AF-alb; for FBs, urinary FB1; for DON, urinary T-DON; and for OTA, urinary OTA. For FBs, a combination of urinary FB1 and red blood cell Sa-Pi/So-Pi is strongly informative, while serum OTA provides a qualitative measure of exposure.

Methods are thin layer chromatography (TLC); high-performance liquid chromatography (HPLC) coupled with FLD, UV, DAD, or MS detection; gas chromatography (GC) coupled with ECD, FID, or MS detection; ultraperformance liquid chromatography (UPLC); enzyme-linked immunosorbent assay (ELISA); and rapid strip screening tests.

References

Alshannaq A, Yu JH (2017) Occurrence, toxicity, and analysis of major mycotoxins in food. Int J Environ Res Public Health 14(6):632

Awuchi CG, Ondari EN, Ogbonna CU, Upadhyay AK et al (2021) Mycotoxins affecting animals, foods, humans, and plants: types, occurrence, toxicities, action mechanisms, prevention, and detoxification strategies-A revisit. Foods (Basel, Switzerland) 10(6):1279

FAO & WHO (2016) Evaluation of certain contaminants in food. Eighty-third report of the joint FAO/WHO expert committee on food additives. FAO, Rome, p 182. https://apps.who.int/iris/handle/10665/254893

Gibb H, Devleesschauwer B, Bolger P M, Wu F et al (2015) World Health Organization estimates of the global and regional disease burden of four foodborne chemical toxins, 2010: a data synthesis. F1000Res 4:1393

Gratz SW, Currie V, Richardson AJ, Duncan G et al (2018) Porcine small and large intestinal microbiota rapidly hydrolyze the masked mycotoxin deoxynivalenol-3-glucoside and release deoxynivalenol in spiked batch cultures *in vitro*. App and Environ Microbiol 84(2):e02106–e02117

Krishnamachari K, Bhat RV, Nagarajan V, Tilac T (1975) Investigations into an outbreak of hepatitis in Western India. Indian J Med Res 63:1036–1048

Lewis L, Onsongo M, Njapau H, Schurz-Rogers H, Luber G et al (2005) Aflatoxin contamination of commercial maize products during an outbreak of acute Aflatoxicosis in eastern and Central Kenya. Environ Health Perspect 113:1763–1767

Lye MS, Ghazali AA, Mohan J, Alwin N, Nair RC (1995) An outbreak of acute hepatic encephalopathy due to severe aflatoxicosis in Malaysia. Am J Trop Med Hyg 53:68–72

Missmer SA, Suarez L, Felkner M, Wang E et al (2006) Exposure to fumonisins and the occurrence of neural tube defects along the Texas-Mexico border. Environ Health Perspect 114:237–241

Pfohl-Leszkowicz A, Manderville RA (2007) Ochratoxin A: an overview on toxicity and carcinogenicity in animals and humans. Mol Nutr Food Res 51:61–69

Turner PC, Snyder JA (2021) Development and limitations of exposure biomarkers to dietary contaminants mycotoxins. Toxins 13:314

Valencia-Quintana R, Milić M, Jakšić D, Šegvić Klarić M, Tenorio-Arvide MG et al (2020) Environment changes, aflatoxins, and health issues, a review. Int J Environ Res Pub Health 17(21):7850

Vidal A, Claeys L, Mengelers M, Vanhoorne V, Vervaet C et al (2018) Humans significantly metabolize and excrete the mycotoxin deoxynivalenol and its modified form deoxynivalenol-3-glucoside within 24 hours. Sci Rep 8(1):5255

Watson S, Moore SE, Darboe MK, Chen G, Tu YK, Huang YT et al (2018) Impaired growth in rural Gambian infants exposed to aflatoxin: a prospective cohort study. BMC Pub Health 18(1):1247

Chapter 72
Rhinosporidiosis

Synonyms

Rhinosporidiosis of mucosal membranes, Conjunctival rhinosporidiosis, Water mould.

Rhinosporidiosis is characterized by friable polyps or masses and a chronic granulomatous infection of mucosa, such as the tongue, oropharynx, nasopharynx, rectum, and external genital organs. The first reported case of rhinosporidiosis was in 1900 by Guillermo Seeber from Buenos Aires, who described a highly vascular nasal polyp. In 1923, Ashworth described the established nomenclature, *Rhinosporidium seeberi*, after describing its life cycle (Wesberry et al. 2023).

72.1 Aetiology

Rhinosporidium seeberi is classified under mesomycetozoa. Mesomycetozoea is in the middle ("meso-") of the fungi ("-myceto-") and the animals ("-zoea").

Rhinosporidium seeberi is dimorphic. Saprophytic form occurred in soil and water and yeast form in infected tissues. Infection of distant sites may be through haematogenous spread. It affects a range of species of farm, domestic, and wild animals such as dogs, cats, horses, cattle, ducks, and swans (Wesberry et al. 2023) and is a zoonotic infection in human. The common sources are water and dust.

72.2 Epidemiology

Rhinosporidiosis affects orofacial region, involving in decreasing order the nasal cavity, nasopharynx, oropharynx, and nasolacrimal duct, and may disseminate to the viscera, trachea, bones, brain, and orbit. It can affect any age, commonly adult in 20 s–40 s; more males than females suffer. Recurrence is common following autoinfection.

It is endemic in some Asian region. Sporadic cases are reported from other regions because of socio-cultural phenomenon of migration (Das et al. 2011). Rhinosporidiosis has been reported from 70 countries including Africa and sometimes the United States. The highest number of cases occurred in India and Sri Lanka. Prakash and Johnny (2015) compared the physiochemical properties of water in India with that of the United States and the United Kingdom where rhinosporidiosis is infrequent. Indian water is more acidic, and the content of sodium chloride is less, possibly favourable for the fungus. Bathing in ponds contaminated by animal faeces is positively related with endemicity. Increased humidity and high temperature, as in tropical countries, aid in spore formation of the fungus. The climatic conditions in India and physiochemical properties of water in India and Sri Lanka favour fungal growth. Some ponds and water bodies in India are used both for washing cattle and for bathing by human.

Nasal mucosa coming in direct contact with infected material while bathing in ponds caused infection. Autoinoculation caused satellite infection in the skin and conjunctiva.

According to Sudarshan et al. (2007), rhinosporidiosis is endemic in Chhattisgarh. During 1994–Dec 2005, 465 cases in age group of 21–30 years occurred. The nose and nasopharynx were affected in 81% and ocular in 14%. Only seven cases presented a generalized infection. Involvements of the viscera, bone, subcutaneous layers, genitals, tracheobronchial tree, and skull have been reported. Three cases of nasopharyngeal, sino-nasopharyngeal, and nasal rhinosporidiosis from migrants in Delhi were reported (Capoor et al. 2009). One gave the history of bathing in stagnant water. Surgical excision and cauterization treated them. Ghosh et al. (2021) reported a primary disseminated rhinosporidiosis involving the skin and respiratory system in a barber from Bardhhaman, India. He had possibly a transdermal infection through abraded skin as a part of professional exposure. He never used gloves during work.

Arseculeratne et al. (2010) examined 143 cases treated in 2 major hospitals of Sri Lanka during 1995–2009. The commonest source was lacustrine water (84%), river (11%), and domestic well water (5%) in Sri Lanka. No animal cases were reported in Sri Lanka. Animal cases were reported in India. No outbreaks occurred in Sri Lanka and India.

72.3   Mode of Infection

Bathing in stagnant pool of water shared with animals is common.

72.4   Infection, Symptoms, and Pathology

The mucous membrane is penetrated by endospores. There is cylindrical cell-type papilloma. Mucosal and submucosal cysts of 10–300 microns diameter form and sporangia mature. Sporangia contain innumerable endospores and these are released in the tissues around.

Commonly, the turbinates, larynx, tracheobronchial tree, less so oesophagus, conjunctiva, and ears show more than one sessile or pedunculated polypoids. These cause nasal obstruction, rhinorrhoea, and epistaxis. On examination, pink to red polyps that look like strawberry are seen, and these easily bleed on manipulation.

Dey et al. (2016) presented a case report of a 36-year-old rice field worker with 1-year-long history of proptosis of the right eye accompanied with foul smelling nasal discharge since 2 months. He reported spells of nasal itching. Examination showed proptosis of the lower eyelid with firm round swelling near medial canthus of the right eye. Friable polypoid reddish mass in inferior turbinate was extending into opening of the nasolacrimal duct. Multiple polypoid reddish friable mass tending to bleed on touch was observed originating from the base of the skull. The extent of pathology was better appreciated by CT scanning, such as intensely enhancing extraconal mass lesion in the inferior portion of the eye, small foci of calcification, enlarged nasolacrimal duct, rarefication of bony walls, and few specs of calcification.

A 35-year- old female had a slow growing soft tissue swelling and ulceration over the thigh. Histopathological examination showed closely packed cysts with innumerable endospores (Jain et al. 2020)

Ghosh et al. (2021) described a case of dermal rhinosporidiosis. The patient had slow-growing multiple subcutaneous lumps for the last 4 months distributed over the trunk and extremities. Lumps grew in size and became painful. Examination revealed tender swelling over the anterior upper chest, waist, hip, thighs, legs, both arms, and forearms. The lesions were subcutaneous sessile/pedunculated-polypoid without local lymphadenopathy. This case appeared unique because disseminated dermal rhinosporidiosis is uncommon, had no contact with stagnant pond water, and responded a novel multidrug regimen (cycloserine-ketoconazole-liposomal amphotericin B) for 5 months.

72.5   Diagnosis

The extent of pathology was better appreciated by CT scanning, such as intensely enhancing extraconal mass lesion in the inferior portion of the eye, small foci of calcification, enlarged nasolacrimal duct, rarefication of bony walls, and few specs of calcification.

Specimen for laboratory investigation is smear or biopsy.

Simple histopathological diagnosis is affordable in resource-poor settings and is useful for early diagnosis and appropriate therapeutic intervention (Ghosh et al. 2021).

Histopathology—Haematoxylin-eosin stain of specimen tissue sections shows chronic inflammation and sporangia containing endospores. HE stained *R. seeberi.* Sporangia and spores are better appreciated by periodic acid-Schiff and Mayer's mucicarmine.

72.6   Treatment

Response to most of the antimicrobials treatment is poor. The treatment of choice is local surgical excision and cauterization of the base of the lesion and chemotherapy like Dapsone, which prevents the maturation of the sporangia and promotes fibrosis in the stroma, thereby preventing a recurrence.

References

Arseculeratne SN, Sumathipala S, Eriyagama NB (2010) Patterns of rhinosporidiosis in Sri Lanka: comparison with international data. Southeast Asian J Trop Med Pub Health 41(1):175–191

Capoor MR, Khanna G, Rajni BK, Nair D et al (2009) Rhinosporidiosis in Delhi, North India: case series from a non-endemic area and mini-review. Mycopathologia 168(2):89–94

Das S, Kashyap B, Barua M, Gupta N, Saha R et al (2011) Nasal rhinosporidiosis in humans: new interpretations and a review of the literature of this enigmatic disease. Med Mycol 49(3):311–315

Dey AK, Sharma R, Mittal K, Kumar P, Murumkar V et al (2016) Case report Rhinosporidiosis: a rare cause of proptosis and an imaging dilemma for Sinonasal masses. Case reports. Otolaryngology 2016:3573512. 5 pages

Ghosh R, Mondal S, Roy D, Ray A, Mandal A et al (2021) A case of primary disseminated rhinosporidiosis and dapsone-induced autoimmune hemolytic anemia: a therapeutic misadventure. IDCases 24:e01076

Jain K, Sarfaraj SM, Sengupta M, Datta C, Chatterjee U (2020) An unexpected host in a soft-tissue lesion of thigh. Indian J Med Microbiol 38(3&4):478–480

Prakash M, Johnny JC (2015) Rhinosporidiosis and the pond. J Pharm Bioallied Sci 7(Suppl 1):S59–S62

Sudarshan V, Goel NK, Gahine R, Krishnani C (2007) Rhinosporidiosis in Raipur, Chhattisgarh: a report of 462 cases. Indian J Pathol Microbiol 50(4):718–721

Wesberry J, Bunya VY, Dryden SC, Mukti FA, Ahmad S (2023) Rhinosporidiosis. American Academy of Ophthalmology. https://eyewiki.aao.org/Rhinosporidiosis

Chapter 73
Sporotrichosis

Synonyms

Rose handler's disease.

Sporotrichosis is caused mainly by *Sporothrix schenckii* and others. It is characterized by localized or disseminated nodular lesions that ulcerate, affecting a number of tissues.

Sporotrichosis presents lesions of heterogenous morphology like subcutaneous swelling or masses, plaques, nodules, nodulo-ulcerative, ulcerative, nodulocystic, warty, and discharging sinuses. Clinical diagnosis is confounding and difficult particularly in non-endemic areas leading to delay in specific treatment. Consequently, clinical course is protracted that impacted morbidity.

73.1 Aetiology

Sporothrix schenckii is found naturally in soil, hay, sphagnum moss, decaying wood, and plants.

Sporothrix schenckii complex are mammalian pathogens. *S. brasiliensis*, *S. schenckii* sensu stricto, *S. globosa*, and *S. luriei* cause animal and human sporotrichosis.

Orofino-Costa et al. (2017) summed up the human pathogenic *Sporothrix* spp. into two: (a) *clinical clade* that includes *S. schenckii*, *S. brasiliensis*, *S. globosa*, and *S. luriei* and (b) *environmental clade* and human pathogen that include *S. chilensis*, *S. mexicana*, *S. pallida*, and *S. stenocercas*.

Species under environmental clade are found in soil and organic matter and are less virulent to warm-blooded vertebrate hosts. These are opportunistic human pathogens. Traumatic inoculation of fungal propagules causes infection. Of the five *S. pallida* complex, three, viz., *S. chilensis*, *S. mexicana*, and *S. pallida*, are human

© Springer Nature Singapore Pte Ltd. 2024
K. G. Narayan et al., *Handbook of Management of Zoonoses*,
https://doi.org/10.1007/978-981-99-9885-2_73

pathogens. Another environmental clade includes *S. stenocercas* detected in cutaneous lesions in human. Of the species under clinical clade, *S. schenckii* and *S. globosa* are common in human, animal, and soil while *S. brasiliensis* in human and feline. *S. luriei* was detected in a single clinical case in South Africa.

The fungus is dimorphic. The saprophytic mycelial form is environmental state of the fungus that prefers atmospheric temperature, 25 °C. These pathogens are able to change to yeast form at temperatures 35°–37 °C in warm-blooded mammals.

Yeasts of Sporothrix are more virulent than longer-term culture conidia. Transmission of Sporotrichosis occurs due to asexual spores. Yeast cells possibly cause zoonotic transmission.

73.2   Epidemiology

Sporotrichosis has hyperendemic foci distributed worldwide. It is common in tropical and subtropical areas and also warm and humid areas in temperate zone favouring the saprophytic growth of the fungus. It is most frequently reported from Japan, China, Australia, India (sub-Himalayan region), Central and South America (Brazil, Colombia, Mexico, and Peru), Guatemala, and South Africa. Sporotrichosis outside tropical countries does occur among the travellers and workers. Immunosuppression due to various reasons, HIV infection, therapy, autoimmune diseases, and organ transplant has contributed to increased prevalence (Mahajan 2014).

The geographic distribution is as follows: *S. brasiliensis* in Brazil, *S. mexicana* in Mexico and *S. globosa* in the United States, the United Kingdom, Italy, Spain, India, China, and Japan.

Epidemiology of sporotrichosis has been changing; From Rosebush mycosis/ gardener's mycosis (source plant material) to zoonotic mycosis (primarily feline), as well as less frequent cases of systemic mycosis due to inhalation of infective fungal propagules caused by environmental- soil manipulation activities whether for occupational (gardeners, foresters) or leisure reasons like trekking (Orofino-Costa et al. 2017). Forest and agricultural workers handling contaminated bales of hay, sphagnum moss, plants, etc. have suffered. The setting is commonly rural. Cats and horses among domesticated and wild mammals most frequently suffer with sporotrichosis. Cats suffer with severe cutaneous form. The exudates from skin lesions are infectious and are source of zoonotic infection among handlers. This zoonotic aspect expanded the area beyond rural areas.

Some epidemics of the past have been cited by Orofino-Costa et al. (2017) wherein infected pine trees and moss seedling infected reforestation workers. Participants of a *Halloween* party in an abandoned house got infected with where contaminated hay had been stored. A large epidemic among 3000 miners in South Africa was reported, and the contaminated wood supporting beams was the source. Endemic in north-east China recorded 457 cases during 2007–2009.

According to the US CDC (2020), the suggested rate of cases per one million populations was less than one. In other parts of the world, Latin America, it was high. In the state of Rio de Janeiro, 2200 cases were reported during 1998–2009.

In the South central highlands of Peru, the suggested rate of sporotrichosis was 40–60/100,000.

Important factor is exposure and occupation the most important determinant. Age, gender, and race are not the primary determinants. More males than females and working age group (20–50 years) are victims primarily because of occupational exposure. The extremities are exposed body parts and hence most likely involved in traumatic inoculation.

Gremião et al. (2017) have discussed zoonotic sporotrichosis. In Brazil, *S. brasiliensis* causes feline sporotrichosis. The infection tends to escalate to epizootics with high zoonotic potential.

It is an emerging disease. The epizootic and zoonotic epidemics occurring in Rio de Janeiro, Brazil, required a joint veterinary and human health approach to intercept transmission chain. Surveillance for sporotrichosis in feline population in endemic areas is key to zoonotic transmission.

73.3 Mode of Infection

Infection occurs by direct contact with contaminated soil, plants, and organic matter. The fungi enter through the traumatized skin and mucosa. Traumatic implantation may occur via contaminated thorns, hay stalks, barbs, splinters, soil, etc.

Outbreaks have occurred among forest workers in the United States as they touched sphagnum moss or hay. Fungi are also transmitted between cats and cat to dog, and man gets zoonotic infection from cats. Animal source includes bites of cats, dogs, birds, rats, reptiles, horses, insects, and handling fish.

Breathing fungal spores causes lung infection. Sporotrichosis is an occupational disease occurring among farmers, agricultural workers, gardeners, veterinarians by handling cats, and cat owners.

73.4 Pathogenesis

Feline response to invasion by *Sporothrix* spp. is increased in CD4 cells associated with single lesions, inflammation, and reduction in fungal burden.

Pathogenesis is less determined. This fungal infection may cause severe disease. Co-infection with retroviruses in cats is known to cause immunosuppression and may lead to severe sporotrichosis. Stray cats are likely to be infected with parasites also, and this might increase the susceptibility. Increased virulence of *S. brasiliensis* is suspected to be a factor in the sporotrichosis outbreak in Rio de Janeiro. As compared to other species under *S. schenckii* complex, *S. brasiliensis* appears to be more invasive, causing extensive damage to hosts' tissues and display higher fungal burden (Gremião et al. 2017).

Virulence factors: Sensitivities to oxidative stress between *S. brasiliensis* and *S. schenckii* differed—the former is resistant to oxidative stress. Melanin production by *S. brasiliensis* and cell wall lipids enable it to evade phagocytosis. Fungal wall compounds (particularly 3-carboxymuconate cyclase Gp70 and Gp60) are important for adhesion to extracellular matrix. The glycoprotein Gp60 is associated with virulent isolates of *Sporothrix*, especially *S. brasiliensis.* These cause specific and protective humoral response. These compounds thus present potential antigens for serological assay and also a vaccine for feline sporotrichosis.

73.5   Disease in Cats

Feline sporotrichosis has been reported from Australia, Spain, Japan, and Germany. Sporadic cases and small outbreaks of cat-transmitted sporotrichosis occur in American and Asian continents. Sporothrix has been detected in nasal cavity and and/or nails of 2.38% of showing no signs and symptoms of disease in an endemic region of Peru. *S. schenckii* sensu stricto is the predominant aetiologic agent in Mexico. Zoonotic transmission has occurred in Malaysia and India.

Gremião et al. (2017) cite an epidemic in Rio de Janeiro, Brazil. There were 4188 cases recorded during 1997–2011. A high incidence of feline sporotrichosis was diagnosed in 2015, considered hyperendemic for cat-associated sporotrichosis. Cases of zoonotic transmission occurred in other states also. Canine sporotrichosis also occurred, but zoonotic transmission was not reported in Rio de Janeiro epidemic.

73.6   Symptoms

Incubation period may be over a week to months. It is a slowly progressing chronic disease. Patients often do not feel that they are ill. The skin, lungs, bone, and joints are affected, and dissemination could be wide. Lesions appear as nodules that later ulcerate. Immunocompromised ones suffer with complications. Depending upon the tissue affected, sporotrichosis may be grouped as dermal (cutaneous), pulmonary, or disseminated forms. Skin lesions may be grouped as lymphocutaneous, fixed cutaneous, and multiple inoculation. Mucous membrane of the eyes, nose, and others may show lesions. Systemic infection involves tissues such as osteoarticular, neurological, pulmonary, skin but may disseminated to others and even causes sepsis. Immunoreactive manifestation may include reactive arthritis, erythema nodosum, erythema multiforme, and Sweet's syndrome (Orofino-Costa et al. 2017).

Dermal—Nodules form at the point of entry and are seen along the lymphatic channels and nodes. Common sites are the finger, hand, and arms. These begin as small painless pink to purple-coloured bumps. If not cared or treated, these become larger (look like boil), increase in number, and ulcerate.

Pulmonary—A case presents in the form of productive cough. Sporotrichosis may lead to pneumonia and tuberculosis. Examination may reveal nodules, fibrosis, cavitation, and enlarged hilar lymph node.

Disseminated—Patients report loss of appetite and weight. Infection spreads from primary to secondary sites and rarely disseminates affecting bones and joints (osteoarticular) and the CNS (meningitis).

There may be spontaneous regression.

73.7 Diagnosis

Symptoms are overlapping and a differential diagnosis is required. Some of the confounding diseases are tuberculosis, leprosy, nocardiosis, leishmaniasis, and cat scratch fever. Diagnosis is difficult.

Pus/secretion is processed for mycological examination by (a) direct microscopy for yeasts (oval-, round-, cigar-shaped) and (b) culture. The growth is further processed for phenotypic and molecular identification. Direct microscopy is more sensitive compared to culture in case of animals, particularly feline infection due to high fungal concentration in tissues. Sporothrix grows well at 25–30 °C. Culture of the specimens, such as exudate from ulcers, sputum, synovial fluid, cerebrospinal fluid, and cytology, yields reliable results.

Cigar-shaped yeasts are seen in pyogranulomatous exudates and phagocytic cells.

Biopsy material collected in sterile saline in sterile container is directly processed for molecular typing. The formalin-fixed tissue is processed for histopathology. PAS or GMS staining shows asteroid bodies, yeasts in positive cases. Asteroid bodies consist of fungal cells surrounded by eosinophil material, probably immunoglobulin attached to the wall of microorganism, generally observed in infectious or granulomatous disease.

Histopathology: Diffuse chronic granulomatous dermatitis with central abscess; histological sections showing hyperkeratosis, acanthosis, and intraepidermal microabscesses; dermal granuloma present in the centre neutrophils and eosinophils surrounded by mononuclear cells in the intermediate layer and lymphocytes and plasmacytes externally.

Serology: A crude antigenic fraction has been characterized and standardized for a fast non-invasive test, proposed serological diagnosis used as supplemental test for sporotrichosis.

The antigen SsCBF (*Sporothrix schenckii* ConA-binding fraction) is a cell wall antigen from yeasts.

The glycoproteins of 60 kDa (3-carboxy-muconate cyclase gp60–gp70) is a virulence factor. Monoclonal antibody mAb P6E7 produced against gp70 passively protected *S. schenckii*-infected mice and proposed for therapeutic use.

Molecular: DNA sequencing PCR, species-specific PCR.

73.8   Treatment

Antifungal drugs, surgery, and heat therapy may be used.

Antifungal drugs are effective and applied topically for skin lesion. Long term treatment with Itraconazole, Potassium iodide, amphotericin B is required. Drug resistance strains pose problem.

Thermal treatment/heat therapy is based on the premise that growth of fungus is inhibited at high tissue temperature. A "pocket warmer" applied locally for 1–2 h for 5–6 weeks leads to cure. A temperature of 44–45 °C is maintained.

73.9   Prevention

Use dresses with long sleeves, and wear gloves while working with soil, plants with thorny/sharp-edged leaves such as rose plants and bushes, and soil-laden/contaminated plants/parts/products like sphagnum moss, hay bales, and pine seedlings.

References

CDC, USA (2020). https://www.cdc.gov/fungal/diseases/sporotrichosis/index.html
Gremião ID, Miranda LH, Reis EG, Rodrigues AM, Pereira SA (2017) Zoonotic epidemic of Sporotrichosis: cat to human transmission. PLoS Pathog 13(1):e1006077
Mahajan VK (2014) Review article sporotrichosis: an overview and therapeutic options. Dermatol Res Pract 2014:272376. 13 pages
Orofino-Costa R, Macedo PM, Rodrigues AM, Bernardes-Engemann AR (2017) Sporotrichosis: an update on epidemiology, etiopathogenesis, laboratory and clinical therapeutics. An Bras Dermatol 92(5):606–620

Part V
Parasitic Zoonoses

This section comprises of 42 chapters, viz., Epidemiology of Parasitic zoonoses 01; Epidemiology of Fishborne Trematodiasis 01; Fish-borne nematodiasis 01; Protozoal -10; Trematodes 09; Cestodes 08; Nematodes 12.

A wide spectrum of parasites has been covered delineated into anthropozoonoses, zooanthroponoses, metazoonoses, cyclozoonoses and saprozoonoses. Taxonomically, represented are protozoa, trematodes, cestodes and nematodes.

Control and prevention of soil- and water-transmitted parasites are a part of sustainable development goals. Soil-transmitted helminths common among children growing in poverty in under-developed and developing countries cause impairment of physical, intellectual and cognitive development.

Fish-borne parasites are globally important impacting economy of health of such countries where fish is an important source of protein. Food animals contribute to economy of nutrition. Parasites affecting these reduce production, affect livelihood of farmers and at the same time cause health hazard to consumers of animal protein, for example, trichinoses. Zoonotic protozoa like *Leishmania* cause serious systemic and skin disease, while *Toxoplasma* infect embryonic stages responsible for foetal death, abortion, premature birth and hydrocephalia, encephalitis, mental retardation among those born alive.

Chapter 74
Epidemiology of Parasitic Zoonoses

Infectious diseases that have spilled over from animals are designated as *zoonoses*. *Zoon* in Greek means animals and *noson* means disease. A range of epidemiological features like relationship between agent-definitive host and agent-intermediate host (s)-definitive host; simple to complex chain of transmission; effect of weather, climate, and ecology; and social and economic status of community are easily appreciable in parasitic infections and diseases.

Parasitic infections like amoebiasis may be simple involving a parasite (*Entamoeba histolytica*), a host (man), and a host's immediate environment (contaminated water). It may be complex and more complex depending upon involvement of a number of intermediate and paratenic hosts. Understanding the epidemiology of parasitic diseases offers a number of sites of interventions to control and prevent these. Epidemiological classification of parasitic zoonotic diseases is therefore important.

74.1 Prevalence of Parasitic Zoonoses

Compilation of the prevalence of zoonotic parasites in a country is rarely done. However, Heejeong Youn (2009) in a mini review compiled the parasites reported in the Republic of Korea, which are as below:

74.1.1 Protozoa

Babesia bovis, *Chilomastix mesnili*, *Cryptosporidium parvum*, *Endolimax nana*, *Entamoeba coli*, *Entamoeba histolytica*, *Giardia lamblia*, *Iodamoeba butschlii*, *Pneumocystis carinii*, *Sarcocystis cruzi*, and *Toxoplasma gondii*.

© Springer Nature Singapore Pte Ltd. 2024
K. G. Narayan et al., *Handbook of Management of Zoonoses*,
https://doi.org/10.1007/978-981-99-9885-2_74

74.1.2 Helminths

Trematodes are *Clonorchis sinensis*, *Echinostoma hortense*, *Echinostoma* spp., *Fasciola hepatica*, *Heterophyes nocens*, *Metagonimus yokogawai*, and *Paragonimus westermani*.

Cestodes are *Diphyllobothrium latum*, *Dipylidium caninum*, *Echinococcus granulosus*, *Hymenolepis nana*, *Raillietina tetragona*, sparganum (*Spirometra* spp.), *Taenia saginata*, *T. solium*, and *T. asiatica*. Nematodes are *Ancylostoma caninum*, *Brugia malayi*, *Capillaria hepatica*, *Dirofilaria immitis*, *Gnathostoma dololesi*, *Gnathostoma spinigerum*, *Loa loa*, *Onchocerca gibsoni*, *Strongyloides stercoralis*, *Thelazia callipaeda*, *Trichinella spiralis*, *Trichostrongylus orientalis*, *Trichuris trichiura*, and *Trichuris vulpis*.

The one arthropod is *Sarcoptes scabiei*.

Many of these parasites have disappeared or were in decline after the 1990s.

Since the late 1990s, the important zoonotic protozoa have been *C. parvum*, *E. nana*, *E. coli*, *E. histolytica*, *G. lamblia*, *I. buetschlii*, *P. carinii*, and *T. gondii*.

The important zoonotic helminths have been *C. sinensis*, *H. nocens*, *M. yokogawai*, *P. westermani*, *D. latum*, *T. asiatica*, *Sparaganum*, *B. malayi*, *T. orientalis*, *T. callipaeda*, and *T. spiralis*.

74.2 Classification of Parasitic Zoonoses

74.2.1 Direct Zoonoses (Orthozoonoses)

Direct zoonoses are human diseases or infections transmitted directly via contact or a mechanical vector or vehicle, and the causative agent is maintained by a single vertebrate animal species (Table 74.1). As an example, *Sarcoptes scabiei* is discussed below, and the rest are described in the following pages.

Sarcoptes scabiei var. *hominis* belongs to the genus *Sarcoptes*, a member of the family of "scab mite". It causes mange in wild and domesticated dogs and cats and also affects ungulates, wild boars, bovids, wombats, koalas, and great apes. Scabies

Table 74.1 Direct anthropozoonotic parasites

Agent	Hosts	Mode of transmission
E. histolytica	Non-human primates	Ingestion, soil, waterborne
Cryptosporidium	Mammals	—Do—
Toxoplasma	Cats	Ingestion, infected meat, contaminated soil, water
Trichinella	Pigs, bears, walrus	Ingestion of infected meat
Sarcoptes scabiei	Wild and domesticated dogs and cats; wild animals affected are boars, ungulates, bovids, koala, great apes	Direct contact

is common in pigs. Elimination of infestation from farm is difficult. Transmission occurs by skin contact with carriers. Hands and wrists are common sites. In 25 min to an hour after contact, the mite burrows into the skin.

S. scabiei has four stages in its life cycle, egg, larva, nymph, and adult.

The infesting female burrows (1) into the outermost layer (stratum corneum) and deposits two to three eggs per day. In 3–4 days, larva hatches out. The six-legged larvae migrate to the surface of the skin to burrow (2) hair follicles, into moulting pouches. Eight-legged nymph appears after 3–4 days. There is another moulting and nymphs enlarge in size and then appear adult mites. Males take 9–11 days to mature and females 17 days because they require more moults. Life cycle takes 2 weeks. Adult male mite penetrates moulting pouch of female. There is only one mating. The impregnated female then searches for a suitable location for creating an S-shaped permanent burrow (3). She continues lengthening the burrow while laying eggs for 1–2 months of her lifespan. 1, 2, and 3 are the sites of damages in the skin caused by the mite.

Only about two dozens of mites infest, but itching is agonizing, and scratches as a response may allow bacterial infection causing impetigo or eczema. Mites, their eggs, or packets of faeces cause delayed type IV hypersensitivity approximately 30 days after infestation.

Examples of such parasites are tabulated (Table 74.1):

74.2.2   Zooanthroponoses

Zooanthroponoses: Causative agents adapted to human beings can infect animals. Examples are listed in Table 74.2.

74.2.3   Metazoonoses or Pherozoonoses

Metazoonotic parasites require both vertebrates and invertebrates for completion of their infectious cycle. Characteristic features include development, propagation, and cyclopropagation of infectious agents in the invertebrates before transmission to vertebrates. The period required for this and spent by infectious agents in the

Table 74.2 Zooanthroponoses—example

Agent	Host	Mode of infection
Diphyllobothrium latum	Canines, felines, bears, pinnipeds, mustelids	Ingestion of plerocercoid-containing fish
Trichuris trichiura (human whipworm)	Non-human primates	Ingestion of embryonated eggs on plant or soil
Clonorchis sinensis (human/Chinese liver fluke)	Dogs, cats, swine, rats, wild animals	Ingestion of raw, partially cooked infected fresh water fish

invertebrate is called extrinsic incubation period. Many parasites pass through intermediate host(s) during development from eggs to infective stage. Depending upon
combination of invertebrate and vertebrates involved, metazoonoses have been subclassed as 1 to 4. Parasites that need a combination of one each of vertebrate and
invertebrate fall under subclass 1 (*B. divergens* and *P. shwetzi* in Table 74.3).
Paragonimus westermani requires one vertebrate and two invertebrates to complete
its life cycle and is classed as subclass 2. A combination of two vertebrates and one
vertebrate requiring *Clonorchis sinensis* is under subclass 3. *Babesia bovis* is transovarially transmitted by vector tick and so it is subclassed as 4.

    Such a classification of parasites illustrates the sites where intervention can be
applied to control the infection.

74.2.4   Cyclozoonoses

Cyclozoonoses require more than one vertebrate species, but no invertebrate host, in
order to complete the developmental cycle of the agent, e.g. taeniases and cestodia-
ses. *T. saginata* is a tapeworm affecting human. The intermediate stage, *Cysticercus
bovis*, develops only in cattle (hence, it is called beef tapeworm (Fig. 74.1)), and
therefore, it is obligatory cyclozoonoses (Table 74.4).

74.2.5   Saprozoonoses

Saprozoonoses have both a vertebrate host and an inanimate reservoir. The non-
animal site serves as a true reservoir or an essential phase of development. The non-
animal/inanimate object reservoir may be organic matter including food, plants, or
soil (called developmental reservoir; Fig. 74.2). Some saprozoonoses are listed in
Table 74.5. Most soil-transmitted zoonoses are saprozoonoses.

74.3   Modes of Infection

Parasites infect human through direct and indirect contact (direct zoonoses).
Ingestion of parasites carried in the flesh of fish and food animals is the most common way of human infection, e.g. *Paragonimus westermani*, *Clonorchis sinensis*,
Trichinella spiralis, and *Taenia saginata*. Soil gets seeded with eggs of some parasites voided in faeces of pet and domestic animals. These undergo development to
infective stage.

Table 74.3 Metazoonotic parasites

Agent	Host	Insect vector/ intermediate host	Mode of transmission	Remarks	Class of metazoonoses
Babesia bovis	Cattle domestic cow, African buff, water buff	Ixodid ticks—*Rhipicephalus* (*Boophilus*) *microplus*	Tick bite Commonly larvae feed upon cattle/human to infect	Adult feed on infected cattle, get infected; mother ticks transmit to eggs; protozoa can remain in ticks for 4 years without infecting vertebrates	Transovarian –class IV
Babesia divergens	Cattle (in Europe)	*Ixodes ricinus*	Tick bite	Infect immunocompromised human causing medical emergencies; there is rapid fulmination, parasitaemia>70%	Class I
Plasmodium schwetzi	Gorilla and chimpanzee	*Anopheles balabacensis*	From gorillas and chimpanzee, mosquito transmits to man through bite; prepatent periods of 24 and 104 days. The infection was passed successfully to nine of ten additional volunteers by the intravenous inoculation of parasitized human blood. The two volunteers in whom patent parasitaemia did not develop were Negroes. Patent infections persisted for up to 145 days with a maximum count of 2750 parasites per cmm of blood. Maximum temperature observed in any of the volunteers was 105.6 °F. The characteristics of the infections were compared with those observed in other simian malaria infections in man. The fact that *P. schwetzi* can be successfully transmitted to man by mosquito bite establishes its potentiality as a zoonosis for Africa (Contacos et al. 1970)		Class I
Clonorchis sinensis	Carnivores and human	Fresh water fish (host 2) Snails (host 1)	Eating fish with metacercaria	Adult in biliary duct; eggs in faeces; snails pick up embryonated eggs that develop to free swimming cercaria that enter fish	Class III

(continued)

Table 74.3 (continued)

Agent	Host	Insect vector/ intermediate host	Mode of transmission	Remarks	Class of metazoonoses
Fasciola hepatica	Sheep, cattle	Snails	Eating metacercaria containing salads, vegetables	Metacercaria on water plants (like paddy stalks) eaten by sheep, cattle; adult in the biliary duct of sheep/cattle/man—Eggs in faeces; miracidia penetrate snails and develop into cercaria that reach water plants to encyst as metacercaria	Class I
Paragonimus westermani; more than ten species infect humans	Pigs, dogs, and variety of felines	Snails	Ingestion of crab, crayfish	Adults in the lungs, eggs in the sputum and also in faeces – embryonate and penetrate snails—Cercaria released taken by crustaceans where metacercaria form	Class II
Dipylidium caninum	Dogs, cats	Dog or cat flea (*Ctenocephalides* spp.)	Ingestion of infected flea	Gravid segments in peri-anal region or faeces of dogs/cats/ human, egg packets released and eaten by larvae of the flea, develop into cysticercoid; larva also develop into adult flea; dogs, cats, and humans accidentally ingest and get infected; parasite develops in the intestine	Class III

Diphyllobothrium latum, less commonly *D. pacificum*, *D. cordatum, D. ursi, D. dendriticum, D. lanceolatum, D. dalliae*, and *D. yonagoensis*	Small fresh water fish (plerocercoid -infective) Eaten by predator fish	Crustaceans, e.g. copepod (procercoid)	Ingestion of infected predator fish (trout, perch, wall-eyed pike)	Adult in the human intestine, pass unembryonated eggs in faeces, embryonated; coracidia swim taken by copepod; procercoid develop; copepod eaten by fresh water small fish, infective stage; plerocercoid develops; small fish eaten by predator large fish — Class III
There are 15 spp. of this roundworm— *Onchocerca* *Onchocerca gibsoni* (forms nodule under skin in cattle)				
Onchocerca volvulus		*Simulium* or black flies breed in fast-flowing (high oxygen) river	Bite of infected flies	Flies get infected by biting a human host; worm larvae spread to its saliva glands. When it bites a human, these pass into the skin. Here, they develop into adults and form nodules under the skin. These adults then breed, producing thousands of larvae which spread throughout the whole body—Including the eye — Class I

(continued)

Table 74.3 (continued)

Agent	Host	Insect vector/intermediate host	Mode of transmission	Remarks	Class of metazoonoses
Sparganum mansoni; genus *Spirometra*	Dogs, cats, and wild carnivores (e.g. raccoons) are definitive hosts and remain infected for 9 years; man is accidental host	Copepods and crustaceans are first intermediate hosts. Birds, reptiles, and amphibians are second intermediate hosts.	(1) drinking water that is contaminated with copepods housing *Spirometra* larvae. (2) consumption of the raw flesh of one of the second infected intermediate hosts, such as frogs or snakes, e.g. for medicinal purposes in some Asian cultures or pigs (3) by placing raw poultices of the infected second intermediate hosts on open wounds, lesions, and/or the eyes for medicinal or ritualistic reasons. (4) contact with infected flesh of an intermediate host Most often occurs following ingestion of infected raw snake, frog, or pig or drinking contaminated water		Class III
Gnathostoma spinigerum and *Gnathostoma hispidum* (nematode) Cutaneous, visceral, ocular, neurological gnathostomiasis	Domestic and wild pigs, cats, dogs, and wild animals are the natural definitive hosts The worm causes tumour in the gastric wall and resides there	First intermediate hosts—Small crustaceans (cyclops) ingest the first-stage larvae that develop into second-stage larvae Fish, frog, and snakes are the second intermediate hosts and ingest cyclops, and the larvae migrate into the flesh to develop into third stage	Mode of infection of the definitive hosts Ingestion of the second intermediate hosts; adult develops into stomach wall Man gets infected by ingesting undercooked fish and poultry, having third-stage larvae Drinking water containing cyclops infected with second-stage larvae		Class III

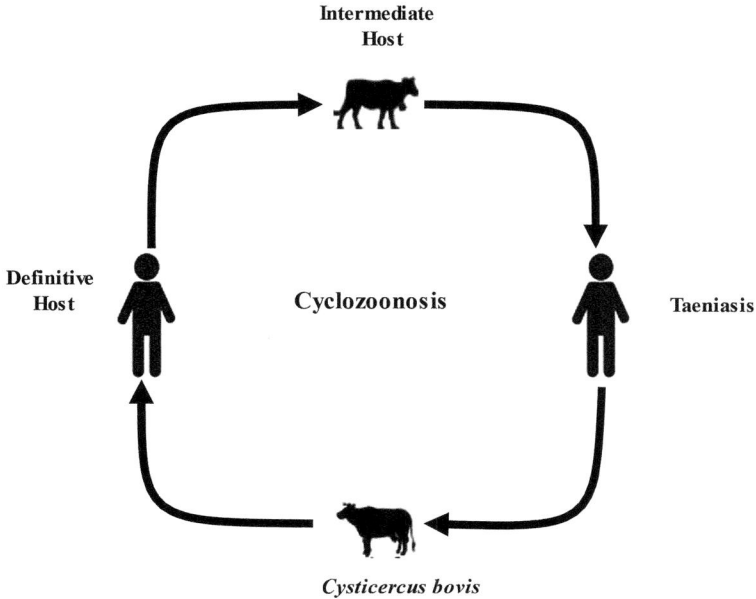

Fig. 74.1 Cyclozoonoses

Table 74.4 Some cyclozoonotic parasites

Agent	Vertebrate 1/ definitive host	Vertebrate 2/ intermediate host	Mode of infection	Remarks
Taenia solium	Man	Pigs	Ingestion of *C. cellulose* containing pork/ autoinfection	Obligate cyclo zoonoses
T. saginata	Man	Cattle	*C. bovis*—Beef	-do-
E. granulosus	Dog	Sheep, horse, etc.	Ingestion of *E. granulosus* eggs—With dust, soil, water	Non-obligatory
T. multiceps	Many canines	Intermediate hosts are many animals, including rodents, rabbits, horses, cattle, sheep, and goats	Embryonated eggs ingested with water/food contaminated with dogs' fomites; fevers cause coenurosis (brain, eyes)	Non-obligatory
T. serialis	Only dogs and foxes			

74.3.1   Soil-Transmitted Parasites

Ascaris, *Toxocara*, *Strongyloides*, *Ancylostoma*, and *Trichuris* are common soil-transmitted helminths causing clinical disorders in human, commonly children living in poverty and in less developed countries. The physical, intellectual, and cognitive developments of children are impaired (Bethony et al. 2006).

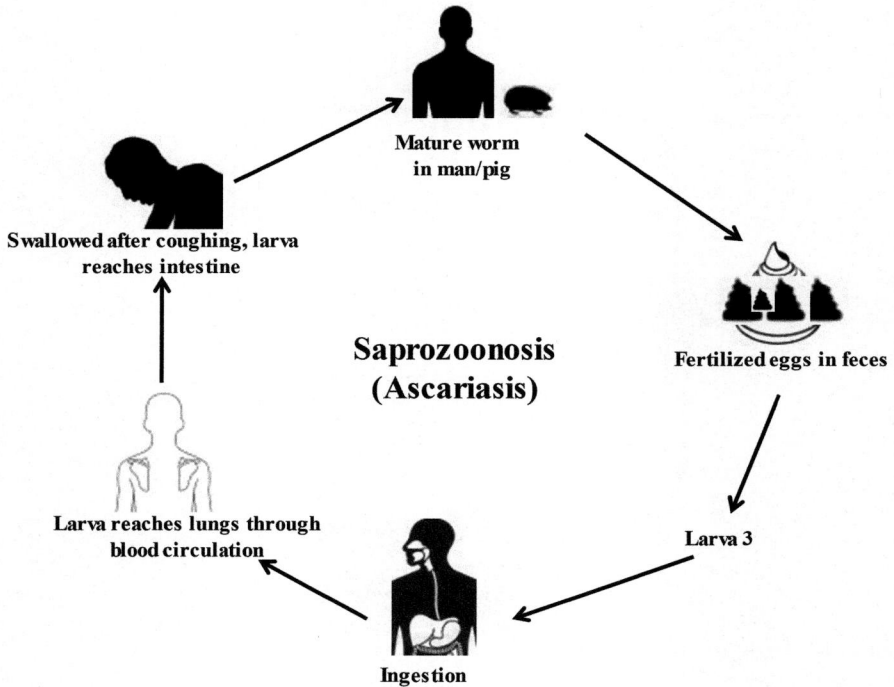

Saprozoonosis (Ascariasis)

Mature worm in man/pig

Swallowed after coughing, larva reaches intestine

Fertilized eggs in feces

Larva reaches lungs through blood circulation

Larva 3

Ingestion

Fig. 74.2 Saprozoonosis

Table 74.5 Some saprozoonoses

Agent	Host	Mode of infection in man
Ancylostoma caninum	Cats, dogs, wild carnivores	Contact with infective-stage larvae that penetrates through the skin
Ascaris suum	Pigs	Ingestion of embryonated eggs
Capillaria hepatica	Small rodents, monkeys	Ingestion of infective eggs
Strongyloides stercoralis	Cats, dogs, sheep	Contact with infective-stage larvae
Trichuris vulpis	Humans, other primates	Ingestion of embryonated eggs on plant foods, soil
Hypoderma bovis	Mammals	

Common ways of infection are

- Eggs attached to vegetables which are ingested without washing, peeling, and adequate cooking.
- Eggs ingested from contaminated water sources.
- Eggs ingested by children who play in the contaminated soil and then put their hands in their mouths without washing them.
- Penetration of the skin by larvae in soil.

Nearly 1.5 billion (or 24%) of the world population are affected with soil-borne helminth parasites. These live in tropical and subtropical areas located mostly in sub-Saharan Africa, the Americas, China, and East Asia. According to the WHO's (2020) estimates, intense transmission of these parasites occurs in areas inhabited by 267 million preschool children and over 568 million school-age children. Risk-associated activities included children playing on contaminated field, farmers walking or working in field barefoot, occupations demanding work in raised buildings such electricians and plumbers, and recreational activities like lying/sunbath on contaminated sand.

An interesting epidemiological study by Traub et al. (2003) in tea-growing community in Assam revealed the role of dogs in dissemination of parasites like hookworm, *Giardia*, and *Ascaris*. The community had heavy infection of hookworms, *Ascaris*, and *Trichuris*. Ninety-nine per cent of dogs in the same locality suffered with at least one of the zoonotic gastrointestinal parasites. Dogs were the significant environmental contaminator and disseminator of *Ascaris lumbricoides* in the area where open defecation existed. Zoonotic transmission of *Giardia duodenalis* (syn. *G. lamblia*) and its worldwide distribution were evidenced by phylogenetic and epidemiological findings.

Zoonotic infection with ascarids and hookworms causes larva migrans in human beings. Most common animal sources are pets such as dogs and cats. Once infected, ascarids start shedding eggs in 2–3 weeks to contaminate the environment. About 100,000 eggs/day are shed by a single female ascarid. Infective stage can survive for years in the environment. *Baylisascaris procyonis* is the common raccoon ascarid but can cause serious disease in other animals and humans. Puppies and kittens of even 2 and 3 weeks age, respectively, pass eggs of *Ancylostoma* that become infective-stage larvae in 5 days in environment.

Humidity and temperature affect the development. Rains and insects spread. During disaster like flood, humans are exposed to contaminated water in various ways such as drinking, inhaling, splashes, or mist, and pathogens enter through the eyes, nose, open wound, and mouth—the most common being drinking contaminated water or eating contaminated food.

Benzimidazole anthelmintics can prevent soil-transmitted helminths and improve children's health.

74.4 Prevention

Parasitic infections are preventable. Hygiene is the most important. It has to be inclusive; personal hygiene, e.g. trimming of nails and frequent handwash particularly before taking meals, prevents giardiasis and amoebiasis. Pure drinking water keeps out cryptosporidiosis. Kitchen, home, or food joints are the most common sources of contamination and cross- contamination. Finally, professional inspection and hygiene of the food processing plants prevent widespread common source food-borne infections, e.g. meat inspection for *Trichinella spiralis*.

Responsible pet owners are expected to practice the following:

- Regular deworming. Choose from drugs such as piperazine citrate, pyrantel pamoate, oxibendazole, fenbendazole, ivermectin, and diethylcarbamazine citrate.
- Clean up pet faeces regularly.
- Unprotected sand boxes are kept away from reach of children.
- Use sanitized water; boiling is most effective.

74.5   Treatment

Most parasitic diseases are treatable with broad-spectrum anthelmintics.

References

Bethony J, Brooker S, Albonico M, Geiger SM, Loukas A et al (2006) Soil-transmitted helminth infections: ascariasis, trichuriasis, and hookworm. Lancet 367:1521–1532
Contacos PG, Coatney GR, Orihel TC, Collins WE, Chin W, Jeter MH (1970) Transmission of *plasmodium schwetzi* from the chimpanzee to man by mosquito bite. Am J Trop Med Hyg 19(2):190–195
Traub RJ, Robertson ID, Irwin P, Mencke N, Monis P, Thompson RCA (2003) Humans, dogs and parasitic zoonoses unravellig the relationships in a remote endemic community in Northeast India using molecular tools. Parasitol Res 90(S156):S157
WHO (2020) Soil - transmitted helminth infections. https://www.who.int/news-room/fact-sheets/detail/soil-transmitted-helminth-infections
Youn H (2009) Review of zoonotic parasites in medical and veterinary fields in the Republic of Korea. Korean J Parasitol 47:S133–S141

Chapter 75
Amoebiasis

Amoebiasis is caused by a protozoan called *Entamoeba histolytica*, which infects human and non-human primates and occasionally dogs and cats.

Amoebiasis is worldwide in distribution, but it is more common in people who live in tropical areas with poor sanitary conditions. Infection occurs through the mouth by swallowing *E. histolytica* cysts (eggs)-contaminated food and water. Some people carry the parasite or cysts in their faeces without symptoms, but they can still pass the disease on to others.

75.1 Symptoms

Only about 10% to 20% of *E. histolytica*-infected people usually develop symptoms within 2 to 4 weeks and show mild symptoms like loose faeces, stomach pain, and cramping. Amoebic dysentery is a severe form of amoebiasis associated with stomach pain, bloody stools, and fever. Rarely, *E. histolytica* invades the liver and forms an abscess. It has been shown to spread to the lungs or brain, but this is uncommon.

75.2 Diagnosis

Faecal microscopic examination helps in diagnosis. A blood test is only recommended for infection spread beyond the intestine to some other organs such as the liver.

© Springer Nature Singapore Pte Ltd. 2024   781
K. G. Narayan et al., *Handbook of Management of Zoonoses*,
https://doi.org/10.1007/978-981-99-9885-2_75

75.3 Treatment

Metronidazole or tinidazole is the drug of choice.

75.4 Prevention

CDC (2021) advised to avoid drinking or eating the following:

- Fountain drinks or any drinks with ice cubes.
- Fresh fruit or vegetables that you did not peel yourself.
- Milk, cheese, or dairy products that may not have been pasteurized.
- Food or drinks sold by street vendors.

Maintenance of personal hygiene like thorough handwashing with soap and water after using the toilet, changing diapers, handling pets, and preparing food.

References

CDC (2021) Division of foodborne, waterborne, and environmental diseases (DFWED)

Chapter 76
Babesiosis

Synonyms

Texas fever, Red water, Cattle tick fever.

Babesiosis is a dangerous, invasive disease of humans and animals and is included among emerging diseases. Cases are increasing, and the infected geographic region is expanding ascribed to changing ecology, increased population, intensified human migration, and invasion of forest biotope.

76.1 Aetiology

The causative agents are apicomplexan parasites of the genus *Babesia*. *B. microti*, *B. divergens*, *B. duncani*, and *B. venatorum* and a currently unnamed strain designated MO-1 (https://www.cdc.gov/dpdx/babesiosis/index.html.) cause human babesiosis.

A splenectomized Yugoslavian farmer was diagnosed as a case of *B. bovis* in 1957. In Europe, most subsequent cases were reportedly caused by *B. divergens*. These were zoonotic and often fatal. In the United States, a series of human babesiosis cases was diagnosed as caused by *B. microti*. These were identified during 1960. Since then, it is the predominant human babesiosis in north-eastern coastal regions and upper Midwestern United States. Other piroplasms identified as causative agents are apicomplexan parasites of the genus *Babesia*, e.g., *B. microti*, *B. divergens*, and *B. duncani*; strains MO-1, WA1 (closely related to *B. gibsoni* of dogs), and CA1 (California protozoan); and *B. microti*-like Hobetsu and Kobe types of Japan. *B. microti* isolates were heterogenous. *B. microti* has been renamed as *Theileria microti* (Uilenberg 2006) because (a) the nuclear small subunit ribosomal DNA (nss-rDNA) sequences are more (91%) similar to *Theileria annulata* than to other *Babesia* (88%, e.g. *B. bigeminy*), (b) transovarial transmission in ticks does not occur, and (c) pre-erythrocytic stage (intra-lymphocytic schizonts) occurs in vertebrate hosts.

© Springer Nature Singapore Pte Ltd. 2024
K. G. Narayan et al., *Handbook of Management of Zoonoses*,
https://doi.org/10.1007/978-981-99-9885-2_76

Study by Tsuji et al. (2001) suggested that new type of *B. microti*-like parasite, namely, the Hobetsu type, is the major species prevalent among Japanese wild rodents. *A. speciosus* served as a major reservoir for both Kobe- and Hobetsu-type *B. microti*-like parasites, and *C. rufocanus* may also be an additional reservoir on Hokkaido Island.

76.2 Epidemiology

76.2.1 Prevalence

The prevalence in human is more than actually reported for understandable reasons such as asymptomatic infection and mild and self-limiting disease. Sporadic occurrence has been reported in parts of the United States, Europe, Asia, Africa, and South America (Vannier et al. 2008). Recent report suggests a worldwide distribution, Asia, Africa, and Oceania, and a significant number of cases in American and European countries and several other countries like Egypt, Mexico, South Africa, Mozambique, Australia, Brazil, Japan, Republic of Korea, Singapore, the United Kingdom, Russia, Spain, etc. The three main species reported in Europe are *B. divergens*, *B. ventorum*, and *B. microti*. The main vector is *I. ricinus* (Chen et al. 2020).

B. divergens is considered endemic in Eurasia (European human babesiosis and bovine red water agent). *Ixodes ricinus* is the vector. In France and British Isles, *B. divergens* is the most common in splenectomized patients. Martinot et al. (2011) reported two clinical cases in immunocompetent humans in France and believed that it occurred also in healthy persons. Infection is considered very serious as it caused 42% mortality. In the United States, most cases of infection with *Babesia microti* are acquired from the bite of the *Ixodes scapularis* tick, the same vector for Lyme disease. Goethert and Telford (2003) observed that 16% of cottontail rabbits on Nantucket Island, Massachusetts, USA, were infected with *Babesia divergens*. *Ixodes dentatus* appeared to be the vector. This is a rabbit-bird feeding tick and may feed on humans causing severe haemolytic syndrome.

According to Chen et al. (2020), >314 cases were reported between 1944 and 2019 from 14 provincial-level administrative divisions in China.

76.2.1.1 The US Surveillance Report

Babesiosis surveillance in the United States (Gray and Herwaldt 2019) explains in brief the epidemiology. Babesiosis is a notifiable disease in the United States since January 2011. It was reported in 33 states in 2015 compared to 22 states in 2011. During 2011–2015, a total of 7612 cases of babesiosis were reported, 82.5% confirmed and 17.5% probable. Cases were reported among residents of 27 states. However, 7194 cases or 94.5% occurred among residents of 7 states (Connecticut,

Massachusetts, Minnesota, New Jersey, New York, Rhode Island, and Wisconsin) with well-documented foci of tick-borne transmission. Maine and New Hampshire, the two states reported <100 cases for 5 years.

Nearly 50% of cases required at least overnight hospitalization. Risk factors are elucidated with the observation of the median age of cases (63 years), 72.6% aged ≥80 years, and the most cases are asplenics. Transfusion-associated cases were 51.

Most cases occurred during June to August in the Northeast and upper Midwest. An indication of expanding foci of infection was the observation of increasing number of cases in Maine and New Hampshire.

76.2.2 Life Cycle (Fig. 76.1)

Most white-footed mice (*Peromyscus leucopus*) in babesiosis-enzootic areas are parasitaemic for life without any threat to their life. Parasitaemia is high (40–50% infected RBC) in susceptible hosts like hamsters and laboratory mice.

The nymphs of *I. scapularis* and white-footed mouse (*P. leucopus*) cycle are essential for maintenance of *B. microti*. Nymph feed indiscriminately on large

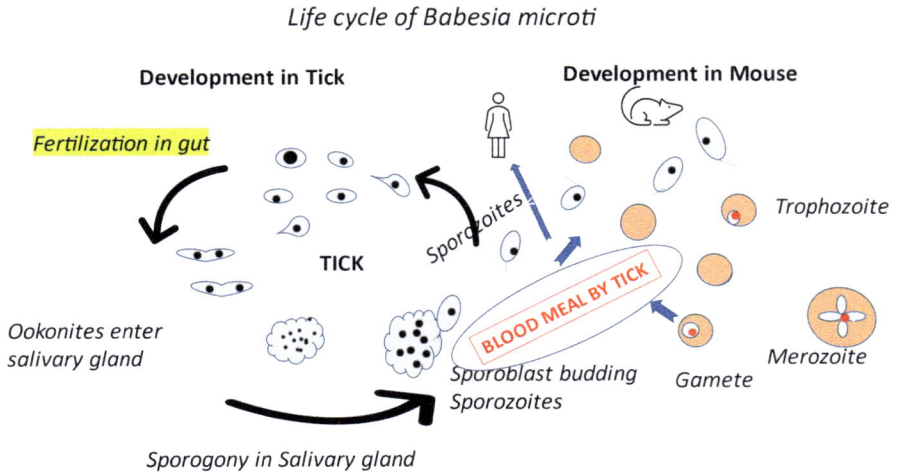

Fig. 76.1 In the blood meal of infected tick parasites are seen gametes and zygotes (*two dots in figure*) in gut tissues of peritrophic membrane, epithelial cells and ookonites entering in salivary gland. Multinucleate undifferentiated sporoblast—specialised organelles of future sporozoites begin to form when the tick begins to feed, finally sporozoites bud off from the sporoblast. Blood meal leads to entry of sporozoites into the reservoir host mouse. Sporozoites invade the lymphocytes and then differentiate into multinucleate schizonts which differentiate in merozoites. Merozoites bud off from schizonts. Merozoites are the pre-erythrocytic form. These invade erythrocyte by invagination. Some of these differentiate into male and female gametes Infection in man is almost a dead end

mammals, including humans, as well as small rodents. The fed nymphs moult into adult during fall.

The adult stage feed primarily on deer (*Odocoileus virginianus*, not a reservoir host but amplify ticks) during fall and spring and lay eggs that hatch in summer (late July). During August and September, larvae feed and acquire infection and overwinter to moult as nymph in spring. Feeding months for nymph are May through July. White-footed mouse *(P. leucopus)* is a reservoir host for two emerging zoonoses also, Lyme disease and human granulocytic ehrlichiosis.

The tick spp. is different in Europe, *I. trianguliceps*, and does not feed on human, so *B. microti* infection is rare.

The ticks are the definitive hosts. The ingested gametes unite in the gut, sporogony occurs, and the sporozoites form in the salivary glands. There is vertical (transovarial) transmission in ticks, from female ticks to its eggs in ovaries in case of large babesiae and not *B. microti*.

Mouse and humans are infected through tick bites that introduce sporozoites. The sporozoites invade erythrocytes and divide by budding (asexual reproduction) into merozoites. Some of these differentiate into male and female gametes. Infection in man is almost a dead end.

B. divergens infection is high when ticks are more active, and most human infections occurred among those who had frequent contact with cattle as *I. ricinus* feeds also on humans.

Almost every mammal who is host for a *Babesia*-infected tick is a potential reservoir. Small terrestrial mammal to subhuman primates acts as host of *B. microti*. Cattle to various rodent species act as host for *B. divergens*.

76.3 Babesia microti

B. microti is common in wild vertebrate species (e.g. *P. leucopus*). In enzootic area, most white-footed mice (*P. leucopus*) in babesiosis are parasitaemic and remain so for life. Man is the most poorly adapted host.

Small mammals, white-footed mice are frequently co-infected with *Borrelia burgdorferi* (Lyme disease agent) and/or *Anaplasma phagocytophilum* and *B. microti*; it means the tick can transfer all the three.

76.3.1 Host-Parasite Interaction

The infection induces both humoral and cell-mediated immune responses. Sporozoites stay in the blood stream for a short duration. The IgG can prevent invasion of target cells by binding and neutralizing sporozoites. Infection succeeds with establishment of intraerythrocytic phase and parasitaemia. Acute disease occurs.

The growth rate of the parasite and the extent of parasitaemia are controlled by cells of the innate immune system. Most likely the gamma interferon (IFN-g) produced by NK cells and tumour necrosis factor-alpha (TNF-a), nitric oxide (NO), and reactive oxygen species (ROSs) by macrophages are responsible.

Non-specific (innate) immune response is also evidenced. The natural killer (NK) cells and macrophages are involved.

76.3.2   Symptoms

It is a self-limiting disease in persons with normal immune function. The symptoms last for 2–4 weeks. The incubation period varies from 1 to 6 weeks and may be long, 3 months. It is 3–7 weeks or longer in case transmitted through blood transfusion. Sporozoites invade erythrocytes and divide to form merozoites that grow and multiply. Erythrocytes lyse resulting into haemolytic anaemia and tissue hypoxia. Lungs are affected in complicated cases causing acute respiratory distress. Severe cases result from excess cytokine release-related immunopathy. Fever (40 °C), chills, fatigue, night sweat, myalgia, nausea and emesis, haemolysis, and haematuria associated with high parasitaemia may be observed. Hepatomegaly and splenomegaly are common pathology. Severe cases are fulminating malaria with haemolytic anaemia lasting for several days to few months, haemoglobinuria, jaundice, respiratory distress renal failure. Parasitaemia lasts for months to years in severe cases and they become source of infection.

Marathe et al. (2005) reported first case from India that was initially diagnosed and treated for malaria. The examination of blood smear demonstrated trophozoites, merozoites, and schizonts.

A 51-year male, with no history of other illness and splenectomy, got high fever and was admitted to hospital. He was examined—high-grade fever, vomiting, profuse sweating, chills, mild headache, and arthralgia. The spleen and liver were palpable. He had scleral icterus, and his urine was dark coloured.

B. microti is responsible for most cases of human babesiosis worldwide. It presents as a malaria-like illness. Severe cases are life-threatening and occur mostly in asplenic, elderly, immunocompromised, and AIDS patients and those with liver and kidney diseases and also in cases with simultaneous infection with other tick-transmitted pathogens (e.g. co-infection with *B. burgdorferi*). Complications are more likely in immunocompromised/AIDS patients. Parasitaemia persist long after acute babesiosis.

B. microti infection is less severe and clinical recovery is common. *B. microti* may affect any individual between 3 and 86 years, most commonly 50 to 60 years.

A 61-year-old woman with chronic lymphocytic leukaemia fell ill and had fever and anaemia 12 days after splenectomy. She had numerous blood transfusions for gastrointestinal bleeding. She developed respiratory failure although she was on clindamycin and quinine. She was put on azithromycin and atovaquone for 12 weeks. The blood smear and polymerase chain reaction findings were negative.

Investigations revealed that one blood donor and another one recipient were positive for *B. microti*. Infective blood on transfusion could result into asymptomatic to fulminant disease causing multiorgan failure and death (Wudhikarn et al. 2011)

Detection of the secreted *B. microti* immunodominant antigen BmGPI12 found to be the most effective method for evaluation of clearance following drug treatment. Gagnon et al. (2022) used a panel of 16 monoclonal antibodies specific against BmGPI12 for detecting secreted BmGPI12 in the plasma of infected humans. Antigen capture assays identified a combination of two monoclonal antibodies, 4C8 and 1E11, to detect active *B. microti* infection. This assay showed 97.1% correlation with RNA-based PCR [transcription-mediated amplification (TMA)] for positive and negative samples on 105 previously characterized human plasma samples.

76.4 *Babesia divergens*

B. divergens causes more severe, fatal disease if not treated. The incubation period varies between 1 and 3 weeks. There is a sudden onset of disease. Haemolysis is severe. There is haemoglobinuria followed by jaundice. Patients suffer with shock, renal failure, and pulmonary oedema.

Transfusion of blood and blood products collected from asymptomatic donors may result in a serious illness that can be fatal (Gubernot et al. 2009). Blood transfusion-associated neonatal babesiosis manifesting hepatosplenomegaly, jaundice, conjugated hyperbilirubinaemia, and anaemia was reported by Fox et al. (2006). It is important to realize that parasitaemia persisted for more than a year in asymptomatic carrier.

Host characters like age and immunocompetence are important. Old age and splenectomized and immunocompromised host are most susceptible and likely to have severe form of disease. *B. microti* infection occurs in age group of 3–86 years, majority in the range of 50–60 years. The mean age of mild or asymptomatic subjects was approximately 30 years less than that of severe cases.

76.5 Transmission

- Tick bites (nymphs of *I. scapularis*, called black-legged or deer ticks, are tiny of the poppy seed size, found on grass, brush, and wood); 24- and even 36-h attachment is required for transmission.
- Blood transfusion.
- Congenital (transfer from infected mother to baby during pregnancy or delivery) are the only means of human-to-human transmission.

76.6   Diagnosis

- Clinical manifestation, history of travel to endemic areas, and exposure to ticks are helpful.
- Clinical laboratory findings in patients are related to parasitaemia: increased transaminases, alkaline phosphatases, unconjugated bilirubin, lactic dehydrogenase, normochromia, normocytic anaemia, and leucopoenia (Homer et al. 2000).
- Blood smear stained with Giemsa to see intraerythrocytic parasite (merozoites) seen as ring forms with blue cytoplasm and red chromatin.
- Laboratory animal inoculation: hamster and gerbil develop parasitaemia in 1–4 weeks.
- HU-RBC-SCID mice and splenectomized hamster were most sensitive (Wei et al. 2001).
- Serological—IFA, CFT.
- Antigen capture assay for detecting secreted BmGPI12 in the plasma of infected humans (Gagnon et al. 2022).
- Molecular methods—PCR for detailed characterization of strains.

Diagnosis is required for specific treatment without which a case may progress to serious or persistent one. Such a case is likely to transmit through blood transfusion. The disease is treatable with specific drugs that are normally not used for febrile cases.

76.7   Treatment

Treatment for 7–10 days with either of the following combination is effective: clindamycin plus quinine and atovaquone plus azithromycin.

76.8   Prevention

The findings of the 5-year surveillance in the United States (Gray and Herwaldt 2019) suggested the following public health measures:

1. For travellers to endemic areas to avoid tick-infected areas, use repellent and clothing for personal protection.
2. Full-body inspection. Remove tick from body with tweezers.
3. Regions showing increase in number of cases warranted investigation to find out contributing factors.

References

Chen M, Liu Q, Xue J, Chen S, Huang D et al (2020) Spreading of human Babesiosis in China: current epidemiological status and future challenges. China CDC Weekly 2(33):634–637

Fox LM, Wingerter S, Ahmed A, Arnold A et al (2006) Neonatal babesiosis: case report and review of the literature. Pediatr Infect Dis J 25(2):169–173

Gagnon J, Timalsina S, Choi JY, Chand M, Singh P et al (2022) Specific and sensitive diagnosis of *Babesia microti* active infection using monoclonal antibodies to the Immunodominant antigen BmGPI12. J Clin Microbiol 60(9):e0092522

Goethert HK, Telford SR 3rd. (2003) Enzootic transmission of *Babesia divergens* among cottontail rabbits on Nantucket Island, Massachusetts. Am J Trop Med Hyg 69(5):455–460

Gray EB, Herwaldt BL (2019) Babesiosis surveillance - United States, 2011–2015. MMWR Surveill Summ 68(SS-6):1–11

Gubernot DM, Nakhasi HL, Mied PA, Asher DM, Epstein JS, Kumar S (2009) Transfusion-transmitted babesiosis in the United States: summary of a workshop. Transfusion 49(12):2759–2771

Homer MJ, Aguilar-Delfin I, Telford SR 3rd, Krause PJ, Persing DH (2000) Babesiosis. Clin Microbiol Rev 13(3):451–469

Marathe A, Tripathi J, Handa V, Date V (2005) Human babesiosis--a case report. Indian J Med Microbiol 23(4):267–269

Martinot M, Zadeh MM, Hansmann Y, Grawey I, Christmann D et al (2011) Babesiosis in immunocompetent patients, Europe. Emerg Infect Dis 17(1):114–116

Tsuji M, Wei Q, Zamoto A, Morita C, Arai S et al (2001) Human babesiosis in Japan: epizootiologic survey of rodent reservoir and isolation of new type of *Babesia microti*-like parasite. J Clin Microbiol 39(12):4316–4322

Uilenberg G (2006) Babesia--a historical overview. Vet Parasitol 138(1–2):3–10

Vannier E, Gewurz BE, Krause PJ (2008) Human babesiosis. Infect Dis Clin N Am 22(3):469–488. viii–ix

Wei Q, Tsuji M, Zamoto A, Kohsaki M, Matsui T et al (2001) Human babesiosis in Japan: isolation of *Babesia microti*-like parasites from an asymptomatic transfusion donor and from a rodent from an area where babesiosis is endemic. J Clin Microbiol 39(6):2178–2183

Wudhikarn K, Perry EH, Kemperman M, Jensen KA, Kline SE (2011) Transfusion-transmitted babesiosis in an immunocompromised patient: a case report and review. Am J Med 124(9):800–805

Chapter 77
Balantidiasis

Balantidiasis is caused by *Balantidium coli*. It is a common ciliated protozoan parasite of 50 mammalian hosts including swine, monkeys, great apes, and human. *B. coli* is cosmopolitan. Balantidiasis is common in the Philippines and occurs in Latin America, Bolivia, South Asia, New Guinea, Southeast Asia, the Western Pacific Islands, rural South America, or communities where close contact with domestic swine occurs.

77.1 Epidemiology

Domestic pigs are generally considered to be the most important natural reservoir for human balantidiasis. *B. coli* causes reduced production in animals and impact economy.

B. coli has been identified in vegetables and pigs in Ghana. The study involved farmers and their exposed household members of two pig-rearing communities. The overall prevalence (10.4%) among farmers was significantly higher than among the exposed household members (5.8%). *Entamoeba histolytica*, *Giardia lamblia*, or *Schistosoma mansoni* were other co-infecting parasites in 20.9%. The factors responsible for human balantidiasis were free-range farming, improper disposal of pig faeces, lack of use of protective farming clothing, and unavailability of dedicated farming clothing (Aninagyei et al. 2021). Swine breeders and slaughterhouse workers are at risk of getting infection.

Countries/regions where pig farming and pork eating is prohibited still report *B. coli* infection. Alternate source, the wild boar is found in rural areas of different parts of Iran, has close contact with farmlands, and is considered a natural source of infection in Iran (Soleimanpour et al. 2016). Persistent diarrhoea in travellers who visited endemic countries or regions is suggestive of balantidiasis.

© Springer Nature Singapore Pte Ltd. 2024
K. G. Narayan et al., *Handbook of Management of Zoonoses*,
https://doi.org/10.1007/978-981-99-9885-2_77

B. *coli* occurs in two forms, trophozoites and cyst. The former replicates and encysts due to dehydration of faeces. Cyst protects against desiccation and other environmental stresses. Humidity and shade offer best protection. Trophic ciliates probably do not survive stomach acidity. The process of encystment begins in host's colon and rectum and is found in faeces.

Route of infection and transmission is faecal-oral. Ingestion of trophozoites or cysts in contaminated water and food causes human infection. Human-to-human transmission occurs.

Poor waste management, opportunities of contaminating water and food, and warm and humid (tropical and/or subtropical) conditions favour contamination, survival of B. *coli*, and transmission.

Outbreak is rare and has occurred under unprecedented situation, such as typhoon in a place where swine herds are common, source of drinking water (catchment and collection) is damaged, and people are compelled to use contaminated water. It happened in typhoon-hit island of truck in the Caroline Islands (Western Pacific). Simultaneous infection with E. *histolytica* and *Ascaris* occurred (Schuster and Ramirez-Avila 2008).

77.1.1   Infection

B. *coli* penetrates the mucosa of the large intestine causing inflammation and ulcers. Caecum and colon seem to be natural location/habitat. Balantidial dysentery results. Rectosigmoidoscopy shows oedema and hyperaemia of mucosa often with ulcers and haemorrhage. B. *coli*-associated appendicitis, intestinal perforation, peritonitis and often deaths have been reported. Immunocompromised individuals may get infected even without contact with pigs, perhaps contact with rats or contaminated produce. Extra-intestinal spread may occur. Infection may spread to the appendix, peritoneum, and genitourinary tract. In females, genitourinary tract infection may also occur by spread/infection from anal area or because of recto-vaginal fistula.

Malnutrition, low stomach acidity, and immunocompromised state predispose.

77.2   Symptoms

Balantidiasis may manifest in any of the following forms:

- Asymptomatic and mild form presents intermittent diarrhoea alternating with constipation.
- Acute form presents dysentery, stool containing blood and mucus, dehydration, and weight loss.
- Fulminant form occurs rarely. There is ulceration and perforation of the colon with haemorrhage and even death.

- Chronic form is characterized by non-bleeding diarrhoea alternating with constipation and abdominal pain.

Untreated cases may dehydrate due to persistent diarrhoea. Case fatality rate may be 30% (Schuster and Ramirez-Avila 2008). In *B. coli* infection, mild to moderate anaemia together with a reduction in levels of platelet, albumin, sodium, chloride, and bicarbonate ions was observed. However, white blood cells were significantly elevated in infected states (Aninagyei et al. 2021).

Soleimanpour et al. (2016) described a case of urinary tract infection in a woman who was drug addict and suffered from diabetes and hypothyroidism. She was admitted for spontaneous abortion and temporary loss of consciousness. Examination revealed severe anaemia, biological inflammatory syndrome (C-reactive protein positive), hypernatremia, hypokalaemia, metabolic acidosis, and an initial functional renal deficiency. Urine examination showed red blood cells (50–60), pus cells (20–25), tubular casts, and *B. coli.*

77.3 Diagnosis

Trophozoites or cyst in infected stool is diagnostic.

77.4 Treatment

Tetracycline, ampicillin, and metronidazole are effective.

77.5 Prevention

Protection of water supply from contamination is important as cysts survive usual sanitation. Good waste management and water sanitation should keep out *B. coli* infection.

References

Aninagyei E, Nanga S, Acheampong DO, Mensah R, Boadu MN et al (2021) Prevalence and risk factors of human *Balantidium coli* infection and its association with haematological and biochemical parameters in Ga west municipality, Ghana. BMC Infect Dis 21(1):1047

Schuster FL, Ramirez-Avila L (2008) Current world status of *Balantidium coli*. Clin Microbiol Rev 21(4):626–638

Soleimanpour S, Babaei A, Roudi AM, Raeisalsadati SS (2016) Urinary infection due to *Balantioides coli*: a rare accidental zoonotic disease in an addicted and diabetic young female in Iran. JMM Case Rep 3(1):e000102

Chapter 78
Chagas Disease

Synonyms

American trypanosomiasis.

Chagas disease or American trypanosomiasis disease is a potentially life-threatening illness caused by the protozoan parasite *Trypanosoma cruzi*. About six to seven million people worldwide are estimated to be infected (WHO 2020).

Chagas disease is named after Carlos Ribeiro Justiniano Chagas, a Brazilian physician and researcher who discovered the disease in 1909. In May 2019, following up on decision of the 72nd World Health Assembly, the World Chagas Disease Day was established to be celebrated on 14 April (the date of the year 1909 when Carlos Chagas diagnosed the first human case in a 2-year-old girl named Berenice).

It is one of the "neglected tropical diseases" listed by the WHO. According to Robertson et al. (2016), the estimated global burden is 300,000 to over 800,000 disability-adjusted life years (DALYs) with a prevalence of 9–10 million and estimated cost of US$ 7.19 billion/year. It caused death of 10,000/year. In Brazil, it accounted for 11% of heart failure.

78.1   Aetiology

Trypanosoma cruzi is a flagellated protozoan parasite, bore tissues in definitive host and feed primarily blood and lymph, and requires haematophagus insect vector.

© Springer Nature Singapore Pte Ltd. 2024
K. G. Narayan et al., *Handbook of Management of Zoonoses*,
https://doi.org/10.1007/978-981-99-9885-2_78

78.2 Vector

T. cruzi replicates in the *Triatomine* vectors' intestine and shed in faeces. The insect vector lives in the cracks in the wall or roof of homes and peri-domiciliary structures, such as chicken coops, pens, and warehouses, in rural or suburban, hidden in day and active at night. They come out of hides, bite an exposed area and moist surface of the skin such as the eyes and face (hence its common name "kissing bug"), and defecate or urinate close to the bite. The infected vector pierces the skin while taking blood meal defecating at the same time. Although the bite is painless, it causes itching and scratch at the site introducing *T. cruzi*-laden faeces into the bite wound.

78.3 Life Cycle

There are two infective life cycle stages, trypomastigotes and amastigotes of *T. cruzi*. The trypomastigotes that actively enter mammalian cells are the infective flagellated form of the parasite found in the blood of the mammalian hosts (blood trypomastigote) and in the hindgut of vectors (metacyclic trypomastigote).

The amastigote forms are usually found in the cytoplasm of infected cells but can also be generated by extracellular differentiation of trypomastigotes.

The extracellular amastigotes (EAs) are capable of invading and sustaining infections in mammalian cells of different hosts. These are infective to both phagocytic and non-phagocytic cells. These relied upon actin-mediated uptake by phagocytes. The EAs are potent inducers of phagocytosis in non-phagocytic phagocytes, and this helps in persistence in infected hosts (Fernandes et al. 2013).

These extracellular amastigotes (EAs) and intracellular amastigotes share morphological and immunochemical markers. However, amastigotes from each successive wave of production bear a different antigenic marker enabling the escape from the antibodies. The parasites stay one step ahead of the host's defence in the form of specific antibody.

78.4 Modes of Infection

Infected triatomine faeces are infective. The trypanosome enters the human body through the bite wound, intact mucosa, and conjunctiva. Oral infection in human occurs through ingestion of drinks and foods contaminated with the infected insects' faeces. Uncooked meat of infected mammalian sylvatic hosts is infective on ingestion. Laboratory accidents may also transmit.

Further human-human transmission may be

- Congenital (15–22.5%).
- Transfusion of contaminated blood and its products (10–25% of the time).
- Transplantation of the heart (75–100%), kidney (19%), and liver (29%) from infected donor.

78.5   Host-Parasite Interaction: Pathogenesis

78.5.1   Invasion

Bite of infected triatomine or "kissing bug" introduces the protozoan in the human host. The motile *T. cruzi* forms trypomastigotes at the site of bite.

The trypomastigotes use different receptors/linkers to get into host cells (internalization). The process may be (a) fusion of *lysosomes* at the site of entry, participation of components of the plasma membrane, (b) actin-dependent pathway, (c) lysosome-independent pathway, entry through plasma membrane. The invasion leads to the formation of parasitophorous vacuole (PV).

The trypomastigote gradually transforms into *amastigote* via an epimastigote-like intermediate stage in the parasitophorous vacuole (PV) a few hours after internalization. The amastigotes are located in PV.

The PV is disrupted by a series of chemical processes to release amastigotes. Following this, the amastigote enters direct to the host cell cytoplasm and starts a process of binary division.

78.5.2   Dissemination

These disseminate and invade various hosts' cells. After several rounds of intracellular replication, amastigotes start the process of transforming into trypomastigotes. The cells burst open and release these into intercellular space which eventually reach the bloodstream to disseminate to various tissues throughout the body and invade cells.

The interval between waves of parasitaemia may vary from 1 to 2 weeks, with clinical symptoms accompanying each bout of parasitaemia.

78.5.2.1   Acute Phase

In the acute phase, the parasite is found in tissues throughout the body and circulating blood. In the early phase of infection, specific IgG and lytic antibodies against trypanomastigotes are widely detected. After 15 days of infection, IgM antibodies are highly abundant in the sera of acute chagasic patients.

Activated macrophages and natural killer cells produce cytokines that might activate CD4+, CD8+, and other T-cell population to produce TNF-alpha and IFN-y molecules and nitric oxide targeting intracellular pathogens. IL10 and other anti-inflammatory molecules might influence or control the response to decrease tissue damage.

Controlled level of parasite is observed in late-acute and throughout chronic phase because of antibodies produced by plasma cells and activation of inflammatory response.

The production of inflammatory cytokines and the activation of cytolytic cells may be critical for parasite control during early stages of infection. The disease enters in chronic stage, associated with cardiac and digestive symptoms (Andrade et al. 2014).

78.5.2.2   Chronic Phase

In chronic Chagas disease, the pathological changes occur due to the combined effect of continued parasite replication and immune response. Cardiac pathology may be explained as follows: striated cardiac muscle fibres invaded during the early phase caused scars scattered throughout the cardiac muscle. Each scar housed inflammatory immune cells, macrophages, and natural killer immune cells. *T. cruzi* may be absent or in low level. The heart is enlarged. Nerve tissues in the heart, oesophagus, and colon are also lost, resulting in dysfunctions such as arrhythmia and intestinal motility (cause of blockage).

78.5.2.3   Reactivation of Chronic Chagas

There is reactivation of chronic Chagas disease cases due to immunosuppression as in "transplant" and HIV patients. Parasitaemia and resulting myocarditis and meningoencephalitis and deaths occur like in acute phase. A patient may undergo a transplant without knowing that he is suffering with asymptomatic/chronic form of Chagas disease. Similar recurrence may happen in lymphoreticular neoplasias, especially acute lymphocytic leukaemia or Hodgkin's.

78.6   Epidemiology of Chagas Disease

It spreads through stercorarian transmission, which occurs through contact with vectors' faeces, and the biting wound or mucosa requires extraordinary combination of somewhat unlikely events.

78.6.1   Vector

T. cruzi is naturally maintained by 11 native triatomine species and animal reservoirs. Over 130 species of bloodsucking triatomine insects (Figs. 78.1 and 78.2) belonging to the genera *Triatoma*, *Panstrongylus*, and *Rhodnius* act as vectors.

Fig. 78.1 *Rhodnius prolixus* taking a blood meal, and defaecate, Mexico- (Isaisa Montilla, WHO 2020)

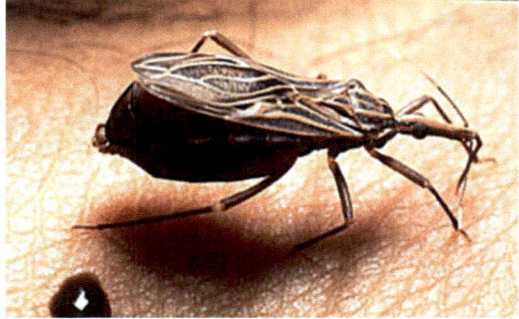

Fig. 78.2 A house colonized with triatomine bugs. Mexico- (Isaisa Montilla, WHO 2020)

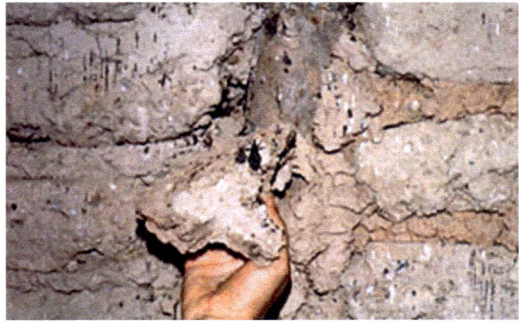

The synanthropic species are important in transmission, and these vary in different geographic locales. In Latin America, *Triatoma infestans*, *T. brasiliensis*, and *Rhodnius prolixus* are epidemiologically important. *T. dimidiate* and *Panstrongylus megistus* colonize peridomestic environments in different regions.

T. cruzi circulates in wild and domestic animals, and Chagas disease occurs exclusively in rural areas. There are two distinct supporting ecological zones: (a) the Southern Cone region (the vector lives in and around human dwellings) and (b) the Central American Mexico (the vector lives inside human dwellings and in uninhabited areas).

78.6.2   Reservoir

All mammals are susceptible to infection, and > 100 mammalian species across Latin America are reservoir hosts. Regional ecology and biology of mammals and vectors and their interaction determine the epidemiology. Opossums, armadillos, marmosets, various rodents, wood rats, raccoons, and bats are important reservoirs and can be infected both by vectors and eating triatomine vectors and infected animals.

78.6.3   Transmission Cycle

The trypanosome is maintained in mammalian host-vector-mammalian host cycle. Stercorarian transmission is relatively inefficient because of the natural barrier like skin and fur of animals to cutaneous penetration of the parasite yet contributed to spill over to domestic fauna.

The bloodsucking triatomine insects get infected with *T. cruzi* while biting infected animal or man. While biting and sucking blood, the insects pass *T. cruzi* in poop which enters the host's body through bite injuries, scratch during rub near the site of bite, and cut in the skin, eyes, and mouth.

The triatomine insects are found in houses that use materials like palm thatch, mud, and straw and hidden in crevices during day. These emerge during night when inhabitants are sleeping and bite, commonly on faces, hence called "kissing bugs".

78.6.4   Spread

Population movement to urban (urbanization) has resulted into most infected people living in urban setting and spread to other countries.

Altered ecology and host behaviour due to man-made environmental imbalance may exacerbate the potential for transmission both oral and vector. The invasion and deforestation of woodlands result in reduction of the biodiversity of mammals available as food sources for triatomines. The species *Triatoma dimidiata*, *Panstrongylus rufotuberculatus*, *Rhodnius stali*, *Eratyrus mucronatus*, and *Panstrongylus geniculatus* have all been reported as being domiciled in urban areas.

Chagas disease is a serious public health problem. Absence of classical symptoms (a skin chagoma or Romaña's sign) in many infected and ignorance about the presence of vector delay diagnosis and treatment. Consequential human sufferings are great. There is increased risk of congenital transmission, intermediate chronic Chagas disease manifesting decades later, and added to these are serious pathology if immunocompromised.

Increasing migration is continuously introducing it to non-endemic areas. In 2010, the 63rd World Health Assembly passed resolution WHA63.20, highlighting the seriousness of Chagas disease in both endemic and non-endemic countries (Andrade et al. 2014). Epidemiological control, efficient diagnosis and treatment, and clinical management are important.

Treatment efficacy of acute cases is around 80%; failure in early diagnosis and treatment leads to the development of chronic form. Given 30% of chronic form will develop severe disease and die, the search for prognostic markers for disease progression is critical (Andrade et al. 2014).

Chagas disease is a complex socioeconomic, environmental (multidimensional) health problem. It has been endemic in Latin America for >9000 years and has spread to non-endemic areas during past decades.

78.6.5 The Endemic Regions

These extend from southern United States to northern Chile and Argentina. Twenty-one countries of Latin America are home to Chagas disease with highest prevalence in Bolivia, Argentina, and Paraguay. The death and infection rates by vector control and screening of blood donation have been reduced from peaks during the 1980s to 2010 and totally in Brazil, Chile, Uruguay, and from most provinces in Argentina. Insecticide resistance in vectors and oral transmission and re-emergence in parts of Venezuela are recent challenges.

78.6.6 Non-endemic Regions

Chagas disease has spread to new areas, mainly the United States and Europe. Nearly 300,000 infected live in the United States. Most (30,000 to 40,000) have cardiopathy, as of 2020. Chagas disease is most common among Latin American immigrants.

Local transmission is possible but locally acquired infections are rare (28 cases during 1955–2015). *Immigration* from Latin America brought Chagas disease to Europe; cases varied with immigration pattern. Spain has 75% of all cases in Europe, followed by Italy, the Netherlands, the United Kingdom, and Germany. It has been reported also from Canada and some African, Eastern Mediterranean, and Western Pacific countries (WHO 2020).

78.7 Symptoms

The symptoms vary with modes of transmission disease.

78.7.1 Vector Bite-Borne

Commonly known vector-bite borne, Chagas disease occurs in two forms:

The *acute form* develops 1–2 weeks after the insect bite. There is parasitaemia. The disease enters into asymptomatic after about 4–8 weeks. The *chronic form* lasts for over many years.

78.7.1.1 Acute Form

It lasts for few weeks to months of infection. There may be no symptoms. Mild cases show fever, fatigue, body aches, headache, rash, loss of appetite, diarrhoea, and vomiting. Such cases may pass undiagnosed. Its characteristic includes swollen nodule on skin "chancre (chagoma)" or on the eyelid unilateral/purplish orbital oedema (Romaña's sign) with local lymphadenopathy and fever.

Symptoms of acute Chagas disease are swelling at the site of bite, headache, myalgia, multiple adenopathy, rashes, painful nodules; oedema, generalized or localized to the face or inferior extremities; dyspnoea; cough; abdominal pain; splenomegaly; myocarditis; and rarely meningoencephalitis.

Severe acute form is rare (1–5%) and can be life-threatening. There is accumulation of fluid (effusion), ascites, pericardial effusion, and inflammation of the heart, brain, and other tissues.

78.7.1.2 Intermediate Chronic Form

Intermediate chronic Chagas disease is detected by the presence of antibodies to *T. cruzi* with few or no parasite in blood.

78.7.1.3 Chronic Form

Chronic Chagas disease appears in the following decades (10–30 years). It lasts for decades to entire life of patients. Nearly 20% to 30% develop complications, like cardiac or gastrointestinal. Cardiopathy may be arrhythmia, myopathy, palpitation, aneurysm, thromboembolism, fainting sometimes, and even heart failure. Digestive lesions include megaoesophagus and megacolon in up to 21% and damage of nerves in 10%.

There is difficulty in swallowing food in megaoesophagus. It may be associated with problems related to acid reflux, dysphagia, cough, and loss of body weight.

Megacolon is manifested as constipation. There may be intestinal blockage or blockage of its blood supply.

Nerve damage caused altered reflexes and movement and numbness.

78.7.2 Congenitally Acquired

Congenital transmission occurs in 1%–10% of children born to infected mothers. Newborns are often asymptomatic. About 10%–40% newborns present mild nonspecific symptoms, low birth weight, low Apgar scores, hepatosplenomegaly, respiratory distress, anasarca, cardiac failure, or meningoencephalitis. Severe cases may die. According to the CDC (2012), estimated 300,000 persons including women with chronic form in the United States had migrated from endemic areas.

A caesarean delivery was performed at 29 weeks of gestation because of foetal hydrops on a 31-year-old mother who had recently moved from Bolivia. The newborn boy had ascites (non-exudative fluid), pleural effusion, and pericardial effusion. He was tested for possible infectious agents but not for trypanosomes and put on antibiotics. It was revealed in the child's second week of life that the mother had Chagas disease at the time of previous pregnancy in Bolivia and had not been treated for it. All antibiotics were stopped. The peripheral blood smear was positive for *T. cruzi*, further confirmed by serological and PCR tests. Clinical investigations revealed only pericardial effusion. A 60-day course of benznidazole resolved ascites and effusions. A follow-up review at his 10 months age found that he was negative to PCR and serological tests.

78.7.3 Blood Transfusion and Transplant Acquired

The presentation is similar to those of vector bite-borne disease, but the symptoms may not manifest for anywhere from a week to 5 months.

Chronically infected individuals who become immunosuppressed can suffer with severe and distinct disease, commonly characterized by inflammation in the brain and surrounding tissue. The size and location of the inflammation in the brain determine the symptoms. Symptoms include fever, headaches, seizures, loss of sensation, and others associated with neurological disorder. Inflammations of other tissues like skin, heart, or gastrointestinal manifest symptoms accordingly.

78.7.4 Oral Transmission (Foodborne)

78.7.4.1 Prevalence

Foodborne Chagas disease caused by *T. cruzi* is an emerging problem documented from 1966. Brazilian Amazon regions recorded 70% foodborne Chagas disease during 2000–2010 (Alarcón et al. 2015). Climate change-related environmental factors probably resulted into a change in the distribution of *Triatoma*, the vector from tropical to temperate areas.

The morbidity, mortality, and socioeconomic impact are high. Foodborne disease is being increasingly reported with control of vectors and blood transfusion-transmitted disease. More than 66% of 73 reports that included 959 acute cases were oral-transmitted and rest congenital and vector-borne.

In foodborne Chagas disease, the contaminating metacyclic trypomastigotes may be available in the vector triatomine insects' faeces, whole insects, or secretions of reservoir hosts such as opossum. It is therefore relevant in endemic countries.

78.7.4.2 Infection: Bite Vs Oral

The insects rapidly defecate following feeding. Frequency of defecation following biting is important for transmission. *P. geniculatus* is the most widely distributed species in the Americas. The small-sized immature forms (nymphs) are common in homes. These are suitable for foodborne transmission, but not for cutaneous vector-borne transmission (Robertson et al. 2016).

Infection progressing to morbidity is more efficient in foodborne transmission. The morbidity and mortality in early stages of foodborne infections are high as compared to vector-borne.

Higher parasite load and more efficient entry through stomach mucosa are possible reasons. *T. infestans* can harbour 684,000 infective trypomastigotes and can infect hundreds by the oral route. The triatomine faeces perhaps contain 3000–4000 metacyclic trypomastigotes per µl. In vector-bite form of infection, only a proportion of this succeeds in penetrating the epidermis. The gp82, stage-specific surface glycoprotein is expressed and binds to gastric mucin and epithelial cells triggering the signalling cascades leading to intracellular Ca^{2+} mobilization and promoting parasite's entry.

78.7.4.3 Vehicles/Foods

Common vehicles are drinks, such as fruit juice. Contamination occurs most likely during processing. The protozoan parasite does not multiply in foods. Tracing back to detect the critical point the parasite made, an entry in the incriminated food is difficult.

Outbreaks of chagas disease due to the consumption of contaminated fruit, palm wine or sugar cane juice, sugar cane, and açaí palm have frequently been reported from Brazil, Colombia, and Venezuela. There are more severe acute morbidity and higher morbidity.

Drying, low moisture content of food, heating but not freezing, and refrigeration inactivate metacyclic trypomastigotes. Risk management includes good food hygiene, pasteurization (of açaí pulp, palm pulp), and cooking, especially in areas with triatomine bugs.

78.7.4.4 Symptoms

Numbness and altered reflexes or movement appear within 3 weeks (5–22 days) of consumption of contaminated food or drink. Other symptoms include fever, gastric irritation, bloody diarrhoea, and jaundice. The patients report pain in the abdomen and muscle. There may be chest pain, shortness of breath, and cough. There is prolonged high fever in 80–100% cases. Cardiac pathology is more frequent and severe.

Consequential severe myocarditis and meningeal irritation occur in many patients. Many die, and average CFR is 7.1%, which may go up to 35.2%.

78.8   Diagnosis

- In early stage, finding the parasite in the blood, buffy coat, or smear (34–85%) of instances.
- PCR detects even low level of parasites.
- Chronic disease is diagnosed by serological tests to detect antibodies to *T. cruzi* in the blood. The tests are ELISA, indirect immunofluorescence (immunohisto-chemistry for tissues), and indirect haemagglutination.
- Western blot.
- Xenodiagnosis: Triatomine insects are made to feed on person's blood; 30–60 days later, faeces are examined. Test is slow and less sensitive.
- Blood culture.
- Animal inoculation.

78.9   Treatment

Early infections are treatable with the medications with benznidazole or nifurtimox.

In chronic disease, medication may delay or prevent the development of end-stage symptoms.

Fexinidazole has shown activity against Chagas disease in animal models and has been approved for treating African trypanosomiasis.

Drugs and vaccines are under various stages of trial.

78.10   Prevention and Control

Depending upon geographical area, the WHO (2020) recommended the following:

- Spraying of houses and surrounding areas with residual insecticides.
- House improvements and house cleanliness to prevent vector infestation.
- Personal preventive measures such as bed nets.
- Good hygiene practices in food preparation, transportation, storage, and consumption.
- Screening of blood donors and testing of organ, tissue, or cell donors and receivers.
- Access to diagnosis and treatment of people with medical indication or recom-mendation to do anti-parasitic treatment, especially children and women of child-bearing age before pregnancy.
- Screening of newborn and other children of infected mothers without previous antiparasitic treatment to do early diagnosis and provide treatment.

The cost of spraying residual insecticide to control vectors and prevent infection is cheaper (<80%) than the medical cost of patients with chronic cardiac, digestive, neurologic, or mixed forms of the disease.

To attain the goal of elimination of Chagas disease transmission and provide health care for infected or people suffering from the disease, both in endemic and non-endemic territories, the WHO aims to increase networking at the global level and reinforce regional and national capacities, focusing on the following:

- Strengthening world epidemiological surveillance and information systems.
- Raising awareness about Chagas disease and affected populations.
- Preventing transmission by blood transfusion and organ transplantation.
- Promoting the identification of most adequate diagnostic tests and algorithms/ protocols to increase screening and diagnosis of infections.
- Expanding primary prevention of congenital transmission and case management of congenital and non-congenital infections.
- Promoting consensus on adequate updated case management.
- Promoting the development of multidimensional approaches.

References

Alarcón de Noya B, Noya O, Robertson LJ (2015) *Trypanosoma cruzi* as a foodborne patho- gen *springer briefs in food, health and nutrition.* Springer, New York, Heidelberg, Dordrecht, London. ISBN: 978-3-319-23409-0

Andrade DV, Gollob KJ, Dutra WO (2014) Acute Chagas disease: new global challenges for an old neglected disease. PLoS Negl Trop Dis 8(7):e3010

CDC (2012). Centres for disease control and prevention. Congenital transmission of Chagas dis- ease — Virginia, 2010. MMWR 2012; 61 (26 July 6, 2012)

Fernandes MC, Flannery AR, Andrews N, Mortara RA (2013) Extracellular amastigotes of *Trypanosoma cruzi* are potent inducers of phagocytosis in mammalian cells. Cell Microbiol 15(6):977–991

Robertson LJ, Devleesschauwer B, Alarcón de Noya B, Noya González O, Torgerson PR (2016) *Trypanosoma cruzi*: time for international recognition as a foodborne parasite. PLoS Negl Trop Dis 10(6):e0004656

WHO (2020). Chagas disease (also known as American trypanosomiasis) 11 March 2020. https:// www.who.int/news-room/fact-sheets/detail/chagas-disease-(american-trypanosomiasis)

Chapter 79
Cryptosporidiosis

Cryptosporidiosis is a highly infectious enteric disease of human caused by pathogenic spp. of protozoa of *Cryptosporidium* genus. It is characterized by watery diarrhoea, similar to cholera. It is an amphixenosis. It affects all age group, mainly children below 5 years of age, and diarrhoea is persistent. Consequential malnourishment may lead to cognitive and fitness problems persisting for years. Cryptosporidiosis in children in developing countries is a serious disease. It causes persistent and life-threatening diarrhoea among immunocompromised/immunodeficient persons.

According to Helmy and Hafez (2022), the World Health Organization's "Neglected Disease Initiative" includes *Cryptosporidium* and *Giardia*. There is no effective chemotherapeutic agent for treatment of cryptosporidiosis. Therefore, effective preventive measures only can reduce prevalence. Specific identification based on genotyping and understanding transmission is important. Innes et al. (2020) discuss the burden of cryptosporidiosis and suggest one health approach for managing it. The disability-adjusted life years lost in children <5 years are estimated at 4.2 million, long sequence, cognitive defects, and retarded growth. Cryptosporidia cause major diarrhoeal disease in neonatal calves and other animals, leading to loss in form of death, production loss and cost of diagnosis, treatment, supportive therapies, etc.

79.1 Aetiology

A protozoan identified in 1907 in the stomach of mice was named *Cryptosporidium* in 1912. There are 18 valid species of *Cryptosporidium* family *Cryptosporidiidae*, order *Eucoccidiorida*, subclass *Coccidiasina*, class *Sporozoasida*, and phylum *Apicomplexa*. There are more than 157 mammalian species listed as hosts for *Cryptosporidium* infection (Helmy and Hafez 2022).

Morphological similarities between the species make molecular genotyping important for precise differentiation. Molecular analyses have now identified 22 *Cryptosporidium* spp. and > 40 cryptic species (i.e. genotypes) across all vertebrate classes. According to Cacciò (2005), *C. parvum* and *C. hominis* (syn. *C. parvum* anthroponotic genotype or genotype 1) are the most common and of great public health concern as >90% of human infections are caused by these. The genotype 1 is found almost exclusively in humans, while the type 2 infects humans and various mammalian species.

C. bovis, C. suis, C. scrofarum, C. tyzzeri, C. erinacei, C. andersoni, C. canis, C. muris, C. felis, C. baileyi, C. meleagridis, C. viatorum, C. cuniculus, C. ubiquitum, chipmunk genotype I, *Cryptosporidium* horse, *Cryptosporidium* mink genotype, and *C. parvum* are considered zoonotic species. *C. felis* has been found in faeces of cats, cows, and human patients. *C. parvum* includes a complex of subspecies that specifically infect cattle, pigs, kangaroos, ferrets, or monkeys. The frequency of *Cryptosporidium* spp. crossing the host barrier and becoming zoonoses seems great. *C. hominis* is maintained by human-to-human transmission cycle mostly in urban settings. *C. parvum* affects pre-weaned calves and also human beings mostly in rural settings.

On the basis of GP60 sequence typing of 115 isolates, Chalmers et al. (2008) concluded that the strains of *C. hominis* in the United Kingdom appeared to be highly conserved. Of the nine subtypes identified, the IbA10G2 predominated and was significantly linked to recent travel outside Europe. The subtype family Ib is the predominant *C. hominis* allele associated with waterborne outbreaks, occurs worldwide, and seems to be predominant in human sewage.

The surface antigen, glycoprotein 60 (GP60), was used to study 37 *C. hominis* and 32 *C. parvum* isolates from cases of cryptosporidiosis in New South Wales, Australia. Isolates were distributed into families and 24 different subtypes. It was concluded that the identified subtypes had a global distribution and anthroponotic and zoonotic transmission contributed to sporadic cryptosporidiosis in NSW (Waldron et al. 2009). According to Ryan et al. (2021), there are 44 recognized *Cryptosporidium* species, and > 120 genotypes, 19 species, and 4 genotypes have been reported in humans with *C. hominis, C. parvum, C. meleagridis, C. canis,* and *C. felis* being the most prevalent. They suggested whole-genome sequencing (WGS) and amplicon next-generation sequencing (NGS) for specific identification and more accurate tracking of transmission. This should help in understanding the mechanisms behind host specificity also.

79.2   Life Cycle

There are two types of oocysts of *Cryptosporidium*.

A. Thick-walled, survive (e.g. −10 °C for 7 days) and persist in environment for months, many disinfectants, chlorine-based, in particular.

B. Thin-walled oocysts are about 20%. The thin-walled oocysts break open in the intestine during passage releasing sporozoites to reinvade more epithelial cells. These may also invade epithelia of biliary and respiratory tracts.

Upon infection, oocysts excyst, and four sporozoites are released. These attach to microvilli and brush border on the surface of epithelial cells of the small intestine and become trophozoites. Trophozoites reproduce asexually by multiple fission, a process known as schizogony. Trophozoites develop into two: Type 1 meronts contain eight daughter cells called type I merozoites which are released by meronts. *Some of these merozoites* cause autoinfection attach epithelial cells. *Other merozoites* become type 2 meronts. These contain type II merozoites which after release from meronts attach epithelial cells. These may become microgametes and macrogametes. Gametogenesis takes place by the fusion of microgametes and macrogametes. Zygotes are formed after gametogony. Zygotes develop into two types of oocysts, thick-walled and thin-walled. The predominantly thick-walled oocysts are expelled with faeces 2 weeks after the symptoms have ceased to contaminate environment and infect other hosts. Long-time asymptomatic carriage is reported.

79.3 Pathogenesis

There is no defined laboratory animal model. Therefore, knowledge about host-parasite relationship is sketchy. *C. muris* parasitizes fundic areas in stomach mucosa as observed by Certad et al. (2007) in their adult severe combined immunodeficient (SCID) mice model. They also observed *C. parvum* causing cystic polyps and intraepithelial neoplasia and intramucosal adenocarcinoma in dexamethasone-treated SCID mice.

The process of host cell penetration and inclusion is not fully understood. Sporozoites are equipped with secretary apical organelles, such as rhoptries, micronemes, and dense granules each designed for invading host cell by modifying host cells and providing anchor sites for cell adhesion. *Cryptosporidium* is able to rearrange host cell skeleton with actin-polymerizing factors to embrace them with a host cell-derived membrane. The parasite hides, proliferates, and differentiates in parasitophorous vacuole membrane under the brush border which is connected to the host cells to protect itself from hostile gut environment yet getting nutrients and energy through feeder organelle (Sunnotel et al. 2006).

Cryptosporidium sporozoite antigens trigger both antibody and cell-mediated responses in an immune response in immunocompetent mammals.

79.4 Pathology

The parasite has intracellular and extra-cytoplasmic location in the host's intestine, mainly jejunum and ileum. The pathogenic process and pathology are not well understood. A combination of increased permeability of intestinal cells, chloride secretion, and malabsorption (of fluids and electrolytes) and also damage due to intracellular replication and development of the parasite may explain the pathology. Histopathological changes seen are villous atrophy, flattening of the epithelium, increased lymphocytes in the lamina propria, and infiltration of lymphocytes, plasma cells, and neutrophils. Narayan (2004) summed up the then available information as (a) displacement of brush border mainly of the ileum (entire intestine in neonates and immunocompromised hosts); (b) disruption of membrane-bound enzymic functions, such as glucose-coupled Na-transport enzymes, sucrase, and lactase secretions; (c) loss of vacuolated villus tips; (d) increased macrophages; (e) reduced xylose and B12 absorption; and (f) disruption of intestinal barrier functions (secondary infection is facilitated). Speculated mechanisms are (1) enterotoxin- and (2) prostaglandin-dependent secretory effect. Subsequent described pathology reviewed by Helmy and Hafez (2022) described epithelial cell degeneration, metaplasia villus epithelium, hyperplastic crypt epithelium, and displacement of microvilli in the infected host in the zone of intracellular parasitic attachment, the pathology causing reduction in intestinal absorption and consequent malabsorption. The activity of brush border membrane enzymes is impacted resulting into reduction of carbohydrate digestion, osmotic diarrhoea, and impeding water resorption.

79.5   Clinical Disease

The incubation period is 5–21, average 10 days in immunocompetent people. It is a self-limiting disease. The disease is characterized by watery diarrhoea associated with one or all of the following: dehydration, stomach-ache, nausea, vomiting, flatulence, fatigue, anorexia, and fever as well as symptoms like cramp, abdominal pain, intermittent and scant or continuous watery copious diarrhoea, sometimes great fluid loss, dehydration, low-grade fever in about 30–60%, nausea and vomiting in 50% lasting for 3–12 days, and cough and short breath. Respiratory symptoms are associated with inhalation of oocysts from contaminated air. Asymptomatic cases also occur. Duration of illness varies between few days and a month or so. It is short (1–2 weeks) in immunocompetent individuals. In some, there may be recurrence of symptoms for a brief period and such events last for a month. Most commonly invaded tissues are the small intestine, and the parasite may invade other parts of the digestive system (gall bladder, biliary duct) also, besides respiratory and possibly conjunctiva.

The immunocompromised individuals such as HIV-infected, transplant, and cancer cases and those on immunosuppressive drugs suffer with serious disease that may even be fatal and chronic (especially in cases with CD4 counts <200/micro litre). Infection in AIDS patients may cause persistent diarrhoea and complications like malabsorption and biliary tract infection. T-cell-mediated immunity seems to be central (Morales et al. 2004). Stool may be bulky and foul-smelling; there may be high fluid loss (15 l/d), significant weight loss, and biliary tract involvement may result in acalculous cholecystitis, sclerosing cholangitis, or pancreatitis. Respiratory infection may manifest as bilateral infiltration. According to Rao Ajjampur et al. (2007), cryptosporidiosis caused by *C. hominis* or zoonotic spp. *C. parvum* was important cause of morbidity in HIV-positive Indians. It caused chronic diarrhoea, fever, and nausea.

79.6   Epidemiology

Human cryptosporidiosis is a global public health problem affecting young, elderly, immunocompromised, and immunocompetent persons residing in both industrialized and developing nations.

Cryptosporidia are most prevalent in Africa. Anthroponotic transmission predominates in a landscape of generally extensive and pastoral husbandry. There are also human-adapted subtypes that seem to be transmitted without animal involvement (Robertson et al. 2020).

According to Helmy and Hafez (2022), diarrheal diseases have caused up to 1.6 million deaths worldwide every year. One-third of these deaths have been reported in children less than 5 years due to contaminated drinking water and poor hygiene. *Cryptosporidium* is responsible for up to 20% of all cases of diarrhoea in children in developing countries and fatal complications in HIV-infected persons. Neonatal infection is high because of their immature immune system, and they can become infected by ingestion of low doses of the parasite's oocysts. Over eight million food-borne illness worldwide per year is caused by *Cryptosporidium*. Rural and urban slums present risk of transmission and spread of cryptosporidiosis.

Although >95% of human *Cryptosporidium* infections are caused by multiple subtypes of *C. hominis* and *C. parvum*, many other species are potential human pathogens.

The oocysts are resistant to adverse environmental conditions such as salinity and the presence of chemicals. These survive outside the host for several months and retain infectivity. The epidemiology is complex. Transmission cycles are multiple. Conventional criteria based on morphology of oocysts fail to identify species. Only molecular methods can distinguish these species, genotypes, and subtypes.

79.6.1   Prevalence

Since first reported human infection in 1976, cryptosporidiosis has been reported throughout the world. With the recognition of AIDS, it became important as a complicating agent. It is a notifiable disease in the United States and European Union.

Prevalence rate commonly determined by faecal examination was 1–3% in developed and 7–8.5% in developing countries. In developed countries, seroprevalence was 25–35% compared to 64% in developing countries. Cryptosporidiosis accounts for 5–10% of acute diarrhoeal diseases in developing countries and 8% of acute food poisoning outbreaks in the United States. An estimated annual case report 748,000 cryptosporidiosis occurs in the United States. There has been a more than threefold rise since 2004.

Cryptosporidiosis is the leading cause of diarrhoea (moderate-to-severe diarrhoea and less-severe diarrhoea) in children globally. There were 2.9–4.7 million cryptosporidiosis cases among children of <2 years of age in sub-Saharan Africa and South Asia (Kotloff et al. 2013; Sow et al. 2016).

According to Semenza and Nichols (2007), there were 7960 cryptosporidiosis cases reported in 16 countries; crude incidence rate was 1.9 cases/lac in 2005 with peak incidence in autumn (August–November accounted for 59% cases); spring and summer were the peak seasons in Northwest England, Ireland, and Spain. In 2001 in England, 97% *C. parvum*, 1% *C. meleagridis*, 0.2% *C. felis*, and < 0.1% *Cryptosporidium* dog type were observed; however, greater proportion of non-*C. parvum* species and both types of *C. parvum* occur in immunocompromised cases (Pedraza-Diaz et al. 2001). It is prevalent both in man and in animals in Indian states and Bangladesh (Narayan 2004).

79.6.2   Source

Infected human, cattle, and sheep shed very high number of oocysts, especially when infected early in life, and contribute to environmental contribution. There may be 3–23% symptomless shedders. A patient begins shedding oocysts 5 days after infection. The infectious stage (sporulated oocyst) of *Cryptosporidium* is excreted in large numbers (10^{10}) in the faeces and continues shedding for 50 days after cessation of diarrhoea. Overcrowding, poverty, and disaster contribute to infection.

79.6.2.1   Environment

Cryptosporidia may be found in soil, water, municipal water supply, foods, and articles contaminated with infected faeces. Natural disasters (storms, earth erosions, floods) often damage overall sanitation including water supply.

79.6.2.2   Water

Issac-Renton et al. (1999) reported association of contaminated community water supply with epidemic diagnosed by serological testing of 1944 sera. While deep water samples were negative, surface water from possibly unprotected watershed were positive.

Discharges of treated and untreated sewage and run-off of manure contaminate surface water and also impact groundwater. Rivers and lakes receive treated and untreated domestic waste water and agricultural run-off discharge.

Irrigation with contaminated water and manure and infected food handlers contaminate foods like raw vegetables, salads, raw milk, fermented milk, meat, oysters, shell fish, and farm-made apple cider, implicated in outbreaks.

79.6.2.3 Food

Macarisin et al. (2010) detected *C. parvum* oocysts strongly adhered to spinach plants, infiltrating into leaves through stomatal openings, such that washings possibly would fail to dislodge.

79.6.2.4 Hands

Commonly, hands get contaminated by a variety of activities that demand touching contaminated surfaces, like changing diapers, caring infected person, plumbing, and handling of infected animals by farmers, veterinarians, hunters, sweepers, vaccinators, debeaking staff, and others responsible for direct and indirect transmission.

The infection cycle follows the oral-faecal route. Infection is acquired by swallowing of contaminated water—drinking/recreational beverages—raw vegetables and fruits, and uncooked food. Autoinfection and horizontal spread from person to person occur.

79.6.3 Transmission (Fig. 79.1)

- Direct contact with infected human (human-human)—as in hospitals, day care centres, schools, and anal sex.
- Water (pristine, ground, surface, large rivers, lakes) to human through drinking, swimming, recreation, and irrigation.
- Ingestion of contaminated food, like contaminated fruits and vegetables.
- Inhalation of oocysts from contaminated air with aerosolized droplets or fomites.
- Zoonotic transmission from animals (wild, domestic, pet) to human while handling infected dogs, cats, rodents, wild animals, dirty shoes, clothes. *C. parvum* is the most prevalent species in calves up to 8 weeks old, while *C. bovis* is dominant in calves ranging between 2 and 11 months of age.
- Synanthropic insects like flies, cockroaches, and beetles, as mechanical spreader to human.

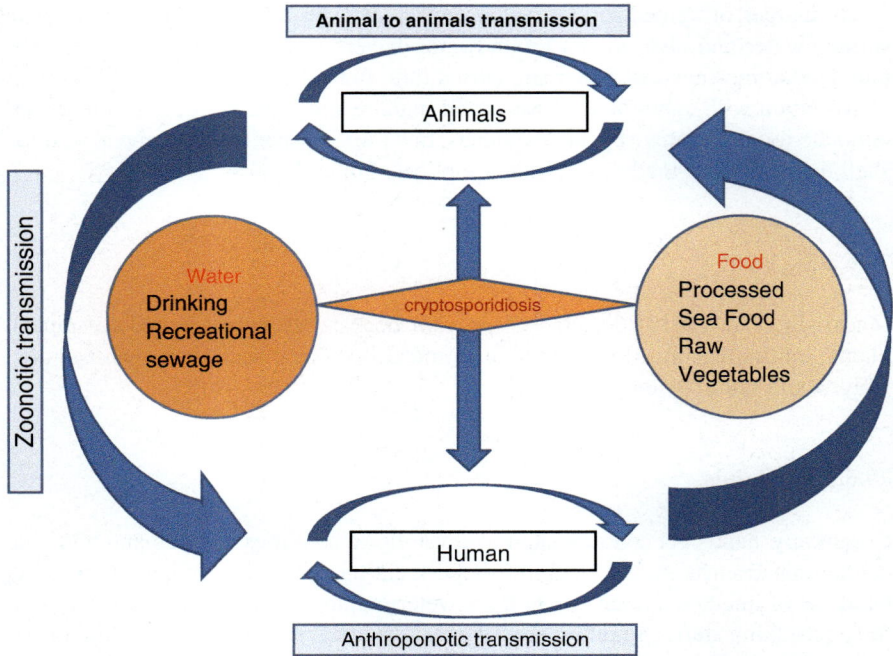

Fig. 79.1 Transmission of *Cryptosporidium* spp.

79.6.4   Epidemiological Factors

79.6.4.1   Risk Factors

According to FAO/WHO (2014), of the waterborne, human-to-human, and zoonotic transmission, foodborne transmission of cryptosporidiosis is less common. It is about 8% of the domestically acquired cases in the United States.

Fresh foods are generally implicated—green onions, sandwich bar ingredients, parsley, carrots, red peppers, lettuce, and chicken salad. Infected food handlers were responsible in some cases. In the United Kingdom, an outbreak caused by precut bagged salad products affected some 300 people in 2012. Outbreaks were caused by drinking unpasteurized apple cider and milk.

Worldwide survey reported contamination with oocysts of *Cryptosporidium* of a wide variety of fresh food items including aquatic foods—gills and tissues of oysters, molluscan shell fish, clams, cockles, and mussels.

79.6.4.2 Agent

The WHO (2009) listed characteristics of *Cryptosporidium* that make it the most dangerous waterborne pathogen. These are high infectivity; infective dose of 10^1–10^3 oocysts, presumably even one; wide range of hosts (human and livestock, pets, and wild animals); high excretal shedding; thick- and thin-walled oocysts being infective; persistence in environment; and resistance to chemical disinfectants (cresylic acid 3%, hypochlorite 2–5%, benzalkonium chloride 5%, sodium hydroxide 0.02 M). There are large percentage of (3.0 – 40.0%) samples of treated drinking water were positive, and the number of oocysts ranged from 0.001 to 1.5 per litre.

79.6.4.3 Host

Males experience higher rate of infection possibly related with professional exposure such as contact with infected animals, poor hygiene, age (> 75 years), immune and transplant status, and recreational activities like swimming, hiking, and camping.

79.6.4.4 Weather

Warm and humid months appear to be favourable, prevalence high during end of rainy season. Outbreaks are most commonly waterborne (recreational, pool, drinking, etc.) and reported during and post summer. The secondary attack rate is high.

79.6.4.5 Outbreak Settings

Cryptosporidiosis epidemics occur in two different settings, urban and urban slum/ endemic.

– *Urban Setting.*

The Milwaukee (Wisconsin) waterborne outbreak was linked to drinking water. The Utah outbreak affected the community but drinking water was rule out as the cause. Recreational water and venue were associated. Childcare centres and contact with patients resulted into infection.

– *Urban Slum and Endemic.*

Newman et al. (1994) conducted an epidemiological study in 31 households in the setting of an urban slum of Fortaleza City in Brazil, where cryptosporidiosis is endemic. Forty-five per cent of index cases had persistent diarrhoea for >14 days. Fifty-eight per cent of secondary cases were identified. Cryptococcus was detected in 18 (58%) with an overall 19% of secondary transmission. Of 202 persons in the study, 94.6% had IgM/IgG antibodies to *Cryptosporidium*. 25% secondary cases had diarrhoea and 25% had persistent diarrhoea.

During a period of 12 months, one student experienced three times infection with *C. parvum* while working with heavily infected calves. The first resulted in severe watery diarrhoea lasting for 9 days. Four and ten months, later he had second and third exposures which were no more than a minor bowel upset with a soft stool for 2–3 days (Current 1994).

Korpe et al. (2019) carried case-control study in urban and rural communities in Bangladesh using molecular genotyping. The person-to-person transmission with the same subspecies of *Cryptosporidium* within families was high in young children of urban communities, suggesting secondary attack rate. The secondary attack rate in urban communities was 35.8% compared to 7.8% in rural.

Ayers Hutter et al. (2020) reported a total of 201 cases of cryptosporidiosis were notified in Québec, Canada, during a 2-year period (January 1, 2016, to December 31, 2017). The end of summer had the maximum cases. Adjusted rates were available for Nunavik, in the north of Québec. Higher incidence was observed among females (20–34 years) than in males. The number of cases in both sexes peaked twice, the first among children <5 years and the second between 20 and 30 years of age. *C. hominis* was the cause for 23% and *C. parvum* for 74% as revealed by molecular typing. Subtyping detected gp60 sequencing. All *C. parvum* subtypes belonged to the IIa family, and *C. hominis* belonged to Ia, Ib, and Id families.

79.6.5   Zoonotic Cryptosporidiosis

Anthroponotic transmission predominates in a landscape of generally extensive and pastoral husbandry. There are also human-adapted subtypes that seem to be transmitted without animal involvement (Robertson et al. 2020). According to the OIE (2022), *C. hominis* is considered to be anthroponotic, rarely detected in animals, possibly due to human activity. *C. parvum* is the main zoonotic species. Cryptosporidia are most prevalent in Africa.

79.6.5.1   Cryptosporidia Species

The most significant zoonotic threat for humans is from *C. parvum* and *C. meleagridis*. Additional zoonotic species are *C. andersoni*, *C. suis*, *C. canis*, *C. felis*, and *C. muris* and genotypes cervine, skunk, chipmunk genotype 1, and *C. hominis* genotype monkey. Two *Cryptosporidium* genotypes can infect humans and may be linked to clinical disease both in immunocompetent and immunocompromised individuals (Cacciò 2005). Waterfowls and insects (flies) are suggested vectors.

Bovine cryptosporidiosis: The prevalence may be as high as 100%. It tends to decrease with age. *C. parvum* is common in calves up to 8 weeks of age while *C. bovis* in 2–11 months of age (Helmy and Hafez 2022).

Companion animal cryptosporidiosis: Santin and Trout (2008) described the role of companion animals—dogs, cats, and horses—as possible source of zoonotic cryptosporidiosis. Cat cryptosporidiosis was first reported in 1979 in Japan and has since then been found to have a worldwide prevalence of 0–12% based on conventional diagnosis. *C. parvum*, *C. felis*, and *C. muris* have been identified—the latter two have been confirmed also by molecular studies in naturally infected cats. *C. parvum* has been found to infect domestic cats experimentally. *Cryptosporidium* infection in dogs was identified in 1981—the clinical cases detected 2 years later. The worldwide infection ranges between 0.23% and 40%. Genotyping of 36 isolates identified 26 *C. canis*, 1 *C. meleagridis*, and 9 *C. parvum*. All are pathogenic to man but the first two infect primarily dogs and birds, respectively. The dog genotype was designated as new species *C. canis* in 2001 on the basis of genomic and cross-transmission studies. Further genomic studies reported 30 asymptomatic human infection with *C. canis* in England both in immunocompetent and immunocompromised. The first *Cryptosporidium* infection identified was in five immunodeficient Arabian foals. Since then, it is known to occur worldwide with a prevalence rate of 1–47%. *C. parvum* has been identified on the basis of the size of oocyst as the cause of diarrhoea in foals. Of the four molecular studies, three reported *C. parvum* and the fourth a novel *Cryptosporidium* horse genotype besides *C. parvum*.

Prevalence of shedders among cats and dogs has been reported variously. According to Abe et al. (2002), prevalence of oocyst shedders varied from 2 to 15%, up to 20% in stray dogs. In cats, Abe et al. (2002) reported simultaneous infection in brother, sister, and a dog with *C. canis* in longitudinal cohort diarrhoea study in Peru, Lima. The dog was asymptomatic.

According to the WHO (2009), the prevalence of *C. felis* was 2.4–8.2% in cats and 1.5–45% of *C. canis* in dogs. Cryptosporidia from dogs and cats usually do not infect human beings except those who are immunodeficient/immunocompromised. Transmission of cattle genotype, *C. parvum*, however occurs. The prevalence in sheep and goats were 10–78% and 28–100%, respectively. Most commonly infected were lambs of 1–2 weeks and kids of 5–15 days age.

Wildlife species: *C. fayeri* was isolated from faeces of a 29-year-old woman suffering with prolonged gastrointestinal illness. The woman resided in national forest on the east coast of New South Wales where marsupials abound, and *C. fayeri* has been isolated from six marsupial species (Waldron et al. 2010). This raises concern on the main water supply for Sydney, Warragamba Dam. This dam covers 9050 km^2 and is surrounded by national forest inhabited by diverse and abundant marsupials (Fig. 79.2).

Other species: *C. viotorum*, *C. tyzzeri* (previously mouse genotype 1), *C. ubiquitum* (previously cervine genotype), *C. scrofarum* (previously pig genotype II), *C. sciurinum* (syn. Ferret genotype), and *C. occultus* are zoonotic species, rarely or occasionally reported from human.

Transmission of *Cryptosporidium*

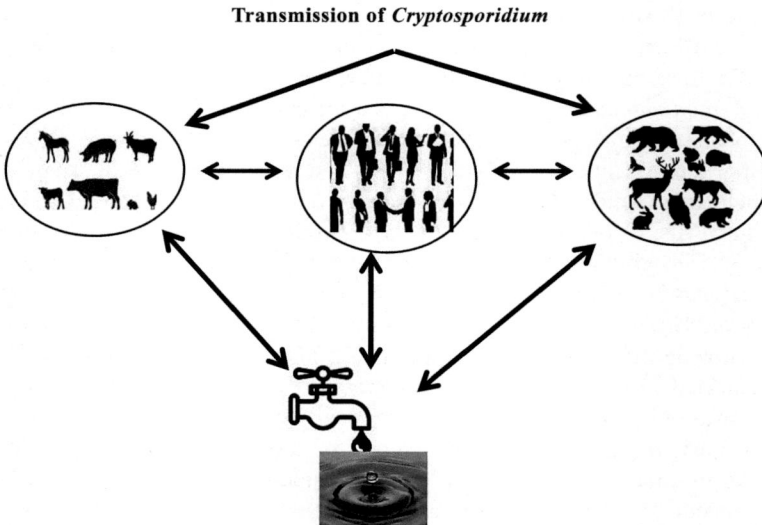

Fig. 79.2 Transmission of *Cryptosporidium* spp.

79.7 Epidemics/Outbreaks

Helmy and Hafez (2022) summed up the outbreak in human.

The 1993 in Milwaukee outbreak caused an estimated 403,000 people affected, 4400 hospitalizations, and more than 100 deaths. The outbreaks between 2009 and 2017 resulted in 7465 infected cases with 287 hospitalizations and 1 death.

Milwaukee outbreak was linked to drinking water. 156 outbreaks between 2009 and 2017 were caused by swimming pool water and water parks. During the same period, 12.8% of outbreaks were linked to contact with infected persons in childcare settings and 14.6% linked to contact with cattle. Among the 22 foodborne outbreaks, 40.9% were linked to unpasteurized milk, and 18.2% were linked to unpasteurized apple cider.

The most predominant identified *C. hominis* during the past 10 years were subtype IfA12G1 in the United States; IbA10G2 in the United Kingdom, Sweden, and Australia; and IbA9G2 in French Guiana and Germany. The most predominant identified *C. parvum* subtype was IIaA15G2R1 in the United States and the United Kingdom and IIaA19G1R1 in Norway. *C. parvum* subtype IIa caused the majority (64.3%) of foodborne outbreaks followed by IId (35.7%). These subtypes are common in livestock. The link between cattle cryptosporidiosis and foodborne outbreaks is suggested.

According to Rolfs et al. (2008), during 2004 and 2006–2007, the CDC reported 719 and 26 outbreaks, respectively. A sudden spurt in cryptosporidiosis cases in all localities between May 23 and December 19, 2007 (an increase by 143% from 2004), was reported to Utah Department of Health. It was a community cryptosporidiosis. The median age of patients was 9 years (range < 1 year to 101 years). Patients aged <5 years constituted 32%. Females accounted for 51%. The overall rate of incidence was 411.8/lac person-years among <5 years. The incidence peaked during the week beginning of August 19.

The distribution of exposure: 80% to recreational water venues (all chlorine-sanitized) within 14 days of the onset of illness; 33% to multiple water venues; 43% had exposure to both –water venue and contact with patients, 37% had exposure to recreational water venue only; 12% had exposure to patients only; 7% had exposure to childcare centres.

Drinking water as source was ruled out.

Plutzer et al. (2019) reported an outbreak related to treated recreational water at a hotel in Somogy County, Hungary. Paediatric organ transplant patients (n = 49) and their families were staying on a residential rehabilitation holiday. There were 35 cases (23 probable and 12 laboratory-confirmed) among 191 attendees in outbreak of June 2015. The overall attack rate was 18%. The odd ratio for swimming in the children's swimming pool was 7.17 and using jetted whirlpool was 5.25. Most of the cases were transplanted children who suffered with acute diarrhoea and required adjustment to their tacrolimus immunosuppression.

79.8   Diagnosis

Clinical cases, especially in AIDS patients and suspected bile duct infection, require imaging. Dilated or irregular intrahepatic and extrahepatic bile ducts and thickened gall bladder seen on abdominal ultrasonography are indicative of cryptosporidial infection. Endoscopic retrograde cholangiopancreatography (ERCP) shows sclerosing cholangitis or papillary stenosis. Examination of bile or biopsy should reveal oocysts to confirm.

Laboratory diagnostic methods have been described in an OIE Terrestrial Manual (2008).

The diagnosis of cryptosporidiosis depends upon demonstration of oocysts, cryptosporidial antigens and cryptosporidial DNA in faeces, bronchial lavage, etc. However, species and subtype identification require molecular methods. These are useful to confirm cryptosporidiosis, identify causative species in less time, and consequently facilitate early action to prevent further exposure.

- Faeces Examination.

Preservation of stool specimen may be done in 2.5% potassium dichromate or 10% formalin. The oocysts are rendered inactive. Such a specimen needs to be washed thrice with deionized water to remove potassium dichromate for DNA analysis. Smears may be air dried and fixed in absolute methanol for examination later.

Faeces examination requires concentration techniques like Sheather's sugar solution (1.18)/zinc sulphate (1.2)/sodium chloride (1.27 specific gravity). Examination may be done by

a) Nomarski differential interference contrast microscopy.
b) Staining—using Ziehl-Nielsen/Kinyoun acid fast staining.

Repeated examination is required as shedding is not continuous:

- Histological examination of intestinal tissue collected at post-mortem.
- Serological tests for detection of coproantigens are useful for sero-epidemiological studies may be done using IFAT and ELISA. Commercial kits are available for IFT (use FITC-C-Mabs) and also for ELISA.
- Lateral flow immunochromatography (IC) has 98–100% specificity (OIE Terrestrial Manual 2008).

Colostral antibodies interfere in the diagnosis of calf cryptosporidiosis. Direct microscopy, most tinctorial and fluorescent stains, and also detection of antigens by ELISA or IC are relatively less but useful in clinical cases. Sensitivity of Kinyoun and modified ZN is up to 10^6 oocysts in unconcentrated faecal smear. Most antigen-capture ELISA and ICs can detect antigen when oocysts in faeces are 3×10^5 to 10^6 /ml. Concentration of faecal specimens increased the threshold of detection. The OIE document (OIE 2022) describes the laboratory methods in detail.

- Molecular diagnostics: These can distinguish species, genotypes, and subtypes to elucidate the complex transmission of *Cryptosporidium*.

Molecular detection included analysis of 18S rRNA and one more locus suitable for both species identification and further subtyping such as GP60 sequencing and analysis of double-stranded RNA element. More discriminatory fingerprinting methods for detecting genotypes/subtypes are PCR-RFPL of ssu rRNA gene and dual TaqMan assays. The latter (Jothikumar et al. 2008) is a real-time PCR TaqMan assay for rapid detection and identification of *C. hominis* and *C. parvum* in stool specimens with 94% specificity. The generic assay detects 1–10 oocysts in 300 microl of stool, and specific assay identifies the species (24/31 *C. hominis*, 21/24 *C. parvum* in the experiment, and 66/67 of either or both in outbreak study in the United States and Botswana).

It is claimed that Cryptonet (CryptoNet_fact_sheet508c) improves detection, investigation, and waterborne zoonotic and person-to-person transmission and foodborne cryptosporidiosis outbreaks. Geographical and temporal changes in distribution are elucidated. It is useful in identifying traditional and novel epidemiological links and risk factors, outbreak sources, and sources of contamination.

79.9   Treatment

Disease is self-limiting in immunocompetent persons. Fluid loss is rapid. Electrolyte replacement is essential. Nitazoxanide is the recommended drug. Its usefulness in immunosuppressed is unclear. In AIDS patients, antiretroviral therapy reduces oocysts excretion and also decreases diarrhoea.

79.10   Prevention

The basic principle of controlling zoonoses is to eliminate/control infection in animals. *C. parvum* is a serious diarrhoeal disease of newborn calves. Immunizing pregnant cows can protect calves through colostral antibodies. Oocyst antigens CP15/60, P23, and rC7 are immunogenic. Ebrahimzadeh et al. (2009) demonstrated recombinant *C. parvum* p23 was an important candidate vaccine.

Regulatory—According to the WHO (2009), in the United Kingdom, monitoring of treated drinking water is embedded in drinking water regulation. The requirement is treated water should have an average concentration of oocysts less than 1 per 10 litre. Approximately 1000 litres are tested in 23 h; between 2000 and 2004, 84% samples tested negative and maximum number of oocysts detected was 0.49/l; the per cent positive samples declined from 8 to 1.0.

HIV-infected persons should not bring in their house dogs and cats under 6 months of age and should not allow stray dogs and cats and animals suffering with diarrhoea in their house.

In the face of outbreak—Cryptosporidiosis is categorized as biohazard grade 2 and requires personal and laboratory safety accordingly. Once detected either by a physician/health provider/diagnostic laboratory, the local/state/central health authority needs to be informed.

In the Utah community outbreak, state-wide press release was made. The directions included banning of swimming for those ill, < 5 years, and anyone needing diaper, hyperchlorination + display good swimming behaviour, and child care centres to ban water plays and enforce "diarrhoea-exclusion" policies like banning children with diarrhoea. This led to a decline from 564.4 in the week beginning August 19 to 313.1 in week September 3–8 to 153.9 in week September 9–15.

General hygienic measure—Realizing that the oocysts may be present on their skin in the anal and genital areas, thigh, and buttocks, hygienic habits need to be inculcated such as handwashing with soap; thorough washing after animal contact and/or visit to animal premises; changing diapers before eating; use of sanitized water—if not accessible, boil or filter it; and kitchen hygiene to prevent cross-contamination especially for food items consumed fresh and uncooked.

References

Abe N, Sawano Y, Yamada K, Kimata I, Iseki M (2002) *Cryptosporidium* infection in dogs in Osaka, Japan. Vet Parasitol 108(3):185–193

Ayres Hutter J, Dion R, Irace-Cima A, Fiset M, Guy R, Dixon B et al (2020) *Cryptosporidium* spp.: Human incidence, molecular characterization and associated exposures in Que'bec, Canada (2016–2017). PLoS ONE 15(2):e0228986

Cacciò SM (2005) Molecular epidemiology of human cryptosporidiosis. Parassitologia 47(2):185–192

Certad G, Ngouanesavanh T, Guyot K, Gantois N, Chassat T et al (2007) *Cryptosporidium parvum*, a potential cause of colic adenocarcinoma. Infect Agent Cancer 2:22

Chalmers RM, Hadfield SJ, Jackson CJ, Elwin K, Xiao L, Hunter P (2008) Geographic linkage and variation in *Cryptosporidium hominis*. Emerg Infect Dis 14(3):496–498

Current WL (1994) *Cryptosporidium parvum*: household transmission. Ann Intern Med 120(6):518–519

Ebrahimzadeh E, Shayan P, MokhberDezfouli MR, Rahbaris. (2009) Recombinant *C. Parvum* p23 as a candidate vaccine for cryptosporidiosis. Iranian J Parasitol 4(1):1–7

FAO/WHO. (2014) Multi criteria - based ranking for risk management of food borne parasites. Microbiological Risk Assessment Series No. 23. Rome, p 302

Helmy YA, Hafez HM (2022) Cryptosporidiosis: from prevention to treatment. Narrat Rev Microorganisms 10(2456):1–22

Innes EA, Chalmers RM, Wells B, Pawlowic MC (2020) One health approach to tackle cryptosporidiosis. Trends Parasitol 36(3):290–303

Isaac-Renton J, Blatherwick J, Bowie WR, Fyfe M, Khan M et al (1999) Epidemic and endemic seroprevalence of antibodies to *cryptosporidium* and *giardia* in residents of three communities with different drinking water supplies. Am J Trop Med Hyg 60(4):578–583

Jothikumar N, da Silva AJ, Moura I, Qvarnstrom Y, Hill VR (2008) Detection and differentiation of *Cryptosporidium hominis* and *Cryptosporidium parvum* by dual TaqMan assays. J Med Microbiol 57(Pt 9):1099–1105

Korpe PS, Gilchrist C, Burkey C, Taniuchi M, Ahmed E, Madan V et al (2019) Case-control study of *cryptosporidium* transmission in Bangladeshi households. Clin Infect Dis 68(7):1073–1079

Kotloff KL, Nataro JP, Blackwelder WC et al (2013) Burden and aetiology of diarrhoeal disease in infants and young children in developing countries (the global enteric multicenter study, GEMS): a prospective, case-control study. Lancet 382:209–222

Macarisin D, Bauchan G, Fayer R, Spinacia oleracea L. (2010) Leaf stomata harboring *Cryptosporidium parvum* oocysts: a potential threat to food safety. Appl Environ Microbiol 76(2):555–559

Morales MAG, Mele R, Ludovisi A, Bruschi F, Tosini F, Riganò R, Pozio E et al (2004) Cryptosporidium parvum-Specific CD4 Th1 Cells from Sensitized Donors Responding to Both Fractionated and Recombinant Antigenic Proteins. Infect Immun 72(6):3696. https://10.1128/IAI.72.6.3696.2004

Narayan KG (2004) Epidemiology, diagnosis and management of zoonoses. ICAR Publisher, New Delhi

Newman RD, Zu SX, Wuhib T, Lima AA, Guerrant RL, Sears CL (1994) Household epidemiology of *Cryptosporidium parvum* infection in an urban community in Northeast Brazil. Ann Intern Med 120(6):500–505

OIE (2022). OIE terrestrial manual 2022. Chapter 3. 10.2. Cryptosporidiosis. First adopted in 2004. Most recent updates adopted in 2022

Pedraza-Díaz S, Amar C, Iversen AM, Stanley PJ, Mclauchlin J (2001) Unusual *cryptosporidium* species recovered from human faeces: first description of *Cryptosporidium felis* and *cryptosporidium* 'dog type' from patients in England. J Med Microbiol 50(3):293–296

Plutzer J, Kelen K, Varga E, Kucsera I, Reusz G et al (2019) First *cryptosporidium* outbreak in Hungary, linked to a treated recreational water venue in 2015. Epidemiol Infect 147(e56):1–6

Rao Ajjampur SS, Asirvatham JR, Muthusamy D, Gladstone BP et al (2007) Clinical features & risk factors associated with cryptosporidiosis in HIV infected adults in India. Indian J Med Res 126(6):553–557

Robertson LJ, Johansen ØH, Kifleyohannes T, Efunshile AM, Terefe G (2020) *Cryptosporidium* infections in Africa—how important is zoonotic transmission? A review of the evidence. Front Vet Sci 7:575881

Rolfs RT, Beach MJ, Hlavsa MC, Calanan RM (2008) Communitywide cryptosporidiosis outbreak –UTAH, 2007. Morb Mortal Wkly Rep 57(36):989–993

Ryan U, Zahedi A, Feng Y, Xiao L (2021) An update on zoonotic *cryptosporidium* species and genotypes in humans. Animals (Basel) 11(11):3307

Santin M, Trout JM (2008) Cryptosporidiosis in companion animals. In: Fayer R, Xiao L (eds) "Cryptosporidium and cryptosporidiosis" 2nd edn. CRC Press, Boca Raton, FL, pp 437–449

Semenza JC, Nichols G (2007 May) Cryptosporidiosis surveillance and water-borne outbreaks in Europe. Euro Surveill 12(5):E13–E14

Sow SO, Muhsen K, Nasrin D et al (2016) The burden of cryptosporidium diarrheal disease among children < 24 months of age in moderate/high mortality regions in sub Saharan Africa and South Asia utilizing data from global enteric multicenter study (GEMS). PLoS Negl Trop Dis 10:e000472

Sunnotel O, Lowery J, Moore JE, Dooley JSG et al (2006) *Cryptosporidium.* Journal compilation [a] 2006 The Society for Appl Microbiol. Lett Appl Microbiol 43:7–16

Waldron LS, Cheung-Kwok-Sang C, Power ML (2010) Wildlife-associated *cryptosporidium fayeri* in human, Australia. Emerg Infect Dis 16(12):2006–2007

Waldron LS, Ferrari BC, Power ML (2009) Glycoprotein 60 diversity in *C. Hominis* and *C. Parvum* causing human cryptosporidiosis in NSW, Australia. Exp Parasitol 122(2):124–127

WHO (2009) Risk assessment of Cryptosporidium in drinking water, WHO_HSE_WS_09.04 https://www.who.int/publications/i/item/WHO-HSE-WSH-09.04

Chapter 80
Giardiasis

Giardia lamblia (syn. *Giardia intestinalis*, *Giardia duodenalis*) is a flagellated unicellular pear-shaped eukaryotic cell 12 to 15 µm long and 5 to 9 µm wide. The trophozoites of *G. lamblia* have widely varying immunodominant cysteine-rich surface antigens. Possibly, this enables its survival in different intestinal environment. Adam (2001) reported the biology of *G. lamblia* and observed that molecular classification tools would enable the understanding of the host range and pathogenesis.

A wide range of animals, commonly dogs, cats, beavers and rodents, and gibbon and apes among wild animals, are infected with *Giardia* and can be source of infection of human. The infection is commonly waterborne and occasionally foodborne. It is highly prevalent in developing countries and is commonly associated with poor sanitation. It is associated with tourism affecting tourists. Infection and persistence may be related with unhygienic habit. Giardiasis occurs throughout the world.

Giardia follows faecal-oral route of transmission. After ingestion with contaminated water or food, there is excystation after passage through acidic environment of the stomach and exposure to the contents of the proximal small intestine. The vegetative form, trophozoites are released. The cells of the upper gastrointestinal tract are invaded by trophozoites where these replicate in the proximal part of the small intestine. Exposure to bile leads to the formation of cyst in jejunum which are passed in the faeces. This cyst-trophozoites-cyst cycle makes cyst available for contaminating water and food for continued transmission.

This causes malabsorption. Infected man and animals develop chronic intermittent diarrhoea, bloat, abdominal cramp, and fatigue lasting for weeks with spontaneous recovery. There is loss of weight. It may cause growth retardation.

Diagnosis requires examination of faeces which is mucoid, soft, light-coloured, and not watery.

It is treatable with quinacrine.

© Springer Nature Singapore Pte Ltd. 2024
K. G. Narayan et al., *Handbook of Management of Zoonoses*,
https://doi.org/10.1007/978-981-99-9885-2_80

References

Adam RD (2001) Biology of *Giardia lamblia.* Clin Microbiol Rev 14(3):447–475

Chapter 81
Leishmaniasis

Synonyms: Variously known, "valley sickness", "Andean sickness", or "white leprosy" (in fifteenth–sixteenth century) are likely the cutaneous forms, papalomoyo, papa lo moyo, úlcera de los chicleros, and chiclera in Latin America, Visceral form has been known as kala-azar or black fever in India.

History: *In 1901, Leishman found certain organism in spleen smear from a patient of dumdum fever (Dum Dum, Kolkata, India). Shortly after this, Captain Charles Donovan confirmed this finding in smears from people in Madras. Ronal Ross proposed Leishmania donovani, name for Leishman-Donovan bodies. Charles Donovan suggested these were linked with kala-azar. Charles Bentley showed L. donovani in patients with kala-azar. Scientists of the School of Tropical Medicine at Kolkata proved its transmission by the sandfly.*

Geographical Distribution

Leishmaniases are vector-borne (metazoonosis) protozoal diseases occurring in every continent in the world except Australia and Antarctica. The patients suffer for long (duration running for months to year) with mutilation, stigma, and stress besides weakness, prostration, and eventual death if left untreated.

It has been reported from about 89 countries. It is mainly a jungle zoonosis in the American continent, transmitted by sandflies. The 83 endemic countries accounted for visceral leishmaniasis (VL) in 2018 and 92 for cutaneous leishmaniasis (CL). Today, > 1 billion people live in areas endemic for leishmaniasis and are at risk of infection; an estimated 30,000 new cases of VL and > 1 million new cases of CL occur annually (https://www.who.int/health-topics/leishmaniasis#tab=tab_1). In Asia, Africa, South and Central America, and southern Europe, leishmaniasis is common and a "neglected tropical disease". The disease has high morbidity and mortality rates.

81.1   Aetiology

Leishmania consists of four subgenera. These are *Leishmania*, *Sauroleishmania* (reptile-infecting), *Mundinia*, and *Viannia*.

Over 20 *Leishmania* species cause a group of diseases, leishmaniases. The infected female phlebotomine sandfly is the vector. Over 90 sandfly species are known to transmit these. Disease may occur in a number of animals including dogs and rodents. Some 70 animal species including humans have been found as natural reservoir hosts.

The *Leishmania* spp. are as follows:

L. donovani complex—*L. donovani* and *L. infantum* (syn. *L. chagasi* in the New World).

L. mexicana complex—*L. mexicana*, *L. amazonensis*, and *L. venezuelensis* (three main species).

L. tropica, *L. major*, and *L. aethiopica*.

Subgenus *Viannia*—*L. [V.] braziliensis*, *L. [V.] guyanensis*, *L. [V.] panamensis*, and *L. [V.] peruviana*.

Morphologically, these species are indistinguishable. Isoenzyme analysis, molecular methods, or monoclonal antibodies are used for identification (https://www.cdc.gov/parasites/leishmaniasis/biology.html).

According to Reithinger et al. (2007), the *Leishmania* spp. may be grouped according to geographic distribution and the type of disease caused (Table 81.1).

Table 81.1 Distribution of *Leishmania* species and the form of leishmaniases caused (Reithinger et al. 2007)

Leishmania (subgenus)	*Leishmania* spp.	Country/region	Type of leishmaniasis
New World (Western hemisphere)			
L. (Leishmania)	*L. mexicana*	Central America, Mexico, the United States	LCL[a], DCL[a]
	L. amazonensis	South America	LCL, DCL
	L. venezuelensis	Northern South America	LCL
	L. Garnhami	South America	LCL
	L. pifanoi	South America	LCL
L. (Viannia)	*L braziliensis*	South America, parts of Central America, Mexico	LCL, MCL
	L. panamensis	Northern South America, Southern Central America	LCL, MCL
	L. peruviana	Peru	LCL
	L. guyanensis	South America	LCL
	L. Lainsoni	South America	LCL
	L. colombiensis	South America	LCL

Table 81.1 (continued)

Leishmania (subgenus)	Leishmania spp.	Country/region	Type of leishmaniasis
Old World (Eastern hemisphere)			
L. (Leishmania)	L. aethiopica	Ethiopia, Kenya	LCL, DCL
	L. Killicki	North Africa	LCL
	L. major	Central Asia, North Africa, Middle East, East Africa	LCL
	L. tropica	Central Asia, Middle East, parts of North Africa, Southeast Asia	LCL anthroponotic
	L. donovani	Africa, Central Asia, Southeast Asia (Indian subcontinent and China)	Visceral, LCL anthroponotic
Old and New World			
Leishmania (Leishmania)	L. infantum	Europe, North Africa, Central America, South America	Visceral, LCL zoonotic

[a]LCL, localized cutaneous leishmaniasis; DCL, disseminated cutaneous leishmaniasis

Cutaneous leishmaniasis (CL) is caused by >15 species. *L. major*, *L. tropica*, and *L. aethiopica* are common in the countries of Eastern Hemisphere. *L. mexicana*, *L. amazonensis*, *L. braziliensis*, *L. panamensis*, and *L. guyanensis* are common in the countries of Western Hemisphere.

Generally, *L. donovani* and *L. tropica* are associated with anthroponotic infection. *L. infantum* and other CL-causing species are zoonotic.

81.2 Life Cycle (Fig. 81.1)

Two developmental stages of *Leishmania* are amastigotes and promastigotes. The former is intracellular, non-motile seen in the vertebrate host, particularly in reticuloendothelial cells (in the spleen, liver, and bone marrow), called Leishman-Donovan body. These are round or oval bodies with a large nucleus and rod-shaped kinetoplast and divided by longitudinal binary fission at 37 °C.

Promastigotes or leptomonads are found in the digestive tract of sandflies and in culture medium, as an elongated body with single flagellum arising close to the kinetoplast at the anterior end. These appear in old culture as clustered in the form of rosettes with flagella centrally directed.

The female sandflies usually feed at night when the prey is sleeping. Sandflies become infected during blood meal on infected mammal. They ingest macrophages infected with amastigotes and release in the mid-gut (1). The protozoan that reproduces asexually in the gut extra-cellularly differentiates into metacyclic promastigotes (2). These migrate to proboscis, reaching the pharyngeal valve. These are poised for the regurgitation transmission to mammalian hosts when the flies are feeding.

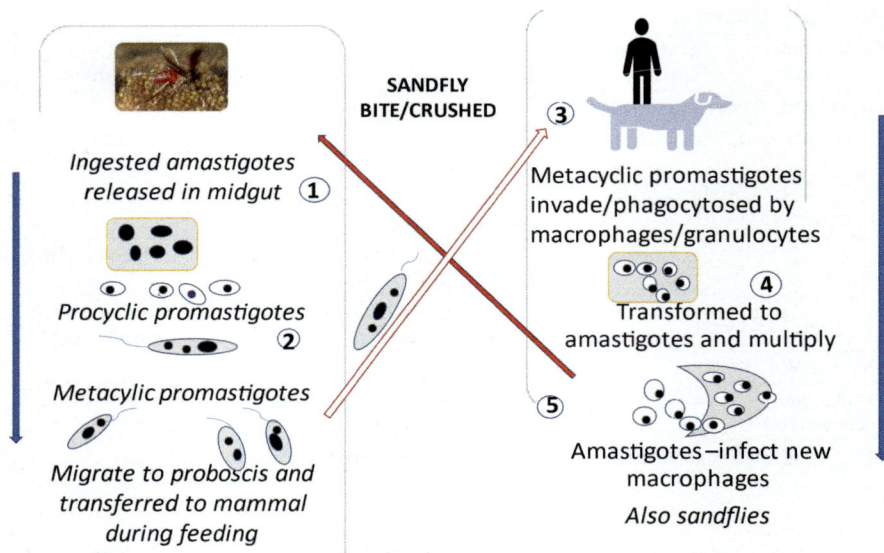

Fig. 81.1 Life cycle of *Leishmania* spp.

   The infected female sandflies transmit *Leishmania*. The infective stage metacyclic
promastigotes (which have anterior flagellum) are deposited with saliva at the site of
puncture by regurgitation transmission (3). These are phagocytosed or these invade
macrophages and granulocytes (4). These are transformed to amastigotes (no flagellum) and multiply by simple division in the infected cells. The cells are then lysed (5).
Daughter protozoans migrate with blood to find other new macrophages to invade
(amastigotes in macrophages). Sandfly is infected during blood meal (cycle back to 1).
   The period after feeding on infected hosts to be able to transmit infection to
another susceptible host (extrinsic incubation period) is 7–10 days.

81.3   Modes of Transmission (Fig. 81.2)

The two important modes of transmission determine the types of leishmaniasis as
zoonotic and anthroponotic.

81.3.1   *Zoonotic Leishmaniasis*

Leishmania are maintained in dogs and rodents with sandflies in many geographic
areas. Spillover to human causes zoonotic leishmaniasis. Zoonotic leishmaniasis of
the New World occurs in some parts of Mexico, Central America, and South
America. It is not found in Chile or Uruguay. In the Old World, these occur in some

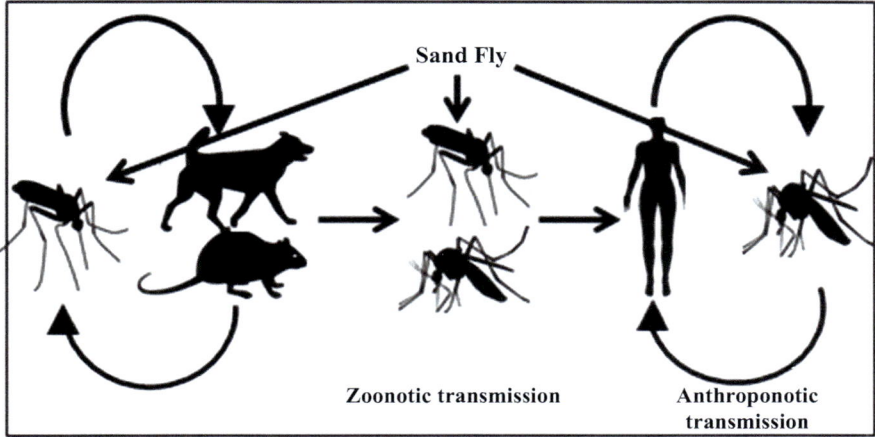

Transmission of Leishmaniasis

Fig. 81.2 Tansmission of leishmaniasis

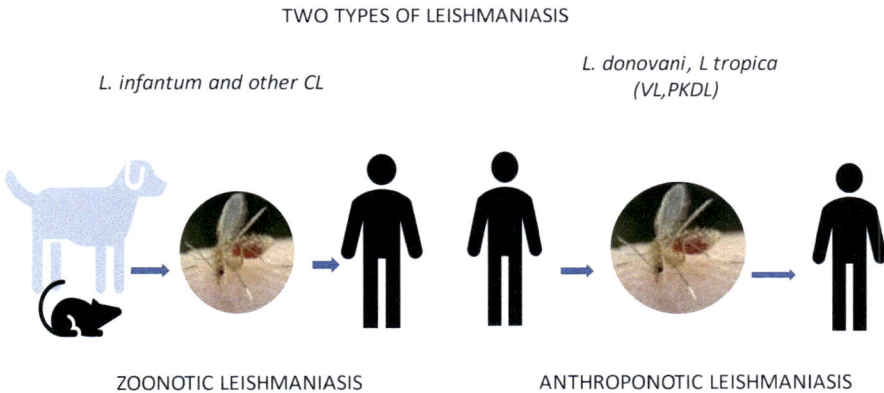

Fig. 81.3 Types of leishmaniasis

parts of Asia, the Middle East, Africa (particularly in the tropical region and North Africa, with some cases elsewhere), and southern Europe. It is not found in Australia or the Pacific Islands.

L. braziliensis is the cause of a more severe form of disease which is distributed throughout the Brazil. CL is now endemic in the north-eastern region and emerging in the south-western region of State of Santa Catarina, Brazil, with case profiles varying significantly by region. *L. (Viannia) braziliensis* has been identified as the predominant species in the State of Santa Catarina. The rate of relapse cases and mucosal cases is high in the southwest region and is an important public health concern. The mucocutaneous is a more virulent form leading to serious disfiguration and difficult to treat. *L. (V.) braziliensis* was commonly associated with this form (Marlow et al. 2013).

81.3.2   Anthroponotic Leishmaniasis

In some other parts of the world, infected people are needed to maintain the cycle of transmission, "anthroponotic" (Fig. 81.1). Using a high cure rate therapy, kala-azar has been targeted for elimination from India, Bangladesh, and Nepal.

Two anthroponotic species are *L. donovani* and *L. tropica*. The former causes visceral (kala-azar) and post-kala-azar dermal (PKL) leishmaniasis in Africa, Central Asia, and Southeast Asia, while the latter causes LCL in Central Asia, Middle East, parts of North Africa, and Southeast Asia. Disseminated visceral and LCL caused by *L. infantum* have a wide distribution, both in the New World and Old World—Europe, North Africa, Central America, and South America.

81.3.3   Other Modes of Transmission

Other modes of transmission are as follows:

Bites by infected female sandflies transmit the parasite. Sandflies make no noise. These are small, about one-fourth the size of a mosquitoes or even smaller. The bite may or may not be painful but pass unnoticed. The flies are active from dusk to dawn—twilight, evening, and night. Exception and accidental bite may occur during hottest part of the day when sandflies are resting under and around tree shed if a man rubs/brushes against the trunk of a tree.

Crushed sandflies release promastigotes that may enter through bite injury.

Non-bite transmission: Needle puncture/inoculation by needle sharing, transfusion, sexual intercourse, and intrauterine during pregnancy, though rare but may happen.

Felinto de Brito et al. (2012) reported accidental inoculation by a contaminated needle while handling American cutaneous leishmaniasis lesion and another during a field study on bird.

81.4   Leishmaniasis-The Disease

Leishmaniasis refers to the disease due to a *Leishmania* infection, differentiating from being infected with the parasite without any clinical manifestation. Most infected people do not develop any symptom during their lifetime. Of the three forms of leishmaniasis, CL, VL (kala-azar), and mucocutaneous leishmaniasis (MCL), CL is the most severe, and MCL is the most disabling.

Leishmaniasis is a mild and slowly progressing condition. Seeking medical care and diagnosis is delayed. The physician may not be familiar with the disease. Atypical manifestations of leishmaniasis add to the problem.

Atypical cases are defined as appearing in non-endemic areas or clinical presentations that are difficult to diagnose by clinicians and require the inclusivity of differential diagnosis, caused by atypical causative species, rare morphological variants, and unusual numbers and sites of lesions (Yadav et al. 2023).

81.4.1 Pathogenesis

Leishmaniasis is a complex disease. Major forms are visceral (VL) and cutaneous (CL). Lesser forms are mucocutaneous (MCL)—ulcers of the skin, mouth, and nose—diffuse cutaneous (DCL), and post-kala-azar (PKDL).

81.4.1.1 Leishmania-The Parasite

Leishmania are genetically diverse and tackle the host's immune system differently. Reithinger et al. (2007) grouped the *Leishmania*—virulence factors that evade hosts' immune system:

(1) Invasive or evasive determinants (e.g. lipophosphoglycans, leishmanolysin, or cysteine proteases) are crucial for infection.
(2) Pathoantigenic determinants (e.g. histones, chaperones, or proteasomes) contribute to immunopathology and clinical symptoms.
(3) Protective determinants contribute to clinical cure.

The macrophages internalize the promastigotes through a range of macrophage receptors. The phagocytosed or invading parasite survives, transforms into amastigotes, and multiplies in the phagolysosomal compartment of host cells. Saliva of sandfly is vasodilatory and influences causation of erythema and its size, parasite burden, and persistence. It is protein in nature and induces antibodies that have protective effect. *Leishmania* use lipophosphoglycans, leishmanolysin, or cysteine proteases for infection. Histones, chaperones, or proteasomes lead to host immunopathology as the principal cause of clinical symptoms.

In murine model, *L. major* infection caused (a) symptomless, subclinical, self-limiting localized cutaneous leishmaniasis (LCL), (b) chronic diffuse cutaneous leishmaniasis (DCL), and (c) mucosal leishmaniasis recidivans (LR). Cellular immune response led to the outcome of infection-triggered inflammatory response. Activated macrophages (mediated by Th1) killed the parasite and resulted into clinical recovery and prevented recrudescence of latent chronic infection. Deactivation of macrophages promotes intracellular infection by the parasite and is mediated by Th2 (Reithinger et al. 2007). LCL cases show Th1 response and delayed-type hypersensitivity. In DCL cases, Th2 response predominates and there is larger DTH response. Patients of mucosal leishmaniasis show a mixture of Th1 and Th2 cytokine responses. Th2-type response tends to dominate when both types of responses are activated, hence non-resolution of disease.

The balance between the pro- and anti-inflammatory mediators plays a vital role in the clinical presentation and outcome of the disease. *Leishmania* infection can transition from one form of the disease to another depending upon the immune response.

81.4.1.2   Forms of Leishmaniasis

There are six forms of leishmaniasis, anergic diffuse cutaneous leishmaniasis (ADCL), disseminated leishmaniasis (DL), leishmaniasis recidivans (LR), self-healing localized cutaneous (SHLC), post-kala-azar dermal leishmaniasis (PKDL), and mucocutaneous leishmaniasis (MCL).

The anergic diffuse cutaneous leishmaniasis (ADCL) and MCL are severe forms, and the rest between these are moderate. According to Volpedo et al. (2021), an exaggerated Th1, or alternatively Th2, response is equally detrimental for leishmaniasis patients as it results in enhanced disease severity. For instance, an uncontrolled Th2 response in ADCL can lead to cell anergy and increased disease pathology. On the other hand, an unrestrained Th1 response in mucocutaneous leishmaniasis (MCL) can cause sustained inflammation and tissue damage. A balance between a Th1 and a Th2 response is necessary for controlling the infection (Fig. 81.4).

The balance between the pro- and anti-inflammatory mediators plays a vital role in the clinical presentation and outcome of the disease. *Leishmania* infection can transition from one form of the disease to another depending upon the immune response.

81.5   Epidemiology

81.5.1   Prevalence and Disease Burden

Leishmaniases are endemic in many tropical and temperate countries and occur in focal areas, generally in peri-urban and rural areas. These occur in the tropics, subtropics, and southern Europe, in rainforests, and in desert.

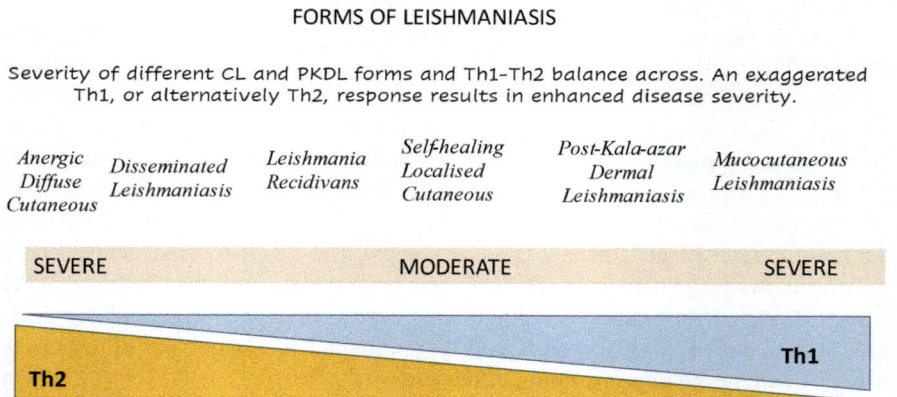

Fig. 81.4 Pathology of Leishmaniasis (Source: Volpedo et al., 2021)

An estimated 700,000 to 1 million new cases of leishmaniasis occur annually. The distribution of different forms varies in the WHO regions (WHO 2023).

Three symptomatic forms of leishmaniases and their distribution (WHO 2020; https://www.who.int/news-room/fact-sheets/detail/leishmaniasis) are as follows:

Visceral leishmaniasis is the main form of the disease in Southeast Asia. Most cases are in Brazil, in East Africa, and in India. An estimated 50,000 to 90,000 new cases of VL occur worldwide annually. It remains one of the top parasitic diseases with outbreak and mortality potential. >95% of new cases reported to WHO occurred in ten countries: Brazil, China, Ethiopia, India, Iraq, Kenya, Nepal, Somalia, South Sudan and Sudan.

Cutaneous leishmaniasis is the most common form. About 95% of CL cases occur in the Americas, the Mediterranean basin, the Middle East, and Central Asia. Over 85% of new CL cases occurred in ten countries: Afghanistan, Algeria, Bolivia, Brazil, Colombia, Iran (Islamic Republic), Iraq, Pakistan, the Syrian Arab Republic, and Tunisia in 2018. In the WHO regions of the Americas, CL is the main form of leishmaniasis with complex epidemiology involving multiple species of *Leishmania*, numerous reservoirs, and types of sandflies in the same geographical area.

Mucocutaneous leishmaniasis begins as sores in the skin, spread to the mucosal membranes of the nostrils and mouth causing profound inflammation and erosion. Over 90% of mucocutaneous leishmaniasis cases occur in Bolivia (the Plurinational State), Brazil, Ethiopia, and Peru.

CL and VL: Both CL and VL are endemic in the WHO European region. Cases are imported mainly from Africa and the Americas.

All forms are endemic in East Africa with outbreaks of visceral leishmaniasis occurring frequently.

According to Glans et al. (2018), there has been an increase in the number of diagnosed cases of leishmaniasis in Sweden from 1996 to 2016, mainly in migrants from endemic countries (81.52%), Syria and Afghanistan, Swedish tourists (25%), and returning workers (13%). Most cases (96%) were of cutaneous leishmaniasis, 44% due to *L. tropica*. Rest were mucocutaneous (4.3%), visceral (2.1%), and post-kala-azar dermal leishmaniasis (1.1%).

The disability-adjusted life years (DALYs) from CL and MCL are estimated to have increased to 43.5% between 1990 and 2016 and 12.5% between 2006 and 2016 and decline in DALYs from VL 77.4% and 61.1%, respectively (Hotez 2018).

81.5.2 Human Host Factor

Malnutrition and immunosuppression increase susceptibility to leishmaniasis. Human genetic appears to influence susceptibility and resistance based on observations of occurrence of MCL caused by *L. braziliensis* in different ethnic groups, familial cluster, and LCL caused by *L. major* among natives and migrants. Whether host genetic determinants of leishmaniasis will be the same for different *Leishmania* spp. remains to be established.

Poor nutrition weakened immunity, and concomitant infections increased the possibility of infected one to progress to clinical leishmaniasis. HIV cases infected with *Leishmania* are most likely to suffer with full-blown disease, high relapse, and mortality. *Leishmania*-HIV co-infection has been reported from 45 countries, as of 2021. High rates of co-infection have been reported from Brazil, Ethiopia, and the State of Bihar, India (WHO 2023). Often, appropriate health service is wanting.

81.5.3   Socioeconomic

Leishmaniasis is associated with poor environmental sanitation and housing conditions, poverty, and economically driven migration and employment. There is an increased possibility of contact with infected sandflies. Poor nutrition weakened immunity, and concomitant infections increased the possibility of infected one to progress to clinical leishmaniasis. HIV cases infected with *Leishmania* are most likely to suffer with full-blown disease, high relapse, and mortality.

VL appears as focal cluster of cases in a hamlet as was observed by Kumar et al. (2020) in southern hamlet of Kosra Village, Sheikhpura District (Bihar, India), where socio-economically disadvantaged migrant population lived (attack rate of 19% vs 0.5% for the rest of the village). Delayed diagnosis of index case and treatment (> a year in this outbreak) increases the number of cases.

81.5.4   Reservoir Hosts

Non-human mammal hosts are mainly marsupials, rodents, edentates, and carnivores. The parasite is maintained endemically in animal reservoirs. Wild animals do not suffer with disease. Dogs however suffer with clinical disease as humans. Infection in human is incidental.

81.5.5   Vector

The sandfly saliva is crucial in the establishment of infection and disease pathogenesis. It acts as vasodilator and increases parasite burden, the size of erythema, and lesion and persistence. The saliva proteins possibly can shift the adaptive immune response from a Th1 to a Th2 cell-mediated immune response (Reithinger et al. 2007).

Transmission of *Leishmania* spp. specific to each disease form is carried out by 98 species of phlebotomine sandflies coming from the genus *Phlebotomus* and *Lutzomyia*. In the Old World, 42 *Phlebotomus* species are found to be involved in the transmission of *L. infantum*, *L. donovani*, *L. major*, *L. tropica*, and *L. aethiopica*.

In almost all cases, each species of *Phlebotomus* transmits only one species of *Leishmania*. In the New World, 56 *Lutzomyia* species transmit 15 species of *Leishmania*, including *L. infantum* (= *Leishmania chagasi*), *Leishmania guyanensis*, *Leishmania mexicana*, *L. amazonensis*, *L. braziliensis*, and *L. panamensis*. Contrary to the genus *Phlebotomus*, *Lutzomyia* spp. have been shown to transmit more than one species of *Leishmania*.

Phlebotomus spp. of sandflies is widely distributed—Europe, North Africa, the Middle East, and Asia. *Lutzomyia* spp. is common in southern United States to northern Argentina. The female phlebotomine flies feed on blood to produce eggs.

Species of sandflies and *Leishmania*, local ecology, human behaviour, and past exposure of human population to parasite determine epidemiology.

Sandflies are found in tropical or temperate regions. The preferred sites for breeding are warm and moist soil rich in organic matter, like near cattle sheds and around mud houses. Resting sites are crevices, cracks of thatched mud houses, old trees, house walls, and scattered waste (i.e. poor sanitation). Climate directly affects the rate of multiplication and thereby abundance of sandflies. Chaves and Pascual (2007) used data on climate and CL in Costa Rica to build a statistical model that can predict incidence of CL 1 year in advance with an accuracy of 72–77%. Climate change favouring vector habitat may increase the area of endemicity. Newer tools like GIS and remote sensing may help better understand the relationship between environmental factors, distribution of sandflies, and prevalence of disease.

81.6   Visceral Leishmaniasis (Kala-Azar/Dumdum Fever)

Visceral leishmaniasis is infectious, chronic, and highly fatal. It begins with skin lesions and irregular bouts of fever (Fig. 81.3). It takes about 2–8 months for appearance of gross inflammation of the viscera (liver and spleen in particular). If untreated, it may be fatal in 95% of cases.

VL is caused by *L. donovani* and *L. infantum*, *L. chagasi* (in S. America), and *L.* (*Mundinia*) *martiniquensis* in parts of Thailand and Myanmar. Atypical VL is caused by *L. tropica* (Yadav et al. 2023).

Pathologies vary with these species, and even same species, *L. donovani* causes different pathologies in India and Sudan. Some strains of *L. infantum* cause CL and some *L. donovani* DCL and PKDL. The liver, spleen, and bone marrow are invaded.

In Sudan, it occurs predominantly during October to February with peak in November because in the preceding months June to August there is population surge of sandflies. Epidemiological pattern differs in different locale. The vector-reservoir host combination and their behaviour determine. *Phlebotomus argentipes* and *Ph. papatasi* are vectors, while jackals and dogs are reservoir hosts in China and Mediterranean countries. VL is zoonotic.

In India, VL is anthroponotic. VL, CL, and PKDL are endemic. MCL is non-endemic. VL caused by *L. donovani* is endemic in lower and middle Gangetic Plain.

It is prevalent in four states with approximately 130 million populations living in the endemic areas and at the risk of acquiring infection. Of the four states, namely, Bihar, Jharkhand, West Bengal, and Uttar Pradesh, Bihar alone contributes more than 60% of the cases. Kala-azar occurs in rainy season in India.

Historically, VL caused by *L. donovani* was widely prevalent in India, and it was almost eliminated as a result of extensive DDT spraying under the national malaria eradication programme in the 1960s.

Ph. argentipes is anthrophilic in India and appears to be an inefficient vector, and therefore VL in India is anthroponotic. Dogs, though susceptible, are not natural non-human vertebrate to maintain the parasite. Bhunia et al. (2013) reviewed VL, a serious public health problem in Indian subcontinent.

81.6.1   Epidemiology

An estimated 50,000 to 90,000 new cases of VL occur worldwide annually, with only 25–45% reported to WHO.

Kala-azar is endemic in Bangladesh, India, and Nepal, in the south-eastern region. Bhutan, Sri Lanka, and Thailand report sporadic cases. *L. donovani* causes kala-azar in the Indian subcontinent ((Bangladesh, Bhutan, India, Nepal, and Sri Lanka). There is no animal reservoir and the disease is anthroponotic. The vector is a peridomestic sandfly, *Phlebotomus argentipes.* It breeds mainly indoors, such as in cracks and holes of mud walls in rural houses and cattle shed. In Sri Lanka, *L. donovani* is believed to be an attenuated strain with visceralizing potential and causes both CL and kala-azar. In Thailand, autochthonous kala-azar is caused by two causative agents, *L. martiniquensis* and *L. siamensis.* The sandfly vector has not yet been identified. Most cases occur in Brazil, East Africa, and India. It has out-break and mortality potential (WHO 2023).

The prevalence and transmission dynamics of VL are closely interrelated to socioeconomic, climatic, and environmental factors including land use/land cover, topography, rainfall, temperature, and vegetation coverage. The expanding endemic areas in Nepal in recent years are attributed to climate change.

It occurs in rainy season. Ecological conditions favouring vector are alluvial soil, humid, warm (as in rainy season), and large-scale vegetation. Rural thatched mud houses and cattle sheds offer a desired combination for promoting vector density.

Indigenous cases occur in non-endemic state Kerala, reported earlier in 2003 and the present report from the foothills of Western Ghats during 2015–2019 (Saini et al. 2020). An outbreak occurred in Kosra village, Sheikhpura district (Bihar, India), a low endemic district in Bihar (Kumar et al. 2020). Tropical, conserved forest, humid, shady microhabitat, and mud unplastered house favoured breeding and resting sites for vector in Kerala.

81.6.2 Symptoms

The prevalence increases with age up to 15 years and then levels off probably with developing immunity in endemic areas. Most cases fall between 5 and 14 years. Familial cluster may be explained as (a) short flight range of sandflies, (b) genetic susceptibility, and (c) anthroponotic transmission. Behavioural/occupational exposure influences the prevalence in any sex. VL is associated with malnutrition, deprivation, poverty, slum, famine, unsanitary, stress, immunosuppression, HIV, and comorbidities weakening the body defences.

The amastigote forms spread to internal organs through systemic circulation. *Leishmania* affect the reticuloendothelium system mainly and are located in cells of the lymph nodes, spleen, liver, and bone marrow.

Incubation period ranges from 10 days to 2 years. In India, it may be 4 months to 1 year. Extrinsic incubation period may vary from 4 to 25 days.

VL is characterized by irregular bouts of fever, weight loss, enlargement of the spleen and liver, and anaemia. Fever usually lasts for >2 weeks. Patients complain chills, fatigue, vomiting, and loss of appetite and weight; there is hepatosplenomegaly, mucosal ulcer. Skin is earthy grey in colour. Hematologic changes include anaemia, leucopenia, and hypergammaglobulinemia. There are extensive wasting and bleeding due to thrombocytopenia in untreated cases. Furthermore, leukocytopenia leads to the suppression of the host's immune system, leading to bacterial infections.

Duration of VL is variable, from 1 to 20 weeks, 12–16 weeks with Sudanese strain.

Yadav et al. (2023) presented atypical manifestation of VL observed particularly in the Indian subcontinent. Atypical presentation may involve the pulmonary or gastric system and occasionally the skin in immunocompetent geriatric or immunocompromised cases. There may be nonspecific duodenitis. The gastrointestinal tract and no other visceral organs were affected in a young immunocompetent person. It was diagnosed by PCR, and he responded to liposomal amphotericin B (LAmB) therapy. VL and HIV mutually reinforce each other. Lesions may be located in gastrointestinal, pulmonary, or laryngeal in immunocompromised and HIV cases.

Morbidity is high, and mortality may be >95% if untreated, largely because of misdiagnosis and neglect. Leishmaniases is not always the direct cause of death.

81.6.2.1 Post-Kala-Azar Dermal Leishmaniasis (PKDL)

Transition to PKDL appears to be affected by genetic polymorphism/changes of parasite, geographical regions, and environmental and host-related factors. The Th1 response increases and is believed to contribute to disease pathogenesis of PKDL. The parasite burden in lesions is lower in East Africa and higher in South Asia (Volpedo et al. 2021).

PKDL is not life-threating. It negatively affects the quality of life of the patients due to disfiguring and disability. It represents a socioeconomic burden in the endemic regions.

It is reported from East Africa, mainly Sudan, Bangladesh, Nepal, and India. It is uncommon in Brazil and also in HIV co-infected VL cases caused by *L. infantum* (WHO 2023).

It is usually a sequel of visceral leishmaniasis in 5–10% of patients appearing earlier or more than 2–3 years after apparent cure in South Asia. The incidence is 50–60%, and the clinical manifestations appear either after VL remission or even during the treatment in East Africa (primarily Sudan and also Ethiopia, Kenya, and Uganda).

The cases serve as reservoir and are potential source of infection, accessible to sandflies during blood meals.

Patients can be categorized into two different subgroups: (a) Polymorphic PKDL is characterized by the development of papules and/or nodules, as well as hypo-pigmented macules. The parasitic burden is high. (b) Monomorphic PKDL patients develop only one type of lesion, mostly papulonodes. In South Asia, PKDL manifests as papulonodular lesions (polymorphic), while in East Africa it causes hypo-melanotic (macular) lesions. Hypopigmentation or erythematous macules, papules, or nodules are seen usually on the face, upper arms, trunks, limbs, and other parts of the body. The papules and nodules on the face resemble those of lepromatous lesions, hypo-pigmented or erythromatous. Blackening of the skin seen in India led to the name kala-azar.

In Asia, PKDL lesions become chronic, rarely resolve, and are associated with CD8+ T-cell infiltration into the cutaneous lesions. Most cases in Africa appear sooner after remission of VL; lesions show self-healing and are characterized by the reactivation of the immune response.

Atypical PKDL presented an unusual combination of healed leprosy sequelae and active PKDL lesions. The nodules involving the mucosa may appear in the corners of the mouth, dorsum of the tongue, and buccal mucosa or soft palate, and sometimes involving the upper respiratory tract leading to ulcerations (Yadav et al. 2023).

81.6.3 Control

The National Vector Borne Disease Control Program (NVBDCP) covers surveillance that began in 2005. The strategy to eliminate kala-azar includes (i) early diagnosis and complete case management; (ii) integrated vector management and vector surveillance; (iii) supervision, monitoring, surveillance, and evaluation; (iv) strengthening capacity of human resource in health; (v) advocacy, communication, and social mobilization for behavioural impact and inter-sectoral convergence; and (vi) programme management (KA_Road-Map-NVDBCP-Nov 2014).

The number of annually reported cases has shown a drop by 90% in 2019. It is targeted to achieve <1 case /10,000 annually at block PHC level, so that kala-azar ceases to be a public health problem. The Southeast Region is poised to achieve this target, with countries aiming to have WHO validate elimination by 2023.

81.7 Cutaneous Leishmaniasis (CL)

CL is caused by *L. major*, *L. tropica*, *L. mexicana*, *L. amazonensis*, *L. braziliensis*, and *L. (Mundinia) orientalis*. Atypical CL is caused by *L. donovani* and *L. infantum* (Yadav et al. 2023). A variety of factors including the species of the parasites and the host's immune response determine the different clinical manifestations of CL. CL causes skin lesions, mainly ulcers, on exposed parts of the body, leaving lifelong scars and serious disability or stigma.

CL is the most common form. It is considered as a severely neglected, emerging, and uncontrolled disease. Endemic cutaneous granulomatous leishmaniasis is divided as Old and New World forms. The former is caused by *L. major*, *L. tropica*, or *L. aethiopica*. The latter is caused by *L. mexicana* or *L. viannia*. According to Valencia et al. (2013), American (New World) cutaneous leishmaniasis is endemic in Peru. Over 1000 cases/year are reported. It causes significant disability and economic loss.

81.7.1 Epidemiology

The abundance, distribution, and infectiousness of reservoir hosts to vectors are important factors that influence epizootiology. The natural ecological settings for Old World CL are open arid or semi-arid or even desert conditions, and for the New World CL, it is mostly forest.

The natural habitat of sandflies is cool, shaded, humid microhabitats—provided by rock crevices, caves, rodent burrows, tree buttress roots, or leaf litter. These microhabitats are available in the environmental settings of both New World and Old World.

Man-made settings that favour CL prevalence, endemicity, and spread are (a) settlement adjacent to forests and intensive agriculture, e.g. coffee plantation, and (b) loss of mammalian biodiversity due to deforestation, intensive agriculture, and urbanization forcing the vector to feed on human beings and few species of synanthropic reservoirs. The Health Ministry in Brazil list cutaneous and mucocutaneous leishmaniasis as occupationally acquired diseases. The risk groups including those engaged in agriculture, forestry, hospitals/laboratories, and biological research are exposed to *L. braziliensis* (Marlow et al. 2013).

Owino et al. (2019) reported the CL epidemic that occurred in Gilgil, Nakuru County, Kenya, and it became a public health issue. *L. tropica* was isolated from *Ph. saevus s.l.* suggesting that there are at least three potential vectors of this parasite species in Gilgil: *Ph. guggisbergi*, *Ph. aculeatus*, and *Ph. saevus s.l.* Sandfly host preference analysis revealed the possibility of zoonotic transmissions of *L. tropica* in Gilgil since the main vector (*Ph. guggisbergi*) does not feed exclusively on humans but also other vertebrate species. *L. major* infections in *Ph. guggisbergi* were detected suggesting this species as a potential permissive vector of *L. major*.

The prevalence is attributed to urbanization; deforestation resulting into proximity with domestic animal reservoirs; travels, tourism, and migration; and disasters—natural and political conflicts. Increased exposure in endemic areas leads to epidemic; new foci emerge.

CL appears in rural and urban settings. The urban CL is anthroponotic and caused by *L. tropica minor*. It is dry and late ulcerative. It is common in man and sometimes dogs in urban and peri-urban locale.

The rural CL is zoonotic and caused by *L. tropica major* affecting rural folk and rodents in desert and semi-desert areas. Poor people who are undernourished, have weak immunity, and are living in poor housing are at risk. It is wet/rural/early ulcerative.

Narayan (2004) summed up the studies (Sharma et al. 1973a, 1973b; Mohan and Suri 1975) on the isolation of *L. tropica* from gerbils, sandflies, and human in India. It is endemic in the north-western half of the Indo-Gangetic Plain bordering Pakistan, covering Amritsar in Punjab, Gujarat, Rajasthan (most in Bikaner), Delhi, and part of Uttar Pradesh. CL emerged in dogs and human beings during the early 1970s in and around Bikaner. Investigation established for the first time that Indian desert gerbil (*Mariones hurrianae*) was the natural reservoir and *Sergentomyia clydei* and *Phlebotomus* spp. natural biological vectors. Endemic areas mapped included Fazilka (Punjab), Canal Zone at Hanumangarh, Sri Ganganagar District, Jodhpur City, and rural and urban areas in Bikaner District of Rajasthan. In the urban locale, man seems to connect one transmission season to another and *Phlebotomus papatasi* for human-dog-human transmission during epidemic. Prevalence was higher in hamlets close to rodent burrows and in the community occupationally exposed. *Phlebotomus salehi* feeding upon gerbils in burrows transmitted *Leishmania* to humans. The endemic area appears expanding. The endemic focus in Sutlej River Valley in Himachal Pradesh (India) lies in the north-western Himalayas, 30°N and 70° E. LCL and VL coexist, *L. donovani* is predominant, and cases due to *L. tropica* are few. *Phlebotomus (Adlerius) chinensis longiductus* seems to be the main vector. *P. major* and *P. (Larroussius) kandelakii burneyi* may also be responsible for some cases.

A clinic-epidemiological study was done by Aara et al. (2013) upon a total of 1379 patients with 2730 lesions reported during 2001–2011. Predominantly male aged 3 months to 86 years were the patients, representing lower middle socio-economic group and located in urban areas. Smear and skin biopsies were positive. *L. tropica* was detected by PCR. Mixed granulomas consist of macrophages, lymphocytes, and epitheloid and plasma cells.

81.7.2 Symptoms

It manifests with limited cutaneous lesions, mainly ulcers that self-cure within 6–18 months leaving scarred tissue in most patients. CL impacts more socially. The disease is stigmatizing as most lesions and the scars therefore are on exposed regions of the skin, for example, the face, arms, and legs.

Small erythema appears at the site of bite and proceeds as follows: papule-nodule-ulcer in 2 weeks to 6 months. DCL is non-ulcerative. It may cover the whole body disseminating from the initial site of infection. The spread is through lymphatics involving the lymph gland. Severity, appearance, and time to spontaneous cure vary. There is no self-cure and also the treatment is difficult. Self-cure, if occurs, may occur within 2–6 or more months. The scar lasts lifelong and is thus psychologically traumatic depending upon the size and location. Recovery is accompanied with immunity that may not be restricted to the infecting species of *Leishmania*.

81.7.2.1 HIV-CL

Immunosuppression due to HIV allows atypical presentation and widespread progression of CL. It also weakens response to classic treatment. Chaudhary et al. (2008) described an HIV-leishmaniasis co-infection. CL was disseminated (diffuse); there were multiple (>200), atypical, widespread infiltrations of skin lesions. Chusri et al. (2012) described two cases of HIV infected with a novel species of *Leishmania* that resembled *L. colombiensis* in Thailand. Diagnosis was difficult because (a) macrophages containing *Leishmania* disappear in the late stage of CL, (b) amastigotes escape from necrotic tissues, (c) *Leishmania* lesions may be found in unusual sites, (d) these cases presented overlapping CL and VL lesions, and (e) distinguishing from *Histoplasma capsulatum* and *Penicillium manefeii* (other common opportunistic pathogens) was required. Bone marrow macrophages were culture-positive, whereas *Leishmania* DNA was detected in these and discharge from ulcer, urine, and oral fluid (saliva).

As per Volpedo et al. (2021), cutaneous *Leishmania* infections can manifest as self-healing localized cutaneous leishmaniasis (LCL), anergic diffuse cutaneous leishmaniasis (ADCL), disseminated leishmaniasis (DL), leishmaniasis recidivans (LR), and mucocutaneous leishmaniasis (MCL).

81.7.3 Localized Cutaneous Leishmaniasis (LCL)

Volpedo et al. (2021) described the epidemiology of LCL and LR. LCL is the most common form, and most cases (>70%) are reported from Afghanistan, Algeria, Brazil, Colombia, Costa Rica, Ethiopia, Iran, Syria, North Sudan, and Peru. Small red papules appear at the site of the bite by sandfly, which progress into painless nodules that ulcerate. The circumscribed ulcers may be invaded by bacteria or fungi (secondary infection). The asymptomatic incubation period ranges from few days to 3 years (typically 2–8 weeks). The common sites are mostly the exposed body parts like the face, arms, and legs. Each lesion represents an independent site of bite, and parasite remains localized for years despite self-healing and clinical cure. Consequently, there is resistance to reinfection. Mucosal lesions or severe disease may develop.

81.7.4   Anergic Diffuse Cutaneous Leishmania (ADCL)

ADCL is characterized by T-cell anergy. This distinguishes it from other forms of CL (Reithinger et al. 2007). It is a less common manifestation of CL caused by *L. aethiopica* in the highlands of Ethiopia and Kenya, Namibia, and Tanzania. *L. amazonesis* and *L. mexicana* cause ADCL in Ecuador, Venezuela, Brazil, Dominican Republic, Mexico, Honduras, Nicaragua, Peru, Bolivia, Colombia, and the United States (southern Texas). It is a chronic disease often refractory to standard treatment. There is suppression of Th1 response as indicated by negative delayed-type hypersensitive (DTH) skin test. There is high level of Th2 cytokines in ADCL patients. ADCL is commonly observed in immunocompromised patients, such as HIV cases. It begins as papule usually on the face and extremities and does not ulcerate. ADCL may persist for decades. The spread is slow by peripheral lymphohaematogenic route leading to the development of further papules and tubercles (Volpedo et al. 2021).

81.7.5   Disseminated Leishmaniasis (DL)

DL is caused by rapid spread (within days to weeks) of parasite from the original site to other skin and mucosal sites through the bloodstream. Parasites are few at the site of lesion. The developing lesions ulcerate. DL patients exhibit strong positive *Leishmania* skin test. Multiple lesions in two or more non-contiguous body regions characterize DL. Lesions may present a mixed pathology: a mixture of acneiform, papular, nodular, and ulcerative involving nasal mucosa. DL may present increased epidermal hyperplasia and follicular pattern in the acneiform-type lesions. It is believed that certain parasite strains account for active DL foci.

It affects commonly males >19 years of age occupied in agriculture.

DL is endemic almost exclusively in northern and north-eastern Brazil and accounts for 1.9% of all CL cases, compared to 0.2% in the past decades. The causative agent primarily is *L. braziliensis*. *L. amazonensis*, *L. panamensis*, and *L. guyanensis* have also been reported as the causative agents of DL in Brazil and Colombia.

It is suggested that early T-cell response and peripheral Th1 response are temporarily impaired allowing the dissemination of parasite. Later, the immune response of the host controlling the infection explains the low number of parasites observed in DL lesions. Delayed inflammatory response explains the observed ulcers in DL. DL has been observed in young and immunocompetent individuals, and hence development of DL cannot be linked to immunosuppression.

81.7.6 Leishmaniasis Recidivans (LR)

It is a chronic form of CL. The parasite remains at the site of the scar over time to get reactivated by some stimulus. Relapsing papules appear within months to years after and around or within the scar on an old cutaneous lesion and resemble a skin TB. There are intense granuloma and fibrinoid necrosis without caseation with frequent satellite lesions considered as extreme form of cellular immune response. It occurs in about 3 to 10% of CL patients. Marovich et al. (2001) described a case recurring after 43 years. *L. tropica* and rarely *L. major* are the cause in Ethiopia, India, and Pakistan. *L. braziliensis*, *L. amazonensis*, *L. panamensis*, and *L. guyanensis* are the causative agents in Brazil, New World. It is notoriously difficult to treat, hence known also as chronic relapsing cutaneous leishmaniasis.

81.7.7 Mucocutaneous/Mucosal/Espundia/Uta of the New World

Mucocutaneous leishmaniasis (MCL) is a rare clinical manifestation caused by the progression of CL into a more severe disease.

Mucocutaneous leishmaniasis is caused by *L. amazonensis*, *L. braziliensis*, *L. panamensis*, and *L. guyanensis*. Atypical MCL is caused by *L. donovani*, *L. infantum*, *L. aethiopica*, and *L. major* (Yadav et al. 2023). *Leishmania* parasites can metastasize and cause MCL lesions. Up to 20% of all CL cases may develop MCL. It depends upon several factors such as the species of *Leishmania* and its virulence; patient's immune response, age, sex, and nutritional status; and size and number of cutaneous lesions. MCL may occur after direct bite of sandfly as seen in *L. major* infection. The site of bite is the mouth or nose.

Metastatic lesions may appear simultaneously with CL lesions or months to years after resolution of the primary CL lesions. The new or latent parasites are likely to spread from one location to another via the blood or lymphatic system. The initial cutaneous lesions develop into chronic, progressive, metastatic lesions in nasal, pharyngeal, and buccal cavities causing destruction of tissues and deformity. It is a most serious, disfiguring, and life-threatening condition or disability preventing the patient from working and earning. Espundia may occur with the LCL or in 1–10% of LCL cases may develop 1–5 years after LCL have healed. This metastasis may be haematogenous or lymphatic. Mild form presents as nasal inflammation and stuffiness. Ulceration of the mucosa and perforation of the septum may follow. Severe cases show extension of lesions to the lips, cheeks, soft palate, pharynx, or larynx. Healing is never spontaneous. Treatment is difficult. Bacterial secondary infection is common and potentially fatal.

RNA viruses that infect *Leishmania* have been abundantly found in the human MCL lesions but infrequent in CL lesions. *Leishmania* RNA virus 1 (LRV1), harboured by *L. guyanensis* and *L. braziliensis*, has been shown to promote autophagy in the host and ultimately to the development of MCL. The MCL causing *Leishmania* spp. uses adaptive mechanisms to survive and persist in the human mucosa, like thermal resistance and ability to spread through the blood stream to new location and establish infection. The exacerbation of MCL is mediated by immunopathology and an exaggerated cellular response, compared to other forms of CL driven by parasitic burden and a limited Th1 response (Volpedo et al. 2021).

81.8 Diagnosis

Operational Guidelines on Kala-azar (Visceral Leishmaniasis) Elimination in India 2015, NVBDCP, GOI, is based on WHO recommendations and should be followed for diagnosis and treatment. Summary follows:

- Complete blood count (pancytopenia), serum plasma electrophoresis (elevated immunoglobulins), and liver function tests (alkaline phosphatase, aspartate aminotransferase, alanine aminotransferase elevated).
- Demonstration of amastigotes (their kinetoplast and nuclei) in aspirate from the spleen/lymph node or bone marrow, skin lesions, buffy coat of peripheral blood stain with Giemsa/Leishman's for 20 min; needle scraping or slit skin biopsy in PKDL.
- Serologic tests—(a) Detection of antibodies to recombinant K39 antigen (rK39) quoted dipstick or rapid detection test. The Kala-azar Detect rK39 rapid test kit was used by Saini et al. (2020). The test is not useful for CL and ML but useful for VL in Brazil and India. Sudan strain differs and so the test is not useful in Sudan. (b) Direct agglutination test (DAT) and (c) latex agglutination test (KAtex).

These tests become negative after the patient is cured and hence have limitation—cure, reinfection, or relapse cannot be diagnosed. These tests may give false negative results in case of immunocompromised (e.g. HIV):

- Isolation and culture of the protozoa.
- PCR.
- Delayed hypersensitivity test—Montenegro skin test (similar to PPD of TB)—a 5-mm area of induration area is considered positive.

81.9   Treatment

- Single-dose single-day treatment with liposomal amphotericin B injection.
- Capsule miltefosine (28 days).
- Injection amphotericin B (15 injections on alternate days).
- Combination of miltefosine and paromomycin injection.

WHO treatment guidelines described in this document should be followed for management of special conditions like relapse, HIV-VL co-infection, and others.

81.10   Control and Prevention

A "suspect" case is defined as history of fever of more than 2 weeks with spleno-megaly and hepatomegaly not responding to antimalarial and antibiotics in a patient from an endemic area. "Early diagnosis and prompt treatment" are important strat-egy to reduce (a) transmission, prevalence, and disease burden and prevent, (b) dis-abilities, and (c) death.

People participatory epidemiology is important for quick reporting and access to health provider. Education and community participation are required for dealing with the following risk factors:

- Waste accumulation, open sewerage, and poor sanitation offer sites for breeding and resting of sandflies. Crowded housing, dense population, and sleeping out-side attract sandflies for feast—blood meal.
- Food deficient in protein, vitamin A, iron, and zinc increases the risk of full-blown disease.
- Occupational exposure—related with activities including incursion and defores-tation in forest. Migration and movement spread.
- Leishmaniasis is climate-sensitive as these can have strong effects on vectors and reservoir hosts; developmental cycle of *Leishmania* promastigotes in sandflies may be profoundly affected by small fluctuation in temperature.
- Natural calamities—drought, famine, and flood—may affect immunity and mas-sive displacement and migration of people to areas with transmission of *Leishmania*.
- Environmental changes—deforestation, urbanization, irrigation schemes, and dam building.
- Vector control—insecticide spray, use of insecticide-treated nets, environmental management, and personal protection.
- Control of animal reservoir hosts—such as treatment/culling of infected dogs, insecticide-impregnated dog collars, insecticide spray of shelters and houses.
- Effective disease surveillance is important to promptly monitor and act during epidemics and situations with high case fatality rates under treatment.

For long-term effect, "detection and elimination of reservoir" are necessary. Singh et al. (2020) recommend xenodiagnoses as it provides direct proof of infectiousness. Their concern is possible infectious status of asymptomatic, self-resolving cases. The target set for the Southeast Region is <1 case/10,000 annual, and this is likely to leave behind undetected infectious people likely to infect sandflies posing problem for emergence in the future.

References

Aara N, Khandelwal K, Bumb RA, Mehta RD, Ghiya BC et al (2013) Clinco-epidemiologic study of cutaneous leishmaniasis in Bikaner, Rajasthan, India. Am J Trop Med Hyg 89(1):111–115

Bhunia GS, Kesari S, Chatterjee N, Kumar V, Das P (2013) Review article: the burden of visceral Leishmaniasis in India: challenges in using remote sensing and GIS to understand and control. ISRN Infect Dis 2013:675846. https://doi.org/10.5402/2013/675846

Chaudhary RG, Bilimoria FE, Katare SK (2008) Diffuse cutaneous leishmaniasis: co-infection with human immunodeficiency virus (HIV). Indian J Dermatol Venereol Leprol 74:641–643

Chaves LF, Pascual M (2007) Correction: climate cycles and forecasts of cutaneous Leishmaniasis, a nonstationary vector-borne disease. PLoS Med 4(3):e123

Chusri S, Hortiwakul T, Silpapojakul K, Siriyasatien P (2012) Consecutive cutaneous and visceral leishmaniasis manifestations involving a novel Leishmania species in two HIV patients in Thailand. Am J Trop Med Hyg 87(1):76–80

Felinto de Brito ME, Andrade MS, de Almeida EL, Medeiros AC et al (2012) Occupationally acquired American cutaneous leishmaniasis. Case Rep Dermatol Med 2012:279517

Glans H, Dotevall L, Söbirk SK, Färnert A, Bradley M (2018) Cutaneous, mucocutaneous and visceral leishmaniasis in Sweden from 1996–2016: a retrospective study of clinical characteristics, treatments and outcomes. BMC Infect Dis 18(1):632

Hotez PJ (2018) The rise of leishmaniasis in the twenty-first century. Transactions of The Royal Trans R Soc Trop Med Hyg 112(9):421–422. https://doi.org/10.1093/trstmh/try075

KA_Road-Map-NVDBCP-Nov (2014). 6. National road map for kala-azar elimination. Directorate of National Vector Borne Disease Control Programme (NVBDCP)

Kumar A, Saurabh S, Jamil S et al (2020) Intensely clustered outbreak of visceral leishmaniasis (kala-azar) in a setting of seasonal migration in a village of Bihar, India. BMC Infect Dis 20:10

Marlow MA, da Silva MM, Makowiecky ME, Eger I et al (2013) Divergent profile of emerging cutaneous Leishmaniasis in subtropical Brazil: new endemic areas in the southern frontier. PLoS One 8(2):e56177

Marovich MA, Lira R, Shepard M, Fuchs GH et al (2001) Leishmaniasis recidivans recurrence after 43 years: a clinical and immunologic report after successful treatment. Clin Infect Dis 33(7):1076–1079

Mohan K, Suri JC (1975) Studies on cutaneous leishmaniasis in India. Isolation of Leishmania tropica from gerbils, sandflies and human. J Commun Dis 7:353–357

Narayan KG (2004) Epidemiology, diagnosis and management of zonnoses. ICAR, New Delhi

Owino BO, Matoke-Muhia D, Alraey Y, Mwangi JM, Ingonga JM et al (2019) Association of Phlebotomus guggisbergi with Leishmania major and Leishmania tropica in a complex transmission setting for cutaneous leishmaniasis in Gilgil, Nakuru county, Kenya. PLoS Negl Trop Dis 13(10):e0007712

Reithinger R, Dujardin JC, Louzir H, Pirmez C, Alexander B, Brooker S (2007) Cutaneous leishmaniasis. Lancet Infect Dis 7(9):581–596

Saini P, Kumar NP, Ajithlal PM, Joji A et al (2020) Visceral Leishmaniasis caused by Leishmania donovani Zymodeme MON-37, Western Ghats, India. Emerg Infect Dis 26(8):1956–1958

Sharma MID, Suri JC, Kalra NL, Mohan K, Swami PN (1973a) Epidemiological and entomological features of outbreak of cutaneous leishmaniasis in Bikaner, Rajasthan during 1971. J Com Dis 5:54–72

Sharma MID, Suri JC, Kalra NL, Mohan K (1973b) Studies on cutaneous leishmaniasis III. Detection of zoonotic focus of cutaneous leishmaniasis in Rajasthan. J Com Dis 5:149–153

Valencia BM, Miller D, Witzig RS, Boggild AK, Llanos-Cuentas A (2013) Novel low-cost thermotherapy for cutaneous Leishmaniasis in Peru. PLoS Negl Trop Dis 7(5):e2196

Volpedo G, Pacheco-Fernandez T, Holcomb EA, Cipriano N et al (2021) Mechanisms of Immunopathogenesis in cutaneous Leishmaniasis and post kala-azar dermal Leishmaniasis (PKDL). Front Cell Infect Microbiol 11:685296

WHO (2023). Key facts Leishmaniasis (who.int)

Yadav P, Azam M, Ramesh V, Singh R (2023) Unusual observations in leishmaniasis-an overview. Pathogens 12(2):297

Chapter 82
Sarcocystosis

Synonyms

Sarcosporidiosis.

Sarcocystosis is an intracellular protozoan infection that is generally chronic and asymptomatic but may have serious neural, reproductive consequences even fatal myocarditis in cattle. Comparative pathology is suggestive of similar pathology in human. Low estimated burden may be due to difficult diagnosis and poor reporting. Several outbreaks involving large number of people have been cited by Fayer et al. (2015) in their review. Trade impact is unknown. Visible cysts are rare; if visible, the carcass is declared unfit. It causes economic loss and affects the livelihood of backyard pig rearers in such situation.

82.1 Aetiology

Sarcocystis hominis, S. suihominis, S. nesbitti, S. cruzi, and *S. hirsuta* are the common pathogenic species of human, primates, pigs, cattle, dogs, and cats. *Sarcocystis* spp. belong to phylum *Apicomplexa*, family *Sarcocystidae*, genus *Sarcocystis*.

   Sarcocystis species are ubiquitous in nature and are found worldwide. These infect virtually all warm-blooded vertebrates, and species of *Cystoisospora* infect humans and a variety of animals. *Sarcocystis* requires a combination of intermediate (prey) and definitive (predator) hosts for completing life cycle. Intermediate hosts including human carry asexual stages, cysts (sarocysts) containing zoites in infected muscle. The final (predator) hosts ingest the cysts and get infected. The stages of development of the parasite occur in the intestine, and finally oocysts or sporocysts are excreted into the environment.

© Springer Nature Singapore Pte Ltd. 2024
K. G. Narayan et al., *Handbook of Management of Zoonoses*,
https://doi.org/10.1007/978-981-99-9885-2_82

Two species, *Sarcocystis hominis* and *S. suihominis*, have been identified in humans and non-human primates serving as definitive hosts. *Sarcocystis nesbitti* has been identified in humans and non-human primates serving as intermediate hosts, with a snake possibly serving as the definitive host. *Sarcocystis* spp. are intracellular protozoan parasites which may involve humans either as definitive or as intermediate hosts.

82.2 Mode of Infection

Sarcocystis spp. are intracellular protozoan parasites. Human beings suffer with two forms of sarcocytosis depending upon the infective stage of the parasite: sarcocyst and sporocyst—sarcocyst containing beef (*S. hominis*) or pork (*S. suihominis*) ingested by human, the definitive host causing intestinal sarcocytosis.

Ingestion of food or water contaminated with faecal sporocysts by human, the intermediate host causing hematogenous dissemination, can occur with invasion of muscle and causing extra-intestinal or muscular sarcocytosis. According to Fayer et al. (2015), there may be seven or more species for which human may act as intermediate host.

82.3 Intestinal Sarcocystosis

Intestinal sarcosystosis has been reported worldwide. It has been reported from the Netherlands, Germany, Poland, Slovakia, France, Spain, China, Tibet, Laos, Thailand, Australia, Argentina, and Brazil (Fayer et al., 2015).

In India, *S. suihominis* infection was high in economically deprived for whom backyard pig rearing and slaughter was livelihood. Children ate raw offal and pig tail with salt and complained abdominal pain and diarrhoea and excreted sporocysts.

Humans get infected with *Sarcocystis hominis* from beef and with *Sarcocystis suihominis* from pork.

82.3.1 Life Cycle

Life cycle explains the pathology. Here under the intestinal form of sarcocystosis is explained in Fig. 82.1.

Humans, the definitive hosts, eat meat containing mature sarcocysts. The wall of sarcocyst is broken/digested releasing bradyzoites. Cells of small intestinal villi are invaded. Bradyzoites are found intracellular. These transform into microgametocytes and become multinucleate and a sperm-like microgamete forms around each nucleus. Male microgamete is flagellated and finds and fuses with female macrogamont. Their nuclei combine. The fertilized macrogamont develops into an oocyst that sporulates in situ, forming two sporocysts that each contains four sporozoites.

examination diagnosed *Sarcocystis nesbitti* infection suggesting that sporocysts in snake faeces were the probable source of infection (Italiano et al., 2014).

Humans and macaques are intermediate hosts for *Sarcocystis nesbitti* (a species with a reptilian definitive host; cobra) and possibly for other unidentified species.

82.4.2   Symptoms

Clinical signs include fever, headache, and myalgia, episodic weakness or fatigue, and arthralgia in the beginning associated with early phase of development in vascular endothelium and difficult to diagnose. Subsequent development of intramuscular cysts is characterized by myositis.

82.5   Diagnosis

Tentative diagnosis may be arrived on the basis of (a) symptoms, various combinations of fever, myalgia, myositis, muscle tenderness, headache, cough, episodic weakness or fatigue, and arthralgia, and (b) certain laboratory tests, nonspecific and slightly elevated levels of hepatic enzymes, inflammatory markers [C-reactive protein and erythrocyte sedimentation rate (ESR) or markers of general cell damage (lactic dehydrogenase (LDH))], elevated serum creatinine phosphokinase, and eosinophilia.

It also includes detection of oocysts and/or sporocysts in the stool of cases of intestinal sarcocystis as well as enteritis and a history of having consumed undercooked meat.

Muscular sarcocystosis is often detected by incidental biopsy and on autopsy.

82.6   Treatment

Neither prophylactic nor curative therapy is available. Anti-coccidial drug is ineffective after sarcocysts are formed.

82.7   Prevention

Meat inspection (unless heavily infected)—It is time-taking and expensive and may be effective to some extent. Sarcocysts remain viable at 4 °C for days to weeks. Meat must be cooked well. Freezing kills bradyzoites in sarcocysts.

The use of untreated sewage water for irrigation of fodder/pasture for free-ranging domesticated food animals should not be permitted.

Scavenging by pigs should not be allowed.

Hygienic handling of meat and precaution to prevent cross-contamination hygiene between handling of pork (butcher to kitchen) should be practiced.

Use sanitized drinking water. Chemical disinfection with chlorine or other agents used for water treatments is not effective in killing sporocysts of *Sarcocystis*.

References

Fayer R, Esposito DH, Dubey JP (2015) Human infections with *Sarcocystis* species. Clin Microbiol Rev 28(2):295–311

Italiano CM, Wong KT, AbuBakar S, Lau YL, Ramli N et al (2014) *Sarcocystis nesbitti* causes acute, relapsing febrile myositis with a high attack rate: description of a large outbreak of muscular Sarcocystosis in Pangkor Island, Malaysia, 2012. PLoS Negl Trop Dis 8(5):e2876

Chapter 83
Toxoplasmosis

Toxoplasmosis is one of the most widely distributed protozoal zoonoses causing serious disease among pregnant women, developing foetuses, and those immuno-compromised due to HIV or chemotherapy. The classical triad "congenital toxoplasmosis" includes hydrocephalus, retinochoroiditis, and encephalitis. Other organs affected may be the heart, liver, and ear. Recently, toxoplasmosis has been linked with attention deficit disorder, obsessive compulsive disorder, schizophrenia, and suicidal tendency.

It may be subclassified as saprozoonosis and cyclozoonosis.

83.1 Aetiology

Toxoplasma gondii was first identified over 100 years ago in the tissues of birds and mammals (Kim and Weiss 2008). Nicolle and Manceaux (1908) reported first the asexual tachyzoite form in the gundi (*Ctenodactylus gundi*), a North American hamster-like rodent. Splendor (1908) in Brazil simultaneously identified the parasite in tissues of rabbits. Nicolle and Manceaux (1908) named the genus *Toxoplasma* for its bow-like shape (Greek: *Toxo* bow or arc; *plasma* creature). It is a coccidian parasite, and the full life cycle was not discovered until the 1960s and 1970s. Cat was identified as the definitive host by several groups working independently (Frenkel et al. 1970). All non-feline warm-blooded animals (including humans) act as intermediate hosts.

Toxoplasma gondii is a member of the phylum *Apicomplexa*. It is an intracellular parasite and has probably a widest range of hosts, all warm-blooded animals including human, livestock, birds, and marine mammals.

There are clonal lineages I, II, and III differing in virulence and pathogenicity (Sibley and Boothroyd 1992; Howe and Sibley 1995). Type I is lethal to mice, while the other two are not. Atypical strains have also been isolated from AIDS patients

© Springer Nature Singapore Pte Ltd. 2024
K. G. Narayan et al., *Handbook of Management of Zoonoses*,
https://doi.org/10.1007/978-981-99-9885-2_83

and pigs in Brazil (Belfort-Neto et al. 2007; Ferreira et al. 2008) besides man (Demar et al. 2007). Majority of ocular cases are caused by type II and congenital by type I. In France and the United States, type II and atypical strains are responsible for majority of asymptomatic cases in man, and about 10% type I and 9% type III were isolated from patients. However, in Brazil, type I strains caused ocular infections (Jones et al. 2006). The genotypes of *T. gondii* strains isolated from São Paulo and Erechim (Brazil) were highly atypical compared to the previously described cloning lineages (Khan et al. 2006). Such diversity was also reported by Dubey et al. (2006). Unusual genotypes of *T. gondii* in domesticated pigs are also found in Brazil (Belfort-Neto et al. 2007).

Ferreira et al. (2008) observed that 40/87(46%) patients of cerebral toxoplasmosis and AIDS treated in Sao Paulo State, Brazil, were infected with strains type I, 4 (4%) with type III, 13 (15%) with polymorphic strains (unusual genotype), and 6 patients with type I or II alleles and 15 (17%) patients had strains not classified for any marker. PCR-RFLP classified nine (11%) clinical isolates as type II, which is uncommon in South America. However, the sequencing of the nested PCR products (of SAG3 marker) of type II and polymorphic isolates (of 5'-SAG2, SAG3, and GRA6 markers) showed a nucleotide polymorphism compared with the archetypal clonal genotypes (types I, II, and III), and these isolates were considered as polymorphic strains. These data confirm other studies showing the high rate of genetic polymorphism in *T. gondii* strains isolated in Brazil.

The molecular analysis of isolates from the 11 patients of multivisceral toxoplasmosis in Patam, a Surinamese village near the French Guianan border by Demar et al. (2007), demonstrated that identical isolates of only 1 atypical strain were responsible for at least 5 of the 11 cases of toxoplasmosis in the outbreak. No epidemiological sources could be linked to this severe community-wide outbreak of toxoplasmosis.

83.1.1   Resistance

The discovery of the environmentally resistant stage of the parasite, the oocyst, made it possible to explain its worldwide prevalence (Dubey 2009).

Dubey (1998) reported that the oocysts stored at 10 °C, 15 °C, 20 °C, and 25 °C for 200 days retained infectivity. Retention of infectivity was dependent upon exposure temperature and period, 32 days at 35 °C, 9 days at 40 °C, 1 day at 45 °C, and 1 h at 50 °C. There was a 100-fold loss of infectivity of oocysts stored at 30 °C for 107 days. Oocysts remained infective up to 54 months at 4 °C, and there was no loss of infectivity in oocysts stored for 106 days at −5 °C and at −10 °C and for 13 months at 0 °C.

T. gondii oocysts survive up to 54 months in cold water.

The effect of gamma irradiation was studied by Dubey et al. (1998). *T gondii* oocysts irradiated at 0.5 kGy fed to mice were detected in histologic sections of mice up to 5 days but not at 7 days after feeding. Sporozoites from irradiated oocysts appeared normal ultrastructurally and formed a typical parasitophorous vacuole containing a well-developed tubulovesicular membrane network and penetrated enterocytes and all cells in the lamina propria except for red blood cells. Irradiation at 0.5 kGy seems effective in "killing" coccidian oocysts on fruits (studied on raspberries) and vegetables.

83.2   Life Cycle

T. gondii has a facultatively heteroxenous life cycle with members of family Felidae, genera *Felis* and *Lynx* as definitive host (Dubey et al. 1998; Frenkel 2000) and warm-blooded animals (some 200 species of mammals and birds) as intermediate host (Tenter et al. 2000; Dubey 2004).

   T. gondii has three infectious stages for both intermediate host (IH) and definitive host (DH): tachyzoites, bradyzoites (in tissue cysts), and sporozoites (in oocysts) in environment.

   In IH, it undergoes two phases of asexual development (Fig. 83.1). The first stage is initiated by active penetration of the cell membrane by fast dividing tachyzoites (or endozoites, crescent-shaped, 2–6 μm in size). It undergoes repeated binary divisions in a variety of host cells until they rupture. This proliferative phase is followed by the second phase when encystment as tissue cysts (5–70 μm in size) in muscle

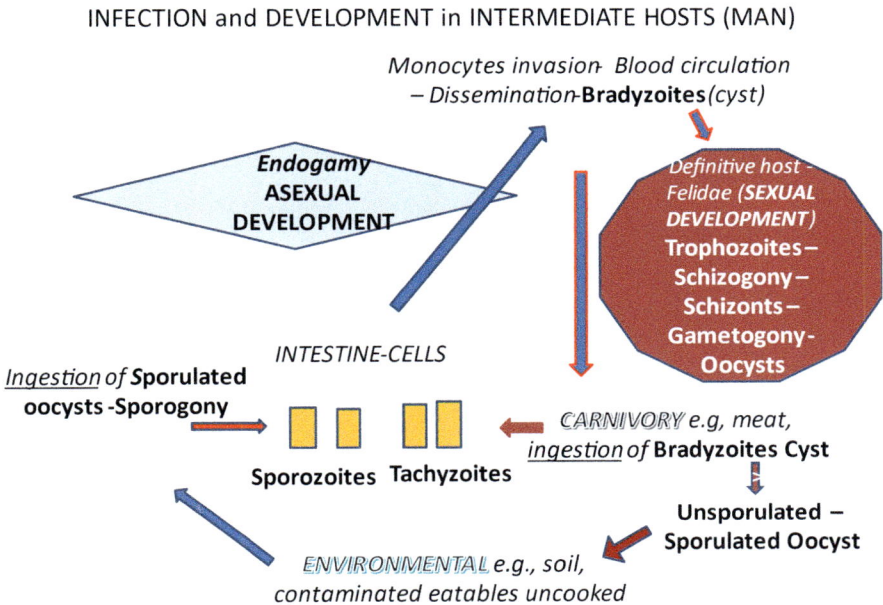

Fig. 83.1   Life cycle of *Toxoplasma gondii*

and neural tissues occurs. Cysts contain bradyzoites that multiply slowly. The cysts remain intracellular.

These tissue cysts may contain a few to several hundred crescent-shaped slender bradyzoites (or cryptozoites). These cysts are predominantly present in the brain, eye, and skeletal and cardiac muscles. However, they may also be found in visceral organs such as the kidney, lung, and liver (Dubey et al. 1998). These bradyzoites measure 7×1.5 µm differing slightly from tachyzoites. The bradyzoites are little more resistant to destruction by proteolytic enzymes (Dubey 2004). These may persist for life in the host and are terminal stage of life cycle in the IH and are infectious (Tenter et al. 2000).

Upon ingestion by the DH, cats, the bradyzoites are released from the tissue cysts by the action of the proteolytic enzymes in the stomach and small intestine, penetrate the lamina propria, and multiply as tachyzoites before getting disseminated to the extra-intestinal tissues. Many enter the epithelial cells of the small intestine initiating several generations of asexual (types A–E schizonts). The merozoites released from the schizonts form male and female gametes, which mate and oocysts form. Upon maturation, these are released into the intestinal lumen following the rupture of the epithelial cells and passed with faeces. These oocysts are formed only in cats—both domestic and wild. The cats shed oocysts after ingesting tachyzoites, bradyzoites, or oocysts (Dubey 2000, 2004). While nearly all cats shed oocysts following ingestion of tissue cysts, less than 50% shed oocyst after consuming tachyzoites or oocysts (Dubey and Frenkel 1976). The unsporulated oocysts (10×12 µm) in freshly passed faeces are non-infective. Depending on the environmental conditions, the oocysts get sporulated within 1–5 days, which contain two ellipsoidal sporocysts each having four sporozoites (2×6–8 µm) in size (Dubey et al. 1998).

83.3 Epidemiology

83.3.1 Prevalence

T. gondii genotype II was endemic in Finland (Jokelainen et al. 2012). Sero-reactors are more common than clinically diseased persons. Almost one-third of the world population have *T. gondii* antibodies. It is estimated to vary between 30% and 65%. According to Pappas et al. (2009), the approximate prevalence among women of childbearing age were 50–80% in Latin America, 20–60% in parts of Eastern and Central Europe, 30–50% in the Middle East, 20–60% in parts of Southeast Asia, and 20–55% in parts of Africa. The average rate of infection in China was 7.9%; higher rate was observed in Guizhou, Guangxi, and Jiangxi provinces. Many animal species including cats (infection rate up to 79.4%) were infected (Zhou et al. 2008). *T. gondii* isolates were different from type I, II, and III lineages that predominate in North America and Europe. Sero-positivity increases with age. 10.8% persons of age 6–49 years and 11% of women of 15–44 years tested IgG antibody positive (Jones et al. 2007). *T. gondii* antibody positivity was high in aborting women and higher among recurrently aborting women.

Demar et al. (2007) reported a community outbreak of multivisceral toxoplasmosis involving 11 cases that occurred in Patam, a Surinamese village near the French Guianan border. Eight were immunocomptetent yet suffered with multivisceral toxoplasmosis and one died; two cases had lethal congenital toxoplasmosis in a neonate and a foetus and one symptomatic child.

Molecular analysis demonstrated that identical isolates of only 1 atypical strain were responsible for at least 5 of the 11 cases of toxoplasmosis in the outbreak. No epidemiological sources could be linked to this severe community-wide outbreak of toxoplasmosis.

A study by Belfort-Neto (2007) indicated high prevalence of infection in domesticated pigs caused by unusual genotypes of *T. gondii* in Brazil (Belfort-Neto et al. 2007). Ferreira et al. (2008) studied 87 cases of cerebral toxoplasmosis and AIDS treated in Sao Paulo State, Brazil.

83.3.2 Sources of Infection

As observed by Zhou et al. (2008), approximately 150 million people are suffering from FBPZs including *T. gondii*, and more people are at risk. It is a worldwide public health problem.

Hebbar et al. (2022) reported Felidae (domestic cats and other felids) and Canids (domestic dogs and wild dogs—coyotes, dingoes, and wolves) are definitive hosts for *T. gondii* and *Neospora caninum*, respectively. They made a seroprevalence study in goats. *T. gondii was* 56.9% prevalent compared to 10.9% *Neospora caninum*. The cut-off serological cross reaction between the two was found to be the serum dilution of $\geq 1{:}200$ for ELISA and IFAT and $\geq 1{:}25$ for MAT/NAT.

The risk factors for infection were abortion, age of animals (> 2 years), extensive rearing system, and reservoir hosts.

83.3.2.1 Animals

According to Elmore et al. (2010), the global seroprevalence in cats is estimated to be around 30–40%. In the United States, it varies between 16% and 80%. However, most cats shed oocysts for a brief period of 1–2 weeks and once in its lifetime, but millions of oocysts can be shed with each oocyst capable of spreading and surviving for months.

Add to this a large number of intermediate hosts, global prevalence of toxoplasmosis could be enormous.

Definitive Host (DH)

The definitive host cats suffered with asymptomatic to generalized fatal infection. Infective dose for cats may be as low as ten sporocysts. Cats with compromised immunity, such as feline immunodeficiency and feline leukaemia infected ones, are more likely to suffer with a clinical disease. These manifest nonspecific symptoms—lethargy, anorexia, and fever. Symptoms vary with tissues parasitized—pneumonia, blindness, uncoordinated movement, circling, etc.—and behaviour/personality change. Post-mortem examination revealed generalized pathological lesions and parasite burden (Jokelainen et al. 2012).

Cats are the only hosts that shed oocysts. Others carry tissue cysts. Feline infection is usually asymptomatic and hence the cat owners are directly at risk.

Ingestion of oocysts, bradyzoites in cysts, or tachyzoites by cat sets up enteric infection. Cats and other members of Felidae are the only species that can excrete oocysts. Systemic infection followed by immune response stops excretion of oocyst. A high seroprevalence for toxoplasmosis in cats may not be accompanied with high prevalence of oocysts in their faeces (Tenter et al. 2000). The proportion of cats shedding oocysts at any time is usually no more than 1% in most countries (Dubey 2004). Cats continue to shed oocysts for 3–15 days in one cycle. The prepatent periods upon ingestion of bradyzoites varies from 3 to 5 days, tachyzoites 5 to 10 days, and sporocysts 20 to 24 days.

The overall prevalence was 48.8%. The study is based on examination of 445 purebred pet and 45 sheltered cats. 2/131 cats' faeces were positive for oocysts. Cats in Switzerland shed oocyst of *T. gondii* with clonal type II alleles and Apico I allele which was also predominant in sheep (Berger-Schoch et al. 2011). According to Al-Kappany et al. (2010), seroprevalence in cats in Egypt was 97.4%. The brain, heart, and tongue of 115/137 cats had *T. gondii*. None of the cats examined had oocysts in rectal content suggestive of high environmental contamination with oocysts.

Dabritz and Conrad (2010) observed that (a) cats' population in the United States has increased significantly, pet cat owners from 50 to 90 million with permission to allow their cats to deposit faeces outside, and (b) cats maintained in colonies also defecate outside. These have added to the toxoplasma burden of the environment significantly.

Wild cat faeces, litter from domestic cats flushed in latrines carried by surface run-off and freshwater outflows containing oocysts, are carried by water infected and even caused death of marine mammals.

Intermediate Hosts (IH): Food Animals

Reviewing literatures, Petersen et al. (2010) mention detection of tachyzoites in almost all body fluids, saliva, sputum, urine, tears, semen, and milk of several intermediate hosts including sheep, goats, and cattle, and of tissue cysts (bradyzoites) in meat, meat-derived products, and also offal. High seroprevalence rate among free-ranging grazing animals, sheep and goats, and outdoor pig rearing is an indication of wide extent of environmental contamination. Similarly, examination of marine mammals—sea otters, dolphins, and whales—also suggested that *T. gondii* oocysts were being washed into the oceans via freshwater run-off contaminated with cat faeces.

Man is thus surrounded by overwhelmingly burdened T. gondii—all three forms of which are dangerous.

Sheep and goat—It may be recognized by spate of abortions and congenital infection. All ages of ewes, especially maidens, are susceptible. Infection during early pregnancy, 45–55 days, leads to death and expulsion of foetus. Infection occurring during middle of gestation causes abortion or death and mummification of foetus to be expelled later. Cotyledons and foetal tissues carry characteristic white lesions of about 2.0 mm. The lesions carry the parasites. Gestation is carried to full term; lamb born may be still born or very weak. Infection at 3 months of pregnancy may not be serious.

T. gondii is widely distributed in the body of infected goats. It can be seen in the skeletal muscles, heart, diaphragm, liver, kidney, brain, milk, semen, placenta, and foetus.

Pigs—Added mode of infection in pigs are *c*annibalism and tail biting. Toxoplasmosis is characterized by pneumonia, encephalitis, and abortion. Fatal cases reveal necrosis and haemorrhage in visceral organs.

Cattle—Toxoplasmosis in cattle is rare, though neonatal infection and even fatal cases occur. Neural syndrome and respiratory symptoms arouse suspicion if other aetiologies have been ruled out.

Dogs—Four clinical forms of toxoplasmosis are known: (a) neuromuscular, (b) pulmonary necrotic lesions in neuromuscular and lungs, (c) gastrointestinal with lesions in the intestine and mesenteric lymph glands, and (d) generalized toxoplasmosis which present generalized necrosis of the hepatocytes, renal glomeruli and tubules, myocardium, spleen, and pancreas.

Birds—Clinical toxoplasmosis occur in chicken, ducks, pigeons, mynahs, canaries, and other passerine birds. Many avian species suffer with subclinical infection. Encephalitis and chorioretinitis are common in chicken. The post-mortem examination of chicken revealed ulceration of the intestine, necrosis of the liver and spleen, pneumonia, and enlargement of the heart (pericardium and myocardium).

83.3.2.2 Foods

Encysted *T. gondii* is found in pig, sheep, and goat tissues; viable cysts are rare in cattle. In Europe, pork is considered a major source of infection to human, and tissue cysts have been found quite often in commercial pork (Dubey 1986). *Meat from camel and wild animals including hare, wild boars, deer, and other cervids, kangaroo, and bears are potential sources* (Tenter et al. 2000; Dubey and Jones 2008). Meat from camel and kangaroo is very lean and is usually served undercooked in restaurants that are available to European consumers (Tenter 2009).

Dubey et al. (2002) studied the prevalence of viable *T. gondii* in meat used for human consumption in the United States. Viable *T. gondii* was isolated from 51 out of 55 pigs destined for human consumption. Cats (55) were fed hearts and tongues (500 g) from 55 six months old pigs from a farm in Massachusetts. Fifty-one of 55 cats fed pig tissues each shed 25–810 million *T. gondii* oocysts in their faeces. Results suggested examination of pork in slaughterhouse. Positive pork should be cooked according to industry guidelines before human consumption.

83.3.2.3   Environment

A large human outbreak is linked to contamination of a municipal water reservoir in Canada by wild felids and the widespread infection of marine mammals in the United States (Jones and Dubey 2010).

Sporocysts are very resistant to environmental conditions and survive for 1–1.5 years in damp soil/sand under shade (Frenkel 2000). These remain infectious in drinking/recreational/irrigation water for long resisting freezing and moderately high temperature. However, the oocysts are killed at 55–60 °C within 1–2 min (Dubey 1998). The sporulated oocysts are highly impermeable and thus very resistant to disinfectants (Kuticic and Wikerhauser 1996). *Toxoplasma gondii* oocysts are not killed by physical and chemical treatments currently applied in water treatment plants including chlorination, ozone treatment, and UV rays (Jones and Dubey 2010).

83.3.3   Transmission and Associated Factors

The infection can be transmitted to the susceptible hosts including the felids by consumption of undercooked meat from infected animal that carries tissue cysts or food or drink contaminated with sporulated oocysts (Fig. 83.2). Alternatively and very important is transplacental transmission of infection. The congenital transmission in man, sheep, and goats may cause death of the foetus when parasitaemia occurs in pregnant mother. Exposure to infected cats is important. Cat owners are thus at risk. Blood transfusion and organ transplant are other modes of infection. Occupational exposure is common among butchers, meat inspectors, housewives, gardeners handling soil contaminated with cats' faeces, and laboratory workers. Paratenic hosts may transport and spread infections—these may be coprophagous insects and flies.

Infection, prevalence, and transmission are dependent upon several factors. These are virulence of strains, number of parasites and route of infection, host species, age, conditions of host (especially immune status), food habits (high prevalence among the whites than blacks), and general sanitation.

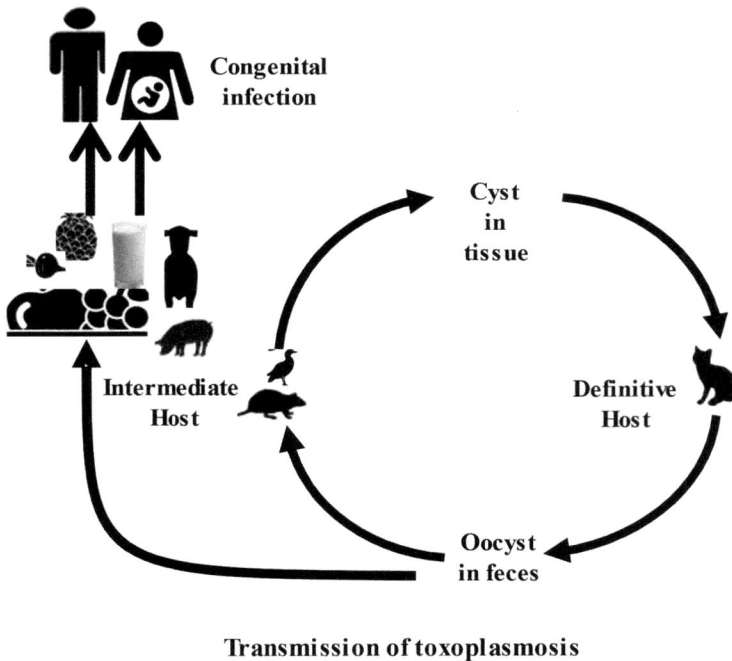

Transmission of toxoplasmosis

Fig. 83.2 Transmission of toxoplasmosis

83.3.3.1 Climate

Prevalence of toxoplasmosis has been found to be higher in moist and hot countries compared to dry or cold countries with higher prevalence in tropical areas which decreases with the increasing latitudes (Petersen et al. 2010). Its prevalence is low in the arctic areas (Tenter et al. 2000). Climate change is causing unprecedented damage to our ecosystem. Warming of ocean possibly transported *T. gondii* to new territories, the Norwegian Arctic archipelago of Svalbard, and beluga whales in western Canada to infect arctic fox, which has social and health impact as the Inuit population depends upon the arctic animals for sustenance. The prevalence increased between 2000 and 2006 with an increase of temperature by 0.6 °C in Mexico (FAO 2020).

83.3.3.2 Contaminated Environment

Innes (2010) has cited *contaminated environment* as a serious source of human toxoplasmosis. Heavy rainfall and contaminated drinking water supply led to acute toxoplasmosis in 110 people in Canada. Contaminated drinking water or ice made from it caused a disseminated outbreak in Brazil. 408 case-patients had *Toxoplasma* IgM and IgG antibodies of which 10% had ocular lesions and 4.4% had retinal lesions. The strain identified was genotype SAG 2 type 1 (de Moura et al. 2006).

83.3.3.3   Region: Rural and Urban

In the rural areas, shallow well located in farm area, contact with soil, sandpits used by children as playground, geophagia, and washing of vegetables and fruits may be strongly associated with toxoplasmosis. In the urban areas, pet cats and unawareness of owners stand exposed and infected. In the urban and rural areas, tissues from food animals may cause infection.

83.3.3.4   Food Animals

Reviewing literatures, Petersen et al. (2010) mention detection of tachyzoites in almost all body fluids, saliva, sputum, urine, tears, semen, and milk of several intermediate hosts including sheep, goats, and cattle, and of tissue cysts (bradyzoites) in meat, meat-derived products, and also offal. High seroprevalence rate among free-ranging grazing animals, sheep and goats, and outdoor pig rearing is an indication of wide extent of environmental contamination. Similarly, examination of marine mammals—sea otters, dolphins, and whales—also suggested that *T. gondii* oocysts were being washed into the oceans via freshwater run-off contaminated with cat faeces.

Multivariate analysis of risk factors studied in Brazil (Jones et al. 2006) suggested *working in garden (odd ratio (OR) 2.35), eating frozen lamb (OR 2.06), and women having children (OR 14.94)*. Risk increased in women as follows: women with no child (17.4%), one child (68.8%), and two or more children (79.3%). Other risk factors identified are poor hand hygiene; consumption of undercooked beef and lamb; cured, dried, or smoked meat; frequent consumption of raw vegetables; drinking unfiltered water; poor socioeconomic state; association with pet cats; and working in slaughter house.

Edelhofer and Prossinger (2010) studied seroprevalence in pigs during pregnancy in Austria. There has been a decline in toxoplasmosis over the years. This is explained—(a) improved management and hygiene in pig herds raised in confinements reducing contact with cats reflected in decreased prevalence in pigs in a decade, (b) decreased infection in cats as these were raised mainly on processed foods, and (c) eating cooked meat commonly. Seroprevalence in goats (69%) and in sheep (66%) kept on small farms was attributed to abundance of cats around these.

83.4   Infection

T. gondii is an intracellular protozoan parasite. It is capable of multiplying in almost any nucleated cell. Upon ingestion of sporocysts, sporozoites are liberated in the gut lumen, enter epithelial cells, and become tachyzoites. These tissue cysts contain bradyzoites. The infection persists throughout the life and so also the parasites till being eaten by the definitive host.

Formation of tissue cysts is related with host's immune response, and it generally occurs 1–2 weeks after infection. Tissue cysts are located preferentially in cells of the central nervous system, skeletal muscle, and heart. Hundreds and thousands of bradyzoites are found in a tissue cyst. Infection elicits both humoral and cell immune responses. IgG antibodies are formed and these persist for long. This is useful in seroepidemiological studies. Responses like formation of interferon-gamma, interleukin 2, CD4+ and CD8+, and T-helper cells enable the host in its battle against infection. Cytokines have a role in killing. Hosts may be stimulated by *Listeria*, *Besnoitia*, *Corynebacterium*, and BCG to produce non-specific protection.

In its fight to establish in the host, the parasite prevents lysosome fusion with parasitophorous vacuoles. This way, it is able to hide and survive in the macrophages, except when coated with antibodies.

Robert-Gangneux and Darde (2012) explained the process of infection by *T. gondii* that can invade a wide range of host cells. It uses motility and ability to secretory organelles like micronemes, the rhoptries, and the dense granules.

Adhesion—The calcium-dependent secretion of adhesins from micronemes like the microneme protein MIC2 that recognize host cell receptors and promote parasite *reorientation and attachment.*

Invasion of host cells depends upon a complex host cell surface-parasite interaction. It is facilitated by an intricate linear motor system promoted by actin-myosin interactions and dynamic rearrangements of the parasite cytoskeleton. The process is called *gliding motility.*

The process of entry is rapid, 15–30 s, and involves association between the apical end of *T. gondii* and host cell membrane—*the moving junction.*

Internalization process involves the "moving junction" to move around the parasite, apical to posterior end, and results into parasitophorous vacuole. This formation of "moving junction" around the invading parasite requires insertion into the host cell membrane of secretory micronemes, apical membrane antigen, and secretion of rhoptry neck proteins.

The nascent parasitophorous vacuole membrane (PVM)—Secretory proteins from rhoptries (ROPs) are rarely required. ROP18 is associated with cytosolic face of the PVM and initiates protein kinase activity required for the growth and virulence of the parasite, while ROP16 manipulate host gene expression that influences secretion of interleukin. The *dense granular proteins support the development of a complex network of membrane tubules from the PVM. This extends into the vacuolar lumen for exchanges between the parasite and the host. Within the PV, tachyzoites divide by endogamy.*

Lei Wang et al. (2023) studied the mechanism of apoptosis of murine Leydig tumour cells (MLTC-1) to elucidate the damage of the reproductive system. The *testis Leydig cell* is the main *testosterone synthesis* cell in male mammals. *T. gondii* entered the cells and caused lesions at 12 h. The *apoptosis rate* of the experiment group increased with time and was significantly higher ($P < 0.05$) than the control group. P53, caspase-3, and Bax expression increased significantly at 12 h. The expression of Bcl-2 and CHOP was significantly increased at 12 h ($P < 0.05$). The *ER stress* (ERS) pathway was important in cell apoptosis. The results indicated that *T. gondii*-induced MLTC-1 cell apoptosis may occur via the ERS pathway.

83.5   Pathology

Pathology is associated with the development of the parasite, especially in extraintestinal organs. Invasion of practically all types of cells, except erythrocytes, occurs. The intracellular growth of tachyzoites produces necrosis in organs. In heavy infection, vital organs like the myocardium, liver, lungs, and brain are affected. Early death may occur due to necrosis of the intestine and mesenteric lymph nodes.

Tissue cysts are distributed in the muscles, lungs, CNS, and other parts of the body. Large-sized (60 microns) cysts survive almost through the life of the hosts. The parasite persists within cyst for lifetime and is likely to recrudesce and actively multiply when the immune system is compromised. Tachyzoites in the brain and spinal cords survive longer as these are left unaffected by the developing immunity.

Acute toxoplasmosis coincides with the proliferative phase of the parasite. This phase is amenable to treatment with drugs. Chronic infection can be detected by the presence of bradyzoites only as there is no manifested symptom. Latent cysts are important in immunocompromised hosts, such as the case of AIDS, transplant patients developing foetus, and those suffering from lymphatic cancers including Hodgkin's disease.

83.6   Symptoms

Most infections in immunocompetent is subclinical. The patients with acute clinical infection may manifest symptoms resembling influenza, muscular pain, and swelling of lymph nodes lasting for a month or more. Immunocompromised individuals suffer severe infection that can damage the eyes (chorioretinitis), brain (encephalitis), heart, and liver.

83.6.1 Immunocompetent

Majority of pregnant mothers show no sign and symptoms of infection, so also the most of infected infants at birth. Intrauterine transmission occurs in approximately 25%, 54%, and 65% of untreated women who developed acute toxoplasmosis during first, second, and third trimesters of pregnancy, respectively. This is of great concern. Foetal infection acquired during first trimester is serious causing foetal parasitaemia, abortion, and premature birth. Congenital infection may manifest few days or several weeks after birth in form of encephalitis, hydrocephalia, calcification of occipital and parietal regions, chorioretinitis, loss of vision and hearing, mental retardation, and even death. Depending upon the tissues parasitized, there may be hepatomegaly, splenomegaly, respiratory symptoms, fever, eruptions, and convulsive attacks. In the United States, about 3000 infants are born with congenital deformities each year costing 31–40 million dollars.

The tragedy is that serious end result of infection may be manifested months and years later in life—such as neuropsychic retardation, chorioretinitis, hydrocephalia, microcephalia, epilepsy, and deafness. Examination of CSF shows xanthochromia and mononuclear pleocytosis. Eye lesions from congenital infection are often not identified at birth but occur in 20–80% of infected persons by adulthood in contrast with <2% of persons infected after birth who develop eye lesions in the United States.

Suresh Babu et al. (2007) observed *mental retardation* (hypogonadotropic hypogonadism) due to congenital toxoplasmosis detected in a 17-year boy, whose development was retarded to the extent of 4 years developmental age. His IQ was 50. He failed to attain secondary sexual character; had short stature, obesity, microencephaly, and low levels of growth and luteinizing and follicular-stimulating hormones in blood; and had healed choroiditis in macula of both eyes a characteristic lesion of congenital toxoplasmosis.

Toxoplasmosis may affect behaviour and perhaps contributes to or may be a cause to various psychiatric disorders such as depression, anxiety, and schizophrenia. The parasite possibly affects dopamine levels (Flegr 2013).

In a recent review, Petersen et al. (2010) observed that in non-pregnant and immunocompetent women, *T. gondii* is emerging as an important cause of retinochoroiditis.

Postnatal infection may be (a) serious, (b) less serious, and (c) ocular forms. Serious form is not very common except in immunodeficient and immunocompromised individuals. They suffer with enlargement of lymph glands, ocular and CNS disturbance, and respiratory and heart diseases. Relapses of disease and high mortality are common.

83.6.2 Immunocompromised

In the United States and Western Europe, 10–30% of seropositive AIDS patients die of toxoplasma encephalitis, and it is the predominant presentation in these countries. Clinical toxoplasmosis manifests as fever, maculopapular eruption, malaise, myalgia, arthralgia, fever, and pneumonia. Pathology includes myocarditis, myositis, cephalalgia, meningoencephalitis, splenomegaly, and lymphadenopathy. Re et al. (1999) recorded toxoplasmic encephalitis in acute T-cell leukaemia and lymphoma cases. The two cases were HIV-negative and were receiving fludarabine or methotrexate combination therapy.

In less serious form, there is lymphadenopathy of one or more lymph glands with or without associated fever. There is lymphocytosis. Such cases may pass unnoticed or undiagnosed.

The *ocular form* is characterized by retinochoroiditis, strabismus, nystagmus, and microphthalmia. Generally, both eyes are affected in infants.

Berdoy et al. (2000) observed *altered behaviour* of infected rats. Some of these sought cat-urine-marked areas and thus easily fell prey to cat. *Toxoplasma gondii* thus got opportunity to continue its life cycle. This prompted studies on association of *T. gondii* infection with altered human behaviour. Based on the review of papers on schizophrenia and toxoplasmosis, Torrey and Yolken (2003) concluded that *T. gondii* infection may contribute to schizophrenia in some cases. Supporting evidences were as follows:

(a) The parasite produced tyrosine hydroxylase that affected the production of dopamine and thus might cause psychological disorder.
(b) Raised dopamine levels and concentrated in the amygdala in infected mice.
(c) Some medications used to treat schizophrenia inhibited the replication of *T. gondii* in cell culture.
(d) Altered neurotransmitter function.

Zimmermann et al. (2013) reported cutaneous toxoplasmosis which is a rare finding in immunocompromised patients. A 60-year-old patient with aplastic pneumonia presented vesicular varicella-like skin lesions on her face, arms, legs, back, and abdomen. Skin biopsy led to a tentative histologic diagnosis of toxoplasmosis and was confirmed by immunohistochemistry and PCR as infection with *Toxoplasma gondii.*

83.7   Diagnosis

Specimens to be examined may be blood, spinal fluid, amniotic fluid, placenta, lymph nodes, bone marrow, or other body tissues and serum. The approaches to diagnosis may consist of demonstration of *T. gondii* by

1. Microscopic examination:

   • Direct.
   • Stained smear Giemsa stain.
   • Indirect fluorescent test.

2. Biological—Trypsin-digested specimens injected intraperitoneally in mice; peritoneal fluid examined by any of the above methods after a week.
3. Serological—Serum from the suspected cases or serum from the mice (biological test above) taken after 6 weeks of inoculation may be tested by any of the following tests for specific antibodies:

- Sabin-Feldman test—Live culture-derived tachyzoites + test serum + complement. Incubate the mixture; add dye. Lysed tachyzoites appear as unstained ghosts microscopically. Intact tachyzoites stain uniform blue in case of negative.
- Complement fixation test.
- ELISA.
- Indirect haemagglutination test—It lacks specificity at titre <1:64.
- Latex agglutination test.
- Indirect fluorescent antibody test

4. Intradermal test
5. Histological—Examine brain tissue of mice after sacrificing/autopsy for cyst.
6. Molecular diagnostic methods—Phylogenetic (molecular) method: Multilocus-nested polymerase chain reaction analysis combined with direct sequencing of a polymorphic intron (Khan et al. 2006).

83.8 Treatment

Toxoplasmosis is most serious in patients with weak immunity, and treatment is recommended. Useful drugs are azithromycin, clindamycin, and sulphonamides.

Sulfadiazine—Pyrimethamine combination is effective against tachyzoites. Pyrimethamine- clindamycin is another combination of choice for those who do not tolerate sulfadiazine.

Spiramycin is useful in pregnant women to prevent infection of their child. Pyrimethamine is generally not recommended. Clindamycin is used mostly in HIV cases.

Drugs do not reach bradyzoites in cyst in concentration sufficient to kill. Clindamycin and atovaquone appear to kill cyst in experimental mice; atovaquone has been used to kill *Toxoplasma* cysts inside AIDS patients.

83.9 Prevention and Control

- *Approaches directed to environment.*

Environmental hygiene and prevention of contamination of animal feed should keep out infection in farm and food animals. Reduction in number of infected cats and consequential reduction of contamination of environment. According to Innes (2010), California passed a legislation requiring "All cat litters sold carry a warning label to advice owners of cats "not to dispose cat faeces into toilets or in the outdoor - to help prevent contamination of environment". Control of coprophagous insects like flies and cockroaches reduce dissemination of oocysts.

• *Approaches directed to animals.*

Monitoring and surveillance of meat food animals for *T. gondii* have been recommended by the European Food Safety (EFSA 2007) to help planning protection of humans.

Detection of tissue cysts in grazing animals (especially sheep) and in wild boars is indicator of environmental contamination with oocysts (Edelhofer and Prossinger 2010) and a potential threat to human infection consuming meat from meat food animals and also wild animals.

• *Approaches directed to meat.*

Cooking >56 °C for 10 min, freezing at −12.8 °C for 2 days, curing with >2.0% salt or 1.4% lactate salts for at least 1 day, and kitchen hygiene should ensure safety to consumers (Kijlstra and Jongert 2009).

• *Approaches directed to high-risk group.*

Pregnant women, cat owners, those working in gardens and exposed to soil, butchers, and those working in kitchen including housewives stand at risk of getting infection. General instructions for them are as follows:

1. Avoid contact with cats' faeces, dirt, and sand used for cats to defecate.
2. Dispose off cats' faeces properly.
3. Wash pan with boiling water.
4. Wash sand boxes used for cats' defecation with boiling water.
5. Never feed uncooked food to cats.
6. Spaying owned cats to reduce overpopulation.
7. Use gloves while working in garden.
8. Eat properly cooked meat.
9. Fruits and vegetables should be thoroughly washed before eating.
10. Butchers and women must use gloves or wash hands well after handling raw meat. Detergents are effective in killing tissue cysts and tachyzoites, and so washing of hands and utensils with soap and hot water is recommended.

References

Al-Kappany YM, Rajendran C, Ferreira LR, Kwok OC et al (2010) High prevalence of toxoplasmosis in cats from Egypt: isolation of viable *toxoplasma gondii*, tissue distribution, and isolate designation. J Parasitol 96(6):1115–1118

Belfort-Neto R, Nussenblatt V, Rizzo L, Muccioli C, Silveira C et al (2007) High prevalence of unusual genotypes of *toxoplasma gondii* infection in pork meat samples from Erechim, Southern Brazil. An Acad Bras Cienc 79(1):111–114

Berdoy M, Webster JP, Macdonald DW (2000) Fatal attraction in rats infected with *toxoplasma gondii*. Proc Biol Sci 267(1452):1591–1594

Berger-Schoch AE, Herrmann DC, Schares G, Müller N, Bernet D et al (2011) Prevalence and genotypes of *toxoplasma gondii* in feline faeces (oocysts) and meat from sheep, cattle and pigs in Switzerland. Vet Parasitol 177(3–4):290–297

Dabritz HA, Conrad PA (2010) Cats and *toxoplasma*: implications for public health. Zoonoses Public Health 57(1):34–52

de Moura L, Bahia-Oliveira LM, Wada MY, Jones JL et al (2006 Feb) Waterborne toxoplasmosis, Brazil, from field to gene. Emerg Infect Dis 12(2):326–329

Demar M, Ajzenberg D, Maubon D, Djossou F et al (2007) Fatal outbreak of human toxoplasmosis along the Maroni River: epidemiological, clinical, and parasitological aspects. Clin Infect Dis 45(7):e88–e95

Dubey JP (1986) A review of toxoplasmosis in pigs. Vet Parasitol 19(3–4):181–223

Dubey JP (1998) *Toxoplasma gondii* oocyst survival under defined temperatures. J Parasitol 84(4):862–865

Dubey JP (2000) The scientific basis for prevention of *Toxoplasma gondii* infection: studies on tissue cyst survival, risk factors and hygiene measures. In: Ambroise-Thomas P, Petersen E (eds) Congenital toxoplasmosis: scientific background, clinical management and control. Springer-Verlag, France, Paris, pp 271–275

Dubey JP (2004) Toxoplasmosis - a waterborne zoonosis. Vet Parasitol 126(1–2):57–72

Dubey JP (2009) History of the discovery of the life cycle of *Toxoplasma gondii*. Int J Parasitol 39(8):877–882

Dubey JP, Frenkel JK (1976) Feline toxoplasmosis from acutely infected mice and the development of *toxoplasma* cysts. J Protozool 23(4):537–546

Dubey JP, Jones JL (2008) Toxoplasma gondii infection in humans and animals in the United States. Int J Parasitol 38(11):1257–1278

Dubey JP, Lindsay DS, Speer CA (1998) Structures of *toxoplasma gondii* tachyzoites, bradyzoites, and sporozoites and biology and development of tissue cysts. Clin Microbiol Rev 11(2):267–299

Dubey JP, Gamble HR, Hill D, Sreekumar C et al (2002) High prevalence of viable *toxoplasma gondii* infection in market weight pigs from a farm in Massachusetts. J Parasitol 88(6):1234–1238

Dubey JP, Su C, Cortes JA, Sundar N, Gomez-Martin JE et al (2006) Prevalence of *Toxoplasma gondii* in cats from Colombia, South America and genetic characterization of *T. gondii* isolates. Vet Parasitol 141:42–47

Edelhofer R, Prossinger H (2010) Infection with *toxoplasma gondii* during pregnancy: seroepidemiological studies in Austria. Zoonoses Public Health 57(1):18–26

EFSA (2007) European food safety authority. Scientific opinion of the panel on biological hazards on a request from EFSA on surveillance and monitoring of *toxoplasma* in humans, foods and animals. EFSA J 583:1–64

Elmore SA, Jones JL, Conrad PA, Patton S et al (2010) *Toxoplasma gondii*: epidemiology, feline clinical aspects, and prevention. Trends Parasitol 26(4):190–196

FAO (2020). *Climate change: unpacking the burden on food safety*. Food safety and quality series No. 8. Rome. https://doi.org/10.4060/ca8185en

Ferreira IM, Vidal JE, Costa-Silva TA, Meira CS, Hiramoto RM et al (2008) *Toxoplasma gondii*: genotyping of strains from Brazilian AIDS patients with cerebral toxoplasmosis by multilocus PCR-RFLP markers. Expt Parasitol 118:221–227

Flegr J (2013) How and why *toxoplasma* makes us crazy. Trends Parasitol 29(4):156–163

Frenkel JK (2000) Biology of *Toxoplasma gondii*. In: Ambroise-Thomas P, Petersen PE (eds) Congenital toxoplasmosis. Springer, Paris. https://doi.org/10.1007/978-2-8178-0847-5_2

Frenkel JK, Dubey JP, Miller NL (1970) *Toxoplasma gondii* in cats: fecal stages identified as coccidian oocysts. Science 167(3919):893–896. https://10.1126/science.167.3919.893. PMID: 4903651

Hebbar BK, Mitra P, Khan W, Chaudhari S et al (2022) Seroprevalence and associated risk factors of Toxoplasma gondii and Neospora caninum infections in cattle in Central India. Int Parasitol 87:102514

Howe DK, Sibley LD (1995) *Toxoplasma gondii* comprises three clonal lineages: correlation of parasite genotype with human disease. J Infect Dis 172(6):1561–1566

Innes EA (2010) A brief history and overview of *Toxoplasma gondii*. Zoonoses Public Health 57(1):1–7

Jokelainen P, Simola O, Rantanen E, Näreaho A, Lohi H, Sukura A (2012) Feline toxoplasmosis in Finland: cross-sectional epidemiological study and case series study. J Vet Diagn Invest 24(6):1115–1124

Jones JL, Dubey JP (2010) Waterborne toxoplasmosis--recent developments. Exp Parasitol 124(1):10–25

Jones LA, Alexander J, Roberts CW (2006) Ocular toxoplasmosis: in the storm of the eye. Parasite Immunol 28(12):635–642

Jones JL, Kruszon-Moran D, Sanders-Lewis K, Wilson M (2007) *Toxoplasma gondii* infection in the United States, 1999-2004, decline from the prior decade. Am J Trop Med Hyg 77(3):405–410

Khan A, Böhme U, Kelly KA, Adlem E, Brooks K, Simmonds M et al (2006) Common inheritance of chromosome Ia associated with clonal expansion of *Toxoplasma gondii*. Genome Res 16(9):1119–1125

Kijlstra A, Jongert E (2009) Toxoplasma-safe meat: close to reality? Trends Parasitol 25(1):18–22

Kim K, Weiss LM (2008) Toxoplasma: the next 100 years. Microbes Infect 10(9):978–984. https://10.1016/j.micinf.2008.07.015. PMID: 18672085; PMCID: PMC2596634

Kuticic V, Wikerhauser T (1996) Studies of the effect of various treatments on the viability of *Toxoplasma gondii* tissue cysts and oocysts. Curr Top Microbiol Immunol 219:261–265

Nicolle C, Manceaux LH (1908) Sur uen infection a corps de Leishman (ou organisms voisons) du gondii. C R Acad Sci 1908(147):763

Pappas G, Roussos N, Falagas ME (2009) Toxoplasmosis snapshots: global status of *Toxoplasma gondii* seroprevalence and implications for pregnancy and congenital toxoplasmosis. Int J Parasitol 39(12):1385–1394

Petersen E, Vesco G, Villari S, Buffolano W (2010) What do we know about risk factors for infection in humans with *toxoplasma gondii* and how can we prevent infections? Zoonoses Public Health 57(1):8–17

Re D, Reiser M, Bamborschke S, Schröder R, Lehrke R et al (1999) Two cases of toxoplasmic encephalitis in patients with acute T-cell leukaemia and lymphoma. J Infect 38(1):26–29

Robert-Gangneux F, Darde M-L (2012) Epidemiology of and diagnostic strategies for toxoplasmosis. Clin Microbiol Rev 25(2):264–296

Sibley LD, Boothroyd JC (1992) Virulent strains of *toxoplasma gondii* comprise a single clone lineage. Nature 359:82–85

Splendor A (1908) un nuovo parassita deconigli incontrato nelle lesioni anatomiche d'une malattia che ricorda in molti punti il kalaazar dell'uomo. Noter preliminare pel Rev Sco Sci Sao Paulo 3:109–112

Suresh Babu PS, Nagendra K, Navaz RS, Ravindranath HM (2007) Congenital toxoplasmosis presenting as hypogonadotropic hypogonadism. Indian J Pediatr 74(6):577–579

Tenter AM (2009) *Toxoplasma gondii* in animals used for human consumption. Mem Inst Oswaldo Cruz 104(2):364–369

Tenter AM, Heckeroth AR, Weiss LM (2000) *Toxoplasma gondii*: from animals to humans. Int J Parasitol 30(12–13):1217–1258

Torrey EF, Yolken RH (2003) *Toxoplasma gondii* and schizophrenia. Emerg Infect Dis 9(11):1375–1380

Wang L, Wang H, Wei S, Huang X, Chunchen Y et al (2023) *Toxoplasma gondii* induces MLTC-1 apoptosis via ERS pathway. Exp Parasitol 244:108429

Zhou P, Chen N, Zhang RL, Lin RQ, Zhu XQ (2008) Food-borne parasitic zoonoses in China: perspective for control. Trends Parasitol 24(4):190–196

Zimmermann S, Hadaschik E, Dalpke A, Hassel JC, Ajzenberg D et al (2013) Varicella-like cutaneous toxoplasmosis in a patient with aplastic anemia. J Clin Microbiol 51(4):1341–1344

Chapter 84
Human African Trypanosomiasis

Human African trypanosomiasis (HAT), also known as sleeping sickness, is a vector-borne parasitic infection of human and animals caused by extracellular protozoa, *Trypanosoma brucei gambiense* (TbG) and *Trypanosoma brucei rhodesiense* (TbR).

84.1 Aetiology

These are haemoflagellates of the genus *Trypanosoma*. Two subspecies, *T. b. gambiense* and *T. b. rhodesiense*, are pathogens, distinguishable genetically. The serum resistance-associated (*SRA*) gene is always present in all *T. b. rhodesiense* isolates. The *TgsGP* gene is found in type 1 *T. b. gambiense* (the classical form of *gambiense* HAT). Type 2 *T. b. gambiense* (genetically different) occurs in Western and Central Africa and causes a more acute form of *gambiense* HAT. *T. b. brucei* is non-pathogenic for humans but parasitizes domestic (*Bovidae*, *Suidae*, *Canidae*) and wild animals.

84.2 Life Cycle

84.2.1 In Vector (Glossina *spp.*)

Development of the parasite proceeds only in the compatible vector species (see later).

© Springer Nature Singapore Pte Ltd. 2024
K. G. Narayan et al., *Handbook of Management of Zoonoses*,
https://doi.org/10.1007/978-981-99-9885-2_84

Trypomastigote from the blood stream of host ingested by tsetse fly (*Glossina* spp.) moves to the mid-gut, differentiates into procyclic forms which replicate there, and crosses the peritrophic membrane to arrive in proventriculus. Here, these become mesocyclic trypomastigotes and later epimastigotes. These travel through the oesophagus, proboscis, and hypopharynx to salivary gland. These multiply and then transform into infectious metacyclic forms. This takes 18–35 days. Such tsetse fly is infective throughout its life. The variant surface glycoprotein (VSG) of the infective metacyclic form protects it from host's defence.

84.2.2   *In Mammalian Host*

Infected tsetse fly injects subdermally the metacyclic form during blood meal. These multiply at the site of bite and transform into slender forms. The draining lymph nodes carry these to blood stream. Long slender replicative trypomastigotes are maintained and found in blood stream. In the blood stream, the non-proliferative, short, stumpy trypomastigote forms are also found. This is adapted to differentiate into the replicative procyclic form in the tsetse fly, ensuring transmission.

The long slender, short stumpy, and intermediate transitional forms are found in the lymph, blood stream, different body fluids, and cerebrospinal fluid and can cross the placenta.

Sexual reproduction in trypanosomes may occur in salivary glands, possibly for genetic exchange of characters such as virulence and drug resistance. Genetic exchange is relatively frequent in *T. b. rhodesiense*.

84.3   Epidemiology

84.3.1   *Prevalence*

Human African trypanosomiasis is a life-threatening disease mainly of poor rural people (agriculture, fishing, animal husbandry, hunting) and travellers, endemic in sub-Saharan African countries. According to the WHO (2023), the Democratic Republic of the Congo, Angola, Central African Republic, Chad, Gabon, Guinea, Malawi and South Sudan, Cameroon, Côte d'Ivoire, Equatorial Guinea, Uganda, Tanzania, Ethiopia, Zambia, Burkina Faso, Ghana, Kenya, Nigeria, and Zimbabwe reported HAT with varying prevalence rates. Benin, Botswana, Burundi, Gambia, Guinea Bissau, Liberia, Mali, Mozambique, Namibia, Niger, Rwanda, Senegal, Sierra Leone, Swaziland, and Togo have not reported cases for over a decade. The intensity of disease varies from one village to other. Single to a series of villages may be affected.

84.3.2 Favourable Factors

Human African trypanosomiasis threatens mainly populations of remote rural areas with limited health services.

Generally, fatality may be cent per cent if untreated. It is mainly a chronic disease and affects the income-generating capacity of families, worsening the economic situation of impoverished groups. In this way, the disease contributes to maintain the poverty cycle in these neglected communities.

84.3.3 Disease Burden and Distribution

Epidemics over the last century:

- One between 1896 and 1906, mostly in Uganda and the Congo Basin.
- One in 1920 in a number of African countries.
- The most recent epidemic started in 1970 and lasted until the late 1990s.

These epidemics were mainly linked to increased population movements and changes in the environment (e.g. deforestation or the introduction of intensive agriculture for cash crops, war, forced displacement) and poverty.

Control efforts brought down the number of reported cases to <5000/year in the continent by the 1960s. Relaxed surveillance and resurgence brought the cases to epidemic proportion in several regions by 1970 reaching almost 40,000 cases in 1998 amidst 300,000 undetected and untreated cases. HAT was first or second cause of mortality in several communities of villages in Angola, the Democratic Republic of the Congo (DRC), and South Sudan where the prevalence was 50% in several villages. With the joint efforts by the WHO, national control programmes, bilateral cooperation, and nongovernmental organizations, HAT cases dropped to <2000 in 2017 and < 1000 in 2018 and continues below that threshold as of 2022. The estimated population at risk was 55 million with only 3 million at moderately high risk during the period 2016–2020 (WHO 2023).

84.3.4 Vector

The vector tsetse flies look like houseflies. Tsetse flies fold their wings while resting completely so that one wing rests directly on top of the other over their abdomen, and they have a long proboscis which extends directly forward and is attached by a distinct bulb to the bottom of their heads. Tsetse flies are found in sub-Saharan region. Only certain spp. are vectors.

84.3.4.1   Habitat

The temperature and humidity requirements for survival of the vector tsetse flies are 16 °C–38 °C and 50%–80%. Vegetation/forest near water bodies, riverbanks, lakes, swamps and mangroves, coffee or cocoa plantations, and agriculture are favourable and also attract animals. These adapt to environmental changes and are found in areas of agriculture, around cities/townships.

The vector tsetse flies are found in sub-Saharan Africa between 14°N and 29°S between two deserts, Sahel and Namibian Kalahari. *G. morsitans* and *G. fuscipes* have been described in some pockets of South-Western Saudi Arabia.

The subgenus *Nemorhina* or the *palpalis* group includes the main vectors of sleeping sickness: *G. palpalis palpalis* and *G. p. gambiensis* for *T. b. gambiense*. These are found on the Atlantic coast from Senegal to Angola.

G. fuscipes, vector for both *T. b. gambiense* and *T. b. rhodesiense*, are spread over Central Africa from Cameroon and Congo to the Rift Valley.

The subgenus *Glossina* sensu stricto or the *morsitans* group includes *G. morsitans*, *G. swynnertoni*, and *G. pallidipes (T. b. rhodesiense)* abound in woodland savannah of East Africa and is linked to the presence of wild fauna and cattle.

Some areas in South-Western Saudi Arabia have *G. morsitans* and *G. fuscipes*. In nature, the infection is carried almost exclusively by *G. fuscipes*, *G. palpalis*, and *G. morsitans*.

84.3.4.2   Vector Efficiency

Only 2%–5% of the flies ingesting trypanosomes produce metacyclic (infective) forms. The mature infection rate among tsetse flies is quite low. An average of less than 1% of tsetse flies is infective for *T. brucei* spp. However, even low ingestion of parasite by the vector and a single bite can result into transmission. Factors that may influence transmission include vector density, longevity, susceptibility to infection, infestation rate, frequency, and intensity of contact with host.

84.3.4.3   Vectors' Life Cycle and Infection

Tsetse flies have a lifespan of 7 months, varying with season, 3–5 months in rainy and 1–2 months in dry. After 20–80 days (temperature- and humidity-dependent) of larviposition of the mature larva in humid soil under a shade, the pupa living on food reserve a few centimetres deep in sand/soil emerges as adult. The adult needs immediate blood meal. The first meal is most likely infective. The flies take meals every 2–4 days up to 10 days. Blood meal lasts for 20–30 seconds. Saliva delays coagulation of blood and causes vasodilation helping the transfer of infective trypanosomes either/both ways—from flies to mammalian host or reverse. Both male and female can transmit infection. Mating occurs days after emergence. Female remains fertile after single mating. More sexual unions leave spermatozoides in spermathecae that survive for nearly 200 days. Fertile female lays larva approximately every 10 days.

Tsetse flies have great dispersal capacity, maybe 20–30 km distance in successive days. Passive dispersal through cattle herds and vehicles presents risk of invading areas free of tsetse.

84.3.5   Reservoir Hosts

The preferred hosts for *G. morsitans* and *G. palpalis* are pigs, warthogs, and bush pigs. Reptiles (monitor lizards, crocodiles, and snakes) are preferred by many species. Humans are occasionally bitten by the *G. morsitans* group. Human odour seems to attract *G. fuscipes* and *G. palpalis*. Tsetse flies are able to adapt to host availability.

Glossina is practically the only vector responsible for transmitting the parasite. Detection and treatment of cases of infection combined with vector control may result into a sustained control of HAT.

84.3.5.1   Significance of Reservoir Hosts

- *T. b. rhodesiense.*

T. b. rhodesiense is zoonotic. The usual transmission cycle is "wild and domestic animal – tsetse". The parasites spill over from this to human. The "man-tsetse-man" cycle is observed during epidemic. Study in Uganda proves cattle as reservoir, and control measures directed to this reservoir reduced the number of infected cattle and consequentially in humans.

Uganda is home to both chronic *T. b. gambiense* (gHAT) and the acute zoonotic form *T. b. rhodesiense* (rHAT). Import of infected cattle into tsetse-infested but previously HAT-free districts introduced *T. b. rhodesiense* resulting in a considerable human health burden in these newly affected districts. Fyfe et al. (2017) reported that a single intervention in form of treatment of cattle reservoir of human infective *T. b. rhodesiense* with a trypanocidal drug is a promising and cost-effective approach for the control of rHAT. Treatment of cattle before relocation could prevent possible merger of the two HAT foci; else, it would complicate diagnosis and treatment of both gHAT and rHAT. The study was carried out in high-risk sub-counties of Kamuli District (endemic for rHAT) and Soroti District (where rHAT has been recently introduced). The prevalence of *T. brucei s.l.* and the human infective subspecies *T. b. rhodesiense* in cattle (n = 1833) was assessed before and 3 and 12 months after intervention using PCR-based methods.

- *T. b. gambiense.*

T. b. gambiense is known largely as anthropophilic with "tsetse-human" cycle. *T. b. gambiense* has been detected in domestic animals such as pigs, sheep, and goats. A wide range of animals have been experimentally infected with *T. b. gambiense*, some of which were shown to be infective to tsetse. According to Mehlitz and Molyneux (2019), metacyclic transmission of *T. b. gambiense* has been reported in antelope-*G. p. palpalis*-antelope and pig-*G. p. gambiensis*-pig cycles. These animal-*Glossina*-animal cycles (antelopes and pigs) retain infectivity for 3 years. The human infectivity markers (human serum resistance, zymodeme, DNA) are stable in non-human hosts for the same period as observed experimentally. It is important to understand the latent infection in human and animal reservoirs—wild and domesticated are targeted—while planning for achieving the WHO set goal of zero transmission by 2030.

Is T. b. gambiense also zoonotic? Tsetse flies caught from areas with no human case of T. b. gambiense HAT have been found infected with this parasite suggesting possible role of cryptic animal reservoir.

Search for potential animal reservoir led Vourchakbé et al. (2020) to examine domestic animals in all HAT foci. It was found that pigs, dogs, sheep, and goats appeared to be potential reservoir hosts for *T. b. gambiense* in Chad. *T. b. gambiense* were identified by PCR.

Study by Cunningham et al. (2020) found that pigs, cattle, and tsetse were negative for T. *b. gambiense* HAT and probably accounted for low prevalence in human in North-West Uganda. However, the study highlighted the limitations of current methods of detecting and identifying *T. b. gambiense* which relies on a single-copy gene to discriminate between the different subspecies of *T. brucei s.l.*

In Côte d'Ivoire, HAT is still present in several foci, e.g. Bonon and Sinfra. Blood samples from animals (goats, pigs, cattle, and sheep) were tested. This study shows that domestic animals are highly infected by trypanosomes in the studied foci. This was particularly true for pigs, possibly due to a higher exposure of these animals to tsetse flies. Whereas *T. brucei s.l.* was the most prevalent species, discordant results were obtained between PCR and trypanolysis (TL) regarding *T. b. gambiense* identification. It is therefore crucial to develop better tools to study the epidemiological role of potential animal reservoir for *T. b. gambiense* (N'Djetchi et al. 2017). Free-ranging pigs were identified as a multi-reservoir of *T. brucei* and/or *T. congolense* with mixed infections of different strains. This trypanosome diversity hinders the direct detection of *T. b. gambiense* with the available tools and to prove or exclude with certainty its presence (Traoré et al. 2021).

84.4   HAT Disease

Human African trypanosomiasis (HAT) or sleeping sickness has two distinct forms, caused by *T. b. gambiense* and *T. b. rhodesiense*, respectively.

The geographical separation appears clearly defined by Rift valley. On the eastern side, *T. b. rhodesiense* is endemic in 13 countries of Eastern and Southern Africa, accounts for 8% of reported cases, and causes an acute disease. *T. b. gambiense* is found on the west, is endemic in 24 countries of West and Central Africa, and accounts for 92% of the reported cases. It causes a chronic form of disease (WHO 2023).

This separation is reducing in North-West Uganda and on the border between the United Republic of Tanzania and the Democratic Republic of the Congo may vanish in the future.

According to Sudarshi and Brown (2015), 94 cases were reported between 2000 and 2010 in non-endemic countries. Of these, 72% were East African form (*rhodesiense* HAT) and 28% due to the West African form (*gambiense* HAT). The response to infection differed in migrants and travellers. *Rhodesiense* HAT positive group were tourists who recently visited game parks in Eastern or Southern Africa, whereas *gambiense* HAT group were migrants from West or Central Africa who left many years (29 years) earlier. The travellers presented acute febrile illness similar to *rhodesiense* HAT with an incubation period of few days to 3 weeks. Many (84%) recalled being bitten by tsetse flies and had a trypanosomal chancre. African migrants presented symptoms of *gambiense* HAT like low-grade fever and neuropsychiatric symptoms like typical sleep disorder, motor and sensory disturbances, abnormal reflexes, and psychiatric symptoms. During 2011–2020, a total of 49 cases of HAT were reported by Franco et al. (2022) in 16 non-endemic countries across 4 continents. These were distributed as 50% in Europe, 22% in South Africa (a non-endemic country), 14% in North America, and 12% in Asia. Only one case was detected in South America. 35 cases were caused by *T. b. rhodesiense*, mainly in tourists visiting wildlife areas in Eastern and Southern Africa, and 14 cases were due to *T. b. gambiense, mainly in African migrants originating from or visiting endemic areas in Western and Central Africa.* HAT in non-endemic countries is rare but can be challenging.

84.4.1 *HAT* T. b. gambiense

HAT *T. b. gambiense* occurs in 24 countries West and Central Africa, accounting for 98% cases. *Gambiense* HAT is considered a rural disease. Occasionally, it occurs in urban settings because of travels to neighbouring rural areas for agricultural activities.

The infection slowly progresses and is chronic for several years even without major signs and symptoms. When more evident symptoms emerge, the patient is often already in an advanced stage of disease where the central nervous system is affected.

84.4.1.1 Epidemiology

It is anthroponotic and humans are the main epidemiological reservoir. Transmission cycle is "infected man-tsetse-susceptible man". Animal has a minor role.

The long duration of human infection with an extended paucisymptomatic period is considered sufficient to maintain a "human-fly-human transmission cycle". Asymptomatic human beings who were parasitaemia-negative but positive for PCR and trypanosome-lysis tests (followed for 5–15 years) and trypanotolerant animals could be chronic carriers. These could be a source of vector infection that maintains the transmission of HAT *gambiense*. Other reservoirs are a number of domestic and wild animals (mammals and reptilians).

T. b. gambiense group 1 parasite infection has been found in domestic livestock (mainly pigs) in some *gambiense* human foci. In other foci where the same human infection prevails, domestic animals are not found infected. Trypanosome genotypes circulating in pigs and humans are different in some other foci. More data are required for clarity.

Reservoir role for *T. b. gambiense* is not clear even when pigs, sheep, dogs, goats, and many different wild animals have been found infected (Franco et al. 2014).

84.4.2   *HAT* T. b. rhodesiense

HAT *T. b. rhodesiense* occurs in 13 countries of Eastern and Southern Africa and represents only 2% of cases. The parasite invades the CNS. Symptoms appear rapidly. The disease is mainly acute lasting weeks to several months after infection.

84.4.2.1   Epidemiology

The peak in the *Glossina* population densities is usually seen after the rainy season. The peak in the human cases can be detected in 1–3 months after the rainy season. Activities like hunting, fetching firewood, timber-related activities, and forest clearing for farming require working in areas where wildlife reservoir and tsetse flies abound. Therefore, rangers and park wardens, visitors of national parks (tourists), or herdsmen grazing their animals in forest are at risk of acquiring *rhodesiense* HAT. Short-term travellers from non-endemic areas can also be exposed.

T. b. rhodesiense is zoonotic. Reservoir role of human is limited and may be occasional. The usual transmission cycle is "wild and domestic animal-tsetse". The parasites spill over from the animal-tsetse fly-animal cycle to human. The "man-tsetse-man" cycle is observed during epidemic.

The wild animal reservoirs are bushbuck, duiker, giraffe, hartebeest, hyena, impala, lechwe, lion, oribi, reedbuck, warthog, waterbuck, and zebra, with bushbucks considered as the most frequently described reservoir. Domesticated animal reservoirs are bovine and porcine species.

The factors responsible for transmission between human and wild animal reservoirs are change in land use, social forestry, animal grazing, and human activity encroachment in forest, ecotourism.

Contact with domestic animal reservoir and those at the forest-human habitat interface is easier. HAT *rhodesiense* can be transmitted from wildlife to humans, either directly or through livestock. Cattle infection accounted for around 1% of livestock infections in areas where human cases are rarely reported and can reach 18% during human outbreaks (Franco et al. 2014).

Only Uganda presents both forms of the disease but in separate zones. Animals can host both the species and play a reservoir role for HAT *rhodesiense* and an unknown role for HAT *gambiense*.

84.5 Modes of Transmission

Cyclic—The tsetse fly is considered as a cyclical vector as the transmission requires a transformation process of the parasite in the fly.

Mechanical—Rare but is possible in the case of high parasitaemia.

Vertical—Congenital.

Accidental mechanical—laboratory accidents.

Blood transfusion.

Transplant—theoretically possible.

Sexual transmission has occurred.

84.6 Parasite-Host Interaction

After an infective bite, the trypanosomes multiply in the subcutaneous tissue, blood, and lymph. This is the first or the haemolymphatic stage. The meningoencephalitic or second stage follows when the blood barrier is crossed by the invading parasites.

Parasitaemia occurs following infection. The level of parasitaemia is influenced by hosts' immune response and antigenic variation in parasite. Generally, parasitaemia in *T. b. gambiense* is <100 /ml and higher in *T. b. rhodesiense*.

Variant surface glycoprotein (VSG) protects from antibodies and complement system. VSG is immunogenic and induces development of IgG and IgM antibodies. The antibodies reduce the number of parasites. The coat protein turnover is rapid, and it binds to the antibodies, permitting parasites to escape the immune response.

New variants of VSG are possibly produced. "Stumpy induction factor" triggers the production of nonreplicating stumpy forms adapted to re-establish the life cycle upon ingestion by the vector fly.

84.7 Signs and Symptoms

Sleeping sickness runs into two stages.

Trypanosomal chancre develops at the site of infectious bite within 2 days. It occurs commonly in cases of *T. b. rhodesiense*, rarely in *T. b. gambiense* among those from non-endemic areas. A trypanosomal chancre consists of a tender, purplish, indurated area of erythema appearing after 1 week of the tsetse fly bite at the same site.

Stage 1 or haemolymphatic stage: The incubation period is 1–3 weeks (after bite) for *T. b. rhodesiense* and longer for *T. b. gambiense*. The parasite multiplies in subcutaneous tissues, blood, and lymph. Bouts of fever, headaches, enlarged lymph nodes, hepatosplenomegaly, joint pain, and itching are manifested. Febrile episode is followed by appearance of a non-itchy, transient maculopapular rash on the torso in some. High fever, headache, gastrointestinal complaints (nausea, vomiting, and jaundice), lymphadenopathy, and headache are the initial symptoms. Bouts of fever last from a day to a week with intervals of a month or longer. The frequency of bouts decreases over time. The lymph nodes swell to tremendous size in sleeping sickness. Commonly cervical, axillary, inguinal, and epitrochlear lymph nodes show inflammation. The chain of posterior cervical lymph nodes is swollen and may be suggestive of cerebral infection. The patients may develop myocarditis and arrhythmias as the disease progresses. Following peaks of parasitaemia, multiorgan failure may happen.

Stage 2 or neurological/meningoencephalic phase: This phase begins weeks to months (21–60 days in case of *T. b. rhodesiense* and 300–500 days in case of *T. b. gambiense*) later. The parasites cross blood-brain barrier to enter the CNS. Generally, HAT is evident at this stage. Sleeping sickness (disturbed sleep cycle) is manifested as sleep inversion, daytime sleep, somnolence, night-time period of wakefulness and insomnia, and episodes of sudden sleepiness. Neurological symptoms are weakening muscles; tremor; hemiparesis and paralysis; ataxia, sensory disturbance, and poor coordination; disturbed speech, vision, and gait; paraesthesia, hyperaesthesia, and anaesthesia; and seizures. Behavioural and psychiatric changes include apathy, confusion, attention deficit, aggressiveness, irritability, anxiety, hallucination, mania, and delirium.

Neurological damage is irreversible. Condition may deteriorate if not treated and progresses to coma, systemic organ failure, and death, within months in case of *T. b. rhodesiense* and after several years in case of *T. b. gambiense*.

The two stages may be clinically indistinguishable. Lumber puncture and demonstration of trypanosomes in cerebrospinal fluid are diagnostic.

Atypical symptoms observed for reasons unknown in people from non-endemic areas, e.g. travellers, include mainly fever with gastrointestinal symptoms and rarely lymphadenopathy.

84.8 Diagnosis

Screening needs to be exhaustive in order not to miss a relatively long asymptomatic stage of infection.

Diagnosis plays a significant role in the control and prevention of infection as well as in the treatment of infected ones. Early diagnosis is important to prevent the progression of infection to the neurological stage with more complex and risky treatment.

Active screening of exposed population to detect cases at an early stage and its removal as reservoir are important to control HAT:

- Swollen cervical lymph gland is suggestive.
- Microscopic test for parasites in blood, chancre fluid, body fluids, and CSF after lumbar puncture—wet or dry—and Giemsa or Field's stain-stained preparation.
- Serologic test (available for *T. b. gambiense* only) for antibodies—the micro-CATT (card agglutination test for trypanosomiasis uses dried blood), wb-CATT, and wb-LATEX use wet blood.

The serologic tests may be used for tracking the disease progression via clinical examination and analysis of cerebrospinal fluid obtained by lumbar puncture. These are used for screening for potential infection.

84.9 Treatment

There is a better prospect for cure if treated in the first stage. A follow-up for 24 months of cases is required as the parasite may remain viable for months after treatment. Clinical and laboratory examinations are done. Drugs pentamidine and suramin may cause allergic side- effects and affect the urinary tract. Drugs for treatment of second stage have to cross blood-brain barrier.

Drugs for *rhodesiense* HAT are suramin and melarsoprol. Drugs for *gambiense* HAT are pentamidine, eflornithine, nifurtimox, and fexinidazole.

The WHO supplies all anti-trypanosome medicines worldwide gratis thanks to donations from Sanofi and Bayer and collaboration with MSF Logistics for conditioning and shipment (WHO 2023).

84.10 Prevention

- Individuals may protect himself by using insect repellents, wearing long-sleeved clothing, and avoiding tsetse-dense areas.
- Bush clearance and wild game culling for the areas.

For the community, detection and prompt treatment of new infections and tsetse fly control:

1. Regular active surveillance: Mobile clinics or fixed screening centres carry out systematic screening of community at risk.
2. Eradication of the tsetse vector population.

Insecticide-impregnated targets, fly traps, insecticide-treated cattle, and ultra-low-dose aerial/ground spraying of tsetse resting sites may be carried out. Raising and release of sterile insects are another approach. Sustained control efforts have reduced the number of new cases by 97% in the last 20 years (WHO 2023).

References

Cunningham LJ, Lingley JK, Tirados I, Esterhuizen J, Opiyo M et al (2020) Evidence of the absence of human African trypanosomiasis in two northern districts of Uganda: analyses of cattle, pigs and tsetse flies for the presence of Trypanosoma brucei gambiense. PLoS Negl Trop Dis 14(4):e0007737

Franco JR, Simarro PP, Diarra A, Jannin JG (2014) Epidemiology of human African trypanosomiasis. Clin Epidemiol 6:257–275

Franco JR, Cecchi G, Priotto G, Paone M, Kadima Ebeja A, Simarro PP et al (2022) Human African trypanosomiasis cases diagnosed in non-endemic countries (2011–2020). PLoS Negl Trop Dis 16(11):e0010885

Fyfe J, Picozzi K, Waiswa C, Bardosh KL, Welburn SC (2017) Impact of mass chemotherapy in domestic livestock for control of zoonotic *T. b. rhodesiense* human African trypanosomiasis in eastern Uganda. Acta Trop 165:216–229

Mehlitz D, Molyneux DH (2019) The elimination of *Trypanosoma brucei gambiense*? Challenges of reservoir hosts and transmission cycles: expect the unexpected. Parasite Epidemiol Cont 6:e00113

N'Djetchi MK, Ilboudo H, Koffi M, Kaboré J, Kaboré JW et al (2017) The study of trypanosome species circulating in domestic animals in two human African trypanosomiasis foci of Côte d'Ivoire identifies pigs and cattle as potential reservoirs of Trypanosoma brucei gambiense. PLoS Negl Trop Dis 11(10):e0005993

Sudarshi D, Brown M (2015) Human African trypanosomiasis in non-endemic countries. Clin Med (Lond) 15(1):70–73

Traoré BM, Koffi M, N'Djetchi MK, Kaba D, Kaboré J et al (2021) Free-ranging pigs identified as a multi-reservoir of *Trypanosoma brucei* and *Trypanosoma congolense* in the Vavoua area, a historical sleeping sickness focus of Côte D'ivoire. PLoS Negl Trop Dis 15(12):e0010036

Vourchakbé J, Tiofack ZAA, Kante TS, Mpoame M, Simo G (2020) Molecular identification of *Trypanosoma brucei gambiense* in naturally infected pigs, dogs and small ruminants confirms domestic animals as potential reservoirs for sleeping sickness in Chad. Parasite 27:63

WHO. (2023). Trypanosomiasis, Human African (sleeping sickness). 2 May 2023 Key facts. https://www.who.int/news-room/fact-sheets/detail/trypanosomiasis-human-african-(sleepingsickness)

Chapter 85
Epidemiology of Fish-Borne Zoonotic Trematodiasis

The World Health Organization has added fish-borne zoonotic trematodes (FZTs) infections to its list of emerging infectious diseases (Clausen et al. 2012). A review by Chai et al. (2009) mention that an estimated 40–50 million people (though an underestimate) are likely to be infected with foodborne trematodes worldwide. Most of them are located in Southeast Asia, including Korea, China, Thailand, Vietnam, Lao PDR, the Philippines, Indonesia, and India. The number of fish-borne zoonotic trematodes (FZTs), currently known to be involved in this area, is counted at least 59. FZTs' life cycle involve first intermediate host (freshwater snails), second intermediate host (freshwater fish), and definitive host (human or other animals). These trematodes can be grouped into two main categories, the liver fluke group (Opisthorchiidae: 12 species) and the intestinal fluke group (Heterophyidae, 36 species; Echinostomatidae, 10 species; and Nanophyetidae, 1 species) (Qiu et al. 2017). They are primarily related to liver and biliary disorders and intestinal diseases, causing severe disease and economic burden (Yu and Mott 1994).

Metacercariae of trematodes are infectious, which is transmitted by aquatic/semi-aquatic plant, crustacean, fish, and fish products (Hop et al. 2007). If these are consumed raw or undercooked, the consumers get infected. The sources may be natural or freshwater aquaculture if quality is compromised. Some 70 species of trematodes are fish-borne and are zoonoses. Prevalence of species differs from country to country. Important ones are listed in Table 85.1.

85.1 Mode of Human Infection

Ingestion of metacercariae by eating raw or insufficiently cooked freshwater fish (*C. sinensis*, *Opisthorchis* spp., *Echinostoma* spp., heterophyids, *Metagonimus* spp.), freshwater crab or crayfish (*Paragonimus* spp.), aquatic plants (*Fasciola* spp.,

Table 85.1 Important fish-borne flukes

Trematodes	Vehicle	Parasite	Predilection site tissues
Liver flukes	Plants	Fasciolidae—*F. hepatica, F. gigantica*	Liver, bile duct
	Fish	Opisthorchiidae—*C. sinensis, O. viverrini*	Biliary duct, liver, pancreas
Intestinal flukes	Fish	*Heterophyidae—Haplorchis taichui, Metagonimus yokogawai, Fasciolopsis buski*	Small intestinal mucosa
Lung fluke	Crayfish, crabs	Troglotrematidae—*Paragonimus westermani. P. kellicoti*	Lungs, pleural cavity, brain

Fasciolopsis buski), and snails or tadpoles (*Echinostoma* spp.) or by drinking contaminated water (*Fasciola* spp.) leads to infection.

85.2   Life Cycle

Sexual reproduction occurs in definitive hosts—human. Eggs pass out in faeces, reach fresh or brackish water, hatch, and infect the intermediate hosts—snails. Further development takes place in snails, and numerous cercariae are released which swim around, get suitable plant or animal to attach, and encyst as metacercariae.

Foodborne trematodes do not show host specificity for either definitive or intermediate hosts. These have widespread zoonotic reservoirs like domestic and pet animals, dogs, cats, cattle, sheep, goats, and buffaloes and even others like rodents, foxes, birds. These act as definitive hosts like humans. Cats, dogs, foxes, pigs, and rodents are definitive hosts for *C. sinensis*, and domestic ruminants serve as reservoirs for *Fasciola hepatica* infections. More than one species of snails, plants, crustaceans, and freshwater fish carry metacercariae. More than 80 crustacean species have been reported to be second intermediate hosts of *Paragonimus* spp. in China (Anonym 2004). Over 100 fish species are secondary intermediate hosts for *C. sinensis* and > 35 for *Opisthorchis* (Keiser and Utzinger 2005).

This impacts control and preventive measures.

85.3   Epidemiology

Foodborne trematodes, *Opisthorchis viverrini, O. felineus,* and *Clonorchis sinensis,* in the family *Opisthorchidae* have long been recognized as the cause of major human health problems.

Geographic distribution of these (Table 85.2) trematodes and population at risk has been compiled and tabulated by Keiser and Utzinger (2005); part is reproduced below.

Table 85.2 Geographic distribution of some foodborne trematodes

Parasite	Geographical distribution and population at risk
C. sinensis	China, Republic of Korea, Taiwan, Vietnam
O. viverrini	Cambodia, Lao PDR, Thailand, Vietnam
O. felineus	Kazakhstan, Russian Federation, Siberia, Ukraine
F. hepatica, F. gigantica	Bolivia, Cuba, highlands of Ecuador and Peru, Nile delta of Egypt, Iran, Portugal, Spain
P. westermani	South-Western Cameroon, China, Ecuador, Eastern Nigeria, Peru, the Philippines, Republic of Korea
F. buski	Bangladesh, India, China, Indonesia, Taiwan, Thailand
Echinostoma spp.	China, Indonesia, Malaysia, the Philippines, Republic of Korea, Taiwan, Thailand
Heterophyes heterophyes	China, Egypt, India, Indonesia, Iran, the Philippines, Sudan, Taiwan, Tunisia, Turkey
M. yokogawai	The Balkans, China, the Philippines, Iran, Israel, Japan, Republic of Korea, Spain, Taiwan

These parasites are important avoidable causes of morbidity and mortality. Additionally, the aquaculture industry employing many gets affected adversely—a huge loss to commodity, market, and employment.

Factors that affect transmission of fish-borne trematodiasis fall under (1) ecologic and environmental, (2) behavioural, and (3) socioeconomic and cultural. Large number of species constitutes first and second intermediate hosts. This presents a great number of opportunities for transmission. Ecological and environmental factors like rainfall, temperature, and quality of water, clean or polluted, affected the species of intermediate hosts—snails. Irrigation schemes, particularly for paddy cultivation and aquaculture, are suitable habitats. Open defecation, unsanitary habits and use of human or animal excreta as fertilizer and enriching aquaculture, and traditional food and cooking habits are important determinants. Dangerous local dishes cited by Keiser and Utzinger (2005) are raw crab soaked in soy sauce (*ke-jang*) in the Republic of Korea, raw drunken crabs and raw grass carp in China, and raw fish (*larb pla* and *plasom*) in Thailand which are considered delicacies and attract tourists.

The distribution of infection is highly focal. The disease is often misdiagnosed. Eggs are not always detected in specimens of stool and sputum. Other tools like serology and ultrasound are most often not available. Foodborne trematodiasis has significantly declined in some settings but is an emerging public health problem in Southeast Asia and Western Pacific regions, affecting the health of more than 40 million people throughout the world.

Keiser and Utzinger (2005) made a comprehensive analysis of the relationship between foodborne trematodiasis and development of aquaculture. They estimated that 601.0, 293.8, 91.1, and 79.8 million people were at risk of infection with *Clonorchis sinensis*, *Paragonimus* spp., *Fasciola* spp., and *Opisthorchis* spp., respectively. Proximity to freshwater bodies to human habitation was a risk factor with RR of 2.15. Growth of aquaculture in foodborne trematode endemic areas may constitute a risk of emergence of this important public health problem. To illustrate, grass carp (*Ctenopharyngodon idellus*) is a major intermediate host of foodborne trematodes. Its production increased many folds in 2002 from 1950 and accounted for 15.6% of freshwater aquaculture production. China is a major producer. Chinese eat raw as sushi or *yusheng zhou*. The prevalence of clonorchiasis has more than tripled in the past decade.

Anh et al. (2009) domestic animals served as reservoir hosts and contributed to the sustained endemicity. The fish-borne zoonotic trematode spp. prevailing in dogs, cats, and pigs in Vietnam had been linked with human infections. Public health efforts must consider this.

85.4   Aquaculture

World production of aquatic organisms, especially fish, is increasing tremendously. The total fishery production in the world in 2004 was 140 million tonnes of which aqua culture contributed almost one-third. Annual growth rate of aquaculture has been maintained at 8% over the past 30 years. Aquaculture market touched $86 billion in 2009. Global production of shrimp and freshwater prawns (excluding crayfish and crabs) in 2003 was 1.6 million tonnes and 280,000 tonnes, respectively. Asia, particularly China and Thailand, produced the maximum (http://en.wikipedia.org/wiki/Aquaculture).

Commercial fishing is harvesting wild fish. Aquaculture is farming of aquatic organisms like fish, crustaceans, molluscs, and aquatic plants and involves cultivating freshwater and saltwater populations under controlled conditions. Farming implies some form of intervention in rearing process to enhance production, such as stocking, feeding, protection from predators, etc., as well as "ownership" that may be individual or corporate. Kinds of farming may be fish/oyster/shrimp, aquaculture, etc. There are two methods of farming—*aquaponics* and *integrated multi-trophic aquaculture*—both integrate fish farming and plant farming. Mariculture is an aquaculture practiced in marine environment and in underwater habitats. Fish farming most commonly uses carp, salmon, tilapia, and catfish world over (http://en.wikipedia.org/wiki/Aquaculture).

Aquaculture provides nutritional food, generates employment, alleviates poverty, is a source of cash income and food to the poor, and is a low-risk route to rural development. It is an important economic activity in China. Indian aquaculture contributes to 55% of total fish production and is classed as (a) freshwater and (b) brackish water. Indian major carp and shrimp are the important species produced (http://indianfisheries.icsf.net/en/page/624-Aquaculture.html). According to Ayyappan (2012), total fish production in 2011–2012 in India was 8.3 million tonnes, with an annual growth rate of 4.5%. India is placed only after China in global fish production. It meets domestic needs, engages 14.5 million people, and earned foreign exchange of Rs.129.0 billion during 2010–2011. Aquaculture has an annual growth rate of 6.0–7.0%.

Forms of aquaculture are commercial, village ponds, backyard ponds, and family ponds as source of food. Crayfish and crabs are often not cultured but caught wild. However, the freshwater aquaculture trade is complex. It is difficult to separate commercially produced from family-owned pond produced. Exception is "Tilapia export from Asia is reasonably well documented" (Anonym 2004).

85.4.1   Risk Assessment

Trung Dung et al. (2007) made risk assessment in Vietnam. There is a strong tradition of eating raw fish. Intestinal fish-borne trematodes—metacercariae—in wild and farmed fish were detected, and this prompted to make "risk assessment" to the community that ate raw fish. 615 people were examined, and 64.9% tested positive; they were treated to expel liver and intestinal parasites for specific identification. *Clonorchis sinensis* (54.5%), ≥ 1 of 4 intestinal species of the family *Heterophyidae* was recovered from 100% of patients. *Haplorchis* spp. was most common (90.4%). The authors consider that the possible factors that contributed may be intensification of aquaculture, use of human and animal faeces to enrich ponds, and increased consumption as a result of affluence.

Last one to two decades, minute intestinal flukes have been increasingly recognized as a widely distributed cause of illness. Snail vectors (e.g. *Melanoides tuberculata*) and suitable vertebrate intermediate (fish) and reservoir hosts (fish-eating birds, dogs, cats, and pigs) are common in Vietnam. *Haplorchis taichui*, *H. pumilio*, *H. yokogawai*, and *Stellantchasmus falcatus* are endemic in neighbouring countries such as Thailand, Lao People's Democratic Republic, and the People's Republic of China.

85.4.2   Approaches to Preventive Measures

85.4.2.1   Inspection and Trace Back

Commercial crab farming, harvesting, and supply to lake-side restaurants may be tied up with inspection and control. A metal tag on the crab would carry identification number of the farmer so that back tracing from restaurant to the farmer is possible. The tags on the crabs can be pinned with the cash memos so that it becomes possible to connect with the consumer. In the event of consumer falling sick, it should be possible to trace back.

85.4.2.2   Approaches

- Faeces containing parasite eggs should not be allowed to flow in freshwater environment—snail's habitat. Often, faeces of human or animals are added to ponds for nutrient enrichment to increase the size, weight of fishes, and overall throughput. It is important to check at this stage that these are free from eggs of trematodes.
- Chemotherapy to reduce production of eggs by reservoirs to be practiced on large scale, triclabendazole for fascioliasis and praziquantel for others.
- Strong veterinary services (detection and treatment, large-scale chemotherapy in endemic areas) to reduce/eliminate infection in animal reservoirs.
- Reduce waterborne/foodborne metacercariae transmission by.

  1. Educating consumers—Raw, pickled, and undercooked are potential threats.
  2. Freezing at −20 °C for 7 days or cooking (60 °C) to eliminate metacercariae.
  3. Practicing good hygiene for housewives and restaurants.
  4. Improving general environmental hygiene and sanitation.

- Aquaculture—where all precaution is taken that produce is "free from parasite". A system of "tracing back" and "recall" should be in built in the market system.
- A system based on "intersectoral or one health" principle of interventions—mass chemotherapy (medicine and veterinary services), inspection and recall (food safety), preservation/cooking practices (inspection, education for restaurant and housewives), preventive efforts at the level of aquaculture (education, control of production, and trade). The activities should have government/legal support.

References

Anh NTL, Phuong NT, Murrell KD, Johansen MV, Dalsgaard A et al (2009) Animal reservoir hosts and fish-borne zoonotic trematode infections on fish farms, Vietnam. Emerg Infect Dis 15(4):540–546

Anonym (2004) Report joint WHO/FAO workshop on Foodborne Trematode Infections in Asia. Ha Noi, Viet Nam 26–28 Nov.2002. (WP)MVP/ICP/MVP/ 1.2/001-E. Report Series Number: RS/2002/GE/40(VTN) English only

Ayyappan S (2012) Indian fisheries on fast track. The Economic Times 28 September 2012. Edition: New Delhi. http://www.icar.org.in/node/5112

Chai J-Y, Shin E-H, Lee S-H, Rim H-J (2009) Foodborne intestinal flukes in Southeast Asia. Korean J Parasitol 47(Suppl):S69–S102

Clausen J, Madsen H, Murrell K, Van P, Thu H, Do D et al (2012) Prevention and control of fish-borne zoonotic trematodes in fish nurseries, Vietnam. Emerg Infect Dis 18(9):1438–1445

Hop NT, De NV, Murrell D, Dalsgaard A (2007) Occurrence and species distribution of fishborne zoonotic trematodes in wastewater-fed aquaculture in northern Vietnam. Trop Med Public Health 12:66–72. https://doi.org/10.1111/j.1365-3156.2007.01943.x

Keiser J, Utzinger J (2005) Emerging foodborne trematodiasis. Emerg Infects Dis 11(10):1507–1514

Qiu J, Zhang Y, Zhang X, Gao Y et al (2017) Metacercaria infection status of fishborne zoonotic trematodes, except for *Clonorchis sinensis* in Fish from the Heilongjiang province, China. Foodb Pathog Dis 14:440–446

Trung Dung D, Van De N, Waikagul J et al (2007) Fishborne zoonotic intestinal trematodes, Vietnam. Emerg Infect Dis 13(12):1828–1833

Yu S, Mott KE (1994) Epidemiology and morbidity of food-borne intestinal trematode infections. World Hlth Org 91:R125–R152

Chapter 86
Clonorchiasis

James McConnell published, in The Lancet on 21 August 1875, his findings from a postmortem examination—undertaken at the Medical College Hospital in Calcutta, India—of a 20-year-old Chinese man, in whom he found *Clonorchis sinensis* in the bile ducts (Qian et al. 2016).

86.1 Aetiology

Clonorchiasis is a disease caused by a trematode—*Clonorchis sinensis*, also known as Chinese or oriental liver fluke. *C. sinensis* is a common parasite of fish-eating mammals, including cats, dogs, and humans.

86.2 Life Cycle

The life cycle includes one invertebrate host (snail) and two vertebrate hosts: freshwater fish and fish-eating mammals (cat, dog, and human). Snails, including *Bithynia fuchsiana*, *Alocinma longicornis*, and *Parafossarulus striatulus*, are important intermediate hosts.

The faeces of infected mammals contain the eggs of *C. sinensis*, which when they enter the water environment are consumed by the first intermediate hosts, the freshwater snails, in which the eggs release miracidia. These miracidia undergo a series of developmental stages: first, sporocyst, followed by rediae, and subsequently cercariae, which are released from the snails and are freely swimming in the water until they penetrate freshwater fish. In the flesh of the freshwater fish, cercariae encyst and continue to mature to metacercariae. On ingestion of the infected fish by a higher mammal such as humans, the metacercariae excyst as juvenile

© Springer Nature Singapore Pte Ltd. 2024
K. G. Narayan et al., *Handbook of Management of Zoonoses*,
https://doi.org/10.1007/978-981-99-9885-2_86

flukes in the duodenum and migrate to the common bile duct along the epithelial lining; mature to hermaphroditic adult worm in 30 days; parasitize the intrahepatic bile duct, the gall bladder, the common bile duct, and occasionally the pancreatic duct; and lay eggs, which pass in faeces. The life cycle can take up to 3 months.

86.3   Mode of Infection

Eating raw freshwater fish or salted, pickled, smoked, marinated, dried, under-cooked, or poorly processed fish causes infection. The contamination of utensils and food with pond water containing metacercariae is also a potential route of infection, which is especially seen in children and women.

86.4   Pathophysiology and Symptoms

C. sinensis can live in humans for 20–30 years. Protracted episodes of re-infection over time result in chronic infection, which may be severe; fibrosis of the biliary duct and destruction of the adjacent liver parenchyma may result. Mechanical injury is caused to the mucosa by suckers of the parasite. The fluke induces chronic inflammation and hepatobiliary complications like biliary obstruction, pyogenic cholangitis, and cholangiosarcoma. *C. sinensis* eats bile and thus affects fat digestion in the host.

Infection may lead to any symptom. If illness results, it may manifest as lasting epigastric pain, dark-coloured urine, reduced appetite, fatigue, and loss of weight, as were seen in a 34-year-old male Thailander (Papachristou et al. 2005). Heavy infection may result in acute illness characterized by fever, right upper quadrant abdominal pain, intermittent colic pain, nausea, diarrhoea, and jaundice. Heavy chronic cases show complications. The International Agency for Research on Cancer (IARC) classifies *C. sinensis* as a Group 1 agent (*carcinogenic to humans*—http://www.who.int/foodborne_trematode_infections/clonorchiasis/en/).

Park and Son (2008) described the clinical and laboratory observation of a 62-year-old who ate raw pond smelt (*Hypomesus solidus*) and experienced fatigue, fever, and cramping abdominal pain for 7 days. The laboratory examination revealed elevated aspartate aminotransferase, alanine aminotransferase, alkaline phosphatase, γ-glutamyl transferase, total bilirubin and conjugated bilirubin, and white cell count, and there was eosinophilia. This prompted a computed tomography (CT) scan of the abdomen. Dilatation of the common bile duct was observed. This led to the detection of duodenoscopy and prominent major papillae. Many *C. sinensis* were removed through the cannulation of the common bile duct.

86.5   Epidemiology

Clonorchiasis is endemic in Southern China, Korea, Taiwan, and Vietnam, as well as in far eastern regions of Russia (Locke et al. 2022). More than 200 million people are at risk of infection in these regions due to the frequent ingestion of improperly cooked fish; the World Health Organization (WHO) therefore listed *C. sinensis* among the most neglected tropical diseases globally (Sripa 2008).

It is estimated that about 35 million people are globally infected with these parasites. Of these, 15 million are in China. It impacts greatly public health in China because of the greater consumption of raw freshwater fish (Lun et al. 2005). An epidemiological study made by Zhang et al. (2007) in China elucidated the factors explaining the transmission and endemicity of *C. sinensis* in the Shenzhen area. Nearly 1500 individuals were studied. It revealed that 54% did not know of fluke disease or its transmission; 12% of such persons believed that slight to no harm is caused by flukes; 27% of the interviewed individuals ate raw fish at least twice a month; the same utensils were used for both cooked food and raw fish by 5% families; and 40% of fish pond owners used faeces of domestic animals and humans as fertilizer. Lin et al. (2011) observed that *C. sinensis* prevalence in humans was high in Guangdong province, China. They studied prevalence in dogs and cats and found 20.5% and 41.8%, respectively.

Climate change impacts the helminths population, but this is detectable after some time. Cercarial quality and production are affected, and the duration of production increases as a result of changes in temperature. The size of the snail host and host mortality are affected.

According to Xue-Ming et al. (2011), the overall prevalence in China was 0.58%. Of the total infected, 29.14% had moderate and 11.52% had heavy infection in Guangxi. The prevalence increased with age, <35 years, and there is a high prevalence in the age group 25–60 years; also, more males (1.64x) than females were infected. Prevalence was high among fishermen, businessmen, physicians and teachers. Out of 38 ethnic groups, Han (3.2%) and Zhuang (3.15%) had the highest prevalence. Infection was prevalent in the hilly part and plains of northeast and south-central China. There was an increasing trend in prevalence in endemic areas. Educated and high-income groups showed high prevalence. The ingestion of raw or undercooked fresh fish or shrimp was the main risk of transmission.

86.6   Diagnosis

Clinical presentation, history of eating raw fish, endemic area or return from endemic area, eosinophilia are strongly suggestive of infection. This is supplemented by imaging—like ultrasound, CT, or magnetic resonance imaging (MRI).

Confirmatory tests include the following:

- Eggs in stool, drained bile, biopsy through parasitological techniques like Kato-Katz thick smear, and the quantification of the intensity or severity of infection.
- Immunological techniques:

    (a) Intradermal—low specificity, especially when treated with anthelmintics.
    (b) Enzyme-linked immunosorbent assay (ELISA), immunoblotting using antigens—ESP (excretory-secretary products), cysteine proteases and glutathione *S*-transferase, and the 7-kDa molecule of *C. sinensis* ESP for serum antibodies.
    (c) Detection of parasite-specific antigen in the stool/serum: Zhao et al. (2004) evaluated the EX7-kDa recombinant protein of *C. sinensis* in ELISA and immunoblots. The sensitivities (71.9 and 81.3%, respectively) and specificities (89.7 and 92.6%, respectively) showed cross-reaction with paragonimiasis.

- Molecular techniques, like PCR.

86.7   Treatment

Praziquantel is the treatment of choice; however, triclabendazole, bithionol, albendazole, and mebendazole are also effective.

86.8   Control

Choi et al. (2010) evaluated a clonorchiasis control programme. It was concluded that repeated mass or selective treatment with praziquantel every 6 to 12 months is highly effective for controlling clonorchiasis in heavily endemic areas. In contrast, one or two selective treatments with health education are effective in moderately endemic areas.

References

Choi MH, Park SK, Li Z, Ji Z, Yu G, Feng Z et al (2010) Effect of control strategies on prevalence, incidence and re-infection of clonorchiasis in endemic areas of China. PLoS Negl Trop Dis 4(2):e601

Lin RQ, Tang JD, Zhou DH, Song HQ, Huang SY et al (2011) Prevalence of *Chlonorchis sinensis* infections in dogs and cats in subtropical southern China. Parasit Vectors 19(4):180

Locke V, Kusnik A, Richardson MS. (2022). Clonorchis sinensis. [Updated 2022 Dec 19]. In: StatPearls [Internet]. Treasure Island, FL: StatPearls Publishing; 2023 Jan. https://www.ncbi.nlm.nih.gov/books/NBK532892/

Lun ZR, Gasser RB, Lai DH, Li AX, Zhu XQ, Yu XB, Fang YY et al (2005) Clonorchiasis: a key foodborne zoonosis in China. Lancet Infect Dis 5(1):31–41

Papachristou GI, Schoedel KE, Ramanathan R, Rabinovitz M (2005) *Clonorchis sinensis*-associated cholangiocarcinoma: a case report and review of the literature. Dig Dis Sci 50(11):2159–2162

Park DH, Son HY (2008) Clonorchis sinensis. N Engl J Med 358:e18. http://www.who.int/foodborne_trematode_infections/clonorchiasis/en/

Qian MB, Utzinger J, Keiser J, Zhou XN (2016) Clonorchiasis. Lancet 387(10020):800–810

Sripa B (2008) Concerted action is needed to tackle liver fluke infections in Asia. PLoS Negl Trop Dis 2(5):e232

Xue-Ming L, Ying-Dan C, Yi O, Hong-Man Z, Rui L, Weil M (2011) Overview of human *Clonorchiasis sinensis* in China. Southeast Asian J Trop Med Public Health 42(2):248–254

Zhang R, Gao S, Geng Y, Huang D, Yu L et al (2007) Epidemiological study on *Clonorchis sinensis* infection in Shenzhen area of Zhujiang delta in China. Parasitol Res 101(1):179–183

Zhao Q-P, Moon S-U, Lee H-W, Na B-K, Cho S-Y et al (2004) Evaluation of *Clonorchis sinensis* recombinant 7-Kilodalton antigen for Serodiagnosis of Clonorchiasis. Clin & Diagn Lab Immunol 11(4):814–817

Chapter 87
Dicrocoeliasis

Geographic Distribution

Dicrocoeliasis is reported throughout Europe, the Middle East (Iran), Asia, North Africa, North and South America, and Australia. *Dicrocoelium hospes* is endemic to sub-Saharan West Africa; cases have been documented in Ghana, Senegal, Sierra Leone, and Mali. The parasite tends to be found in areas that favour the intermediate hosts, such as fields with dry, chalky, and alkaline soils.

87.1 Aetiology

It is caused by the lancet liver fluke *Dicrocoelium dendriticum* and *D. hospes*.

87.2 Hosts

Ruminants, especially cattle and sheep, are the normal definitive hosts of *Dicrocoelium* spp. Humans, various species of non-human primate, and domestic dogs are accidental hosts.

The terrestrial snail species of the genera *Cochlicopa*, *Helix*, *Xerolenta*, and *Zebrina* serve as first intermediate hosts, while second intermediate hosts are ants, especially members of the genus *Formica*.

87.3   Life Cycle (Fig. 87.1)

Ruminants are definitive hosts. Adult *D. dendriticum* parasitizes the liver of ruminants. The terrestrial snails and ants are the first and second intermediate hosts,
respectively. Interestingly, the parasite takes control of the infected ants, enabling
the grazing ruminants to ingest ants along with grass, facilitating the entry of metacercaria in the grazing ruminants as well as invasion.

The eggs of *D. dendriticum* are excreted with ruminant faeces. The first intermediate hosts—the terrestrial snails—consume faeces and thus get infected with the
embryonated eggs. Miracidia are hatched, which drill through the gut wall, settle in,
and develop into the juvenile stage in the digestive tract. The infected snails create
a defensive wall around the parasite to protect themselves and excrete these on grass
or substrate. Ants—the second intermediate hosts—use the trail of snail slime as a
source of moisture and swallow the cysts. Each cyst has hundreds of juvenile lancet
flukes. The parasite drifts through the body from the gut. Most cercariae encyst in
haemocoel and mature to metacercaria. Some move to the sub-oesophageal ganglion. This is a cluster of nerve cells underneath the oesophagus. The parasite takes
control of such ants. The infected ants are driven away from the ants' colony when
the air is cool in the evening. These ants move up on the top of grass blades, clamp
with mandible, and stay till dawn. The process may be repeated night after night.
Grazing animals eat ants containing metacercaria, along with grass, to get infected.
Infected ants may carry 100 metacercaria. A large number of ants may be carrying
metacercaria. Tens of thousands of adult worms may be found in infected cattle
(Ekstam et al. 2011). The invading metacercaria develops into an adult, and the life
cycle continues (Holmes 1993; Callahan 2002).

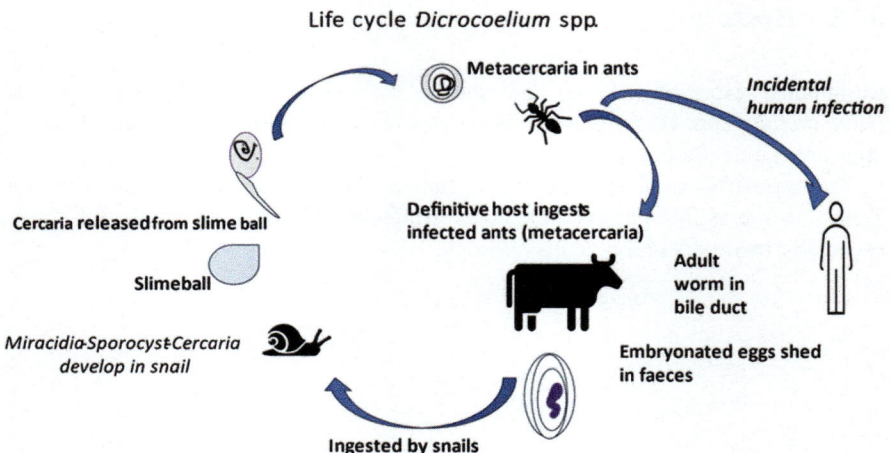

Fig. 87.1 Life cycle of *Dicrocoelium* spp.

87.4 Symptoms

Infections, especially in cows, are asymptomatic, but the effect on the liver depends on the number of flukes and the length of infection and may show anaemia, oedema, emaciation, and liver cirrhosis (Otranto and Traversa 2002).

Human infection is rare and is incurred through the ingestion of undercooked liver and not by eating infected ants. In a cross-sectional study in peri-urban area of Kyrgyzstan, on 138 children of 2–15 years, prevalence 8.0% with 95% confidence interval (4.5–13.7%) was found which probably related with the prevailing animal husbandry system, the diet and hygienic conditions of the study area; suggest that the social-ecological system in Kyrgyzstan is conducive for human transmission of *D. dendriticum* (Jeandron et al. 2011).

In human, fluke infections are generally confined to the distal parts of the bile ducts; therefore, they produce only mild symptoms like biliary colic and general digestive disturbances, including bloating and chronic constipation or diarrhoea. However, in heavier infections, bile ducts and the biliary epithelium may become enlarged and, due to the generation of fibrous tissue surrounding the ducts, result in enlarged liver (hepatomegaly) or inflammation of the liver (cirrhosis) (Cengiz et al. 2010). In one unique case, an infection with *D. dendriticum* was associated with a skin rash (urticarial) (Sing et al. 2008).

Paranjpe et al. (2020) reported a case of dicrocoeliasis in an 82-year-old woman having epigastric and right upper quadrant abdominal pain, nausea, and vomiting lasting for 3 days without fever and with a bilirubin level of 2.9 mg/dL without leukocytosis or eosinophilia. Peak aspartate aminotransferase, alanine aminotransferase, alkaline phosphatase, and lipase levels were 675, 708, 236, and 7366 U/L, respectively. Computerized tomography (CT) scan with contrast showed mild gallbladder wall thickening and no stones or pericholecystic fluid. Bile ducts and pancreas appeared normal. Endoscopic ultrasound (EUS) of the distal common bile duct revealed a 5-mm thin hyperechoic lesion without shadowing and no pancreatic abnormalities. Endoscopic retrograde cholangiopancreatography (ERCP) revealed poor contrast drainage but showed no filling defects. Sphincterotomy and sweeping with a balloon retrieved a live 3- × 3- × 1-mm fluke, which was identified as *Dicrocoelium dendriticum* by the Centers for Disease Control and Prevention (CDC). The patient was discharged after symptomatic improvement and downtrending liver enzymes while on empiric nitazoxanide and 2 doses of triclabendazole for suspected *Fasciola hepatica*. Notably, the patient emigrated from China 20 years earlier after working in the fields and construction; she last visited 4 years earlier and might have been infected during one of those trips.

87.5 Laboratory Diagnosis

- Microscopic identification of eggs in the stool, duodenal, and/or bile fluid.
- Post-mortem examination of the livers.

- In Italy, ELISA using a *D. dendriticum* antigen was developed, which identified cases of dicrocoeliasis in sheep 28 days earlier than traditional methods (Otranto and Traversa 2002).

Eggs may be detected in stool following the consumption of liver infected with adult flukes; additional specimens should be collected to distinguish this spurious passage from true infection.

87.6   Prevention

The condemnation of contaminated livers to eliminate any possibility of food-borne infection is recommended.

87.7   Treatment

Suggested treatment is anthelmintic, such as praziquantel, triclabendazole, or Mirazid.

References

Callahan GN (2002) Infectious madness: disease with a past and a purpose: mental illness may not be just craziness, but have a parasitic, fungal, or viral etiology. Emerg Med News 24(11):52–54

Cengiz ZT, Yilmaz H, Dulger AC, Cicek M (2010) Human infection with *Dicrocoelium dendriticum* in Turkey. Ann Saudi Med 30(2):159–161

Ekstam B, Johansson B, Dinnétz P, Ellström P (2011) Predicting risk habitats for the transmission of the small liver fluke, *Dicrocoelium dendriticum* to grazing ruminants. Geospat Health 6(1):125–131

Holmes B (1993) Evolution's neglected superstars: there is nothing glamorous about fleas, flukes or intestinal worms. So why are they suddenly attracting so much attention? New Scientist

Jeandron A, Rinaldi L, Abdyldaieva G, Usubalieva J, Steinmann P et al (2011) Human infections with *Dicrocoelium dendriticum* in Kyrgyzstan: the tip of the iceberg? J Parasitol 97(6):1170–1172

Otranto D, Traversa D (2002) A review of dicrocoeliosis of ruminants including recent advances in the diagnosis and treatment. Vety Parasitol 107(4):317–335

Paranjpe V, McCabe P, Mollah F, Bandy A, Hamerski C (2020) A fluke catch: biliary obstruction and pancreatitis from dicrocoeliasis. Video Case Rep 5(11):P567–P568

Sing A, Tybus K, Fackler I (2008) Acute urticaria associated with *Dicrocoelium dendriticum* infestation. Indian J Med Microbiol 26(1):97–98

Chapter 88
Echinostomiasis

Echinostomiasis is a food-borne parasitic disease caused by intestinal trematodes belonging to the genera *Echinostoma*, family Echinostomatidae (Toledo and Esteban 2016), which includes numerous spiny-collared intestinal flukes known to infect humans.

88.1 Aetiology

Infections are documented mostly from *Echinostoma hortense*, *E. trivolvis*, *E. macrorchis*, *E. revolutum* sensu lato, *E. ilocanum*, *E. cinetorchis*, *E. echinatum* (= *lindoense*), and *E. fujianensis*.

88.2 Geographic Distribution

Echinostomes occur in wildlife and domestic animals worldwide, but human cases are seen most frequently in Southeast and East Asia, where undercooked or raw freshwater snails, clams, fish, or amphibians are eaten.

88.3 Life Cycle

Echinostoma spp. have a three-host life cycle with aquatic snails (families Planorbidae, Lymnaeidae, and Bulinidae) as first intermediate hosts in which a sporocyst, two generations of rediae, and cercaria develop. Emerged cercariae freely swim and infect the second intermediate hosts, such as snails, frogs, clams, and fish.

© Springer Nature Singapore Pte Ltd. 2024
K. G. Narayan et al., *Handbook of Management of Zoonoses*,
https://doi.org/10.1007/978-981-99-9885-2_88

The definitive host (human and other animals, viz. birds, carnivores, rodents) becomes infected after ingestion of the second intermediate host harbouring the encysted metacercariae. In the definitive host, adult worms mature in the gastrointestinal tract and produce eggs that are released with the host's faeces (Toledo et al. 2014).

88.4 Symptoms

Patients are usually asymptomatic. However, with heavy infections, the worms can produce catarrhal inflammation with mild ulceration, causing abdominal pain, anorexia, nausea, vomiting, diarrhoea, and weight loss.

88.5 Case Report

Shah et al. (2018) reported a case of echinostomiasis from Nepal in a 62-year-old male with a complaint of abdominal pain and distension with vomiting on and off for 3–4 months and was presented to Tribhuvan University Teaching Hospital, Kathmandu. He had a history of consumption of insufficiently cooked fish and snails with alcohol. During endoscopy, an adult flatworm was seen with mild portal hypertensive gastropathy (McCormack's classification) and erosive duodenopathy. The adult worm was identified as *Echinostoma* species based on its morphology and the characteristic ova found on a stool routine microscopic examination of the patient. The patient was treated with praziquantel. He improved, and on follow-up, the stool examination after 2 weeks revealed no ova of *Echinostoma* species.

88.6 Prevention

 (i) Human infection can be prevented by avoiding eating raw, insufficiently cooked fish and snails.
(ii) To cut disease dissemination at the human level, three main initiatives should be taken: apply appropriate pharmacological treatment to infected subjects after proper diagnosis, avoid promiscuous defecation near water bodies, and prohibit using unsterilized "human night soil" as fertilizer.

88.7 Treatment

Praziquantel (40 mg/kg body weight, single dose) is the drug of choice.

References

Shah R, Khadka S, Hamal R, Pouyal S (2018) Human echinostomiasis: a case report. BMC Res Notes 11(17):1–6

Toledo R, Esteban JG (2016) An update on human echinostomiasis. Trans R Soc Trop Med Hyg 110(1):37–45

Toledo R, Muñoz-Antoli C, Esteban JG (2014) Intestinal trematode infections. Adv Exp Med Biol 766:201–240

Chapter 89
Fascioliasis

Fascioliasis is caused by *Fasciola hepatica* and *F. gigantica*, which are also called liver flukes and are leaf-shaped worms, large enough to be visible to the naked eye; adult *F. hepatica* measures 20–30 mm × 13 mm, and adult *F. gigantica* measures 25–75 mm × 12 mm. They both cause a similar disease.

89.1   Geographic Distribution

Fascioliasis is widespread throughout the world, especially in regions where sheep and/or cattle production is common. The World Health Organization WHO (2020) estimates that at least 2.4 million people are infected in more than 75 countries globally, with several million at risk. No continent is free from fascioliasis, and it is likely that where animal cases are reported, human cases also exist. Over the past few decades, *F. hepatica* is increasing in Europe, the Americas, and Oceania, and the two species, *F. hepatica* and *F. gigantica*, are increasing in Asia and Africa. Chand et al. (2009) observed that there was no firm evidence of indigenous zoonotic fascioliasis in England and Wales; despite the parallel rise in animal and human fascioliasis, most cases originated from the Horn of Africa and Yemen. Parkinson et al. (2007) made a meta-analysis of epidemiological surveys from 38 communities in the Bolivian Altiplano and found that fascioliasis was zoonosis of rural communities and has been endemic since 1984. The highest level of *Fasciola hepatica* was found in the indigenous Aymaran people of northern Bolivian Altiplano.

Besides the zoonotic transmission from livestock to humans, human-to-human transmission is often reported in endemic areas. The reservoir hosts are a number of animals classed as domestic (cattle, buffalo, sheep, goats, pigs, horses, donkeys, camels, dromedaries, and llamas) and sylvatic (rabbit, hare, and rodents).

89.2 Life Cycle

The definitive hosts of *Fasciola* spp. are animals and humans. The immature eggs are shed in the bile ducts. These are passed out with faeces/stool. The eggs embryonate in fresh water, which takes about 2 weeks. Then miracidia are released. Snails, the intermediate hosts, are invaded. Miracidia undergoes a series of developments: sporocyst, rediae, and cercaria. The snails shed out cercaria, which encyst on aquatic vegetation or other substrate and are called metacercaia, which are infective and eaten with contaminated vegetation (e.g., watercress) by animals and humans. The cyst is shed out by metacercaria in the duodenum. The parasite penetrates through the intestinal wall to reach the peritoneal cavity. The immature *Fasciola* migrates through the parenchyma of the liver to reach its destination, the biliary ducts. These mature into adult liver flukes. The development from metacercaia to adult fluke takes about 3–4 months in humans. Compared to *F. hepatica*, *F. gigantica* may take longer time.

89.3 Clinical Disease

Humans are infected accidentally by ingesting metacercariae on watercress or from kitchen utensils washed with water carrying metacercariae. The incubation period is wide—from days to months.

The immature worms penetrate the intestinal (duodenal) wall, peritoneum, or Glisson capsule to reach the biliary tree. The acute larval, hepatic, and invasive stages of human infection are initiated. Larvae sometimes also travel to ectopic body sites.

1. Acute phase or liver phase is manifested as fever; malaise; abdominal pain, frequently localized to the right hypochondrium; respiratory disturbances; headache; pruritus; urticaria; and weight loss; a laboratory investigation reveals eosinophilia. Severe anaemia occurs among children. Imaging showed multiple, small, clustered, necrotic cavities or abscesses in the peripheral parts of the liver; also, tunnels and caves are suggestive of parasite migration in the liver parenchyma.
2. The chronic or biliary phase is rare—the worm reaches the bile duct. There is no or non-specific symptom; progressive inflammation leads to fibrosis of the walls of the gall bladder; the stricture of the bile duct, which gets clogged with a parasite, its fragments, and debris; obstruction, and cholestasis (Patil et al. 2009); biliary colic pain is a characteristic symptom. Persisting infection may result in biliary cirrhosis and fibrosis of the liver. Growth is affected. Imaging demonstrated flukes as small flat objects, sometimes floating in the intra- and extrahepatic bile ducts and the gall bladder.
3. Ectopic or pharyngeal—a syndrome called *halzoun* in Lebanon and *marrerra* in the Sudan occurs after consuming raw livers of infected sheep, goats, or cows.

The parasite adheres to the posterior walls of the pharynx. Severe pharyngitis and laryngeal oedema result. In Japan, the sashimi of bovine liver contaminated with liver fluke, generally served in Yakitori bars, cause a similar syndrome (Tolan 2009).

89.4   Diagnosis

- During the acute stage, the stool may be negative for eggs; serological tests such as enzyme-linked immunosorbent assay (ELISA) has 100% sensitivity and 97% specificity during the first 3–4 months of infection. Using partially purified antigen of *Fasciola gigantica* with 1:800 dilution of serum as cut-off titre, sensitivity of Dot-ELISA was found to be 94.23% and its specificity as 99.36%. (Dalimi et al. 2004). Western immunoblot is another test.
- Chronic biliary infection can be diagnosed by stool examination, but multiple concentrated samples need to be examined as the excretion of eggs is sporadic.
- Imaging such as endoscopic retrograde cholangiopancreatography (ERCP) is helpful in diagnosis (Patil et al. 2009).

89.5   Treatment

Triclabendazole 10 mg/kg body weight, single dose, is the choice for drugs.

89.6   Prevention

Mass drug administration (MDA) should be followed if the prevalence is high. However, treatment should be complemented by implementing measures that aim to reduce transmission rates:

  i. Education and communication to communities to promote the cultivation of vegetables in water free from faecal pollution and the thorough cooking of vegetables before consumption.
 ii. Veterinary public health measures, including treating domestic animals and enforcing separation between husbandry and humans, and.
iii. Environmental measures such as the containment of snail intermediate hosts and drainage of grazing lands.

References

Chand MA, Herman JS, Partridge DG, Hewitt K, Chiodini PL (2009) Imported human fascioliasis, United Kingdom. Emerg Infect Dis 15(11):1876–1877

Dalimi A, RamtinHadighi R, Madani R (2004) Partially purified fraction (PPF) antigen from adult *Fasciola gigantica* for the serodiagnosis of human fascioliasis using dot-ELISA technique. Ann Saudi Med 24(1):18–20

Parkinson M, O'Neill SM, Dalton JP (2007) Endemic human facsiolosis in Bolivian Altiplano. Epidemiol Infect 135(4):669–674

Patil K, Kulkarni S, Gorad K, Panchal A, Arora S, Gautam R (2009) Acute fascioliasis-rare cause of obstructive jaundice—a case report (2009). Bombay Hosp J 51(3):398–400

Tolan Jr Robert W (2009) Fascioliasis. eMedicine Specialties>Pediatrics: General Medicine>Parasitology updated Jan 22. 2009

WHO (2020). https://www.who.int/news-room/questions-and-answers/item/q-a-on-fascioliasis

Chapter 90
Gastrodiscoidiasis

It is an intestinal trematodiasis caused by *Gastrodiscoides hominis*—the only common amphistome of man (Mas-Coma et al. 2005), which was first discovered from the caecum of an indigenous Assamese man in India in 1876 by two British medical doctors, Timothy Richard Lewis and James McConnell.

90.1 Geographical Distribution

First described from an Indian patient, *G. hominis* was initially believed to be restricted to India and Southeast Asia. However, later it was also reported in Africa, in countries like Zambia (Hira 1983) and Nigeria (Dada Adegbola et al. 2004).

Gastrodiscoidiasis distribution covers India, especially the states of Assam, Bengal, Bihar, Madhya Pradesh, Meghalaya, Odisha, and Uttar Pradesh (Shrivastav and Shah 1970; Murty and Reddy 1980; Roy and Tandon 1992), and countries like Nepal, Pakistan, Burma, Thailand, Vietnam, the Philippines, China, Kazakhstan, Russia, Zambia, and Nigeria (Buckley 1939; Ahluwalia 1960; Kumar 1980; Harinasuta et al. 1987; Yu and Mott 1994; Ivanov and Semenova 2000; Dada-Adegbola, et al. 2004; Sah et al. 2019). A high prevalence of *Gastrodiscoides* in children (≈41%) in the Kamrup district of Assam (India) was reported (Buckley 1964). Roy and Tandon (1992) reported seasonal prevalence of *G. hominis* in Meghalaya (India).

© Springer Nature Singapore Pte Ltd. 2024
K. G. Narayan et al., *Handbook of Management of Zoonoses*,
https://doi.org/10.1007/978-981-99-9885-2_90

90.2   Life Cycle

Pig is the main animal reservoir of *G. hominis*. The parasite is commonly found in the caecum and colon (Ahluwalia 1960; Kumar 1999). Animals such as Napu mouse deer (*Tragulus napu*; Khalil 1923), common field rat (*Rattus brevicaudatus*), rhesus monkey (*Macaca mulatta*), other species of monkey (Buckley 1964; Fox and Hall 1970; Herman 1967), and American muskrat (*Ondatra zibethica*) in Volga Delta, Russia (Ivanov and Semenova 2000), have also been found to be infected. Wild boar is also a definitive host for this parasite in Thekaddy forest, Kerala, India (Easwaran et al. 2003).

   G. hominis is transmitted by small freshwater snails of the species *Helicor biocoenosis* of the family Planorbidae, which acts as intermediate hosts. Humans and animals get infected after swallowing encysted metacercariae through the ingestion of vegetation (aquatic plants) or animal products such as raw or undercooked crustaceans (crayfish), squid, molluscs, or amphibians (frogs, tadpoles).

   Man is the accidental host of *G. hominis*. It causes inflammation of the mucosa of caecum and ascending colon, leading to diarrhoea. This infection causes ill health in a large number of persons and deaths among untreated patients, especially children.

90.3   Diagnosis

The diagnosis of gastrodiscoidiasis is done by coprology, and human infection by *G. hominis* is easily diagnosed by finding the characteristic eggs in faeces. The egg is operculated and non-embryonated and measures about $150 \times 70 \text{ mm}^2$ (Mas-Coma et al. 2005, 2006; Esteban et al. 2019; Toledo et al. 2019).

90.4   Treatment

Praziquantel is the drug of choice. However, a single dose of mebendazole (500 mg) is also efficient.

90.5   Prevention and Control

The following control measures should be applied:

  (i) Prevent human infection by avoiding eating raw water-derived foods. Implement strong community therapy planning.

(ii) To cut disease dissemination at the human level, three main initiatives should be taken: apply appropriate pharmacological treatment to infected subjects after proper diagnosis, avoid promiscuous defecation near water bodies, and prohibit using unsterilized "human night soil" as fertilizer.

(iii) To control the disease at the animal reservoir level, measures should be adopted to restrain pigs from having access to ponds and canals. Avoid feeding pigs with raw vegetables and aquatic green fodder, which are sources of metacercaria. A routine parasitological examination of pig faeces, followed by appropriate treatment of pigs, is also necessary.

(iv) Control activities at the intermediate molluscan host (snail) level include the application of molluscicides in ponds and prohibiting the contamination of ponds with human and pig excreta.

(v) Educational programmes should be directed primarily towards school-age children because they are less entrenched in their food and eating habits, behaviour, and customs. These programmes should emphasize the importance of immersing vegetables in boiling water for a few minutes, peeling them, and washing them in running water to wash away the metacercarial cysts, if any, and boiling drinking water before consumption.

References

Ahluwalia SS (1960) *Gastrodiscoides hominis* (Lewis and McConnell, 1876) Leiper, 1913-the amphistome parasite of man and pig. Indian J Med Res 48:315–325

Buckley JJC (1939) Observations on *Gastrodiscoides hominis* and *Fasciolopsis buski* in Assam. J Helminthol 17:1–12

Buckley JJC (1964) The problem of *Gastrodiscoidesominis* (Lewis and McConell, 1876) Leiper, 1913. J Helminthol 38(1/2):1–6

Dada-Adegbola HO, Falade CO, Oliwatoba OA, Abiodun OO (2004) *Gastrodiscoideshominis* infection in a Nigerian—case report. West African J Med 23:185–186

Easwaran KR, Reghu R, Pillai KM (2003) Parasitic infection of some wild animals at Thekkady in Kerala. Zoos' Print J 18:1030

Esteban JG, Muñoz-Antoli C, Toledo R, Ash LR (2019) Diagnosis of human trematode infections. Adv in Exptal Med & Biol 1154:437–471

Fox JG, Hall WC (1970) Fluke (*Gastrodiscoides hominis*) infection in a rhesus monkey with related intussusception of the colon. J Am Vet Med Assoc 157:714–716

Harinasuta T, Bunnag D, Radomyos P (1987) Intestinal fluke infections. Bailliere'sClin Trop Med Commun Dis 2(3):695–721

Herman LH (1967) *Gastrodiscoides hominis* infestation in two monkeys. Vet Med Small Anim Clin 62:355–356

Hira PR (1983) Further spurious parasitic infestations of man in Zambia. Central African J Med 29:33–40

Ivanov VM, Semenova NN (2000) Parasitological consequences of animal introduction. Russian J Ecol 31:281–283

Khalil M (1923) A description of *Gastrodiscoideshominis* from the Napu mouse deer. Proc R Soc Med 16(1):8–14

Kumar V (1980) The digenetic trematodes, *Fasciolopsis buski*, *Gastrodiscoides hominis*, *Artyfechinostomum malayanum*, as zoonotic infections in South Asian countries. Ann Soc Belge Med Trop 60:331–339

Kumar V (1999) Trematode infections and diseases of man and animals. Kluwer; Antwerp: Institute of Tropical Medicine, Dordrecht; Boston

Mas-Coma S, Bargues MD, Valero MA (2005) Fascioliasis and other plant-borne trematodezoonoses. Int J Parasitol 35:1255–1278

Mas-Coma S, Bargues MD, Valero MA (2006) Gastrodiscoidiasis, a plant-borne zoonotic disease caused by the intestinal amphistome fluke *Gastrodiscoides hominis* (Trematoda: Gastrodiscidae). Rev Iber Parasitol 66:75–81

Murty CV, Reddy CR (1980) A case report of *Gastrodiscoideshominis* infection. Indian J Pathol Microbiol 23:303–304

Roy B, Tandon V (1992) (1992) seasonal prevalence of some zoonoticdigenean infections in cattle and pigs in a humid subtropicalmontane zone in India. Vet Parasitol 41:69–76

Sah R, Acosta L, Rafael T (2019) A case report of human gastrodiscoidiasis in Nepal. Parasitol Int 71:56–58

Shrivastav HO, Shah HL (1970) On *Gastrodiscoideshominis* (Lewis and McConnell, 1876) Leiper, 1913 from pigs (*Sus scrofadomestica*) in Madhya Pradesh, its pathology and public health importance. Indian J Pathol Bacteriol 13:68–72

Toledo R, Alvárez-Izquierdo M, Muñoz-Antoli C, Esteban JG (2019) Intestinal trematode infections. Adv Exp Med Biol 1154:181–213

Yu SH, Mott KE (1994) Epidemiology and morbidity of food-borne intestinal trematode infections. Trop Dis Bull 91(7):R125–R152

Chapter 91
Intestinal Flukes

Food-borne intestinal flukes are highly diversified, consisting of at least 74 species with diverse global distribution. Taxonomically, they include 28 species of heterophyids, 23 species of echinostomes, and 23 species of miscellaneous groups (Chai and Jung 2020). Of the intestinal flukes, *Fasciolopsis buski* is the most common, followed by *Heterophyes heterophyes*, *Metagonimus yokogawai*, and *Echinostoma ilocanum*. *Gastrodiscoides hominis*, *Phaneropsolus bonnei*, and *Prosthodendrium molenkampi* rarely cause human intestinal infections (http://emedicine.medscape. com/article/219662-overview). More than 70 species of fish, including both freshwater and marine species, are intermediate hosts susceptible to invasion by metacercariae and can thus potentially infect food. These are a variety of freshwater and brackish-water fish and snails, reptiles (amphibians and certain snakes), aquatic plants, and insects. There is a wide variety of reservoir hosts for these flukes, including fish-eating birds and wild and domestic mammals, especially cats, dogs, and pigs. Human fondness for raw or lightly prepared fish foods is the primary human risk factor and is responsible for the wide geographical distribution of human infections. An estimated 40–50 million people get infected by intestinal flukes, and nearly 600 million are at risk the world over, especially in Asia and also in Europe, Africa, the Near East, and North and South America (FAO/WHO 2014).

The parasites cause pathology in three ways: (a) mechanical irritation, blockage, or perforation; (b) toxaemia/allergies; and (c) malabsorption—protein and vitamin (B12) deficiency.

91.1 *Fasciolopsis buski*

Fasciolopsis buski, commonly known as a giant intestinal fluke because of its size, is a trematode of the Fasciolidae family and was first discovered by George Busk in 1843 in the duodenum of an Indian sailor (Cook 1996). It infects humans, pigs,

© Springer Nature Singapore Pte Ltd. 2024
K. G. Narayan et al., *Handbook of Management of Zoonoses*,
https://doi.org/10.1007/978-981-99-9885-2_91

dogs, and rabbits in Asian countries like Bangladesh, Cambodia, China, India, Indonesia, Laos, Malaysia, Pakistan, Taiwan, Thailand, and Vietnam, where pigs are reared and freshwater plants are fed. It does not occur in other parts of the world. Living in endemic areas and travelling to endemic areas are likely to cause exposure.

Its prevalence in India and China is 60%; about 10 million people are infected, mostly children in impoverished areas, where there is a lack of sanitation. It is endemic in central Thailand. Aquatic plants like water caltrops are a common vehicle of infection. Infection in different districts was associated with water pollution. More females than males and children of 10–14 years were infected.

Deka et al. (2023) reported a case of heavy infection of *Fasciolopsis buski* in a 4-year-old girl with severe acute malnutrition (SAM). Many adult worms came out with the stool following the consumption of some herbal concoction. A wet mount of the stool revealed the ova of *Fasciolopsis buski*. She was treated successfully with praziquantel and food supplements.

91.1.1 Clinical Manifestation

Water plants eaten raw that are risky are water chestnuts, bamboo shoots, water caltrops, morning glory, and other water plants. Peeling parts of these raw plants with teeth and consuming contaminated water containing infective metacercariae lead to infection.

The severity of pathogenicity is dependent upon parasitic load. The parasites cause mechanical damage, mucosal destruction, erosion, ulcer, abscess, and catarrhal inflammation. Toxic metabolites cause facial/orbital oedema and ascites. Infection has a wide range of outcomes—sub-clinical to fatal.

Heavy infection is symptomatically manifested as pain in the abdomen, epigastric, chronic diarrhoea, obstruction of the bowel, intestinal perforation, skin swelling, and allergic reaction caused by allergenic metabolites. The reaction may even be fatal. Light infection is manifested as headache, dizziness, gastric pain, loose motion, anaemia, and eosinophilia.

91.2 *Echinostoma ilocanum*

Echinostoma ilocanum was first described in five prisoners in Manila, Philippines, in 1907. *Gyraulus* or *Hippeutis* is a freshwater snail that sheds cercariae. Human infection occurs after eating large snails, *Pila conica* (Philippines) and *Viviparus javanicus* (Java), harbouring metacercariae. Rats and dogs are reservoirs. Countries where humans are known to be infected are Indonesia (Celebes, Java), China, Thailand, the Philippines, and India. A fatal case due to *Artyfechinostomum malayanum* (*A. mehrai*) was reported in India. The autopsy revealed several hundred parasites. *Echinostoma malayanum* (Leiper 1911), another species of *A. mehrai* Faruqui

1930, later synonymized with *A. malayanum*, was recovered from a Hindu girl patient. *Echinostoma malayanum* is endemic in Malaysia, Thailand, Indonesia, and the Philippines. Snail intermediate hosts are *Indoplanorbis exustus* or *Gyraulus convexiusculus*, and cercariae encyst in various species of snails, i.e. *Pila scutata*, *Lymnaea (Bullastra) cumingiana*, and *Digoniostoma pulchella*. The definitive hosts are humans, pigs, rats, cats, dogs, mice, hamsters, and house shrews (Chai et al. 2009).

91.2.1 Clinical Manifestation

Intestinal flukes are located in the upper small intestines. Pathological changes are located at the site of attachment to the mucosa, which is pinched and even eaten by the flukes. The parasite causes mechanical irritation. When they are numerous, these are seen also in the lower part of the intestine and stomach and cause blockage or even perforation of the intestine. Their toxic metabolites induce allergic reactions. A histological examination revealed a range of changes in focal areas—destruction and detachment of villi, loss of mucosa, and ulceration. The parasite causes malabsorption. This leads to hypoalbuminemia and vitamin B12 deficiency. Immunity leads to the spontaneous expulsion of primary infecting worms. The dynamics of expulsion differ with the species of the parasite and host.

Infection with *Echinostomes* is more severe than with other intestinal flukes, such as *Heterophyids*. *E. ilocanum* causes intestinal colic and diarrhoea. Generally, patients suffer abdominal pain, chronic diarrhoea and tenesmus, anorexia, headache, nausea, vomiting, and hematemesis. There is a loss of body weight and a feeling of fatigue. Severe epigastric discomfort may be consistent and persistent for long. Endoscopy reveals presence of ulcerative lesions in stomach or duodenum , if any, and even an adult fluke attached to mucosa.

91.3 *Metagonimus yokogawai* (earlier *Heterophyes yokogawai*)

It is the most common intestinal fluke in humans in the Far East and has been reported in Japan, China, Taiwan, Korea, Siberia, the Balkan states, Israel, and Spain. Endemicity is generally in regions along the coasts, streams, river basins, and water bodies. Prevalence is high in villagers and certain ethnic groups, such as observed in Russia.

Cercariae are shed by freshwater snails, *Semisulcospira coreana* or *Semisulcospira libertina*. The second intermediate hosts include the sweetfish *Plecoglossus altivelis*, the dace *Tribolodon* spp., and the perch *Lateolabrax japonicus*. Natural definitive hosts are dogs, rats, and cats.

Heterophyes heterophyes is the most common species in this genus to infect humans orally. It is a small fluke that parasitizes the small intestine and causes mild inflammation, superficial necrosis, and shallow ulcers. Eggs are small and sometimes enter the blood vessels to cause embolism and cerebral haemorrhage if brain vessels are involved. Myocarditis, chronic congestive heart failure, and death may result if eggs enter lymphatics and travel to the heart.

91.4   Diagnosis

- Examination for the detection of parasite eggs, at times adults in the stool and sometimes vomitus.
- Endoscopy
- Serology in the case of *F. buski*
- The Merthiolate- iodine- formalin (MIF) method: Concentrate the Specimen using MIF method, which simultaneously preserves and stains the eggs. sensitivity is increased to identify *F. buski*, *Heterophyes* species, and *Echinostoma* species in stool specimens.
- Polymerase chain reaction: Various polymerase chain reaction (PCR) methods have shown potential in detecting intestinal fluke parasites.

91.5   Treatment

Praziquantel is the drug of choice. However, other anthelmintics, like thiabendazole, mebendazole, and levamisole, can be used.

91.6   Preventive Measures

- Decontaminate vegetables by dipping them in boiling water for a few seconds or heating them at 60°C or freezing them at −10° C for a few days
- Prohibit use as fertilizer—untreated night soil/animal excreta
- Improve sanitation and hygiene.

References

Chai JY, Jung BK (2020) Foodborne intestinal flukes: a brief review of epidemiology and geographical distribution. Acta Trop 201:105210
Chai JY, Shin EH, Lee SH, Rim HJ (2009) Foodborne intestinal flukes in Southeast Asia. Korean J Parasitol 47(Suppl):S69–S102

Cook GC (1996) George Busk, FRS (1807–1886): surgeon, zoologist, parasitologist and palaeontologist. Trans R Soc Trop Med Hyg 90:715–716

Deka S, Kalita D, Hazarika NK (2023) Heavy load of intestinal fluke in a four-year-old child with severe acute malnutrition: a case report. J Lab Physicians 15:139–141

Leiper RT (1911) Notes of the occurrence of parasites presumably rare in man. J London School Trop Med 1:16–19

FAO/WHO (2014) Multi criteria - based ranking for risk management of food borne parasites. Microbiological Risk Assessment Series No. 23. Rome. 302 pp S133–S141, October 2009. https://doi.org/10.3347/kjp.2009.47.S.S133

Chapter 92
Opisthorchiasis

Opisthorchiasis is a major public health problem in many parts of Southeast Asia, Europe, and Russia. The two important species of *Opisthorchis* are *O. viverrini* and *O. felineus*. *O. viverrini* is highly endemic in Southeast Asia, including Thailand, Lao PDR, Vietnam, and Cambodia, while *O. felineus* in Europe and Russia (Ogorodova et al. 2015).

Opisthorchiasis is underestimated as a public health problem. Its spread is related to globalization-driven people movement and trade in fish (aquaculture). Metacercariae can remain viable in fish muscle even when pickled or fermented. *O. viverrini* is regularly carried by tourists and Thai labourers. Climate change may impact the epidemiology. The developmental time of the immature stage, and hence the time for searching a host, is likely to be reduced with increased temperature. Similarly, increased rainfall/melting glaciers will enhance wetlands and the expansion of habitat for the intermediate hosts—snails and fish.

92.1 *O. viverrini*

A conservative estimate is that 10 million people in Thailand and Laos are infected with *O. viverrini* (Andrews et al. 2008). No prevalence data are available for Vietnam and Cambodia. This fluke has been recognized as a type 1 carcinogen. The infection occurs in young children; it may not be life-threatening immediately, but cholangiocarcinoma (CCA) may develop 30–40 years later, and death follows within 3–6 months. The age is productive. Social, community, family, and economic costs are enormous. Family earning is affected as more males are affected. Opisthorchiasis

© Springer Nature Singapore Pte Ltd. 2024
K. G. Narayan et al., *Handbook of Management of Zoonoses*,
https://doi.org/10.1007/978-981-99-9885-2_92

is estimated to cost US\$ 120 million in a year in Thailand alone, including the cost of medical care and the loss of wages.

92.1.1   Life Cycle

The life cycle of *O. viverrini* involves cats, dogs, and various fish-eating mammals, including humans, as definitive hosts. Freshwater snails like *Bithynia goniompharus*, *B. funiculate*, and *B. siamensis* are the first intermediate hosts. The ingested ova develop into cercaria in these. The second intermediate hosts are freshwater fish (*Cyclocheilichthys* spp., *Puntius* spp., *Hampala dispar*) and have metacercariae in their muscles and under scales. At least 18 species of cyprinoid freshwater fish are intermediate hosts in Thailand, and 90% of them are infected.

Opisthorchiasis is a major public health problem in the northeastern and northern regions of Thailand. Many traditional raw or uncooked fish products are popular in rural areas in these regions and are incriminated as the cause. The infection presents a variety of hepatobiliary pathologies—cholangitis, obstructive jaundice, hepatomegaly, cholecystitis, cholelithiasis, and cholangiocarcinoma.

Opisthorchiasis as a public health problem in Thailand has been reviewed by Kaewpitoon et al. (2008b). There is a causal relationship between the frequency of consumption of traditional fish preparation and prevalence and also between the metacercarial loads in these. Small and medium-sized fish are used in the preparation of (1) *Koi pla*, (2) *plasom*—moderately fermented for a few days to weeks and eaten several times a week, and (3) *plara* –extensively fermented and salted and stored for 2–3 months. The frequency of consumption of *Koi pla* every week is about 80% in some communities. *Koi pla* had the highest prevalence of liver fluke. The prevalence of opisthorchiasis is relatively less among people consuming other types of preparations—preserved for <7 days, *plara* and *jeow bong* in which viable metacercariae are rare. The prevalence and intensity of infection are greater in rural than urban dwellers and seem to be strongly related to the habit and frequency of eating *koi pla*. Most cases occurred among those engaged in agriculture. The infection is observed as early as in the age group of 0–4 years. As the age advances to adulthood, the prevalence of infection increases, and subsequent prevalence is related to the consumption of *koi pla*. Most cases are recorded in the age group 35–65+ years, peaking at 55–64 years. The intensity of infection is measured as a faecal egg output and rises steadily in early life and is the maximum in the age group 55–64 years in both males and females. Generally, more metacercariae are seen on fish before the dry season, September to February, and this coincides with increased human infection.

Opisthorchiasis is widespread in Laos, and more than half of the population is infected. In highly endemic villages, 70% of the population is infected with *O. viverrini*, with an increasing prevalence of infection with age (Forrer et al. 2012). There is a close correlation between the consumption of fish and the prevalence of *O. viverrini* in communities in rural Laos. In some villages of Laos, up to 60% of fish species carry metacercariae (Sayasone et al. 2007). An examination of cats and dogs revealed that 30% of them were infected with *O. viverrini*, which can contribute to intensifying the transmission of these parasites to humans. Moreover, the deeply culturally rooted habit of raw fish dish consumption is a major public health challenge (Xayaseng et al. 2013).

92.2   *O. felineus*

Armignacco et al. (2008) described opisthorchiasis as being caused by *O. felineus* (cat liver fluke) in Europe. The estimated number of human infections is 1.2 million globally. Sporadic cases in Germany and Greece and a high prevalence in Byelorussia, Russia, and Ukraine have been reported. *O. felineus* has been endemic in Italy. Cases were few because customarily cooked fish was consumed. In the last four outbreaks investigated since 2003, observations were as follows: 2–4 weeks of incubation period; 100% attack rate in three outbreaks; 58.8% in the fourth, where not all participants ate marinated tench filets (*Tinca tinca*); 59% were asymptomatic; and none had severe symptoms. These differed from those observed in the endemic regions of Eastern Europe and Asia. People who like eating raw fish get infected and manifest severe symptoms. The liver, pancreas, and gall bladder are affected, and cirrhosis may be caused. Epidemiologic surveys on stray cats in the areas of Lakes Bolsena and Trasimeno reveal that 23.5% to 40.0% had eggs of *O. felineus* in their faeces. Cats ate garbage from restaurants and fish carcasses discarded by fishermen and thus were infected. It was determined that 83.1% of the tenches (fish) tested had metacercariae. Freezing at −10°C for 5 to 70 days or −28°C for 24 h killed metacercariae, depending upon the size of the fish. In the outbreak of August 2007, fish had been frozen at −10°C for 3 days. The internal temperature of fish frozen in home freezers cannot be assessed.

92.3   Pathogenesis, Pathology, and Clinical Symptoms

Kaewpitoon et al. (2008a) discussed the pathogenesis and pathology, especially, of cholangiocarcinoma caused by *O. viverrini*.

Opisthorchiasis may be either the following:

- Asymptomatic.
- With mild symptoms: constipation or diarrhoea, dyspepsia, and abdominal pain.
- Chronic: severe manifestation—malnutrition and hepatomegaly; rarely cholangitis, cholecystitis, and cholangiocarcinoma (CCA).

It is suggested that mechanical damage, the secretion of fluke, and immune pathological response contribute to CCA. Nitrosamine, a carcinogen, may lead to or contribute to CCA, and several *N*-nitroso compounds and their precursors occur at low levels in fermented food such as preserved mud fish paste, like *plara*, which is commonly used in Thailand and Laos.

Acute changes are primarily due to the parasite, while progressive ones are due to immunopathological mechanisms.

Severity is related to the intensity and duration of infection. The fluke inhabits the intra- and extra-hepatic ducts, the gall bladder, the bile ducts, and the pancreas. The liver is enlarged, maybe 3.0–3.5 kg during heavy infection. Large and medium-sized bile ducts are dilated and fibrosed. Histopathological changes include inflammation, desquamation of the epithelia, metaplasia of goblet cells, epithelial and adenomatous hyperplasia, and periductal fibrosis. There may be granulomatous inflammation entrapping eggs. Fibrosis of the wall of the gall bladder is the most common.

Both humoral and cellular immune responses are observed in human and hamster models. The parasite antigen may be detected as early as 3 days after infection in epithelial cells lining the intra- and extra-hepatic bile ducts. Humoral antibodies to excretory-secretory and egg antigens may be detected in the serum. IgG, IgE, and IgA antibodies may be detected in the bile and serum of patients.

92.4   Diagnosis

Reliable clinical and parasitological diagnostic tools are required. There is no tool for the early detection of CCA.

- Standard faecal examination for the detection of fluke eggs—eggs may not be detected in cases of light infection and obstruction of the bile ducts.
- Detection of *Opisthorchis* antigen in faeces—may be difficult.
- Immunodiagnostic method—e.g. indirect enzyme-linked immunosorbent assay (ELISA) is a highly sensitive technique. Cross-reaction is a problem. Antigens used are Ov-CP-1, somatic extracts, excretory-secretory products, and eggs. The recombinant cysteine proteinase-based ELISA with Ov-CP-1 antigens is good as cross-reaction with hookworms and minute intestinal flukes was nil, sensitivity 94.66% and specificity 95.55%.
- Deoxyribonucleic acid (DNA) detection.
- PCR-based amplification of parasite DNA from stools was more sensitive compared to formalin-ether and Stoll's egg counting.

92.5   Control

Liver fluke control strategies are as follows:

- Eliminate host reservoirs—stool examination and treatment of the infected with praziquantel.

- Health education—awareness campaign to promote the cooking of fish to prevent infection.
- Sanitation—hygienic defecation; stop defecation in the open.
- Regulate the use of human/animal faeces in aquaculture.

Intensive and continuous control activities in Thailand have led to a reduction from 34% in 1992 to 10% in 2002 (Andrews et al. 2008).

References

Andrews RH, Sithithaworn P, Petney TV (2008) *Opisthorchis viverrini*: an underestimated parasite in world health. Trends Parasitol 24(11):497–501

Armignacco O, Caterini L, Marucci G, Ferri F, Bernardini G et al (2008) Human illnesses caused by *Opisthorchis felineus* flukes, Italy. Emerg Infect Dis 14(12):1902–1905

Forrer A, Vounatsou P, Sayasone S, Vonghachack Y et al (2012) Spatial distribution of, and risk factors for, *Opisthorchis viverrini* infection in southern Lao PDR. PLoS Negl Trop Dis 6:e1481

Kaewpitoon N, Kaewpitoon SJ, Pengsaa P (2008a) Opisthorchiasis in Thailand: review and current status. World J Gastroenterol 14(15):2297–2302

Kaewpitoon N, Kaewpitoon SJ, Pengsaa P, Sripa B (2008b) *Opisthorchis viverrini*: the carcinogenic human liver fluke. World J Gastroenterol 14(5):666–674

Ogorodova LM, Fedorova OS, Sripa B, Mordvinov VA, Katokhin AV et al (2015) TOPIC Consortium. Opisthorchiasis: an overlooked danger. PLoS Negl Trop Dis 9(4):e0003563

Sayasone S, Odermatt P, Phoumindr N, Vongsaravane X et al (2007) Epidemiology of *Opisthorchis viverrini* in a rural district of southern Lao PDR. Trans R Soc Trop Med Hyg 101:40–47

Xayaseng V, Phongluxa K, van Eeuwijk P, Akkhavong K, Odermatt P (2013) Raw fish consumption in liver fluke endemic areas in rural southern Laos. Acta Trop 127:105–111

Chapter 93
Paragonimiasis

Paragonimiasis is among the food-borne zoonotic trematodes with a very broad geographical distribution (tropical and some subtropical regions of Asia, Africa, and the Americas), a large number of causative *Paragonimus* species, and a range of clinical signs and symptoms, which mimic especially tuberculosis and cancer (Blair 2022). More than ten species of *Paragonimus*—the lung fluke (Table 93.1)—infect human beings, but *P. westermani* is the most common.

93.1 *Paragonimus westermani* (the Oriental Lung Fluke)

Starting with eggs in the human or feline sputum or stool (if sputum is swallowed), it takes 2 weeks for the miracidium to develop in the eggs and hatch. The first intermediate hosts are freshwater snails—*Semisulcospira* spp. Miracidia seek and penetrate the first intermediate hosts, snails. A series of development takes place inside the snails. Mother sporocyst forms and produces a number of mother rediae. A number of cercariae develop and are released. Cercariae invade the second intermediate hosts—crustaceans such as crayfish and crabs—and encyst. Human infection occurs when inadequately cooked or pickled infected crayfish or crab is eaten. The metacercariae excyst in the small intestine and duodenum and penetrate through the intestinal wall, reach the peritoneal cavity, and move through the abdominal wall and diaphragm to enter the lungs, where they become adult. It takes 65 to 90 days from the date of infection to oviposition. Adult worms may be seen in other tissues, like striated muscles or the brain, but eggs laid do not find an exit, and so the parasites' life cycle cannot continue. The worms may persist for as long as 20 years.

Other animals, like pigs; carnivores, including felids, canids, viverrids, and mustelids; and some rodents may be infected, harbour the parasite, and act as reservoirs. A number of mammals and birds may act as paratenic hosts too, which when eaten can cause human infection.

© Springer Nature Singapore Pte Ltd. 2024
K. G. Narayan et al., *Handbook of Management of Zoonoses*,
https://doi.org/10.1007/978-981-99-9885-2_93

Table 93.1 Zoonotic species of *Paragonimus* and their geographical distribution

Species of *Paragonimus*	Geographical distribution
P. uterobilateralis, P. africanus, P. gondwanensis	Africa
P. mexicanus, P. kellicotti, P. mexicanus	The Americas
P. westermani, P. heterotremus, P. philippinensis, P. skrjabini	Asia

An estimated 22.0 million people are affected globally. The prevalence is high in Southeast Asia, Japan, China, and countries where eating raw seafood is popular. It is recorded in the USA because of immigrants. Boland et al. (2011) described four cases of *P. westermani* in the USA. Lane et al. (2009) described three cases of paragonimiasis (*P. kellicotti*), where the patient acquired infection by consuming raw crayfish from the rivers of Missouri. This species seems to be endemic in areas of the Mississippi River drainage basin. The boiling of crayfish before eating is suggested (Diaz 2011). According to Lane et al. (2012), seven autochthonous cases were reported in 40 years (1968–2008). They described three new cases in 2009, which were caused by *P. kellicotti*. In the following 18 months, six more cases were identified and intervention methods suggested.

Other species of *Paragonimus* are prevalent in parts of Asia, Africa, and South and Central America.

About 80% of freshwater crabs are infected in Asia. Crab collection and trade in areas miles away spread, e.g. collected in sea and brought inland in for sale in Taiwan markets. Metacercariae survive crab preparations—marination, pickling in vinegar or wine, immersing in wine for 3 min (so-called drunken crabs), smashing rice eating crabs in rice paddies, splashing and using fresh crab juices for medicinal purposes. While handling and crushing crabs, metacercariae contaminate the fingers and utensils, and thus other ready-to-eat food may get contaminated too.

93.2 Symptoms

Beginning from metacercariae invasion to developing into adult parasites, the host's response determines the symptoms. These may be described into the following phases:

- Acute—while migrating, the parasite moves through different organs, and symptoms may follow accordingly, such as diarrhoea and abdominal pain, fever, urticaria, hepatosplenomegaly, cough, pulmonary symptoms (dyspnoea and eosinophilia).
- Chronic—pulmonary symptoms usually begin 6 months after infection, with the parasite settling in the lungs: cough, bronchitis, bronchiectasis, pleuritic chest pain, discoloured sputum, haemoptysis, and pathology-detected on radiography.

Extra-pulmonary-located parasites cause a variety of symptoms depending upon the tissues:

- Severe symptoms may appear if the parasite gets to the brain. These include headache, vomition, neurological signs, facial palsy, and hemiplegia.
- Abdominal pain, palpable abdominal mass, and bloody diarrhoea may occur when the parasite is located in the abdomen and arrested in the form of cysts in the liver, spleen, and mesenteric lymph glands and haematuria if located in the kidney.
- Abscess and granuloma may appear if the parasite is located in the subcutaneous tissues.

93.3 Diagnosis

- X-ray.
- Haematology—eosinophilia.
- Detection of eggs in the sputum, stool, effusion fluid, or biopsy; eggs may not be detected until 2–3 months after infection.
- Serology—enzyme-linked immunosorbent assay (ELISA).

93.4 Treatment

Praziquantel, bithionol.

References

Blair D (2022) Lung flukes of the genus Paragonimus: ancient and re-emerging pathogens. Parasitology 149(10):1286–1295

Boland JM, Vaszar LT, Jones JL, Mathison BA, Rovzar MA et al (2011) Pleuropulmonary infection by *Paragonimus westermani* in the United States: a rare cause of eosinophilic pneumonia after ingestion of live crabs. Am J Surg Pathol 35(5):707–713

Diaz JH (2011) Boil before eating: paragonimiasis after eating raw crayfish in the Mississippi River basin. J La State Med Soc 163(5):261–266

Lane MA, Barsanti MC, Santos CA, Yeung M, Lubner SJ, Weil GJ (2009) Human paragonimiasis in North America following ingestion of raw crayfish. Clin Infect Dis 49(6):e55–e61

Lane MA, Marcos LA, Onen NF, Demertzis LM, Hayes EV et al (2012) *Paragonimus kellicotti* flukes in Missouri, USA. Emerg Infect Dis 18(8):1263–1267

Chapter 94
Schistosomiasis

Synonyms

Bilharzia, Bilharziasis, Snail fever.

Schistosomiasis is an acute and chronic waterborne parasitic disease characterized by blood in the urine and/or faeces and hepatomegaly commonly affecting children. They get anaemic and debilitated. Growth may be stunted. People at risk are those exposed to infested water such as agricultural, fishing, occupational (washerman), recreational, and swimming.

94.1 Geographical Distribution

Schistosomiasis was reported in Gimvi village, Ratnaagiri, Maharashtra, India. The World Health Organization (WHO) team collaborating with the government of India eliminated the infection from Gimvi village (Agrawal and Rao 2011). The disease occurs in tropical and subtropical areas and is endemic in Africa, South America, and Asia. Most of the infection (>90%) is reported in Africa, and it is estimated to cause 200,000 deaths in sub-Saharan Africa (WHO 2013). It is prevalent in 78 countries, 52 of which have moderate to high transmission. In 2018, at least 290.8 million people required preventive treatment (WHO 2020).

© Springer Nature Singapore Pte Ltd. 2024
K. G. Narayan et al., *Handbook of Management of Zoonoses*,
https://doi.org/10.1007/978-981-99-9885-2_94

94.2   Aetiology

The parasite *Schistosoma haematobium*, a blood fluke, was first identified by Theodor Maximilian Bilharz, a German pathologist working in Egypt, as a cause of haematuria in the 1850s (Schadewaldt 1962). Male worms are robust and tuberculate and measure 6–12 mm in length. Females are longer (7–17 mm in length) and slender. The lateral edges of the male fluke are enfolded to form a groove, which is inhabited by the female worm. There are two major forms of schistosomiasis: intestinal and urogenital. These are caused by five main species of blood fluke (Table 94.1).

Table 94.1 Parasite species and the geographical distribution of schistosomiasis (WHO 2020 modified)

Form	Species	Tissue parasitized	Intermediate host	Definitive host	Geographical distribution
Intestinal schistosomiasis	*Schistosoma mansoni*	Inferior mesenteric veins	Freshwater snails, genus *Biomphalaria*	Humans, baboons, raccoons, and rodents.	Africa, the Middle East, the Caribbean, Brazil, Venezuela, and Suriname
	S. japonicum	Superior mesenteric veins	Freshwater snails, genus *Oncomelania.*	Humans, cats, dogs, rats, pigs, water buffaloes, and horses.	China, Indonesia, and the Philippines
	S. mekongi	Superior mesenteric veins, CNS	Snail *Neotricula aperta*	Humans, dogs, and pigs.	Several districts of Cambodia and the Lao People's Democratic Republic
	S. guineensis and related *S. intercalatum*[a]	Central nervous system disorders, one with a liver disorder and another with cardiopulmonary	Freshwater snail *Bulinus forskalii*		Rainforest areas of Central Africa
Urogenital schistosomiasis	*S. haematobium*	Vesical plexus of the urinary bladder	Freshwater snails, genus *Bulinus* (*B. truncates*)	Humans are common. Baboons and monkeys are rare.	Africa, the Middle East, Corsica (France)

[a]Phylogenetic results clearly treat *Schistosoma intercalatum* and *S. guineensis* as separate taxa, with each more closely related evolutionarily to *S. haematobium* than to each other

The **mode of infection** is contact with pond and dam water and stagnant water infested with the larval stage (cercariae) of *Schistosoma* spp.

94.3   Life Cycle (Fig. 94.1)

The *S. haematobium* larval stage (cercaria) emerges from an infected snail; *Bulinus truncates* and swims until it penetrates the skin of the human in contact with water. After entry through skin penetration, the cercaria remains in the skin for 2 days, locates, enters the capillary venule, and travels to the lungs, simultaneously developing to a form necessary for migration to the liver. It takes 8–10 days post-skin penetration to reach the liver sinusoids. The parasite develops oral suckers and begins to feed on red blood cells. Male and female worms of intestinal schistosomes relocate to the mesenteric or rectal veins (multiplication sites) and urinary schistosomes to the perivesical venous plexus of the bladder, ureter, and kidneys. Worms mature in 6–8 weeks and begin laying eggs—300 (*S. mansoni*) to 3000 (*S. japonicum*) every day. The pairs may remain for four and half years on average but may continue for 20 years. The eggs may pass through the walls of the blood vessels to the lumen—intestine or urinary bladder—to be excreted by the host. Eggs hatch, and freely swimming miracidia penetrate the snails (intermediate hosts) and develop into mother sporocysts. Two weeks later, daughter sporocysts form, and 4 weeks after initial entry into snails, cercariae are released.

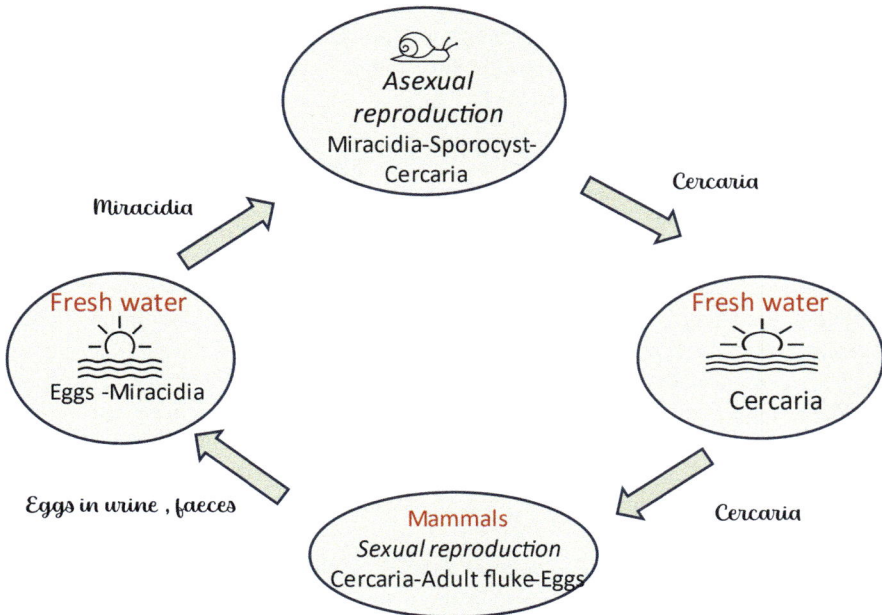

Fig. 94.1 Life cycle of schistosomes- Asexual reproduction in snails and sexual reproduction in mammals

94.4 Epidemiology

Schistosomiasis is a chronic 'blood fluke' disease known to infect more than 230 to 250 million people annually (Alemu et al. 2018; Wei et al. 2018), and 779 million people are at risk of infection (Chala and Torben 2018). This disease causes 280,000 deaths annually (Sundaraneedi et al. 2017) and a worldwide burden of 3.3 million disability-adjusted life years (Alemu et al. 2018; Braun et al. 2018). Human schistosomiasis is among the most prevalent human parasitic infections, which ranks second beneath malaria on the list of parasitic diseases (Alemu et al. 2018; Mohamed et al. 2018).

The impact of schistosomiasis on children in endemic areas provides guidelines for implementing control at the community level through treatment. Three situations may happen: (a) >50% of children have blood in the urine—all in the village need to be treated, (b) 20–50% of children have blood in the urine—treatment is limited to school-aged children, and (c) <20% of children have blood in the urine—no mass treatment.

The overall prevalence is 34.4%. For the age group 6–8 years, it is 30%; 9–11 years, 24.2%; 12–14 years, 48%, and 15–17 years, 50%. Children of self-employed parents showed a significantly higher prevalence than children of salaried employed. Subjects had low knowledge of the disease (Okanla et al. 2003).

The factors favouring infection are poverty; poor living conditions; poor awareness of environmentally acquired infections naturally at a young age; deprivation of sanitary conditions, like sanitized water; and available water bodies enjoyed for swimming by children, resulting in maximum cases of infection in the growing age of 5–14 years. People engaged in agricultural, domestic (washing clothes and utensils and fishing in canals, rivers, ponds, lakes, and other natural water bodies), and recreational activities stand at risk.

94.5 Symptoms

The antigens secreted by the invading cercariae elicit a strong immune response, initiating pathology. Local acute inflammation and light rash (swimmers' itch) develop within 12 h and may ulcerate. These may be seen in the feet and hands. Response of individuals differs with the three phases of the parasitic invasion, migratory phase and penetration into host to maturity. These are acute phase—when production of eggs begins and the chronic phase. Repeated infection in children leads to anaemia, retarded growth, and impaired cognitive function.

After 1 to 2 months of infection, common symptoms like fever, chills, cough, and pain in the muscles appear.

Urinary schistosomiasis (*S. haematobium*) damages the bladder and kidneys, resulting in painful urination, blood in the urine, and abdominal pain. Adults are located in the venous plexus around the urinary bladder. The migrating eggs cause fibrosis of the wall of the bladder, even calcification. There is reverse pressure on the ureters and kidneys, resulting in hydronephrosis. There is haematuria. Complications like squamous cell carcinoma may happen. Urogenital schistosomiasis presents vaginal lesions, painful intercourse, and bleeding and adds to the risk of human immunodeficiency virus (HIV) infection. In males, the prostate and seminal vesicles may be affected and may lead to irreversible consequences, including infertility.

Intestinal schistosomiasis (*S. mansoni*, *S. japonicum*) damages the intestines and liver, resulting in abdominal pain, fever, and rectal bleeding. *S. mansoni* and *S. japonicum* infections range from asymptomatic to acute (known as Katayama's fever). The manifestations depend upon the tissues invaded. Commonly, it is intestinal—abdominal pain, diarrhoea, fever, and cough. Occasionally, the ectopic location of the parasite may lead to cerebral granuloma, transverse myelitis, and flaccid paraplegia. Colonic polyposis with bloody diarrhoea, haematemesis, and splenomegaly may be seen in cases of long-continued infection.

Human pathology due to schistosomes is mainly caused by the process of immunological reaction to eggs deposited in tissues. Immune reaction to eggs deposited in tissues causes pathology. Sites may vary. Eggs in the intestinal wall cause an immune granulomatous reaction, leading to obstruction of the colon and blood loss. Lodgement in the liver and spleen leads to hepato- and splenomegaly, respectively. *S. guineensis* infection first causes dysentery. Eggs are swept back to the liver with portal blood flow and lodge in the narrow branches of the portal system. Granuloma develops around and becomes fibrous. Clinical manifestations may be a pot belly—fluid accumulation in the abdomen—and portal hypertension. Life-threatening oesophageal varices (profuse bleeding caused by dilations and swollen areas) may occur. Rare cases of pathology in other organs, the central nervous system, and cardiopulmonary are due to ectopic migration (Murinello et al. 2006).

94.6   Diagnosis

- Urine/stool examination—detection of eggs.
- Antigen detection in the blood and urine.
- Intradermal injection of a schistosome antigen produces wheal—useful in chronic infection when eggs are not detected.
- Complement fixation and other serological tests for the detection of exposure.

94.7   Treatment

Praziquantel is the drug of choice. It can reverse 90% of the damage caused by the parasites.

94.8   Prevention and Control

The assisted programme of The Carter Center (The Carter Center • One Copenhill, 453 Freedom Parkway, Atlanta, GA 30307 • (404) 420–5100 • www.cartercenter. org) is an example worth imitating. The Carter Center has been working in Nigeria since 1999. Its approach is (a) health education and (b) treatment. The Carter Center has been treating over 1 million patients, mostly children, every year in the programme area. Nigerians are benefitting from the programme. The reduction of blood in the urine is 94% in the Plateau and Nasarawa states and nearly 88% in the Delta area.

In 2008, WHO and Merck KGaA (Germany) donated 1.5 million tablets of praziquantel to The Carter Centre, enabling it to expand the programme's reach.

Schistosomiasis was successfully eliminated in Tunisia (WHO 2009). The last autochthonous case detected was in 1981–1982. The population at risk was 150,000. The overall prevalence in 1973 was 70.2%. Urine examination of children detected the transmission site. *Bulinus truncatus* was a vector restricted to oases. Endemic areas thus defined were visited by locally employed workers (hence, communication was effective) to educate. Two-prong attacks included (a) the use of a molluscicidal agent and (b) treatment with praziquantel or metrifonate, mostly at home. The first application of the molluscicidal agent eliminated 75% of the sites; the rest of the sites required a number of applications. All treated cases were cured. Surveillance continued. Initially, the entire population in the ten oases was covered. Samples of the urine of the selected were examined annually, later every 2 years, and finally limited to school children. By 1994, most oases dried, and the principal source of water was an artesian well.

The experience is educative may be multiplied. The estimated requirement is >500 million tablets per year to treat cases worldwide.

The snail population may be controlled by acrolein, copper sulphate, and niclosamide. Predation by crayfish may be exploited.

Human waste (urine/faeces) must not be allowed to contaminate water supplies. Adherence to this (hygienic disposal) may also eliminate schistosomiasis. The irrigation system may also be so planned as to keep out or limit the population of snails. Praziquantel is the drug of choice for preventive/adjusted preventive chemotherapy. Complementary interventions are access to safe water, improved sanitation, hygiene education and behaviour change, and snail control and environmental management.

94.9   Elimination of Schistosomiasis and Proposed Timelines from the World Health Organization (WHO)

WHO has recommended strategies for the control of schistosomiasis by means of preventive chemotherapy, with the use of complementary interventions where possible, and the elimination of the disease as a public health problem by means of adjusted preventive chemotherapy, with the use of complementary interventions

being strongly recommended. The elimination of transmission by means of intensi-
fied preventive chemotherapy in residual areas of transmission and complementary
interventions is considered to be essential. The time lines are as below:

1. *Disease Control Target: 2020 (up to 5–10 yr.) 100% Geographic and 75%*
   national coverage. Prevalence of heavy-intensity infection.
2. *Elimination of Schistosomiasis as a Public Health Problem Target: 2025 (up to*
   3–6 yr.) Prevalence of heavy-intensity infection.
3. *Elimination of Transmission Target: 2025 (up to 5 yr.) Reduction of incidence of*
   infection to zero.

The most recent assessment was made by Deol et al. (2019). Data from nine national schistosomiasis control programmes (in eight countries in sub-Saharan Africa and Yemen) were analyzed according to schistosome species, *Schistosoma mansoni* or *S. haematobium*.

These included a number of treatment rounds impacting the overall prevalence and the prevalence of heavy-intensity infection. Disease control and elimination were defined:

– Prevalence of heavy-intensity infection of less than 5% and the elimination target of less than 1% aggregated across sentinel sites.
– Heavy-intensity infection was defined as at least 400 eggs per gram of faeces for *S. mansoni* infection or as more than 50 eggs per 10 ml of urine for *S. haemato-bium* infection.

RESULTS: Except for one country programme (Niger), all achieved the disease-control target by two treatment rounds or less, earlier than projected, 5 to 10 years. The elimination target was reached only for *S. mansoni* infection (in Burkina Faso, Burundi, and Rwanda within three treatment rounds).

The study suggested the need to re-evaluate progress and treatment strategies in national schistosomiasis control programmes more frequently.

References

Agrawal MC, Rao VG (2011) Indian schistosomes: a need for further investigations. J Parasitol Res 2011:250868

Alemu M, Zigta E, Derbie A (2018) Under diagnosis of intestinal schistosomiasis in a referral hospital, North Ethiopia. BMC Res Notes 11:245

Braun L, Grimes JET, Templeton MR (2018) The effectiveness of water treatment processes against schistosome cercariae: a systematic review. PLoS Negl Trop Dis 12(4):e0006364

Chala B, Torben W (2018) An epidemiological trend of urogenital schistosomiasis in Ethiopia. Front Public Health 6:60

Deol AK, Fleming FM, Calvo-Urbano B, Walker M et al (2019) Schistosomiasis - assessing Progress toward the 2020 and 2025 global goals. N Engl J Med 381(26):2519–2528

Mohamed I, Kinung'hi S, PNM M, Onkanga IO et al (2018) Diet and hygiene practices influence morbidity in schoolchildren living in schistosomiasis endemic areas along Lake Victoria in Kenya and Tanzania-a cross sectional study. PLoS Negl Trop Dis 12(3):e0006373

Murinello A, Germano N, Mendonca P, Campos C, Gracio A (2006) Liver disease due to Schistosoma guineensis- a review. GE - J Port Gastrenterol 13:97–104

Okanla EO, Agba BN, Awotunde JO (2003) *Schistosoma haematobium*: prevalence and socioeconomic factors among students in Cape Coast Ghana. Afr J Biomed Res 6:69–72

Schadewaldt H (1962) Theodor BILHARZ (1825–1862), one of the founders of German tropical medicine research. Munchener Medizinische Wochenschrift 104:1730–1734

Sundaraneedi MK, Tedla BA, Eichenberger RM, Becker L et al (2017) Polypyridylruthenium (II) complexes exert anti-schistosome activity and inhibit parasite acetylcholinesterases. PLoS Negl Trop Dis 11(12):e0006134

Wei Y, Huang N, Chen S, Chen D, Li X, Xu J et al (2018) The diagnosis and treatment introspection of the first imported case of atypical cerebral schistosomiasis in Guangzhou city. PLoS Negl Trop Dis 12(3):e6171

WHO (2009) Elimination of schistosomiasis from low-transmission areas. Report of a WHO Informal Consultation. Salvador, Bahia, Brazil 18–19 August 2008 WHO_HTM_NTD-PCT_2009.2_eng.pdf

WHO (2013) Schistosomiasis. Fact sheet No115, updated March 2013. http://www.who.int/mediacentre/factsheets/fs115/en/

WHO (2020) Schistosomiasis. https://www.who.int/news-room/fact-sheets/detail/schistosomiasis

Chapter 95
Coenurosis

Coenurosis is a zoonotic cestode infection. It is a rare disease reported mainly in developing countries. It occurs in the sheep-raising areas of Europe, South Africa, South America, the USA, Canada, Russia, and Asian countries, including India (Varma and Malviya 1989). The larval stage, metacestode (coenurus), causes cerebral multilocular coenuri that are rarely intra-parenchymal. Mortality used to be high before the advent of modern neuroradiological techniques like computed tomography (CT) and magnetic resonance imaging (MRI) and surgery.

95.1 Aetiology

Taenia multiceps and *T. serialis*.

95.2 Life Cycle

The definitive hosts for *Taenia multiceps* and *T. serialis* are members of the family Canidae. Many canids (dogs, wolves, coyotes, and red and grey foxes) can serve as definitive hosts for *T. multiceps* but only dogs and foxes for *T. serialis*.

Many animals (rodents, rabbits, horses, cattle, sheep, and goats) may serve as intermediate hosts. Humans, like other intermediate hosts, become infected by ingesting eggs.

The tapeworm develops and resides in the small intestine. This sheds eggs or proglottids in faeces, which are available in the environment to infect intermediate hosts by ingestion. Eggs hatch in their intestine, and oncospheres migrate through circulation and lodge in suitable organs—skeletal muscles, subcutaneous tissues,

© Springer Nature Singapore Pte Ltd. 2024
K. G. Narayan et al., *Handbook of Management of Zoonoses*,
https://doi.org/10.1007/978-981-99-9885-2_95

eyes, and the brain. It takes about 3 months for metacestodes or coenuri to develop. Tissues containing coenuri infect definitive hosts upon ingestion.

Human beings are infected by the accidental ingestion of eggs on fomites or in contaminated food and water. The coenuri of *T. multiceps* usually are found in the brain and eyes (choroids, retina), causing cerebral coenurosis, while those of *T. serialis* are found in the subcutaneous tissue of infected human beings.

95.3   Symptoms

Most cases are detected in children, with an average age of 7.2 years (Khaldi et al. 2000). Three forms are described: (1) subcutaneous, (2) cerebral, and (3) ocular.

The skin and subcutaneous form present as painless nodules, similar to lymphomas, pseudotumors, and neurofibromas, seen commonly on the trunk, neck, shoulders, head and limbs, or sclera and subconjunctiva, causing difficulty in swallowing and movement of muscles. The cerebral form manifests as headache, vomition, fever, epileptic fits, hemiplegia, paraplegia, and localized neurological symptoms like nerve palsies, and intracranial arteritis with transient hemiparesis. Benfila et al. (2007) reported an unusual case of huge intraparenchymal cyst in the brain of a 4-year-old girl, successfully operated in Israel. Ocular infection may be intra and orbital. There is a varying degree of visual impairment. Uncared cases suffer from painful inflammation, glaucoma, and blindness.

Recently, Labuschagne et al. (2022) reported a case of disseminated subarachnoid coenurosis caused by *T. serialis* in South Africa, where a 5-year-old male patient had acute hydrocephalus with a 1-month history of intermittent vomiting, headaches, regression of milestones, and recent onset seizures. MRI revealed multiple cysts in the cerebrospinal fluid (CSF) spaces with a predominance of clumped grape-like cysts in the basal cisterns with resultant acute obstructive hydrocephalus. The child underwent an emergency ventriculoperitoneal (VP) shunt. A presumptive diagnosis of neurocysticercosis racemosus was made. Despite prolonged antihelminthic therapy, the child continued to deteriorate. This case involved a single parenchymal lesion in the occipital lobe, which recovered following complete surgical excision. It was confirmed to be *T. serialis* by mitochondrial gene sequencing.

95.4   Diagnosis

- CT scan.
- Biopsy or autopsy reveals coenuri.

95.5   Treatment

Surgical hydrostatic expulsion of the complete cyst without rupture is recommended. Praziquantel is effective.

95.6   Prevention

Maintaining pet dogs free from infection and not letting dogs move uncontrolled outside besides personal and environmental hygiene.

References

Benfila M, Barrelly R, Shelef I, El-on J, Cohen A, Cagnano E (2007) Huge hemispheric intra-parenchymal cyst caused by *Taenia multiceps* in a child- case report. J Neurosurg (6 Suppl Pediatr) 107:511–514

Khaldi M, Mohamed S, Kallel J, Khouja N (2000) Brain hydatidosis: report on 117 cases. Child Nerv Syst 16(10–11):765–769

Labuschagne J, Frean J, Parbhoo K, Mutyaba D, Pillay T, Boughan S, Nkala H (2022) Disseminated human subarachnoid Coenurosis. Trop Med and Infect Dis 7(12):405

Varma TK, Malviya HC (1989) Prevalence of coenuriosis in sheep, goat and pigs in Bareilly. Utar Pradesh J Vet Parasitol 3:69–71

Chapter 96
Taeniasis–Cysticercosis

Zoonotic tapeworms are *Taenia saginata*, *T. solium*, *T. multiceps*, and *T. serialis*, all species of *Echinococcus*, *Dipylidium caninum*, *Hymenolepis nana*, and *Spirometra* (sparganosis).

Taeniasis–cysticercosis is one of the 'neglected tropical zoonotic diseases (NTDs)', which are a diverse group of 20 conditions that are mainly prevalent in tropical areas and mostly affect impoverished communities and disproportionately affect women and children. These diseases cause devastating health, social, and economic consequences to more than one billion people (https://www.who.int/health-topics/neglected-tropical-diseases#tab=tab_1). Poor and marginalized farmers have taken to pig farming (it is low input but economically profitable) to meet the increasing demand for pork. However, they do not or cannot prioritize disease control. Despite global distribution, real prevalence in men and cattle is difficult to assess because of asymptomatic infection, imperfect diagnosis, and poor reporting.

Taeniasis is an obligatory cyclozoonosis.

96.1 Life Cycle (Fig. 96.1)

96.1.1 Taenia solium

The gravid segments or eggs of *T. solium* passed in the stool by infected human beings are ingested by scavenging pigs. The embryos or oncospheres are released in the intestine, penetrate the intestinal wall, reach the circulatory system, and are thus disseminated in different tissues and organs. It takes 9–10 weeks for the larvae to develop into *Cysticercus cellulosae*. These are located in the muscles, heart, and even brain. The body system of the definitive host, the human being, is required for development beyond this. The *Cysticercus cellulosae* in pork is ingested by man.

© Springer Nature Singapore Pte Ltd. 2024
K. G. Narayan et al., *Handbook of Management of Zoonoses*,
https://doi.org/10.1007/978-981-99-9885-2_96

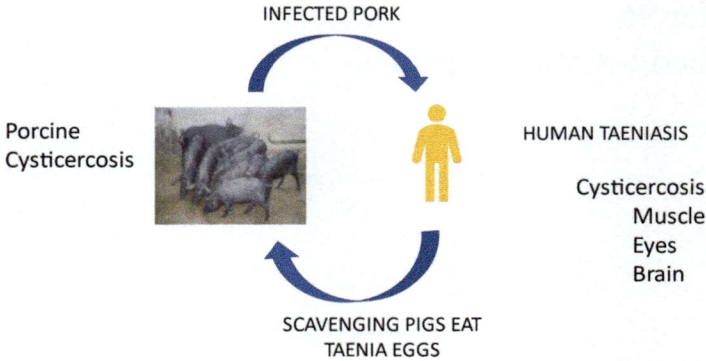

Fig. 96.1 Life cycle of *Taenia solium*

The larvae emerge in the human intestine. Through the evaginated scolex, the tapeworm attaches to the intestinal wall and grows into an adult tapeworm in 5–12 weeks. The gravid segments/eggs are passed out with stool to begin a fresh cycle.

Human beings also act as intermediate hosts for *T. solium*, and therefore, *C. cellulosae* also develops in them.

96.1.2   T. saginata

Events in the life cycle of *T. saginata* are similar to those of *T. solium*.

The gravid segments of *T. saginata* in the human intestine get detached one after the other and move to come out through the anus. Open defecation scatters these, and pasture is contaminated. The gravid segments disintegrate, and about 1 lakh eggs are scattered. Cattle get infected while grazing. The larvae, *Cysticercus bovis*, develop in the muscles. A man consuming such beef ingests the larvae and get infected. *T. saginata* develops in an infected human intestine in 10–12 weeks to begin the next cycle.

Man does not act as an intermediate host of *T. saginata*.

96.2   Mode of Infection

Taeniasis occurs after the ingestion of larvae, i.e. *Cysticercus bovis*/*C. cellulosae*. This may happen with the ingestion of under-processed, undercooked meat, sausage, or minced meat and the accidental ingestion of a ruptured cyst during meat cutting and handling in the kitchen.

The ingested larvae develop into adult tapeworms, about 3 m long. These shed eggs in faeces, which can in turn infect pigs and also the same or other human beings. The shortest route of infection is reverse peristalsis in a tapeworm carrier (auto-infection). Another and more common route is the ingestion of tapeworm eggs through contaminated food and water.

Taeniasis is mostly sub-clinical which is detected on faecal examination, may be for other parasites.

The ingested eggs of *T. solium* develop into larval worms, which migrate to different parts of the human and pig body and form cysts (cysticercosis). Pigs can harbour thousands of cysts, making the pork from these pigs unsafe to eat and often resulting in the total condemnation of the carcass. Depending upon the tissues of the infected human invaded and parasitized by *Cysticercus cellulosae*, manifestation varies. The brain is the principal site, hence neurocysticercosis, which is the most frequent preventable cause of epilepsy. Some 50 million people are affected, and 50,000 die in the world (World Health Organization 2009). The disease is chronic and may cause disability and even death.

Human infection presents two forms of illnesses: cysticercosis and taeniasis. Cysticercosis is caused by *C. cellulosae* only. Intestinal illness or taeniasis is caused by adult tapeworms of both species.

96.3   Symptoms

96.3.1   Taeniasis

The incubation period is 8–14 weeks. Most cases are sub-clinical, and there is hardly any indication. Detection is based on microscopic stool examination—may be examined for other intestinal parasites. Often, a single worm is present in the intestine, though there may be more, and infection may be caused by multiple parasites. There is a loss of body weight, debility, nausea, abdominal pain, anorexia, flatulence, diarrhoea, and constipation—which may be associated with nervousness and insomnia. One or more of these are seen in a patient. The disease may turn serious if mobile gravid segments of the parasites get lodged into unusual sites, such as the bile duct or appendix, and may cause ileus, cholecystitis, cholangitis, and pancreatitis. More females than males (2:1) are affected, possibly because of the nature of work and exposure in the kitchen.

96.3.2   Cysticercosis

The ingested eggs of *T. solium* hatch in the small intestine. Cysticerci develop in the subcutaneous tissues, striated muscles, heart, ear, eye, and central nervous system. Cysticercosis is more serious a disease than that caused by an adult tapeworm.

The incubation period may vary from a minimum of 15 days post-ingestion to years. The clinical forms recognized are as follows:

1. Myocysticercosis
2. Ocular cysticercosis
3. Neurocysticercosis

96.3.2.1 Myocysticercosis

The pathology is attributed to the pressure caused by the cyst in vital tissues and organs or inflammatory changes initiated by the degenerating larvae. Muscular cramps, pain, and fatigue are experienced. Accumulated fluid and subcutaneous large nodules can be palpated.

96.3.2.2 Ocular Cysticercosis

Cysticerci located in the vitreous humour and the anterior chamber of the eyes cause uveitis, iritis, retinitis, palpebral conjunctivitis, and affection of motor muscles.

96.3.2.3 Neurocysticercosis (NCC)

The World Health Organization (2022) reported *Taenia solium* as the cause of 30% of epilepsy cases, which may be as high as 70% in high-risk communities where people and pigs live in close proximity. In 2015, the WHO Foodborne Disease Burden Epidemiology Reference Group identified *T. solium* as a leading cause of death from food-borne diseases, resulting in a considerable total of 2.8 million disability-adjusted life years (DALYs). The total number of people suffering from NCC, including symptomatic and asymptomatic cases, is estimated to be between 2.56 and 8.30 million based on the range of data available on epilepsy prevalence (World Health Organization 2022).

In non-clinical and a large number of cases, *Cysticercus cellulosae* may be detected only at autopsy. The clinical manifestation of neurocysticercosis is pleomorphic. The determining factors are type, stage, location, and the number of lesions in the nervous system and also the hosts' age and response. The cysts are generally located in the meninges, cerebral cortex, and ventricles. The clinical manifestations are meningitis, epileptic encephalitis, epileptic attacks, focal deficit, intracranial hypertension, cognitive impairment, headache, ataxia, nausea, vomiting, and visual disturbances.

The association of neurocysticercosis with epileptic seizures was strongly evidenced by the use of computed tomography (CT) scan histopathology, serology, and nucleotide-based diagnostics. In a study of two villages in Guatemala,

Garcia-Noval et al. (1996) observed 2.8–2.9% epilepsy cases. Prasad et al. (2008b) reported that 26.3–53.8% of active epilepsy cases in the developing world, including India and Latin America, are due to NCC. Single to multiple punctuate calcified lesions, possibly calcified cysts or single hypo-densities of the size and shape of cysts suggestive of viable cysts were seen by CT scan. Brain tumours and haematological malignancies associated with neurocysticercosis (Herrera et al. 2000), a higher frequency of chromosomal aberration, and micronuclei in the peripheral blood lymphocytes of cysticercosis patients than in healthy and praziquantel-treated ones have been reported. Chronic inflammatory response to the cysticercus possibly caused damage to the deoxyribonucleic acid (DNA) in the surrounding cells.

96.4   Epidemiology

96.4.1   Taeniasis

The epidemiology and management of taeniasis caused by *T. solium* and *T. saginata* are similar. The differences lie in the species of intermediate hosts. Bovine is the intermediate host of *T. saginata* and porcine for *T. solium*. The larval stages are cysts—called *Cysticercus bovis* for *T. saginata* and *C. cellulosae* for *T. solium*. Infection in a 3-week calf is suggestive of antenatal infection. *C. bovis* survives for 9 months in live animals and 2 weeks in carcasses, whereas *C. cellulosae* survives for several years in pigs and over a month in carcasses. *T. solium* infection therefore is more persistent. This also enables the parasite to infect more people.

A *T. solium* carrier may carry the worm for years and thus constitutes a source of infection for long. Eggs in carriers' stool can survive long in the environment—2 months in summer and 5 months in winter in England and 1 year in the highlands of Kenya. *T. saginata* eggs remain viable for 6 months, 8 weeks on pasture, and 71 days in liquid manure, as observed in Kenya.

Open defecation is still observed in some settings. Untreated sewage is used for irrigation sometimes. The dispersal of eggs is possible with river water and irrigation channels. Short- to long-distance dispersal is possible through scavenging pigs, coprophagous beetles, and some birds like starlings and seagulls. *Taenia* eggs may get ingested with salads and other fresh eatables washed with contaminated water.

High prevalence is seen in rural settings and is frequently associated with poverty, illiteracy, poor personal and community hygiene, drainage, and unsanitized drinking water. *T. solium* infection should almost be absent among Moslems and Jews and, similarly, *T. saginata* infection among Hindus because of their respective religious precepts.

The natural transmission cycle of *T. saginata* is man–bovine–man and of *T. solium* is man–pig–man. Man–man transmission appears as an aberration. It is not in the interest of the parasite as it meets its dead end.

The cyst developing in human tissues does not find an opportunity to develop into an adult, except in the case of cannibalism—which is unlikely in humans.

Taeniasis occurs in India and has been reported in Tamil Nadu, West Bengal, Sikkim, Maharashtra, and other places (Narayan 2004). Prasad et al. (2007) reported an 18.6% prevalence of *T. solium*—taeniasis in the Mohanlalganj block of Lucknow, Uttar Pradesh, India, and the factors associated were age above 15 years, history of passage of taenia segments in the stool, consumption of undercooked pork, and poor hand hygiene. They cited earlier reports of 0.5–2% prevalence in hospitalized patients in northern India and 12–15% in labour colonies where pigs were raised.

Cysticercosis in swine in India is widely prevalent. The recent study in Mohanlalganj block, Lucknow, showed that 26% were positive for *C. cellulosae*, and 40% of these pigs had the cyst localized in the brain. Singh et al. (2018) found that out of 642 pigs reared in Punjab, nine had *T. solium* cysts (1.40% prevalence), while in 450 pigs imported from outside the state, 15 were positive (prevalence: 3.33%). A meta-analysis, spanning the period 2000–2019, on the prevalence of porcine cysticercosis in India showed a pooled prevalence of 5.21% (Bhangale 2021).

96.4.2   Cysticercosis

Taeniasis–cysticercosis is endemic in many developing countries. Developed countries no longer consider it 'exotic' because of increased immigration from endemic countries. Cysticercosis is uncommon, not reportable in the USA, and so true prevalence is not known. However, it is estimated that more than 1000 cases of cysticercosis are annually diagnosed in the United States alone (García et al. 2002). Immigrants from taeniasis-/cysticercosis-endemic countries, Americans travelling to endemic countries, and focal endemicity in the United States contribute.

DeGiorgio et al. (2005) documented the seroprevalence of *T. solium* cysticercosis and *T. solium* taeniasis in rural southern California to be 1.8% and 1.1%, respectively, after a serum-immunoblot test done on 449 farm workers and Hispanic residents in the region.

Sorvillo et al. (2007) used 'multiple cause-of-death' data to study cysticercosis-related deaths for the period 1990–2002. A total of 221 cysticercosis deaths were identified. Percent death according to race were 84.6 Latinos, 6.8 Whites, 5.9 Blacks, 2.3 Asians, and 0.5 in Native Americans. Sex and age distribution was 62% males and 38% females, with mean age at death 40.5 years (range 2–88 years, >60% in age <45 years). Higher rates among males and in the working age group may be related to travel—in search of jobs. Sixty-one per cent had <12 years of education. Most were born in foreign a country. Sixty-two per cent had emigrated from Mexico, and 77% of the Black and all of Asians were foreign born. The 33 Native American cases were distributed in 21 states—mostly in California (highest

57%, mostly Los Angeles County) and the southern states bordering Mexico. One death of a US-born person at least each year of the study was recorded. They had a higher level of education. Hydrocephalus (26.2%), cerebral oedema (10.4%), cerebral compression (7.2%), and epilepsy/convulsions (5.4%) were recorded as concurrent conditions contributing to death. These were significantly more common conditions among cysticercosis deaths than in matched controls.

Estimated global deaths due to cysticercosis were 700 in 1990 and 1200 in 2010 (Lozano et al. 2012). The ingestion of a large number of eggs by a human being may cause fatal acute infection with CNS pathology. In racemose cysticercosis, cysticerci grow and proliferate through tissues. Such cases have a poor prognosis.

Cysticercosis and taeniasis are widely prevalent in many Latin American countries. Garcia-Noval et al. (1996) studied prevalence. A faecal examination determined the prevalence of taeniasis in Mexico bordering Guatemala (0.3–3.1%), in Honduras on the east of Guatemala (0–6.2%), and in two villages of Guatemala (1 and 2.8%, respectively). Seroprevalence via the immunoblot method using metacestode glycoprotein detected 10 and 17%, respectively, in the two villages. However, tongue palpation revealed cysticercosis in 4 and 14% of pigs in the two villages. Autopsy studies conducted in Mexico have reported cysticercosis prevalence of 2.8–3.6%, and serosurveys have demonstrated infection rates of ≥20% in some areas of Peru, Guatemala, and Bolivia (Schantz et al. 1998).

The spatial distribution of porcine cysticercosis in 13 villages of the Sierra de Huautla in Central Mexico was studied on 562 pigs (Aug–Dec 2003). Pig tongue cysticercosis ranged between 0 and 33.3%, averaging 13.3%. GPS was applied to the plot distribution of cysticercotic pigs and risk factors in the villages. The distribution of healthy and cysticercotic pigs did not differ. The risk factors significantly associated were (a) free-roaming pigs, (b) the drinking of stagnant water, and (c) the absence of a latrine (Morales et al. 2008).

According to Rajshekhar et al. (2003), cysticercosis is widely prevalent in Asian countries, including India, China, Indonesia, Taiwan, Thailand, Korea, and Nepal. Neurocysticercosis has been known in Indonesia since the 1970s. Epileptic seizures in 11 districts were studied during 190–195 by histopathology and the DNA analysis of cysts (Wandra et al. 2000). There has been a rapid increase since the 1990s. Nearly 67% of epileptic seizures and 65% of subcutaneous nodule cases had highly specific antibodies to cysticercosis. Nearly half of the epilepsy cases in India are due to cysticercosis presenting as partial seizures. Cysticercosis-caused epilepsies are also prevalent in Bali (Indonesia), Vietnam, China, and Nepal. Seroprevalence ranges from 0.02 to 12.6% in several countries, indicating high rates of exposure. It was associated with unhealthy pig-rearing practices, poor sanitation, low hygienic standards, and unusual customs such as the consumption of raw pork in some countries.

Prasad et al. (2008a) have reviewed neurocysticercosis in general and its status in India in particular. Cysticercosis is mentioned in the ancient Indian medical book Charak Samhita. Early reports mention cysticerci in the muscles, heart, and brain at autopsy and epilepsy as being related to cysticercosis in the British army deployed in India. Neurocysticercosis caused 26.3–53.8% of active epilepsy cases in developing countries, including India and Latin America. An estimated 3/4 of the estimated 50 million active epilepsy cases live in poor countries in the world. The prevalence before and after the advent of diagnostic tools like CT scans and magnetic resonance imaging (MRI) was 2% in unselected series of epilepsy and 31% of CT-scanned patients at the National Institute of Mental Health and Neuro Science, Bangalore, India. A CT scanning survey in South India revealed 3.83/1000 active epilepsy, and of these, 28.4% were neurocysticercosis. Based on the information available, neurocysticercosis was more prevalent in the northern states of India, Bihar, and Uttar Pradesh through Panjab. In a study of the community in Mohanlalganj block, Lucknow (Prasad et al. 2007), active epilepsy was identified and clinically confirmed in 5.8%, and a door-to-door survey revealed that 48.3% met the definitive or probable diagnostic criteria of neurocysticercosis. In another study (Prasad et al. 2008a), families having no separate housing for pigs were identified as a risk factor for the clustering of neurocysticercosis as epilepsy cases were found clustered in such families.

Lescano et al. (2009) made interesting studies on the clustering of seroprevalent cases of cysticercosis surrounding current tapeworm carriers. In seven rural communities in Peru, 11 tapeworm carriers were identified by stool microscopy. Enzyme-linked immunoelectrotransfer blots (EITBs) were used on 803 persons living in a radius of 50 m from a tapeworm carrier. Those showing one or more positive bands were considered positive. They numbered 196, a prevalence of 24%, indicating the transmission of infection. Seroprevalence gradient from 21% (>50 m distance) increasing to 32% (1–50 m) was observed. Based on clinical, neuroimaging and serological diagnosis the cysticercosis related seizure prevalence was 3%. The seizures, however, did not cluster around the carriers, obviously as they developed later than the antibodies; i.e. seropositivity reflected recent infection. Thirty to fifty per cent of late-onset epileptic cases were cysticercosis in endemic countries.

96.5   Diagnosis

96.5.1   Taeniasis

- Examination of anal swab and human stool.
- Serological method—detection of coproantigen through a dipstick dot ELISA (Allan et al. 1993): purified glycoprotein antigen from *C. cellulosae* is run on SDS-PAGE and transferred onto the nitrocellulose membrane. Using human anti-serum, anti-human IgG-peroxidase conjugate, and 3,3′-diaminobenzedine substrate, one or more of the seven antigens are detected in a positive case. The advantage is that it detects even microscopically negative cases.

- Immunoblot method for the detection of serum antibody to *T. solium* metacestode glycoprotein antigen: in search for a suitable serodiagnostic antigen for the detection of antibody to *Cysticercus cellulosae* glycoprotein, cyst fluids from the two genotypes of *T. solium*, viz. African/American and Asian (division based on mitochondrial DNA), were purified and compared with those of the recombinant (chimeric) *T. solium* (Rec-Ag1V1/Ag2) proteins—Ag1V1/Ag2. The glycoproteins of the two genotypes differed in their immunoblot patterns. However, the antigens did not differ significantly in their sensitivity, as observed through an immunosorbent assay, indicating that Rec-Ag1V1/Ag2 can be used as an alternative antigen (Sato et al. 2006).
- Molecular method: according to Yamasaki et al. (2003), it is possible to identify and differentiate *Taenia* mitochondrial DNA in faecal samples from carriers through polymerase chain reaction (PCR). Excision sequence scanning thymine-base analysis is the molecular method for identifying human cestodes. There are four thymine-base peak profiles unique for Asian and American/African genotypes of *T. solium*, *T. saginata*, and *T. asiatica*, and differentiation even without DNA sequencing is possible.

96.5.2   Cysticercosis

The methods are as follows:

1. Clinical presentation.
2. Examination of biopsied tissue for cysts.
3. Radiography.
4. Computed axial tomography (CAT) scanning of the brain and muscles.
5. Magnetic resonance imaging (MRI) to detect small intra-parenchymal lesions missed on CAT scan.
6. The serodiagnostic tests used are indirect hemagglutination assay (IHA), complement-fixation test (CFT), and enzyme-linked immunosorbent assay (ELISA) to detect antibodies in the serum and antigen in cerebrospinal fluid.
7. *Taenia solium* cyst fluid antigen-based lymphocyte transformation test: Prasad et al. (2009) developed this test and observed a sensitivity of 93.7% (87.5% in cases of single cyst infection) and a specificity of 96.2%. It used radioactive thymidine but has the potential of modification using non-radioactive techniques like bromodeoxyuridine-ELISA LTT.
8. The Institute of Health Carlos III in Madrid has developed highly sensitive and specific PCR-based assays for diagnosing *T. solium* infections as well as identifying *T. solium* antigens of a diagnostic and protective potential.
9. Objective and holistic evaluation of observation and test results: Del Brutto et al. (2001) proposed the objective and holistic evaluation of clinical, imaging, immunological, and epidemiological data.

96.6 Treatment

Albendazole and praziquantel are the recommended anthelmintics.

García et al. (2002)) presented the following treatment guidelines for neurocysticercosis. There appears to be no generalized principle for treatment. Each case has to be assessed individually. The factors to be considered are (a) types—parenchymal or extra-parenchymal (ventricular/subarchanoid/spinal/ophthalmic), (b) the status of the larvae—live or degenerating or calcified cysts, (c) infection burden—mild, moderate, or heavy.

The approaches to the treatment of neurocysticercosis may be (a) anti-parasitic drugs, (b) surgery, and (c) symptomatic treatment and the use of anti-inflammatory drugs.

Although anti-parasitic therapy may not be equivocally accepted, it is advantageous. One undisputed advantage is the ultimate reduction of incidence. Drugs killing adult tapeworms and/or larvae reduce worm burden. The number of severe cases is reduced. There are fewer seizures and fewer cases of residual calcification. The latter two require more authentication. Anti-parasitic therapy kills the larvae. The death of the larvae results in temporary inflammation. A non-symptomatic case may manifest symptoms, or there may be an exacerbation of symptoms on the second and fifth days (short, severe, and acute) of the start of therapy due to the death of the larvae and consequential inflammation. A combination of albendazole–praziquantel–steroids is suitable in such a situation.

Symptomatic and anti-inflammatory treatment is another approach. Anti-parasitic drugs do not have any role in cases with calcified lesions.

Prior to the advent of anti-parasitic drugs, open surgery was used for the excision of large cysts or ventricular cysts. Hydrocephalus secondary to neurocysticercosis or intracranial hypertension required aggressive management. The placement of ventricular shunts is required. Shunt blockage and dysfunction are common. These require multiple surgical shunt revisions. The combination of anti-parasitic drugs and surgery reduces shunt failure. Neuroendoscopic resection for ventricular cysts is less invasive and promising.

96.7 Prevention and Control

Taeniasis–cysticercosis has been identified as one of six potentially eradicable diseases. Powerful and inexpensive control tools are currently available. Well-developed implementation strategies are feasible. Preventive chemotherapy makes control and prevention and also elimination possible. The reduction of infection rates in the human carriers of adult tapeworms is ultimately the best way to reduce environmental contamination.

Intercepting the transmission of *T. solium* is required to control it. Transmission is known to be associated with poverty, the lack of sanitary services, and practices of rearing backyard pigs with free access to the areas that villagers use as toilets, as well as cultural behaviour. Add to these the increase of migration and tourism, leading to the emergence of cysticercosis in industrial countries also.

96.7.1 The Basic Methods

(a) Detection and anthelmintic treatment of the human carriers of *T. solium*, supplemented with public health education; personal hygiene, like washing hands after ablution and before eating; kitchen hygiene; the stoppage of defecation in the open; and sewage treatment.
(b) Measures to control/eliminate the larval stage of the worm (cysticerci)—such as detection by palpation of the tongue of live pigs (25–70% sensitivity, 100% specificity)
(c) Rigorous post-mortem examination and carcass inspection—total condemnation or freezing at −6.5 °C for 3 weeks or -10 °C for 2 weeks or thorough cooking of the pork.
(d) Stopping scavenging by pigs.

Taeniasis/cysticercosis has focal prevalence (high prevalence in one location but sparse in the neighbourhood)—spatial distribution is difficult to understand and assess.

Target groups for mass treatment should be identified; these may be pork eaters, slaughter men, pig farmers (pig–human transmission), and immigrants from taeniasis-/cysticercosis-endemic areas.

96.7.2 Preventive Chemotherapy

Preventive chemotherapy of carriers (Taeniasis and non-symptomatic cysticercosis) should be tried. Mass chemotherapy of the human population to remove the carriers of *T. solium* may not be adequate to control the source of infection—cysticercosis in pigs and human beings—because of increased human mobility and immigration.

96.7.3 Vaccination

The simultaneous vaccination of all pigs at risk may lead to eradication (Lightowlers 1999). Flisser et al. (2004) observed that *Taenia solium* oncosphere antigens, TSOL18 and TSOL45-1A, induced very high levels of protection (up to 100%) in three independent vaccine trials in pigs against experimental challenge infection with *T. solium* eggs, which were undertaken in Mexico and Cameroon. The TSOL18/ TSOL45 vaccine has the potential to control and eradicate human neurocysticercosis (Lightowlers 2004). A study by Kyngdon et al. (2006) found complement fixing antibodies in serum of pigs immunized with TSOL18 and TSOL451A recombinant vaccine against *T. solium* cysticercosis, which are believed to induce protection.

Of the oncospheral-stage-specific 45W proteins, a recombinant 45W-4B protein was used for vaccination. Two animal trials showed a significant reduction in parasite burden (Luo et al. 2009). Wu et al. (2005) observed 83% protection in pigs challenged after 2 weeks of vaccination with DNA vaccine pVAX-S-deltaC-3n. This vaccine is a construct of deltaC-3n, a polymer peptide, and the signal peptide sequence of IL-2 cloned in a vector pVAX3.0. The deltaC-3n protein was expressed by hepatitis virus HBc149 after epitopes KETc1, KETc12, and GK-1 (three promising vaccine candidates for *Taenia solium* cysticercosis) had been introduced into its immunodominant loop.

96.8   International Concern

International agencies and institutions, such as the World Health Organization, the Food and Agriculture Organization, and the International Livestock Research Institute, are concerned and involved. The WHO Global Plan to combat 'Neglected Tropical Diseases (NTDs) 2008–2015' and recommendations of the Second International Meeting on the Integrated Control of Neglected Zoonoses in Africa, Nairobi, Kenya, 13–15 Nov, 2007 (World Health Organization 2007), include this disease. WHO is organizing a global campaign for combating cysticercosis. The inaugural meeting of the cysticercosis working group in Europe (Willingham 3rd et al. 2008) is an effort in this direction. It has social, economic, and trade impacts.

References

Allan JC, Mencos F, Garcia-Noval J, Sarti E, Flisser A et al (1993) Dipstick Dot ELISA for detection of coproantigens in human. Parasitology 107:79–85

Bhangale G (2021) Prevalence of porcine cysticercosis in India: a meta-analysis. Res Square. https://doi.org/10.21203/rs.3.rs-565544/v1

DeGiorgio C, Pietsch-Escueta S, Tsang V, Corral-Leyva G, Ng L et al (2005) Seroprevalence of *Taenia solium* cysticercosis and *Taenia solium* taeniasis in California, USA. Acta Neurol Scand 111:84–88

Del Brutto OH, Rajshekhar V, White AC Jr, Tsang VC, Nash TE et al (2001) Proposed diagnostic criteria for neurocysticercosis. Neurology 57:177–183

Flisser A, Gauci CG, Zoli A, Martinez-Ocaña J, Garza-Rodriguez A et al (2004) Induction of protection against porcine cysticercosis by vaccination with recombinant oncosphere antigens. Infect Immun 72(9):5292–5297

García HH, Evans CA, Nash TE, Takayanagui OM, White AC Jr et al (2002) Current consensus guidelines for treatment of neurocysticercosis. Clin Microbiol Rev 15(4):747–756

Garcia-Noval J, Allan JC, Fletes C, Morena E, DeMata F et al (1996) Epidemiology of *Taenia solium* taeniasis and cysticercosis in two rural Guatemalan communities. Am J Trop Med Hyg 55:282–289

Herrera LA, Ramirez T, Rodriguez U, Corona T, Sotelo J et al (2000) Possible association between *T. solium* cysticercosis and cancer: increased frequency of DNA damage in peripheral lymphocytes from neurocysticercosis patients. Trans R Soc Trop Med Hyg 94:61–65

Kyngdon CT, Gauci CG, Gonzalez AE, Flisser A, Zoli A et al (2006) Antibody responses and epitope specificities to the *Taenia solium* cysticercosis vaccines TSOL18 and TSOL45-1A. Parasite Immunol 28(5):191–199

Lescano AG, Garcia HH, Gilman RH, Gavidia CM, Tsang VC, Cysticercosis Working Group in Peru et al (2009) *Taenia solium* cysticercosis hotspots surrounding tapeworm carriers: clustering on human seroprevalence but not on seizures. PLoS Negl Trop Dis 3(1):e371

Lightowlers MW (1999) Eradication of *Taenia solium* cysticercosis: a role for vaccination of pigs. Int J Parasitol 29(6):811–817

Lightowlers MW (2004) Vaccination for the prevention of cysticercosis. Dev Biol (Basel) 119:361–368

Lozano R, Naghavi M, Foreman K, Lim S, Shibuya K, The Working Group (2012) Global and regional mortality from 235 causes of death for 20 age groups in 1990 and 2010: a systematic analysis for the Global Burden of Disease Study 2010. Lancet 380(9859):2095–2128

Luo X, Zheng Y, Hou J, Zhang S, Cai X (2009) Protection against Asiatic *Taenia solium* induced by a recombinant 45W-4B protein. Clin Vaccine Immunol 16(2):230–232

Morales J, Martínez JJ, Rosetti M, Fleury A, Maza V et al (2008) Facultad de MedicinaVeterinaria y Zootecnia, Universidad Nacional Autónoma de México, Ciudad d. PLoS Negl Trop Dis 2(9):e284

Narayan KG (2004) Epidemiology, diagnosis and management of zoonoses. ICAR, New Delhi

Prasad KN, Prasad A, Gupta RK, Pandey CM, Uttam S (2007) Prevalence and associated risk factors of *T. solium* taeniasis in a rural pig farming community of North India. Trans R Soc Trop Med Hyg 101:1241–1247

Prasad KN, Prasad A, Verma A, Singh AK (2008a) Human cysticercosis and Indian scenario: a review. J Biosci 33(4):571–582

Prasad A, Prasad KN, Yadav A, Gupta RK, Pradhan S et al (2008b) Lymphocyte transformation test: a new method for diagnosis of neurocysticerosis. Diagn Microbiol Infect Dis 61:198–202

Prasad KN, Prasad A, Gupta RK, Nath K, Pradhan S et al (2009) Neurocysticercosis in patients with active epilepsy from the pig farming community of Lucknow district, North India. Trans R Soc Trop Med Hyg 103(2):144–150

Rajshekhar V, Joshi DD, Doanh NQ, van De N, Xiaonong Z (2003) *Taenia solium* taeniosis/cysticercosis in Asia: epidemiology, impact and issues. Acta Trop 87(1):53–60

Sato MO, Sako Y, Nakao M, Yamasaki H, Nakaya K et al (2006) Evaluation of purified *Taenia solium* glycoproteins and recombinant antigens in the serologic detection of human and swine cysticercosis. J Infect Dis 194:1783–1790

Schantz PM, Wikins PP, Tsang VCW (1998) Immigrants, imaging, and immunoblots: the emergence of neurocysticercosis as a significant public health problem. In: Scheld WM, Craig WA, Hughes JM (eds) Emerging infections. ASM Press, Washington, DC, pp 213–242

Singh SP, Singh BB, Kalambhe DG, Pathak D et al (2018) Prevalence and distribution of *Taenia solium* cysticercosis in naturally infected pigs in Punjab, India. PLoS Negl Trop Dis 12(11):e0006960

Sorvillo FJ, DeGiorgio C, Waterman SH (2007) Deaths from cysticercosis, United States. Emerg Infect Dis 13(2):230–235

Wandra T, Subahar R, Simanjuntak GM et al (2000) Resurgence of cases of epileptic seizures and burns associated with cysticercosis in Assologaima, Jayawijaya, Irian Jaya, Indonesia, 1991–95. Trans R Soc Trop Med Hyg 94:46–50

World Health Organization (2007) 2nd International meeting on the integrated control of neglected Zoonoses in Africa, Nairobi, Kenya 13–15 Nov, 2007

World Health Organization (2022) Taeniasis/cysticercosis. https://www.who.int/news-room/fact-sheets/detail/taeniasis-cysticercosis

Papers Recommended for Reading

Willingham AL 3rd, Harrison LJ, Fèvre EM, Parkhouse ME, Cysticercosis Working Group in
   Europe (2008) Inaugural meeting of the cysticercosis Working Group in Europe. Emerg Infect
   Dis 14(12):e2
World Health Organization (2009) Seven neglected endemic zoonoses—some basic facts
Wu L, Diao Z, Deng X, Gao J, Zhou Z, Liu Y, Wang Y (2005) DNA vaccine against *Taenia solium*
   cysticercosis expressed as a modified hepatitis B virus core particle containing three epitopes
   shared by *Taenia crassiceps* and *Taenia solium*. J Nanosci Nanotechnol 5(8):1204–1210
Yamasaki H, Sato MO, Sako Y, Nakao M, Nakaya K et al (2003) Cysticercosis/taeniasis: recent
   advances in serological and molecular diagnoses. Southeast Asian J Trop Med Public Health
   34(Suppl 2):98–102

Chapter 97
Diphyllobothriasis

According to Cong and Elsheikha (2021), diphyllobothriidean tapeworms are one of the four important fish-borne parasitic zoonoses. Others are anisakid, intestinal heterophyid, and opisthorchid. Fish is a major source of protein in Asia. Raw, mildly cooked, and other unheated preparations are liked by certain communities. Raw or minimally cooked fish preparations, such as sashimi, sushi, ceviche, carpaccio, and fish tartare, are considered delicacies, which are served in Korean restaurants and have entered Western countries. Fish trade requires transportation of intact fish, i.e., fish without evisceration on ice. Parasites thus enter regions otherwise free from these. The liking for exotic fish and travel contributes to the distribution of fish-borne parasites.

The plerocercoid larvae of diphylobothria in fish is minced and infect the consumer. Diphyllobothriasis (*D. latum*/*D. latus*) and dicrocoeliasis (*Dicrocoelium dendriticum*, *D. hospes*, and *D. chinensis*) are food-borne zoonoses responsible for an estimated 20 million human infections worldwide (Shamsi et al. 2020) and are the most frequent fish-borne zoonosis in Europe (Králová-Hromadová et al. 2021). They impact the fish trade.

The most important foci of diphyllobothriosis have been Fennoscandia, the Baltic region, France, Scandinavia, Switzerland, the Alpine Lakes region, the Danube River region, and several endemic regions of Russia in Europe and North America. Clinical cases have been reported also in Asian countries, like Japan and South Korea, and in South America, such as Brazil, Chile, and Peru.

According to Králová-Hromadová et al. (2021), the prevalence of the broad fish tapeworm is either nil or low in Fennoscandia and the Baltic and Danube regions but circulates in the natural environment and in humans in the Alpine Lakes region.

Table 97.1 Some species of *Diphylobothrium* and distribution

Species	Country/region
D. latum and *D. pacificum*	*Chile, Peru, Argentina*
D. latum	India, China, Malaysia, Taiwan
D. dentriticum	Europe, Asia, Iran, northern Africa, and North America
D. hospes	Sub-Sahara and West Africa
D. chinensis	Eastern Asia and Europe
D. nihonkaiense	*Japan, Republic of Korea*
D. klebanovskii	Russia

97.1 Aetiology

Fourteen of 50 species of *Diphylobothrium* infect humans. The disease is mild and not reportable; some are listed in Table 97.1.

The consumption of raw, marinated, smoked, or inadequately cooked fish products caused infection.

97.2 Life Cycle

Diphyllobothrium latum is a human tapeworm also known as broad fish tapeworm. It infects non-human fish-eating mammals like canids, felines (carnivores), bears, and birds. It is an example of zooanthroponoses and also metazoonoses, and this offers two details—(a) the definitive host is man, and (b) the parasite has to pass through non-vertebrate hosts (for development).

It takes about 4–6 weeks from the infection of a man to the appearance of eggs of *D. latum* in his faeces (range: 2 weeks to 2 years). Once infected, the tapeworm can live for 20 years; i.e. man is infective for these long years.

D. latum reproduces in human intestines. Immature eggs are passed in the stool. Freshwater crustaceans, like copepods, are the first intermediate hosts. These ingest eggs. Coracidia develop into procercoid larvae. Small freshwater fish, like a minnow, is the second intermediate host, which eats the infected copepod. The procercoid larvae from the copepod migrate to the flesh of the fish. They develop into plerocercoid larvae (spargana), the infective stage larvae, capable of infecting definitive hosts.

Large predator/paratenic fish, like salmon, trout, pike, and perch, may eat the minnow and similar small freshwater fish, which are generally not eaten by man and, that too uncooked. The definitive hosts, mammals eating these infected predator fish, raw or undercooked (not likely by man), ingest the infective stage larvae,

ZOOANTHROPONOSES, METAZOONOSES
– e.g. *D. latum*

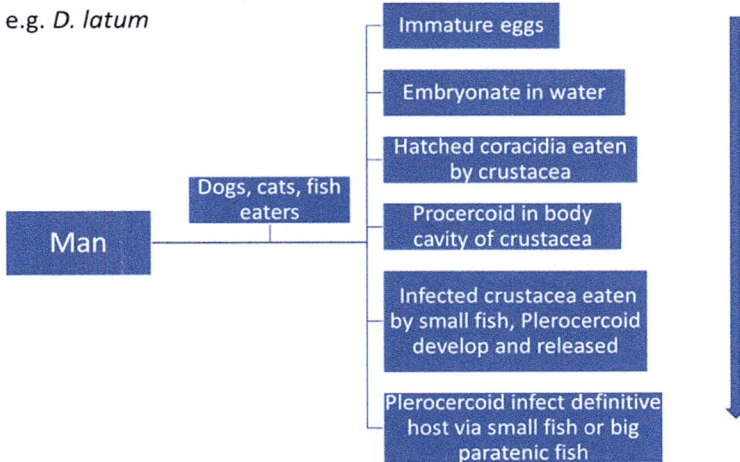

Fig. 97.1 Life cycle of *Diphylobothrium* spp.

plerocercoids, and get infected. Adult *D. latum* develops and resides in the small intestine (ileum), attached to the mucosa. The adult worm may be as long as 30 ft.— probably the longest parasite. The proglottid segments regularly detach from the main body of the worm and release immature eggs as many as 1.0 million per day per worm. The eggs in faeces discarded in fresh water begin the life cycle (Fig. 97.1).

97.3 Symptoms

Tapeworms of *Diphylobothriidium* spp. affect the small intestine, and some segments may be seen in the upper part of the colon. The incubation period (following the ingestion of infected fish) is about 3 weeks. Mild bowel symptoms include fatigue, myalgia, anorexia, fever, anxiety, depression, intermittent pain, abdominal distension, dyspepsia, indigestion, vomiting, and diarrhoea.

   D. latum appears to be a real parasite causing minimal harm to the host. It causes vitamin B12 deficiency and megaloblastic anaemia through parasite-mediated dissociation of the vitamin-B12-intrinsic factor complex within the gut lumen, making B12 unavailable to the host. Approximately 80% of the B12 intake is absorbed by the worm, with a differential absorption rate of 100:1 in relation to absorption by the host. Nearly 2% of the acutely infected show clinical anaemia, which is hyperchromic and macrocytic and may be associated with low platelets or low white blood cell counts. For the chronically infected, about 40% may show only low levels of B12. The deficiency may damage the central nervous system (CNS), e.g. peripheral neuropathy and/or CNS degenerative lesions.

97.3.1   Outbreak

Jackson et al. (2007) reported an outbreak affecting members of a wedding party in Switzerland. Perch fillets harvested from Lake Geneva the same day were marinated. Seven out of the 26 who ate raw marinated perch were confirmed, and there was one probable case (30.8% attack rate). The median age of the cases was 34 years (range: 24–60 years), which were more likely females. The stool of the seven participants who ate (raw fish preparation) tested positive for characteristic eggs or proglottids of *D. latum*. Most (75%) reported symptoms 20–91 (median 56) days after the wedding. Symptoms included diarrhoea, fatigue, abdominal pain, nausea, loss of weight, vomiting, or dizziness.

97.4   Diagnosis

- *Proglottids appear in the faeces*; faecal examination shows eggs that are ovoid with an operculum on a narrowed pole.
- Molecular methods are available in research labs only.
- *Colonoscopy shows motile creamy-white proglottids in the sigmoid colon.*

97.5   Treatment

A single dose of praziquantel 10 mg/kg body weight is effective.

97.6   Prevention

The inactivation of larvae (plerocercoids) requires cooking fish at 55 °C for at least 5 min or freezing it at −18 to −20 °C for at least 24 h before consumption.

References

Cong W, Elsheikha HM (2021) Biology, epidemiology, clinical features, diagnosis, and treatment of selected fish-borne parasitic zoonoses. Yale J Biol Med 94:297–309

Jackson Y, Pastore R, Sudre P, Loutan L, Chappuis F (2007) *Diphyllobothrium latum* outbreak from marinated raw perch, Lake Geneva, Switzerland. Emerg Infect Dis 13(12):1957–1958

Králová-Hromadová I, Radačovská A, Čisovská Bazsalovicsová E, Kuchta R (2021) Ups and downs of infections with the broad fish tapeworm *Dibothriocephalus latus* in Europe from 1900 to 2020: Part I. Adv Parasitol 114:75–166

Shamsi L, Samaeinasab S, Samani ST (2020) Prevalence of hydatid cyst, *Fasciola* spp. and *Dicrocoelium dendriticum* in cattle and sheep slaughtered in Sabzevar abattoir. Iran Ann Parasitol 66(2):211–216

Chapter 98
Dipylidium caninum

Synonyms

Dog tapeworm, Cucumber tapeworm, Flea tapeworm, Double-pored tapeworm.

98.1 Aetiology

Dipylidium caninum belongs to class Cestoda, order Cyclophyllidea. It is a common dog and cat tapeworm and also infects human beings, especially toddlers and children, through the ingestion of an infected flea. Natural infection occurs in members of the dog and cat families, occasionally in wild animals like fox, jaguar, wildcat, hyena, dingo, and others acting as reservoirs. Infection is commonly without any symptoms. *Ctenocephalides canis*, *C. felis*, and dog louse *Trichodectes canis* and human flea *Pulex irritans* act as intermediate hosts. Dogs and cats get infected by biting and eating infected fleas.

Climate change affects the prevalence and endemicity of the intermediate hosts. Additionally, increased urbanization, coupled with an increased number of pets per family, leading to more closeness with their owners, especially toddlers and children due to their playing habits and proximity with dogs and cats, causes a high prevalence of diseases like dipylidiasis (Dantas-Torres and Otranto 2014; Rust 2017; Abdullah et al. 2019). Infection is common in dogs as stray dogs' population is high. Parasite load is high in dogs over 1 year old. Cats have a lower parasite load. Adult worms live for 1 year.

© Springer Nature Singapore Pte Ltd. 2024
K. G. Narayan et al., *Handbook of Management of Zoonoses*,
https://doi.org/10.1007/978-981-99-9885-2_98

98.2   Geographical Distribution

Dipylidium caninum is ubiquitous, being reported from every continent. The prevalence of canine dipylidiasis varies from country to country; viz., in Mexico, the prevalence is up to 60%; in Chile, 2–54%; in Kenya, 45%; in Jordan, 20%; in Brazil, 1–15%; in Spain and Uruguay, around 13%; in the UK, 9%; and in Germany, only 1% (García-Agudo et al. 2014).

Human infections, like 'diplydiasis,' though rare have been reported in Europe, the Philippines, China, Japan, Argentina, India, Spain, and the United States (Narsimham et al. 2013; Jiang et al. 2017).

98.3   Mode of Infection

Faecal-oral transmission is common, more specifically the ingestion of vectors. The cysticercoid (infective larva) sticks to the teeth of dogs and cats; therefore, the saliva is contaminated. Infection among toddlers may be through contact and the caressing of pets or if their food gets contaminated.

98.4   Life Cycle

The definite hosts (dogs, cats) pass gravid proglottids containing egg packets in the faeces (Fig. 98.1). The larvae of dog or cat fleas, *Ctenocephalides*, ingest these egg packets. The oncospheres hatch from the eggs within them, penetrate the intestine, reach the haemocoel, and develop into cysticercoids. The larvae of the fleas

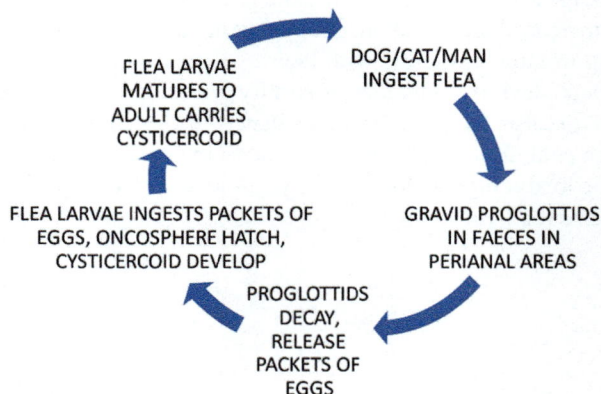

Fig. 98.1 Life-cycle of *Dipylidium caninum*

continue to grow to adulthood with cysticercoids in them. Dogs and cats eating such fleas get infected, and adult tapeworms develop in the small intestine after about a month. The dog louse *Trichodectes canis* may be an occasional intermediate host. Canids and felids are natural hosts; man is incidental.

98.5   Clinical Features

The incubation period is about 20 days. Infection may be asymptomatic. The clinical manifestations are abdominal pain, mild diarrhoea, anorexia, restlessness, constipation, and anal pruritis. In infants, parents may, with astonishment, observe small, white, rice-like bodies in the stool. These are proglottids and contain egg packets. The proglottids can crawl from the anus to the exterior of the host, where they contract and expand vigorously—this may be a process to release the egg packets. Proglottids may be found in the perianal region, diapers, and occasionally on the floor and carpet and furniture.

98.6   Diagnosis

Watching pets' behaviour may be helpful in arriving at a diagnosis, as well as taking pre-emptive precautionary measures. To relieve anal pruritis, pets scrape their anal region across grasses or carpets. Proglottids are motile when freshly laid and may be mistaken for maggots or fly larvae.

   A macroscopic examination of the stool is recommended for the presence of rice-like bodies. Stool specimens on several different days may be necessary for the detection of the packets of eggs in proglottids. Egg-cluster in packets is typical of dipylidiasis and diagnostic. The treatment of *Enterobius vermicularis* (confounding infection) will not eliminate *D. caninum*.

98.7   Treatment

Praziquantel is the drug of choice.

98.8   Prevention

It requires a regular examination of the pet dogs and cats, as well as treatment, to keep them free from *Dipylidium* infection.

98.9 Case Reports

Case Report 1

Narsimham et al. (2013) reported a case in a 4-year-old boy from Odisha. For 6 months, the boy complained of anal itching, and there was a passage of small structures resembling rice grains in the stool and recurrent abdominal pain. The mother had a history of handling pet cats and street dogs. The authors opined that diagnosis was difficult. A precise history of the case and caretaker of the child is important. Clinical diagnosis must be supported by a laboratory diagnosis of the stool, lest error is likely, such as misdiagnosis as threadworm (*Enterobius vermicularis*).

In another case, the mother of a 17-month-old boy observed for over a month small, white, active worms in her son's faeces. The son had mild diarrhoea. The authors observed three tapeworms looking like cucumber seeds in the stool. A laboratory examination identified the worm as *D. caninum*. The boy was successfully treated with praziquantel. The family had a pet dog for years. The infected pets should also be treated.

Case Report 2

A Spanish girl of 9 months contracted a *D. caninum* infection, possibly from her pet dog while playing with it. The mother reported that small worms, about 1 cm long, ivory white, and with rice-like structure, were observed in her daughter's stool on three different occasions for over-a-month period. The stool sample showed six proglottids; each segment was about 8–9 mm long and 2–3 mm thick (Fig. 85.3). The dog too was found infected (García-Agudo et al. 2014).

References

Abdullah S, Helps C, Tasker S, Newbury H, Wall R (2019) Pathogens in fleas collected from cats and dogs: distribution and prevalence in the UK. Parasit Vectors 12:71

Dantas-Torres F, Otranto D (2014) Dogs, cats, parasites, and humans in Brazil: opening the black box. Parasit Vectors 1:22

García-Agudo L, García-Martos P, Rodríguez-Iglesias M (2014) *Dipylidium caninum* infection in an infant: a rare case report and literature review. Asian Pac J Trop Biomed 4(2):S565–S567

Jiang P, Xi Z, Liu RD, Wang ZQ, Cui J (2017) A human case of zoonotic dog tapeworm, *Dipylidium caninum* (Eucestoda: Dilepidiidae), in China. Korean J Parasitol 55(1):61–64

Narsimham MV, Panda P, Mohanty I, Sahu S, Padhi S, Dash M (2013) *Dipylidium caninum* infection in a child: a rare case report. Indian J Med Microbiol 31:82–84

Rust MK (2017) The biology and ecology of cat fleas and advancements in their pest management: a review. Insects 8:118

Chapter 99
Hydatidosis

Synonyms

Human echinococcosis, Hydatidosis, Hydatid disease.

Geographical Distribution

Human echinococcosis is a zoonotic disease. The 2015 WHO Foodborne Disease Burden Epidemiology Reference Group (FERG) estimated echinococcosis to be the cause of 19,300 deaths and around 871,000 disability-adjusted life years (DALYs) globally each year. The World Health Organization (2020) estimates over one million affected at any one time. The incidence rate can reach more than 50 per 100,000 person-years in endemic regions, and prevalence levels as high as 5–10% may occur in parts of Argentina, Peru, East Africa, Central Asia, and China. The cystic echinococcosis cost/year was estimated at US$3.0 billion—the cost of treatment of cases + loss to the livestock industry. On average, there were 2.2% post-operative deaths and 6.5% relapses after intervention for cystic echinococcosis.

The prevalence of cystic echinococcosis in livestock detected in slaughterhouses in hyper-endemic areas of South America varies from 20 to 95% of slaughtered animals. It is the highest in rural areas where older animals are slaughtered. The condemnation of organs, commonly the liver; a reduction in carcass weight; a decrease in hide value; a decrease in milk production; and reduced fertility contribute to economic loss, the value of which will vary with the species of animals.

Hydatidosis in man is emerging or re-emerging cyclozoonosis caused by the larval stages (metacestodes) of *Echinococcus granulosus*, *E. multilocularis*, *E. oligarthus*, and *E. vogeli* after accidental ingestion of their eggs through close contact with untreated infected dogs, drinking contaminated water, and eating raw or uncooked contaminated food.

© Springer Nature Singapore Pte Ltd. 2024
K. G. Narayan et al., *Handbook of Management of Zoonoses*,
https://doi.org/10.1007/978-981-99-9885-2_99

99.1   Forms of Human Hydatidosis

There are three forms, manifesting a wide range of symptoms and also death (Table 99.1).

Of these, CHD (also called cystic echinococcosis or CE) and AHD (also called alveolar echinococcosis or AE) are common. The two differ in morphology, pathology, clinical manifestations, and epidemiology.

Table 99.1   Three forms of human hydatidosis (hydatid disease)

Agent	Disease	Characteristics pathology	Distribution
Echinococcus granulosus	Cystic hydatid disease (CHD), cystic echinococcosis (CE)	Unilocular cysts; enlarging cysts in the liver, lungs, and other organs Rupture leads to urticaria, anaphylactic shock, and further dissemination	Widespread, globally common, except Antarctica
E. multilocularis, small fox tapeworm	Other names of Alveolar Hydatid Disease are - Alveolar echinococcosis, Alveolar colloid of the liver, Alveolococcosis, Multilocular echinococcosis	Multilocular cysts and alveolar colloids of the liver; the larvae remain in the proliferative stage indefinitely in the liver, leading to invasion of the surrounding tissues	China, the Russian Federation, and countries in continental Europe and North America (rarely diagnosed, not as widespread; serious, high fatality rate; the potential of an emerging disease in many countries in the north hemisphere)
E. vogeli, E. oligarthrus	Polycystic hydatid disease (PHD), neotropical echinococcosis *E. oligarthrus* causes unicysts (World Health Organization 2020)	Polycystic; the larval stage (in the liver, lungs, and other organs) develops both externally and internally, resulting in multiple vesicles—a slow-growing tumour	Rare, relatively new
E. shiquicus	Unilocular minicyst hydatid disease	Zoonotic transmission is unknown	Tibetan plateau, China
E. felidis[a]	Unilocular cysts		Africa

[a]The public health impact may be minimal. Most of the exposed are pastoralists in East Africa as they are synanthropos with wildlife; human activity is minimal in national parks and game reserves where lions are kept

99.1.1   Cystic Echinococcosis

Cystic echinococcosis (CE) is a serious public health problem, persistent in one location, emerging and re-emerging at another. It may be a silent infection in some and a serious and disabling disease in others and may even be reoccurring after treatment. It is highly prevalent in many developing countries, especially in poor communities.

CE probably accounts for more than 95% of the estimated three million global cases, with human AE causing only 0.3–0.5 million cases (Zhang et al. 2008).

In humans, the incidence of surgical cases ranges from 0.1 to 45 cases per 100,000, and the real prevalence ranges between 0.22 and 24% in endemic areas (World Health Organization 2006). The cysts (or metacestodes) are unilocular and expansile and have an inner germinal layer (endocysts) and an outer acellular laminated layer (parasite-derived ectocyst or exocyst). A pericyst is an outer fibrous capsule made by the host's response. This contains blood vessels that provide nutrients to the parasite. Endoproliferation or internal budding produces scolices, brood capsules, and daughter cysts from the germinal layer.

99.1.2   Alveolar Echinococcosis

Alveolar echinococcosis (AE) or alveolar hydatid disease (AHD) is a serious human infection manifested as slow-growing destructive tumour-like proliferation and infiltration in the liver (associated symptoms: abdominal pain, biliary obstruction), less so in the lungs, the brain, and other organs, and often fatal if left untreated. The cysts (or metacestodes) in AE are multilocular and infiltrative, seen in rows by external budding from the germinal membrane with progressive infiltration of the surrounding tissues. The laminated layer is very thin, pericyst is absent, and this enables tissue invasion.

99.1.3   Polycystic Hydatid Disease

Polycystic hydatid disease (PHD) is less progressive than AHD and is rarely reported in Central and South America (Panama, Peru, Ecuador, Columbia, Venezuela, and Brazil). This is mostly due to *E. vogeli* and a small number of cases due to *E. oligarthrus*. PHD is a slow-growing tumour mainly in the liver. Secondary cysts develop commonly. The cysts are large with multiple vesicles separated by septa lined with the germinal epithelium and surrounded externally by fibrous tissue. These are located primarily in the liver, spreading in contiguous areas and appearing as a relatively large tumour-like mass filled with fluid, brood capsules, and numerous protoscoleces.

99.2   Aetiology

Hydatidosis caused by the members of genus *Echinococcus* of family Cyclophyllidea. The species are summarized in Table 99.2.

The cyst-containing organs of intermediate hosts are ingested by the definitive hosts; the protoscolices evaginate, attach to the intestinal mucosa, and develop into adult tapeworms (32–80 days in the case of *E. granulosus*). Hunting dogs are often fed the raw viscera of pacas and thus get infected with *E. vogeli* and become a potential source of human infection. Human beings and other intermediate hosts get infected by ingesting the eggs of a tapeworm—shed in the faeces. Oncospheres released in the intestine get disseminated to various organs, where they develop into cysts.

The parasite perpetuates itself in nature with a combination of canids as definitive hosts and small mammals, mainly rodents, as intermediate hosts. It is the intermediate stage which causes a tumour-like proliferation leading to infiltration in affected organs.

99.2.1   Genotypes of E. granulosus

While genetic variability in *E. vogeli*, *E. oligarthus*, or *E. shiquicus* seems to be low and information is limited, it is wide in *E. granulosus*. Genotyping has important public health implications.

There are ten distinct genotypes identified through polymerase chain reaction (PCR) amplification by sequencing mitochondrial markers in *cytochrome c oxidase*

Table 99.2   Species of *Echinococcus* and the respective hosts and intermediate hosts

Species	Definitive host	Intermediate host
E. granulosus (3–6 mm)	Dogs, other canids Dingo in Australia and black-backed jackal in South Africa	Sheep, goat, swine, cattle, horses, camel, kangaroos, and other wild herbivores
E. multilocularis (1.2–3.7 mm)	Polar foxes (*Alopex lagopus*), red foxes (*Vulpes vulpes*), arctic foxes, coyotes, wolves, and other wild canids; dogs; cats	Small rodents, deer, moose, reindeer, bison *Clethrionomys*, *microtine*, and *arvicolid*
E. oligarthus (up to 2.9 mm)	Wild felids, pumas, jaguars	Rodents, rabbits
E. vogeli (up to 5.6 mm)	Bush dogs, dogs	Rodents, paca (*Cuniculus paca*), agoutis, and spiny rats
E. shiquicus[a]	Tibetan fox (*Vulpes ferrilata*)	Liver of plateau pika (*Ochotona curzoniae*)
E. felidis	African lion	Wild ungulate

[a]Xiao et al. (2006)

1 (CO1) and *nicotinamide adenine dinucleotide dehydrogenase 1* (ND1) genes, of which seven infect human beings. These are two sheep strains (G1 and G2), two bovid strains (G3 and G5), a horse strain (G4), a camelid strain (G6), a pig strain (G7), and a cervid strain (G8). A ninth genotype (G9) has been described in swine in Poland and a tenth strain (G10) in reindeer in Eurasia.

According to Santivanez et al. (2008), the genotype G1 (sheep strain) is widely reported as a cause of human infection in Southern and Eastern Europe, Northern and Eastern Africa, parts of Asia, Australia, Tasmania, Jordan, Lebanon, Holland, Kenya, China, Spain, and South America (Argentina). In Peru, 95% of strains were G1, and control measures should focus on the sheep-dog cycle. The same was true for Chile (Manterola et al. 2008). According to Moro and Schantz (2009), the 'cervid', or northern sylvatic genotype (G8), is prevalent in North America and Eurasia. It is perpetuated in nature, involving wolves and dogs as definitive and moose and reindeer as intermediate hosts. Pulmonary localization in humans is predominant. Compared to other forms, its growth is slower and more benign, and clinical complications are fewer. Sadjjadi (2006) presented the current status of CE and AE in dogs, sheep, cattle, goats, and camels in countries in the Middle East and Arabic North Africa, from Morocco to Egypt.

The strains of G2, G5, and G6 have shortened the maturation time of the adult form of the parasite in the intestines of dogs. Therefore, the interval period for administering anti-parasite drugs to infected dogs will have to be shortened.

Not all genotypes cause infections in humans. The genotype causing the great majority of cystic echinococcosis infections in humans is principally maintained in a dog–sheep–dog cycle, yet several other domestic animals may also be involved, including goats, swine, cattle, camels, and yaks.

99.3 Epidemiology

The prolificity of the agent (say *Echinococcus granulosus*) is an important factor in determining worm burden. Assuming a dog is carrying 35 adult tapeworms, 175,000 eggs (35×5000 eggs per gravid segment) would be voided in faeces to contaminate the environment. The viability of eggs may be 3 months (up to about 1 year in a moist environment at lower ranges of temperatures of about +4 to +15 °C), and they are alive also at freezing temperatures. Eggs are sensitive to desiccation—they die in 4 days and 1 day at 25% and 0% humidity, respectively. Further, each cyst may contain as many as 2.0 million fertile scolices—dispersed as hydatid sand in the cyst. Additionally, any shred of detached germinal layer in the cyst is capable of generating daughter cysts and scolices. The persistence of the parasite in nature is almost assured, with 92% and 80% fertile cysts in sheep and goats, respectively. Even after the slaughter of sheep, the cysts may remain viable for 9 and 7 days, respectively, in the lungs and liver.

The relative capacity of the definitive hosts to contaminate the environment (i.e. their relative susceptibility to infection, a carrier state, and the number of gravid segments/eggs released per unit of faeces) matters. Foxes and dogs are highly and cats less susceptible to infection with *E. multilocularis*. Carriers of *E. granulosus* and *E. multilocularis* can contaminate public grounds, recreational areas, and gardens with infective eggs of the parasite, with a potential risk of human infection. Geological and geoclimatic conditions, land use, etc. influence the distribution and transmission pattern of the parasites.

99.3.1   Source, Mode of Infection, and Spread

Domestic dogs and cats acquire infection by ingesting rodents from the sylvatic cycle and harbouring the metacestode stage with protoscoleces of the parasite. Infected dogs pass eggs in their faeces. Eggs adhere to hair strands around an infected dog's anus and also are found on the muzzle and paws. *Direct transmission to humans occurs through the faecal (dogs)-oral (human) route*, particularly in the course of playful and intimate contact between children and dogs. An indirect transfer of eggs may occur either through contaminated water and uncooked food or through the intermediary of flies.

The spread of infection is determined mainly by the movement of definitive hosts—natural or translocation. The distance of spread may be influenced by the movement of definitive and/or intermediate hosts. While infected rodents and cockroaches may lead to short-distance spread, birds may be responsible for long-distance (>60 km) spread.

Disease transmission may be influenced by factors such as agricultural occupation, dog and cat ownership, hunting, outdoor activities, eating raw garden products or wild berries and herbs, etc. The high incidence of *E. granulosus* infection is often coincidental with rural, grazing areas where dogs are able to ingest organs from infected animals.

Climatic factors such as intermediate temperature, rainfall, permanent grassland surface, and some other factors may contribute to an ecosystem for increased grassland rodent population and favour the survival and transmission of *E. multilocularis* eggs.

There are opportunities in synanthropy that promote human-dog contact, such as:

- Children playing with dogs added with their relatively poor personal hygienic habits.
- Dog owners (risk factor 20x).
- Hand washing after handling/fondling with dogs (Christians stand 2x at risk than Moslems).
- Occupational exposure of tanners using dog feces as cheap source of enzyme for tanning.
- Shepherds (Turkana tribe in Kenya using dog-sheep) and foods getting contaminated with dust laden eggs.

99.3.2 **E. granulosus**

E. granulosus occurs in all geographical zones—circumpolar, temperate, subtropical, and tropical. It occurs in all continents. Parts of Africa, Australia, Eurasia, and South America have the highest prevalence. The prevalence is low in several countries in Central Europe and North and Central America. It constituted a major public health problem in the People's Republic of China. It is endemic and prevalent in 87% of the entire territory of the country. In South America—Argentina, Uruguay, and Chile—>2000 cases of CE are operated annually. The real number of cyst carriers would be much higher in endemic areas.

Sporadic autochthonous transmission is currently recognized in Alaska, California, Utah, Arizona, and New Mexico.

E. granulosus perpetuates mainly in the synanthropic cycle with domestic dogs as definitive hosts and livestock as intermediate hosts. Cystic echinococcosis (CE) occurs predominantly among those engaged in raising sheep. The dog-sheep cycle and the sheep strain of *E. granulosus* constitute a significant public health problem. There is a spectrum of intermediate host species of livestock, and the cycle depends upon the genotype of *E. granulosus*.

Sylvatic cycles in some regions serve as a source of infection for both man and domestic animals. The ingestion of the eggs of *E. granulosus* by the intermediate hosts—man and livestock animals—leads to the development of a metacestode cyst. CE may develop in any organ of the human being, but the liver and lungs are most frequent.

Eckert et al. (2000) summed up the most important factors that influence persistence, emergence, and re-emergence:

- Dog population, especially stray dogs in *E. granulosus* endemic areas.
- Easy access of dogs to the viscera of livestock containing *E. granulosus* cysts.
- Inadequate measures of parasitic control in dogs.
- Uncontrolled animal slaughter—the lack of municipal slaughterhouses.
- Increased home/road-side illegal uninspected slaughter.
- Meat inspection—non-existent or inefficient.
- Lack of facilities for the destruction of infected viscera.
- Poor education, especially health education and awareness.
- Specific control measures not yet been initiated in some areas/by some states.
- Inadequate state public health, resources, and financing as against the requirement for a long-term programme.

The failure to sustain the control programme led to re-emergence in Bulgaria (Todorov and Boeva 1999). The incidence of CE in children increased from 0.7 to 5.4/100,000 between the 1970s and 1990s in Bulgaria. In Wales, the prevalence in dogs doubled from 3.4% in 1993 to 8.1% in 2002 due to a change in policy—favouring health education over weekly praziquantel dosing (Moro and Schantz 2009).

99.3.3   E. multilocularis *[Alveolar Echinococcosis (AE)]*

In Central Europe, infected foxes—rodents—dogs cycle of infection is considered a source of infection to human beings. The endemic areas appear to be increasing as infected red foxes have been observed, from four countries (Austria, France, Germany, and Switzerland) by the end of the 1980s to seven more countries (Belgium, the Czech Republic, Liechtenstein, Luxembourg, Poland, the Slovak Republic, and the Netherlands). *E. multilocularis* in red foxes spread from 8 to 90% of the area in Hokkaido, Japan—from the earlier-known eastern part to the central and western parts of Hokkaido, with a concurrent increase in the number of human cases. The endemic areas in North America are the northern tundra zone (NTZ) of Alaska (USA) and Canada, with arctic foxes as the definitive hosts, and the North Central Region (NCR) further south, where red foxes, other wild canids, or rodents (microtine and arvicolid) are definitive hosts.

Eckert et al. (2000) reviewed the problem of AE in China. It is an important disease as (a) new endemic areas have been detected in recent years, (b) treatment is difficult and expensive, (c) it is life-threatening, and (c) efficient control measures are not available.

The fatality due to AE used to be high. Early diagnosis and radical surgery, plus chemotherapy, have reduced it considerably since the mid-1970s, yet this continues to be a life-threatening zoonosis.

The annual incidence of AE is not well documented. In Central Europe and Japan, it varied between 0.3 and 1.2/lakh, although in the highly endemic areas of Alaska, northern Siberia, and China, it was 98 ± 170/lakh. AE has focal distribution. Three major epidemiological situations have been observed. This is an emerging infection as in Poland and Belgium; stable as in Switzerland and increasing incidence per lakh such as in Japan (4.2 during 1937–1964 to 11.2 during 1985–1994) and in endemic areas of Europe (from mean of 0.1 during 1993–2000 to 0.26 per lakhs during 2001–2005).

Authentic information on the population density of foxes is not available. However, radiotelemetry may be helpful in estimating it. Epidemiological surveys use the method of examination of intestinal smears for the diagnosis of infection in foxes. It is 78% sensitive. Foxes harbouring a low number of parasites are not detected. However, epidemiological evidence suggests that humans and other aberrant/intermediate hosts get infected by ingesting the eggs of a parasite released in faeces by infected foxes. Dry environmental conditions are detrimental to the survival of oncospheres. Winter seems to be favourable. The parasite may jump over from the sylvatic cycle to the synanthropic cycle. Adjacent urban and rural cycles of the parasite may exist.

Several studies (Budke et al. 2005; Tiaoying et al. 2005; Wang et al. 2008) confirm the prevalence in China. Using ultrasonography and serology, Yu et al. (2008) found 25.8% seropositivity, morbidity 16.6% in pastor and 15% in Buddhist priests. This study was supported by finding stray dogs positive for adult tapeworm and yaks and sheep for hydatid cysts. According to Li et al. (2008), the predominant genotype was G1 (sheep–dog strain) of *E. granulosus*. In general, prevalence appeared to increase with age, more females than males were infected, and pastoral herdsmen were at the highest risk. The number of dogs owned, the frequency of contact with dogs, and the sources of drinking water were associated with prevalence. Buishi et al. (2006) identified the risk factors in north Turkana and northwester Lokichoggio in Kenya: the non-restraint of dogs, feeding raw offal, less than 5 years of age of dogs, the improper disposal of slaughter offal, the lack of knowledge among dog owners about the transmissibility of echinococcosis, and dogs not given anthelmintic treatment. In Eastern European countries, CE is a major emerging zoonosis (Bruzinskaite et al. 2009). Their observation is significant as it is related to (a) pigs and (b) the type of pig husbandry with G6/7 (pig/camel) strains.

99.4 Clinical Disease

The life span of the hydatid cysts of *E. granulosus* can be as long as 53 years in humans and 16 years in horses (Zhang et al. 2003), which is suggestive of the parasite's ability to survive in hosts with a potential to infect. The parasite is able to subvert or avoid the hosts' protective immune responses, possibly by escaping/avoiding the damaging effect of the hosts' response (impregnable tissues and capsules around the cyst) and immunomodulation.

CE can occur in any sex and age; the most common age group is 20–40 years. Most infections are acquired during childhood. Small encapsulated and calcified cysts may not induce any major pathology throughout life. Thirty-six to 60% of cases may remain asymptomatic.

In humans, *E. granulosus*, *E. multilocularis*, *E. oligarthus*, and *E. vogeli* are localized in the liver (75% of cases), the lungs (5–15% of cases), and other organs in the body, such as the spleen, brain, heart, and kidneys (10–20% of cases).

99.4.1 *Cystic Echinococcosis*

Cystic echinococcosis (*E. granulosus*) manifests into silent to serious, even disabling (blindness, paralysis), morbidity and high recurrence. The enlarging cysts cause symptoms, depending upon the size and organ infected.

99.4.1.1 Liver

Generally, the right lobe of the liver is the site of CE. The cyst is slow growing and spherical and has a typically *single compartment*, and *growth is expansive*, usually found in one area. There may be pressure atrophy, adhesions with the diaphragm, and secondary infection. The manifestations are abdominal pain, a lump/mass in the hepatic area, and biliary duct obstruction (colic). Other related symptoms may be hepatomegaly, liver abscess, jaundice, cholangitis, pancreatitis, portal hypertension, and ascites with litres of fluid. Alveolar and polycystic echinococcosis usually have cysts with *multiple compartments* and *infiltrative growth.*

99.4.1.2   Pulmonary echinococcosis

Pulmonary echinococcosis occurs when the cyst is located in the lungs, pleura, mediastinum, or chest wall. General manifestations are chest pain, cough, fever, dyspnoea, pneumothorax, pleural effusion, and haemoptysis. Mediastinal cysts may press into adjacent structures, causing bone pain, haemorrhage, or airflow limitation. The rupture of the cysts may lead to the escape of fluid into the trachea, causing the expectoration of a clear salty or peppery-tasting content, with fragments of the hydatid membrane and scolices.

99.4.1.3   Cysts in Other Organs

Cysts may be found in *other organs* too—the brain and spinal cord (neurologic symptoms—paralysis, serious if vital organs are involved), orbit, heart (pericardial effusion), kidneys, ureter, adrenal glands, spleen, uterus, fallopian tube, mesentery, pancreas, diaphragm, muscles, and bones (deformity, fracture). Abu-Eshy (1998) listed seven unusual presentations of hydatidosis recorded during an 8-year period at Asir Central Hospital, Abha, Saudi Arabia: (1) brain; (2) pericardial; (3) simultaneous multiple organs in the abdominal cavity; (4) liver, right diaphragm, and pleura; (5) left diaphragm—presenting as pleurisy; (6) right thigh; and (7) multiple abdominal and pelvic in a woman complaining chronic ill health, abdominal pain, and primary infertility.

Most cases of *cerebral hydatid* disease experienced headache (83.3%) and vomiting (66.6%). Other signs and symptoms observed are seizures, visual disturbance, papilloedema, hemiparesis, dysphasia, cranial nerve palsy, facial palsy, and ataxia (ArBukte et al. 2004).

99.4.1.4   Rupture of Cysts

Rupture into the peritoneal or pleural cavity, pericardium, bile ducts, gastrointestinal tract, or even blood vessels leads to embolism, extraordinary manifestations, and severe complications. Metastases (the generation of further cysts) may occur. The rupture of the cysts releases antigenic materials, inducing immune responses with a range of manifestations. Hypersensitivity reactions like fever, eosinophilia, urticaria, wheezing to life threatening anaphylactic shock, immune-complex disorders like glomerulonephritis or nephritic syndrome, secondary amyloidosis may be seen.

99.4.2 Alveolar Echinococcosis

Alveolar echinococcosis (*E. multilocularis*) is a slow-growing destructive tumour in the liver, which may be accompanied by abdominal pain and biliary obstruction. The larval mass proliferates indefinitely by exogenous budding and invades the surrounding tissues, thus resembling malignancy in appearance and behaviour. Protoscolices are rarely observed in infections in humans. The liver is the primary site. Metastasis may occur with lesions in the lungs and brain.

The initial symptoms are vague. The patient may complain of mild pain in the upper quadrant and epigastric region. It may progress to hepatomegaly and obstructive jaundice. Mortality may be due to hepatic failure, the invasion of contiguous tissues, and, less frequently, metastases to the brain. In progressive and clinically manifest cases, mortality may be high—50–75% (Moro and Schantz 2009).

E. vogeli causes a slow-growing tumour, mainly in the liver. Secondary cysts develop commonly.

99.5   Diagnosis

99.5.1   Diagnosis in Intermediate Hosts

One may find the basic approaches and methods of diagnosis in Zhang et al. (2003). The methods of detection of metacestodes in the intermediate hosts and adults in the definitive hosts are dealt with by the Organisation for Animal Health (OIE 2008). The *E. granulosus* larval form can be visually detected in organs. If *E. granulosus* and *Taenia hydatigena* in sheep are co-endemic, differentiation will require a histological examination of formalin-fixed tissues stained by conventional methods. Periodic –Acid- Schiff positive acellular laminated layer can be regarded as specific for metacestodes of *Echinococcus*. The following are the methods:

- Suggestive clinical presentation and epidemiology.
- Percutaneous aspiration and examination of the aspirate, of pleural fluid, bronchial washings or sputum for protoscolices, hooklets or hydatid membranes (considered risky for lung cysts but useful for diagnosis and treatment of hepatic cysts).
- Imaging—radiology, ultrasonography, computed tomography (CT) scanning, and magnetic resonance.

Macpherson et al. (2003) discuss the usefulness of ultrasonography in the diagnosis, treatment, and epidemiology of CE and AE.

In order to promote uniform standards of diagnosis in diagnostic surveys and patients and treatment, the sonographic appearances of cysts have been classified (active-transitional-inactive) by the World Health Organization Informal Working Group on Echinococcosis (Anonym 2003).

- Immunodiagnosis: the tests used are intradermal (ID) test, complement fixation test (CFT), indirect haemagglutination (IHA), latex agglutination (LA), indirect fluorescent antibody (IFA), enzyme-linked immunosorbent assay (ELISA), immunoelectrophoresis (IEP), counter-immunoelectrophoresis (CIEP) or immunoelectrodiffusion (IED), and arc double diffusion (DD5). A positive result in more than one test is often desired.

Immunodiagnostics are specific, complementary, and useful as primary and also follow-up tests post surgery and chemotherapy. The detection of circulating antibodies is more sensitive than the detection of antigens. The desired test should be specific and highly sensitive. Cassoni intradermal, CFT, indirect HA, and latex agglutination tests are insensitive and non-specific. The enzyme-linked immunosorbent assay (ELISA), the indirect immunofluorescence antibody test, immunoelectrophoresis (IEP), and immunoblotting (IB) have been adopted in routine laboratories.

The IgG1 assay for CE in endemic areas seems better than IgG, IgG2, and IgG4. The most widely used antigens are HCF (hydatid cyst fluid), lipoprotein antigen B (Ag B), and antigen 5 (Ag 5) in the immunoassay of CE.

Serologic tests have limitations. Only about half of pulmonary cyst patients are detected through these. In cases of intact cysts at any site, cysts in the brain or eyes, and no-viable or calcified cysts or in the case of children and pregnant subjects, serological tests often give negative results.

- PCR and DNA probes

PCR was useful in diagnosing atypical echinococcosis (both CE and AE)—extra-hepatic osseous tissue involvement (Georges et al. 2004).

99.5.2 Diagnosis of Infection in Definitive Hosts

- Necropsy and search for the smallest tapeworm in the intestine.
- Faecal examination for eggs after arecoline purgation and coproantigen or coprogen by PCR.

Handling infected materials presents a risk of contracting a potentially fatal disease to the operator.

Lahmar et al. (2007) made a comparison of tests for screening dogs for *E. granulosus* in experimentally infected dogs. Of the tests—arecoline purgation, copro-ELISA, and copro-PCR and necropsy in pre-patent infection in dogs—copro-ELISA was found more sensitive than arecoline purgation for the detection of pre-patent *E. granulosus* infection in dogs.

Infection in dogs and cats can be detected through a combination of tests—ELISA as a screening test for coproantigen, followed by necropsy or PCR for the detection of DNA as confirmatory tests.

99.6 Treatment

The rational treatment of hydatid disease requires diagnosis, location of the cyst, surgically reaching the cyst, and killing the protoscolices.

PAIR (puncture, aspiration, injection, re-aspiration), PAIRD (PAIR plus drainage), or PPDC (percutaneous puncture with drainage and curettage) are the procedures.

The recommended procedure to prevent recurrence is as follows:

- Aspiration of cystic fluid.
- Injection of 15–20% w/v sodium chloride solution into each cyst for 10 min and re-aspiration.
- Removal of the endocyst.
- Scrubbing of the exocystic wall with a small gauze soaked in 70% v/v ethanol three times.
- Suture of the wall.

Other common protoscolicidal agents that have been used in hydatid surgery are 4–10% v/v formalin, 3–5% v/v hydrogen peroxide, 95% v/v ethanol solution, 1% w/v cetrimide, and hypertonic sodium chloride solution.

The oral administration of albendazole or other anti-hydatid drugs should be also considered before and after surgery.

99.7 Control

Anthelmintics, a change in lifestyle, and vaccination are the tools to control the transmission of *E. granulosus*. Most of the programmes have adopted the first two—activities are directed to cut the transmission; the third is in the experimental stage, though with encouraging results.

1. Praziquantel administered to dogs monthly prevented the release of *E. granulosus* eggs in the environment—four times/year (World Health Organization 2020).
2. Culling unwanted and stray dogs—the programme, which was run for 4 years, resulted in a reduction in the prevalence of infection in dogs, from 14.7 and 18.6% to 0, and consequently a reduction by 90–100% CHD in sheep born after the commencement of the programme (Zhang et al. 2009).
3. Add to these the improved meat inspection and slaughterhouse hygiene/management.
4. Health education.

The vaccination of livestock is a recent new realistic option—though not yet widely available. Vaccine as a control measure has been described by Zhang et al. (2003). Intercepting transmission to either host can reduce and even eliminate infection in human beings. The vaccination of either host is thought to accelerate the control of infection. The vaccination of intermediate hosts—sheep and others—may be helpful in the control of *E. granulosus*, but the sylvatic nature of the cycle of *E. multilocularis* makes it less likely.

PSC, cyst membrane, cyst fluid, adult worm extract, and worm secretions are possible promising antigens.

Another one is 16.5-kD, a recombinant protein, termed EG95. The vaccine contains 50 micrograms of fusion protein [glutathione S-transferase (GST) fusion protein] formulated in oil adjuvant or made up with saponin, Quil A, or ISA70 adjuvant—it elicited significant protection (mean: 96–98%) in sheep against the development of hydatid cysts. Two injections given in a 1-month interval induced protection for 12 months; an annual booster is recommended. Immunity was transferred to neonates passively with a colostral antibody from vaccinated dams. Trials in New Zealand, Australia, China, and Argentina showed 96–100% protection in challenged sheep. A major mechanism responsible for protection induced by the vaccine is antibody- and complement-mediated lysis of oncospheres. The number of viable cysts was reduced by 99.3% (Lightowlers et al. 2000). The vaccine (EG95) offers encouraging prospects for prevention and control; it is registered in China and Argentina and is being extensively used in China (World Health Organization 2020).

A similar protein—EM95—has been observed to induce a significant level of protection in mice against a challenge with the eggs of *E. multilocularis*.

5. The most effective intervention against Echinococcosis is a combination of vaccination of 75% of sheep and 6 monthly anthelmintic treatments of dogs, as revealed by mathematical modelling. It is expected to have easy compliance and low cost (Moro and Schantz 2009). If this is combined with culling of older sheep, it could lead to elimination of cystic echinococcosis disease in humans in less than 10 years (World Health Organization 2020).

Long-term control measures resulted in the eradication of *E. granulosus* or the reduction of parasite prevalence to very low levels in a few island situations, including Iceland, New Zealand, Tasmania, and southern Cyprus. In the endemic regions of several countries (Argentina, Chile, Uruguay, Spain, Bulgaria, some North African countries, Australia, and others), control measures have been taken. A reduction of parasite prevalence in animal populations and a decrease in disease transmission to humans have been achieved but not eradication in Argentina, Chile, Uruguay, and Spain.

99.7.1   Suggested Control Measures for AE

- Sero-epidemiological and ultrasound screening of the human population, especially the high-risk group.
- Continuous surveillance of definitive hosts for infection with *E. multilocularis*.
- Praziquantel-containing baits to treat foxes in highly endemic areas.
- Empowering the local public health management system.
- International coordinated countermeasures.

World Health Organization (2020) suggested improving the data on cystic echinococcosis (CE), which is important for epidemiology, risk evaluation, setting priorities, action, and evaluation. The indicators defined are (a) the number of endemic countries for CE and (b) the number of countries with intensified control in hyperendemic areas. A hyper-endemic area has been defined as an area with an annual incidence of five human cases/100,000 people. The epidemiological indicators include a combination of passive and active surveillance. The control indicators include impact and outcome indicators.

99.8 Case Report

Fasihi Karami et al. (2022) reported a case of primary disseminated intra-abdominal hydatidosis with multiple organ involvement in a 51-year-old Iranian man with abdominal pain. Ultrasound and computed tomography revealed six cystic lesions in the patient's liver, sub-hepatic region, pelvic, and omentum. The cystic lesions were completely removed surgically. Post-operatively, the patient received albendazole (400 mg/kg/day) for 4 months.

References

Abu-Eshy SA (1998) Case report: some rare presentations of hydatid cyst (*Echinococcus granulosus*). J R Coll Surg Edinb 43:347–352

Anonym (2003) WHO Informal Working Group. International classification of ultrasound images in cystic echinococcosis for application in clinical and field epidemiological settings. Acta Trop 5(2):253–261

ArBukte Y, Kermanog S, Nazarog H, Ozkan U, Ceviz A, Masum S (2004) Cerebral hydatid disease: CT and MR imaging findings. Swiss Med Wkly 134:459–467

Bruzinskaite R, Sarkūnas M, Torgerson PR, Mathis A, Deplazes P (2009) Echinococcosis in pigs and intestinal infection with *Echinococcus* spp. in dogs in southwestern Lithuania. Vet Parasitol 160(3–4):237–241

Budke CM, Campos-Ponce M, Qian W, Torgerson PR (2005) A canine purgation study and risk factor analysis for echinococcosis in a high endemic region of the Tibetan plateau. Vet Parasitol 127(1):43–49

Buishi I, Njoroge E, Zeyhle E, Rogan MT, Craig PS (2006) Canine echinococcosis in Turkana (North-Western Kenya): a coproantigen survey in the previous hydatid-control area and an analysis of risk factors. Ann Trop Med Parasitol 100(7):601–610

Eckert J, Conraths FJ, Tackmann K (2000) Echinococcosis: an emerging or re-emerging zoonosis? Int J Parasitol 2000(30):1283–1294

Fasihi Karami M, Bahreini A, Rafiei A et al (2022) Primary disseminated intraabdominal hydatidosis: a case report. J Med Case Rep 16:35

Georges S, Villard O, Filisetti D, Mathis A, Marcellin L, Hansmann Y, Candolfi E (2004) Usefulness of PCR analysis for diagnosis of alveolar echinococcosis with unusual localizations: two case studies. J Clin Microbiol 42(12):5954–5956

Lahmar S, Lahmar S, Boufana B, Bradshaw H, Craig PS (2007) Screening for *Echinococcus granulosus* in dogs: comparison between arecoline purgation, copro-ELISA and coproPCR with necropsy in pre-patent infections. Vet Parasitol 144(3–4):287–292

Li T, Ito A, Nakaya K, Qiu J, Nakao M et al (2008) Species identification of human echinococcosis using histopathology and genotyping in northwestern China. Trans R Soc Trop Med Hyg 102(6):585–590

Lightowlers MW, Flisser A, Gauci CG, Heath DD et al (2000) Vaccination against Cysticercosis and hydatid disease (review). Parasitol Today 16(5):191–196

Macpherson CN, Bartholomot B, Frider B (2003) Application of ultrasound in diagnosis, treatment, epidemiology, public health and control of *Echinococcus granulosus* and *E. multilocularis*. Parasitology 127:S21–S35

Manterola C, Benavente F, Melo A, Vial M, Roa JC (2008) Description of *Echinococcus granulosus* genotypes in human hydatidosis in a region of southern Chile. Parasitol Int 2008(57):342–346

Moro P, Schantz PM (2009) Echinococcosis: a review. Int J Infect Dis 13:125–133

OIE (2008) OIE terrestrial manual—Ch 2.1.4 Echinococcosis/hydatidosis. 175–89.2.01.04_ ECHINOCOCCUS.pdf

Sadjjadi SM (2006) Present situation of echinococcosis in the Middle East and Arabic North Africa. Parasitol Int 55(1):S197–S202

Santivanez SJ, Gutierrez AM, Rosenvit MC, Muzulin PM, Rodriguez ML, Cysticercosis Working Group in Peru et al (2008) Human hydatid disease in Peru is basically restricted to *Echinococcus granulosus* genotype G1. Am J Trop Med Hyg 79(1):89–92

Tiaoying L, Jiamin Q, Wen Y, Craig PS, Xingwang C et al (2005) Echinococcosis in Tibetan populations, western Sichuan Province, China. Emerg Infect Dis 11(12):1866–1873

Todorov T, Boeva V (1999) Human echinococcosis in Bulgaria: a comparative epidemiological analysis. Bull World Health Organ 77:110–118

Wang Z, Wang X, Liu X (2008) Echinococcosis in China, a review of the epidemiology of *Echinococcus* spp. EcoHealth 5(2):115–126

World Health Organization (2006) The control of neglected zoonotic diseases: a route to poverty alleviation; combating a hidden threat: cystic echinococcosis in Morocco [report of a joint WHO WHO (2006) WHO/DFID-AHP meeting with the participation of FAO and OIE Geneva, 20 and 21 September 2005, Geneva, 2006

World Health Organization (2020) Echinococcosis. https://www.who.int/news-room/fact-sheets/detail/echinococcosis. Accessed 23 Mar 2020

Xiao N, Qiu J, Nakao M, Li T, Yang W et al (2006) *Echinococcus shiquicus*, a new species from the Qinghai–Tibet plateau region of China: discovery and epidemiological implications. Parasitol Int 55(Suppl):S233–S236

Yu SH, Wang H, Wu XH, Ma X, Liu PY et al (2008) Cystic and alveolar echinococcosis: an epidemiological survey in a Tibetan population in Southeast Qinghai, China. Jpn J Infect Dis 61(3):242–246

Zhang W, Li J, McManus DP (2003) Concepts in immunology and diagnosis of hydatid disease. Clin Microbiol Rev 16(1):18–36

Zhang W, Ross AG, McManus DP (2008) Mechanisms of immunity in hydatid disease: implications for vaccine development. J Immunol 181:6679–6685

Zhang W, Zhang Z, Yimit T, Shi B, Aili H, Tulson G et al (2009) A pilot study for control of hyperendemic cystic hydatid disease in China. PLoS Negl Trop Dis 3(10):e534

Chapter 100
Hymenolepiasis

Hymenolepiasis is a rare tapeworm infection associated with bad personal hygiene. It occurs in children and in persons living in institutional settings and in areas where sanitation is inadequate. It has a wide distribution but is most common in temperate areas.

100.1   Aetiology

- *Hymenolepis nana* (the dwarf tapeworm)—adults measure 15–40 mm in length, and eggs have polar filaments and rostellar hooks. It infects rats, mice, and man and has worldwide distribution. The incidence of hymenolepiasis is high in children and institutionalized groups in warm and temperate climates.

  - *Hymenolepis diminuta* (rat tapeworm)—adults measure 20–60 cm in length. It is distributed worldwide, but it occurs less frequently in crowded environments.
  - *Hymenolepis fraterna* is a morphologically identical variant—*H. nana* var. *fraterna*. It infects rodents, particularly mice, and uses arthropods as intermediate hosts. It is known in South Europe, Africa, the Middle, and the Far East. Infection may last for 2 months to years, the latter due to recurrent or auto-infection.
  - *Hymenolepis microstoma* (rodent tapeworm/mouse bile duct tapeworm) is prevalent worldwide, infecting rodents but rarely humans.

H. nana, *H. diminuta*, and *H. microstoma* are well-known zoonotic tapeworms. Other species may occasionally infect humans. Nkouawa et al. (2016) reported a *Hymenolepis hibernia* adult worm from a 52-year-old Tibetan woman.

© Springer Nature Singapore Pte Ltd. 2024   987
K. G. Narayan et al., *Handbook of Management of Zoonoses*,
https://doi.org/10.1007/978-981-99-9885-2_100

H. microstoma has a cosmopolitan distribution. According to Cunningham and Olson (2010), it is most commonly reported as a mixed infection with *H. nana*. The natural hosts are a large range of rodent genera, which include mice, gerbils, and voles. Infections in rats are controversial; rats become refractory with age, probably golden hamsters. Auto-infection in congenitally athymic mice has been experimentally observed. The common shrew (*Sorex araneus*) and the European hamster (*Cricetus cricetus*) have been found to be definitive hosts in the urban and natural ecosystems of national parks in Slovakia out of 186 small mammals studied (Jarošová et al. 2020). *H. microstoma* has the potential to infect humans directly without requiring an intermediate host. This is more likely in immunocompromised persons such as, HIV-infected, alcoholics, malnourished, comorbidities like cancer and diabetes type II.

NOTE: A study by Arai et al. (2018) *on H. diminuta has demonstrated a **positive side of infection**. Its antigen triggers an immunological memory response in previously infected mice, and this limits the severity of colitis, an example of 'Helminth therapy' for inflammatory bowel disease (IBL). The study is useful, considering an alarming increase in inflammatory bowel disease (IBD) in children.*

100.2   Life Cycle (Fig. 100.1)

Note: Direct, H. nana; indirect (two host life cycle), H. microstoma.

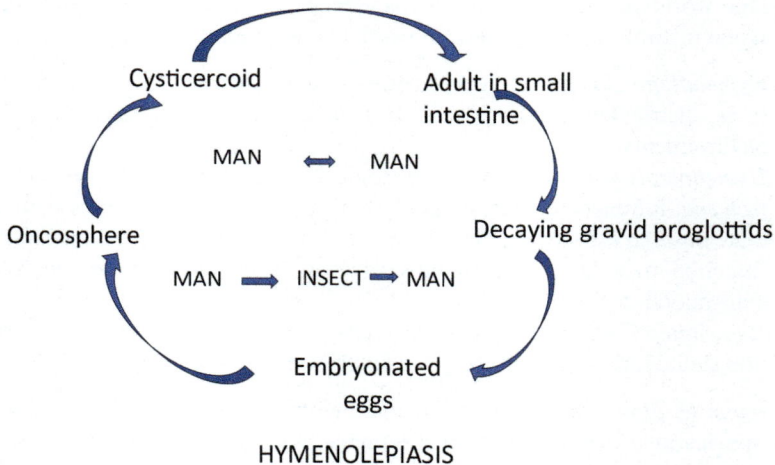

Fig. 100.1 Life cycle of *Hymenolepis* spp.

100.2.1 H. nana

The life cycle may be direct as in *H. nana*, which does not require an intermediate host. Rodents or men harbouring adult tapeworms pass eggs in faeces.

The most common way of infection is the ingestion of eggs in the faeces of an infected individual contaminating food. Eggs hatch in the duodenum. Oncosphere is released. It penetrates the mucosa and reaches and lies in the lymph channels of the villi. An oncosphere develops into a cysticercoid, which has a tail and a well-formed scolex. Cysticercoids emerge in 5–6 days into the lumen of the small intestine, where they attach and mature.

H. nana can follow an indirect life cycle, developing normally within larval fleas and beetles. An indirect life cycle requires arthropods/insects (beetles and fleas for *H. nana* and *Tribolium* for *H. diminuta*) for development. These are ingested, and cysticercoid larvae develop.

Ingestion of such insects (in precooked cereals, or other food items) by rodents and directly from the environment e.g., oral exploration of the environment by children causes infection of rodents and man.

The parasite attaches to the intestinal mucosa through scolex, and the worm grows into an adult in 2 weeks. The tapeworm matures in 20–30 days in the small intestine and is ready to release eggs.

100.2.2 H. microstoma

H. microstoma follows a life cycle typical of other hymenolepid species, except that its location is in the bile duct of the mammalian host.

The eggs containing patent oncospheres are expelled with faeces into the environment. These may be ingested by either an adult or larval stage of an appropriate beetle host (e.g. *Tribolium confusum*, *T. castaneum*, *Tenebrio molitor*, and *Oryzaephilus surinamensis*). Oncospheral larvae are released from their thin shells with the help of their hooks and enzymes. These penetrate the gut of the beetle to enter the haemocoel, where metamorphosis occurs. Cysticercoid larvae develop in approximately 7 days.

Ingested by the definitive hosts, the larval membranes are dissolved by the combination of pepsin and hydrochloric acid (HCl) in the stomach. The juvenile worms are activated in the duodenum in response to trypsin and bile salts in the first 3 days to move through the upper 20% of the small intestine and duodenum before establishing permanently in the bile duct, where they commence strobilation.

The terminal segments are gravid, and most of their strobila extends outside of the bile duct and into the duodenum in about 2 weeks. The entire life cycle, from an egg to a gravid adult, can be completed in the laboratory in only 3 weeks.

H. microstoma persists for an average of 6 months in mice and in the intermediate host beetle can remain infective for the life (>1 year).

Rodents (mice) get infected by eating beetles. These are reservoirs for *H. microstoma* that parasitizes the bile duct. It takes nearly a week for worms to mature and pass eggs. Eggs are dispersed in the environment passively. The life of the worm in mice is nearly 6–12 months, as observed in the laboratory.

100.2.3   Direct/Indirect Life Cycle

The direct life cycle of *H. nana* makes person-to-person spread possible and rapid. It is probably the most common route of human infection. The short period from infection to patency facilitates the spread and ready availability of the worm. The dependence of the parasite on insects for development is bypassed. An indirect life cycle, like that of *H. microstoma*, requires arthropods, like flour beetles (*Tribolium* spp.), as intermediate hosts.

The differences between *H. microstoma* and *H. nana* cysticercoid development in mouse intestinal tissues include the following: the time course for the development of infective cysticercoids was approximately 11 days for *H. microstoma* but only 4 days for *H. nana*, and *H. microstoma* cysticercoids that developed in mice had tails, while those of *H. nana* had no tails (Ito and Budke 2021).

All developmental stages, including oncospheres, cysticercoids, and adult tapeworms, appear to be immunogenic, resulting in stage-specific immunity to re-infection. The mature *H. nana* produces eggs. The protective immunity developed does not allow auto-infection. Oncospheres from re-infection may invade the intestinal tissue but do not develop into cysticercoids. Usually, within 1 month of infection, the adult tapeworms become stunted and disappear. This varies with hosts.

The life span of *H. nana* is less than 1 month. Infective *H. nana* cysticercoids develop in mouse intestinal tissue within 4 days and escape into the intestinal lumen to develop into adult tapeworms.

The life span of *H. microstoma* in the bile duct is at least 6 months but likely less than a year. The life span is possibly related evolutionarily to direct and indirect life cycles for *H. nana* and *H. microstoma*, respectively, and other species.

There is a similarity between *H. nana* and the zoonotic taeniid *T. solium*, which completes its entire life cycle between pigs (intermediate hosts) and humans (definitive host); humans can also be infected with eggs through auto-infection or from other tapeworm carriers. *T. solium* exclusively causes cysticercosis in humans.

100.3   Epidemiology

Hymenolepiasis (*H. nana*) occurs worldwide. It is common in South Europe, Russia, India, Latin America, and the southern United States, especially in dry and warm areas. There is a large number of carriers. It is prevalent in 5–25% of children. The prevalence is linked to poor sanitation and personal hygiene. Crowded settings, like refugee camps, usually compromise sanitation.

A study by Yang et al. (2017) detected 6.1% (7/114) and 14.9% (17/114) of *H. nana* and *H. diminuta*, respectively, in faecal samples of brown rats in Heilongjiang Province, China, suggesting the risk of zoonotic transmission of hymenolepiasis.

Jarošová et al. (2020) studied a possible transmission from pet rodent shops and breeding clubs in Slovakia. Pooled samples from 119 boxes with 228 mice, 191 rats, 124 hamsters, and 25 Mongolian gerbils collected from different shops were examined. *H. nana* eggs [polymerase chain reaction (PCR) identified] were detected in 25 (21.0%) boxes. Compared to breeding clubs, the infection was higher in animal pet shops. The highest prevalence was recorded in rats from pet shops (41.7%), followed by mice (25%) and hamsters (23.8%). The prevalence in mice was the highest (40%), followed by rats and hamsters, in the breeding clubs.

Panti-May (2020) considered *Hymenolepidid* cestodes of synanthropic rodents as a public health risk, particularly in children. In a survey in two rural villages of Yucatan, Mexico, samples of stool from children and *Mus musculau* and *Rattus rattus* were examined. *Hymenolepis nana* in 7.8% of children and *Hymenolepis diminuta* in 15.3% of *R. rattus* were detected. Molecular characterization and phylogenetic analysis confirmed the identity. Thus, epidemiological evidence of non-zoonotic transmission of *H. nana* and possible zoonotic transmission of *H. microstoma* and *H. diminuta* in synanthropic rodents was suggested.

100.4   Mode of Infection

It is faecal-oral transmission. It may happen by accidental ingestion of eggs of *H. nana* by ingesting faeces/soil contaminated food and water or hand to mouth by contaminated fingers. Auto-infection may occur; i.e., the tapeworm may reproduce inside the body. If it happens, the infection persists for long, beyond the normal 4–6 weeks life of an adult tapeworm.

The eggs of these worms are ingested by insects, the intermediate hosts. Eating material containing infected arthropods—intentionally or unintentionally—causes infection.

100.5   Symptoms

Infection may be asymptomatic but may cause weight loss. Severe cases manifest as headache, nausea, gastrointestinal discomfort, colic and diarrhoea, poor appetite, weakness, and itchy anus. There is enteritis and atrophy of the villi.

100.6   Diagnosis

- Stool examination.
- PCR for the confirmation of identification based on morphology.

100.7   Treatment

Praziquantel, albendazole, and mebendazole.

100.8   Prevention

Good hygiene, public health and sanitation programmes, and the elimination of synanthropic rodents help prevent the spread of hymenolepiasis.

Personal hygiene involves washing hands with soap and water after using the toilet and before handling food.

In a childcare centre, workers must wash their hands thoroughly with plenty of soap and warm water after every diaper change, even if wearing gloves.

While in endemic regions or countries, it is advised to wash, peel, or cook all raw vegetables and fruits with safe water before eating.

References

Arai T, Lopes F, Shute A, Wang A, McKay DM (2018) Young mice expel the tapeworm *Hymenolepis diminuta* and are protected from colitis by triggering a memory response with worm antigen. Am J Physiol Gastrointest Liver Physiol 314(4):G461–G470

Cunningham LJ, Olson PD (2010) Description of *Hymenolepis microstoma* (Nottingham strain): a classical tapeworm model for research in the genomic era. Parasites Vectors 3:123

Ito A, Budke CM (2021) Perspectives on intestinal tapeworm infections: an evaluation of direct and indirect life-cycles with a special emphasis on species of *Hymenolepis*. Curr Res Parasitol Vector Borne Dis 1:100023

Jarošová J, Antolová D, Šnábel V, Miklisová D, Cavallero S (2020) The dwarf tapeworm *Hymenolepis nana* in pet rodents in Slovakia-epidemiological survey and genetic analysis. Parasitol Res 119(2):519–527

Nkouawa A, Haukisalmi V, Li T, Nakao M, Lavikainen A et al (2016) Cryptic diversity in hymenolepidid tapeworms infecting humans. Parasitol Int 65(2):83–86

Panti-May JA, Servían A, Ferrari W, Zonta ML et al (2020) Morphological and molecular identification of hymenolepidid cestodes in children and synanthropic rodents from rural Mexico. Parasitol Int 75:102042

Yang D, Zhao W, Zhang Y, Liu A (2017) Prevalence of *Hymenolepis nana* and *H. diminuta* from Brown rats (*Rattus norvegicus*) in Heilongjiang Province, China. Korean J Parasitol 55(3):351–355

Chapter 101
Raillietina spp.

Raillietina is a genus of parasitic tapeworms that have chicken, turkey, geese, and numerous other domestic and wild birds, as well as rats, as definitive hosts. In the year 1920, the genus was named in honour of a French veterinarian and helminthologist, Louis-Joseph Alcide Railliet. It has a worldwide distribution of traditional and free-ranging poultry.

Geographical Distribution

In Asia, human cases of *Raillietina* infection have been reported in Indian Ocean countries, China, Japan, and Thailand. While most cases of *Raillietina celebensis* occurred in East and Southeast Asia, the Pacific islands, and once in Australia, those caused by *R. siriraji were* reported exclusively from Thailand. *R. demerariensis* is a New World species, with cases described from isolated pockets in South America (primarily Ecuador), Central America, and the Caribbean (https://www.cdc.gov/dpdx/raillietina/index.html).

Two cases of *Raillietina* infection in infants in Thailand were reported by Chandler and Pradatsundarasar (1957). Rougier et al. (1981) reported four cases from French Polynesia. They were young ones, 2 years to 3½ years old. One was asymptomatic. The others reported diarrhoea, gastrointestinal disturbance, abdominal distension, and pain lasting for 2 weeks. Moving white segments of the worm were visible in the stool of one case. The infection was focal. The distribution of 13/16 earlier cases was as follows: Philippines (three), Thailand (nine), and Australia (one). Several different rodents are natural hosts. Recently, Davis et al. (2019) reported Raillietiniaisis in a toddler from Hawaii.

© Springer Nature Singapore Pte Ltd. 2024
K. G. Narayan et al., *Handbook of Management of Zoonoses*,
https://doi.org/10.1007/978-981-99-9885-2_101

101.1   Aetiology

Raillietina is a complex genus of cestodes, family Davaineidae. Hundreds of species with a wide range of vertebrate hosts are described. *Raillietina* spp. are medium-sized tapeworms. These parasitize birds, rodents, and sometimes humans.

Human infection is rare, accidental, and innocuous. *R. celebensis* and its many synonyms (e.g. *R. formosana*, *R. garrisoni*, and *R. madagascariensis*) have been mostly reported. *R. demerariensis* and *R. siriraji* have also been reported.

R. celebensis, *R. demerariensis*, and *R. siriraji* are zoonotic. The natural hosts are rodents and not birds. *R. celebensis* and *R. siriraji* are primarily found in peri-domestic rats (*Rattus norvegicus* and *R. rattus*) and some other Southeast Asian murid rodents. *R. demerariensis* has been found in various Neotropical rodents and occasionally in monkeys. The intermediate hosts for the zoonotic *Raillietina* species are not precisely known. *Raillietina celebensis* infection is considered a medical curiosity rather than a public health problem. *Raillietina* spp. can be misidentified as *Inermicapsifer madagascariensis* (=*cubensis*) (=*arvicanthis*) infects many species of rodents and is rarely found in humans (https://www.cdc.gov/dpdx/raillietina/index.html).

According to de Oliveira et al. (2017), *R. celebensis* is a cestode that parasitizes the small intestine of rats and humans. Cestodes were collected from *Rattus norvegicus* in the municipality of São Gonçalo, state of Rio de Janeiro, Brazil. The number and size of testes, the number and shape of rostellar hooks, the cirrus sac length, the capsules and eggs per capsule, and the morphology of the mature proglottid allowed for the conclusion that the present specimens constitute a new record of *R. celebensis* in South America. Genetic and phylogenetic analyses, based on the partial small sub-unit 18S rRNA gene, revealed *R. celebensis* to be in the family *Davaineidae* within the genus *Raillietina*.

101.2   Life Cycle

Chicken, turkey, geese, and numerous other domestic and wild birds, as well as several rodent species, act as definitive hosts. Several insects (e.g. houseflies, ants, and beetles), slugs, and snails are intermediate hosts.

The gravid segments of adult tapeworms are shed with the rodents'/birds' faeces. They are motile and capable of climbing upwards on the vegetation. The eggs can remain infective for insects, slugs, and snails for several days in mild and humid weather. The intermediate hosts ingest the gravid segments, which release the eggs in their gut after digestion. The development of the juvenile stage in the intermediate host comprises five stages: (1) the oncosphere stage, (2) the lacuna stage, (3) the cystic cavity stage, (4) the scolex formation stage, and (5) the infective stage cysticercoid, which is an inflated sphere with distinct rostellar hooks. The cysticercoid migrates into the body cavity of the intermediate hosts. The rodents/birds ingest such contaminated insects or molluscs. After digestion, the cysticercoid releases the young tapeworms, which attach to the wall of the small intestine. The time between the infection and the shedding of the first eggs (pre-patent period) is 2–3 weeks.

101.3 Rodents as Hosts of Zoonotic *Raillietina*

Surveillance elucidating potential helminth and rodent reservoir species, different habitats, and their impact on human–rodent–helminth interaction is useful in understanding their epidemiology.

In a study on the potential rodent-borne zoonotic helminths, Chaisiri et al. (2015) examined 2478 wild-caught murid rodents from four different habitats: forests, non-flooded land, irrigated land, and human settlement in seven localities in Thailand, Cambodia, and Laos PDR. *Echinostoma malayanum*, *Echinostoma ilocanum*, *Plagiorchis muris*, *Raillietina* spp., *Hymenolepis diminuta*, *Hymenolepis nana*, *Cyclodontostomum purivisi*, and *Moniliformis moniliformis* were detected in 29.7% of rodents. Season and host maturity influenced the intensity of total zoonotic helminths. *Rattus tanezumi* was found host to seven zoonotic helminth species. This species is ubiquitous and is found in all the habitats and can possibly act as bridge hosts carrying parasites across different habitats. Sithay et al. (2020) detected zoonotic helminth species in 54.2% of three rodent species—*Bandicota indica*, *Bandicota savilei*, and *Leopoldamys edwardsi*—in Vientiane capital, Laos PDR. *Raillietina* spp. (30.7%), followed by *Hymenolepis diminuta* (17.7%), *Hymenolepis nana* (2.6%), *Echinostoma ilocanum* (1.9%), *Echinostoma malayanum* (1.3%), and *Angiostrongylus cantonensis* (1%) were the six highest prevalent.

101.4 Diagnosis

Diagnosis can be done upon an autopsy of rodents/birds. Microscopy of mucosal scrapping for the presence of tapeworm is diagnostic.

Gravid segments can be detected in faeces.

101.5 Prevention and Control

Most cases have been in toddlers. Mothers have to be vigilant and careful to prevent accidental infection.

References

Chaisiri K, Siribat P, Ribas A, Morand S (2015) Potentially zoonotic helminthiases of murid rodents from the Indo-Chinese peninsula: impact of habitat and the risk of human infection. Vector Borne Zoonotic Dis 15(1):73–85

Chandler AC, Pradatsundarasar A (1957) Two cases of Raillietina infection in infants in Thailand, with a discussion of the taxonomy of the species of Raillietina (Cestoda) in man, rodents and monkeys. J Parasitol 43(1):81–89

Davis RE, Mathison BA, Couturier MR (2019) Raillietiniaisis in a toddler from Hawaii: a case of mistaken tapeworm identity. Clin Infect Dis 69(6):1053–1055

de Oliveira SR, Simões SBE, Luque JL, Iñiguez AM, Júnior AM (2017) First record of *Raillietina celebensis* (Cestoda: Cyclophyllidea) in South America: redescription and phylogeny. J Parasitol 103(4):359–365

Rougier Y, Legros F, Durand JP, Cordoliani Y (1981) Four cases of parasitic infection by *Raillietina* (R.) *celebensis* (Kanicki, 1902) in French Polynesia. Trans R Soc Trop Med Hyg 75(1):121

Sithay P, Thongseesuksai T, Chanthavong S, Savongsy O et al (2020) Zoonotic helminthiases in rodents (*Bandicota indica*, *Bandicota savilei*, and *Leopoldamys edwardsi*) from Vientiane capital, Lao PDR. Am J Trop Med Hyg 103(6):2323–2327

Chapter 102
Sparganosis

Sparganosis is a neglected food-borne disease caused by the larval form of the parasite. Most human cases occur in Eastern and Southeast Asian countries.

102.1 Aetiology

The genus *Spirometra* belongs to pseudophyllid cestodes affecting canines and felines. The species are *S. mansoni*, *S. ranarum*, *S. mansonoides*, and *S. erinacei*, as well as the aberrant *Sparganum proliferum*. Human infection is termed sparganosis.

102.2 Life Cycle

Dogs and cats are the natural definitive hosts. Eggs shed in their faeces, embryonate, and hatch in water. Coracidia are released and are ingested by the first intermediate hosts, copepods. Coracidia develop into procercoid larvae. The second intermediate hosts are fish, reptiles, and amphibians, which ingest infected copepods. The procercoid larvae develop into plerocercoid larvae (spargana). Predators like dogs or cats eat an infected second intermediate host, and adult worm develops in them.

© Springer Nature Singapore Pte Ltd. 2024   997
K. G. Narayan et al., *Handbook of Management of Zoonoses*,
https://doi.org/10.1007/978-981-99-9885-2_102

102.3   Mode of Infection

Drinking water contaminated with infected copepods or the consumption of the flesh of an undercooked second intermediate or paratenic host—fish or frogs—causes human infection. Spargana can live up to 20 years in humans.

Humans act as paratenic or second intermediate hosts and suffer sparganosis.

102.4   Symptoms

The incubation period may be 20 days to 3 years. Infection in man causes many varied symptoms depending on the tissues invaded by the migrating spargana and the final location of the parasite. This may involve the subcutaneous tissue, urinary tract, orbit, pleural cavity, lungs, breast, central nervous system (CNS), and abdominal viscera. The location of the parasite in the CNS (brain or spine) causes neurological symptoms, seizures, hemiparesis, memory flashbacks, and strange smells. Although migration is painless, if spargana is located in the skin, it causes an abnormal sensation, numbness, or tingling. If located in the ear, it causes deafness or vertigo. Ocular sparganosis manifests as eye pain, excessive watering and/or ptosis, and periorbital oedema. It may lead to blindness.

Sparganum proliferum can cause proliferative lesions in the infected tissue, with multiple plerocercoids present in a single site.

Saksirisampant et al. (2020) reported ocular sparganosis in a 22-year-old Thai man. He had acute swelling of the left eye, itching, and discharge. It was not diagnosed and treated with albendazole and prednisolone. After a few years, he developed a painless moveable mass at the left eye's upper lid. Recurrent pseudotumor oculi was suspected. A surgical removal of the mass was performed. A white pseudo-segmented worm revealed a definite diagnosis of ocular sparganosis by a plerocercoid larva. The sequencing of the polymerase chain reaction (PCR)-amplified *cox*1 fragments showed 99.0% sequence homology to *Spirometra ranarum*.

102.5   Epidemiology

The parasite *Spirometra* has worldwide distribution. Southeast Asian countries report most human cases. Sparganosis is endemic in North America in animals. Human cases from this area are uncommon. According to Liu et al. (2015), more than 1600 cases have been reported worldwide, mostly from East and Southeast Asia. Sporadic reports were recorded from South America and Europe. Travellers returning from endemic regions reported sick. This was attributed to greater consumption of fresh/partially cooked freshwater frogs and snakes.

Zhang et al. (2020) made a large-scale survey (July 2013–September 2018) of *Sparganum* infection in wild frogs from 145 locations covering 88.9% of endemic regions of human sparganosis because frogs play an important role in spread of sparganosis in China. The consumption of undercooked/raw frog meat causes human infection. Chinese use raw frog flesh in traditional 'poultices'. The number of reported human sparganosis is >1300 in 26 of 34 provinces/autonomous regions/municipalities in China. Most cases are clustered in southern and eastern China. A total of 4665 wild frogs belonging to 13 species were collected in paddy fields or other wild environments and euthanized. Sparagna isolates were identified by a multiplex PCR assay and evaluated through cluster analysis. For each specific locality, one *Sparganum* was selected for PCR analysis. *Sparganum* infection rates in wild frogs were >10%, especially in South and Southwest China. Eight out of 13 frog species were infected. The most frequently infected species was *Pelophylax nigromaculatus* (the infection rate was up to 14.07%). The most common site of infestation was the thigh muscles of frogs, and the number of spargana per frog ranged between 1 and 49. Phylogenetic analyses identified the isolates similar to *S. erinaceieuropaei.*

According to Kuchta et al. (2021) cases have been reported from 17 European countries in wildlife. Human clinical cases are autochthonous (17) and imported (eight) have been reported. There is molecular evidence of the prevalence of *Spirometra erinaceieuropaei* and *Spirometra mansoni* in Europe. The latter is distributed across Asia and Oceania. The parasite is prevalent in Eastern Europe and has the potential to expand, along with its invasive or migrating mammal hosts and the risk of human infection.

102.6   Diagnosis

The examination of suspected infected tissue is recommended for the detection of *Sparganum.*

102.7   Treatment

Praziquantel is effective.

102.8   Prevention

Water and food sanitation is important, as well as avoiding the ingestion of raw/undercooked fish, reptiles, and amphibians.

References

Kuchta R, Kołodziej-Sobocińska M, Brabec J, Młocicki D et al (2021) Sparganosis (Spirometra) in Europe in the molecular era. Clin Infect Dis 72(5):882–890

Liu Q, Li MW, Wang ZD, Zhao GH, Zhu XQ (2015) Human sparganosis, a neglected food borne zoonosis. Lancet Infect Dis 15(10):1226–1235

Saksirisampant W, Eamudomkarn C, Jeon HK, Eom KS et al (2020) Ocular Sparganosis: the first report of *Spirometra ranarum* in Thailand. Korean J Parasitol 58(5):577–581

Zhang X, Hong X, Liu SN, Jiang P, Zhao SC, Sun CX, Wang ZQ, Cui J (2020) Large-scale survey of a neglected agent of sparganosis Spirometra erinaceieuropaei (Cestoda: Diphyllobothriidae) in wild frogs in China. PLoS Negl Trop Dis 14:e0008019. https://10.1371/journal.pntd.0008019

Chapter 103
Fish-Borne Nematodiasis

Increased travel and global trade are associated with increasing fish borne-nematodiasis. In humans, fish-borne nematodiasis occurs when raw or undercooked fish is eaten. The same may happen when eating the raw meat of mammals, birds, amphibians, and reptiles, which may act as intermediate or paratenic hosts in the life cycle of fish-borne nematodes. Cultural mixing, a change in eating habits, travel and global trade, the expansion of fishing areas, and cold transportation have led to changes in the epidemiology of fish-borne parasitic zoonoses. Incidence and geographic distribution are difficult to derive from the 'travel-based' study by Eiras et al. (2018) because the symptoms of food poisoning may appear almost immediately or later, even sometime after return. However, it is safe to state that these infections are emerging zoonotic nematode diseases.

Certain preparations of fish are delicious and traditional and are considered delicacies but use raw or undercooked fish. Examples are **sushi** and **sashimi** (Japanese preparations), popular in Japan and several other countries; **koi pla**, **plara**, **plasom**, and **somfak** (Thai preparations), common in Thailand, Laos, and Cambodia; **Kinilaw** and **Sabaw (soup)** - traditional foods in Philippines; **ceviche** in Peru; **gravlax** in Nordic countries; **boquerones in vinegar** in Spain; and **crudo** in Italy.

Eiras et al. (2018) identified nematodes reportedly affecting travellers. These are *Gnathostoma spinigerum*, *G. binucleatum*, *Capillaria philippinensis*, *Anisakis simplex*, *A. physeteris*, *A. pegreffii*, *A. cantonensis*, *Pseudoterranova decipiens* (previously known as *Phocanema decipiens*), *Contracaecum* spp., *Hysterothylacium* spp., *Raphidascaris* spp., *Thynnascaris* spp., *Eustrongylides*, *Hystrichis*, and *Dioctophyma renale*. The incidence of gnathostomiasis was high.

© Springer Nature Singapore Pte Ltd. 2024
K. G. Narayan et al., *Handbook of Management of Zoonoses*,
https://doi.org/10.1007/978-981-99-9885-2_103

103.1   Prevention

Travellers must avoid activities that expose them to infection. Physicians and health authorities should advise travellers on the risks associated with eating behaviour.

References

Eiras J, Pavanelli G, Takemoto R, Nawa Y (2018) An overview of fish-borne nematodiases among returned travelers for recent 25 years—unexpected diseases sometimes far away from the origin. Korean J Parasitol 56:215–227

Chapter 104
Angiostrongyliasis

Angiostrongyliasis is a potentially fatal food-borne nematode zoonosis manifested as eosinophilic meningitis. It is endemic in South Asia, the Pacific islands, Australia, and the Caribbean islands. It has also been reported in Africa, Hawaii, and, recently, the southern United States.

104.1 Aetiology

The causative parasites are *Angiostrongylus cantonensis* and *A. costaricensis* of the genus *Angiostrongylus* (*Morerastrongylus*), superfamily Metastrongyloidea.

104.2 Life Cycle (Fig. 104.1)

Angiostrongylus cantonensis is a rat lungworm. It resides commonly in the pulmonary arteries and heart of domestic rats. Rats are definitive hosts and are infected by ingesting L3 larvae. The larvae move to the central nervous system (CNS) through circulation and moult twice to become adults in 2 weeks. The adults then move to the pulmonary arteries, where they attain sexual maturity. A female lays around 15,000 eggs daily. Eggs are carried to the capillaries, break into air space, and hatch. The young larvae migrate to the trachea and get swallowed, to finally be excreted with faeces. It takes 6–8 weeks, from ingestion by rats to the excretion of larvae L1. Molluscs, the intermediate hosts, pick them up, and development in them proceeds to L3 in 12 days. L3 are then transferred to the paratenic hosts.

A. *costaricensis* causes abdominal disease. The adult parasite is located in the mesenteric arteries and the branches of the intestine of the definitive host, the cotton rat (*Sigmodon hispidus*). Eggs laid in the arteries develop into first-stage larvae,

K. G. Narayan et al., *Handbook of Management of Zoonoses*,
https://doi.org/10.1007/978-981-99-9885-2_104

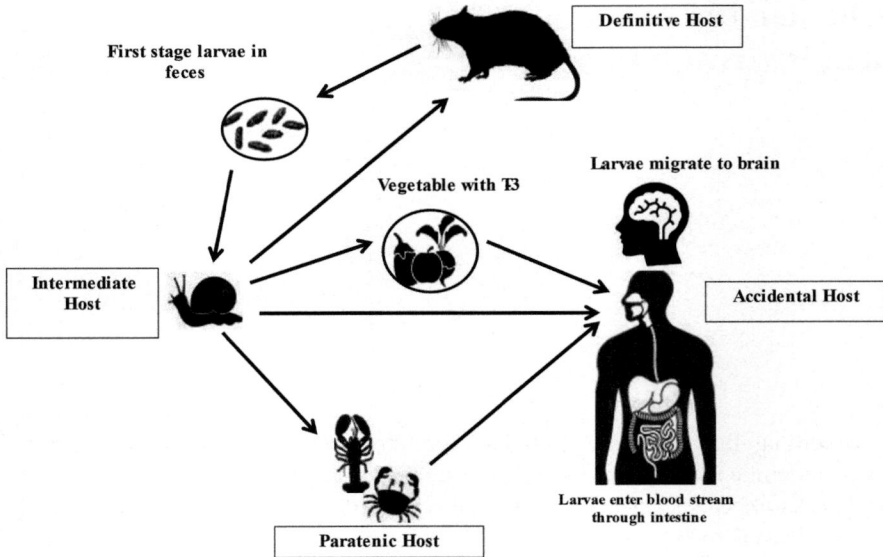

Fig. 104.1 Life cycle of *Angiostrongylus* spp.

which penetrate the intestinal wall to enter the lumen and get expelled in faeces. Slugs (*Vaginulus ameghini*) ingest the first-stage larvae. Development occurs through L2 and L3. The latter is infective. The cotton rat ingests the infected slug, and the L3 seeks the ileo-caecal region, penetrates the mucosa, and localizes in the lymph vessels. There are two further moults, and the worm reaches the mesenteric arteries near the caecum. Oviposition begins after 18 days, and the first-stage larvae appear in faeces within 24 days of infection.

Abdominal angiostrongylosis is a relatively new disease reported in Central and South America - Costa Rica, El Salvador and Brazil. Rodents with adult parasite have been reportrd in Panama, Texas, and Columbia and slugs with larval stage in Ecuador (PAHO 2003).

104.3   Epidemiology

Angiostrongyliasis (eosinophilic meningitis/meningoencephalitis) is a global, emerging disease of increasing public health importance. Globalization contributes to geographical spread, and more international travellers encounter the disease.

104.3.1   Prevalence

According to Wang et al. (2008), there are at least 2827 documented cases globally. China, Taiwan, and the USA have experienced several outbreaks. Angiostrongyliasis occurs among tourists/travellers returning from the parasite-endemic region. It has spread from the traditional endemic areas of Asia and the Pacific Basin to the American continent, including the USA, Brazil, and the Caribbean islands. Incidence has increased rapidly, especially in Thailand, Taiwan, and mainland China (Eamsobhana 2014). It is endemic in Hawaii, and there are sporadic cases in the southern continental United States.

104.3.2   Expanding Endemicity

Although *A. cantonensis* is considered a tropical parasite, it appears to expand to temperate regions by adapting to gastropod hosts. The distribution of gastropods, the intermediate hosts, is affected by climate change and average temperatures. The area is likely to expand, especially for non-native species, influencing the epidemiology of *A. cantonensis*. On the other hand, climate change, including humidity and precipitation, may have a different effect on the transmission and life cycle of the parasite.

104.3.2.1   Definitive Hosts—Rodents

Rats, the definitive host, are ubiquitous. The spatial distribution of reservoir rodents determines the endemic areas, as observed in ten provinces in mainland China with 650 million people at risk. The apple snail, *Pomacea canaliculata*, a large freshwater snail, is native to South America, was imported into Taiwan as a source of food, and then was introduced to mainland China. Most cases had eaten water snails. The unintentional importation of infected rodents is extending the endemic areas beyond the Pacific islands and South Asia. Additionally, travellers also facilitate importation. Once imported, *A. cantonensis* establishes and spreads, as happened in Cuba. Cases increased and were reported in Jamaica and Costa Rica. US travellers returning from Jamaica reported angiostrongyliasis.

The prevalence and intensity of *A. cantonensis* infection varied with environmental and rodent (host)-related factors, such as body mass (Niebuhr et al. 2021), as was observed in a study on *Rattus exulans* and *R. rattus* in Hawaii.

104.3.2.2 Intermediate Hosts

Lv et al. (2009) studied angiostrongylosis in Dali, China, and concluded that importing and selling *Pomacea canaliculata* led to human infection. They reviewed the records from 1 October 2007 to 31 March 2008 and investigated an outbreak lasting for 8 months. Approximately 1.0% of *P. canaliculata* from the market was positive for *A. cantonensis*. The patients had eaten raw/undercooked snails. Severe headache was reported by 97%, and high eosinophils in circulating blood and cerebrospinal fluid (CSF) were observed in 84.8% of cases. Patients responded well to the combined therapy of albendazole and corticosteroids.

A study by Stockdale Walden et al. (2017) detected adult and larval stages of *A. cantonensis* in definitive hosts and intermediate hosts throughout Florida, thus establishing its endemicity. They found 22.8% of 171 *Rattus rattus*, 16.2% of rat faecal samples, and 1.9% of 1437 gastropods, representing 32 species collected from multiple sites in Florida as positive. The three non-native gastropod species were *Bradybaena similaris*, *Zachrysia provisoria*, and *Paropeas achatinaceum*. The native gastropod species, *Succinea floridana*, *Ventridens demissus*, and *Zonitoides arboreus*, were newly recorded intermediate hosts for *A. cantonensis*.

Howe and Jarvi (2017) reported a study on 16 cases of angiostrongyliasis in Hawaii, including an outbreak in Maui. Angiostrongyliasis cases were reported from January to April 2017 in Maui, where invasive semi-slug has been recently documented. Angiostrongyliasis has been reported since 1950 in Hawaii. There has been an increase in the number of cases, and angiostrongyliasis is considered an important disease in Hawaii. There has been unregulated, widespread use of rainwater catchment to supply household and agricultural water. The study demonstrated that drowned gastropods can be found in catchment tanks. These are capable of shedding live L3 parasites, which can live for weeks. A single gastropod has the potential to harbour thousands of *A. cantonensis* parasites. Five cases of angiostrongyliasis were detected among children under the age of 1 from 2010 to April 2017. Some cases among babies from east Hawaii Island were reported to have no direct exposure to slugs or snails. One baby subsequently died. It is possible that they were infected in contaminated bathwater.

Several species of gastropods are reported as potential intermediate hosts of *A. cantonensis*, both native and non-native to the islands.

The natural definitive host is a rat, commonly *Rattus rattus* and *R. norvegicus* and cotton rats (*Sigmodon hispidus*), besides other species of rats in rural and forest areas. A natural nidus of *A. cantonensis* is defined by the establishment of infection in rats. The area is then considered endemic. Humans and non-human primates are accidental hosts and are dead ends as the larvae die in the brain or with the patients. Canines, opossums, equines, and birds are also infected.

Generally, molluscs and slugs (intermediate hosts) are susceptible to infection with *A. cantonensis* and one or two species of terrestrial and aquatic snails, and slugs (*Biomphalaria* spp., *Bulinus* spp., *Lymnaea* spp., *Pomacea* spp., and more) are intermediate hosts, capable of transmitting this parasite in certain regions.

For example, the giant African snail *Achatina fulica* is a major source of infection worldwide, which is responsible for the dispersion of *A. cantonensis* from Africa to the Pacific islands and South Asia. Another snail, *P. canaliculata*, is highly susceptible, is a good intermediate host, and has a wide distribution in Asia—Taiwan, mainland China, and Japan. However, the *Pila* spp. snail in Taiwan is a poor vector and carries fewer numbers of parasites, and so infected humans suffer from mild disease.

Frogs are a major source of human infection among paratenic hosts in China, Japan, and the USA. Eating monitor lizards caused human infection in Thailand, Sri Lank, and India.

In their review, Wang et al. (2008) described pathology based on autopsy studies and clinical features observed in adults and children.

104.3.2.3 Determinants of Infection

Lv et al. (2008) reviewed angiostrongyliasis in China. Eating raw food, including snails and seafood, has been common in the south-eastern coastal areas. Socio-economic changes led to the popularity of similar dishes among the urban middle and upper classes. *A. fulica* and *P. canaliculata* were imported for food, and these invaded and got established in the southern part of China and expanded to new areas. *P. canaliculata*, *A. fulica*, *Cipangopaludina chinensis*, and *Bellamya aeruginosa* are the predominant freshwater and land snails available in the Chinese market. While *P. canaliculate* and *A. fulica* accounted for the most cases of angiostrongyliasis in mainland China, *C. chinensis* was important in Taiwan. *B. aeruginosa* was associated with most of the recent cases. The endemic area is rapidly expanding.

Local customs and popular dishes are also determinants of infection. Young adults in the northeastern provinces of Thailand relish a popular typical snail dish called *koi hoi*. It is made from chopped raw snail meat, usually the *Pila* spp., and flavoured with seasoning and vegetables, e.g. minced roasted rice, onion, lime or lemon juice, chilli, fish sauce, parsley, and mint leaves. The dish is consumed immediately after preparation, along with a local alcoholic drink. Most cases were reported from this region. The popularity of exotic food, including snails (raw/undercooked), is increasing in mainland China, explaining the increasing cases/outbreaks of angiostrongylosis.

104.4 Transmission and Human Infection

Humans get infected through the ingestion of raw or undercooked snails or slugs or, indirectly, through vegetables and paratenic hosts carrying infective larvae. Prawns, land crabs, frogs, monitor lizards, and predacious land planarians may act as paratenic hosts, which may be consumed by humans. After ingestion, the transport hosts are digested, and the larvae released cause enteritis. The infected human experiences cough, sore throat, rhinorrhoea, malaise, and fever when the larvae move through the lungs. On reaching the CNS in 2 weeks, eosinophilic meningitis and pleocytosis are caused. Larvae may move to the eyes to cause ocular angiostrongyliasis.

There are many routes of spread and transmission mentioned by Stockdale Walden et al. (2017). The transportation of non-native gastropod intermediate hosts via plant nurseries and horticultural products spreads the parasite. The mucus secreted by snails and faeces from snails containing infectious L3 or contaminated water may be potential sources of infection. Larvae could come from dead snails also. Street vendors used a single bucket of water to rinse vegetables; cross-contamination and spread are possible in this case. Infective larvae from *A. cantonensis* can contaminate water if terrestrial snails fall into the water and drown. Chlorine/iodine treatment is ineffective.

Paratenic hosts such as freshwater prawns and frogs play an important role in the transmission. Predatory flatworms can transmit the infection to humans. *Platydemus manokwari*, a flatworm, can be a predatory or paratenic host after ingesting infected snails and slugs, as observed in Florida, USA. It is considered a major way of transmitting *A. cantonensis* in Japan.

Transmission to humans occurs by eating infected raw or undercooked molluscs, poorly cleaned contaminated vegetables and their juice, or other paratenic hosts such as freshwater prawns, crabs, frogs, or monitor lizards.

Accidental ingestion of the infected molluscs, contaminated vegetables not properly washed and cooked and contaminated vegetable juice leads to infection in human.

104.5 Pathology

The larvae or developing parasites induce local reactions. The dead and dying worms provoke inflammation. There is no change or haemorrhage on the surface of the brain and spinal cord. Conspicuous changes are observed around the dead worms, and there are micro-cavities and lesions along the migratory routes. The infiltration of eosinophils, plasma cells, and lymphocytes in meninges and around intra-cerebral vessels is common. Granuloma, eosinophils, and sometimes Charcot-Leyden crystals are seen around the dead worms.

104.6 Clinical Features

There is a local inflammatory reaction at the site of larvae or developing worms that cause eosinophilic meningitis/meningoencephalitis. *A. cantonensis* is the main but not the only cause of eosinophilic meningitis.

The incubation period is variable, ranging from 1 day to several months, depending on the number of worms. The condition is eosinophilic meningitis/meningoencephalitis. The frequencies of symptoms vary in children and adults and differ in some respects.

The main symptoms are severe headache, neck stiffness, paresthesia, vomiting, and nausea. Based on combined data from Thailand, Taiwan, mainland China, and the United States of America, headache is the most common (95%), followed by a mild stiff neck (46%), persistent paresthesia (44%), vomiting (38%), and nausea (28%) in adults (Wang et al. 2012). Nausea and vomiting were more frequent symptoms among children, and neck stiffness and paresthesia were less common.

Adults experience pain in the muscles and weakness. Increased cranial pressure caused headache, nausea, and vomiting, often relieved by lumber puncture. Headache may be intermittent, frequent, and severe in the beginning. The stiffness of the neck may be mild. Paraesthesia symptoms lasted for nearly 2 weeks and manifested as pain, numbness, itching, or a sensation of a worm crawling under the skin. Fever ranged between 38 and 39 °C.

Most cases are mild and self-limiting; however, severe cases without therapeutic intervention may enter into a coma and die.

Howe and Jarvi (2017) reported their observations on patients in Hawaii. The symptoms may be mild to seriously irreversible. There are flu-like symptoms, such as *nausea, diarrhoea, fever, muscle aches, general malaise, paresthesia, headache, stiff neck, eosinophilic enteritis, hydrocephalus, encephalitis, coma, and death*. Patients complain of pain in the areas of previous injury, possibly due to further damage to the previously injured nerves. The vagus nerve controls the functions of a number of organs—the heart, lungs, and digestive tract. Damage/demyelination could explain heart, lung, and other seemingly disassociated complications observed with angiostrongyliasis. An adult parasite has been found in the heart and lungs of several infected children on autopsy, which is possibly responsible for the irregularities of the heart and lungs, continued damage of the tissues parasitized, larval longevity/survivability, and possible migration within the body.

Ten individuals diagnosed with acute neuro-angiostrongyliasis between 2009 and 2017 sustained residual symptoms for many years. They suffered from troubling sensory paresthesia, which meant abnormal spontaneous sensation of the skin experienced as 'burning, pricking, pins and needles'. It is also described as allodynia or hyperesthesia. They had diffused muscular pain, insomnia, and accompanying emotional distress (Meyer 2021).

104.7   Diagnosis

A presumptive diagnosis is possible on the basis of clinical features, a history of eating molluscs, eosinophilic pleocytosis in the cerebral spinal fluid, and advanced imaging, such as computed tomography. Confirmation may be made by examining the CSF and ocular chamber fluid for recovering/demonstrating *A. cantonensis* or its antigen, though the success rate is low. Elevated white cells, eosinophils in blood and protein in CSF which appear turbid resembling coconut juice is pathognomonic of angiostrongyliasis (Sawanyawisuth and Sawanyawisuth 2010). An elevated protein level is more common than a low glucose level (Punyagupta et al. 1975). Advanced imaging, such as computed tomography and magnetic resonance imaging (MRI), of the brain shows lesions and helps rule out cysticercosis, paragonimiasis, gnathostomiasis, and schistosomiasis. Tests that may be used are the following:

- Serological tests using an *A. cantonensis* antigen or a corresponding antibody.
- PCR.

104.8   Treatment

- Surgery to remove worms from the eyes.
- Lumber puncture to reduce intra-cranial pressure and headache.
- Analgesics without corticosteroids.
- Anthelmintics like albendazole and mebendazole.

104.9   Prevention

The definitive and intermediate hosts are very widely distributed; hence, eradication is impossible. Preventive infection and disease in human beings is possible by interrupting the transmission of the parasite.

Thoroughly washing each leaf of produce, like vegetables, should effectively remove snails and slugs. Washing with bleach, vinegar, and salt solutions is as effective as water.

The public, in general, and many physicians and veterinarians may not be aware of this parasite or its presence. An awareness campaign in endemic areas is recommended:

- Kitchen hygiene: food preparation techniques to kill the parasites in snails, slugs, frogs, crabs, monitors, etc. and washing of vegetables.
- Washing of hands frequently, particularly after gardening.
- Making travellers to endemic regions aware of this disease.
- Preventing the spread of snails from endemic to non-endemic areas.
- Control of rodents in snail farms.
- Regulating trade of wild rodents and snails.

References

Eamsobhana P (2014) Eosinophilic meningitis caused by *Angiostrongylus cantonensis*—a neglected disease with escalating importance. Trop Biomed 31(4):569–578

Howe K, Jarvi SI (2017) Angiostrongyliasis (rat lungworm disease): viewpoints from Hawaii Island. ACS Chem Neurosci 8(9):1820–1822

Lv S, Zhang Y, Steinmann P, Zhou XN (2008) Emerging angiostrongyliasis in mainland China. Emerg Infect Dis 14(1):161–164

Lv S, Zhang Y, Chen S-R, Wang L-B et al (2009) Human angiostrongyliasis outbreak in Dali, China. PLoS Negl Trop Dis 3(9):e520

Meyer BC (2021) Chronic neuroangiostrongyliasis: case study of chronic presentations in Hawaii. Parasitology 148(2):221–226

Niebuhr CN, Siers SR, Leinbach IL, Kaluna LM, Jarvi SI (2021) Variation in Angiostrongylus cantonensis infection in definitive and intermediate hosts in Hawaii, a global hotspot of rat lungworm disease. Parasitology 148(2):133–142

PAHO (2003) Zoonoses and Communicable Diseases common to Man and Animals (Scientific and Technical Publication No. 580). Third Edition, Volume III, Parasitoses. Washinton DC, USA

Punyagupta S, Juttijudata P, Bunnag T (1975) Eosinophilic meningitis in Thailand. Clinical studies of 484 typical cases probably caused by Angiostrongylus cantonensis. Am J Trop Med Hyg 24:921–931

Sawanyawisuth K, Sawanyawisuth K (2010) Drug target in eosinophilic meningitis caused by Angiostrongylus cantonensis. Infect Disord Drug Targets 10:322–328

Stockdale Walden HD, Slapcinsky JD, Roff S, Mendieta Calle J et al (2017) Geographic distribution of *Angiostrongylus cantonensis* in wild rats (*Rattus rattus*) and terrestrial snails in Florida, USA. PLoS One 12(5):e0177910

Wang QP, Lai DH, Zhu XQ, Chen XG, Lun ZR (2008) Human angiostrongyliasis. Lancet Infect Dis 8(10):621–630

Wang QP, Wu ZD, Wei J, Owen RL, Lun ZR (2012) Human *Angiostrongylus cantonensis*: an update. Eur J Clin Microbiol Infect Dis 31(4):389–395

Chapter 105
Anisakiasis

Synonyms

Herring worm disease.

Anisakiasis is a parasitic disease caused by anisakid nematodes (worms), which can invade the stomach wall or intestine of humans. The infective larvae are ingested by fish or squid, which humans eat raw or undercooked, causing inflammation, perforation in the stomach, intestine, mesentery, and ascites. The cases are treated by the removal of the larvae via endoscopy or surgery.

105.1 Aetiology

The term anisakidosis/anisakiasis refers to a disease caused by any member of the family Anisakidae. Anisakiasis is caused by members of the genus *Anisakis*. Pseudoterranovosis is caused by the *members of the* genus *Pseudoterranova*. These invade the walls of the stomach or intestine of humans.

Anisakidosis is the most common fish-borne nematodiasis occurring in coastal areas. Over 90% are reported from Japan; the rest are from the coastal areas of the Netherlands, Germany, and France and the west coast of the USA and Hawaii. It impacts trade and the economy.

Herring or fish worms, *Anisakis simplex* and *A. physeteris*, and the cod worm, *Pseudoterranova decipiens* (previously known as *Phocanema decipiens*), are the common causes. Among the less common causes, *Anisakis pegreffii* is reported from anisakiasis cases in Korea. *Contracaecum* spp., *Hysterothylacium* spp., *Raphidascaris* spp., and *Thynnascaris* spp. are less commonly linked with human infections.

© Springer Nature Singapore Pte Ltd. 2024
K. G. Narayan et al., *Handbook of Management of Zoonoses*,
https://doi.org/10.1007/978-981-99-9885-2_105

Pseudoterranova decipiens complex is distributed as *A. simplex* (sensu stricto) and occurs in the northern Atlantic; *A. simplex* C in the northern Pacific, the southern waters below 30 °N; and *A. pegreffii* in the Mediterranean Sea.

The distribution of the *Pseudoterranova decipiens* complex is as follows: *P. decipiens* A in the northeast Atlantic and Norwegian Sea, *P. decipiens* C in the northwest Atlantic and Barents Sea, and *P. decipiens* B throughout the northern waters.

Anisakiasis or herring worms are found attached to the wall of the oesophagus, stomach, or intestine to cause the disease.

105.2 Life Cycle

The life cycle of *Anisakis simplex* involves fish and marine mammals (Fig. 105.1). Humans are incidental hosts, who ingest the infective stage larvae (L3) through raw/undercooked fish, and they suffer from intestinal or allergic anisakiasis.

The first case of anisakiasis was detected in the Netherlands in 1960. A patient diagnosed with acute local enteritis of the terminal ileum had a small nematode penetrating the mucous membrane detected on surgery, and this was L3 of *A. simplex.*

Studies in Japan showed that it was common in the north as most marine caught in large volumes in this area were paratenic hosts. These are mackerel, sardines, and squids. Anisakis larvae are always found on the surface of internal organs and

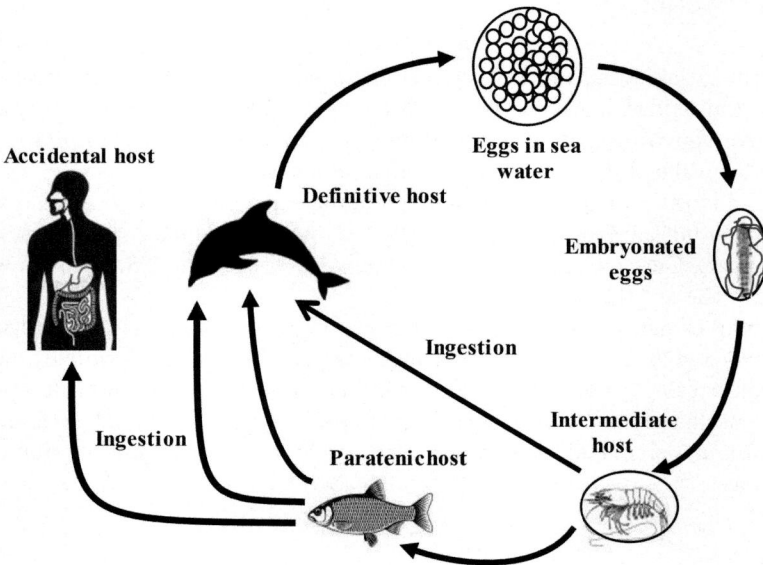

Fig. 105.1 Life cycle and transmission of *Anisakis* spp.

muscles. The cases presented as chronic granuloma and a phlegmonous intestinal type [anisakiasis (tmd.ac.jp)].

Marine mammals shed unembryonated eggs in water, which embryonate. Larva 2 (L2) is released and becomes a free-swimming larva, which is ingested by crustaceans (usually euphausids), wherein it matures into L3, which is infective, burrows into the gut wall, and forms a protective coat (encysts). The cyst is usually located outside the visceral organ but occasionally in the muscle or beneath the skin of fish and squid. This is eaten by marine mammals, such as whales, seals, sea lions, or dolphins, or other animals, like seabirds or sharks. The life cycle is then complete. The nematode excysts, moults twice in the intestine, matures to an adult, mates, and releases eggs into seawater in the host's faeces.

The gut of a marine mammal is functionally very similar to that of a human. *Anisakis simplex* is able to infect humans who eat raw or undercooked fish. Humans being the dead end of *Anisakis*, the worms do not survive.

105.3 Mode of Infection

Humans get infected through the ingestion of raw or uncooked marine fish and its preparations. Salmon, sardines, squids, and cuttlefish are common.

105.4 Epidemiology

Anisakis is absent from fish of water with low salinity because it is not favourable for crustaceans, usually euphausids. Anisakis is not found in the southern part of the North Sea, where cetaceans are rare.

The prevalence is worldwide.

Raw/undercooked marine fish preparations are getting popular in Japan (sushi, sashimi), Scandinavia (cod liver), the Pacific coast of South America (ceviche), and the Netherlands (fermented herrings called maatjes), so also the reported cases of anisakiasis are increasing.

The inadvertent ingestion of the *Anisakis* larvae when eating raw/undercooked fish, squid, or eel also causes anisakiasis. Shweiki et al. (2014) added the ingestion of raw clams to the list.

In a case-control study, Caballero and Moneo (2002) observed that detecting specific IgE directed to *Anisakis simplex* major allergen Ani s 1 is a useful tool for diagnosing hypersensitivity and intestinal anisakiasis. Measuring the specific IgG directed to *Anisakis simplex* major allergen Ani s 1 is only valid for an *Anisakis simplex* allergy.

Puento et al. (2008) used *Anisakis simplex*-specific IgE ELISA, which did not show cross-reactivity for a study in Spain. High prevalence was found to be associated with the ingestion of fish. The prevalence was 11.7% among healthy subjects and 16% among patients with non-digestive non-allergic pathologies. According to Anadón et al. (2009), the t-Ani s 7 polypeptide, secretory/excretory (ES) *Anisakis simplex* allergen, recognized in 100% infected patients, is specific and does not cross-react even with *Pseudoterranova decipiens*.

Occupationally, fish-processing workers have experienced asthma, conjunctivitis, and contact dermatitis.

According to Yera et al. (2018), all French laboratories notified a total of 37 cases during 2010–2014. Seven cases had evidence of a worm. Twelve cases had abdominal pain after the consumption of raw fish, plus anti-*Anisakis* precipitin, and 18 cases presented with acute symptoms after consuming fish and showed specific anti-*Anisakis* specific IgE. Significantly, more females (67%) were affected. The median age was 42 years (11–69).

105.5   Pathology

Orally administered larvae may be found dead in faeces. The infecting larvae penetrate the walls of the abdominal and intestinal cavities, and a histopathological examination shows the larvae migrating into the digestive tract. About 1/3–1/4 of larvae penetrate the abdominal cavity. There are numerous eosinophilic cell granulomas.

In extra-intestinal anisakiasis, the larvae may be found distributed in all organ tissues—the abdominal wall, small and large intestines, omentum, muscles and fats, pancreas, liver, spleen, testicle, ovary, uterus, urinary bladder, thyroid gland, and mesentery. In the abdominal cavity, the larvae reach the serous membranes of organs and often produce eosinophil cell granuloma.

The larvae penetrate the digestive wall and reach the abdominal cavity, leaving perforation detectable by endoscopy. Penetration takes a short time and is accompanied by subjective symptoms, which are over soon and pass unnoticed by the patient. There is a strong cell reaction at the second infection and perforation outside the stomach and intestine with extensive bleeding and internal bleeding in the mucous membrane, possibly resulting from localized reactions to secretion and excrement (ES) antigens.

Infection and second/re-infection carried out on experimental rabbits revealed, respectively, (a) foreign body reaction with live larvae and (b) surrounding acute exudative inflammation; infiltration of immune cells, neutrophils, and eosinophils; and oedema, which subsided quickly, leaving abscess and granuloma around the dead larvae. Re-infection (third) using a soluble fluid fraction of larvae caused an instantaneous allergic reaction. Re-infection (third) using sedimented antigen caused a delayed allergic reaction.

Immunity in cases where larvae penetrated the wall of the digestive tract and died was weak compared to those in whom larvae infected the abdominal cavity.

The fate of *Anisakis* larvae ingested with infected marine organisms is as follows: (a) 1/3 pass out with stool, (b) 1/3 die in the walls of the stomach and intestine, and (c) 1/3 die forming granuloma or after penetrating the abdominal cavity. The penetration of the digestive tract and entry into the abdominal cavity is more common in the intestinal form than in the gastric form. The invasion of the abdominal cavity is accompanied by secondary bacterial infection, indicated by the clear abdominal fluid changing to lemon yellow, opaque, and turbid.

105.6 Symptoms

Some may experience a tingling sensation in the mouth and throat while eating because of the moving worm. The incubation period is short, less than 48 h. The duration of the illness is 1–5 days. The anisakid larvae penetrate the gastric and intestinal mucosa. There is violent abdominal pain and nausea within hours after ingestion of the infected fish. Larvae may be coughed up. There is history of intermittent abdominal pain, nausea, and vomiting lasting for weeks to years. Larvae entering the bowel elicit symptoms mimicking Crohn's disease after 1–2 weeks. The larvae migrate from the stomach to other tissues, and severe IgE-mediated allergic reactions, such as urticaria and anaphylaxis, can occur. The reaction may be with or without accompanying gastrointestinal symptoms. A number of allergens (biochemicals) are released by anisakids and related species, like seal worm (*Pseudoterranova decipiens* spp.) and cod worm (*Hysterothylacium aduncum*), which are often consumed accidentally. These lie inside a fish fillet, so even thoroughly cooked fish food (where larvae are killed) poses an allergic reaction. Fish processors may exhibit occupational allergies, like contact dermatitis, conjunctivitis, and asthma.

105.7 Some Illustrative Case Reports

These case reports point out that anisakiasis (a) is difficult to diagnose on clinical examination, (b) requires endoscopy, and may require (c) exploratory laparoscopy and even (d) laparotomy. Treatment requires the simple removal of the worm from the oesophagus/stomach and surgery.

1. According to Ahmed et al. (2016), enteric and ectopic anisakiasis is rare and is often challenging, from diagnosis to treatment. Of the 201 cases of anisakiasis in Japan, 56% had abdominal complications. Seven per cent required open surgery. They reported that a 37-year-old female was admitted to emergency with severe epigastric pain progressing towards the periumbilical area, nausea, multiple vomiting, abdominal tenderness, and a temperature of 100.4 °F. Abdominal computed tomography showed free pelvic fluid collection. Diagnostic laparoscopy revealed yellowish fluid in all quadrants and some induration in the lesser and greater curvature of the stomach and the ligament of Treitz. Scattered exudates were seen along the small bowel and mesentery without any perforation.

Open laparotomy revealed a 2 cm long and 4 mm wide, white, wriggling worm in the peritoneal exudate. This was an anisakid nematode.

2. Carmo et al. (2017) reported a case of an otherwise healthy 32-year-old man with severe epigastric pain, vomiting, and low-grade fever for a week. He had eaten sushi recently. Upper gastrointestinal endoscopy detected a filiform parasite attached to a swollen hyperaemic mucosa with its end penetrating the gastric mucosa. It was removed with Roth Net, and the symptoms resolved immediately.

3. A 26-year-old woman had eaten squid a week earlier. She was admitted to an emergency with acute abdominal pain. Contrast-enhanced computed tomography showed ascites, localized submucosal oedema of the intestinal wall, and a dilated small bowel segment with oedema. Laparoscopy showed bloody ascites and severe inflammation in a part of the ileum. A live *Anisakis* larva was found in the inflamed mesentery after it had perforated the intestinal wall. The ileum was highly ischemic (Shibata et al. 2020).

4. Carlin et al. (2018) presented a case of intestinal intussusception in a 30-year-old male, causing complete small intestine blockage, which required surgery. He suffered from severe abdominal pain 3 days after eating home-cured salmon gravlax. He had to be operated upon. He had to be treated with albendazole plus prednisone for the inflammation proximal to the surgical anastomosis. Prophylactic treatment was given to family members as they shared the home-cured salmon gravlax. The worm passed out with stool.

Differential diagnosis: anisakiasis (nematode), clonorchiasis (trematode), and diphyllobothriasis (cestode) are fish-borne gastrointestinal parasitic diseases but with distinct symptoms. Anisakiasis presents sudden severe abdominal pain. Clonorchiasis presents jaundice. The examination of the eyes, skin, abdomen (tender), and liver (enlarged) may detect jaundice. Diphyllobothriasis patients report irritability, tingling and numbness of the skin, muscular weakness, and abdominal discomfort (increased heart rate on examination).

105.8   Diagnosis

- Fibre optic gastroscopic examination, during which the 2 cm larvae are visualized and can be removed.
- Histopathologic examination of tissue—biopsy during surgery.
- Skin prick test is a hypersensitivity test.
- Levels of *Anisakis*—a specific IgE antibody rises during the first several days of infection. The t-Ani s 7 polypeptide is a useful target for differentiating from other possible cross-reacting antigens.
- X-ray and ultrasonography.
- Immuno-serodiagnostics are being increasingly perfected.

105.9 Treatment

The infection may be resolved with symptomatic treatment. Small intestinal obstruction may occur and may require the surgical/endoscopic removal of the larvae. Intestinal perforation is an emergency but is possible. The anthelmintic albendazole may be useful.

105.10 Prevention

Cooking fish at 63 °C or freezing it at −20 °C for 7 days or −35 °C until solid and then stored at −35 °C or below for 15 h or −20 °C for 24 h kills anisakid helminths.

References

Ahmed M, Ayoob F, Kesavan M, Gumaste V, Khalil A (2016) Gastrointestinal Anisakidosis—watch what you eat. Cureus 8(11):e860

Anadón AM, Romarís F, Escalante M, Rodríguez E et al (2009) The *Anisakis simplex* Ani s 7 major allergen as an indicator of true *Anisakis* infections. Clin Exp Immunol 156(3):471–478

Caballero ML, Moneo I (2002) Specific IgE determination to Ani s 1, a major allergen from *Anisakis simplex*, is a useful tool for diagnosis. Ann Allergy Asthma Immunol 1:74–77

Carlin AF, Abeles S, Chin NA, Lin GY et al (2018) Case report (2018). A common source outbreak of Anisakidosis in the United States and postexposure prophylaxis of family collaterals. Am J Trop Med Hyg 99(5):1219–1221

Carmo J, Marques S, Bispo M, Serra D (2017) Anisakiasis: a growing cause of abdominal pain! BMJ Case Rep 2017:bcr2016218857

Puento P, Anadon AM, Rodero M, Romaris F et al (2008) *Anisakis simplex*: the high prevalence in Madrid (Spain) and its relation with fish consumption. Exp Parasitol 118(2):271–274

Shibata K, Yoshida Y, Miyaoka Y et al (2020) Intestinal anisakiasis with severe intestinal ischemia caused by extraluminal live larvae: a case report. Surg Case Rep 6:253

Shweiki E, Rittenhouse DW, Ochoa JE, Punja VP et al (2014) Acute small-bowel obstruction from intestinal Anisakiasis after the ingestion of raw clams; documenting a new method of marine-to-human parasitic transmission. Open Forum Infect Dis 1(2):ofu087

Yera H, Fréalle É, Dutoit E, Dupouy-Camet J (2018) A national retrospective survey of anisakidosis in France (2010–2014): decreasing incidence, female predominance, and emerging allergic potential. Parasite 25:23

Chapter 106
Ascariasis

Soil-transmitted parasites cause major burden of disease world over. Ascariasis is one of them.

106.1 Aetiology

Ascariasis is cause by *Ascaris* spp. There are two species, *Ascaris lumbricoides* and *A. suum*, which are difficult to distinguish. There is a host preference—*A. lumbricoides* for humans and *A. suum* for pigs, the latter being zoonotic. In places where human infection with *A. lumbricoides* does not occur, human infection with *A suum* occurs, attributed to being acquired from pig farms. However, the Centers for Disease Control and Prevention (CDC 2020) reported that an estimated 807 million–1.2 billion people in the world are infected with *Ascaris lumbricoides*. Ascariasis occurs in tropical and subtropical areas of Asia, sub-Saharan Africa, and the Americas, particularly where open defecation prevails or faeces are used as fertilizers. *Ascaris suum* is found wherever pigs are found.

Warm and moist conditions favour the viability and development of eggs to infectivity. Ascariasis may be more common in arid areas when periodic rains mobilize dormant *Ascaris* eggs from soil and other sources, such as latrines, resulting in a high level of contamination of water and food supplies.

106.2 Life Cycle

Ascaris is an intestinal roundworm: *A. lumbricoides* in humans and *A. suum* in pigs' intestines. The eggs are passed in faeces and deposited in the soil. Eggs undergo development to become infective in days' to weeks' time. The ingestion of infective

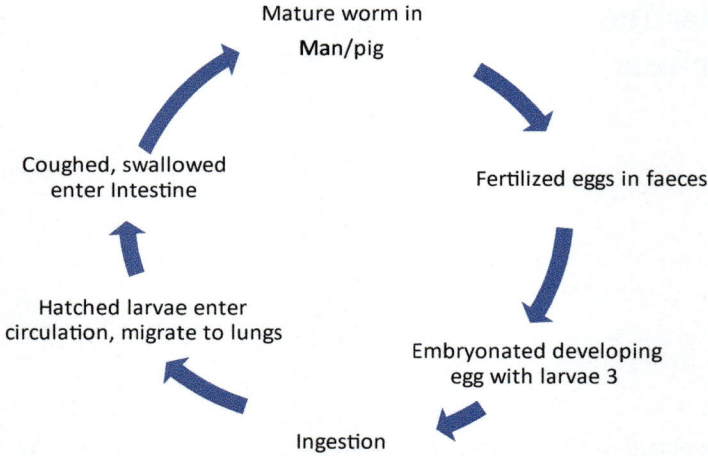

Fig. 106.1 Life cycle of *Ascaris* spp.

eggs causes infection (Fig. 106.1). This is possible when hands or fingers are contaminated with soil containing infective eggs and are put in the mouth. The ingestion of unwashed, unpeeled, or uncooked vegetables or fruits can lead to infection.

106.3 Symptoms

The most infected show no symptoms. Large numbers of worms reside in the intestines, which cause discomfort, abdominal distension, dehydration, fever, pain, and even intestinal blockage. Parasites may invade and damage the biliary or pancreatic ducts and cause obstruction and even death. Consequently, jaundice and hepatic abscess pancreatitis follow. Ascariasis causes malabsorption and affects the growth of children. The worm may migrate to the respiratory system to cause a severe immune hypersensitivity response (Loeffler's syndrome[1]), which may be life-threatening. Severe pulmonary reactions can be caused by exposure to the eggs of either *A. lumbricoides* or *A. suum*. Ascaris allergens may cause an allergic response.

Infected pigs may have difficulty in breathing (called thumps). Slow weight gain, loss of weight, and unthrifty are indicative.

Pig farmers; pig handlers; farm workers, especially those cleaning manure; gardeners using raw pig manure; and those with poor hygienic habits are at risk.

---

[1] In response to soil-borne parasitic infection, eosinophiles accumulate in the lungs and manifest as difficult breathing, cough, and fever; it may also include irritable bowel, abdominal pain, cramps, skin rashes, and fatigue.

106.4 Diagnosis

It is based on the demonstration of the worm (sometimes the whole worm comes out through the anus)/eggs in faeces and/or the larvae in throat swab or sputum.

In parasitic infections, there is an increase in IgE and eosinophils in the blood as well as eosinophils and mast cells in tissues.

106.5 Prevention

- Washing hands thoroughly after handling pigs, cleaning pig pens, or handling pig manure is recommended.
- The washing/peeling/cooking of fruits and vegetables grown in gardens where pig manure has been used or kept is suggested.
- Preventive chemotherapy is one of the largest and most successful public health interventions in history, benefitting a billion people worldwide.

Soil-transmitted helminths and four 'neglected tropical diseases' (river blindness, lymphatic filariasis, schistosomiasis, and trachoma) are treatable, and that, too, at the population level without stool examination. The method is "preventive chemotherapy or Mass drug administration (MDA)" through school-health programmes and health clinics. It involves administering six medicines in seven different combinations, making it possible to treat more than one disease at a time. The WHO-identified group includes preschool and school-age children, women of childbearing age (including pregnant women in the second and third trimesters and lactating women), and adults in occupations where there is a high risk of heavy infection (https://www.who.int/data/gho/data/themes/neglected-tropical-diseases).

Approximately 1.6 billion—one-sixth of the world's population—are at risk of infection with helminths. The soil (and water) around the village or community becomes contaminated and transmits infection with parasite eggs. The infected show non-specific symptoms in adults and impede children's physical growth and cognitive development due to malnutrition and increased anaemia, contributing significantly to school absenteeism.

Preventive chemotherapy delivery tied up with (a) the Expanded Program on Immunization (EPI) in preschool and school children, alongside (b) pro-poor policies—e.g. the introduction of basic public health measures, such as access to clean water and sanitation, as well as health education—is cost-effective, sustainable, and more focused. The coverage increased to 69.5% by 2017 with >600 million treated, morbidity was eliminated in seven countries, and an additional 21 countries would have ≥75% coverage for 5 years (World Health Organization 2019).

106.6   Treatment

Anthelminthic drugs such as albendazole and mebendazole are the drugs of choice.

References

CDC (2020). https://www.cdc.gov/parasites/ascariasis/index.html
World Health Organization (2019) Twelfth report of the Strategic and Technical Advisory Group for Neglected Tropical Diseases (STAG-NTDs). 30 April 2019. | Meeting report. https://www.who.int/publications/m/item/twelfth-report-of-the-strategic-and-technical-advisory-group-for-neglected-tropical-diseases-(stag-ntds)

Chapter 107
Capillariasis

Capillariasis is a roundworm disease manifesting in three forms, depending upon the nematode species *Capillaria*: hepatic capillariasis, intestinal capillariasis, and pneumonic capillariasis.

107.1 Hepatic Capillariasis

107.1.1 Aetiology

Capillaria hepatica (or *Calodium hepaticum*) is a nematode belonging to the family *Capillariidae* under the superfamily *Trichinelloidia*. It has global distribution. This infection is reported in Japan, India, America, Canada, Brazil, and temperate and tropical zones.

107.1.2 Life Cycle

C. hepatica has a direct life cycle. A single host is required. The adult worm and ova are present in the liver of the host. The female worm lays eggs in the surrounding tissue of the liver of the host, e.g. a rodent, for 30–40 days (adult life span), and further development is arrested. The ova are not embryonated and thus non-infective. These may remain dormant and viable for some months. Eggs must escape from the host (rodent) and spend 6 weeks to 5 months in the air and damp soil in the environment for embryonation, becoming infectious.

The mechanism of release of eggs into the environment: The escape from the first host (rodent) is possible when it dies and decomposes (eggs released to the soil) or is eaten by secondary hosts or predators or scavengers.

© Springer Nature Singapore Pte Ltd. 2024
K. G. Narayan et al., *Handbook of Management of Zoonoses*,
https://doi.org/10.1007/978-981-99-9885-2_107

Cannibalism may be one of the mechanisms of transmission among rodents. The process of release of unembryonated eggs into the environment and becoming infectious makes human infection uncommon.

Spurious infection occurs when unembryonated eggs that are not infectious are ingested and passed into the faeces.

True infection occurs when the embryonated ova are ingested by rodents. The larvae hatch in the small intestines and penetrate the portal vein to reach the liver, where they form adult worms and copulate. The fertilized female deposits unembryonated eggs in the hepatic parenchyma.

107.1.3   Hosts

The hosts of *C. hepatica* are rodents (>70 species), rabbits, eastern chipmunks, squirrels, moles, shrews, opossums, weasels, skunks, foxes, prairie dogs, dogs, cats, pigs, monkeys, and humans. Approximately 90% of rats are infected with *Capillaria* species (Yadav et al. 2016). Humans are the accidental hosts.

107.1.4   Mode of Infection in Humans

Humans are incidental hosts and get infected by ingesting infective embryonated eggs in contaminated soil, water, and food. Soil-to-mouth contact is common in children (1–5) years, so infection is common in children.

Upon ingestion of embryonated eggs (infectious) by a suitable mammalian host, e.g. human, the eggs hatch; release larvae, which invade the intestinal mucosa; and migrate through the mesenteric and portal veins to the liver, where maturity takes place in about 4 weeks (true infection). Following mating, females lay eggs, which remain in the liver.

107.1.5   Infection

Poor hygienic conditions and the presence of rodents increase the risk of infection. Sixty per cent of cases reported are in children less than 8 years of age, the youngest being an 11-month-old male. Frequent soil-hand-mouth contact explains the increased susceptibility in children (Misra et al. 2019). Pica is a risk factor. Misra et al. (2019) reported both pica and exposure to rodent-infested granaries in a case in a village in India. The ages of the cases in the three reports were 14, 18, and 24 months (Nabi et al. 2007; Yadav et al. 2016; Misra et al. 2019). Females are more infected than males, and most patients are from a very low socio-economic class.

According to Misra et al. (2019), over 78 human cases of spurious infection have been reported from South America and China. *C. hepatica* eggs in human stool do not indicate true infection. The ingestion of liver from infected animals might harmlessly result in the passage of eggs. Only six of 74 cases of true infection reported worldwide have been from India, five from Maharashtra and one from Uttar Pradesh (Misra et al. 2019).

According to Nabi et al. (2007), 16/37 cases were children (mostly 1–5 years), including two from India. Pica is an important accompanied complaint, possibly also contributing to soil exposure and consequential infection. Anaemia and hypergammaglobulinemia occur. The case described by them was a 14-month-old child diagnosed with pyrexia of unknown origin running for a month.

C. hepatica invades the liver, lays eggs, and induces an inflammatory response. Granuloma forms around the worm.

In 40–60 days, the adult worms die. The disintegrating worms release cytokines, which induce an eosinophil-rich inflammatory and fibrotic response in the liver.

107.1.6 Pathogenesis

C. hepatica induces granuloma in the liver parenchyma. The granulomas are eosinophilic multifocal, discrete, and confluent. Dense mononuclear cells and eosinophils are seen surrounding the granulomas. The wandering nematode damages the liver tissue and causes consequential functional loss. Massive necrosis of the liver parenchyma and advanced fibrosis could be lethal. In early cases, only immature worms are seen. In advanced cases, adult parasites and eggs are seen scattered in the liver parenchyma. The adult worms disappear over time, and multifocal fibrosis is seen.

107.1.7 Symptoms

According to Yadav et al. (2016), hepatic capillariasis presents with a typical triad of symptoms: persistent fever, hepatomegaly, and leukocytosis with eosinophilia. Pica is an important presenting complaint.

Symptoms include persistent fever, 40 °C (pyrexia of unknown origin); leucocytosis; eosinophilia; anaemia; hypergammaglobulinemia; hepatomegaly; hepatitis; hepatolithiasis; liver dysfunction [high serum levels of alanine amino-transferase (ALT), aspartate amino-transferase (AST), and lactic dehydrogenase (LDH)]; and loss of body weight. The presence of non-specific symptoms causes difficulty in identifying hepatic capillariasis. Sometimes larvae may migrate to the lungs, kidneys, and other organs.

Wang et al. (2019) systematically analyzed 16 cases of *C. capillariasis* recorded during 2011–2017 in China. Clinical presentation included sustained fever (56.25%), respiratory disorder (37.5%), abdominal pain (37.5%), diarrhoea (25%), leukocytosis (93.75%) and eosinophilia (100%). On investigation, >60% had elevated hepatic enzymes and proteins, suggestive of cirrhosis of the liver. Scattered parasitic granuloma in the liver was detected on ultrasound and magnetic resonance imaging (MRI). A liver biopsy revealed parasite eggs, necrotized parasitic granulomas, and septal fibrosis.

The prognosis depends upon the amount of damage to the liver tissues. Hepatic failure and death may take place if a liver transplant is not undertaken.

C. hepatica infection can be serious and lethal. Persistent febrile hepatomegaly with eosinophilia should alert and need an aggressive search for the liver lesion and cause be made.

107.1.8 Diagnosis

Kazemi Aghdam et al. (2015) reported a case of hepatic capillariasis in a 4-year-old boy in Iran. It illustrates the process of diagnosis. He was admitted to the hospital with high-grade fever, chills, and a weight loss of about 1.5 kg in 2 months. Physical examination detected hepatomegaly. A liver ultrasound was done. It showed a relatively well defined but irregular isoechoic mass with a hypoechoic periphery measuring 58 × 51 × 47 mm in the VII segment of the right lobe, suggestive of an abscess. Core needle biopsy strongly suggested parasitic infection.

Definite diagnosis is through liver biopsy and the identification of *C. hepatica* ova (Misra et al. 2019). It is based on finding adults and eggs in biopsy or autopsy specimens. A serological test using an immunofluorescence test (IFT) is also recommended.

107.1.9 Treatment

Thiabendazole, albendazole, and ivermectin are useful. Treatment may be long—3 months. Steroids may be required sometimes to resolve hepatitis.

107.1.10 Prevention

Proper hygiene and proper disposal of faecal matter are important, as well as washing hands with soap and water after touching soil or working in the garden, washing fruits and vegetables, and cooking fish before eating.

107.2   Intestinal Capillariasis

Intestinal capillariasis is a zoonotic parasitic gastrointestinal (GI) disease. The first human case of intestinal capillariasis was diagnosed in 1963 by Chitwood et al. (1964) during an autopsy of a male patient from Ilocos Norte province, northern Luzon, in the Philippines. This disease can take a serious turn if not treated because of auto-infection and protein-losing enteropathy with consequential complications like severe emaciation, cachexia, cardiomyopathy, and death.

107.2.1   Aetiology

Intestinal capillariasis is caused by a tiny nematode, *Capillaria philippinensis*; females measure 2.5–5.3 mm, and males are 1.3–3.9 mm.

Auto-infection may lead to hyper-infection (a massive number of adult worms). Other embryonated eggs are evacuated with faeces in water, which are eaten by freshwater fish, wherein they develop into the infective stage larvae in 3 weeks. Birds and humans get infected upon the ingestion of fish. Adults develop in 2 weeks in the human gut, mate, and produce thick-shelled eggs.

107.2.2   Geographical Distribution

Intestinal capillariasis is a zoonosis commonly infecting those consuming raw or undercooked fish containing the larvae of *C. philippinensis*.

The Philippine epidemic in 1967–1968 involved 1300 cases and the death of 90 confirmed cases. Also, in an outbreak in 1978–1979, 50 persons were infected. It is endemic in the Philippines and Thailand but has also been reported in Egypt, Korea, Taiwan, Iran, India, Japan, Italy, and Spain. However, the major outbreaks have occurred in the Philippines and Thailand. The annual epidemiological reports of Thailand from 1994 to 2006 had 82 accumulated cases of intestinal capillariasis (Saichua et al. 2008). A rapid lateral-flow immunochromatographic test was used for screening 292 patients with chronic diarrhoea for intestinal capillariasis in a hospital in Thailand, and 22.6% were positive (Prasongdee et al. 2022). According to Abdelsalama et al. (2012), cases have also been reported from Egypt, Iran, India, and Colombia.

Buri Ram in Thailand presented a high prevalence of intestinal capillariasis, totalling 24 cases from 1994 to 2006. About half of all cases had consumed raw or undercooked fish (Saichua et al. 2008). In a study of patients during 2001–2013 in Thailand, Limsrivilai et al. (2014) observed that the affected people were from rural areas of Thailand and habitually ate raw freshwater fish. An increasing rate of immigration from rural to urban explained the detection of infection among those living in urban areas. Cases have occurred in individuals who denied ever eating raw or undercooked fish, especially from non-endemic areas. A possible explanation is a contamination in the kitchen with the uncooked visceral content of fish. The patient is usually a 20–50-year-old. Adiraju et al. (2015) reported a case of a woman agricultural labourer of 40 years.

C. philippinensis was first described in Egypt in 1989. About 84% of Egyptian patients were women, mostly housewives. Some reportedly consumed partially cooked fish. However, the largest group reported preparing fish, and this raises the possibility of carrying the infective stage under the fingernails after fish evisceration (Abdelsalama et al. 2012).

107.2.3   Pathogenesis-Pathology

The definitive hosts are fish-eating birds. Humans are infected when they ingest raw or insufficiently cooked freshwater fish. The parasite is a tiny nematode that can multiply fast. Thousands of worms invade the intestine to cause enteropathy (large number/litre of intestinal content in autopsy). Jejunum is the most affected. A heavy cellular infiltration around the adult worm and larvae may be observed.

The parasite has the unusual ability to multiply within the host, and female parasites can produce infectious larvae, which can lead to auto-infection and massive parasite burden in the small bowel. The adult nematodes cause induration and villous atrophy, leading to protein-losing enteropathy and cachexia. There is chronic non-specific inflammation, partial villous atrophy of crypts, and flattening of the villi as these invade and denude the villi mucosa and mucosal glands and infiltrate the lamina propria. Inflammatory cells infiltrate. Adiraju et al. (2015) observed erosive antral gastritis through upper GI endoscopy. Colonoscopy revealed sub-epithelial haemorrhages in the ascending and transverse colon, scattered erosive mucosal lesions with loss of villi, and whitish exudates in the distal ileum. Worms can be seen in the intestinal mucosal surface and lumen in sections stained with haematoxylin and eosin.

107.2.4   Symptoms

Chronic diarrhoea may extend for months. The frequency of loose, watery yellowish stools per day may be 10–15 times. There may be colicky abdominal pain, distension and borborygmus, vomiting non-bilious, non-projectile, and swelling of feet, which gradually progresses to generalized body swelling, anasarca, ascites, cachexia, and dehydration. There is malabsorption, protein and electrolyte loss, and hypoalbuminemia. Electrolyte loss may result in heart failure and/or septic shock.

Based on a retrospective study of 26 patients at Siraj Hospital, Bangkok, Thailand, Limsrivilai et al. (2014) reported that 93% had chronic diarrhoea and 70%

had chronic abdominal pain. All had hypoalbuminemia (most had <2 g/dL), 92% experienced a loss of weight, and 50% had anaemia. The duration of illness ranged between 1 and 60 months, with a median of 5.5 months. The parasite was detected in 57% of the patients' stools. The remaining patients were diagnosed by tissue biopsies from endoscopies, esophagogastroduodenoscopies, colonoscopies, enteroscopies, and balloon-assisted enteroscopies. The jejunum and proximal ileum had a scalloping appearance, mucosal cracking, and redness of the mucosa. Fold thickening, fold effacement, and increased luminal fluid are seen in 80% of the patients, mainly at the distal jejunum and ileum. Sixty per cent of the patients showed clinical features of generalized malabsorption. Fifty per cent had anaemia.

Carmel Kasher et al. (2022) reported the first case from Israel. He was a Thai. He had severe leg oedema, which appeared 1 year earlier. This case was working for 2 months in 2019 when he was admitted. He had anasarca and progressive weakness. Examination revealed that he had severe hypoalbuminemia and microcytic anaemia without eosinophilia, and liver and renal functions were within normal ranges. Ascites were detected by computed tomography (CT) scan. Colonoscopy and histology showed terminal ileitis with erosions and villi flattening. Additional biopsies demonstrated active inflammation, severe atrophy of the intestinal villi, infiltration of plasma cells, eosinophils in the lamina propria, and round small diameter bodies (30–50 µ) suspected as a helminth's larvae. Polymerase chain reaction (PCR) confirmed it was capillariasis.

107.2.5 *Diagnosis*

- Radiographic (barium), conventional endoscopic, and video capsule endoscopic methods have assisted in definitive diagnosis.
- Stool examination, though less sensitive, showed numerous peanut-shaped eggs with flattened bipolar plugs; the subsequent examination of stools showed dead adult worms.
- Eggs, larvae, and/or adult worms are also found in intestinal biopsies.
- Enzyme-linked immunosorbent assay (ELISA): Abdel-Rahman et al. (2019) evaluated a *Capillaria* spp. adult worm crude antigen extracted from freshwater fish in the serodiagnosis of human capillariasis using enzyme-linked immunosorbent assay (ELISA). This antigen was able to detect anti-*Capillaria* antibodies in the sera of infected cases but showed no reactivity with any of the healthy control sera. However, Khalifa et al. (2020) found ELISA for the detection of copro-antigen to be a sensitive test but not specific.
- Lateral-flow immunochromatographic test: Prasongdee et al. (2022) suggested that a rapid lateral-flow immunochromatographic test (available as a kit) was useful for the detection of intestinal capillariasis among chronic diarrhoeal cases in endemic areas.

- Nested PCR to identify parasite copro-DNA offers a satisfactory sensitive and specific method for the detection of infection in clinically suspected patients, which is superior to coproscopy and copro-ELISA antigen detection (Khalifa et al. 2020).

107.2.6   Treatment

Albendazole or ivermectin has a good response in curing patients.

107.2.7   Prevention

The health education campaign aims to promote the consumption of cooked fish, the avoidance of defecation into a water resource, and the early diagnosis of cases, which are necessary to minimize and eliminate *C. philippinensis* infection.

107.3   Pulmonary Capillariasis

Pulmonary capillariasis is an infection of the lungs and airways. It is also known as bronchial capillariasis (Capillaria aerophila) or sometimes referred as Thominxosis (Thominx aerophilum).

It is a zoonotic diagnostically challenging disease caused by *Capillaria aerophila*, which is widely distributed. It is a parasite found in dogs, cats, and other carnivores and omnivores, causing pulmonary capillariasis. The occurrence is rare (https://www.bibliovet.net/node/247).

107.3.1   Life Cycle

The tiny worm is about 2.4–3 cm long. The females lay eggs, which are coughed up and swallowed and reach the pharynx. The non-embryonated eggs travel the entire gut and escape with faeces. These embryonate (internal larvae) in an external environment in 5–7 weeks and remain viable for up to 1 year. Facultative hosts, like earthworms, and receptive vertebrate hosts ingest them; the latter can ingest earthworms, too. The infective larvae cross the gastrointestinal mucosa and travel through the lymphatics to reach the lung parenchyma. It takes them 1–2 months after infection to mature into adult worms. The life cycle is completed without the facultative host, earthworm. The parasite has a direct life cycle.

107.3.2   Epidemiology

Pulmonary capillariasis is extremely rare. It is also an under-diagnosed, poorly recognized human infection due to clinicopathological mimicry and the lack of accurate, robust laboratory diagnostics.

It is prevalent in Europe and North America. Cases from Australia and New Zealand, Asia, Russia, and South America have been reported.

A wide range of wild and domesticated animals, including dogs, cats, foxes, coyotes, racoons, etc., are infected, usually without symptoms. Infected animals (pets) suffer from nasal discharge, sneezing, breathing difficulty, dry or productive cough, and chronic bronchitis and may die of bronchopneumonia and secondary bacterial infection.

C. aerophila is likely to be more common in areas where there are increased chances of infection in cats and dogs. Soil is seeded with worm's eggs. These survive in the external environment and the facultative host, earthworm. Such environmental conditions increase the chance of infection of more cats, dogs, and foxes. These animals abound in peri-urban and even urban zones.

107.3.3   Mode of Infection

The ingestion of eggs contained in an infected animal's sputum or faeces causes infection. Human exposure to infected dogs or cats, certain wild animals' faeces, or soil contaminated by their faeces, salivary secretions, or sputum may cause infection. Drinking untreated water and the consumption of soil-contaminated water and unwashed raw fruits and vegetables are likely modes of infection.

Human-to-human transmission may rarely happen through exposure to the sputum or faeces of infected humans. Poor sanitation and toilet facilities and poor personal hygiene are risk factors.

107.3.4   Pathogenesis

The parasite can infect all age groups and both sexes. There is no racial or ethnic predilection. Upon ingestion, the eggs develop into larvae in the human intestine. These migrate to the respiratory system. *C. aerophila* parasitizes the mucosa of the trachea, bronchi, bronchioles, lungs, and rarely the frontal sinus and nose. It causes inflammation, tracheitis, bronchitis, rhinitis, and sinusitis. Secondary bacterial infection may occur.

107.3.5   Symptoms

Fever, runny nose, sneezing, dyspnoea, cough, catarrhal expectorates, and haemoptysis may occur. It may result in pneumonia, episodes of asthma, and eosinophilia. Medical examination reveals vesicular murmur, nasal discharge, dry cough, bronchial-vesicular breath sounds, and wheezing.

Aftandelians et al. (1977) reported a case of a 9-year-old boy in Tehran, Iran. He had asthma, a productive cough, and moderate eosinophilia. A lung biopsy detected a nematode- *Capillaria aerophila* in a granulomatous lesion.

A Serbian woman patient was considered for bronchial sarcoma on computed tomography. A pulmonary biopsy revealed parasite eggs to confirm the diagnosis (Laloševic et al. 2001).

Complications are rare. There may be acute bronchitis, hyper-infection (repeat infection by the host larvae present in the body), and secondary bacterial infection (https://www.dovemed.com/diseases-conditions/pulmonary-capillariasis/).

107.3.6   Diagnosis

• Demonstration of the typical eggs of the parasite in the mucus, bronchial lavage fluid.
• A microscopic examination of stool samples may also reveal eggs.
• Semi-nested PCR—sensitivity 97–100% and specificity 100% (Di Cesare et al. 2012).

107.3.7   Treatment

Administration of broad-spectrum anthelmintics, such as ivermectin, fenbendazole, or levamisole, kills the parasite.

References

Abdel-Rahman SM, Bakir HY, Othman RA, Khalifa MM (2019) Evaluation of fish *Capillaria* spp. antigen in diagnosis of human intestinal capillariasis. J Adv Parasitol 6(1):1–6

Abdelsalama N, Hassanya SM, Medhata A, Husseinb HI, Blum HE (2012) *Capillaria philippinensis*: a cause of chronic diarrhoea in upper Egypt. J Arab Soc Med Res 7:10–13

Adiraju K, Yarlagadda PH, Kalwa D (2015) Human intestinal capillariasis: a case report. Inter J Sci Res 4(1):2558–2560

Aftandelians R, Raafat F, Taffazoli M, Beaver PC (1977) Pulmonary capillariasis in a child in Iran. Am J Trop Med Hyg 26(1):64–71

Chitwood MB, Valesquez C, Salazar NG (1964) Physiologic changes in a species of Capillaria (Trichuroidae) causing a fatal cases of human intestinal capillariasis. Proc Int Congr Parasitol 2:797

Di Cesare A, Castagna G, Otranto D, Meloni S, Milillo P et al (2012) Molecular detection of *Capillaria aerophila*, an agent of canine and feline pulmonary capillariosis. J Clin Microbiol 50(6):1958–1963

Kasher C, Grossman T, Vainer J, Yanovskay A et al (2022) First case of imported *Capillaria philippinensis* in Israel. J Travel Med 29(1):taab132

Kazemi Aghdam M, Karimi A, Amanati A, Ghoroubi J, Khoddami M et al (2015) *Capillaria hepatica,* A case report and review of the literatures. Arch Pediatr Infect Dis 3(2):e19398

Khalifa MM, Abdel-Rahman SM, Bakir HY, Othman RA, El-Mokhtar MA (2020) Comparison of the diagnostic performance of microscopic examination, Copro-ELISA, and Copro-PCR in the diagnosis of *Capillaria philippinensis* infections. PLoS One 15(6):e0234746

Laloševic D, Dimitrijevic S, Jovanovic M, Klun I (2001) Pulmonary aelurostrongylosis in cats. Vet Glas 55:181–185

Limsrivilai J, Pongprasobchai S, Apisarnthanarak P, Manatsathit S (2014) Intestinal capillariasis in the 21st century: clinical presentations and role of endoscopy and imaging. BMC Gastroenterol 14:207

Misra S, Nanda P, Nandan D, Sakhuja P (2019) Casee report: *Capillaria hepatica*: report from North India. Trop Gastroenterol 40(3):118–120

Nabi F, Palaha HK, Sekhsaria D, Chiatale A (2007) *Capillaria hepatica* infestation. Indian Pediatr 44(10):781–782

Prasongdee TK, Seesui K, Sadee P et al (2022) Prevalence of intestinal capillariasis in chronic diarrhoea patients in Thailand: serologic screening using a rapid lateral-flow immunochromotagraphic assay. Am J Trop Med Hyg 107(2):370–372

Saichua P, Nithikathkul C, Kaewpitoon N (2008) Human intestinal capillariasis in Thailand. World J Gastroenterol 14(4):506–510

Wang L, Zhang Y, Deng Y, Li X, Zheng X, Wang F, Zou Y (2019) Clinical and laboratory characterizations of hepatic capillariasis. Acta Trop 193:206–210

Yadav SC, Sathe PA, Ghodke RK (2016) Hepatic capillariasis: a rare parasitic infection. Indian J Pathol Microbiol 59:124–125

Chapter 108
Dracunculiasis

Synonyms

Dracunculosis, Dracontiasis, Guinea worm disease, Medina vein, Medina worm disease.

Dracunculiasis is classified as a neglected tropical disease. The name dracunculiasis is derived from the Latin word 'affliction with little dragons', while the name 'guinea worm' appeared after Europeans saw the disease on the Guinea coast of West Africa in the seventeenth century. Guinea worm disease (GWD) is one of the oldest known human parasitic diseases. It is a painful and debilitating disease widespread in humans in sub-Saharan Africa and southern Asia. It primarily affects poor, rural communities and has an enormous adverse impact on agricultural production and school attendance. Infection is close to being eradicated. Guinea worm disease derived its common name from its prevalence in the Gulf of Guinea.

108.1 Aetiology

Dracunculiasis is caused by the nematode *Dracunculus medinensis*, which has been known since Egyptian times. The life cycle of the parasite was fully described by Alexei Fedchenko in 1870.

Dracunculus medinensis, one of the 14 valid species of the genus *Dracunculus*, superfamily Dracunculoidea, family Dracunculidae, is one of the longest (female worm up to 100 cm, males 16–40 mm) known nematodes that parasitizes subcutaneous tissues of mammals and reptiles. The males are rarely seen in patients as they die immediately after copulation. Persian physicians called it by a variety of names, including Medina vein, considering it a rotten vein. Bastian in 1863 conclusively demonstrated that it was a worm and gave the scientific name *Dracunculus*

© Springer Nature Singapore Pte Ltd. 2024   1037
K. G. Narayan et al., *Handbook of Management of Zoonoses*,
https://doi.org/10.1007/978-981-99-9885-2_108

medinensis, incorporating the word for dragon with Medina, and Sir John Tennent in 1868 gave the common name Guinea worm (Tayeh et al. 2017).

108.2   Life Cycle

Historically, it has been reported that *Cyclops* is the only intermediate host and water is the only source of infection to man.

The female *Dracunculus* matures in definitive vertebrate hosts. In the subcutaneous tissue of the definitive hosts (human), these form blisters primarily on the distal extremities. When the host places the affected area in water, the blister will erupt and the female will release nearly 500,000 first-stage larvae (L1) into the water. The process of release occurs many times and during different events.

The intermediate hosts are cyclopoid copepods, which consume L1. The L1 larvae mature (moult) to L3, which is the infective stage.

The definitive hosts get infected upon ingesting L3 within the copepods. Domestic dogs, domestic ferrets, and humans are definitive hosts.

108.3   Transmission

Humans become infected when they drink water contaminated with intermediate hosts, *Cyclops* or water fleas (copepods), harbouring the infective larvae. After a prolonged pre-patent period of approximately a year, the under-skin migrant female of *D. medinensis* (Guinea worm) causes, first, a blister and then an ulcer, mainly in the lower limbs. At the infection site, one or more worms emerge, giving a burning sensation. To soothe this, patients often immerse the infected part of the body in water, or when an infected person enters water, through the ulcer, a milky fluid is exuded from the female uterus containing hundreds of thousands of first-stage larvae, which remain alive for about 72 h in the water. These are ingested by cyclopoid crustaceans, also called water fleas. The larvae develop best between 25 and 30 °C in about 12–14 days and will not develop at all below 19 °C (Muller 1979).

108.4   Disease

In the course of the disease, burning blisters follow the subcutaneously located mature female worm. The blisters burst following the immersion of the legs in the water. The ulcers heal rapidly. The disease is incapacitating. There is severe cellulitis, especially when worms are damaged in tissues around the joints. Abscesses and ulcers continue for months if the number of worms is large. Permanent disability is a possibility from ankylosis of joints or contraction of tendons. Secondary infection is common. Repeated infection year after year may occur (Muller 1979).

108.5 Epidemiology

Infective stage larvae (L3) of *D. medinensis* in cyclops ingested with drinking water by human resulted in emmergence resulted in emergence of adult female worm after a prolonged prepatent period which produces painful ulcers that can impair mobility for up to several weeks. This disease occurs annually when agricultural activities are at their peak. A large proportion of economically productive individuals may be affected simultaneously, resulting in decreased agricultural productivity and economic hardship. Infection is limited to tropical and subtropical regions.

108.5.1 Geographical Distribution

D. medinensis was historically widespread in Africa and South Asia. During the mid-1980s, an estimated 3.5 million cases of dracunculiasis occurred in 20 countries worldwide, 17 countries of which were in Africa. The number of reported cases fell to fewer than 10,000 cases for the first time in 2007, dropping further to 542 cases (2012). Over the past 8 years, human cases have stayed at double digits: 28 in 2018 and a slightly higher number of 54 human cases in 2019. Infection is currently limited to Sudan, Ghana, Mali, Nigeria, and Niger. The majority of infections are in Sudan, where continuing civil disturbance has caused a problem in operations, and Ghana.

108.5.2 Source of Infection

Chippaux and Massougbodji (1991) conducted a prospective study in four villages in the central part of Benin. Dracunculiasis could be introduced or maintained by a few patients in a community. The duration of Guinea worm latency in humans lasted from 10 to 13 months. The smallest density of cyclopids able to induce steady transmission was evaluated to ten cyclopids per 10 L of water. There is no transmission when there is less than one susceptible copepod per litre in the pond. It was observed that village ponds acted as sites, which extended transmission over the dry season (from November to April). Reservoir dams induced a short-period transmission at the beginning of the dry season (from October to January). Dracunculiasis is not transmitted in flowing water sources such as rivers or streams.

Drinking water taken from stationary water bodies like ponds, large open wells, step wells, or rain-filled cisterns offers suitable conditions for infection.

Stagnant sources of drinking water such as ponds, cisterns, pools in dried-up riverbeds, temporary hand-dug wells, and step wells, commonly harbour populations of copepods and are sites of infection and transmission. The infected *Cyclops* become less and less active. At this stage, they are not able to move more than a few centimetres from the bottom of the water source, which, in turn, favours the completion of the life cycle of the parasite (Galán-Puchades 2019).

Seasonal variation closely related to rainfall has been reported. In arid areas, the incidence is higher during the rainy season, when surface water is available, whereas in wet regions, transmission occurs more during the dry season, when sources of drinking water are limited.

The incidence varies by sex, age, and occupation and by village and country, which relates to sources of drinking water.

108.5.3   Changing Epidemiology

The epidemiology appears changing. Domestic dogs and domestic ferrets are added to the list of definitive hosts of *D. medinensis*. The infective stage larva L3 was recovered from a wild-caught frog (*Phrynobatrachus francisci*) in Chad. Green frogs (*Lithobates clamitans*) have been experimentally infected with *D. medinensis* worms. The frogs can serve as natural paratenic hosts in endemic countries in Africa (Eberhard et al. 2016; Cleveland et al. 2018), increasing the environment and opportunity for human exposure and infection. According to Galán-Puchades (2019), dracunculiasis would be a food-borne zoonosis in addition to being exclusively a waterborne anthroponosis. Animal reservoirs, mainly dogs but also cats and baboons, and possibly a new food-borne route of transmission through the ingestion of paratenic (frogs) or transport (fish) hosts have been identified. A large number of infected dogs, mainly in Chad, and a low number of infected humans have given rise to this potential food-borne transmission. Dracunculiasis is on the verge of eradication. The measures have exclusively aimed at the waterborne route. Control measures aimed at dogs (or at other potential reservoirs) should be added in the form of detection of infection and treatment.

108.6   Prevention, Control, and Eradication

108.6.1   Community Level Measures

The foci of infection of dracunculiasis in the Middle East and South Asia have been eliminated using the following strategies at the community level:

- Heightening surveillance to detect every case within 24 h of the emergence of worms.
- Preventing transmission from each worm by treatment and regular cleaning and bandaging of the affected areas of the skin until the worm is completely expelled from the body.
- Preventing the contamination of drinking water by not allowing infected people with emerging worms to wade into water.

- Ensuring wider access to improved drinking water supplies.
- Filtering or boiling water from open water bodies before drinking.
- Implementing vector control by using the larvicide temephos.
- Promoting health education and behavioural change.

108.6.2 Intensive Control

Intensive control efforts for dracunculiasis began in 1981, and early success led to a World Health Assembly resolution to eradicate the disease. The eradication strategy is to interrupt transmission to humans by preventing the ingestion of the minute cyclopoid crustacean containing the larval parasites. Continued active surveillance and the mapping of infected villages, followed by implementation of the eradication strategy, are required in order to complete eradication.

The main strategies of the Global Dracunculiasis Eradication Campaign rely on identifying communities with endemic diseases, restricting the movement of active cases (thereby preventing the contamination of drinking water sources), and educating the population to avoid drinking contaminated water. Vector control through the use of insecticide on unsafe sources of drinking water to control the copepod population (the intermediate host) also helps.

108.6.3 The Road to Eradication

In May 1981, the Interagency Steering Committee for Cooperative Action for the International Drinking Water Supply and Sanitation Decade (1981–1990) proposed the elimination of dracunculiasis as an indicator of the success of the decade. In the same year, the World Health Organization (WHO) decision-making body the World Health Assembly adopted resolution WHA 34.25, recognizing that the International Drinking Water Supply and Sanitation Decade presented an opportunity to eliminate dracunculiasis. In 1986, The Carter Center joined the battle against the disease and, in partnership with WHO and the United Nations Children's Fund (UNICEF), has since been at the forefront of eradication activities. This led the WHO and the United States Centres for Disease Control and Prevention to formulate the strategy and technical guidelines for an eradication campaign. To give it a final push, in 2011, the World Health Assembly called on all Member States where dracunculiasis is endemic to expedite the interruption of transmission and enforce nationwide surveillance to ensure the eradication of dracunculiasis.

Seven countries have already eradicated the disease, namely Pakistan (1993), Kenya (1994), India (1996), Cameroon, Senegal and Yemen (1997), and Chad (1998), since the beginning of the Global Dracunculiasis Eradication Campaign in 1981 (Greenaway 2004).

References

Chippaux JP, Massougbodji A (1991) Aspects épidémiologiques de la dracunculose au Bénin. 2. Relations entre la périodicité des émergences et l'origine de l'eau de boisson [epidemiological aspects of dracunculosis in Benin. 2. Relationship between periodicity of worm eruptions and the origin of drinking water]. Bull Soc Pathol Exot 84(4):351–357

Cleveland CA, Garrett KB, Cozad RA, Williams BM et al (2018) The wild world of Guinea Worms: a review of the genus *Dracunculus* in wildlife. Int J Parasitol Parasites Wildl 7(3):289–300

Eberhard ML, Cleveland CA, Zirimwabagabo H, Yabsley MJ et al (2016) Guinea worm (*Dracunculus medinensis*) infection in a wild-caught frog. Chad Emerg Infect Dis 22(11):1961–1962

Galán-Puchades MT (2019) Dracunculiasis: water-borne anthroponosis vs. food-borne zoonosis. J Helminthol 94:e76

Greenaway C (2004) Dracunculiasis (Guinea worm disease). CMAJ 170(4):495–500

Muller R (1979) Guinea worm disease: epidemiology, control, and treatment. Bull World Health Organ 57(5):683–689

Tayeh A, Cairncross S, Cox FEG (2017) Guinea Worm: from Robert Leiper to eradicaion. Parasitol 144:1643–48

Chapter 109
Gnathostomiasis

This nematode has been reported from East Asia, especially Thailand and Japan, also from Korea, Cambodia, Laos, Indonesia, the Philippines, Malaysia, India, Australia, Mexico, Ecuador, Guatemala, and Peru. Gnathostomiasis is uncommon, though increasingly reported because of common international travel and the popularity of raw and undercooked/fish or meat preparations. The number of reports of autochthonous cases is increasing.

109.1   Aetiology

According to Diaz (2015), the six zoonotic species of *Gnathostoma*, their endemic distribution, and the hosts are as follows:

1. *G. binucleatum*: Central and South America—wild and domestic cats and dogs.
2. *G. doloresi*: Japan and Southeast Asia—wild and likely domestic pigs.
3. *G. hispidum*: China, Korea, Japan, Southeast Asia, Australia, and Central America—wild and domestic pigs.
4. *G. malaysiae*: Japan and Southeast Asia—rats.
5. *G. nipponicum*: Japan and Korea—weasels.
6. *G. spinigerum*: China, Japan, Southeast Asia, India, Central America, South America, and East Africa (Botswana, Zambia)—wild and domestic cats and dogs.

Of these, *G. spinigerum* is the most commonly reported and is usually isolated from cats and dogs in Asia. The condition has been named variously—the migratory/wandering swellings have been referred to as Yangtze River oedema in China, tuao chid in Japan, and paniculitis nodular migratoria eosinophilica in Latin America (Diaz 2015). Other names are larva migrans profundus, nodular migratory eosinophilic panniculitis (Ecuador), and wandering swelling.

© Springer Nature Singapore Pte Ltd. 2024
K. G. Narayan et al., *Handbook of Management of Zoonoses*,
https://doi.org/10.1007/978-981-99-9885-2_109

G. binucleatum is endemic in some Latin American countries (Mexico, Ecuador, and Peru). It is a public health problem in Mexico, where a large number of cases were reported in 2010 (Eiras et al. 2018).

109.2   Life Cycle

Gnathostomes have a complex life cycle. Three hosts are required: (1) a freshwater copepod ingests eggs shed by adults, (2) the larvae mature in a wide range of fish and other aquatic intermediate hosts, and (3) the adult worm develops in definitive vertebrate hosts.

Natural definitive hosts are cats, dogs, wild carnivores, and adult worms residing in their gastric mucosa. In the gastric mucosa, a tumour is formed with an opening, through which eggs pass out into water and faeces. Eggs develop into L1 in a week, and hatched larvae are eaten by minute crustaceans, *Cyclops* (also called copepods, the first intermediate hosts). The L1 larvae penetrate the gastric wall, migrate through the body cavity, and mature into L2 and early L3 larvae. The second intermediate hosts—fish, frogs, snakes, poultry, and pigs—consume the copepods. The L2 and early L3 larvae penetrate the gastric wall and migrate to reach the muscles, wherein they all mature to infective stage L3 and encyst. The definitive hosts eating an infested muscle get infected. The larvae excyst in the stomach, penetrate the gastric mucosa, and migrate, passing through the liver to the connective tissues and muscles, finally returning to the stomach in 4 weeks, and forming a tumour. It takes 6–8 months (or 8–12 months after initial ingestion) for worms to mature, mate, and pass eggs.

It is postulated that fishermen feed their domestic animals (cats and dogs) with decaying fish, not suitable for human consumption but contaminated with L3 larvae. The parasite matures, mates, and passes eggs in their faeces to contaminate rivers and estuary water.

109.3   Mode of Infection

Humans get infected by ingesting the L3 of the nematode present in the undercooked meat of pigs, chickens, freshwater fish, snails, or frogs or contaminated water. The infective dose is as small as a single infective stage larva.

Though rare, penetration of the skin is another mode of infection. There is a possibility of prenatal transmission in humans. The larvae continue to migrate in the body for several years (10–12) without returning to the stomach, and hence, faecal examination does not reveal eggs.

109.4 Epidemiology

There is an increasing array of such infections that were not known in temperate regions because of international travel. One such infection is *Gnathostoma spinigerum*, which is acquired by eating uncooked food infected with the third-stage larva of a helminth; such food typically includes fish, shrimp, crab, crayfish, frog, or chicken (Moore et al. 2003).

Diaz (2015) reviewed the reports on gnathostomiasis. Citizens of various countries get infected when travelling to places where *G. spinigerum* is endemic. These are Laos, Thailand, Hong Kong, Myanmar, Bangladesh, Peru, Mexico, Central America, Zambia, Botswana, and South Africa. Autochthonous cases have been reported from Japan, China, Korea, Mexico, the United States, and Brazil, suggesting new areas or the expansion of the parasite.

According to Bravo and Gontijo (2018), the highest incidence is observed in Japan, China, India, Sri Lanka, and Southeast Asian countries like Indonesia, the Philippines, Malaysia, and Vietnam. Travelers to Africa are likely to get infected. Infection was reportedly associated with low socio-economic group; in contrast most cases in Peru consumed ceviche in high-class neighbourhood.

The parasite could be imported with fish; e.g., swamp eels imported from Asia to the United States infected the freshwater eels raised in the United States, explaining the occurrence of autochthonous cases in non-endemic areas.

109.5 Pathogenesis

The infective larva has a round mouth with hooks and a grinding apparatus. The parasite perforates the gastric or intestinal mucosa and reaches the peritoneal cavity, causing mechanical tissue damage, inducing acute abdominal pain, or migrating through the liver. It secretes compounds such as analogues of acetylcholine, a hyaluronidase-containing spreading factor; proteolytic enzymes; and haemolytic substances. There is a combined pathophysiological effect. The characteristic haemorrhagic 'worm track' is thus formed, seen in the liver and brain during imaging studies and post-mortem examinations. The larva has the potential to perforate the pleura and lungs, causing pleurodynia, hemoptysis, and pneumothorax. Migration through tissues causes trauma, inflammatory reactions, and eosinophilia. They wander (1 cm/h) either in the deep fat tissue level or at a more superficial dermal level in bouts.

109.6   Symptoms

The incubation period seems to be short. The initial symptoms—malaise, fever, anorexia, nausea, vomiting, and epigastric pain—are followed by painful pruritic erythematous swellings, which appear within 24–48 h of ingestion. The migrating larvae invade the gastric and/or intestinal wall during this time. Eosinophilia develops.

Gnathostomiasis is a long-term infection, 10–12 years, and causes significant morbidity as it can involve any part of the body. The clinical forms in humans are cutaneous, visceral, neurological, and ocular, depending upon the migration of the L3 larvae. Migration through the subcutaneous tissues causes intermittent, painful pruritic, and erythematous swelling (cutaneous larva migrans); through the viscera—cough and hematuria (visceral larva migrans); and through the central nervous system (CNS)—eosinophilic meningitis and myeloencephalitis. Ocular involvement leads to vision disorders.

109.6.1   Cutaneous Form

The migratory subcutaneous swellings with hyper-eosinophilia appear weeks to months after consuming raw seafood, provoking a suspicion of gnathostomiasis. These may also occur months to years later and may recur in untreated cases for up to 10–12 years. The most common manifestation is intermittent migratory subcutaneous swellings.

There are three forms: (a) superficial, like cutaneous larva migrans; (b) deep-seated panniculitis, and (c) a mixed form. Creeping superficial presentation is the most common. Primary sites could be any, from the extremities, like the dorsum of the hand, to the head and neck area and even the scalp; the latter locations have the potential for ocular and CNS forms. Relapsing sites are slightly away from the primary (migratory swelling). About 3–4 weeks after infection, a nodular, lumpy, ill-defined oedematous, erythematous area appears, which may be itchy and painful. The skin feels infiltrated, lumpy, and even hard, and tends to heal in 7–14 days. The biopsy of nodular lesion persisting in a fixed site after therapy may reveal a viable hibernating larva.

Moore et al. (2003) described 16 patients with *G. spinigerum* infection diagnosed at the Hospital for Tropical Diseases, London. All were seropositive and responded to albendazole therapy. They had travelled to China, Hong Kong, Japan, Thailand, Singapore, Bangladesh, India, Sri Lanka, Cambodia, Brazil, and South Africa and fell in the age group of 26–51 years. A 26-year-old woman frequently ate raw fish and had intermittent migratory subcutaneous swellings of 3–6 cm in diameter. There was an episodic appearance of 'irritating' lumps on her limbs. The first of these lumps appeared on the right hand 9 months earlier. A similar lump appeared on her left foot and left hand, lasting for a few days without any visible and palpable sequelae. Nine years earlier, she had a lump near her left knee, which was followed 4 days later by a similar lump on the right thigh, resolving spontaneously.

The systemic manifestations of gnathostomiasis are less common than the cutaneous manifestations.

109.6.2   Visceral Form

Visceral migrans symptoms are episodic, lasting for 1–2 weeks, and may begin 3–4 weeks or several years after ingestion. The migration of the larvae through the liver (right upper quadrant pain), causes abdominal pain, resembling appendicitis and cholecystitis. Pulmonary migration may cause cough, pleuritic chest pain, pleural effusion, dyspnoea, hemoptysis with cough-up worm, and hypereosinophilia.

Genitourinary manifestation is less common. There is haematuria if the kidney and/or ureter are affected. There may be vaginitis, cervicitis, balanitis, and hematospermia. The frequency, intensity, and duration of the episodes decrease over time.

109.6.3   CNS Form

Cerebral gnathostomiasis is associated with altered consciousness and coma. There may be intra-cerebral haemorrhage and subarachnoid haemorrhage. CNS invasion is serious and causes death in 8–25% of patients or leaves permanent damage in about 30%. There is agonizing neuritic pain. This may be followed by temporary reduced sensation or paralysis.

Radiculomyelitis is most common and characterized by spinal syndromes like paraplegia, neurogenic bladder, and quadriplegia. It may progress to myeloencephalitis. Patients present with myelitis, intra-cerebral haemorrhage, and subarachnoid haemorrhage. *Meningitis/meningoencephalitis* is manifested as severe headache interrupted by the passage of the parasite near the root of the nerve. The pain may last for up to 5 days and is frequently followed by a variable motor deficit, from weakness to complete paraparesis. Meningismus (stiff neck), cranial nerve (abducens) palsies, focal neurologic signs, and depressed consciousness are observed.

109.6.4   Ocular Form

There is a sudden unilateral loss of visual acuity. The anterior chamber is invaded. The larva is visible, unlike in any other invaded tissues. Eosinophilia is absent.

There is intense pain in the ocular globe, as well as a decreased visual capacity in up to 40% of cases. Wide-ranging pathology can be caused, such as uveitis, iritis, intra-ocular haemorrhage, glaucoma, and even retinal scarring and detachment.

109.7   Prognosis

The risk of complications is high in the case of involvement of the eye and CNS. Bravo and Gontijo (2018) believe that patients with migratory panniculitis in the head and neck region should be closely monitored since they are more prone to develop such complications.

109.8   Diagnosis

Gnathostomiasis presents a classical triad picture: (a) history of travel to endemic areas, (b) eosinophilia, and (c) intermittent migratory swelling.

G. spinigerum larvae are large and can be visualized through the skin in cases of subcutaneous nodular gnathostomiasis and in the anterior chamber (iris) or retina in ocular gnathostomiasis. Serological tests, such as enzyme-linked immunosorbent assay (ELISA) and the 24-kDa L3 antigen immunoblot, may be negative due to the avascularity of the anterior chamber in an ocular form.

Plain radiography and CT scan of the brain may help locate the worm/tissue damage/both. ELISA and western blot are promising. Immunoblot using a 24-kD diagnostic band is highly sensitive and specific.

109.9   Treatment

The detection of the worm is the final diagnosis, and its surgical removal is the specific treatment. Albendazole and ivermectin are recommended.

109.10   Prevention

Avoid eating raw fish, for travellers in particular. The L3 larva survives for 5 days in lemon juice. Marinating may not be effective. Home-making sushi, sashimi, or ceviche is risky. Quick freezing used in the preparation of these delicacies will kill the larva but enforcing it is difficult.

Gnathostoma is globally distributed; the only effective preventive strategy is to educate persons in endemic and non-endemic areas.

References

Bravo F, Gontijo B (2018) Gnathostomiasis: an emerging infectious disease relevant to all dermatologists. An Bras Dermatol 93(2):172–180

Diaz JH (2015) Gnathostomiasis: an emerging infection of raw fish consumers in Gnathostoma nematode-endemic and non-endemic countries. J Travel Med 22(5):318–324

Eiras JC, Pavanelli GC, Takemoto RM, Nawa Y (2018) An overview of fish-borne nematodiases among returned travelers for recent 25 years—unexpected diseases sometimes far away from the origin. Korean J Parasitol 56(3):215–227

Moore DA, McCroddan J, Dekumyoy P, Chiodini PL (2003) Gnathostomiasis: an emerging imported disease. Emerg Infect Dis 9(6):647–650

Chapter 110
Larva Migrans

Some of the nematodes infect human beings, although they are not the natural hosts. In such a situation, the parasitic larvae move at random in the body system, initiating an inflammatory response. The development of the parasite is arrested. The larvae fail to become a mature worm. The fate of such larvae is eventual death due to the hosts' response. The wandering larvae damage tissues and produce pathology, which may be described as cutaneous larva migrans, visceral larva migrans, and ocular larva migrans.

The following nematodes have been associated with these conditions:

- *Ancylostoma caninum*, *A. braziliense*, *A. duodenale*, *Necator americanus*, occasionally *A. ceylanicum*, and the larvae of other nematodes, such as *Gnathostoma spinigera*, *Strongyloides stercoralis*, *Capillaria* spp., and *Bunostomum phlebotomum*, a cattle hookworm, cause cutaneous larva migrans (creeping eruptions).
- *Toxocara canis*, *T. cati*, *T. leonina*, *Angiostrongylus cantonensis*, *Gnathostoma spinigerum*, *Ascaris suum*, *Capillaria hepatica*, *Lagochilascaris minor*, and *Dirofilaria* cause visceral larva migrans.
- *Toxocara canis* causes ocular larva migrans.

Larva migrans occur mostly in tropical and sub-tropical areas.

110.1 Cutaneous Larva Migrans

Synonyms: Cutaneous larva migrans has been variously named—dermatitis linearis migrans, ground itch, minor itch, sand itch, erythema larva migrans, and hookworm-related cutaneous larva migrans.

© Springer Nature Singapore Pte Ltd. 2024

K. G. Narayan et al., *Handbook of Management of Zoonoses*,

https://doi.org/10.1007/978-981-99-9885-2_110

It is characterized by progressive linear eruptions, causing the thickening of the skin and pruritis.

It is caused by ancylostomes (*Ancylostoma braziliense*, *A. caninum*, and *Uncinaria stenocephala* zoonotic parasites of dogs and cats). The larvae of other nematodes such as, occasionally, *A. ceylanicum*; *Gnathostoma spinigera*; *Strongyloides stercoralis*; *Capillaria* spp.; *Bunostomum phlebotomum*, a cattle hookworm; *Cinaria stenocephala*; *Ascaris* species; and *Bunostomum phlebotomum* larvae also cause cutaneous larva migrans.

The larvae of human hookworms, *Ancylostoma duodenale* and *Necator americanus*, can cause a similar skin eruption; however, the rash associated with these infections is shorter lived as the parasite is able to penetrate the dermis to complete its life cycle. Larvae migrating via hair follicles through the dermis cause cutaneous pili migrans.

110.1.1   Life Cycle

Dog and cat reservoirs shed eggs of the parasite in faeces. Soil is seeded with the eggs of the nematode. The shed eggs that hatch and the larvae undergo developmental stages 1–3 (non-infectious rhabditiform to filariform infectious) in about a week. The third stage is infective and survives in soil for weeks under moist and warm conditions. The exposed animal hosts get infected by the larvae, penetrating through the skin or gut mucosa. These migrate through the blood capillaries to the lungs and are coughed up and swallowed by the host, eventually reaching the intestine, where these mature into adults.

110.1.2   Epidemiology

The condition is typical in sub-tropical and tropical regions; is endemic in the Caribbean, Central and South America, and the southern United States; and may occur among visitors/travellers to the endemic regions. Walking barefoot on the beach is a common form of exposure. The soil contaminated with dog/cat faeces contains excreted eggs, which develop into filariform larvae in hot and humid conditions. Poor environmental hygiene and the high population of stray dogs and cats provide an ecological support system for the parasites, and thus such regions/countries will have a high burden of parasite eggs and a high prevalence.

Infection in human beings occurs when they walk barefoot over contaminated soil. Mostly children are affected because of this unsanitary habit. Occupationally, plumbers, electricians, sweet potato growers, rice field workers, and tea leaf pickers stand at a high risk of getting it.

Sharma et al. (2015) listed 12 cases reported in India. Each had contact with the soil in one way or another, such as walking on the sea beach, gardening, and handling soil and/or compost.

110.1.3 Symptoms

The point of entry by the larvae is marked by a skin scab on the lower extremities. The typical symptoms include rash, pruritis, and a secondary bacterial infection due to frequent itching. The incubation period ranges from 7 days to 7 months. The larvae die within several weeks to months.

The larvae penetrate the corneal layer of the human epidermis, migrate within the epidermis, and spread a few centimetres per day, causing an inflammatory reaction. The larvae may cause an allergic reaction, and there is a reddish papule at the site of penetration, which is itching—the early infection is thus described as 'ground itch'. The migrating larvae produce snake-like markings, referred to as 'creeping eruption' or 'cutaneous larva migrans'. The lesion may proceed to become reticular and erythematous. Intense itching provokes scratching and a consequential pyogenic infection.

Lesions are usually few. Common sites of entry include the feet, areas between the fingers and toes, the thighs, the trunk, and the buttocks in adults.

110.1.4 Diagnosis

It is based on clinical characteristic lesions and epidemiology. Confounding lesions are due to scabies, myiasis, tinea corporis, and contact dermatitis. A microscopic examination shows larvae between the corium and stratum granulosum, with infiltrating eosinophils and round cells. Skin biopsy is generally not recommended.

It is a self-limiting disease, but secondary infections are likely, with a few progressing into Loeffler's syndrome, which warrants treatment with antihistamines and anthelminthics. (*Löffler syndrome is thought to result from a type 1 hypersensitivity reaction related to the pulmonary larval migration phase of various parasites*).

Comparin et al. (2016) reported a case of extensive cutaneous larva migrans in a 32-year-old man living in Midwest Brazil. He developed severe itching skin eruptions after 15 days of exposure while lying on the lawn of an amusement park for a few hours. He had no history of clinical illness or the use of any medicine. The lesion was a large erythematous plaque on the lower part of his back with serpiginous tracks in some areas. Clinical characteristics and a history of exposure strongly suggested a 'cutaneous larva migrans' with severe eczematous reaction. He was treated accordingly with 5% thiabendazole, three times daily for 15 days, and 400 mg of oral albendazole daily for three consecutive days. He responded well; the lesions resolved, supporting the initial diagnosis. Shakir and King (2020) suggested that a rash that follows no pattern and appears after a vacation should be checked for 'cutaneous larvae migrans'. In another case, a 59-year-old male suffered from a pruritic rash for 2 weeks. A worsening spread of infection to his foot was a matter of concern. He was referred to the hospital. The rash was serpiginous and did not follow any superficial veins. It extended beneath the fifth toe. Scabs were seen on the dorsum of the fourth and fifth toes. The searching question was: 'Where did you spend vacation recently?' He had passed a vacation in the Caribbean about 6 weeks prior to presentation. He recalls frequently walking barefoot on the beaches.

110.2   Visceral Larva Migrans (VLM)

Synonyms: Toxocarosis and larval granulomatosis (occurs due to the larvae of *T. canis*, *T. cati*, and *Ascaris suum*).

Extra-intestinal migratory larvae produce chronic granuloma, usually eosinophilic. It is a systemic manifestation of the migration of second-stage larvae of nematodes through the tissue of human viscera. It is not uncommon but is under-diagnosed in developing countries. It has a worldwide distribution with a high prevalence in sub-tropical countries. It is more common in Korea and Japan (Rohilla et al. 2013). It affects people under 20 years of age. Sharma et al. (2015) listed 11 reported cases in India. According to Weller and Leder (2023), approximately 1.4 billion people are infected worldwide. Its prevalence is higher in tropical regions with high humidity than in temperate regions. Infection is more common in the rural population with poor housing and inadequate water supply and is commonly associated with poverty. A meta-analysis estimated 19% global seroprevalence. The distribution was the highest in the African region, followed by Southeast Asia, the Western Pacific, the Americas, Europe, and the eastern Mediterranean region.

110.2.1   Life Cycle

The larvae of canine (*Toxocara canis*) and feline (*Toxocara cati*) *Ascarid* species and others cause this. Dogs act as reservoirs. The worm burden in the soil is high for *Toxocara canis*. The eggs can remain infectious for years in the soil. It takes several weeks for the eggs of both roundworms to become infective. The dogs commonly get infected per os. Most adult dogs have encysted larva L2, which gets reactivated during pregnancy and transplacentally infects the puppies in utero. Puppies may be vertically infected through breast milk also. Approximately 50% of puppies and 20% of adult dogs are infected with *T. canis*. Vertical transmission in cats occurs only through breast milk.

110.2.2   Source of Human Infection

Lactating bitches and female cats and their pups and kittens have high worm loads and hence are the potential sources. Infectious mothers and puppies under 5 weeks can pass eggs in their faeces. Indirectly, flies can spread the eggs. Infected dogs contaminate the soil.

110.2.3   Transmission

The accidental ingestion of embryonated eggs of *T. canis* is the route of infection. The ingestion of raw or undercooked organs and meat, especially giblet and liver, from the paratenic hosts (pigs, lamb, rabbits, chicken) also leads to the disease, as well as the consumption of raw vegetables.

110.2.4   Contributory Factors

Dirty habits, poor personal hygiene, the unsanitary status of the kitchen, and mud eating (pica) are the most likely factors. The most commonly affected age group is 1–5 years, when sanitary habits have not developed. Additionally, they fondle and play with pups and dogs, and thus exposure is high. Visits to contaminated public places such as parks and school grounds may lead to infection. Studies on contaminated soil in public places, such as school grounds in Andhra Pradesh and parks in Uttar Pradesh, India, have been reported (Sharma et al. 2015). Access of dogs to public places should be restricted or not allowed. Many dog owners do not know about VLM.

110.2.5   Infection

After ingestion, the larvae hatch and penetrate the intestinal wall, enter the blood circulation, and flow through the portal vein to reach the liver, lungs, orbit, and brain. Some larvae become encapsulated in the liver and remain there for an indefinite period.

The liver is the most commonly affected, possibly because of its portal drainage. Occlusion or alteration of the microvascular portal blood supply and eosinophilic infiltration appear because larvae are distributed through the portal blood flow. The focal lesion is eosinophilic granuloma.

Three clinical forms are recognized: (a) visceral larva migrans covers diseases associated with major organs, (b) covert toxocariasis is a milder version, and (c) ocular larva migrans affects the eye and optic nerve.

110.2.6 Symptoms

Visceral larva migrans occurs after repeated infection or the ingestion of a large number of embryonated eggs. The fate of infection is resolution within weeks with chronic eosinophilia. The wandering larvae incite inflammatory responses in the internal organs, including sometimes the central nervous system (CNS).

Most infections are asymptomatic. Symptoms vary according to the organs affected. Symptoms depend upon the site of larval migration. The larva may migrate to the liver, lungs, heart, and CNS. Fever, splenomegaly, hepatomegaly, lymphadenopathy, hepatic necrosis, and myocarditis may occur. Pallor, fatigue, weight loss, anorexia, headache, rash, cough, asthma, chest tightness, increased irritability, abdominal pain, nausea, and vomiting may be observed. The cases are often diagnosed as chronic pulmonary inflammation, pneumonia, or bronchospasm as the patient manifests cough, wheeze, dyspnoea, or asthma. Seizures and neuropsychiatric symptoms appear when the CNS is involved.

Those hypersensitive to allergens suffer severely. Epilepsy, carditis, pleural effusion, and death due to respiratory failure are seen.

Rohilla et al. (2013) presented a case of VLM in a 16-year-old vegetarian girl from a rural background. She experienced intermittent abdominal pain, malaise, loss of appetite, and restlessness for 3 months. There were no pets at home but plenty of stray dogs in the neighbourhood. The patient was slightly pale and had hepatosplenomegaly (liver span being 17 cm and spleen being 15 cm) but no significant lymphadenopathy. Dog hair and soil also contain infective-stage eggs. It appears she contracted the infection via either the stray dogs of the neighbourhood or infected soil. This case report highlights the imaging features of hepatic lesions.

Covert toxocariasis results from chronic exposure. Patients experience coughing, fever, abdominal pain, and headaches. Sleep is disturbed. Medical examination may reveal wheezing, an enlarged liver, and inflamed lymph nodes.

110.2.7 Diagnosis

The clinical triad of toxocariasis is unexplained eosinophilia, liver or lung nodules on imaging studies, and a history of eating animal liver. There is chronic production of parasite antigens, continuous stimulation of the host immune system, and concomitant production of eosinophils gamma globulins (IgM, IgG, IgE). Several fragments of myosins of *Toxocara* are highly antigenic and can be used as a potential candidate vaccine. An IgG-ELISA assay based on a recombinant version (rTES-30USM) of the 30 kDa *Toxocara* excretory-secretory antigen (TES-30) has recently been developed. It has a sensitivity of 92.3% and a specificity of 89.6%, compared with a sensitivity of 100% but a specificity of only 55.7% with a commercial kit (Rohilla et al. 2013). Ultrasonography, computed tomography (CT) scan, and magnetic resonance imaging (MRI) may be used as an aid in diagnosis.

110.3   Ocular Larva Migrans (OLM)

Synonym: Toxocara retinitis.

110.3.1   Aetiology

The larvae of *T. canis* and *T. cati* and occasionally, *Baylisascaris procyonis* (raccoon roundworm) are cause of OLM.

It occurs mostly in older children. Sharma et al. (2015) listed 15 cases reported in India. Eleven cases detected in a serological study on 68 patients with ocular manifestations suspected of *Toxocara* infection were <15 years old, and three were >15 years old. Another case of OLM was a 12-year-old girl from Kashmir.

Usually, one of the eyes is affected. There is a decrease in visual acuity, strabismus, or leukocoria. Eosinophilic granuloma is seen around the larva (entrapping it and preventing it from further spread). The eyes may be red and the pupil white or fixed. It is accompanied by pain in the eye, visual disturbance, loss of vision for days or weeks, and strabismus. The lesion is located commonly in the posterior pole of the retina. There may be endophthalmitis, uveitis, and chorioretinitis. The damage may be permanent and may end in blindness. The granuloma may be confounded with retinoblastoma. Generally, there is no eosinophilia.

110.4   Neural Larva Migrans

Neural larva migrans is caused by the migrating larvae of *Baylisascaris procyonis*. It is a serious neurological disease. Raccoons are the reservoir hosts, found in northern and midwestern United States. It can cause severe inflammation, seizures, and an altered mental state (encephalopathy). There is eosinophilic meningoencephalitis seen primarily in children (Sharma et al. 2015).

110.5   Diagnosis

- The presentation of cutaneous larva migrans may be strongly suggestive.
- Ultrasound, CT, and MRI are done to visualize granulomas.
- Observation of leucocytosis, eosinophilia (as high as 90%), gammaglobulinemia, and high titres of isohaemagglutination are supportive.
- Biopsy and demonstration of larvae are a confirmation.
- Complement fixation, indirect immunofluorescence, indirect haemagglutination, and enzyme-linked immunosorbent assay (ELISA) are serologic tests used but are less specific and sensitive. The specificity and sensitivity of ELISA has been enhanced.
- Polymerase chain reaction (PCR) may be done.
- In animals, the examination of the stool for eggs of the parasites is done.

110.6   Treatment

Topical treatment with thiabendazole ointment is very effective in controlling cutaneous larva migrans. Mebendazole is an effective anthelmintic. Corticosteroids are helpful. Surgical removal of the granuloma may be done.

110.7   Prevention and Control

- Dogs as sentinel animals may be used.
- Specific anthelmintics administered to animals would reduce the worm burden in the environment. Pyrantel pamoate, mebendazole, albendazole, levamisole, or tetrachloroethylene is useful.
- Strong salt solution and borax may be used to kill the larvae in soil.
- Sanitary habits—personal (hand washing) and in the kitchen (washing of all fruits and vegetables)—overall reduce the chance of infection.
- Health education, like a reminder to wear shoes, would make people aware of the dangers of soil contamination through the faeces of man and animals. The kennel floor should be kept clean and dry as *Toxocara* eggs may remain infectious for years, being resistant to environmental temperature changes and chemicals. Freshly shed eggs in the faeces of dogs and cats do not cause toxocariasis. It takes about 2 weeks under ideal summer conditions for eggs to mature to the infective stage.
- Picking up pet faeces and proper disposal or burying reduce transmission in public places like parks and beaches.
- Active veterinarian participation, like making owners aware, is important.

References

Comparin C, Rodrigues MM, Santos BC (2016) Extensive cutaneous larva migrans with eczematous reaction on atypical localization. Am J Trop Med Hyg 94(6):1185–1186

Rohilla S, Jain N, Yadav R, Dhaulakhandi DB (2013) Hepatic visceral larva migrans. BMJ Case Rep 2013:bcr2013009288

Shakir H, King L (2020) Cutaneous larva migrans: the rash is not what you think. https://www.emra.org/emresident/article/cutaneous-larva-migrans-case-report

Sharma R, Singh BB, Gill JP (2015) Larva migrans in India: veterinary and public health perspectives. J Parasit Dis 39(4):604–612

Weller PF, Leder K (2023) Toxocariasis: visceral and ocular larva migrans. https://www.uptodate.com/contents/toxocariasis-visceral-and-ocular-larva-migrans

Chapter 111
Strongyloidiasis

The World Health Organization (2020) has alerted healthcare workers in tropical and sub-tropical areas, where soil-transmitted parasites, especially strongyloidiasis, are prevalent, about the use of corticosteroids given to patients suspected of infection with SARS-COV-2. Globally, over 600 million people are estimated to be infected by *Strongyloides stercoralis*.

Millions of marginalized communities that walk barefooted are estimated to be affected. Infection is sub-clinical. Immunosuppression converts the infection into severe deadly 'hyper-infection' syndrome. Immunosuppression may be due to diseases like acquired immunodeficiency syndrome (AIDS), lymphoma, and leukaemia. The continued use of corticosteroids or similar drugs used for transplant and even in new serious infectious diseases, like SARS-COV-2, can similarly be dangerous.

111.1 Aetiology

Strongyloides stercoralis, *S. fuelleborni* (*fülleborni*) subsp. *fuelleborni*, and *S. fuelleborni* subsp. *kellyi* are zoonotic. Species like *S. myopotami* (nutria), *S. procyonis* (raccoons) may produce mild short-lived cutaneous infections (larva currens -recurrent serpiginous maculopapular or urticarial rash along the buttocks, perineum, and thighs, commonly called as "nutria itch") in humans.

The distribution of *Strongyloides stercoralis* is worldwide in tropical and sub-tropical areas. Infection is common in areas with poor sanitation and in rural marginalized groups, and transmission is usual in the summer months. The overall global prevalence is 8%. The burden is the highest in Southeast Asia, the Western Pacific, and African WHO regions (World Health Organization 2020).

S. fuelleborni (*fülleborni*) subsp. *fuelleborni* occurs in non-human primates, apes, and monkeys in the Old World. Most human cases occur in sub-Saharan Africa

© Springer Nature Singapore Pte Ltd. 2024
K. G. Narayan et al., *Handbook of Management of Zoonoses*,
https://doi.org/10.1007/978-981-99-9885-2_111

and are sporadic in Southeast Asia. *S. fuelleborni* subsp. *kellyi* is found in humans in Papua New Guinea. Transmission to infants through breastfeeding often leads to severe or fatal disease. (CDC 2015; https://www.cdc.gov/parasites/strongyloides/biology.html).

111.2   Life Cycle of *S. stercoralis*

S. stercoralis is primarily a human parasite. Domestic dogs and primates such as chimpanzees and monkeys also get patent infection with female parasites. Dogs appear to be infected with *S. stercoralis* of two genetically different types: one infects only dogs, and the other both dogs and humans. All human infections are caused by the second type. Cats' role as reservoirs is not known, although they are experimentally proven susceptible.

111.2.1   Mode of Infection

Contact with soil containing infective larvae, followed by penetration of the skin, is the mode of infection. The larvae migrate to the intestines. The larvae or eggs are excreted back into the environment and may infect a new host. *S. stercoralis* is a unique nematode that can re-infect (auto-infection) its human host without passage through the soil; it has the ability to chronically infect for decades.

111.3   Symptoms

Initial and acute symptoms may be localized pruritis, erythema at the site of entry, tracheal irritation and dry cough due to migratory larvae, abdominal pain, anorexia, diarrhoea, and constipation due to intestinal invasion. Larvae are limited to the gastrointestinal tract and lungs.

Chronic strongyloidiasis is generally asymptomatic to mild eosinophilia and elevated IgE. Rarely do complications develop, such as arthritis, cardiac arrhythmias, chronic malabsorption, duodenal obstruction, nephrotic syndrome, and recurrent asthma.

Hyper-infection syndrome and disseminated strongyloidiasis occur in those receiving immunosuppressants like corticosteroids and sub-clinically infected with *S. stercoralis*. Auto-infection is accelerated in immunologically compromised patients as an overwhelming number of migrating larvae invade. Strongyloidiasis is disseminated. Systemic, gastrointestinal, pulmonary, and neurologic signs/symptoms have been documented. There may be severe complications. Mortality may be as high as 90% if untreated.

111.4   Treatment

Ivermectin is the first-line therapy.

References

CDC (2015) Parasites—Strongyloides. https://www.cdc.gov/parasites/strongyloides/biology.html. Accessed 30 July 2019

World Health Organization (2020) Soil—transmitted helminth infections. https://www.who.int/news-room/fact-sheets/detail/soil-transmitted-helminth-infections

Chapter 112
Toxocariasis

The detection of a nematode in human retinal granuloma in a child in 1950 led to the recognition of human toxocariasis. A severe long-term multi-system disease with eosinophilia in a number of children offered an opportunity to describe the symptoms of visceral larva migrans (VLM) because the juvenile parasite was detected on biopsy. Toxocariasis is considered a major public health problem (Despommier 2003).

112.1 Aetiology

Toxocara canis and *T. cati* are roundworms affecting the gastro-intestines of domestic cats and dogs and wild canines like foxes, wolves, and coyotes. These belong to the order Ascaridida, superfamily Ascaridoidea, family Toxocaridae.

112.2 Life Cycle

Dogs and cats are definitive hosts. Infected cats and dogs pass unembryonated eggs in their faeces. These embryonate in 2–4 weeks, and infective larvae (stage 3) develop in the eggs. The eggs can remain infectious for years in the soil. Dogs and cats get infected by ingesting these directly from contaminated soil and environment. The infective eggs hatch, and the released larvae penetrate the gut.

The parasite adopts four modes of transmission: direct, prenatal, paratenic, and trans-mammary transmission.

Indirectly, dogs and cats are infected by eating the paratenic hosts carrying encysted larvae. Paratenic hosts are a number of mammals (rabbits, rodents including livestock) and birds. Earthworms, ants, and other soil-dwelling invertebrates

© Springer Nature Singapore Pte Ltd. 2024
K. G. Narayan et al., *Handbook of Management of Zoonoses*,
https://doi.org/10.1007/978-981-99-9885-2_112

also act as paratenic hosts. The ingested embryonated eggs containing infective larvae hatch, and the larvae penetrate the gut wall and migrate to various tissues, where they remain encysted.

The infective-stage larvae migrate through the lungs, bronchial tree, and oesophagus, to be swallowed into the gastrointestinal tract. Adults develop in the small intestine and pass eggs in faeces to begin a fresh cycle of development and infection. In older dogs, the development of larvae is commonly arrested in tissues. The reactivation of arrested larval development occurs in bitches during late pregnancy. There is trans-placental (more often) and trans-mammary infection of pups. *T. cati* is transmitted via trans-mammary infection.

Development to the adult stage in the small intestine takes 60–90 days after the infective-stage larvae hatch. Mating ensues. Unembryonated eggs are excreted in the faeces. Embryonation occurs in the soil in a week or so. In regions where environmental temperature is low, the incubation period may be longer. Eggs can remain dormant until the temperature rises in spring, and then embryonation occurs.

Dogs suffer from mild to severe diarrhoea. Pet owners may observe a loss of appetite, poor skin condition and dull hair coat, weakness, and vomiting. Infected cats may manifest poor or loss of appetite, growth disturbance, and diarrhoea alternating with constipation and vomiting, especially after feeding.

Puppies and kittens are better spreaders than older ones because patent infection is more common.

112.3   Human Infection

Toxocara canis and *Toxocara cati*, which infect dogs and cats, respectively, may cause infection in humans. Human beings are accidental hosts. Human toxocariasis is a zoonosis shared with pets and feral dogs, cats, and wild canids with a wide spectrum of clinical symptoms and morbidity. According to Hare and Franco-Paredes (2014), studies on prevalence suggest widespread affliction than indicated by the level of awareness among clinicians in endemic areas. In the USA, seroprevalence estimates identified as high as 22% in some low-income communities. The prevalence in tropical settings is not well known but clearly is under-reported. Considering the wide range of clinical manifestations, severe morbidity and long-term sequelae, human toxocariasis is placed in the category of neglected tropical disease.

112.4   Source of Human Infection

Dogs and cats are reservoir hosts. Pregnant or lactating bitches and female cats and their pups and kittens have a high worm load and hence are potential sources. The worm burden in the soil is high. Eggs can remain infectious for years in the soil. *T. canis* can lay 200,000 eggs/day. Eggs have a resistant outer shell, enabling their survival. Hot and humid regions are favourable for survival, and with sufficient moisture and oxygen, they can remain infectious for years. Eggs are dispersed by earthworms, flies, cockroaches, and peri-domestic mammals like squirrels and chipmunks. Birds that feed primarily on the ground, like pigeons, starlings, and sparrows, can carry eggs on their feet and beaks and deposit them in places far from the original (Despommier 2003).

112.5   Mode of Infection

Infection occurs through the ingestion of infective eggs or under-processed meat/viscera of paratenic hosts. Undercooked contaminated beef, lamb, chicken, and ducks (liver in particular) have been associated with human infection.

Transmission is per os (Fig. 112.1). The embryonated eggs are ingested accidentally. Dirty habits, poor personal hygiene, the unsanitary status of the kitchen, and mud eating (pica) are most likely factors. The most commonly affected age group is 1–5 years, when sanitary habits have not developed. Additionally, they fondle and play with pups and dogs, and thus exposure is high.

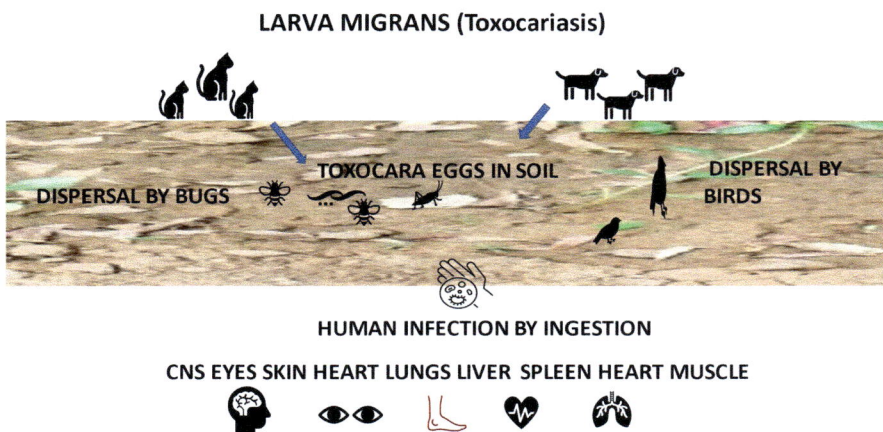

Fig. 112.1 Transmission of *Toxocara* spp.

112.6   Pathogenesis

The infective larvae hatch after the ingestion of eggs. The larvae penetrate the intestinal mucosa, enter the circulatory system, and wander throughout the body for months and years, damaging a variety of tissues, the heart, the lungs, the liver, the brain, the eyes, and the muscles. Survival for long years in a mammalian host by parasites, like the larvae of *Toxocara*, adult schistosomes, the first-stage larvae of *Trichinella spiralis*, and the juvenile stage of tapeworms, is ascribed to their ability to evade the host's immune system. This is the end of the development of the parasite.

The disease is a consequence of the extra-intestinal migration of the larvae of, commonly, *Toxocara canis* and *Toxocara cati* in humans, who act as paratenic hosts. The larvae enter the cardiovascular system and reach the lungs and liver during the first week of infection. This hepato-pulmonary phase constitutes the acute stage of toxocariasis. The chronic stage is characterized by the migration and accumulation of the larvae throughout the somatic tissue. It is the beginning of the chronic myoneurotropic phase.

The larvae may wander through any organ—the liver, lungs, eyes, and brain—and are active nearly for a year till granuloma develops to entrap them. The migration through tissues causes mechanical damage and local reactions. The extent of the damage and pathology is dependent upon the tissues, the number of migrating juveniles, and the age of the host.

The death of the juvenile initiates immediate-type and delayed-type hypersensitivity responses in the viscera (visceral larva migrans) and retinal granuloma and blindness [ocular larva migrans (OLM)]. The two conditions tend to appear independently of each other; i.e., ocular larva migrans occurs without systemic involvement, and the same is true for visceral larva migrans. Inflammation is manifested as eosinophilic granulomas.

112.6.1   Larva Migrans

The extra-intestinal migratory larvae produce chronic granuloma, usually eosinophilic. It has worldwide distribution. It affects people under 20 years of age.

Larva migrans occurs after repeated infection or the ingestion of a large number of embryonated eggs. Mild infection is often asymptomatic and followed by a resolution. The infection resolutes within weeks with chronic eosinophilia. The wandering larvae incite inflammatory responses in internal organs, including sometimes the central nervous system (CNS). Symptoms vary according to the organs affected.

Four clinical forms are recognized: (a) visceral larva migrans covers diseases associated with major organs, (b) covert toxocariasis is a milder version, (c) ocular larva migrans affects the eye and optic nerve, and (d) neurotoxicosis occurs as a result of accumulation and persistence in the CNS.

112.6.2   Visceral Larva Migrans

It occurs commonly among children <5 years old. Patients report loss of appetite and weight, fatigue, headache, and increased irritability. Some report abdominal pain, nausea, and vomiting. Others present with fever and lower respiratory symptoms like asthma (bronchospasm), seizures, and neuropsychiatric symptoms.

There is hepato-splenomegaly. There may be involvement of the heart (myocarditis), kidney (nephritis), and central nervous system (encephalopathy). Investigations reveal eosinophilia and hypergammaglobulinemia (IgM, IgG, and IgE). Increased IgE/anti-IgE complex is seen in cases with pronounced symptoms. Those hypersensitive to allergens suffer severely. Epilepsy, carditis, pleural effusion, and death due to respiratory failure are common.

Cianferoni et al. (2006) presented a case of a 16-year-old girl who ingested an earthworm on a dare. One month later, she had a cough, hypereosinophilia, hypergammaglobulinemia, and multiple non-cavitary pulmonary nodules. Parabronchial biopsy revealed eosinophilic organizing pneumonitis with multiple eosinophilic microabscesses. There was no evidence of ocular larva migrans. Clinical recovery was achieved with albendazole. She had elevated *Toxocara* titres (>1:4096), which continued even 3 months after a 10-day course of albendazole. The earthworm acted as a paratenic host.

112.6.3   Covert Toxocariasis

Long-term exposure (chronic) to larvae migrating in specific target organs causes asymptomatic, subtle, and mild symptoms, with eosinophilia as the only biomarker; this is called covert toxocariasis. It is often linked to cognitive and developmental delays, lung dysfunction, and asthma.

Patients experience coughing, fever, abdominal pain, and headaches. Sleep is disturbed. Medical examination may reveal wheezing, an enlarged liver, and inflamed lymph nodes.

Larvae migrating in the lungs cause asthma and in the brain, idiopathic seizures. Despommier (2003) cited prurigo and urticaria and eosinophilic arthritis linked to *Toxocara* infection.

112.6.4   Ocular Larva Migrans

Hare and Franco-Paredes (2014) reviewed the epidemiology and pathology of ocular larva migrans. The estimation of prevalence is difficult as there is a poor association with toxocariasis, according to serologic studies. A survey between 2009 and 2010 reported more cases in the southern United States, with maximum cases in Georgia and a higher prevalence in urban and suburban communities. *Toxocara* spp. larvae migrate through the choroidal and retinal vessels into the posterior segment of the eye. While migrating through the central nervous system, the larvae enter the eye through the optic nerve. There is considerable variability in the response to intra-ocular infection, as observed in animal experiments. The larvae remained long, for 9 months, in the vitreous, retina, and optic nerve without inflammatory response. A brief stay did not cause any immune response. Even when acute inflammatory granuloma or chronic fibrotic granuloma surrounded the larvae, these remained unaffected as they could move through the ocular tissues and leave the site. Dead larvae caused little reaction, and *Toxocara* proteins injected intra-vitreally caused severe retinal vasculitis.

It occurs mostly in older children (5–10 years) and teenagers, who suffer impaired unilateral vision, pain, significant visual disability strabismus, photophobia, leukocoria, vitritis, ocular injection, and blindness.

Often only one eye is invaded by a single larva encysting within the orbit. The eyes may be red and the pupil white or fixed. It is accompanied by pain in the eye, visual disturbance, loss of vision for days or weeks, and strabismus. The lesion is located commonly in the posterior pole of the retina. Eosinophilic granuloma is seen around the larva (entrapping it and preventing it from further spreading). The vision is distorted. There may be detachment of the macula and blindness. Diffuse endophthalmitis or papillitis and secondary glaucoma may also be caused. There may be endophthalmitis, uveitis, chorioretinitis, and retinal detachment. The damage may be permanent and may end in blindness. The granuloma may be confounded with retinoblastoma. Generally, there is no eosinophilia. The diagnosis depends upon ophthalmic examination and the identification of typical features, Anthelmintics and steroids are effective, but a full return of vision is unlikely.

112.6.5   Cardiac Larva Migrans

Involvement of the cardiac muscles, damaged by invading larvae combined with immunological reaction and systemic eosinophilia, has been reported. Kuenzli et al. (2016) reported 24 cases of toxocariasis involving the heart. Cardiac larva migrans manifested in a range of symptoms, from asymptomatic to mild life-threatening myocarditis, pericarditis with heart failure, or cardiac tamponade leading to death. A combination of clinical, radiological, and laboratory findings led to a diagnosis. Histological examination was done either pre- or post-mortem in three cases. Granuloma and remnants of the parasite were detected in six cases. Anthelmintic combined with corticosteroids was the line of treatment.

112.6.6   Neural Larva Migrans

Neural larva migrans (NVM) is the most serious form. The preferred location for *T. cati* larvae is the cerebellum and muscles, while for *T. canis* larvae, it is the cerebrum, and this is reflected in the severity of the structural brain damage, neurological syndrome, and behavioural changes. There is a progressive encephalopathy with indolent or fulminant onset, causing a delay in development and residual neurologic deficits. The immunoregulatory process induced by the host/parasite or their interaction contributes to pathogenesis. According to Waindok et al. (2019), bioactive regulatory lipids, derived from arachidonic acid and other polyunsaturated fatty acids, are mediators participating in the complex molecular signalling network during infection and inflammation. In experimentally infected mice, they observed only minor changes in the pattern of pro-inflammatory oxylipins and significantly elevated anti-inflammatory metabolites derived from lipoxygenase pathways in the sub-acute phase, as well as in the beginning of the chronic phase of infection. The larvae accumulate and persist in the CNS and may not be trapped by an inflammatory response. The lesions are focally distributed and characterized by haemorrhages and the presence of myelinophages, spheroids, and activated microglia. Severe neurological symptoms included headache, fever, oversensitivity to light, weakness, confusion, tiredness, and visual impairment. Neural larva migrans results in serious neurocognitive deficits, blindness, and developmental delays. The following two cases reported by Gavin et al. (2002) from suburban areas in Chicago after exposure to raccoon faeces carrying infective larvae of the roundworm *Baylisascaris procyonis* illustrate the seriousness of neural larva migrans.

Case 1

Delayed language and motor development was noted in a 9-month-old boy, although he caught up but was slow; during age 2.5–4 years, the boy was less socially interactive; and there was stagnated development, followed by regression. The child became increasingly ataxic and developed worsening spastic quadriparesis. He was unable to sit and stand on his own. An investigation revealed that he had a long history of pica and geophagia. He picked up dirt by his hands from the backyard contaminated by faeces of raccoons and put it into his mouth. A detailed investigation was made. A confirmation of neural larva migrans and ocular larva migrans was arrived at by observing anti-*B. procyonis* antibodies in the serum (1/4096) and cerebrospinal fluid (CSF) (1/64) through immunofluorescence assays (IFAs).

Albendazole alone was not effective. The addition of corticosteroid led to the recovery of alertness and the ability to walk and interact but only temporarily. At 10 years, the child is in a wheelchair, without speech, and being fed through a gastrotomy tube, and he has incontinent urine and faeces.

Case 2

A 2.5-year-old normal Hispanic boy complained of fever (38.5 °C), mild cough, and encephalopathy. He had a history of pica and geophagia, received iron tabs for anaemia, and was in good health at the time of hospitalization. He developed marked lethargy and somnolence 3 days before admission. He was irritable, confused, and ataxic. He developed stiffness of the neck, hypertonicity, and hyperreflexia. Cranial reflexes were normal. A detailed laboratory investigation and scanning for bacterial, viral, and most of the parasitic infections were done. Intravenous cefotaxime and acyclovir were started. However, within 24 h, he went into a coma. Anti-*B. procyonis* larvae antibody was detected by indirect IFA in the serum (titre 1/1024) and CSF (titre 1/4). The respective titre rose to 1/4096 and 1/1024 after 2 weeks of therapy. The combined albendazole-corticosteroid therapy for 4 weeks led to minimal clinical recovery. The boy continued in a semi-comatose state with spastic quadriparesis and extensor posturing and remained unresponsive to visual stimuli. Twenty months after the onset, he had bouts of long agitation and irritability. He suffered from developmental delay severely, with marked general spasticity and cortical blindness. His twin brother and older sister, who did not have pica and geophagia, were well. An epidemiological investigation led to the site of exposure, a small cluster of trees beneath which the patient had played and was seen eating dirt. The area contained active raccoon latrines. The soil samples and raccoon faeces collected from the site examined by centrifugal floatation or a modified detergent wash-floatation method showed numerous *B. procyonis* eggs. Thousands of infective eggs (containing motile infective larvae) were detected from the soil and debris from the site (as many as 3320 infective eggs in a 20 g sample).

112.7   Epidemiology

Children with pica stand at a high risk.

Toxocariasis is the clinical term applied to infection with either *T. canis* or *T. cati* in the human host. It is a neglected but important zoonosis. In the United States, it is one of the five neglected parasitic infections and is possibly the most common after pinworm (*Enterobius vermicularis*).

Toxocariasis has global distribution. A true estimate of prevalence is lacking because of the lack of population-based epidemiological studies and clinical awareness/education. Seroprevalence is disproportionately high in areas of community poverty and suburban and poor neighbourhoods. The recent global seroprevalence was estimated at 19% based on a meta-analysis of the contributions from 71 countries (Rostami et al. 2019). The highest (37.7%) prevalence was in the African region, and the lowest was in the Eastern Mediterranean region. In the other WHO regions, Southeast Asia had 34.1%, the Western Pacific 24.2%, the American region 22.8%, and the European region 10.5%. Factors that could be linked to high prevalence were identified as low income, low human developmental index, lower latitude, higher humidity, higher temperature, and precipitation. The potential risk factors were male; young age; close contact with dogs, cats, or soil (gardens, sandpits/boxes, and playgrounds); living in rural areas; eating raw/under-processed meat; and drinking untreated water. In China, the seroprevalence ranged from 12.14% to 44.83% (Kong and Peng 2020). It increased from 12.14% in children in 1993 to 19.3% in 2015. From 1983 to 2019, 103 cases were reported in China, distributed as 92.23% OLM, 6.80% VLM, and 0.7% NLM. Borecka and Kłapeć (2015) reported that 1.8–76% of 18,367 sera of suspected toxocariasis tested during 1994–2005 were positive. As many as 1022 clinical cases were recognized during 1978–2009 in Poland.

Toxocara infection is very common, and most reliable kennels and pet shops would have adults infected. The opportunity for transmission to humans is enhanced if the litter of puppies is delivered to the home. Children with pica stand at a higher risk than the ones without this habit. They are likely to eat dirt inadvertently from outdoor environments, such as sandboxes, where dog and cat faeces can be found. The soil of parks in urban and semi-urban localities and areas where owners take their pets for a walk is likely a source of infection. Infection with *Toxocara* spp. may be associated with poor personal and social hygiene, especially in low socio-economic habitations. The increasing population of wild cats and dogs in urban areas presents a risk in tropical and semi-tropical regions. Environmental factors affect the survival and development of eggs in the soil. Climate change is likely to have an influence.

112.8 Diagnosis

Symptoms are indicative. For example, child showing fever, eosinophilia, and hepatosplenomegaly with history of pica indicates visceral larvae migrans. Unilateral vision loss with strabismus in a child is suggestive of ocular larva migrans. Hypergammaglobulinemia and an elevated isohaemagglutinin titre is also indicative.

Diagnostic tests like imaging and/or molecular are expensive. Currently diagnosis of human toxocariasis relies on serologic tests that use *Toxocara* excretory-secretory (TES) antigen to detect immunoglobulin G (IgG) antibodies to the larvae. Recombinant antigen made from TES used in ELISA, which enhanced the specificity and sensitivity.

A history of pica, clinical symptoms, eosinophilia, and positive serology together may lead to a diagnosis.

A liver biopsy showing granuloma surrounding the larvae is diagnostic. Polymerase chain reaction (PCR) to detect larval DNA in tissues or body fluid samples is confirmatory.

112.9 Treatment

Anthelmintic like mebendazole alone or with corticosteroid is effective.

112.10 Prevention

- Preventing the indiscriminate deposition of dog and cat faeces in play areas frequented by children is important.
- Fencing of playgrounds can be done.

- Placing clear vinyl plastic covers over sandboxes at night seemed to discourage pets from using them as faecal dump zones in Japan. This raised the temperatures within the sand often to >45 °C during summer (Despommier 2003). Considering that second-stage larvae are sensitive to certain environmental conditions and rapidly degenerate at high temperatures and low moisture, this may render the play area safe.
- Chemoprophylaxis: non-feral dogs and cats may be treated with ivermectin and mebendazole.
- The removal of sandboxes from parks and playgrounds has been practised by some municipalities.
- Reproductive control programmes for owned and stray dogs may reduce the number of young dogs in the population and may have an impact on prevalence.
- Public awareness for prevention is emphasized—children with pica and geophagia should not be allowed in suspected play areas and should be trained to wash their hands frequently, especially after visiting play areas and before eating.
- Surveillance and targeted prevention: samples of soil 3–5 cm below the surface after removing the topsoil layer should be analyzed by soil floatation and molecular methods for eggs and infective-stage larvae in eggs. The deoxyribonucleic acid (DNA) extracted from the soil is tested and quantified for *T. canis* and *T. cati* DNA using a multi-parallel real-time quantitative polymerase chain reaction (qPCR) protocol. This was used to detect environmental contamination in public places in New York City (Tyungu et al. 2020). Prophylactic treatment of domesticated and feral dogs and cats by veterinarians and the other measures suggested above may be used.

References

Borecka A, Kłapeć T (2015) Epidemiology of human toxocariasis in Poland—a review of cases 1978-2009. Ann Agric Environ Med 22(1):28–31

Cianferoni A, Schneider L, Schantz PM, Brown D, Fox LM (2006) Visceral larva migrans associated with earthworm ingestion: clinical evolution in an adolescent patient. Pediatrics 117(2):e336–e339

Despommier D (2003) Toxocariasis: clinical aspects, epidemiology, medical ecology, and molecular aspects. Clin Microbiol Rev 16(2):265–272

Gavin PJ, Kazacos KR, Tan TQ, Brinkman WB, Byrd SE et al (2002) Neural larva migrans caused by the raccoon roundworm *Baylisascaris procyonis*. Pediatr Infect Dis J 21(10):971–975

Hare AQ, Franco-Paredes C (2014) Ocular larva migrans: a severe manifestation of an unseen epidemic. Curr Trop Med Rep 1:69–73

Kong L, Peng HJ (2020) Epidemic situation of human toxocariasis in China. Adv Parasitol 109:433–448

Kuenzli E, Neumayr A, Chaney M, Blum J (2016) Toxocariasis-associated cardiac diseases—a systematic review of the literature. Acta Trop 154:107–120

Rostami A, Riahi SM, Holland CV, Taghipour A, Khalili-Fomeshi M et al (2019) Seroprevalence estimates for toxocariasis in people worldwide: a systematic review and meta-analysis. PLoS Negl Trop Dis 13(12):e0007809

Tyungu DL, McCormick D, Lau CL, Chang M, Murphy JR, Hotez PJ et al (2020) *Toxocara* species environmental contamination of public spaces in New York City. PLoS Negl Trop Dis 14(5):e0008249

Waindok P, Janecek-Erfurth E, Lindenwald D, Wilk E, Schughart K, Geffers R et al (2019) Multiplex profiling of inflammation-related bioactive lipid mediators in *Toxocara canis-* and *Toxocara cati-*induced neurotoxocarosis. PLoS Negl Trop Dis 13(9):e0007706

Chapter 113
Trichinellosis

Synonyms

Trichinosis, Trichiniasis.

Trichinellosis is a helminthozoonosis acquired by humans upon the ingestion of raw or poorly cooked meat of domestic and wild swine, bears, walruses, horses, badgers, dogs, cougars, jackals, and turtles. Meat and meat-derived products of all *Trichinella*-susceptible animals are a risk for humans if consumed raw or semi-cooked. Recent accumulated knowledge suggests that it is an important economic and public health problem. *Trichinella* spp. circulates with a relatively high prevalence in backyard or free-ranging pigs of poor rural areas without the cover of veterinary services. This impacts trade.

Against the single species *T. spiralis* known earlier, there are nine encapsulated and three non-encapsulated species under the two clades, and meat from a variety of sources is known to infect human beings. This has a highly diverse host range, and the sources of infection make it cosmopolitan, spread over all continents, except Antarctica. Besides the domestic pig cycle, the non-pig domestic animal and sylvatic cycles have become more significant. According to Shimshony (2009), the World Organisation for Animal Health (WOAH/OIE) considers it a multi-species notifiable disease due to the severity and high case fatality of the disease. In Europe, Latin America, and Asia, it is recognized as an emerging and/or re-emerging disease. The average incidence worldwide is over 10,000, and mortality is 0.2% (Gottstein et al. 2009).

The International Commission on Trichinellosis (ITC) was created in 1958 in Budapest. There are 110 members drawn from 46 countries. The ITC meets every 4 years. Recently, the Food and Agriculture Organization (FAO), World Health Organization (WHO), and OIE jointly instigated the ITC members to develop a new set of guidelines on surveillance, prevention, and control.

© Springer Nature Singapore Pte Ltd. 2024
K. G. Narayan et al., *Handbook of Management of Zoonoses*,
https://doi.org/10.1007/978-981-99-9885-2_113

113.1   Aetiology

The special features of *Trichinella* are as follows: (a) the infective larva is meat borne, (b) both intermediate and definitive hosts are the same vertebrate, (c) reproducing adult and infective larvae develop in the same host.

Trichinella spp. belong to the family *Trichinellidae*; the genus *Trichinella* is related to *Trichuris trichiura* and *Capillaria* spp.

The biological diversity of *Trichinella* is of major evolutionary significance and reflects substantial genetic diversity, divergent ecology, and host–parasite affiliation.

Korhonen et al. (2016) fully reconstructed a phylogeny and biogeography for the *Trichinella* complex. The encapsulated (collagen surrounding the nurse-cell-larva complex) and non-encapsulated *Trichinella* taxa diverged from their most recent common ancestor ~21 million years ago (mya), with taxon diversifications commencing ~10–7 mya. Currently, based on genetic data, there are nine and three species, respectively, under the two clades.

The nine encapsulated clade (infecting only mammals) includes *T. spiralis*, *T1*; *T. nativa*, *T2*; *T. britovi*, *T3*; *T. murrelli*, *T5*; *T. nelsoni*, *T7*; *T. patagoniensis*, *T12*; and *Trichinella* genotypes *T6*, *T8*, and *T9* taxa.

The three non-encapsulated clade includes *T. pseudospiralis*, *T4* (infecting mammals and birds); *T. papuae*, *T10*; and *T. zimbabwensis*, *T11* (infecting mammals and reptiles). Varying degrees of intra-specific genetic variability (*T. pseudospiralis*), dispersal ability, and host usage are exhibited by these taxa. These often represent a localized population.

Trichinella is distributed widely, from the Arctic to the tropics. *T spiralis* is cosmopolitan in distribution and temperate to equatorial climatic regions. Generally, domestic and sylvan swine maintain the parasite. Synanthropic animals, like brown rats, armadillos, dogs, cats, and a broad range of wild carnivores, are also parasitized. The encapsulated species are generally adapted to colder regions. The aetiology with the respective hosts and geographic distribution (Gottstein et al. 2009) are as follows.

113.1.1   Clade I (Encapsulated) Species

- *T. spiralis* or *T1* is cosmopolitan in distribution, except in the Arctic region. It is endemic in China and Japan, common in certain parts of Southeast Asia and Europe, less common in the USA, and not reported in Africa, except Egypt. It maintains itself in both domestic (domestic pigs, horses, and rats) and sylvatic cycles involving wild boar, bear, and fox. It is highly infective and pathogenic to humans. The nurse cell forms in 16 days and is sensitive to freezing.
- *T. nativa* or *T2* is distributed in the Arctic and subarctic areas of Holarctic (the isotherm 5 °C in January is the southern limit of distribution) regions in North America, Europe, and Asia. The nurse cell forms in 30 days and is highly resistant

to freezing. The sylvatic cycle involves a wide range of terrestrial and marine carnivores—mustelids, Arctic foxes, red foxes, wolves, raccoon dogs, domestic and sylvatic cats, lynxes, Siberian tigers, black bears, brown bears, polar bears, sled dogs, walruses, and several species of seals. The parasite survives for at least 20 years in the muscles of these natural hosts. The parasite has been rarely detected in domestic and sylvatic swine because of its innate low reproductive capacity in them and in laboratory rodents. Eating raw meat from walruses, bears, and other game animals causes human infection. It is highly infective and moderately pathogenic to humans with a long incubation period (IP).

- *Trichinella T6* has been reported from Canada and the USA (Alaska, Idaho, Montana, and Pennsylvania). The sylvatic cycle involves carnivores. The collagen-capsulated larvae are resistant to freezing.
- *T. britovi* or *T3* is distributed in Palearctic (the isotherm 6 °C in January is the northern limit of distribution) regions, temperate zones, and biotopes 500 m above sea level in Europe, America, Asia, and Northern and Western Africa. The sylvatic cycle occurs in wild carnivores, mustelids, Viverridae, brown boars, red foxes, jackals, wild and—seldom—domestic dogs and cats, horses, and—occasionally—pigs. It causes low-muscle invasion. The nurse cell forms in 42 days and is not resistant to freezing. Brown rats foraging in garbage get infected, but the parasite is short-lived in them. Human infection occurs from the meat of red foxes, wild boars, jackals, horses, and domestic pigs. The infectivity and pathogenicity are moderate. Cases show low gastrointestinal symptoms.
- *Trichinella T8* is distributed in South Africa and has a sylvatic cycle in carnivores. The nurse cells form and are encapsulated and are sensitive to freezing.
- *T. murrelli* or *T5* is distributed mainly in temperate areas of the Nearctic region of America, Canada, Mexico, and Central America. Human infections are more common in the USA. The sylvatic cycle is mainly in bears and other carnivores, like bobcats, black bears, coyotes, raccoons, pine martens, and red foxes. Nurse cells form in 4 months and have low resistance to freezing. Infection in domestic dogs, horses, and cats occurs, and meat from horses and black bears is the common cause of infection in humans, although infectivity is low. Domestic swine are not naturally infected.
- *Trichinella T9* has been reported from Japan. It has a sylvatic cycle in carnivores. Nurse cells form, but their sensitivity to freezing is not known.
- *T. nelsoni* or *T7* is distributed in the tropical region—confined to equatorial Africa, viz. Ethiopia. The sylvatic cycle involves mainly carnivores, striped and spotted hyenas, side-striped jackals, black-backed jackals, bat-eared foxes, domestic dogs, lions, leopards, cheetahs, servals, occasionally bush pigs and wart hogs, and seldom swine and rodents. Some of these have been the source of human infection. It is highly infective but lowly pathogenic and non-fatal to humans. Nurse cells form in 40 days and are sensitive to freezing.
- *Trichinella T12* has been detected in a mountain lion (*Puma concolor*) from Trapalco, Patagonia, Río Negro, and Argentina.

113.1.2   Clade II (Not Encapsulated) Species

This species invades other vertebrates in addition to mammals.

- *T. pseudospiralis* or *T4* is widely distributed in Nearctic, Oceania and many foci in Palearctic; Alabama and Texas (North America); Sweden and Slovak Republic in Europe, Asia, Tasmania (Australia—in a mammal 'devil'). It has a sylvatic cycle in birds of prey, wild carnivores, and omnivorous animals, including rats and marsupials. The domestic cycle is seldom. Nurse cells do not form and are sensitive to freezing. Infectivity for humans is moderate. Three outbreaks (in Kamchatka, Thailand, and France) and a case probably acquired in Tasmania are known.
- *T. papuae* or *T10* is restricted to Papua New Guinea. It has a sylvatic cycle in wild and domestic pigs, possibly a wild pig-crocodile cycle. It does not infect birds. Nurse cells do not form and are sensitive to freezing. It caused the Thailand outbreak in 2006. All the case patients had consumed *T. papuae*-infected wild boar meat. They had myalgia (83%) and oedema (70.8%) of the trunk, limbs, and face (Khumjui et al. 2008).
- *T. zimbabwensis* or *T11* is restricted to Zimbabwe, Mozambique, and Ethiopia in Africa and has a sylvatic cycle in crocodiles (reptiles) and mammals/lions. It has low infectivity. Nurse cells form in 40 days and are sensitive to freezing.

113.2   Life Cycle

Animal/human infection begins with the ingestion of an infective-muscle-stage-larva complex. This happens when undercooked or uncooked meat containing a nurse-cell-larva complex is eaten. After ingestion, the stomach enzymes (pepsin, hydrochloric acid) digest the complex and larvae are released in the small intestine. The partial digestion of the epicuticle sends a message to the larvae to select the sites to parasitize. The base of the columnar epithelium in the upper 2/third of the small intestine (duodenum) is the common site (Fig. 113.1). The immature larvae live within a row of these cells—hence, the parasite is considered an intra-multicellular organism. In quick succession, four moultings occur in 30 h and mature males (1.5 mm × 36 micro-mm) and females (3 mm × 36 micro-mm) develop and mate. Five to 7 days after infection, a number of newborn larvae (0.08 mm × 7 micro-mm) are produced. Newborn larvae production continues for 1 to 2 weeks or more. The host responds, and protective immunity develops and forces the adult parasite to descend and relocate further in the intestine. An intestinally immune-mediated host response is established within weeks, and immune effector mechanisms affect the viability of the female parasites. The final egress takes several weeks.

The newly born larvae have stylets in their oral cavity, which help puncture a hole in potential hosts' cells and reach the lamina propria, where they enter either the mesenteric lymphatics or the bloodstream. Once in the bloodstream, they get

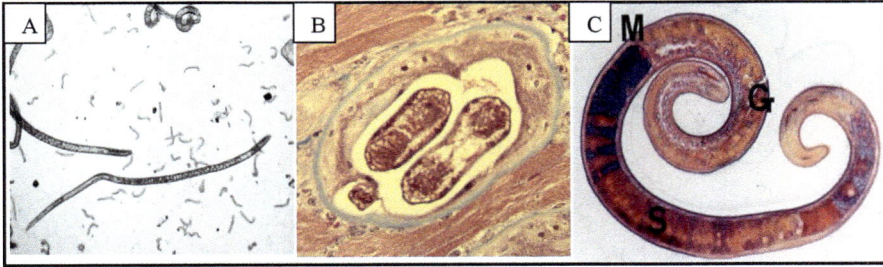

Fig. 113.1 (**a**) Adult worms that developed in the small intestine following oral infection with muscle larvae; the small worms are new born larvae (immature L1), which are infective to muscle. (**b**) Infective muscle larva in altered muscle cell surrounded by a collagen capsule (blue). (**c**) Infective muscle larva, Azan staining of longitudinal section of excysted larvae. *M* Midgut, *G* Genital primordium, *S* Stichocyte. (Source: Mitreva and Jasmer, 2006)

disseminated and then leave the capillaries to enter the hosts' cells. There is no tropism. Most of the invaded cells die, except the striated muscle cells.

The invaded striated muscle cells are forced to transform into a nurse-cell-larva complex. The growth and development of the muscle cells and the larvae proceed in a coordinated fashion. The parasite–cell association is intimate, and this intracellular niche is permanent (Fig. 113.2). Possibly, the larvae/genes cause the muscle cell nuclei to enlarge and create a 'placenta' like structure around the muscle cell, called 'circulatory/capillary rete (network)', and form new blood vessels (angiogenesis) around the muscle cell. The development of the nurse-cell-larva complex thus includes the replacement of myofilaments and cell components with whorls of smooth membrane and clusters of dysfunctional mitochondria, the enlargement of the nuclei and their division, and the amplification of the hosts' genome. There is a shift in cell metabolism from aerobic to anaerobic. Although the larva is infective in 14 days, it continues to grow in size for 20 days; the nurse cell development is completed in 16 days. The life of the nurse-cell-larva complex (the hypobiotic stage) seems to equal the life of the host, waiting to be ingested by another host—for over 20 years in polar bears and 40 years in humans. The nurse-cell-larva complex may calcify after weeks/months/years. The host species; its immune response, which can change among individuals within a given species; and the *Trichinella* species or genotype influence the period of calcification of the collagen capsule, nurse cell, and larva.

The perpetuation of the parasite requires the eating of the nurse-cell-larva complex by another host. Cannibalism of the cadavers of infected hosts or the scavenging of uncooked/undercooked meat containing the nurse-cell-larva complex facilitates this. Most wild and domestic scavenging animals are involved. Herbivorous animals at times get infected as they occasionally ingest meat. Eating horse meat caused trichinosis in France, Italy, and Poland. Infected humans are dead ends.

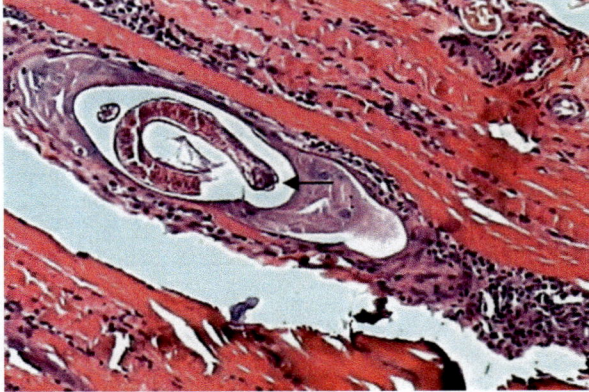

Fig. 113.2 Histopathological slide of one index case of muscle biopsy specimen showing larvae (arrow) of *T. spiralis* with lymphocytic infiltrate surrounding the parasite (H & E ×500). (Source: Mitreva and Jasmer, 2006)

The survival of muscles in a decaying carcass facilitates the transmission of *Trichinella*; the greater the persistence of larval viability, the higher the probability of it being ingested by a scavenging host. It is dependent upon environmental conditions. High humidity and low temperature favour encapsulated larval survival, even when the muscle tissue is completely liquefied. Survival time is greatest between 0 °C and −18 °C. The survival time of larvae in the striated muscles of carnivores is the highest. It is reduced to a few days or weeks for the larvae in striated muscles of swine or rodents.

113.3 Epidemiology

113.3.1 Prevalence and Burden

Trichinellosis is probably the most widely distributed nematode zoonosis. Devleesschauwer et al. (2015) estimated the global number of disability-adjusted life years due to trichinellosis to be 76 per billion persons per year. The burden is shared by the World Health Organization European region (the main contributor), followed by the WHO region of the Americas and the World Health Organization Western Pacific region. The predominant impact of trichinellosis relates principally to acute outbreaks following the consumption of infected raw meat products, with examples in Argentina, China, Laos, Papua New Guinea, Romania, and Vietnam.

According to Dupouy-Camet (2000), there were approximately 11 million human and 10,000 porcine infections worldwide reported particularly in the Balkans, Russia, the Baltic republics, and some parts of China and Argentina.

Horsemeat-related outbreaks were reported in France and Italy involving about 3000 patients in the past 25 years. There were 65,818 cases and 42 deaths reported from 41 countries in 2009, and 87% were located in the European region of the World Health Organization. Romania accounted for 50% of these reported during 1990–1999 (Murrell and Pozio, 2011).

According to Troiano and Nante (2019), trichinellosis has spread to New Zealand and many countries in Europe, East Asia, South America, and North Africa. Outbreaks were reported from 55 countries. The annual global average of cases was 5752 and five deaths. It was most prevalent in Eastern Europe, but outbreaks were reported also in Italy and Spain. The parasite is able to infect virtually all mammals, birds, and reptiles, depending on the involved *Trichinella* species. *T. spiralis* is the most common species adapted to domestic and wild swine, but its life cycle could also include synanthropic rats, and it is globally distributed. *T. britovi* is the second-most common species that may affect human health and is widely distributed within the sylvatic life cycles of Europe, Asia, and Northern and Western Africa. It affects domestic pig populations also mainly via extensive grazing systems or feed with scraps or carrion originating from sylvatic carnivores.

Although France and Italy reported horse-meat-related trichinellosis, most cases are swine related. Animal farming and regulatory systems determine human infections.

113.3.2 Factors Associated

113.3.2.1 Animal Farming

Animal farming influences the entry and propagation of *Trichinella spiralis* in farms. Farming (pigs/horse/sled dogs/fur animals/crocodile) that permits feeding waste containing scraps from slaughtered or hunted or dead pig, game animal, dog, fur animal, wild boar, other wild animal, crocodile, and rat as well as allow to scavenge on garbage dumps are most likely to permit infection with *Trichinella*. The parasite is maintained. Horses and some other herbivores are atypical hosts, and their flesh may contain trichina larvae. In most of the horse-meat-associated trichinellosis, the horse meat originated from areas with high prevalence in domestic swine and/or wildlife, where veterinary control on food safety was rudimentary.

The swine farming system has undergone tremendous improvement. It is now possible to raise *Trichinella*-free swine. A '*Trichinella*-free pig farm' or a '*Trichinella*-free region' is achieved and maintained. The integrated management of swine production and slaughter and meat inspection are important to ensure safety against trichinellosis.

Prevalence in pigs is reflected in human trichinellosis if contaminated pork is sold.

In many parts of the world, both domestic and sylvatic cycles are operative.

113.3.2.2   Sylvatic Cycles and Hunters

The study of the eco-biology of the *Trichinella* species and the host species helps in understanding the epidemiology. Owen et al. (2005) observed that, in all probability, the new species, *T. papuae*, existed among the hunters in Papua New Guinea. They consumed raw or undercooked wild pig meat. A wild-pig-crocodile cycle propagated this parasite (Pozio et al. 2005). A shift from farmed-pig-meat-linked trichinellosis to wild-animal-meat (farmed or hunted)-linked one is observed.

The epidemiology of trichinellosis in developed and developing countries differs.

113.3.2.3   Developing Countries

In developing countries, swine continues to be the main source. Undercooked pork is associated with human trichinellosis. In Thailand, larb is a delicacy, and undercooked pork is an ingredient. Not surprisingly, 200 to 600 cases are annually reported around the Thai New Year celebration. An epidemiological study in China for the period 2000–2003 has been reported by Wang et al. (2006). There were 17 outbreaks, 828 cases, and 11 deaths. The study revealed that most cases were ethnic groups who ate raw meat. Pork was predominant (13/17 outbreaks), followed by dog flesh (2/17), and the rest were game animals—wild bears and boars. According to Wang et al. (2007), trichinellosis in China seems to be widespread in animals. Sheep and cattle are infected, as evidenced serologically. Mutton and beef also contain larvae. The prevalence in dogs is high, averaging 16.2% among slaughtered and 3.5% in dog meat sold in the market. Feline infection is reported in ten provinces, autonomous regions, or municipalities (P/A/M). House and wild rats and wildlife—foxes, bears, wild boars, weasels, raccoon dogs, muntjacs and bamboo rats, shrews, and moles—have been found infected. *T. spiralis* in pigs and *T. native* in dogs have been identified. From 1964 to 2004, 27 outbreaks of human trichinellosis associated with mutton, dog, and game meat occurred.

In India, reported outbreaks in the recent past led to several studies and the citation of earlier reports. Konwar et al. (2017) examined a total of 319 tissue and 279 serum samples collected from 279 slaughter pigs in Assam, Chandigarh (Union territory), Punjab, and Uttarakhand. The overall seroprevalence of trichinellosis was found to be 2.87%. Thirty-eight free-ranging and 94 farm pigs from Uttarakhand were negative on serological and tissue (tongue and diaphragm examined for larvae) examination, 2/40 and 3/38 free-ranging pigs from Ludhiana and Chandigarh were positive.

Trichinellosis is common in Northeast India and is suspected among communities where >75% relish pork. An examination of 865 meat samples collected during 2016–2017 from five different states detected no larvae. Serologically positive samples originated from Meghalaya and Assam but none from Arunachal Pradesh, Tripura, and Mizoram (Acheenta et al. 2019).

In Tehri Garhwal, another outbreak associated with pork was reported (Sharma et al. 2014). The pork was consumed in different forms—uncooked by 24% ($n = 13$), open-fire roasted by 39% ($n = 21$), and fried by 37% ($n = 20$). None who ate fried pork suffered. The study group consisted of 54 (18 males + 36 females) who participated in community feast. One died with a similar clinical manifestation. The participants were aged 5 to 87 (mean 40) years; four were under 12 years. The signs and symptoms conformed to trichinellosis. A biopsy of muscles showed larvae.

Encapsulated larvae of *Trichinella* spp. in domestic cats, wild toddy cat, civet cat and domestic pigs as well as non-encapsulated larvae of *T. pseudospiralis* in Indian mole rat and once in human are documented (Alipuria et al. 1996). Undercooked wild boar meat caused multiple outbreaks in Uttarakhand, India (2008–2011). Of the 49 patients aged 7–60 years, 69% were male and 31% were female. They ate wild boar meat. Seventy were suspected cases, and 11 died. Nineteen per cent of the 42 tracked patient biopsies revealed larvae (Sethi et al. 2012).

113.3.2.4 Developed Countries

Hunters and game animal eaters are considered a high-risk group in developed countries. The relevance of swine appears to be lessening. The US surveillance report (1997–2001) highlights the changing shift from trichina-infected pork from domesticated sources to wild game meat. Eating non-commercial pork from home—raised or directly from a swine farm—accounted for nine (13%) cases, and these were not covered by US regulations and standards. This trend of association with 'meat other than pork' continued from 2002 to 2007, as evidenced by the report (Kennedy et al. 2009).

Wilson et al. (2015) analyzed US surveillance data between 2008 and 2012. A total of 84 cases, including five outbreaks, were recorded in the United States and analyzed. The incidence was 0.1 case/million population. Eating raw or undercooked meat caused 47% of cases, as reported. Pork products were associated with 22 (26%) cases. Meats other than pork were associated with 45 (54%) cases, including 41 (91%) that were linked to bear meat, two (4%) that were linked to deer meat, and two (4%) that were linked to ground beef (deer and herbivores are atypical hosts). Five outbreaks were reported. Bear meat was implicated. Two or more cases, at least one of which was laboratory confirmed, constituted an outbreak. Analyzing this surveillance report, it was observed that (a) the seasonal pattern 'December to March' of occurrence is not observed now. (b) Approximately 400 cases and ten to 15 deaths were reported during 1947–1951. The annual incidence declined to eight cases during 2002–2007 with no deaths. (c) Raw or undercooked *Trichinella*-infected pork accounted for 60–70% of infections. The number of cases associated with eating non-pork products was more than twice (45 cases) as many as those associated with pork products (22 cases), and the majority was linked to eating wildlife meat. The consumption of meat from *Trichinella*-infected wildlife, including wild boar, is now implicated in a greater proportion of cases.

The consumption of walrus (*Odobenus rosmarus*) meat caused the first multiple-case outbreaks during July 2016–May 2017, and this is the first since 1992. These two outbreaks, involving five cases each, add to the concern of increasing non-porcine-wild-game-species-linked trichinellosis (Springer et al. 2017).

In Canada, trichinellosis is endemic, but the domestic swine population is free. The annual incidence in humans is 11/100,000. In an outbreak in Victoria, meat from a hunted black bear was frozen for 3 days, barbequed, and stewed on different occasions and was found to carry 300 larvae per gm; 78 ate, and there were 26 probable cases and 14 patients (McIntyre et al. 2007). A rash was found on the limb of a patient.

113.3.2.5 Glimpses of Other Countries

France and Italy reported horse-meat-related trichinellosis; most cases in Europe were swine related. According to Gari-Toussaint et al. (2005), large outbreaks due to horse meat were getting rare, and cases due to wild boar have been reported regularly since 1975 among hunters and their families. Frozen wild boar meat caused trichinellosis in southern France. The wild boar meat frozen for 7 days at −35 °C caused an outbreak. Six persons were infected. The examination of frozen boar meat revealed encapsulated *Trichinella* larvae identified as *T. britovi*. The French National *Trichinella* Reference Centre reported five cases of trichinellosis among those who sailed from Aleutian Islands to Greenland. They consumed meat from a variety of wild animals, including polar bears and walruses, the most frequent sources of human trichinellosis. According to Gallardo et al. (2007), wild-boar-meat-associated trichinellosis seems to be common in Spain and Sweden. A study of trichinellosis in the past 60 years in Poland suggests a similar pattern—pork replaced with other (boar) meat (Gołab and Sadkowska-Todys 2006). This seems to be happening in other parts of Europe also.

In Italy, Troiano and Nante (2019) observed that 764 cases have been recorded since 1989. *T. spiralis* and *T. britovi* accounted for 84.4% and 13.7%, respectively. The most important sources of infections were horse meat (82.2%), wild boar meat (11.9%), and pig meat (5.9%).

113.3.2.6 Socio-Political-Economic Conditions

Socio-political-economic conditions influenced trichinellosis in Latin America, Asia, and the East European countries. Romania is an example. Romania had the most cases of trichinellosis in the world, according to an International Commission on Trichinellosis survey in 2004. Analyses of epidemiological data for two different periods (1980–1989 and 1990–2004) were done. The incidence was 51.0 cases/10^6/year. It was 86.2 in Transylvanian counties (Blaga et al. 2007). A comparison of the data from the two different periods led the scientists to believe that political upheavals in Romania contributed to the resurgence of swine infection and the corresponding increase in the incidence of human trichinellosis. The incidence rate (cases per lac) in Romania was 51 during 1980–2004. The communist regime ended in 1990. The incidence rate for 1980–1989 was 19.6, compared to 71.8 during 1990–2004. They attributed this increase to (a) the closure of state units of production of swine and pork/pork products in 1989, (b) chaotic veterinary and food safety, (c) the increased circulation of parasites in swine and an increase in infected pork, and (d) the increased consumption of meat because its supply was limited. The high incidence rate observed in Transylvania was a result of the traditional food habit (eating raw meat) of the local population.

According to Neghina et al. (2009), *T. spiralis* and *T. britovi* caused trichinellosis in Romania. More outbreaks/cases were reported in winter. Certain regions reported a higher number of outbreaks. This was explained as due to the following: (a) the cluster of populations of labourers, the unemployed, and low-income groups living under poor hygienic conditions; (b) the consumption of traditional home-made pork preparations (sausages, ham, bacon, blood pudding, and mosaic salami) during winter; and (c) the slaughter of pigs at home without veterinary inspection.

According to Neghina et al. (2010), 95% of human trichinellosis cases originate from specific cultural food practices involving pork consumption, although the sylvatic cycle, such as the consumption of meat from wild boars and bears, has been implicated in human cases.

113.3.2.7 Food Habit/Prejudices

This is the most important determinant. In some countries, like Finland, Sweden, and Switzerland, human trichinellosis is not documented, although prevalence in wildlife and domestic swine is known. The most convincing explanation seems to be the habit of eating cooked meat. Bantu, a predominant ethnic group in Africa, rarely eats meat, and despite the prevailing sylvatic *Trichinella*, human trichinellosis is seldom recorded.

113.3.2.8 Influence of Religion

Islam and Judaism prohibit eating pork, and hence, trichinellosis is rare among Moslems and Jews; game animals may be responsible.

113.3.2.9 Processing

During 1997–2001 (MMWR 25 July 2003) in the United States, 38 of 72 cases identified the cooking method applied for preparing the suspected food. The distribution of 30 cases according to the method of making food was 20 for uncooked, 14—open-fire roasted or barbequed, 13—fried, 6—stewed, 2—baked, and 1—microwaved (certain cases had multiple methods of cooking).

113.4   Source of Infection

A FAO/WHO/OIE (2007) document described the natural *Trichinella* spp. infections in more than 100 species of mammals belonging to 11 orders (Marsupialia, Insectivora, Edentata, Primates, Lagomorpha, Rodentia, Cetacea, Carnivora, Perissodactyla, Artiodactyla, and Tylopoda). Seven species of birds are documented as hosts for *T. pseudospiralis*. Among primates, only humans have been naturally infected with *Trichinella*.

The natural reservoir differs from the species of *Trichinella*. Swine are not suitable hosts for *T. nativa*, *T. murrelli*, and *Trichinella T6* and do not have a reservoir role for these species. *T. nativa* in marine mammals has a circumpolar Arctic distribution. Arctic carnivores like polar bears (*Ursus maritimus*), Arctic foxes (*Alopex lagopus*), and domestic dogs have a high prevalence of *T. nativa* in the Arctic. The carcasses of these animals dumped in the ocean may be scavenged by marine animals, such as walrus. Predation, carrion feeding, and cannibalism have been documented for walruses (*Odobenus rosmarus*). Infections in walruses present a challenging zoonotic hazard, and the testing of harvested walrus meat for *Trichinella* larvae has been implemented. There is a possibility of the existence of the marine cycle (walrus-*Trichinella*) of infection. Seals and whales are likely to be infected. The availability of a potential host species in a region is an important determinant of its role in the cycle of infection. A few suggestive examples are as follows: walrus in Canada and Greenland; wild boar (*Sus scrofa*) in Asia, Europe, and North and South America; horse in France and Italy; dog in the People's Republic of China, Greenland Russia, the Slovak Republic, and Switzerland; and jackal (*Canis aureus*) in Thailand.

The sylvatic cycle of *T. spiralis* includes a broad range of wild carnivores, which may, however, introduce the parasite into a domestic host population, e.g. a domestic pig cycle. Pork scraps from *T. spiralis*-infected pigs are the main source of infection for synanthropic animals, e.g. rats, horses, stray cats, and dogs. When humans fail in the proper management of domestic animals and wildlife, some *Trichinella* spp., like *T. spiralis*, *T. britovi*, *T. pseudospiralis*, *T. papuae*, and *T. zimbabwensis*, are transmitted from the sylvatic environment to the domestic one, sometimes through synanthropic animals.

113.5   Mode of Infection

The ingestion of striated muscle containing the nurse-cell-larva complex is the mode of infection in man and animals.

There is a potential for transplacental infection in men and animals. Dubinský et al. (2001) reported an outbreak in the Slovak Republic affecting 336 people, including a pregnant woman who contracted an infection during the tenth week.

She opted for abortion, which was performed in the 22nd week. The infection was established serologically and larvae were detected in placenta, fluid of body cavities, tissues and organs of the foetus. Saracino et al. (2016) reported a study on six pregnant women and their newborns from different outbreaks of trichinellosis (*T. spiralis*). Transplacental transmission was evidenced. All of them showed helminthocytotoxic activity against newborn larvae, four in a progesterone-dependent manner and the other two by antibodies. Specific antibodies were detected in the newborn (≥ 1 year) from the infected mother. There was a transplacental transfer of IgG, IgE, and IgM.

113.6 Pathology

It is dependent upon the stage of infection, the precise state of parasite development, the number of newborn larvae, and their migration and penetration in tissues, broadly described as the (a) enteral and (b) parenteral phases of the parasite. The former consists of the release from the nurse-cell-larva complex, one to four moultings, the development of adults, mating, and the birth of newborn larvae. It lasts for about 3 weeks or more. The columnar epithelium is damaged.

The parenteral phase consists of (a) the birth of newborn larvae and (b) the invasion, migration, and penetration of tissues. A local inflammatory reaction is appreciated through the infiltration of eosinophiles, neutrophiles, and lymphocytes caused by the presence of a large number of newborn larvae. The epithelial villi are somewhat flattened, leading to reduced absorption. While penetrating the mesenteric lymphatics and/or blood vessels, larvae may injure the intestinal epithelium, causing bacteraemia with the enteric flora and sometimes sepsis and death. The wheat germ receptors are lost from the entire length of the intestine. In search of striated muscle, the larvae may penetrate any tissue—the heart (cardiomyopathy), liver, kidney, and brain [central nervous system (CNS) symptoms], causing cell death. The severity depends upon the number of cells penetrated.

Intestinal motility is retarded, and heavy infection may lead to generalized oedema and proteinuria.

Some ideas on immunological responses, pathology, and the expulsion of the adult parasite emerge from experimental studies on immunologically defined rodents. The strains of a parasite possibly have varying immunological capabilities that determine the number of nurse-cell-larva complexes formed. Interleukins 4 and 13, eosinophiles, and IgE antibodies limit the number of newborn larvae. Local cellular pathology surrounding the worms and the inflammation and the production of local nitric oxide probably contribute to the expulsion of adult worms.

113.7   Symptoms

Clinical manifestations may range from mild to moderate to severe, depending upon the number of nurse-cell-larva ingested, the age, the gender, and host immunity. Similarly, most but not all of the nurse-cell-larva complexes are destroyed during convalescence. More males (72%) than females, from 3–81 years of age (median 45), become patients.

The incubation period observed was 13 (1–50) days. The IP depended upon the number of larvae ingested. The onset of the acute form is sudden, manifesting general weakness, chills, headache, fever (40 °C), excessive sweating, and tachycardia.

Symptoms are related to the enteral and parenteral stages of infection. A few days (1–2 days) post infection and lasting for about 10 days, symptoms of gastroenteritis such as diarrhoea, abdominal pain, heartburn, nausea, and vomition are seen. A history of association with food often leads one to diagnose food poisoning. During 1–3 weeks, there is mild, intermittent fever, chill, myalgia (may be severe causing paralysis), joint pain, bilateral periorbital oedema extending to entire face and petechiae under fingernails, on conjunctiva (also conjunctivitis), mucous membrane, itching and rash. Myalgia develops in the nuchal and trunk muscles, in the muscles of the upper and lower extremities, and, less frequently, in the masseter muscles. Cases in the 2006 Thailand outbreak reported myalgia and oedema of the trunk, limbs, and face (Khumjui et al. 2008). An examination of a patient reveals muscular tenderness, and clinical laboratory findings include enhanced white blood cells and eosinophiles (5–50%). Eosinophilia shows a pattern—rising eosinophiles and a persistent plateau throughout infection.

During the next 2–4 weeks, the above symptoms and signs, particularly myalgia, fever, and cardiac pain, continue. Leucocytosis and eosinophilia persist. The muscle enzymes creatinine kinase and lactate dehydrogenase increase, and the serum antibody IgG appears. The newborn larvae are migrating, invading the tissues, and settling down in striated muscle cells.

Pozio et al. (1993) observed that *T. britovi* infection occurred in south Italy and caused a less severe intestinal pathology, there was a lesser increase in creatine phosphokinase, and the duration of a specific IgG was shorter compared with *T. spiralis* infection. The outbreak caused by the ingestion of *T. spiralis*-infected wild boar meat involved two families. The principal symptoms were fever, myalgia, and diarrhoea, and the laboratory findings included eosinophilia and increased creatine phosphokinase and other muscle enzymes and specific IgG titre. An anti-newborn larva antibody was also observed in 30% of cases. The level of response was related to the number of infective larvae ingested.

The penetration of tissues other than the striated muscle leads to severe disease with serious sequelae. Penetration of cardiac muscle by the newborn larvae induces ECG disorder but not necessarily accompanied by any clinical symptoms to myocarditis. There will be respiratory apnoea in case the diaphragm and accessory muscles are invaded. CNS involvement may also occur manifesting in neurological deficit –ataxia, respiratory failure, death in 10–24% of the reported cases of the rare form of stroke.

Neurotrichinellosis (Madariaga et al. 2007) is rare and is most likely to be misdiagnosed. A woman admitted to the hospital in an unconscious state was neurologically unresponsive. She had a fever, weakness of the upper left extremity, and leucocytosis. Lumbar puncture revealed red blood cells (RBC), neutrophils, and mild elevation of protein and glucose. The examination for bacterial and viral pathogens proved negative, and she did not respond to antibiotics. Magnetic resonance imaging (MRI) showed non-specific changes. After 3 days, she woke up but was disoriented and aphasic. Re-evaluation was done. Periorbital oedema, petechiae, and conjunctivitis in the left eye; leucocytosis; 22% eosinophilia; and increased creatinine kinase (467 against 145 U/L) were recorded. The enzyme-linked immunosorbent assay (ELISA) was positive for the dominant *Trichinella* antigen. She responded to anthelmintic treatment. Wild animal meat was probably the cause. Other neurological symptoms are headache, deafness, aphasia, seizures, and apathy.

Death usually occurs in 4–6 weeks due to myocarditis, encephalopathy, or pneumonia.

Some of the severe cases report problems months and even years after acute illness. They suffer from chronic pain, general discomfort, tingling, numbness, excessive sweating, and signs of paranoia. Conjunctivitis, impaired muscle strength and coordination, and IgG antibodies have persisted for up to 10 years after infection. At the same time, larvae have been detected in muscles without symptoms, even up to 39 years of infection.

113.8   Diagnosis

Diagnosis is based on the detection of *Trichinella* larvae. The OIE recommended that pepsin–HCl digestion assay (OIE 2012) may be used to separate the larvae from the muscle (e.g. pork, biopsied muscle from a human case).

Stereomicroscopy: the *Trichinella* larvae may appear coiled (when cold), motile (when warm), or C shaped when examined by a stereomicroscope. The larvae can be used for genotyping and the preparation of antigens for serological tests to detect specific antibodies in persons infected with any species of *Trichinella*. FAO/WHO/OIE (2007) describes the types of antigens extracted from larvae/infected muscle and the methods of diagnosis.

- History of the consumption of meat (partially/undercooked or processed) of domestic or wide pigs or game animals of suspected species; clinical symptoms (myalgia following gastroenteritis), tenderness of muscle, leucocytosis and patterns of eosinophilia, and an increase in serum creatine phosphokinase and lactic dehydrogenase (muscle enzymes) contribute to arriving at a diagnosis.
- Histological examination of biopsied muscle revealing a nurse-cell-larva complex is diagnostic. Early developmental stages of the parasite and sampling error limit this method, and all positive cases may not be detected.

- The serum antibody appears about 12 days post-infection and can be detected by ELISA.
- PCR to detect *Trichinella* spp.-specific DNA is the latest method with high specificity and sensitivity. All laboratories may not adopt it as the cost is prohibitive.

Western blot (Nöckler et al. 2009) may be useful in distinguishing infections caused by *T. pseudospiralis* from those caused by *T. spiralis* and *T. britovi* (Gómez-Morales et al., 2018).

Genotyping is useful in epidemiological studies. Information on species and genotype distribution and host range can be downloaded from the website of the International Trichinella Reference Centre (www.iss.it/site/Trichinella/index.asp).

113.9   Treatment

Anthelmintics like mebendazole (200–400 mg three times a day for 3 days) or albendazole (twice a day for 8–14 days) are effective but should not be given to pregnant women.

Anti-inflammatory drugs, like prednisolone (20–60 mg per day for the first few days), are useful; antipyretic (aspirin), anti-allergic (corticosteroids), and analgesic drugs may be continued till fever and allergic signs and symptoms persist.

113.10   Prevention

The related provisions of OIE should be followed for international trade. The control of trichinellosis in the United States may be attributed to the following: (a) trichinellosis has been a nationally notifiable disease in the United States since 1966; (b) legislation and changes in the US pork industry reduced the exposure of domestic pigs to *Trichinella*; (c) the 1980 Federal Swine Health Protection Act prohibited the feeding of potentially *Trichinella*-contaminated garbage to swine and preventing access of swine to rodents, raccoons, skunk, opossums as well as cannibalism within a drift/drove; (d) commercial production practices are implemented that ensure swine are raised in bio-secure confinement; (e) the United States Department of Agriculture (USDA) has stipulated specific cooking temperatures and times, freezing temperatures and times, and curing methods for processed pork products to inactivate *Trichinella* larvae in meat; and (f) educating consumers has been successful. The USDA defined pre-harvest and post-harvest procedures. The USDA, the National Pork Producers Council, and the pork processing industry developed the Trichinae Herd Certification Program, with the goal of establishing a system wherein pork production facilities following good practices can be certified as trichinae-safe.

In Europe, countries of the EU employ several strategies for the detection of larvae in muscles. Generally, a pool of meat from a region is examined, and if they are found consistently negative, the region is designated as *Trichinella*-free.

Measures at the level of processing plants are (a) meat inspection, (b) control and destruction of meat found positive for trichinae, (c) the removal and proper disposal of the diaphragm of pigs, and (d) cleaning meat grinders before use.

Public awareness is desired. Swine reared at the interface of human habitation and forests are exposed to the sylvatic cycle and *Trichinella* spp., with the possibility of the introduction of infection to the synanthropic (i.e. ecologically associated with humans) region. Hunters should be educated to avoid leaving animal carcasses in the field. Public awareness of the processing of meat to destroy trichina larvae is important:

- Heating meat to an internal temperature of 165 °F (74 °C) for a minimum of 15 s.
- Freezing pork less than 6 inches thick for 20 days at 5 °F (−15 °C) or 3 days at −4 °F (−20 °C) and thorough cooking of wild game animal meat; in general, one should not depend on curing, drying, smoking, and microwaving.

Sentinel animals: It is important to examine samples of muscles from indicator animal species like foxes and racoons to assess prevalence among wildlife reservoirs and the associated risks of introduction into domestic animals.

References

Acheenta GB, Jyoti CP, Himangshu R, Dharitree S et al (2019) Epidemiological studies on porcine trichinellosis in five states of north East India. Iran J Parasitol 14(2):303–309

Alipuria S, Sangha HK, Singh G, Pandhi S (1996) Trichinosis—a case report. Indian J Pathol Microbiol. 39(3):231–232

Blaga R, Durand B, Antoniu S, Gherman C et al (2007) A dramatic increase in the incidence of human trichinellosis in Romania over the past 25 years: impact of political changes and regional food habits. Am J Trop Med Hyg 76(5):983–986

Devleesschauwer B, Praet N, Speybroeck N, Torgerson PR et al (2015) The low global burden of trichinellosis: evidence and implications. Int J Parasitol 45(2–3):95–99

Dubinský P, Böör A, Kinceková J, Tomasovicová O et al (2001) Congenital trichinellosis? Case report. Parasite 8(2 Suppl):S180–S182

Dupouy-Camet J (2000) Trichinellosis: a worldwide zoonosis. Vet Parasitol 93(3–4):191–200

FAO/WHO/OIE Guidelines for the surveillance, management, prevention and control of trichinellosis (2007). Dupouy-Camet J, Murrell KD (eds). FAO-WHO-OIE_Guidelines%20TRICHENELLOSIS.pdf

Gallardo MT, Mateos L, Artieda J, Wesslen L, Ruiz C et al (2007) Outbreak of trichinellosis in Spain and Sweden due to consumption of wild boar meat contaminated with *Trichinella britovi*. Euro Surveill 12(3):E070315.1

Gari-Toussaint M, Tieulié N, Baldin J, Dupouy-Camet J et al (2005) Human trichinellosis due to *Trichinella britovi* in southern France after consumption of frozen wild boar meat. Euro Surveill 10(6):117–118

Gołab E, Sadkowska-Todys M (2006) Epidemiologia włośnicy w polsce dawniej i dziś [Epidemiology of human trichinellosis in Poland—currently and in the past]. Wiad Parazytol. 52(3):181–187

Gómez-Morales MA, Ludovisi A, Amati M et al (2018) Differentiation of *Trichinella* species (*Trichinella spiralis/Trichinella britovi versus Trichinella pseudospiralis*) using western blot. Parasites Vectors 11:631

Gottstein B, Pozio E, Nöckler K (2009) Epidemiology, diagnosis, treatment, and control of trichinellosis. Clin Microbiol Rev 22(1):127–145

Kennedy ED, Hall RL, Montgomery SP, Pyburn DG, Jones JL (2009) Centers for Disease Control and Prevention (CDC). Trichinellosis surveillance—United States, 2002-2007. MMWR Surveill Summ 58(9):1–7

Khumjui C, Choomkasien P, Dekumyoy P, Kusolsuk T et al (2008) Outbreak of trichinellosis caused by *Trichinella papuae*, Thailand, 2006. Emerg Infect Dis 14(12):1913–1915

Konwar P, Singh BB, Gill JPS (2017) Epidemiological studies on trichinellosis in pigs (*Sus scofa*) in India. J Parasit Dis 41(2):487–490

Korhonen PK, Pozio E, La Rosa G, Chang BC et al (2016) Phylogenomic and biogeographic reconstruction of the *Trichinella* complex. Nat Commun 7:10513

Madariaga MG, Cachay ER, Zarlenga DS (2007) A probable case of human neurotrichinellosis in the United States. Am J Trop Med Hyg 77(2):347–349

McIntyre L, Pollock SL, Fyfe M, Gajadhar A et al (2007) Trichinellosis from consumption of wild game meat. CMAJ 176(4):449–451

Mitreva M, Jasmer DP (2006) Biology and genome of *Trichinella spiralis* (November 23, 2006), WormBook, ed. The C. elegans Research Community, WormBook, https://10.1895/wormbook.1.124.1, http://www.wormbook.org

Murrell KD, Pozio E (2011) Worldwide occurrence and impact of human trichinellosis, 1986–2009. Emerg Infect Dis 17(12):2194–2202

Neghina R, Neghina AM, Marincu I, Moldovan R, Iacobiciu I (2009) Trichinellosis, a threatening and re-emerging disease in a Romanian western county. Vector Borne Zoonotic Dis 9(6):717–721

Neghina R, Neghina AM, Marincu I, Moldovan R, Iacobiciu I (2010) Epidemiology and epizootiology of trichinellosis in Romania 1868–2007. Vector Borne Zoonotic Dis 10(4):323–328

Nöckler K, Reckinger S, Broglia A, Mayer-Scholl A, Bahn P (2009) Evaluation of a Western Blot and ELISA for the detection of anti-*Trichinella*-IgG in pig sera. Vet Parasitol 163(4):341–347

OIE (2012) Trichinellosis. In: Manual of diagnostic tests and vaccines for terrestrial animals 2012, Chapter 2.1.16. World Organisation for Animal Health, Paris, pp 1–9. http://www.oie.int/fileadmin/Home/eng/Health_standards/tahm/2008/pdf/2.01.16_TRICHINELLOSIS.pdf

Owen IL, Gomez Morales MA, Pezzotti P, Pozio E (2005) *Trichinella* infection in a hunting population of Papua New Guinea suggests an ancient relationship between *Trichinella* and human beings. Trans R Soc Trop Med Hyg 99(8):618–624

Pozio E, Varese P, Morales MA, Croppo GP et al (1993) Comparison of human trichinellosis caused by *Trichinella spiralis* and by *Trichinella britovi*. Am J Trop Med Hyg 48(4):568–575

Pozio E, Owen IL, Marucci G, La Rosa G (2005) Inappropriate feeding practice favors the transmission of *Trichinella papuae* from wild pigs to saltwater crocodiles in Papua New Guinea. Vet Parasitol 127(3–4):245–251

Saracino MP, Calcagno MA, Beauche EB, Garnier A et al (2016) *Trichinella spiralis* infection and transplacental passage in human pregnancy. Vet Parasitol 231:2–7

Sethi B, Butola KS, Kumar Y, Mishra JP (2012) Multiple outbreaks of trichinellosis with high mortality rate. Trop Doc 42:243

Sharma RK, Raghavendra N, Mohanty S, Tripathi BK et al (2014) Clinical & biochemical profile of trichinellosis outbreak in North India. Indian J Med Res 140(3):414–419

Shimshony A Trichinellosis: a re-emerging helminthozoonotic infection. Infectious Diseases News. Zoonotic infections (Posted March 1, 2009). https://www.healio.com/news/infectious-disease/20120225/trichinellosis-a-re-emerging-helminthozoonosis

Springer YP, Casillas S, Helfrich K, et al. Two outbreaks of Trichinellosis linked to consumption of walrus meat—Alaska, 2016–2017. Morb Mortal Wkly Rep 2017; 66:692–6

Troiano G, Nante N (2019) Human Trichinellosis in Italy: an epidemiological review since 1989. Prev Med Hyg 60:E71–E75

Wang ZQ, Cui J, Xu BL (2006) The epidemiology of human trichinellosis in China during 2000-2003. Acta Trop 97(3):247–251

Wang ZQ, Cui J, Shen LJ (2007) The epidemiology of animal trichinellosis in China. Vet J 173(2):391–398

Wilson NO, Hall RL, Montgomery SP, Jones JL (2015) Trichinellosis Surveillance—United States, 2008–2012. MMWR Surveill Summaries 64(SS-1)

Chapter 114
Trichostrongyliasis

114.1 Aetiology

Trichostrongyliasis is caused by a small nematode, *Trichostrongylus* spp. commonly found in herbivores. However, several species of *Trichostrongylus* have been known to infect humans, like *T. orientalis*, *T. colubriformis*, and *T. axei* (CDC 2017).

It has a worldwide distribution but is more common where animal husbandry is common.

114.2 Life Cycle

The definitive host (a herbivorous mammal) passes the eggs in the stool. Rhabditiform larvae hatch from the eggs under favourable conditions (moisture, warmth, shade) within several days and grow in the soil or on vegetation. They undergo two moults to become filariform (third-stage) larvae, which are infective and enter the vertebrate hosts, including man, through infected plants and vegetation and mature in 3–4 weeks in the small intestine, where they remain attached to the mucosa.

114.3 Symptoms

Mostly the infections are asymptomatic. Heavy infections can cause gastrointestinal problems (abdominal pain, diarrhoea, anorexia), headache, fatigue, anaemia, and eosinophilia.

© Springer Nature Singapore Pte Ltd. 2024
K. G. Narayan et al., *Handbook of Management of Zoonoses*,
https://doi.org/10.1007/978-981-99-9885-2_114

114.4 Treatment

Stool specimens from infected persons may show eggs and hatched larvae. Recommended drugs for the treatment of trichostrongyloisis are pyrantel pamoate, albendazole, and mebendazole.

114.5 Prevention

Personal hygiene, like washing hands before preparing or eating meals, is important. Vegetables should be thoroughly washed or cooked before eating. Animal manure can be composted to a high enough temperature to kill *Trichostrongylus* eggs and larvae before being used as a fertilizer. *T. orientalis* can be controlled by proper sanitation and the removal of animal faeces from areas occupied by humans. Infections with *Trichostrongylus* spp. of animal origin can be controlled by periodic treatment of domestic livestock with anthelmintics.

References

CDC (2017). https://www.cdc.gov/dpdx/trichostrongylosis/index.html

Chapter 115
Trichuriasis

Trichuriasis is the third most common roundworm infection of human and one of the seven most common neglected tropical diseases. There has been a reduction in the rate of prevalence in some countries. Once an important nematode infection among Koreans, its prevalence has been reduced to below 1.0% in the 1980s and currently almost nil (Youn 2009).

115.1 Aetiology

Trichuriasis is caused by *Trichuris trichura*, also known as the whipworm due to its shape. The parasite originated in Africa and spread to Asia and South America with infected humans in the past (Hawash et al. 2016).

It has a worldwide distribution, infecting an estimated 600 million people, mainly in children aged between 5 and 15 years, especially in tropical and sub-tropical areas, mostly Africa, southern India, China, Southeast Asia, and the Americas. This adds up to the global burden of diseases and disability-adjusted life years (DALYs) (FAO/WHO 2014). Eating raw, unwashed vegetables; drinking contaminated water; or not washing the hands after handling contaminated soil (a common transmission route for children) causes infection.

115.2 Life Cycle

Females produce 2000–10,000 single-celled eggs per day, discharged with human faeces to the soil, where these mature (embryonated) to an infective stage in 2 to 3 weeks under optimal hot and humid conditions. Upon ingestion by humans, they hatch in the small intestines, grow, and moult. The young worms move to the

© Springer Nature Singapore Pte Ltd. 2024
K. G. Narayan et al., *Handbook of Management of Zoonoses*,
https://doi.org/10.1007/978-981-99-9885-2_115

caecum and penetrate the mucosa with the cephalic end, and there they complete their development into adult worms. It takes about 3 months. The life of the parasite is 2–3 years.

115.3   Disease

It is related to the infection load; <100 worms cause no symptoms, and heavy infection may cause bloody diarrhoea, dysentery, and rectal prolapse when severe. It damages the mucosa mechanically and causes vitamin A deficiency and toxic inflammation.

Trichuriasis can be associated with intestinal symptoms, such as abdominal pain, dysentery, nausea, vomiting, anorexia, constipation, and chronic appendiceal syndrome.

115.4   Prevention

Trichuriasis can be prevented through the following:

  (i) Improvement in personal hygiene
 (ii) Thoroughly washing fruits and vegetables before consumption, and
(iii) Educating patients and families about the importance of handwashing

Global initiatives focussed on improving sanitation, poverty reduction, and periodic preventative chemotherapy have been started. The World Health Organization (WHO) has recommended preventative chemotherapy for soil-transmitted helminth (STH) infections through mass drug administration (MDA) to school children. A single dose of albendazole or mebendazole is most effective (Else et al. 2020). Attempts for the development of a vaccine against STH are ongoing (Zawawi and Else 2020), but we have to wait.

References

Else KJ, Keiser J, Holland CV, Grencis RK et al (2020) Whipworm and roundworm infections. Nat Rev Dis Primers 6(1):44
FAO/WHO (2014) Multi criteria-based ranking for risk management of food borne parasites. Microbiological Risk Assessment Series No. 23. Rome. 302 pp
Hawash MBF, Betson M, Al-Jubury A et al (2016) Whipworms in humans and pigs: origins and demography. Parasites Vectors 9:37
Youn H (2009) Review of zoonotic parasites in medical and veterinary fields in the Republic of Korea. Korean J Parasitol 47:S133–S141
Zawawi A, Else KJ (2020) Soil-transmitted helminth vaccines: are we getting closer? Front Immunol 11:576748

Appendix A: Rodent-Associated Zoonoses

Among the mammals, rodents are the most abundant. There are 2220 species. A large number, 224, host (10.7%) as many as 85 zoonoses. Most are found in North America, the Atlantic coast of South America, Europe, Russia, and parts of Central and East Asia (Han et al. 2015, 2016).

Reservoir Rodent-Zoonotic Agent System

Rodents for experiments in laboratories are raised free from pathogens. Those captured from the wild/outdoors or purchased from stores/ratteries/breeders or those living in natural habitats may carry zoonotic agents and constitute a 'rodent-zoonotic agent system'. This system may be recognized if clinical illness and/or death occur, as in the case of a plague. This is not so with many pathogens. Physiological and social behavioural differences between reservoir and non-reservoir rodents have been observed. Reservoir rodents reach sexual maturity early and begin producing offspring at higher rates—mid- to large-sized litters and relatively short gestation periods. Growth post-natal is fast. These are hyper-reservoir species.

Rodent-Associated Zoonoses

Rats and mice, including gerbils, hamsters, guinea pigs, and other rodent-species-associated zoonoses, which are over 35 in number, may be broadly classed as (a) directly transmitted and (b) indirectly transmitted (Table A.1). Direct contact with animals, scratches, bites, and secretions and excretions like their urine, saliva, and faeces or the ingestion of food contaminated with these transmits directly transmitted zoonoses. Indirectly transmitted zoonoses take the

© Springer Nature Singapore Pte Ltd. 2024
K. G. Narayan et al., *Handbook of Management of Zoonoses*,
https://doi.org/10.1007/978-981-99-9885-2

Table A.1 Potential zoonotic diseases from rodents

Zoonoses/agents	Host	Mode of transmission	Disease in humans
A. Transmitted directly			
Leptospira interrogans	Rodents, rabbits, foxes, skunks, raccoons, opossums	Direct or indirect contact with rat urine, ingestion of contaminated water or food	Weil's disease—fever, jaundice, renal failure, and pulmonary haemorrhage, often in sewer workers
Salmonellosis	Rodents	Organisms in faeces contaminate food.	Food poisoning, enteric fever
Streptobacillus moniliformis—rat-bite fever	Rodents	Organisms in the gum and teeth of rodents; hence, bites transfer. Ingestion of food contaminated by rats.	Abrupt onset—fever, chills, headache, muscle ache, pharyngitis, rash on the legs and arms, polyarthritis, sepsis similar to the rat-bite fever of the Orient, called *sodoku*, caused by *Spirillum minus*
Capillaria spp.	Rat liver harbours and is infected.	Rats' faeces/dead rats/predators disperse the parasite's eggs in the environment.	Asymptomatic but can cause hepatitis
Hantavirus pulmonary syndrome (HPS)	Deer mouse (*Peromyscus* spp.), cotton rat (*Sigmodon hispidus*), rice rat (*Oryzomys palustris*), and white-footed mouse (*Peromyscus leucopus*)	Aerosol from rodent excretions and secretions	Most HPS infection manifests fever, body aches, progressing to severe breathing difficulties may require hospitalization. Mortality is 38% of cases.
Hantaviruses—family *Hantaviridae*, order *Bunyavirales* Haemorrhagic fever with renal syndrome (HFRS)	*Apodemus* spp., Deer, mice, rodents, other wildlife	Aerosol, animal bites	HFRS develops about 3 weeks post-exposure; begins suddenly with intense pain in the head, back, and abdomen, fever, chills, nausea, blurred vision, flushing of the face, inflammation or redness of the eyes, or a rash; and progresses to low blood pressure, acute shock, vascular leakage, and acute kidney failure.

Seoul orthohantavirus (SEOV) and other hantaviruses	Apodemus spp., wild, laboratory and pet rats—for hantaviruses Clethrionomys spp., Rattus spp.	Direct contact with rat urine, faeces, or saliva; aerosol	Haemorrhagic fever with renal syndrome (HFRS), acute kidney injury (AKI), hantavirus cardio-pulmonary syndrome (HCPS), febrile illness, chills, flushing of the face, myalgia, headache, shock, renal failure; mortality: 1–2%
Lassa virus	Wild rodents—Mastomys	Contact with rodent's faeces and urine in house, Person-to-person transmission is common in health care settings (called nosocomial transmission)	About 80% of infected do not show any symptoms, and about 20% develop severe illness. The liver, spleen, and kidneys are affected. The incubation period (IP) is 6–21 days; illness opens up gradually—fever, weakness, sore throat, headache, myalgia, chest pain, vomiting, diarrhoea, and cough. Severe/haemorrhagic form—swollen face; bleeding from the mouth, vagina, and gastrointestine; fluid in the lungs; shock; coma for a 2–21 day duration; fatality 1%, may be 15% in severe cases.
Lymphocytic choriomeningitis mammarenavirus	Rodents—house mice, guinea pigs, hamsters	Excretions and secretions	IP 1–2 weeks, biphasic fever. 1st phase—fever, headache, muscle aches, malaise, nausea, and/or vomiting. 2nd phase—after apparent recovery, meningoencephalitis appears, as well as confusion, drowsiness, sensory abnormalities and motor signs for a duration of 1–3 weeks; temporary to permanent damage may result.
Guanarito mammarenavirus (arenavirus)—Venezuelan haemorrhagic fever	Short-tailed cane mice	Saliva, respiratory secretions, urine, blood from infected rodents (Aerosol transmission)	Fever, malaise followed by haemorrhagic manifestations, multiple organ involvement and convulsions; 30% mortality

(continued)

Table A.1 (continued)

Zoonoses/agents	Host	Mode of transmission	Disease in humans
Brazilian mammarenavirus or Sabiá virus (arenavirus)—Brazilian haemorrhagic fever	Brazilian rodents	Excretions and secretions—aerosol	Highly infectious, lethal haemorrhagic fever
Machupo mammarenavirus—Bolivian haemorrhagic fever	Bolivian mice	Excretions	Slow onset—fever, malaise, headache, myalgia, petechiae on the upper body, bleeding from gum and nose, progressing to severe haemorrhagic or neurological form in one-third of cases; mortality about 25%
Junin virus (arenavirus)—Argentinean haemorrhagic fever	Argentina rodents	Rodent's saliva and urine—contact, i.e. skin and mucous membrane, inhalation	Infection more in males between 15 and 60 years of age. Fever, headaches, weakness, loss of appetite. Severe form—vascular, renal, haematological, and neurological alteration; mortality: 15–30%
B. Transmitted indirectly			
Babesia microti –babesiosis	Wild rodents (white-footed mice, meadow vole)	Bites of ticks—*Ixodes scapularis*	Gradual onset—loss of appetite, fever, sweating, fatigue, general muscle aches, prolonged anaemia, sometimes fatal
Cutaneous leishmaniasis	Rodents, canids, marsupials, sloths, wild mammals	Bites of *Phlebotomus* sand flies	Destructive and disfiguring skin lesions may heal and then reappear as satellite lesions around the site of the original lesion or along the route of the lymphatic drainage.
A. phagocytophilum—human granulocytic anaplasmosis	White-footed mice, *Peromyscus leucopus*	*Ixodes scapularis, I. ricinus, I. persulcatus, I. pacificus*	Influenza like symptoms, fever, chills, severe headache, skin rash, vomiting, diarrhoea, myalgia, and confusion.

Angiostrongylus cantonensis—rat lungworm	Cotton rats, slugs	Indirect—molluscs are intermediate hosts. Consumption of intermediate hosts, slugs, contaminated vegetation, or paratenic hosts.	Granulomatous pneumonia, febrile illness, eosinophilic meningitis, ocular angiostrongyliasis—headache, photophobia, stiff neck, vomiting, paraesthesia
Borrelia hermsii, B. turicatae, B. parkerii—tick-borne relapsing fever	Wild rodents—chipmunks, tree squirrels	Soft ticks—Ornithodoros parkeri, O. turicata, O. hermsii	Recurring episodes of fever: ~3 days of non-specific symptoms, afebrile for ~7 days. Symptoms: high fever, 103°; headache; muscle and joint aches. In untreated patients, the alternate episodes may repeat several times.
Borrelia burgdorferi sensu lato—Lyme disease/Lyme borreliosis	Wild rodents (like chipmunks and white-footed mice), racoons, deer, rabbits, white-tailed deer	Hard ticks—Ixodes scapularis, I. pacificus	Fever; headache; fatigue; muscle ache; stiff neck; arthritis; expanding red rash, known as erythema, at the site of bite; cardiac and neurologic manifestation; 10–20% suffer for 6 months from joint pain and memory problems.
Borrelia lonestari—southern tick-associated illness	Peromyscus leucopus—white-footed mouse	Amblyomma americanum	Rash may be accompanied by fatigue, fever, headache, muscle and joint pains.
B. elizabethae	Rats	Blood-sucking arthropods (ticks, fleas, sand flies, lice)—reservoir mammal cycle	Endocarditis
B. grahamii	Mice	Do	Endocarditis, neuroretinitis
B. washoensis	Squirrels	Do	Myocarditis
Bartonella vinsonii	Mice, domestic dogs and cats	Do	Endocarditis
Colorado tick fever	Wild small rodents, ground squirrels, hares, rabbits, marmots, chipmunks, porcupines	Ticks—Dermacentor andersoni, D. occidentalis	High fever, headache, muscle ache, lethargy, biphasic symptoms

(continued)

Table A.1 (continued)

Zoonoses/agents	Host	Mode of transmission	Disease in humans
Rickettsia typhi—murine typhus	Rats	Flea—*Xenopsylla cheopis*. *Rickettsia* in the faeces of infected fleas enter through scratches or is rubbed into a flea-bite wound.	The classic triad of fever, headache, and skin rash; myocarditis
Rickettsia akari—*Rickettsial pox*	House mice	House mouse mite *Liponyssoides sanguineness*	Mild non-fatal disease resembling chicken pox
Rickettsia tsutsugamushi—scrub typhus	Rodents	Bite of infected larval trombiculid mites	Fever; headache; body aches; sometimes rash, a dark, scab-like region at the site of the chigger bite (also known as eschar); enlarged lymph node; and confusion to coma
Rickettsia rickettsii—Rocky Mountain spotted fever	Wild rodents, rabbits, hares, carnivores, birds	Ticks—*Dermacentor andersoni, D. variabilis, Amblyomma americanum, Haemaphysalis leporispalustris, Rhipicephalus sanguineus*	Fever-rash-tick bite history is a classical triad. Fever, nausea, vomiting, headache, muscle aches, maculopapular rash spreading from the extremities to the trunk, petechiae, abdominal pain, loss of muscle control; may even be fatal.
La Crosse virus—encephalitis	Chipmunks and squirrels	*Aedes triseriatus*	IP 5–15 days, fever for 2–3 days, headache, nausea, vomiting, fatigue, reduced alertness, loss of muscle control, severe neuro-invasive disease in <16 years of age
Venezuelan equine encephalomyelitis—VEE virus (alphavirus)	Rodents, equids Outbreak in Columbia 1995 explained—deforestation led to the replacement of rodents, preferring *C. taeniopius* to *Ae. taeniorhynchus* mosquitoes, and these both bite humans and equids. Now, *Ae. albopictus* is a viable carrier.	Mosquitoes—*Monsonia, Aedes, Culex* spp.	Flu-like symptoms; those with weakened immunity, old and young, suffer serious illness and may die.

			Acute disseminated encephalomyelitis
Powassan virus	White-footed mice, white-tailed deer, woodchucks, squirrels, skunks	Ticks—*Ixodes* spp., *Dermacentor* spp.	

C. Transmitted both directly and indirectly

Yersinia pestis	Rats, squirrels, chipmunks, rabbits	Fleas, direct—skinning of animals	Bubonic plague—febrile illness, chills, septicaemia, lymphadenitis, pain in the armpits, groin sepsis, often fatal
Francisella tularensis—tularemia	Wild rodents, rabbits, hares, cats, sheep	Occupational and recreational exposure—insect (tick) bites, ingestion, inhalation, skinning of animals	Clinical disease depends on the site of entry—commonest are ulceroglandular; glandular, oro-pharyngeal, pneumonic, oculo-glandular, and typhoidal. Ulcer at the inoculation site, swollen lymph nodes, mild illness to severe meningitis, pneumonia, death.
Omsk haemorrhagic fever	Rodents, muskrats	Bites of ticks (*Dermacentor* spp.), also directly transmitted through contact and excretions of rodents	Phase 1 - for 1–8 days: chills, headache, pain in the extremities, prostration, conjunctival suffusion, hypotension. Some people may recover in 1–2 weeks. Others suffer from haemorrhage in the gum, uterus, and lungs; soft palate; and cervical lymphadenopathy. Occasional second wave of neurological symptoms in 3 weeks with signs of encephalitis may end in death. Post-recovery: loss of hearing and hair, behavioural and neurological problems.
Hymenolepis spp. and *Rodentolepis* spp.—tapeworms	Rats are the reservoir; they reside in the intestinal tract.	Faeces-contaminated food/ intermediate arthropod hosts	Enteritis

13 directly + 19 indirectly+ 4 both = 36 total

route through insects like ticks, mites, fleas, and intermediate hosts. Nearly 20–30% of those working with and exposed to laboratory animals may suffer from allergies. Inhalation of or contact with allergens like animal dandruff, hair, skin, urine, saliva, serum, contaminated feed, or beddings may lead to allergic reactions.

Factors Favouring Infection

Factors extrinsic to the 'rodent-pathogen-system', such as urbanization, agriculture, and socio-economic standing, control host and human population dynamics. These control the frequency of transmissible contacts. Urban poverty offers an extensive habitat and an opportunity for contact between rats and disadvantaged people (inadequate infrastructure, sanitation, housing, dense population). The ecology of rat-associated zoonoses is changing as both 'urbanization and urban poverty' are dynamic. A number of factors, such as rats, people, pathogens, vectors, climate, and weather, influence the rat population, the rat-pathogen and rat-pathogen-vector associations, and ultimately exposure and infection in humans. The distribution and prevalence of rat-associated zoonoses are heterogeneous, even over a short geographic distance. Estimating the burden of zoonoses associated with urban rats and developing informed and effective strategies to monitor and mitigate those risks is difficult. High rates of under/misdiagnosis arise due to strikingly similar clinical presentations of cases in several zoonoses. Health care practitioners are unaware, and access to specific diagnoses is poor.

Impoverished populations are at the highest risk. Specific conditions, such as chronic illness, immunodeficiency, and pregnancy, increase the risk of infection with zoonoses. Climate/weather affects the ecology of rats, vectors, and pathogens. Heavy rains/the rainy season and floods facilitate the spread of leptospires in the environment and force human contact with bacteria, increasing the incidence of leptospirosis. Incidence is also high in flood plains and in areas proximate to water bodies. Infection with Seoul and Hantavirus is the highest in April and the lowest in September in China, reflecting a seasonal effect on the rat population and rat-human contact. Warm months favour the flea population and influence murine typhus and plague. A temperature of >28 °C clears the blockage (blood clot) in the gut of a flea, and it cannot transmit *Y. pestis*. Plague epidemics tend to subside at high temperatures. The geographic areas of Lyme disease are changing with climate change (Himsworth et al. 2013).

Seoul virus Outbreak

An outbreak of the *Seoul virus* was reported by Kerins et al. (2018). It affected 31 US facilities in 11 states, of which six exchanged rats with Canadian ratteries. Seventeen persons had a recent infection. Eight were ill. Three had to be hospitalized. All recovered. *Seoul virus* is the Old World hantavirus in the Bunyaviridae family. Its natural reservoir is the Norway rat (*Rattus norvegicus*). Rats show no symptoms. The virus is shed in urine or droppings. Humans get infected through contact with or the inhalation of dust from contaminated beddings. Humans suffer from flu-like illness, which may be a severe disease; haemorrhagic fever with renal failure (HFRS); and death.

The owner of an in-home rattery of Norway rats was admitted to the hospital with fever, leukopenia, elevated transaminases, and proteinuria. Another member of the family fell ill with a similar illness. Both tested hantavirus positive.

Suggestions: rat pet owners, breeders, and rattery owners and workers should be made aware of these zoonoses. Flu-like illness with a history of contact with rats leads to a suspicion of *Seoul virus* infection. Laboratory confirmation is made through the Centers for Disease Control and Prevention's (CDC's) enzyme-linked immunosorbent assay (ELISA) and reverse transcription-polymerase chain reaction (Rt-PCR).

Euthanasia for all rats in such facilities is recommended. Newly brought rats need to be quarantined for 4 weeks and should be tested for antibodies to the *Seoul virus* before co-mingling with other rats.

Rat-Bite Fever (*Streptobacillus moniliformis*)

It can be very serious and at the same time most difficult to diagnose. A 59-year-old snake keeper suffered from acute tetraplegia and was admitted to the intensive care unit (ICU) and had to be kept under sedation and ventilation. He had extensive injury, arthralgia, swollen knees and left wrist with effusion of joints, vertebral osteomyelitis, and epidural abscess. Examination of the synovia and serum of the patient and swab and biopsy from rats' mouths yielded genotypically identical *S. moniliformis* (Eisenberg et al. 2017).

Strategy for Prevention

1. Rodent control in and around the home: eliminate all/any food sources, seal all points of entry, use rat trappers, and clean up rat-infested areas.
2. Educate rattery owners and breeders/raise awareness of potential zoonoses.

3. Call/report to a medical officer in the case of a suspected illness; thoroughly wash any bite or scratch to minimize the chances of infection.
4. Call a veterinarian to attend to an illness in pet rodents/rattery.
5. Cages, traps, and areas housing rodents should be maintained clean, and all equipment should be cleaned and disinfected after use.
6. Avoid activities that put you in contact with mouse droppings, urine, saliva, or nesting materials.
7. While handling animals or animal tissue, waste, secretions, and excretions, wear personal protective gear, like masks, gloves, gowns/overalls, etc.
8. Launder the soiled clothing and sanitize gloves, instruments, etc.
9. Do not eat or drink while handling animals or working in animal houses.
10. Avoid sleeping in rodent-infested buildings.
11. To protect against insects like ticks, wear clothing to cover the arms and legs and use DEET-based insect repellents, pesticides, and tweezers to remove ticks. If the removed ticks are full of blood, consult a physician.
12. Observe some measures to prevent ticks on pets and in your yard—grassy, bushy wooded areas favour ticks.

References

Eisenberg T, Poignant S, Jouan Y, Fawzy A, Nicklas W, et al (2017) Acute tetraplegia caused by rat bite fever in snake keeper and transmission of *Streptobacillus moniliformis*. Emerg Infect Dis 23(4):719–21

Han BA, Schmidt JP, Bowden SE, Drake JM (2015) Rodent reservoirs of future zoonotic diseases. Proc Natl Acad Sci USA 112:7039–44

Han BA, Kramer AM, John M, Drake JM (2016) Global patterns of zoonotic disease in mammals—review. Trends Parasitol 32(7):565–77

Kerins JL, Koske SE, Kazmierczak J, et al (2018) Outbreak of Seoul virus among rats and rat owners—United States and Canada, 2017. Morb Mortal Wkly Rep. 67(7):232

Himsworth CG, Parsons KL, Jardine C, Patrick DM (2013) Rats, cities, people, and pathogens: a systematic review and narrative synthesis of literature regarding the ecology of rat-associated zoonoses in urban centers. Vector Borne Zoonotic Dis 13(6):349–59

Important Website

Diseases directly transmitted by rodents. https://www.cdc.gov/rodents/diseases/direct.html

Diseases indirectly transmitted by rodents. https://www.cdc.gov/rodents/diseases/indirect.html

Zoonoses associated with rodents. https://iacuc.wsu.edu/zoonoses-associated-with-rodents/#:~:text=Zoonotic%20diseases%20associated%20with%20rodents%20include%20rat%20bite,virus%2C%20lymphocytic%20choriomeningitis%20virus%2C%20leptospirosis%2C%20salmonellosis%2C%20and%20campylobacterosis

7 Serious Illnesses Carried by Rats and Mice. *https://www.thespruce.com/rats-and-mice-spread-disease-2656481*

Appendix B: Dog-Associated Zoonoses

Dogs-human association is close, because these are used as shepherd dogs, hunting dogs, family pets as companion and home security, therapy, intelligence and security by police and army. Such dogs have definite owners and defined jobs. These contribute to the microbiome around their owners. The owners are expected to have knowledge about dog keeping and responsibilities and the perception of animal welfare. The owners' occupation, cultural background, and knowledge about dog keeping also influence the association.

Warembourg et al. (2021) therefore suggested that the association, which is similar to social distance among the human population, differed from region to region, as well as the use of dogs.

The free-roaming population of dogs uses human habitations for a range of activities, like foraging and breeding and movement around it. There is no human control over this population of dogs, yet they strongly depend upon humans for their habitat (home range). These constitute important reservoirs, sources, and spreaders of a variety of zoonotic infections (Table B.1). The management of the population of such dogs is an important strategy.

References

http://www.phsource.us/PH/ZD/Zoonotic_Disease_Table.htm

Tick borne diseases [**Institutional animal care and use committee of University of California, Santa Barbara]

Table—Dog associated zoonoses [Sources—http://www.phsource.us/PH/ZD/Zoonotic_Disease_Table.htm]

Tick borne diseases [** Institutional animal care and use committee of University of California, Santa Barbara]

Table B.1 Dog-associated zoonoses

Disease	Causative agent	Mode of human infection
***Bacterial diseases* (12)**		
Anthrax	*Bacillus anthracis*	Occupational exposure, food-borne, wounds or insect bites; rarely airborne
Capnocytophaga infection	*Capnocytophaga canimorsus, C. cynodegmi*	Bites or scratches
Campylobacteriosis	*C. jejuni*	Food/water-borne, occupational; exposure to infected dogs and cats
**Ehrlichiosis—tick-borne fever	*Ehrlichia ewingii, E. chaffeensis, E. canis (Rhipicephalus sanguineus)**	Infected tick bites, recreational exposure
Leptospirosis	*Leptospira interrogans* (200 serovars) in 23 serogroups	Occupational and recreational exposure; water- and food-borne
**Pasteurellosis	*Pasteurella multocida*	Bite/scratch/direct contact
Salmonellosis	*Salmonella* serotypes	Food/waterborne, recreational exposure
**Tick-borne relapsing fever *Synonyms: spirochetal fever, vagabond fever, famine fever	*Borrelia hermsii, B. turicatae, B. parkerii*	Infected tick bite, recreational exposure
Tuberculosis	*M. tuberculosis*	Exposure to animals infected with human-type tuberculosis
Tularemia	*Francisella tularensis*	Occupational and recreational exposure, insect bites, ingestion, inhalation
Yersiniosis	*Y. enterocolitica*	Ingestion, recreational exposure
*Zoonotic diphtheria	*Corynebacterium ulcerans*	Direct contact, milk
***Rickettsial diseases* (4)**		
Boutonneuse fever	*Rickettsia conorii, Rickettsia* spp.	Bite of infected ticks
Rocky Mountain spotted fever	*Rickettsia rickettsii*	Bite of infected ticks or their crushing on the skin of *Dermacentor variabilis, D. andersoni*
**Indian tick typhus	*R. conorii*—*Rhipicephalus sanguineus* and also other ticks	Infected tick bite, recreational

	Coxiella burnetii	Aerosol, direct contact, milk, fomites
**Q fever		
***Fungal infections/diseases* (4)**		
Blastomycosis	*Blastomyces dermatitidis*	Environmental exposure; also reported by animal exposure
Histoplasmosis	*Histoplasma capsulatum*	Environmental exposure
Nocardiosis	*Nocardia asteroides,* *N. brasiliensis, N. caviae*	Environmental exposure
Dermatophytosis	*Microsporum,* *Trichophyton,* and *Epidermophyton* spp.	Direct contact with infected animal and fomites
***Parasitic diseases* (31)**		
Chaga's disease	*Trypanosoma cruzi*	Faecal material of *Triatoma* bug, including Reduviidae (also called conenose, kissing, or assassin bug); contaminates bite wounds, abrasions, or mucous membranes
***Cryptosporidiosis	*C. hominis, C. parvum,* *C. andersoni, C. canis,* *C. muris, C. felis, C. baileyi, C. meleagridis*	Ingestion—contaminated water—drinking water, swimming pool, irrigation, river, recreational exposure
Giardiasis	*Giardia lamblia*	Water and less often food; person to person
Leishmaniasis—visceral (kala-azar)	*Leishmania donovani* and others	Bite of Phlebotomine sand flies
Leishmaniasis—cutaneous and mucosal	*L. tropica, L. braziliensis* complex	Bite of Phlebotomine sand flies
Pneumocystis pneumonia	*Pneumocystis carinii* (human strain)	Environmental exposure
African sleeping sickness	*T. brucei rhodesiense,* *T. brucei gambiense*	Bite of infected fly *Glossina*
Clonorchiasis	*Clonorchis sinensis* (Chinese liver fluke)	Ingestion of raw or partially cooked infected freshwater fish

(continued)

Table B.1 (continued)

Disease	Causative agent	Mode of human infection
Echinostomiasis	*Echinostoma ilocanum* and other *Echinostoma* spp.	Ingestion of uncooked/partially cooked fish, shellfish
Heterophyiasis	*Heterophyes*	Ingestion of uncooked fish
Nanophyetiasis	*Troglotrema salmincola*	Ingestion of undercooked fish
Opisthorchiasis	*Opisthorchis felineus, O. viverrini*	Ingestion of undercooked fish containing encysted larvae
	Amphimerus pseudofelineus	Undetermined
Paragonimiasis (Lung fluke disease)	*Paragonimus westermani, P. africanus, P. mexicanus,* and other species	Ingestion of raw or partially cooked, infected freshwater crustaceans
Schistosomiasis (Bilharziasis)	*Schistosoma japonicum, S. mansoni, S. mekongi*	Penetration of unbroken skin by cercariae larvae from infected snails in water
Coenurosis/Coenuriasis	*Taenia multiceps*	Ingestion of eggs of tapeworms in canine faeces
Diphyllobothriasis (Fish tapeworm infection)	*Diphyllobothrium latum (Dibothriocephalus latus), Diphyllobothrium pacificum*	Ingestion of raw or partially cooked infected fish
Dipylidiasis (Dog tapeworm)	*Dipylidium caninum*	Ingestion of infected dog and cat fleas
Echinococcosis (Hydatid disease)	*Echinococcus granulosus, E. multilocularis, E. vogeli*	Ingestion of eggs of tapeworms
Pulmonary capillariasis (roundworm)	*Capillaria aerophila*	Ingestion of infective eggs in soil or contaminated food
Dioctophymosis	*Dioctophyme renale* (Giant kidney worm)	Ingestion of infected fish or frog liver and mesentery
Dracunculiasis (Guinea worm infection)	*Dracunculus insignis*	Ingestion of frogs and other paratenic hosts
Dirofilariasis	*Dirofilaria immitis*	Bite of infected mosquitoes
Malayan filariasis	*Burgia malayi*	Bite of infected mosquitoes
Gnathostomiasis	*Gnathostoma spinigera*	Ingestion of infected fish, poultry

Disease	Causative agent	Mode of human infection
Larva migrans, cutaneous (*see also* Gnathostomiasis above)	*Ancylostoma caninum*, *A. braziliensis, Strongyloides stercoralis*	Contact with infective larvae that penetrate the skin
Larva migrans, visceral (*see also* Angiostrongyliasis and Anisakiasis)	*Toxocara canis*	Ingestion of embryonated eggs shed in the faeces of dogs
Thelaziasis	*Thelazia* spp.	Infected insects
Macracanthorhynchosis	*Macracanthorhynchus hirudinaceus* and other spp.	Ingestion of infected beetles
Mange (scabies)	*Cheyletiella*	Contact with infected individuals or animals
Pentastomid infection	*Linguatula serrata, Armillifer* spp. (tongue worms)	Ingestion of infected animal tissues
Tunga infections	*Tunga penetrans* (sand fleas, jiggers)	Contact with contaminated soil
Tick paralysis	Venom of ticks—*Dermacentor andersoni*, *D. variabilis*, and sometimes *Ixodes, Haemaphysalis, Rhinocephalus,* and *Argas* spp.	Attachment with ticks
Viral infections (2)		
Rabies and rabies-related viral and other Lyssa viral encephalitis	*Lyssavirus, Rabies virus, Duvenhage virus, Mokola virus, Ibadan shrew virus, Obodhiang virus*	Bites of diseased animals; aerosols in closed environments
**Crimean Congo haemorrhagic fever – viremia occurs in dogs.	CCHFV group; family Bunyaviridae, genus *Nairovirus*— Principally *Hyalomma spp.* ticks, transovarial, transstadial and venereal. Other ticks: *Rhipicephalus/Boophilus, Dermacentor* and *Ixodes*	Infected tick bites, recreational exposure

***Narayan (manuscript)—Narayan, K. G Rabies—Most Important Dog Associated Zoonoses. *Lead paper- National Congress on "Strategy for Canine Health Care with Focus on Zoonotic Diseases" and XIth Annual Convention of ISACP 10th–12th February, 2014. Patna. Organisers- Indian Society for Advancement of Canine Practices (ISACP) & Bihar Veterinary College, Patna.*

Warembourg C, Wera E, Odoch T, Bulu PM, Berger-González M et al (2021) Comparative study of free-roaming domestic dog management and roaming behavior across four countries: Chad, Guatemala, Indonesia, and Uganda. Front Vet Sci 8:617900.

Appendix C: Non-human Primate-Associated Zoonoses

There are 365 primate species. Nearly 21% or 77 of these are hosts to at least one of 63 zoonotic agents. Overlapping spatial distribution and a high degree of phylogenetic relatedness between humans and non-human primates (NHP) probably make the transmission/spillover of zoonotic agents to human easy (Table C.1). The equatorial Africa (in central Africa in the Congo Basin and West Africa), Southeast Asia, and the tropical/mixed forest regions of northern Brazil and the Guiana Shield seem to be hotspots and where zoonotic hosts are located.

Non-human primates are a part of the wildlife ecosystem but when petted can be a part of the human ecosystem. Zoonotic infections in non-human primates have great implications, as can be shared with human. Non-human primates are also important players, along with other animals in the ecosystem, such as bats, rodents, and birds in forests and livestock and farm animals in the human ecosystem, acting as intermediates in the transmission of pathogens (Devaux et al. 2019). Some of the parasites and bacteria transmitted by non-human primates to humans are mentioned below.

Parasites

Triatomine-transmitted *Trypanosoma cruzi* and common enteric pathogenic parasites include *Giardia*, *Entamoeba histolytica*, and *Cryptosporidium*.

Bacteria

(a) Bite transmitted—most zoonotic infections occur through monkey bites on hands. Arms and legs causing superficial abrasions to crush wounds are major tissue loss. The risk of infection increases with the amount of tissue damage. A

© Springer Nature Singapore Pte Ltd. 2024
K. G. Narayan et al., *Handbook of Management of Zoonoses*,
https://doi.org/10.1007/978-981-99-9885-2

Table C.1 Monkey (non-human primate)-associated zoonoses

Agent/zoonoses	Host	Mode of transmission	Prevention/protection	Disease in human
Entamoeba histolytica, *Entamoeba polecki*, *Balantidium coli*, *Cryptosporidium*	Monkeys, chimps, apes, gibbons	Soil, water, and food contaminated with protozoa	Sanitation of the environment, prompt removal of faeces, and treatment with anti-parasitic agents of infected animals; personal and environmental hygiene	Enteric disorder
Oesophagostomum bifurcum	Monkeys, sheep, goat, cattle	Infective-stage larvae contaminate fruit, food (eaten raw), or water.	Personal, kitchen, and environmental hygiene	L3 larvae pass the stomach acid barrier. Symptoms confounded with appendicitis, colon cancer, intestinal obstruction
B. studeri, B. mucronate— cestode—Bertielliasis/ Bertiellosis	Non-human primates, rodents, Australian marsupials	Ingestion of orbatid mites present in the soil	Avoid contact with non-human primates (chimpanzees), rodents, and soil in endemic areas.	Common in children; continuous or intermittent post-meal epigastric pain, nausea, diarrhoea, anorexia, loss of weight, and cases of constipation
Malaria of non-human primates; about 20 sp. of *Plasmodium*	Monkeys and chimpanzees	Anopheline mosquitoes	Insecticide spray, release of Mosquitoes with *Wolbachia*, use mosquito-nets, and repellants	Fever, chills, headache, nausea and vomiting, muscle pain and fatigue, sweating—continuous or intermittent
Enterobius vermicularis	Old World primates	Oral and inhalation	Personal and kitchen hygiene	Perianal pruritis, irritability, disturbed sleep
Trichuris trichiura	Old World primates	Oral	Personal and kitchen hygiene	Intermittent abdominal pain, blood in the stool, diarrhoea, may be rectal prolapse
Schistosoma mansoni, Schistosoma mekongi	Baboons and monkeys, respectively	Penetration of the skin by cercariae in water from infected snails	Snail control, management of water bodies, and maintaining animals around free from infection	Itchy maculopapular at the site of entry of the cercariae, systemic hypersensitivity reaction weeks after the initial infection—fever, cough, abdominal pain, diarrhoea

				Enteritis
Campylobacteriosis, salmonellosis, shigellosis	Non-human primates	Ingestion of contaminated water and food	Personal, kitchen, and community hygiene	Enteritis
Mycobacterium tuberculosis	Great apes (African-American and South American)	Respiratory (inhalation), ingestion, direct and indirect contact with infected tissues, and secretions, and excretions	Screening: i/d, thoracic radiography in suspected for early diagnosis. In animals, TB + are euthanized to protect the uninfected. Animal and health care takers need to adopt personal protection and should be screened periodically.	Chronic coughing for more than 3 weeks, haemoptysis, chest pain when breathing or coughing, weight loss, fatigue, fever, night sweats, chills, back pain if the spine is affected
M. leprae	Chimpanzees, sooty mangabey monkeys, rhesus, and African green monkeys	Direct contact	Protectives while caring patients	Pale skin sores, lumps, or bumps persisting for several weeks or months; nerve damage in the skin, eyes, nose, and muscle
Francisella tularensis (tularemia)	Non-human primates, e.g. vervet monkeys, patas monkeys, marmoset, cynomolgus	Air, contact, vector	Personal protection, avoiding contact	
Leptospirosis	Non-human primates	Contact of abraded skin or mucous membrane with urine, tissues, and contaminated equipment	Personal protective and hygiene	

(continued)

Table C.1 (continued)

Agent/zoonoses	Host	Mode of transmission	Prevention/protection	Disease in human
Monkeypox virus	Monkeys, other primates, rodents, pets	Contact with animals' blood or bite	Avoid direct contact; adopt guidelines for the housing and handling of laboratory animals.	• High temperature, headache, muscle aches, backache, swollen glands, chills, and exhaustion
Saimiriine herpesvirus 1 (SaHV1), previously known as *Herpesvirus tamarinus*, or herpes T	Squirrel monkeys and *Saimiri*, *Ateles*, *Cebus*, and *Lagothrix*	Virus in oral secretion, direct, bite, scratch	Avoid contact.	Vesiculation on the skin and mucosa, oral ulcers
Tanapox virus	Monkeys and other reservoir hosts	Mechanical transmission by arthropods	Refer rodent zoonoses.	Febrile illness with localized skin lesions
Yaba monkey tumour pox virus	Rhesus monkeys, baboons	Contact	Handle with protectives.	Histiocytoma, lump under the skin, spontaneous regression in 3–6 weeks
Herpesvirus simiae (B virus)	Old World monkeys, macaque—initial gingivostomatitis followed by latency of virus, then reactivation under stress and shedding in saliva and genital secretions. Monkeys are thus active carriers.	Scratch, bite	Avoid contact with monkeys and follow guidelines for housing and handling laboratory monkeys. Wash under running water with detergent, apply antiseptic, antibiotics, and acyclovir.	Serious neurological disorder—nerve, spinal cord, and brain affected; high CFR; residual nerve-related disorder in survivors; IP 1 month
Yellow fever	Monkeys	Mosquito bite	Protection from mosquitos, vaccination	Haemorrhagic fever, nausea, vomiting, diarrhoea, jaundice; fatality around 50%

Agent/zoonoses	Host	Mode of transmission	Prevention/protection	Disease in human
Measles virus (*Morbillivirus*), disease known as measles/ rubeola/morbilli	Man is the only natural hosts; primates are sometimes infected. Transmission from monkey to man or monkeys, monkeys to monkeys, and man to man	Respiratory—aerosol, direct contact with fluid from the nose and mouth of the infected	MMR (measles mumps, rubella) vaccine; isolating cases till complete recovery, i.e. several days after symptoms have disappeared	Four-day fever and the three Cs—*cough, coryza* (head cold, fever, sneezing), and *conjunctivitis* (red eyes); *maculopapular rash* duration—1 week
Marburg virus and *Ebola*—both are identical structurally, although they elicit different antibodies.	Egyptian fruit bat, green monkeys Cynomolgus monkeys for Ebola-related filovirus in Southeast Asia[a]	Contact with fluids from patients, like blood, saliva, vomit and other excrement, and sperm	Follow guidelines for housing and handling laboratory monkeys. Nurses/those attending cases require barrier infection control measures—like wearing double gloves, impermeable gowns, face shields, eye protection, and leg and shoe coverings.	IP 5–10 days: sudden onset of fever, chills, headache, and myalgia Around fifth day after the onset of symptoms: maculopapular rash on the chest, back, and stomach; nausea, vomiting; chest pain; sore throat; abdominal pain; diarrhoea; severe illness—may be jaundice, pancreatitis, multi- organ dysfunction, death—23–90%
Simian immunodeficiency virus	Chimpanzees (SIVcpz)—HIV1, sooty mangabeys (SIVsmm)—HIV2	Contact with the blood of infected monkeys hunted for meat; accidental cut/ open wound while handling lab monkeys	Avoid contact, particularly with any cut/open wound with blood from monkeys.	HIV appears to have been derived from SIV.

[a]http://www.phsource.us/PH/ZD/Zoonotic_Disease_Table.htm zoonotic diseases Table 1

wide variety of bacteria have been reported from bite injuries. These are *Streptococcus pyogenes, Staphylococcus aureus, Neisseria* spp., and *Haemophilus* spp.

(b) Respiratory bacterial pathogens from non-human primates include *Klebsiella pneumoniae, Streptococcus pneumoniae,* and *Mycobacteria* spp.

(c) Common enteric bacterial pathogens likely to infect humans through the faecal-oral route are *Shigella flexneri, S. sonnei,* enteropathogenic *Escherichia coli, Salmonella enteritidis, S. typhimurium, Campylobacter fetus, C. jejuni,* and *Helicobacter pylori.*

Herpesvirus simiae/B Virus (*Cercopithecine herpesvirus* 1)

The virus causes inflammation of brain and spinal cord. Kaplan et al. (1990) reviewed 25 cases of human B virus recorded till 1987. Thirteen of 18 fully reported cases died (case fatality rate (CFR) >65%), and 3/5 survivors had a neurological disorder. Exposure to clinically ill and healthy monkeys and failure to use chemical and mechanical means to restrain monkeys before handling and using protective gear led to infection.

A case of encephalitis in a monkey handler in 1932 led to the realization that B virus was highly pathogenic. Transmission from man to man also occurred. Twenty of 22 infected resulted in encephalitis; 15 of these died. It caused high morbidity and fatality. It appears that the rate of transmission/infection is low, possibly because of infrequent shedding of the virus and cross-protection due to infection with herpes simplex.

Herpesvirus simiae (B virus) is enzootic in rhesus (*Macaca mulatta*), cynomolgus (*M. fascicularis*), and other Asiatic monkeys of the genus *Macaca.* It is highly prevalent (80–90%) in adult macaques (Ostrowski 1998). It causes gingivostomatitis, blisters, or ulcers in and around their mouth and on their genitalia, often appearing very similar to cold sores or fever and blisters in humans. Recovery follows, but the virus remains latent in the host. On reactivation by factors like stress and immunosuppression, virus is shed in saliva and/or genital secretions. Sexually mature macaques are more likely to be exposed and be shedding virus both in the wild and in captivity.

Non-occupational exposure incidents, such as bites/scratches involving macaques, have also been recorded. Children are three times more likely to be bitten (Ostrowski et al. 1998).

The mode of transmission includes exposure to infected monkeys and tissues and contact with infected saliva through a scratch or bite. Cases of infection while working with contaminated simian cell culture, while handling infected nervous and kidney tissues in the laboratory, and while cleaning monkey skull suggest other ways of exposure through broken skin. Indirect contact exposures may also occur, such as scratches from contaminated equipment, needle-stick injuries, and mucous membrane exposure (i.e. splashes to the eyes, nose, or mouth).

The incubation period may be as short as 2 days or 4–5 weeks (1 month). The progress of virus in the brain and spinal cord is rapid. The disease begins as a flu-like illness (fever, chills, nausea, vomiting, and dizziness), sinusitis, and persistent headaches. At the site of the bite/exposure appear vesicular lesions (blisters, redness). Ascending encephalomyelitis (infection of the brain and spinal cord) eventually results in death.

Preventive Measures

Guidelines for the prevention of B virus infection in monkey handlers have been suggested by the B virus group. There are regulations related to primate trade. The use of macaque monkeys restricted to only those that are B virus free or are maintained so; minimal direct handling; physical or chemical (injection of ketamine hydrochloride) restraining methods before capturing and handling; wearing personal protective gears like gloves, long-sleeved garment, goggles, mask, etc.; quarantining macaques showing oral lesions; and educating animal handlers are the preventive measures.

Post-exposure Care

All bite or scratch wounds incurred from macaques or from cages that result in bleeding should be immediately and thoroughly scrubbed and cleansed with soap and water. Superficial wounds that can be adequately cleansed probably require no further treatment. Cases with deep and penetrating wound require prophylactic treatment with acyclovir.

Simian Immunodeficiency Virus (SIV)

SIVcpz (chimpanzee SIV) and SIVsm (sooty mangabey SIV) are genetically closest to HIV 1 and HIV 2, causing acquired immunodeficiency syndrome (AIDS) in human beings. Evidence suggests that these have been transmitted to humans. Opportunities of frequent contact of humans with primates are great in many parts of sub-Saharan Africa.

The zoonotic transfer of these viruses from primates is possible among persons who hunt primates and prepare their meat for consumption, keep primates as pets or trade, or maintain and handle primates for biomedical research. Zoonotic transmission appears to contribute to the present pandemic of human immunodeficiency virus (HIV).

Peeters et al. (2002) examined 16 primate species, 13 of which were found infected with SIV, suggesting that a substantial proportion of wild monkeys in Cameroon were infected, and hunters and those who handled bush meat were exposed to a plethora of genetically highly variant SIV.

Tuberculosis (*M. tuberculosis*) and Other Mycobacteria

Non-human primates and human beings appear to be equally infected by mycobacteria. The transmission of infection may be both ways, from humans to non-human primates and from non-human primates to humans (anthropozoonoses and zooanthroponoses). Old world monkeys (Africa and Asia) are considered highly susceptible to infection with *M. tuberculosis*. The New World (tamarins, capuchins, marmosets) are fairly resistant. Baboons and apes have intermediate susceptibility (Willis et al. 2007). Rhesus monkey (*Macaca mulatta*) and cynomolgus monkey (*Macaca fascicularis*) are most commonly used in biomedical research. *M. tuberculosis* accounts for most (nearly 75%) and *M. bovis* for about 24% of infections in NHP.

It is difficult to relate species of monkeys with specific mycobacteria. *M. tuberculosis* has been common in spider monkeys, baboons, and orangutans; *M. bovis* in rhesus monkeys and dusky langur; *M. gordonae* in squirrel monkeys; and *M. africanum* in chimpanzees and green monkeys. Other species of mycobacteria infecting monkeys are *M. avium*, *M. kansasii*, *M. scrofulaceum*, *M. intracellulare*, and *M. paratuberculosis* (PHR 420, Zoonoses of Non-human Primates. Tuberculosis and other mycobacterial zoonoses; B. Chomel and N. Lerche, pdf). The transmission of infection to human beings occurs through inhalation and direct contact. It may result in conversion to tuberculin sensitivity measured by the i/d tuberculin test or a clinical case. The population at risk is those occupationally exposed, such as foresters and laboratory animal workers.

Une and Mori (2007) described outbreaks affecting pig-tailed macaques, orangutans, and chimpanzees in an exhibition facility of a zoo in Japan. Tuberculosis was introduced through the import of an infected monkey/animal, or it spread from an already infected animal/man on the premises of the zoo. Tuberculosis was important because it spread to human beings and other animals in the zoo, as was experienced by the authors. In the exhibition facility, two of the infected monkeys died, others that tested positive were euthanized, and four persons, including two veterinarians who conducted post-mortem, were later found tuberculin positive.

Leprosy (*M. leprae*)

Rhesus monkeys and African green monkeys are susceptible. Leprosy has been reported also in chimpanzees, sooty mangabeys, and cynomolgus macaques (PHR 420, Zoonoses of Non-human Primates. Tuberculosis and other mycobacterial zoonoses; B. Chomel and N. Lerche, pdf).

Leprosy has been naturally occurring in chimpanzees and sooty mangabey monkeys in Africa, besides the known nine-banded armadillos in Louisiana and Texas in the wild or in captivity. Experimentally, it has been possible to infect rhesus monkeys (Meyers et al. 1991). African green monkeys and cynomolgus macaques have also been found to suffer with leprosy.

According to Hamilton et al. (2008), rhesus monkeys were more susceptible to leprosy when co-infected with SIV. However, the authors suggested a re-evaluation of rhesus monkeys in zoonotic leprosy because leprosy played a protective role in AIDS in humans.

These non-human primates are naturally infected with leprosy. Co-infection with SIV enhanced susceptibility. The infection is spread through direct contact. These make a strong case for alerting the high-risk group.

Tularemia

Francisella tularensis infects a wide range of hosts, mammals, birds, amphibians, fish, and also invertebrates. Hares, rodents, and rabbits are important mammalian hosts in the terrestrial cycle. Beavers, muskrats, and voles serve as the main hosts in the aquatic cycle. These could shed live bacteria into the environment. This bacterium can persist for a long time in watercourses and at low temperatures in a terrestrial environment. Insects like ticks, mosquitoes, and horseflies are important vectors. The protozoan *Acanthamoeba castellanii* might also be an important environmental reservoir of *F. tularensis* (Abd et al. 2003).

Gyuranecz et al. (2009) reported clinical tularemia in vervet monkeys and patas monkeys in a zoo in Hungary. The most likely route of infection was inhalation, suggested predominantly by lung lesions. Free-ranging wildlife may be reservoirs. Zoo primates frequently prey upon these; rodents and birds frequenting the pens are likely to get infected. Tularemia has also been reported in cynomolgus monkeys and marmosets in Germany and Switzerland zoos.

These reports indicate that infected non-human primates may be potential sources of zoonotic disease for animal keepers and visitors, and appropriate hygienic measures should be taken.

Devaux et al. (2019) reviewed the risk of infection at the human–non-human-primate interface. The hunting of non-human primates, meat consumption, the illegal import of meat, and the legal and illegal import of meat for biomedical research and ecotourism are associated with the infection, transmission, and spread of non-human primate zoonoses. It is important to understand that non-human primates transmit, receive (e.g. polio, influenza, measles, hepatitis, scabies, etc.) and again transmit zoonotic infections to humans. Recommended precautionary measures to protect ecotourists and also wildlife are (a) reducing the duration of visit, (b) limiting the number of tourists, (c) not allowing people with known diseases, (d) not permitting eating at wildlife sites, (e) defining and limiting the distance between tourists and wildlife/prohibiting touching animals in wildlife parks, and (f) wearing face masks.

OIE Regulation

According to the World Organisation for Animal Health (OIE, 2022), there are 376 different species of non-human primates split into three sub-orders and further into 15 families (shrews excluded). Their international transport must be accompanied with permits or certificates. The tests required and the directions for quarantine should be described. Non-human primates are mostly used for research, education, and breeding. Their sourcing should be in accordance with Article 7.8.7. Important considerations include public health safety, welfare, and possible introduction and spread of pathogens.

References

Abd H, Johansson T, Golovliov I, et al (2003) Survival and growth of Francisella tularensis in Acanthamoeba castellanii. Appl Environ Microbiol 69: 600–606

Devaux CA, Mediannikov O, Medkour H, Raoult D (2019) Infectious disease risk across the growing human-non human primate interface: a review of the evidence. Front Pub Hlth 7:305

Guidelines for prevention of Herpesvirus simiae (B Virus) infection in monkey handlers. MMWR.1987;36(41):680–682, 687-89

Gyuranecz M, Fodor L, Makrai L, Szoke I, Janosi K, et al (2009) Generalised tulremia in vervet monkey (*Chlorocebus aethiops*) and a patas monkey (*Erythrocebus patas*) in a zoo. J Vet Diagn Invest. 21(3):384–387

Hamilton HK, Levis WR, Martiniuk F, Cabrera A, Wolf J (2008) The role of the armadillo and sooty mangabey monkey in human leprosy. Int J Dermatol 47(6):545–550

Kaplan JE, Holmes GP, Hilliard JK, Klontz KC, Rupert AH, et al (1990) B virus (Herpesvirus simiae) infection in humans: epidemiologic investigation of a cluster. Health. Ann Intern Med American College of Physicians. ISSN: 0003-4819

Meyers WM, Gormus BJ, Walsh GP, Baskin GB, Hubbard GB (1991) Naturally acquired and experimental leprosy in nonhuman primates. Am J Trop Med Hyg 44 (4 Pt 2):24–27

OIE (2022) Zoonoses transmissible from non-human primates. Terrestrial Animal Health code- 10/08/2022. Chapter 6.12

Ostrowski SR, Leslie MJ, Parrott T, Abelt S, Piercy PE (1998) B-virus from pet macaque monkeys: an emerging threat in the United States? Emerg Infect Dis 4(1):117–121

Peeters M, Courgnaud V, Abela B, Auzel P, Pourrut X, et al (2002) Risk to human health from a plethora of simian immunodeficiency viruses in primate bushmeat. Emerg Infect Dis 8(5):451–457

Une Y, Mori T (2007) Tuberculosis as a zoonosis from a veterinary perspective. Comp Immun Microbiol Infect Dis 30(2007): 415–425.

Willis J, Webb JL, LeRoy BE, Quinn FD (2007) An overview of Tuberculosis in Macaques. http://www.vet.uga.edu/vpp/clerk/willis/index.php

Appendix D: Swine-Associated Zoonoses

The swine industry has increased during the past over 50 years to meet the demands for pork and pork products. Farming systems range from backyard farming to intensive farming system with associated range of exposure to zoonotic and environmental pathogens (Table D.1).

Pigs are monogastric animals. Development in techniques for genetic manipulation led to raising pigs as potential organ donors for humans (xenotransplant). This adds to the list of potential zoonotic infectious agents. Khan et al. (2013) reviewed papers on swine-associated zoonoses and grouped these in 1–5, depending upon the occurrence the world over.

The economic impact of zoonoses associated with meat food animals is great. Emerging and re-emerging zoonoses associated with pigs cause severe economic loss due to mortality, reduced production, fall in prices, and trade sanctions on the export of pigs, pork, and pork products. The protection of public health often demands culling, and the cost is huge. The cost of controlling zoonotic disease in human is additional.

Prevention

Healthy pigs pose no threat. Measures to maintain pigs healthy require biosecurity and other related activities.

1. *Biosecurity*—protecting farm animals, e.g., pigs from infectious agents. Measures include the following:

    (a) Avoid visiting farm/contacting pigs if one had been in contact with other pigs.

    (b) Not allowing visitor wearing boots that he had used to visit other farms during the past 24 h.

© Springer Nature Singapore Pte Ltd. 2024
K. G. Narayan et al., *Handbook of Management of Zoonoses*,
https://doi.org/10.1007/978-981-99-9885-2

Table D.1 Pig-associated zoonoses

Agents	Modes of transmission to humans	Remarks
Hepatitis E virus (HEV)[a]	Poor hygiene, food-borne, xenotransplant	Primates and human (swine farm workers, vets) suffering to hepatitis may transmit
Swine influenza viruses (SIV) (triple reassortment tr H1N1, tr H3N2, and tr H1N1)[a]	Droplet infection	Flu among pig raisers and pork producers; Pigs susceptible to both avian and human influenza virus, hence act as vessel for re-assortment
Influenza B, C[b]		Sporadic distribution
Ebola Zaire (ZEOV)	Humans are likely to get infection by contact or ingestion of pork.	Pigs suffer from REOV. Pigs are susceptible to ZEOV virus experimentally; seropositivity among pig workers is observed.
Nipah virus	Direct contact	Pigs suffer; abattoir workers and pork sellers may get infected.
Menangle viruses	Direct contact	Stillbirth, mummification, congenital defects in pigs; flu-like, non-pruritic rash among farm workers
Japanese encephalitis virus	Mosquito-bite transmitted	Rarely stillbirth in sows
Vesicular stomatitis virus[c]	Direct contact with lesions, nasal secretion, saliva	Flu like symptoms, stomatitis among pig-workers
Norwalk virus	Faecal-contaminated soil/water, food-borne	One genotype of porcine NoVs was genetically and anti-genically related to human NoVs and was replicated in gnotobiotic pigs (Wang et al. 2005). NoVs in swine most similar to human strains observed in Ethiopia (Sisay et al. 2016)
Rota virus G3 G5 G9 (G3 G9 major cause of diarrhoea)	Faecal contaminated soil/water, food-borne	The global importance of genotype G9 rota viruses in humans and pigs is increasing (Wu et al. 2017).
Porcine lymphocytic choriomeningitis virus[d]	Xenotransplant	
Swine torque teno viruses[d]	Xenotransplant	
HeV-genotype 3[d]		
Livestock-associated methicillin-resistant Staphylococcus aureus (LA-MRSA)[a]	Possibly food-borne, direct contact	Development and spread of antibiotic-resistant bacteria

Organism	Transmission	Comments
Streptococcus suis[a]	Direct contact, ingestion	Pig and pork producers and pork consumers are often affected.
Streptococcus porcinus[a]	Direct contact	Lymphadenitis, endocarditis, abortion in swine, infections of female genital tract and stillbirth in women (Martin et al. 2004)
Bacillus anthracis	Direct and indirect contact, transdermal, mucosal, aerosol, food-borne	
Clostridium difficile[a]	Direct and environmental (indirect) contact	Common as nosocomial, colonized humans can also be reservoir.
Burkholderia pseudomallei[a]	Direct contact, faecal-/soil-contaminated food, water	
Brucella suis[e]	Direct contact, transdermal, mucosal	
Campylobacter enteritis[e]	Direct contact, food-borne	
Erysipelothrix rhusiopathiae[e]	Direct contact, damaged skin, mucosa	Pig farm workers are most likely affected.
Escherichia coli infections[e]	Direct/indirect contact, poor hygiene, food-borne	
Francisella tularensis[e]	Direct, aerosol, food-borne, vector-borne	
Leptospira interrogans[e]	Direct, indirect contact with fomites	
Listeria monocytogenes[e]	Direct contact, food-borne	
Pasteurella multocida[e]	Enters through animal bites, scratches	
Pasteurella aerogenes[e]	Bites	
Salmonellosis[e]	Direct contact, food-borne, poor hygiene, faecal-contaminated soil/water	
Yersinia enterocolitica[e]	Food-borne, poor hygiene, faecal-contaminated water/soil, direct contact	
Tuberculosis[e]	Direct contact	Lesions in the pig neck region and mesenteric lymph nodes; TB in humans is non-progressive—sub-clinical but serious in immunocompromised.

(continued)

Table D.1 (continued)

Agents	Modes of transmission to humans	Remarks
Erysipelothrix rhusiopathiae	Damaged skin/mucosa	
Tularemia	Direct, aerosol, vector, and food-borne	
Trichinella spiralis	Food-borne	
Cysticercus cellulosae[a]	Food-borne	
Ecchinococcosis[e]	Parasite is maintained in sheep/pig-dog cycle. Ingestion of parasite eggs infect human.	
Giant intestinal fluke[c]	Ingestion of raw/undercooked aquatic plant carrying encysted *Fasciolopsis buski*	
Asian taeniasis[c]	Ingestion of infected beef or pork	
Gastrodiscoidiasis[c]	Ingestion of metacercaria in fish or contaminated plant infects man and pigs.	
S. japonicum—schistosomiasis[c]	Pigs act as reservoir hosts. Faecal (egg)-contaminated water initiates the life cycle; infective cercariae in water penetrate the human skin.	
Sarcosporidiosis[b] *Sarcocystis hominis*	Faecal-contaminated soil/water, ingestion of uncooked pork	
Toxoplasma gondii	Food-borne	
Balantidium coli[b]	Faecal-/water-/soil-contaminated water/food	
Cryptosporidium suis	Water-/soil-contaminated water/food	
Giardia intestinalis[a]	Oral/poor hygiene	
Dermatophytosis (except *Microsporum canis*)[b]	Contaminated fomites, contact—ringworm	

[a]Emerging swine-associated zoonoses distributed worldwide
[b]Sporadic distribution
[c]Limited distribution
[d]Xenotransplant
[e]Endemic (non-emerging), cluster of cases occur the world over

(c) Ill persons should not enter farms till they had been free from any symptoms for 24 h.
(d) Limit exposure to rodents, wildlife, bird, and pests.
(e) Quarantine for 7 days for new arrivals, animals returning from animal fare/shows, etc. Healthy animals should be attended to first if the same set of farm workers are looking after both. Evaluate the health of animals.
(f) Cleaning and disinfect facilities, feeder, and equipment after every use.

2. *Vaccination of pigs*—plan vaccination with the help of veterinarian.
3. *Personal protective* like boots, gloves, masks, and clothing should be used by farm workers. Frequent washing of the hands must be practised after touching an animal and equipment. Eating, drinking, and sleeping in animal areas are not allowed.

Any sickness in farm workers, exhibitors, and their family should be reported to health care providers and public health officials.

The integration of the swine industry, farmers, veterinarians, clinicians, and public health professionals is required for the sustained availability of nutritious pork and its products and to keep out threatening swine-borne zoonoses.

References

Khan SU, Atanasova KR, Krueger WS, Ramirez A, Gray GC (2013) Epidemiology, geographical distribution, and economic consequences of swine zoonoses: a narrative review. Emerg Microbes Infect 2(12):e92

Martin C, Fermeaux V, Eyraud JL, Aubard Y (2004) *Streptococcus porcinus* as a cause of spontaneous preterm human stillbirth. J Clin Microbiol 42(9):4396–4398

Sisay Z, Djikeng A, Berhe N, Belay G, Abegaz WE, et al (2016) First detection and molecular characterization of sapoviruses and noroviruses with zoonotic potential in swine in Ethiopia. Arch Virol 161(10):2739–2747

Wang QH, Han MG, Cheetham S, Souza M, Funk JA, Saif LJ (2005) Porcine noroviruses related to human noroviruses. Emerg Infect Dis 11(12):1874–1881

Wu FT, Bányai K, Jiang B, et al (2017) Novel G9 rotavirus strains co-circulate in children and pigs, Taiwan Sci Rep 7:40731

Appendix E: Equine-Associated Zoonoses

Equine-associated zoonoses are tabulated below.

Disease in man	Causative agent	Mode of transmission to man
Encephalitis	EEEV	Mosquito bite
	WEEV	Mosquito bite
	VEEV (horses, donkeys, mules)	Mosquito bite
	West Nile virus	Mosquito bite—*Culex* spp.
	JEV	Mosquito bite—*Culex* spp., *Aedes* spp.
Respiratory illness and encephalitis	Hendra virus	Direct contact with nasal secretions
Hydrophobia (rabies)	Rabies virus	Direct contact (generally horses suffer from dumb/paralytic form—gradual lameness)
In immunocompromised or with AIDS—pneumonia, fever, diarrhoea, arthritis	*Rhodococcus equi*	Respiratory disease of foals—man gets it through inhalation.
Anthrax—inhalation, gastrointestinal and cutaneous form	*Bacillus anthracis*	Contact
Glanders	*Burkholderia mallei*	Contact with nasal discharge and skin lesions
Febrile (undulant fever)	*Brucella abortus*	Fistulous wither in horse—contact with lesion
Enteric disease, fever	*Salmonella enterica* sub spp. *enterica*, serotype Typhimurium definitive type 104	Faecal-oral route
Respiratory disease, meningitis	*Streptococcus equi* sub spp. *zooepidemicus*	Contact?

© Springer Nature Singapore Pte Ltd. 2024
K. G. Narayan et al., *Handbook of Management of Zoonoses*,
https://doi.org/10.1007/978-981-99-9885-2

Disease in man	Causative agent	Mode of transmission to man
Colitis—pseudomembranous, perforation of intestine, fatal	*Clostridium difficile*	Colitis in horse—bacteria and toxin in faeces; human infection through the faecal-oral route (?)
Miscellaneous infections	Methicillin-resistant *Staphylococcus aureus*	Contact
Tuberculosis	*Mycobacterium tuberculosis, M. bovis*	Contact
Copious watery diarrhoea	*Cryptosporidium parvum*	Faecal-oral route
Diarrhoea	*Giardia intestinalis*	Faecal-oral route
Dermatophytoses	Dermatophytoses— *Trichophyton equinum*	Contact

Reason, Emotion and Will

Edited by

R. Jay Wallace

Humboldt-Universität zu Berlin, Germany

Ashgate

DARTMOUTH

Aldershot • Brookfield USA • Singapore • Sydney

Published by
Dartmouth Publishing Company Limited
Ashgate Publishing Limited
Gower House
Croft Road
Aldershot
Hants GU11 3HR
England

Ashgate Publishing Company
Old Post Road
Brookfield
Vermont 05036
USA

British Library Cataloguing in Publication Data
Reason, emotion and will. – (The international research
   library of philosophy)
   1. Reason   2. Emotions   3. Will
   I. Wallace, R. Jay
   171.2

Library of Congress Cataloging-in-Publication Data
Reason, emotion and will / edited by R. Jay Wallace.
         p.   cm. — (The international research library of philosophy)
      Includes bibliographical references.
      ISBN 1-85521-970-0 (hardcover)
      1. Ethics.   2. Psychology and philosophy.   I. Wallace, R. Jay.
   II. Series.
   BJ45.R43   1999
   170—dc21   98-44663
                                                                                CIP

ISBN 1 85521 970 0

Printed in Great Britain by Galliards, Great Yarmouth

Reason, Emotion and Will

The International Research Library of Philosophy
Series Editor: John Skorupski

Contents

Acknowledgements

The editor and publishers wish to thank the following for permission to use copyright material.

The American Philosophical Association for the essay: Harry Frankfurt (1991–92), 'The Faintest Passion', *Proceedings and Addresses of the American Philosophical Association*, **66**, pp. 5–16.

The Aristotelian Society for the essays: Jonathan Dancy (1994–95), 'Why There is Really No Such Thing as the Theory of Motivation', *Proceedings of the Aristotelian Society*, **95**, pp. 1–18. Reprinted by courtesy of the Editor of the Aristotelian Society. Copyright © 1995; Derek Parfit (1997), 'Reasons and Motivation', *The Aristotelian Society*, Supplementary Volume **77**, pp. 99–130. Reprinted by courtesy of the Editor of the Aristotelian Society. Copyright © 1997; John Broome (1997), 'Reasons and Motivation', *The Aristotelian Society*, Supplementary Volume **77**, pp. 131–46. Reprinted by courtesy of the Editor of the Aristotelian Society. Copyright © 1997.

Australian Journal of Philosophy for the essay: Amelie Oksenberg Rorty (1980), 'Where Does the Akratic Break Take Place?', *Australasian Journal of Philosophy*, **58**, pp. 333–46.

Blackwell Publishers, USA for the essays: Elijah Millgram (1996), 'Williams' Argument Against External Reasons', *Noûs*, **30**, pp. 197–220. Copyright © 1996 Blackwell Publishers Inc.; J. David Velleman (1992), 'The Guise of the Good', *Noûs*, **26**, pp. 3–26; Robert Audi (1979), 'Weakness of Will and Practical Judgment', *Noûs*, **13**, pp. 173–96. Copyright © 1979 Indiana University.

Cornell University for the essays: Dennis W. Stampe (1987), 'The Authority of Desire', *The Philosophical Review*, **96**, pp. 335–81. Copyright © 1987 Cornell University. Reprinted by permission of the publisher and the author; Gary Watson (1977), 'Skepticism about Weakness of Will', *The Philosophical Review*, **86**, pp. 316–39. Copyright © 1977 Cornell University. Reprinted by permission of the publisher and the author; Robert C. Roberts (1984), 'Will Power and the Virtues', *The Philosophical Review*, **93**, pp. 227–47. Copyright © 1984 Cornell University. Reprinted by permission of the publisher and the author.

International Phenomenological Society for the essay: Michael Smith (1995), 'Internal Reasons', *Philosophy and Phenomenological Research*, **55**, pp. 109–31.

The Journal of Philosophy for the essays: Michael Stocker (1979), 'Desiring the Bad: An Essay in Moral Psychology', *The Journal of Philosophy*, **76**, pp. 738–53. Copyright © 1979 The Journal of Philosophy, Inc.; Richard Moran (1993), 'Impersonality, Character, and Moral Expressivism', *The Journal of Philosophy*, **90**, pp. 578–95. Copyright © 1993 The Journal of Philosophy, Inc.; Rüdiger Bittner (1992), 'Is It Reasonable to Regret Things One Did?', *The Journal of Philosophy*, **89**, pp. 262–73. Copyright © 1992 The Journal of Philosophy, Inc.

Series Preface

The International Research Library of Philosophy collects in book form a wide range of important and influential essays in philosophy, drawn predominantly from English-language journals. Each volume in the Library deals with a field of inquiry which has received significant attention in philosophy in the last 25 years, and is edited by a philosopher noted in that field.

No particular philosophical method or approach is favoured or excluded. The Library will constitute a representative sampling of the best work in contemporary English-language philosophy, providing researchers and scholars throughout the world with comprehensive coverage of currently important topics and approaches.

The Library is divided into four series of volumes which reflect the broad divisions of contemporary philosophical inquiry:

- Metaphysics and Epistemology
- The Philosophy of Mathematics and Science
- The Philosophy of Logic, Language and Mind
- The Philosophy of Value

I am most grateful to all the volume editors, who have unstintingly contributed scarce time and effort to this project. The authority and usefulness of the series rests firmly on their hard work and scholarly judgement. I must also express my thanks to John Irwin of the Ashgate Publishing Company, from whom the idea of the Library originally came, and who brought it to fruition; and also to his colleagues in the Editorial Office, whose care and attention to detail are so vital in ensuring that the Library provides a handsome and reliable aid to philosophical inquirers.

JOHN SKORUPSKI
General Editor
University of St. Andrews
Scotland

Introduction

The last 20 years have seen an explosion of interest in what has come to be referred to as moral psychology. This may be thought of, very roughly, as the study of the distinctively psychological aspects of the ethical life. Characteristic questions addressed within moral psychology include the following: What are the typical objects of moral concern? What structures of thought, perception and feeling enable us to act as morality requires? What is it to have a particular character, and what is distinctive about the character traits regarded as morally admirable? Which are the specially moral emotions, and in what ways do these emotions contribute to the ethical life? To what extent is it possible to do freely what one believes to be wrong or undesirable, and what can we learn from this phenomenon about the nature and etiology of rational action?

Interest in questions of these kinds is coextensive with moral philosophy itself. The major texts from the history of philosophical ethics are all, in one degree or another, treatises in moral psychology. Faced with normative issues about the value of the ethical life or the authority and objectivity of moral norms, philosophers as diverse as Aristotle, Hobbes, Hume, Kant, and Nietzsche all found it necessary to develop interpretations of moral agency and the will. The natural explanation for this is that morality is, in the first instance, a practical matter, defining standards for the regulation of human conduct. It is therefore virtually impossible to say anything interesting about morality without making assumptions about, say, the motives to which human beings are typically subject or the different contributions of reason and sentiment to human behaviour.

Contemporary interest in moral psychology thus represents a return to a set of issues that has traditionally helped to define philosophical ethics as a subject. These issues were pushed out of view by the style of meta-ethical discussion that dominated English-language moral philosophy during the mid-twentieth century. Debates between emotivists, prescriptivists, and descriptivists about the meaning of moral discourse, for example, were often conducted by philosophers who either agreed fundamentally in their conceptions of human agency and moral selfhood or whose disagreements in this area were relegated to an invisible place somewhere beyond public philosophical view. The return of such disagreements to the centre stage reflects a widespread conviction that both meta-ethical and normative controversies in moral philosophy largely hinge on assumptions about moral psychology, which therefore need to be scrutinized directly by anyone interested in the subject.

The essays collected in this volume may all be regarded as contributions to this flourishing area of philosophy. Beyond the unity they exhibit as examples of contemporary moral psychology, however, many of them also share a common focus on a particular set of substantive issues concerning the roles of cognitive and non-cognitive states in relation to agency and the will. These are, of course, ancient philosophical questions – reminiscent of Plato's and Aristotle's depictions of the virtuous soul as one in which reason is sovereign over the appetites, and of Hume's famous counter that 'reason is, and ought only to be the slave of the passions'. Nevertheless, the issues have continued to grip contemporary philosophers, as the essays

collected in this volume attest. A further common thread that links many of the essays is a methodological issue they raise, concerning the proper attitude of the philosopher to the psychological phenomena of the moral life. To what extent, and in what ways, should a philosophical theory take account of these phenomena not only in their standard manifestations, but also in their deviant and irrational forms (such as perverse desires, weakness of will and irrational guilt)? Is it ever appropriate for philosophers to allow their understanding of psychological phenomena to be constrained by their theories, or must philosophers always yield to our pre-philosophical sense of what is possible within the human psychological economy?

The discussions of these questions in this volume have been organized into five Parts, and the remainder of this Introduction sketches in a little more detail the issues tackled within each.

Motivation and Desire

The Humean approach to moral psychology is now associated primarily with a certain thesis about the role of desire in motivating people to act – namely, that motivation is essentially constituted by desire, so that cognitive or rational states are incapable by themselves of generating a motive.

In his essay, 'The Humean Theory of Motivation' (Chapter 1), Michael Smith defends a version of this thesis about the connection between desire and motivation. Smith's argument turns essentially on the following two ideas. First, he suggests that motivating states are distinguished by a particular 'direction of fit' vis-à-vis the world; they are essentially states with which the world is to be brought into alignment, rather than states that aim to conform to the way the world (already) is. Second, he contends that to be in a state with this distinctive direction of fit is, in effect, to be in a state of desire. Hence the Humean conclusion that motivation is essentially constituted by desire. A similar conclusion is defended by Simon Blackburn in 'Practical Tortoise Raising' (Chapter 2). Reflecting on Lewis Carroll's famous discussion of Achilles and the tortoise, Blackburn extracts from it the moral that the will can never be determined to act solely by reason and the facts. Rational influences on action can be represented as the premises from which we deliberate, but no set of premises, however complete, can alone determine us to act. Action in accordance with reason and the facts ultimately depends on an orientation of the agent's will, which cannot itself be represented as the acceptance of a premise.

The strength of this conclusion depends, to a considerable degree, on how the contrast between the rational and the non-rational is understood. For both Blackburn and Smith, the non-cognitive states essential to motivation are not desires in the familiar, colloquial sense of appetite or yearning (in which, for instance, attention is focused on a particular object or possibility for action), but rather pro-attitudes in the broadest possible sense. One question this raises is whether the Humean thesis retains its interest once it is clear that the desires implicated in motivation are to be construed in this broad way. If the non-cognitive states required for motivation include the dispositions that are manifested by any act of inference from premises one accepts, as Blackburn's argument seems to imply, it may be wondered whether there is any interesting philosophical position that is ruled out by that argument. (A Kantian, after all, might be willing to allow that desires are essential to motivation, if these include the general dispositions that underlie any reasoning from premises to a conclusion.)

A second question is whether the very broad understanding of desire undermines the explanatory aspirations of the Humean approach to moral psychology. Traditionally, that approach has been thought to yield a certain schema for explaining intentional action, in terms of non-cognitive states to which the agent is subject, which (in concert with the agent's beliefs) both rationalize and cause the agent's behaviour.[1] But if the non-cognitive states involved in motivation are merely pro-attitudes in the broadest sense, their presence might not tell us anything interesting about how intentional actions are ultimately to be explained. Thus from the fact that I chose to grade some papers this morning it follows that, in the pro-attitude sense, I 'wanted' to grade the papers. But this is compatible with the possibility that the desire itself can be explained in a way that does not presuppose the presence of some further non-cognitive state on my part – say, in terms of my beliefs about what I am obligated to do – and, in that case, the desire that is ascribed to me in motivation will be superficial from the explanatory point of view.[2]

The issue of the explanatory role of desire with regard to motivation is joined in different ways in the essays by Alfred Mele and Jonathan Dancy. In 'Motivational Internalism' (Chapter 3) Mele defends the conclusion that processes of thought can only give rise to motivation and desire by drawing on antecedent motivations, to which the agent was already subject prior to the episode of practical reflection. That this is the case is not, Mele admits, a *conceptual* truth, but he suggests that this Humean approach offers the most plausible account of the etiology of intentional action and points out that the approach does not have the restrictive normative implications often attributed to it. In 'Why There is Really No Such Thing as the Theory of Motivation' (Chapter 4) Dancy takes a very different tack. His point of departure is the familiar thought that normative or justifying reasons, construed as considerations that recommend or speak in favour of acting in a particular way (say, doing x), must be capable of moving the agent to do x in fact: this is one version of what has been called 'internalism' – the general thesis that there is a necessary connection between our reasons and our motivations. Given internalism in this form, Dancy contends that we can only make sense of normative reasons for action if we abandon the Humean assumption that actions are causally explicable in terms of psychological states to which the agent is subject. His discussion thus touches on a subject that is fundamental for moral psychology more generally: to what extent can our image of ourselves as autonomous deliberators be reconciled with the idea that what determines us to act are psychological states, such as beliefs, and desires, with respect to which we are merely passive?

A different challenge to the Humean theory is presented by Michael Bratman in 'Taking Plans Seriously' (Chapter 5). Bratman contests the Humean assumption that all motivational states should be thought of as desires. He favours instead a motivational psychology that makes room for such irreducibly volitional elements as future-directed intentions and decisions, arguing that a motivational psychology of this kind is necessary to account for the forms of planning distinctive of human (as opposed to animal) agency. Our intentions and decisions fix the context for much of our practical deliberation and enable us to coordinate our activities with others who are planning agents like ourselves.[3] Humeans might respond that their notion of desire as generic pro-attitude is sufficiently capacious to accommodate volitional states of these sorts. It must then be asked, however, whether we can really attain an adequate understanding of human motivation by abstracting from the differences between intentions and decisions on the one hand, and more ordinary desires on the other. Bratman's argument suggests that this might not be possible.[4]

Reasons and Desires

In the previous section I adverted to a distinction between two different kinds of reasons: explanatory reasons which serve to explain why we act the way we do; and normative reasons which recommend or speak in favour of acting in a particular way. One might think of explanatory reasons as answering the question, 'Why did A do x?', while normative reasons answer the different question, 'Why should A do x?'. The theme of the essays in Part I of this volume is the role of desires as explanatory reasons; in Part II, the issue is the bearing of desires on our normative reasons.

Of outstanding importance for the recent discussion of this question is an essay by Bernard Williams, 'Internal and External Reasons', which has not been included in this collection because it is readily available elsewhere.[5] Williams defends the thesis that one can have reason to do x only if there is some element in one's 'subjective motivational set' – some *desire*, in a suitably broad and formal sense – that would be served by so acting. Statements about an agent's reasons for action are thus 'internal', in the sense that their truth hinges on the shape of the agent's actual motivational profile. In defence of this conclusion, Williams appeals to a version of the thesis that I referred to above as internalism, to the effect that even normative reasons have a 'dimension of possible explanation'; specifically, if an agent A has reason to do x, then it must be possible for A to acquire a motivation to do x as a result of deliberating correctly. But, Williams contends, rational deliberation can give rise to a new motivation only by proceeding from some motivation to which the agent is already subject. It follows that A's reasons are constrained by the elements already present in A's subjective motivational set.

This argument has sparked a wide-ranging and lively debate.[6] One point of controversy has been the version of internalism that Williams relies on, to the effect that A can have reason to do x only if it would be possible for A to acquire the motivation to do x through a rational deliberative process. If x is, say, the right or best thing to do, then perhaps we should say that there is reason for A to do x even if A could only acquire the corresponding motivation by a non-deliberative process, such as conversion or habituation.[7] But even if we accept Williams' brand of internalism, there is room to question whether his conclusion about the connection between reasons and desires really follows from it. His argument at this point rests on the assumption that deliberation can give rise to a new motivation only if it, in some way, begins from motivations to which the agent is already subject. This assumption, which touches on issues in motivational psychology canvassed in Part I, is challenged in my own essay, 'How to Argue about Practical Reason' (Chapter 6). I point out that Williams offers no clear defence of the thesis that deliberation must begin from motivations to which one is already subject, and suggest that we have no good reason to suppose that practical reasoning could only be motivational efficacious if it conforms to this pattern.[8]

Beyond this, it is not entirely clear what it means to say that rational deliberation must begin from an agent's existing subjective motivational set. Williams refers to the elements of such sets as 'desires', at least in a formal sense; but if the notion of a desire is construed sufficiently broadly, it becomes quite unclear whether his position would exclude any interesting possibilities. Thus, one might say that any agent who is actually moved to do x in a particular set of circumstances must have had a latent disposition to do x in circumstances of that kind – a disposition that was already part of the agent's subjective motivational set. But the claim that reasons

depend on desires of this kind seems vacuous and so uninteresting. On the other hand, attempts to give the claim that deliberation must begin from items in one's existing motivational profile more bite threaten to render that claim correspondingly implausible. Thus, one might suppose that deliberation begins from an agent's existing motivations when the agent expressly takes those motivations into account, reflecting on how the ends they supply may best be attained. Deliberation of the kind of which Williams approves, however, would then acquire a narrowly instrumental character, and it may be doubted whether so narrow an account could possibly be adequate to our understanding of the possibilities for practical reflection. These questions are pressed by Elijah Millgram in 'Williams' Argument against External Reasons' (Chapter 7).

Chapters 8 and 9, by Michael Smith and J. David Velleman, focus on the relativism about reasons that seems implicit in Williams' position. In 'Internal Reasons' (Chapter 8), Smith challenges Williams' contention that normative reasons depend on elements in the subjective motivational profiles of particular agents. His challenge rests on the idea that reasons for action share with other normative concepts an aspiration to intersubjective convergence and stability, and that this aspiration cannot be reconciled with the assumption that a given agent's reasons are relative to that agent's arbitrary motivations. In 'The Possibility of Practical Reason' (Chapter 9), Velleman mounts a different challenge to the thesis that reasons necessarily display a relativity to the motivational sets that distinguish one agent from another. He concedes that normative reasons can only be ascribed to persons who have a suitable desire, but maintains that the desire in question is one that is constitutive of us as agents – namely, the desire for autonomy. The general dependence of reasons on this desire thus does not entail a relativity to the variable contours of one's individual motivational profile.

The exchange between Derek Parfit and John Broome about 'Reasons and Motivation' (Chapters 10 and 11) focuses on two further aspects of the debate about reasons and desires. One of these is its relation to naturalism about normative discourse. Parfit distinguishes between reductionistic and non-reductionistic interpretations of the thesis that all reasons are internal and argues that both are problematic. Reductionistic interpretations hold that facts about a person's reasons ultimately consist in natural facts about what that person would be motivated to do under conditions of procedural rationality. But Parfit contends that no form of naturalistic reductionism about the normative could possibly be correct. On the other hand, a non-reductionistic interpretation of the internal reasons thesis would undermine its own basis. The claim that reasons have their source in our desires derives at least part of its appeal from the thought that intrinsically motivating normative truths about what we have reason to do would be metaphysically extravagant from the perspective of the scientific world-view, but this line of thought loses its cogency, as an argument for the internal reasons thesis, once that thesis has been given a non-reductionistic interpretation.

Parfit himself believes that all normative reasons are external in Williams' sense; their status as reasons in no way depends on facts about whether we would be motivated accordingly under conditions of procedural rationality. In his contribution to the exchange about 'Reasons and Motivation' (Chapter 11), Broome explores the commitments of this kind of position, particularly regarding the motivational effects of practical reasoning. How is it possible that normative reflection about what we ought to do can move us to act accordingly, when such reflection is construed in the cognitivist terms that Parfit favours? Broome's own tentative answer is that normative reflection might give rise to appropriate motivation if one supposes that a disposition to act as one believes one ought to belongs to the natural psychology of

those who are rational. Broome himself notes several grounds for dissatisfaction with this position (which has affinities with Velleman's claim that the desire for autonomy is constitutive of rational agency).[9] But one of the most important of them does not emerge in his discussion. If practical rationality is ultimately traced to the operations of a natural psychological tendency in the way suggested by Broome and Velleman, then our own activity as agents seems to disappear. Doing what is rationally required becomes the result of psychological forces operative in us, and not something for which we ourselves are responsible. Perhaps we can make sense of the practical dimension of normative reasons only in terms of *the will*, construed as a capacity for self-determination in ways that are independent of all our antecedent desires and dispositions.

Desire and the Good

There are two important theses about the connection between desire and the good that have attracted the attention of philosophers interested in moral psychology.[10] The first of these is a thesis about the good, to the effect that there is a constitutive connection between beliefs about goodness and desires. According to one version of this thesis, for example, if an object or state of affairs, *p*, is believed to be valuable, then the agent with that belief must also desire *p*. The second thesis, by contrast, is essentially about the nature of desire. It maintains that there is a constitutive connection between desires and beliefs about the good, such that objects and states of affairs can only be desired *sub specie boni* – that is, under the aspect of the good. Together, the two theses about desire and the good form a systematic package with a long and distinguished philosophical provenance (although it would be possible to endorse either one of the theses without endorsing the other). Recent work in moral psychology, however, has subjected the two theses to strong attack.

Important examples of the sceptical attitude toward the theses are Chapters 12 and 13 of this volume.[11] In 'Desiring the Bad' (Chapter 12), Michael Stocker presents a series of vivid cases in which agents fail to be attracted to things that they take to be good, and in which they are positively attracted to other things that they believe to be bad (indeed, precisely because they believe those things to be bad). Stocker extracts from these cases the general moral that the connections between evaluation and motivation are exceedingly complex, mediated by structures of energy, interest, mood and the like that vary markedly from person to person; a central task of moral psychology, he suggests, is the investigation of such structures. A similar conclusion is defended by J. David Velleman in 'The Guise of the Good' (Chapter 13). He traces the attraction of the discredited theses to deepseated misunderstandings about the nature of intentional action and desire, and he defends the surprising conclusion that the believed badness of a course of action can be not only what is attractive about it to the agent, but also what justifies the action from the agent's point of view.

A rather different perspective is offered by Dennis Stampe in his wide-ranging article 'The Authority of Desire' (Chapter 14). This essay defends a seemingly very strong thesis about the normative significance of desire – namely, that desires have *per se* authority for practical deliberation: the mere fact that one wants something is (ordinarily) a reason to act accordingly. In support of this thesis, Stampe develops an interpretation of the nature of desire that differs interestingly from the conceptions implicit in the essays by Stocker and Velleman. According

to Stampe's interpretation, desires are forms of perception or awareness; in particular, they are attitudes in which a propositional object, *p*, essentially strikes the subject of the attitude in a certain way, as something whose obtaining would be good. Clearly, if this account is correct, then the forms of perverse desire that Stocker and Velleman focus on – in which a state of affairs is allegedly desired because it is taken by the desirer to be bad – will need careful interpretation – if they are to be possible at all. Perhaps the object that is perversely desired may *seem* good to a subject, even while the subject *believes* that very same object to be bad. But this suggestion raises difficult issues, both about the phenomenology of perverse desire and about the meaning of the claim that the objects of desire are perceived as good. For instance, does it really seem to the subject of a perverse desire as if the object of such a desire would be good in any sense? If so, what exactly might this sense be?

These are the sorts of consideration that move some to think, with Stocker and Velleman, that desires are not necessarily connected with thoughts about the good. It does not follow from this position, however, that desire and evaluation are not linked in any way. Even if desires are not in general connected with thoughts or beliefs about the good, there might be a definable subclass of desires that are constitutively connected with evaluation.

A proposal roughly to this effect has influentially been developed by Harry Frankfurt.[12] In his view, desires by themselves do not necessarily have any privileged position in determining what we ought (by our own lights) to do; one can be subject to, and even moved by, a given desire (say, an addiction), while also feeling alienated from the desire and action, as items in one's own biography that one would not endorse. There is, however, a subclass of desires from which one cannot feel alienated in this way. These are our second-order desires, formed after, and as a result of, reflection on the first-order desires to which we happen to be subject. Desires of this kind have – in a way that ordinary first-order desires do not – a special authority when it comes to determining our evaluative perspective on the world. In Frankfurt's own terms, they are expressive of what we care about.

This important proposal raises a host of questions, most saliently about the normative significance that is ascribed to second-order desires.[13] If desires by themselves do not necessarily reflect what an agent cares about, what is so special about second-order desires? How can the mere fact that a desire is reflexive invest it with a kind of authority that other desires do not exhibit? 'The Faintest Passion' (Chapter 15) presents Frankfurt's most recent response to questions of this kind.[14] Here Frankfurt suggests, first, that desires can have authority for a person only if they derive from that person's conscious reflection, which is of necessity a reflexive or higher-order process. Second, he contends that it is sufficient for reflection to yield second-order desires – volitions of higher orders are not required – so long as our second-order desires are ones with which we are *satisfied*. With this analysis in place, Frankfurt identifies an interesting and neglected phenomenon for philosophical investigation – that of wholeheartedness. This involves the absence of ambivalence at the level of second-order evaluation. If Frankfurt's approach is correct, volitional wholeheartedness in this sense is both of decisive importance in fixing what we really care about, and ultimately a matter of luck.

Weakness and Strength of Will

The phenomenon of weakness of will is a crux for many of the issues in moral psychology that

have been touched on so far. In its most striking form, weakness of will is exhibited when persons freely and intentionally do something that they believe, at the time of action, to be worse than the alternatives that are open to them. The classical philosophical problem of weakness of will is whether, and if so how, this phenomenon is even possible. The essays collected in Part IV of this volume offer a representative sample of the work that has been done on this central topic during the past two decades.[15]

Weakness of will, in the striking form just characterized, involves a breakdown in the normal (or rational) connections between one's evaluative judgement about what it would be best to do, on the one hand, and one's intentional action on the other. It is important to bear in mind, however, that practical judgements and intentional actions are typically situated in a broader context of character, values and beliefs, and that the successful translation of one's own values into a suitable and sustained pattern of action is subject to interference at a variety of points along the way. The failure to act in accordance with one's immediate practical judgement about what is to be done may be the philosophically most interesting kind of breakdown that can occur. But it is not the only kind, and attention to the wider range of possibilities can lead to a sharper understanding of the varieties of hazard we encounter in attempting to realize our ends, and of the appropriate means for meeting those threats. So argues Amélie Oksenberg Rorty, in 'Where Does the Akratic Break Take Place?' (Chapter 16).

From a philosophical standpoint, however, the striking form of weakness of will remains the most challenging, because it brings pressure to bear on our understanding of intention, desire, practical judgement, and their various contributions to action. Take the case of our practical judgements, about what it would best to do in a given situation. There is a version of the thesis referred to above as internalism, according to which it is a condition of the genuineness of judgements of this kind that the person to whom they are ascribed be motivated accordingly. This condition finds clear expression in the following principle of Donald Davidson's: 'P2. If an agent judges that it would be better to do *x* than to do *y*, then he wants to do *x* more than he wants to do *y*'.[16] But if practical judgement is linked with motivation in this direct way, there is an apparent difficulty seeing how weakness of will can be so much as possible, at least on the natural assumption that intentional action always accords with one's strongest desires. In response to this difficulty, one might retain P2, but refine one's account of the practical judgements involved in cases of weakness, distinguishing, say, between the conditional judgements against which one acts and the unconditional judgements revealed in one's behaviour, to which P2 properly applies.[17] Alternatively (and perhaps also more straightforwardly), one might modify P2, contending that the connection between practical judgement and motivation is less direct than that principle would entail. This option is explored and defended in Robert Audi's essay 'Weakness of Will and Practical Judgment' (Chapter 17).

On the other side, there are common assumptions about the nature of intentional action that make it seem puzzling how actions of this kind can ever fail to correspond to one's own judgement about what it would be best to do. One such assumption is the Humean theory of motivation discussed in Part I of this collection. Suppose that this theory is true, so that motivation always entails the presence of desire, and suppose, further, that the following assumptions are also true: (a) that desires always aim at what is believed to be valuable, and (b) that all values are ultimately commensurable, in some sense. With these assumptions in place, it becomes very difficult to make sense of intentional actions that conflict with one's sincere judgement about what it would be best to do; from the agent's own point of view,

there seems to be nothing in the weakwilled action capable of engaging one's desires, in the way necessary for intentional action. This is essentially the Socratic argument against weakness of will developed in Plato's *Protagoras* – an argument that can be resisted by weakening the connection between desires and beliefs about the good (as Stocker and Velleman urge in Part III), or by challenging the assumption of the commensurability of values.[18]

A different set of assumptions about intentional action that seems to leave no room for weakness of will is expressed in some versions of modern decision theory. According to this framework for thinking about rational action, value is ultimately a function of an agent's preferences over outcomes, where the strength of one's preferences is in turn understood causally. It follows that intentional action reflects one's strongest desires, together with one's beliefs about the probabilities of outcomes, in such a way that one always does what one believes will be 'best' – a position that apparently leaves no room for the striking form of weakness of will described above. In 'Weakness of Will' (Chapter 18), Frank Jackson sketches this general approach to intentional action, linking it with the Humean conception of reason and the will, and arguing that the approach in fact has the resources to accommodate something like weakness of will. The key, Jackson contends, is to attend to the *dynamics* of value – the ways in which one's preferences change over time in relation to one's evolving beliefs about the probability of outcomes. Weakness occurs when one's present strongest desire cannot be accounted for in terms of one's earlier desires, together with one's new subjective probabilities. Against this, it has been maintained that not all changes in preference that satisfy Jackson's conditions are cases of genuine irrationality and that, even when such changes are irrational, they do not display the element of synchronic conflict between action and better judgement that is the hallmark of true weakness of will.[19] This raises the basic question whether the Humean approach, as elaborated in modern decision theory, is really adequate to account for the full range of phenomena to which a theory of rational action should apply.[20]

A more modest assumption that seems to be called into question by weakness of will is that intentional action is always done for a reason. Depending on how the idea of acting for a reason is interpreted, there is a puzzle about how weakwilled agents can be understood to be doing such a thing, given the judgement that the course of action they are pursuing is not the best available to them. Implicit in Davidson's discussion, for instance, is the idea that acting for a reason has an essentially inferential structure, in which the action can be represented as the conclusion of a piece of practical reasoning. But if the conclusions of such inferences are construed in evaluative terms, there seems little room for full-blooded actions to diverge from one's own better judgement. One will be forced (with Davidson) to posit an *ad hoc* and implausible distinction between two different kinds of evaluative judgement to explain how the weakwilled agent can both believe that x would be better than y, and yet do y for a reason. Two responses to this problem seem to be available. One might abandon the assumption that the practical conclusions implicit in action are evaluative in nature, distinguishing between practical judgements about what it would be good to do, on the one hand, and essentially volitional states of intention on the other (compare Bratman's discussion of such states in Chapter 5). Or, one could question whether intentional action can always accurately be represented as the conclusion of an inference. Perhaps, in especially perverse cases, weakwilled agents can decide to pursue a course of action without doing so for any reason at all that they would endorse.[21]

Until now my discussion has focused on assumptions about the nature of practical judgement and intentional action that apparently render weakness of will problematic. Further difficulties arise when one considers the relation between these two moments in the etiology of weakwilled action. Traditionally weakness of will has been taken to be both free or uncoerced, and also a paradigm of irrationality in action, so an adequate account of it must do justice to these twin aspects. For instance, a norm of rationality must be specified, that is violated in cases of action against one's concurrent better judgement, but not violated in such a way as to entail that the agent is merely stupid or logically obtuse (since weakness of will does not necessarily seem to involve irrationality of *those* varieties).[22]

As for the issue of freedom, it has seemed to many philosophers (such as Audi, Chapter 17) that weakness of will can be distinguished from the different phenomenon of compulsion only if it is true that weakwilled agents are free to do what they believe to be best. In 'Skepticism about Weakness of Will' (Chapter 19), Gary Watson challenges this widespread assumption. He proposes that the distinction between weakness and compulsion properly turns on the question of whether the desires to which an agent gives in are ones that a normal and reasonable level of self-control would enable the agent to resist. If the answer to this question is 'yes', then we may speak of weakness rather than compulsion. It does not follow, however, that weakwilled agents are actually free to do what they believe best. Watson argues that we can only explain the behaviour of such agents if we assume that they are not free to act on their better judgement, on account of a failure to develop and maintain the normal capacities for self-control. This seems correct, but it raises the question as to why we should assume that human action is always fully explicable. What is to rule out the possibility that the behaviour of the weakwilled agent is ultimately inscrutable?

Watson's discussion draws attention to the important connections between weakness of will and self-control. Those who give in to the temptation to do something which they believe to be bad either lack the normal powers of self-control, or fail to exercise them at the crucial juncture. Self-control, or strength of will, is thus the other side of the coin represented by weakness of will. Both weakness and strength of will can be understood either episodically (as when we refer to a single occasion on which one or the other of these phenomena occurred), or as traits of character, woven into the dispositions of the agent (as when we describe someone as having a high or low degree of will power).[23] But what exactly does it mean to ascribe to a person strength of will as a trait of character? This question is addressed by Robert C. Roberts in 'Will Power and the Virtues' (Chapter 20).[24] Roberts distinguishes will power from other kinds of virtue, and defends the view that it is best understood as a kind of skill: it is the skill, namely, of self-management in the face of refractory inclinations. Much recent work in moral psychology reflects a neo-Aristotelian interest in the phenomena of character and the virtues, and Roberts' treatment of will power is a good example of this influential development.

Shame, Guilt, Remorse

A particular focus of concern within moral psychology are the moral sentiments. These may be understood as the emotions to which one is peculiarly susceptible insofar as one has a morally admirable character, and that accompany and reinforce one's acceptance of moral norms. The moral sentiments in this sense include, perhaps most strikingly, the backward-

looking emotions of guilt and remorse, which are typically prompted by one's awareness that one has fallen short of one's own moral standards or ideals. Another backward-looking sentiment, shame, might also be considered a moral emotion in a somewhat broader sense; although it is not connected as tightly with moral standards as guilt and remorse seem to be, shame nevertheless has an important role to play in moral development and it is strikingly expressive of a person's character and values. Shame, guilt and remorse, like the moral sentiments more generally, raise philosophical questions of two distinct but interlocking kinds – questions as to the nature of the emotions, and questions about their rational assessment. The essays in Part V of this volume pursue issues of both kinds.

A good starting point for thinking about these issues is the observation that both shame and guilt can be felt in response to a single action or aspect of oneself. An adequate characterization of these emotions must make clear how they differ from each other, even when they share a common occasion. The now standard approach solves this problem by pointing in two directions.[25] First, it is observed that shame and guilt are typically connected with differing syndromes of behaviour, feeling and response. Guilt leads one to feel ostracized, to expect the resentment of others and to accept their reproof, and to strive to make amends, while shame is expressed in feelings of loss of standing, in the expectation of disdain from those one respects, and in a primitive tendency toward concealment. Second, it is emphasized that shame and guilt are propositional attitudes, tied with distinctive ways of thinking about who one is and what one has done. Guilty agents conceive of an action of theirs as a transgression or a wrongdoing, whereas those subject to shame are responding to what they think of as a failure or shortcoming on their part. Guilt is thus connected to demands or requirements that one accepts, while shame reflects a conception of what is valuable in one's life, as the basis of one's self-esteem.

One way of testing a hypothesis such as this is to see whether it can accommodate the full range of emotional phenomena to which it is meant to apply, including not only the 'normal' cases in which shame and guilt are experienced on occasions on which it seems appropriate to do so, but also the deviant cases of irrational emotion. This test is deployed in Chapters 21 and 22 to raise doubts about the standard characterization of shame and guilt. In 'Subjective Guilt and Responsibility' (Chapter 21), Patricia Greenspan points out that guilt, in many of its familiar if irrational manifestations, does not involve the belief that one has transgressed against a moral norm one accepts. Persons who are subject to survivor guilt, for instance, need not really accept that they have done anything wrong in coming through a horrible accident alive. To account for cases of this kind, Greenspan urges that we see guilt as connected not with *beliefs* about wrongdoing in the fullest sense of the term, but rather with our *thoughts*, which can structure our emotional experience even if we do not really accept them as true.

John Deigh's essay 'Shame and Self-Esteem' (Chapter 22) raises still more fundamental questions about the standard approach to shame. On that approach, shame is linked with our self-esteem, which in turn reflects a conception of the value we impart to our own lives through the successful pursuit of worthwhile ends. Against this approach, Deigh cites cases in which the loss of self-esteem is not in any way accompanied by a sense of shame, and in which shame is occasioned by events that have nothing to do with failures in one's active life pursuits. He draws attention to the natural connection between shame and concealment, and suggests that this manifestation of the emotion only makes sense on the supposition that it is

a kind of self-protective mechanism; shame is not a grieved response to the recognition of a *loss* of worth, but an attempt to *preserve* one's worth in face of a threat. This interesting proposal raises questions both of detail and of methodology. Can we account for the link between shame and concealment while retaining the traditional idea that shame is a response to loss of self-esteem? To what extent is it legitimate or even necessary to attend equally to rational and irrational forms of an emotion in constructing an account of the nature of that emotion?

A rather broader perspective on these issues is provided by Richard Moran's essay 'Impersonality, Character, and Moral Expressivism' (Chapter 23). Moran directs our attention to the fact that the emotions of self-assessment are distinctively *first-personal* phenomena; one can only feel shame, for instance, about some aspect of oneself. Furthermore, emotions of these kinds are totalizing attitudes, involving a complete psychic orientation in which one's attention is focused in a distinctive way. It follows that one cannot really be in a state of self-assessive emotion while also reflecting impersonally on what the fact that one is in that state reveals about one's character. There is thus a form of third-personal judgement that is not accessible to the person in the grip of such first-personal emotions as shame, guilt, or remorse, and Moran urges that this fact needs to be accommodated in an adequate interpretation of impersonality as a moral ideal. But his emphasis on the totalizing character of the emotions of self-assessment seems to rule out ambivalence with respect to them, and one may wonder whether this result is true to our emotional experience.

Finally, there are issues about the rational evaluation of the moral emotions that have importantly attracted the attention of philosophers. Questions of this general kind can take one of two forms – local or global. Local questions of rational evaluation take for granted the basic legitimacy of a certain kind of emotional experience, seeking only to clarify the kinds of circumstance under which an emotion of that general kind would be warranted. Answering such local questions of rational evaluation often goes hand-in-hand with analysis of the nature of the emotion in question. If guilt, for instance, is essentially a response to one's own moral wrongdoing, then episodes of guilt will only be appropriate when one has in fact done something morally wrong. In global assessment, by contrast, the question is not so much about the nature of a given emotion, but about the wholesale point and value of emotions of that kind. With respect to the emotions of self-assessment, the global question would be this: is it justifiable for us to retain our general susceptibility to such feelings as guilt and remorse, or would we be better off without them?[26]

This question is taken up in Chapters 24 and 25. In 'Is It Reasonable to Regret Things One Did?' (Chapter 24), Rüdiger Bittner defends the Spinozistic thesis that such sentiments as regret and remorse cannot survive rational scrutiny. We should by all means face up squarely to the rotten and tawdry things we have done, but there is nothing to be gained by grieving or suffering over them in the way that is characteristic of the emotions of self-assessment. Herbert Morris' essay, 'The Decline of Guilt' (Chapter 25), takes the opposite position. His primary concern is the sense of guilt with respect to the law – a phenomenon that he takes to be under increasing attack in the modern world, both in theory and in practice. Morris sees this as a lamentable development, arguing that the sense of guilt is importantly connected with our conception of ourselves as agents, our attachment to the other persons with whom we live, and our commitment to moral values. Those, such as Bittner, who would have us do without emotions of this kind need to show, for instance, that it is possible for us to take seriously the moral norms that structure our individual and collective deliberations in the absence of

remorse or guilt. Can we clearly acknowledge the *wrongness* of our own actions without these emotional resources?

Acknowledgement

Many thanks to my research assistants, Jacob Klingner and Sigrid Krowas for help in preparing this volume; also to John Skorupski for some constructive suggestions about the moral sentiments.

Notes

1   For a classic formulation of this schema, see Donald Davidson, 'Actions, Reasons and Causes,' reprinted in his *Essays on Actions and Events* (Oxford: Clarendon Press, 1980), pp. 3–19.

2   This possibility is forcefully presented by Thomas Nagel in *The Possibility of Altruism* (Princeton: Princeton University Press, 1978), ch. 5; see also my own essay 'How to Argue about Practical Reason', reprinted as Chap. 6 in this volume.

3   Bratman's position on these issues is presented in more detail in his book *Intention, Plans, and Practical Reason* (Cambridge: Mass.: Harvard University Press, 1987).

4   For further discussion of this general issue, see also G.F. Schueler, *Desire: Its Role in Practical Reason and the Explanation of Action* (Cambridge: Mass.: MIT Press, 1995).

5   The printing most widely cited is in Bernard Williams, *Moral Luck: Philosophical Papers 1973–1980* (Cambridge: Cambridge University Press, 1981), pp. 101–13. Further discussions of this issue by Williams himself include 'Internal Reasons and the Obscurity of Blame', reprinted in Bernard Williams, *Making Sense of Humanity and Other Philosophical Papers 1982–1993* (Cambridge: Cambridge University Press, 1995), pp. 35–45, and 'Replies', in J.E.J. Altham and Ross Harrison, (eds), *World, Mind, and Ethics: Essays on the Ethical Philosophy of Bernard Williams* (Cambridge: Cambridge University Press, 1995), pp. 185–224, esp. at pp. 186–94 and 214–6.

6   Two influential contributions to the debate that could not be included here are Christine Korsgaard, 'Skepticism about Practical Reason', *Journal of Philosophy*, **83** (1986), pp. 5–25 (reprinted as Chapter 9 in Michael Smith (ed.), *Metaethics* (Aldershot: Dartmouth Publishing Company, 1995)) and John McDowell, 'Are There External Reasons?', in Altham and Harrison (eds), *World, Mind, and Ethics*, pp. 68–85. Other important discussions include Brad Hooker, 'Williams' Argument against External Reasons', *Analysis*, **47** (1987), pp. 42–4, and Rachel Cohen, 'Are External Reasons Impossible?', *Ethics*, **96** (1986), pp. 545–56.

7   This is essentially McDowell's suggestion, in 'Might There be External Reasons?' Williams himself responds to McDowell's argument in his 'Replies'.

8   Mele's discussion in Chapter 3 can be read as an attempt to argue for the assumption crucial to Williams' position at this point. For further discussions of this issue, see Korsgaard, 'Skepticism about Practical Reason', Hooker, 'Williams' Argument against External Reasons' and Cohen, 'Are External Reasons Impossible?'.

9   See also Blackburn's reflections about the non-cognitive psychological presuppositions of theoretical inference, in Chapter 2.

10   The theses here discussed are theses in moral psychology, insofar as they postulate connections between *beliefs* about the good and desires. There are also metaphysical issues about the relation between desires and the good, raised, for example, by the claim that the good is what would be desired under certain specified conditions. Arguments for this claim draw on some of the same considerations at play in the debate about the relation between normative reasons and desires (canvassed in Part II of this volume). For discussion of this metaphysical claim, see the contributions by Mark Johnston, David Lewis and Michael Smith to the symposium on 'Dispositional

Theories of Value', *The Aristotelian Society* supplementary volume **63** (1989), pp. 89–174. (The papers by Johnston and Lewis are reprinted in Smith (ed.), *Metaethics*.)

11   A similar challenge is mounted by Gary Watson in 'Free Agency', reprinted in Gary Watson, (ed.), *Free Will* (Oxford: Oxford University Press, 1982), pp. 96–110.

12   In 'Freedom of the Will and the Concept of a Person', reprinted in Watson, (ed.), *Free Will*, pp. 81–95; also in Harry Frankfurt, *The Importance of What We Care about: Philosophical Essays* (Cambridge: Cambridge University Press, 1988), pp.11–25. It should be stressed that I shall only be concerned with one strand of Frankfurt's multifaceted discussion, which also contains important reflections about freedom, autonomy, and the nature of personhood.

13   See Watson, 'Free Agency', s. 3, for an influential presentation of many of these questions.

14   For an earlier and somewhat different response, see his 'Identification and Wholeheartedness', reprinted in Frankfurt, *The Importance of What We Care about*, pp. 159–76.

15   For a more comprehensive overview of recent work on this topic, with copious references, see Arthur F. Walker, 'The Problem of Weakness of Will', *Noûs*, **23** (1989), pp. 653–76 and Alfred R. Mele, *Irrationality: An Essay on Akrasia, Self-Deception, and Self-Control* (New York: Oxford University Press, 1987).

16   Davidson, 'How is Weakness of Will Possible?', reprinted in his *Essays on Actions and Events*, pp. 21–42, at p. 23.

17   This is Davidson's solution, in 'How is Weakness of Will Possible?'.

18   For an important defence of the latter response, see David Wiggins, 'Weakness of Will, Commensurability, and the Objects of Deliberation and Desire', reprinted in David Wiggins, *Needs, Values, Truth: Essays in the Philosophy of Value* (Oxford: Blackwell, 1991), pp. 239–67.

19   See, for example, Christopher Cordner, 'Jackson on Weakness of Will', *Mind*, **94** (1985), pp. 273–80.

20   In response to this problem, it has been suggested that decision theory can be enriched to accommodate synchronic conflict by drawing on the kind of higher-order desires that figure in Frankfurt's hierarchical account of the structure of the will (Chapter 15); see, for example, John Bigelow, Susan Dodds and Robert Pargetter, 'Temptation and the Will', *American Philosophical Quarterly*, **27** (1990), pp. 39–49. For critical discussion of both this strategy and Jackson's, see Jeanette Kennett, 'Decision Theory and Weakness of Will', *Pacific Philosophical Quarterly*, **72** (1991), pp. 113–30.

21   Compare again the remarks of Stocker and Velleman concerning desires for things believed to be bad, in Chapters 12 and 13. (Velleman apparently holds that genuine action is done for a reason, but contends that in the perverse cases, what supplies a normative reason is not a positive evaluative judgement on the part of the agent. But why assume that the agents in these cases take their action to be justified in any sense?)

22   Jackson, for instance, specifies a candidate norm of reason that satisfies these constraints in Chapter 18; see also Davidson, 'How is Weakness of Will Possible?'.

23   Aristotle's discussion of *akrasia* in Book 7 of the *Nicomachean Ethics* treats it primarily as a trait of character. For interesting recent discussions that follow Aristotle in this, see Thomas E. Hill Jr, 'Weakness of Will and Character', reprinted in his *Autonomy and Self-Respect* (Cambridge: Cambridge University Press, 1991), pp. 118–37 and Christine Swanton, *Freedom: A Coherence Theory* (Indianapolis: Hackett Publishing Co., 1992), ch. 10.

24   A revised version of this chapter appears in Christina Sommers and Fred Sommers (eds), *Vice and Virtue in Everyday Life: Introductory Readings in Ethics* (Fort Worth: Harcourt Brace, 1993), pp. 266–87.

25   See, for example, John Rawls, *A Theory of Justice* (Cambridge, Mass.: Harvard University Press, 1971), ss. 67 and 73. For a subtle and qualified elaboration of this position, see Gabriele Taylor, *Pride, Shame, and Guilt: Emotions of Self-Assessment* (Oxford: Clarendon Press, 1985).

26   For an important discussion of the possibility and terms of rational assessment of such emotions, see P.F. Strawson, 'Freedom and Resentment', reprinted in Watson (ed.), *Free Will*, pp. 59–80. See also my book *Responsibility and the Moral Sentiments* (Cambridge, Mass.: Harvard University Press, 1994), especially ch. 4.

Part I
Motivation and Desire

[1]

The Humean Theory of Motivation

MICHAEL SMITH

1. *Two principles*

It has recently been argued that the Humean Theory of Motivation is a
dogma in philosophical psychology, that the dogma is fundamentally
incorrect, and that the Humean theory should therefore be replaced in
philosophical psychology with a more plausible theory of motivation. I am
thinking in particular of recent work by Tom Nagel, John McDowell, and
Mark Platts.[1]

In fact the Humean seems committed to two claims about motivating
reasons, a weaker and a stronger. However, there is no agreement amongst
non-Humeans as to whether the weaker and the stronger are both equally
unacceptable, or whether it is only the stronger that we have reason to reject.
The stronger—the claim that is, as I understand it, constitutive of the
Humean theory—is the claim that motivation has its *source* in the presence
of a relevant desire and means-end belief. This claim finds more formal
expression in the following principle:

> P1. R at t constitutes a motivating reason of agent A to ϕ iff there is some
> ψ such that R at t consists of a desire of A to ψ and a belief that were
> he to ϕ he would ψ.[2]

Non-Humeans are united in their rejection of P1. However, P1 entails the
following weaker principle:

> P2. Agent A at t has a motivating reason to ϕ only if there is some ψ such
> that, at t, A desires to ψ and believes that were he to ϕ he would ψ.

—the principle that motivation requires the *presence* of a relevant desire and
means-end belief—and non-Humeans are not at all united in their rejection
of P2. Thus, for instance, while Tom Nagel, and John McDowell following
him, have argued that P2 is acceptable because consistent with the claim that

---

[1] See Nagel, *The Possibility of Altruism*, Princeton University Press, 1970, Part 2; McDowell, 'Are
Moral Requirements Hypothetical Imperatives?' in *Proceedings of the Aristotelian Society Supplementary
Volume*, 1978, 'Virtue and Reason' in *The Monist*, 1979, and 'Non-cognitivism and Rule Following' in
Wittgenstein: To Follow a Rule, London, Routledge and Kegan Paul, 1981, edited by Holtzman and
Leich; Platts, *Ways of Meaning*, London, Routledge and Kegan Paul, 1979, Chapter 10, and 'Moral
Reality and the End of Desire' in *Reference, Truth and Reality*, London, Routledge and Kegan Paul,
1980, edited by Mark Platts. I shall hereafter refer to the Humean Theory of Motivation as the 'Humean
theory'.

[2] Compare Davidson's 'Actions, Reasons and Causes' in his *Essays on Actions and Events*, Oxford,
Clarendon Press, 1980, p. 5.

the desires and means-end beliefs that must be present whenever there is
motivation are not themselves the *source* of such motivation[3]—other non-
Humeans, such as Mark Platts, have argued that P2 is also unacceptable
because either 'phenomenologically false . . . or utterly vacuous'.[4]

I am inclined to agree with the non-Humeans that the Humean theory is a
dogma in philosophical psychology, a 'dogma' in the sense that both P1 and
P2 seem to find a fair degree of uncritical acceptance. However, unlike the
non-Humeans, I do not believe that the Humean theory, as characterized by
P1, is fundamentally incorrect (and thus I do not think that P2 is either
phenomenologically false or utterly vacuous). My task in the present paper
is thus to offer an explicit argument for the Humean theory, and to defend it
against the objections offered by the likes of Nagel, McDowell, and Platts.
If the argument offered here is correct, then the Humean theory is the
expression of a simple but important truth about the nature of motivating
reasons, a truth that non-Humeans have failed to appreciate either because
they have failed to distinguish motivating reasons from other sorts of
reasons, or because they have an inadequate conception of desire, or because
they have overlooked the implications of the fact that reason explanations
are teleological.

2. *Motivating reasons and normative reasons*

P1 is a principle connecting *motivating* reasons with the presence of desires
and beliefs. We must begin by emphasizing this fact, otherwise it will seem
simply implausible to suppose that P1 provides individually necessary or
jointly sufficient conditions for a state's constituting a motivating reason.

In order to see this, consider the following counterexamples to the claim
that P1 provides necessary conditions:

> (i) Suppose I now desire to purchase an original Picasso, but I do not
> now believe that were I to purchase the painting before me I would do
> so—suppose I don't believe that it is a Picasso. Surely it would be
> appropriate for an outsider to say that I have a reason to purchase the
> painting before me. But I lack the relevant belief.

> (ii) Suppose that I am standing on someone's foot so causing him pain,
> and that I know that this is what I am doing. Surely we can imagine its
> being appropriate for an outsider to say that I have a reason to get off
> his foot even though I lacked the relevant desire, and, indeed, even if
> I desired to cause him pain.

Consider now the following counterexample to the claim that P1 provides
a sufficient condition:

---

[3] *The Possibility of Altruism*, p. 29; 'Are Moral Requirements Hypothetical Imperatives?', p. 15.
[4] *Ways of Meaning*, p. 256.

(iii) Suppose I now desire to drink a gin and tonic and believe that I can do so by mixing the stuff before me with tonic and drinking it.[5] Suppose further that this belief is false—the stuff before me is not gin, it is petrol. Surely it would be appropriate for an outsider to say that I had no reason to mix this stuff with tonic and drink it. Yet I have both the relevant belief and desire.

Do we have, in examples the like of these, the makings of an objection to P1, and hence to the Humean theory? We do not. The reason why was perhaps evident from the start. The outsider's perspective is not irrelevant to the examples.

It has been noticed before that the claim that A has a reason to ϕ is ambiguous. It may be a claim about a *motivating* reason that A has or a claim about a *normative* reason that A has.[6] The crucial feature these reasons have in common is that each purports to justify certain behaviour on A's behalf; for there is an *a priori* connection between citing an agent's reasons for acting in a certain way and giving a partial justification for his acting in that way, that is, a specification of what was to be said for acting in the way in question. This is not to say that the existence of a reason for acting in a certain way, be it motivating or normative, entails that, all things considered, acting in that way is justified. But it is to say that, abstracting away from other considerations, the action is justified from the perspective of the reason (more on this below). However, in virtue of their differences, motivating and normative reasons forge the connection between justification and action differently.

The distinctive feature of a motivating reason to ϕ is that in virtue of having such a reason an agent is in a state that is *potentially explanatory* of his ϕ-ing.[7] (Note the 'potentially'. An agent may therefore have a motivating reason to ϕ without that reason's being overriding.) It is thus natural to suppose that an agent's motivating reasons are, as we might put it, *psychologically real*, for it would seem to be part of our concept of what it is for an agent's reasons to have the potential to explain his behaviour that his having those reasons is a fact about *him*; that is, that the goals that such reasons embody are *his* goals.[8] And it is also natural, therefore, to assign to an agent's motivating reasons the minimal justificatory role possible: the role of

---

[5] The example comes from Williams, 'Internal and External Reasons' in his *Moral Luck*, Cambridge University Press, 1981, p. 102.

[6] I borrow these terms from *The Possibility of Altruism*, p. 4 and p. 18. In his 'Reasons for Action and Desire' in *Proceedings of the Aristotelian Society Supplementary Volume*, 1972, Michael Woods makes room for a somewhat similar distinction when he notes that 'the concept of a reason for an action stands at the point of intersection, so to speak, between the theory of the explanation of actions and the theory of their justification' (p. 189).

[7] It will emerge in section 4 that, in the sense in which we need to think of motivating reasons as being explanatory, we need only think of them as being teleologically explanatory; we do not need to think of them as being causally explanatory.

[8] Compare Christopher Peacocke's objections to instrumentalism in Chapter 8 of his *Sense and Content*, Oxford, Clarendon Press, 1983.

justifying from the perspective of the value that that very reason embodies. For a motivating reason, even when it does explain an agent's behaviour, may reveal little of value in what the agent did even from his own point of view. Consider Davidson's example of the man who has always had a yen to drink a can of paint, and who ultimately yields, but not because he thinks that doing so is really worthwhile.[9] None the less, knowing that he has always had a yen to drink a can of paint does provide us, and him, with a partial justification for his action, albeit a justification that justifies only from a perspective that assigns value to the drinking of a can of paint, a perspective that he himself may occupy only to the extent that he has a yen to drink a can of paint, and that we none of us may actually share.

However, to say that someone has a normative reason to ϕ is to say something different. It is to say that there is some normative requirement that he ϕ's. It is therefore to justify his ϕ-ing from the perspective of the normative system that generates that requirement. For present purposes there is no need to be precise about the kinds of normative requirement, and hence the kinds of normative reasons, that there may be. For all that has been said here there may therefore be as many kinds of normative reason as there are normative systems for generating reasons: normative reasons of rationality, of prudence, of morality, and perhaps normative reasons of other kinds. Nor is there any need to be precise about the relation between the normative reasons an agent has, at a time, and the motivating reasons he has at that time. Rather, the important point to note is that, on any plausible conception of what it is for there to be a normative requirement and the relation that therefore exists between this normative requirement and an agent's motivating reasons, he may well be motivated to do what he is required to do (that is, he may have a motivating reason to do what he has a normative reason to do), he may be motivated to do something that there is no normative requirement for him to do (that is, he may have a motivating reason to do what he has no normative reason to do), and there may be a normative requirement that he do what he has no motivation to do (that is, he may have a normative reason to do what he has no motivating reason to do).[10] Given that motivating and normative reasons may come apart, we must therefore emphasise that P1 purports to give necessary and sufficient conditions for the existence of *motivating* reasons. P1 is silent concerning the conditions under which an agent has some *normative* reason.

Consider now the examples. I said that the outsider's perspective is not irrelevant. The reason is that the outsider's perspective draws our attention

---

[9] 'Actions, Reasons and Causes', p. 4.

[10] Here I assume that the mere existence of the materials with which to construct a partial justification for acting in a certain way from the agent's point of view—that is, the mere existence of a motivating reason to act in that way—does not suffice for the existence of a normative reason to act in that way. If that assumption is wrong, then there will be at least one kind of normative reason for which these claims are false. That will not affect the argument that follows. For the argument requires only that there are some kinds of normative reasons for which these claims are true.

40   *Michael Smith*

to the normative requirement in each case. Thus, note that in (i) the reason that I have to buy the painting in front of me is a normative reason. For it suffices for the truth of the claim that I have such a reason, that there is a requirement—in this case, in the broad sense, a requirement of rationality[11]—that I buy the painting in front of me. For I want to buy a Picasso and the painting in front of me is a Picasso. But the existence such a normative reason does not suffice for my having a motivating reason to buy the painting in front of me. For, since I do not believe that that painting is a Picasso, I am not in a state that is potentially explanatory of my buying it. (I am, of course, in a psychological state that is potentially explanatory of my buying a Picasso, for I desire to buy a Picasso and believe that were I to buy a Picasso I would buy a Picasso. But the Humean will say that this is not to have a motivating reason to buy the painting in front of me. It is rather to have a motivating reason to buy a Picasso. He will thus regard an agent's desire to ϕ together with the trivial belief that were he to ϕ he would ϕ as the limiting case of having a motivating reason to ϕ.) Thus the example in no way undermines the necessity of having a means-end belief for having a motivating reason.

A similar point applies in (ii), the case in which I have a reason to get off someone's foot when I am causing him pain. For it suffices for the truth of the claim that I have a reason to get off his foot that there exists a require-ment—in this case moral—that I do not cause him pain, and that, in the present circumstances, in order to comply with that requirement I have to get off his foot. But, once again, the mere existence of this normative reason is consistent with the claim that I am not in a state that is potentially explanatory of my behaviour. (Indeed, note that this ought to be conceded even by those who think that moral reasons are rational requirements on action. For, as we have seen, rational requiremets are in turn simply further normative reasons, and may thus exist in the absence of motivating reasons.) Thus this kind of example does not by itself show that having a desire is not a necessary condition for having a motivating reason.

Consider now (ii), the counterexample to the sufficiency of the condition. In what sense do I not have a reason to mix the stuff before me with tonic and drink it? Clearly, one thing we can say is that *prudence* would not require that I mix the stuff before me with tonic and drink it, for the stuff before me is petrol, and drinking petrol mixed with tonic would not be in my interests. However, I am in a state that is potentially explanatory of my mixing the stuff before me with tonic and drinking it, for I desire to drink a gin and

---

[11] In suggesting that the requirement is 'in the broad sense' a requirement of rationality I am following Williams in 'Internal and External Reasons', pp. 102-3 and Parfit in *Reasons and Persons*, Oxford, Clarendon Press, 1984, especially note 2a to Part I and pp. 117-20. For both Williams and Parfit think that a theory of rationality would tell us what an agent has reason to do, and both think that what an agent has reason to do from the perspective of rationality will depend on what an agent desires together with the *truth*. It will thus not depend on what he believes given that he may have false beliefs. (What I am calling a 'normative reason of rationality' seems to be what Williams calls an 'internal reason'.)

tonic and believe that the stuff before me is gin. Moreover, if that state did explain my doing so, we would certainly know what was to be said for doing so, from my point of view. Though prudence does not require my mixing the stuff before me with tonic and drinking it, and hence there is a sense in which I do not have a reason to do so, yet it seems entirely correct to suppose that I now have a motivating reason to do just this. So this is no counter-example to the claim that P1 provides a sufficient condition for a state's constituting a motivating reason.

Let me emphasize what little I take myself to have shown here. In the light of the distinction between motivating and normative reasons, I have emphasized the fact that the Humean's is a theory about the nature of *motivating* reasons. His theory may yet be false. But it is not shown to be false simply by showing that P1 fails to give necessary and sufficient conditions for the existence of normative reasons. Though I take this to be a fairly trivial point, it suffices to undermine one of Tom Nagel's principal arguments against the Humean theory in *The Possibility of Altruism*; an objection based largely on consideration of the conditions under which we would ordinarily say of someone that he has a reason. Nagel's objection centres on the Humean's explanation of prudential motivation.

3. *A preliminary objection: Nagel*

Prudential motivation is possible only if an agent's recognition of the fact that he will have a desire to ϕ in the future somehow gives him a reason now to take steps to promote his ϕ-ing then. The task of explaining this pos-sibility takes on a particular form for a Humean. For, as we have seen, he holds that now having a motivating reason to ϕ requires *presently* desiring to ϕ. He must therefore explain how an agent's recognition that he *will* desire to ϕ in the future gives rise to a *present* desire to promote his ϕ-ing then. The Humean's answer is fairly predictable. He says that agents who are moti-vated by prudential considerations each have a quite general present desire to further their future interests.

However Nagel offers the following objection to the Humean's giving this answer:

The two features of the system to which I object are (a) that it does not allow the expectation of a future reason to provide by itself any reason for present action, and (b) that it does allow the present desire for a future object to provide by itself a reason for present action in pursuit of that object.[12]

Thus, as he points out, the following constitute possibilities under the Humean theory:

First, given that any desire with a future object provides a basis for reasons to do what will promote that object, it may happen that I now desire for the future

---

[12] *The Possibility of Altruism*, p. 39.

something which I shall not and do not expect to desire then, and which I believe there will then be no reason to bring about. Consequently I may have a reason now to prepare to do what I know I will have no reason to do when the time comes.

Second, suppose that I expect to be assailed by a desire in the future: then I must acknowledge that in the future I will have a prima facie reason to do what the desire indicates. But this reason does not obtain now, and cannot by itself apply derivatively to any presently available means to the satisfaction of the future desire. Thus in the absence of any further relevant desire in the present, I may have no reason to prepare for what I know I shall have reason to do tomorrow.[13]

The response that Nagel wants to elicit from us, faced by these examples, is that, in the first case, I have no reason to promote the future object despite my present desire, and that, in the second, I do have a reason to promote the object of my future desire despite my lacking a relevant present desire.

Myself I think that we do have this response and that we are right to. But I do not think that this fact counts against the Humean theory. In order to see that this is so, consider Nagel's own summary objection to the Humean theory's licensing such possibilities:

A system with consequences such as this not only fails to require the most elementary consistency in conduct over time, but in fact sharpens the possibilities of conflict by grounding an individual's plottings against his future self in the apparatus of rationality. These are formal and extremely general difficulties about the system, since they concern the relation of what is rational to what will be rational, no matter what source of reasons is operative.[14]

Thus if we accept Nagel's own diagnosis of our response to these examples—and I think we should—it emerges that examples like these fail even to touch the Humean. For, to take just the first (the second follows suit), Nagel's objection to the Humean's claim that an agent may have a *motivating* reason now to promote his φ-ing in the future, despite the fact that he believes that he will have no motivating reason to φ then, is that it would not be *irrational* to do so; that is, that he now has no reason from the perspective of rationality to do so. But this is to conflate the claim that an agent has a motivating reason to φ with the claim that he has a normative reason from the perspective of rationality to φ. The Humean is making only the first claim, not the second.

Moreover, if Nagel is right that it is irrational to promote φ-ing in the future believing that one will then have no motivating reason to φ, then the Humean can accept this on his own terms; by claiming that a theory of rationality requires that agents have the desire to promote their future interests.[15] For, importantly, the tasks of constructing a theory of motivating reasons and a theory of the normative reasons of rationality are

---

[13] *The Possibility of Altruism*, pp. 39-40.   [14] Ibid., pp. 40-1.
[15] Compare *Reasons and Persons*, pp. 131-6.

just different tasks. I therefore do not see that the rationality of prudence makes for an especial difficulty with the Humean's theory of motivation. (It may indeed provide a problem for Hume's own theory of rationality.)[16]

4. *Why believe the Humean theory?*

We have seen that we will find no easy refutation of P1 — the claim that motivating reasons are constituted by the presence of desires and means-end beliefs — by reflecting on those cases in which we would ordinarily say of someone that he has a reason to ϕ. But can we find some reason actually to believe this claim?

John McDowell has attempted to diagnose commitment to the Humean theory in the following terms. He begins by isolating what he takes to be the distinctive feature of the Humean's theory; namely, that 'to cite a cognitive propositional attitude', that is, a belief, 'is to give at most a partial specification of a reason for acting; to be fully explicit, one would need to add a mention of something non-cognitive, a state of the will or a volitional event' or, in the terms in which we have put it, a desire.[17] He then goes on:

I suspect that one reason people find . . . [this claim] obvious lies in their inexplicit adherence to a quasi-hydraulic conception of how reason explanations account for action. The will is pictured as the source of forces that issue in the behaviour such explanations explain. This idea seems to me a radical misconception of the sort of explanation a reason explanation is, but it is not my present concern.[18]

I am not sure that I understand McDowell's diagnosis here. But, in so far as I do, it seems to me to get things entirely wrong.[19]

According to McDowell, one reason people believe the Humean theory is that they have a 'quasi-hydraulic' conception of how reason explanations account for action; that is, in less prolix terms, because they have a *causal* conception of reason explanations. Moreover, in McDowell's view, this lays the Humean theory so supported open to an objection; for, he says, a causal conception of reason explanations is a 'radical misconception'. Let me begin with the second point first.

Those of us who do not agree that causal conceptions are radically mis-conceived may well think that McDowell has here provided *us* with good reasons for believing the Humean theory; for McDowell suggests that the Humean theory is supported by something that we believe to be true. However, it seems to me that we would be conceding too much to McDowell if we were to argue in this way. For, now taking up his first point, I doubt that there is any support to be found for the Humean theory in a causal conception of reason explanations.

[16] This seems to be Nagel's real objection to the Humean on pp. 64-5 of *The Possibility of Altruism*.
[17] 'Non-cognitivism and Rule Following', p. 154.   [18] Ibid., p. 155.
[19] Though, in fairness to McDowell, see my comments on Hume's own view in section 6, and footnote 38 below.

In order to see this we only need ask why a causal conception should
be thought to support especially the Humean theory. To be sure, one who
holds that reason explanations are causal must conceive of some psychological states as possessed of *causal force*. But why, as McDowell seems to
assume, must he think that *desires* are the only psychological state possessed
of causal force? Why mightn't he think instead that only certain *beliefs* are
possessed of causal force? McDowell offers no argument on this point.

Indeed, when we consider the reason causal theorists actually give for
holding a causal conception, it emerges that no such argument is forthcoming. For they reason roughly as follows: 'We ordinarily say of agents that
they φ *because* they have reason to φ. The "because" here may uncontro-
versially be regarded as the "because" of rationalization; or, better, the
"because" of teleological explanation. But now observe that an agent may
have reason to φ and ψ, and yet not φ because he has reason to φ. What then
is the feature that makes the difference between this case and the case in
which the agent φs *because* he has reason to φ? The only illuminating answer
available is that the reasons in the second case *cause* the agent to φ.'[20] It thus
emerges that the argument causal theorists give for a causal conception of
reason explanations makes no substantial assumption about the nature
of the reasons we have. So, it seems, we should be able to accept or reject
this argument quite independently of our views concerning the nature of
reasons. The upshot is that if Humeans and non-Humeans alike may have
a causal conception of reason explanations then it cannot be that holding a
causal conception supports especially the Humean theory.

I think this shows that the Humean is engaged in a debate that is both
independent of and more fundamental than the debate over whether reason
explanations are causal. In short the difference is this. The causal and non-
causal theorist can both accept that reason explanations are teleological
explanations without enquiring further into what it is about the nature of
reasons that makes it possible for reason explanations to be teleological
explanations—that is, explanations that explain by making what they
explain intelligible in terms of the pursuit of a goal. For their disagreement
concerns the further question whether such explanations are themselves in
turn a species of causal explanation; a disagreement which may, as I have
suggested, cut across disagreements concerning the nature of reasons. But,
as I see it, the Humean and non-Humean are precisely engaged in a dispute
concerning what it is about the nature of reasons that makes it possible for
reason explanations to be teleological explanations. If this is right, then it
would seem that there will be only one reason to believe the Humean's theory,
if indeed we should believe his theory at all, and that is that the Humean's
theory is alone able to make sense of motivation as the pursuit of a goal.

I want to argue that this is indeed the case in the remainder of this paper.

[20] This is a summary of the argument in 'Actions, Reasons and Causes', pp. 8-11, the *locus classicus*
of arguments for a causal conception of reason explanations.

My reason for believing this is relatively simple—it seems to me to follow from a proper conception of desire. I therefore proceed by focussing on two different conceptions of desire. One of these gives no support to the Humean theory. I argue that this conception is anyway implausible. Perhaps unsurprisingly, this seems to be the conception of desire held by many opponents of the Humean theory. There is, however, an alternative and more plausible conception. This conception enables us to see that desires must be constituents of reasons given that reasons must themselves be constituted by goals.

5. *Desires and phenomenology*

According to Hume, desires are a species of the passions, and passions are, in turn, a certain kind of *feeling*. Hume seems to hold that this is so not just in the trivial sense that passions are a species of perception and perceptions are a kind of feeling.[21] Rather he seems to be suggesting that when we desire something 'we feel an . . . emotion of aversion or propensity';[22] as though, as Stroud puts it when discussing Hume's conception of desire, his view is that we are '*directly aware*' of the presence of the desires that we have.[23]

Hume's suggestion is not entirely misguided. For there is such a thing as the phenomenology of desire; as, for instance, to use one of Hume's own examples, 'when I am angry I am possest with the passion'.[24] That is, we may agree with Hume that, on occasion, when I have a desire, I am possessed with a psychological feeling; an analogue of a bodily sensation. This may suggest an elaboration of Hume's view. For if we take quite seriously his suggestion that all desires are known by the way they make us feel, then, in an attempt to explain why this is so, we may be led to identify desires with such psychological feelings. And this may in turn lead us to endorse what I shall call the 'strong phenomenological conception' of desires; the view that desires are, like sensations, simply and essentially states that have a certain phenomenological content.

Perhaps unsurprisingly, I think that the strong phenomenological conception of desires ought to be rejected. For it seems to me that there is no way such a conception can be married with a plausible epistemology of desire.[25]

Now I suspect that there will be some who think that this objection doesn't even get off the ground. For they will say: 'Surely the strong

---

[21] See *Treatise of Human Nature*, Oxford, Clarendon Press, 1958, p. 190.

[22] *Treatise*, p. 414.

[23] See Barry Stroud, *Hume*, London, Routledge & Kegan Paul, 1977, p. 163.

[24] *Treatise*, p. 415.

[25] I suspect that there will be some who think that this is all too obvious. They will think that the strong phenomenological conception is a strawman and thus not worth considering. However, I disagree. I think that it is worth working through our objections to strong phenomenological conceptions in order better to understand our objections to phenomenological conceptions quite generally. Those who disagree may prefer to skip the next six paragraphs.

phenomenological conception of desire makes the epistemology of desire unproblematic. For the epistemology of desire becomes like the epistemology of sensation. Thus, just as it is plausible to hold that a subject is in pain if and only if he believes that he is in pain—for we take it that a subject is in a state with a certain phenomenological content if and only if he believes himself to be in a state with that content—so, if we think of desires on the model of sensations, it is plausible to hold that a subject desires to ϕ if and only if he believes that he desires to ϕ.' What exactly is wrong with this? There are two things wrong with it. I begin with an objection that concedes more to the strong phenomenological conception than strictly ought to be conceded. Doing so teaches us a valuable lesson.

As I understand it, the principle that a subject desires to ϕ if and only if he believes that he desires to ϕ is supposed to express a necessary truth; the putative truth that we are infallible about what we desire. But, intuitively at any rate, this principle is simply false. Thus, conceding for the moment that the strong phenomenological conception does entail that a subject desires to ϕ if and only if he believes that he desires to ϕ, it ought to be rejected. I argue by counterexample.

Suppose each day on his way to work John buys a newspaper at a certain newspaper stand. However, he has to go out of his way to do so, and for no apparently good reason. The newspaper he buys is on sale at other newspaper stands on his direct route to work; there is no difference in the price or condition of the newspapers bought at the two stands; and so on. There is, however, this difference between the stands. There are mirrors behind the counter of the stand where John buys his newspaper. Given their placement, one who buys a newspaper there cannot help but look at himself. Let's suppose, however, that if it were suggested to John that the reason he buys his newspaper at that stand is that he wants to look at his own reflection, he would vehemently deny it. And it wouldn't seem to John as if he were concealing anything in doing so. However, finally, let's suppose that if the mirrors were removed from the stand, his preference for that stand would disappear. If all this were the case, wouldn't it be plausible to suppose that John in fact desires to buy his newspaper at a stand where he can look at his own reflection; that, perhaps, he has a narcissistic tendency and that buying his newspaper at that stand enables him to indulge it on the way to work? And wouldn't it also be plausible to suppose that he does not believe that this is so, given his, from his point of view, sincere denials? If this is agreed, then we have reason to reject the principle left to right.[26]

Consider another example. Suppose John professes that one of his fundamental desires is to be a great musician. However, his mother has

---

[26] Indeed, it seems to me that there are more mundane counterexamples to the principle left to right. Consider cases in which you go to the refrigerator convinced that there is something in particular that you want, though you aren't quite sure what it is. Then, while looking at the contents you suddenly, as we should put it, 'realise what it was that you wanted all along'. If we wish to respect this common sense description of such occurrences then we should reject the principle left to right.

always drummed into him the value of music. She is a fanatic with great hopes for her son's career as a musician; hopes so great that she would be extremely disappointed if he were even less than an excellent musician, let alone if he were to give up music altogether. Moreover, John admits that he has a very great desire not to upset her, though he denies that this in any way explains his efforts at pursuing excellence in music. However, suppose now that John's mother dies, and that, upon her death, he finds that all of his interest in music vanishes. He gives up his career as a musician and pursues a career in film as an actor. In such circumstances, wouldn't it be plausible to suppose that John was just mistaken about what he originally wanted to do and that, despite the fact that he believed that achieving excellence in music was a fundamental desire of his, it never was? If so, then we have reason to believe that the principle is false right to left as well.

If this is agreed, then any conception of desires that entails that a subject desires to ϕ if and only if he believes that he desires to ϕ is a conception that is to be rejected, rejected for the simple reason that the epistemology it provides is implausible. Thus, if the phenomenological conception entails such a principle, it ought to be rejected. This teaches us the following lesson. It is an adequacy constraint on any conception of desire that the epistemology of desire it recommends allows that subjects may be fallible about the desires they have.

I said that the first objection concedes more to the strong phenomenological conception than strictly ought to be conceded. What it concedes is that the strong phenomenological conception does entail that a subject desires to ϕ if and only if he believes that he desires to ϕ. But this it most certainly does not do. Here, then, is a second objection.

Let's grant for the moment that desires are like sensations in that they essentially have phenomenological content. It must be noted that they differ from sensations in that they have in addition *propositional* content. For ascriptions of desires, unlike ascriptions of sensations, may be given in the form 'A desires that p', where 'p' is a sentence. Thus, whereas A's desire to ϕ may be ascribed to A in the form *A desires that he ϕs*, A's pain cannot be ascribed to A in the form *A pains that p*.[27]

It is therefore ambiguous to claim that the epistemology of desire is 'like the epistemology of sensation'. To be sure, if desires are essentially phenomenological states, then the epistemology of the phenomenological content of a desire may be based on the epistemology of sensation. But what about the epistemology of the propositional content of desire? This cannot be based on the epistemology of sensation at all, for sensations have no propositional content. It therefore turns out that we have an even stronger reason to reject the strong phenomenological conception of desire. For, according to this conception, there is simply no difference between desires and sensations. Each is a state which simply and essentially has

---

[27] Compare 'Moral Reality and the End of Desire', pp. 74–7.

phenomenological content. The strong phenomenological conception of desires is thus unable to account for the fact that desires *have* propositional content *at all*. Little wonder that it cannot provide a plausible epistemology of the propositional content of desires.

I suspect that, for this very reason, some will have thought that the strong phenomenological conception of desire was a straw man all along. But note that, with our objections to the strong phenomenological conception firmly in place, we are now in a position to argue against all versions of the phenomenological conception, even the more plausible weaker conceptions according to which desires are *like* sensations in that they have phenomenological content essentially, but *differ* from sensations in that they have propositional content as well. For we can now say this about all such conceptions: they in no way contribute to our understanding of what a desire as a state with propositional content is, for they cannot explain how it is that desires have propositional content; they therefore in no way explain the epistemology of the propositional content of desire; and they thus require supplementing by some independent and self-standing account of what a desire is which explains how it is that desires have propositional content and which explains how it is that we have fallible knowledge of what it is that we desire.

The question that immediately arises with regard to weaker phenomenological conceptions is then why we should believe that any such conception is true. The only answer available is that a phenomenological conception is alone true to the phenomenology of desire. But is this answer plausible? Do we really believe that desires are states that have phenomenological content essentially? That is, do we believe that if there is nothing that it is like to have a desire, at a time, then it is not being had at that time?

I should say that, at least as far as common sense opinion goes—and what else do we have to go by in formulating a philosophical conception of folk psychological states?—we evidently have no such belief. Consider, for instance, what we should ordinarily think of as a long term desire; say, a father's desire that his children do well. A father may actually feel the prick of this desire from time to time; in moments of reflection on their vulnerability, say. But such occasions are not the norm. Yet we certainly wouldn't ordinarily think that he loses this desire during those periods when he lacks such feelings. Or consider more mundane cases like those that Stroud mentions in his discussion of Hume, cases in which, as we should ordinarily say, I desire to cross the road and do so, or in which I desire to write something down and so write it down. As Stroud points out, in such cases 'it is difficult to believe that I am overcome with emotion . . . I am certainly not aware of any emotion or passion impelling me to act'; rather 'they seem the very model of cool, dispassionate action'.[28] However, it would be grossly counter to our common sense opinion to conclude that simply because I do

[28] *Hume*, p. 163.

not introspect the presence of desires in such cases so I incorrectly attribute
desires to myself—that I cross the road and write things down even though
I do not want to!

Of course, if we thought that there was nothing for a desire to be, in the
absence of its being felt, then we might, in our role of philosophical theorist,
feel ourselves forced into concluding that some of our common sense
attributions are mistaken, and hence feel ourselves forced into revising our
common sense opinions in favour of a phenomenological conception. But
given that a phenomenological conception is unable to deliver an account of
desire as a state with propositional content, we should feel no such pressure
in our role of philosophical theorist. Rather we should concede that a desire
may be had in the absence of its being felt.

This is significant. For many non-Humeans seem to work with a
phenomenological conception of desire, and then use the fact that we do not
introspect the presence of desires whenever there is motivation against the
Humean theory.

Consider, for instance, the following argument of Mark Platts's:

> The crucial premiss . . . is the claim that any full specification of a reason for an
> action, if it is to be a reason for the potential agent for action, must make reference to
> that agent's desires. At first sight, it seems a painful feature of the moral life that this
> premiss is false. We perform many intentional actions in that life that we apparently
> do not desire to perform. A better description of such cases appears to be that we
> perform them because we think them desirable. The difficulty of much of moral life
> then emerges as a consequence of the apparent fact that desiring something and
> thinking it desirable are both distinct and independent.
>
> The premiss can, of course, be held true by simply claiming that, when acting
> because we think something desirable, we do indeed desire it. But this is either
> phenomenologically false, there being nothing in our inner life corresponding to the
> posited desire, or utterly vacuous, neither content nor motivation being given to
> the positing of the desire. Nothing but muddle (and boredom) comes from treating
> desire as a mental catch-all.[29]

Thus, according to Platts, the Humean may hold that when we believe that
something is desirable we do desire it. However, if he does, then Platts
claims that he is impaled on the horns of a dilemma. But consider the horns
of Platts's dilemma.

If there is no reason why *any* theorist should accept a phenomenological
conception of desire, as we have seen that there is not, then it can hardly be
an objection to the Humean's theory that we are unable to introspect the
presence of each and every desire that he says we have. Thus we should not
force the Humean onto the phenomenological falsehood of the first horn.
Platts might agree. But, he would say, this merely forces the Humean onto
the second horn of his dilemma. Here Platts seems to claim that if we do not
accept a phenomenological conception of desire, then the positing of a desire

---

[29] *Ways of Meaning*, p. 256.

50 *Michael Smith*

must be 'utterly vacuous', or without 'content'.[30] But, as we have seen, given just the assumption that desires are states with propositional content, an assumption that must be accepted even by one who does wish to endorse a phenomenological conception, the *only* way that we can give content to the concept of such a state, and hence to the positing of a desire, is precisely via some independent and self-standing non-phenomenological conception. So, far from non-phenomenological conceptions making ascriptions of desire 'utterly vacuous', non-phenomenological conceptions alone make the ascription of desires with propositional contents possible.

Indeed, even John McDowell, who himself rejects a phenomenological conception, covertly ascribes such a conception to the Humean when arguing against him.[31] This emerges in McDowell's defence of his own view that the virtuous agent may be motivated by his conception of the situation in which he finds himself, something that, according to McDowell, may properly be thought of as a cognitive state. McDowell rightly supposes that the Humean would respond that, if someone who has such a conception is indeed motivated, then getting him to have such a conception must involve getting him to have a certain desire. But he then interprets this as the suggestion that

'See it like this' is really a covert invitation to feel, quite over and above one's view of the facts, a desire which will combine with one's belief to recommend acting in the appropriate way.[32]

And he rightly rejects this suggestion. But, unless it is compulsory to accept a phenomenological conception of desire, why give the Humean's response that interpretation? To be sure, getting someone to have a certain view of the facts may not involve getting him to *feel* a certain desire, but it may involve getting him to *have* a certain desire none the less.[33]

6. *Desires, directions of fit, and dispositions*

We have seen that there must be an alternative to phenomenological conceptions of desire, an alternative that allows us to make sense of desires as states with propositional contents and that thus allows us to make sense of our common sense desire attributions. But what is the alternative to be?

---

[30] I say 'seems', for Platts does in fact consider an alternative characterization of desires. I discuss the alternative characterization in section 6. I discuss Platts's assessment of the support that the alternative characterization gives to the Humean theory in section 8 (ii).

[31] I say McDowell rejects a phenomenological conception. He nowhere says that he rejects such a conception. But given that he thinks that 'consequentially ascribed desires are indeed desires' ('Are Moral Requirements Hypothetical Imperatives?', p. 25), he must. For the point of consequentially ascribed desires is that there may be no phenomenological ground for their ascription. The idea of 'consequentially ascribed desires' derives from the work of Tom Nagel. For a discussion of the idea that some desires are merely consequentially ascribed see section 8 (i).

[32] 'Are Moral Requirements Hypothetical Imperatives?', p. 22.

[33] I briefly discuss McDowell's view further in section 8 (iii).

Surprisingly enough, Platts himself outlines the alternative I favour; a suggestion about the difference between beliefs and desires that he attributes to Anscombe. Platts's own summary is so succinct and makes the idea sound so plausible that I shall merely quote it. (I consider below why Platts is himself subsequently so unsympathetic towards the idea.)

Miss Anscombe, in her work on intention, has drawn a broad distinction between two *kinds* of mental states, factual belief being the prime exemplar of one kind and desire a prime exemplar of the other . . . The distinction is in terms of the *direction of fit* of mental states with the world. Beliefs aim at the true, and their being true is their fitting the world; falsity is a decisive failing in a belief, and false beliefs should be discarded; beliefs should be changed to fit with the world, not vice versa. Desires aim at realisation, and their realisation is the world fitting with them; the fact that the indicative content of a desire is not realised in the world is not yet a failing *in the desire*, and not yet any reason to discard the desire; the world, crudely, should be changed to fit with our desires, not vice versa.[34]

Myself I think that this characterization of the difference between beliefs and desires captures something quite deep in our thought about their nature. Moreover, I want eventually to argue that the idea that desires are states with which the world must fit allows us to bring out an important connection between our concepts of desire and motivation.

However, as Platts notices, talk of the direction of fit of a state is highly metaphorical. This is problematic. For it seems that we would be unjustified in appealing to the concept in characterizing desires, and in illuminating the connection between desires and motivation, if we had no way of understanding it in non-metaphorical terms. Moreover, as once again Platts notices, if we take the characterization quite strictly, it is unclear whether it allows us to characterize desires at all. For, he claims, since 'all desires appear to involve elements of belief', desires are not states whose direction of fit is entirely of the second kind: the question arises whether there are any such states.[35]

It seems to me that Platts is right to highlight these problems with the metaphor, but that we would be wrong to think that the problems he raises are insurmountable. For I want to suggest that the metaphorical characterization of desires as states which are such that the world must fit with them meshes with another, and more plausible, suggestion about the epistemology of desires; a suggestion inspired, ironically enough, by certain other remarks of Hume's.

Hume realized all to well that alongside the 'violent passions' that affect the subject who has them, there are 'calm passions', passions that lack phenomenological content altogether. Hume was therefore cognizant of the fact that his official line on the epistemology of desires—that they are known by their phenomenology—was totally inadequate as an account of

[34] *Ways of Meaning*, pp. 256-7.   [35] Ibid., p. 257.

the epistemology of the calm passions, and that he therefore needed an alternative account of the epistemology appropriate for them. As a result, Hume suggested that, by contrast with the violent passions, the calm passions 'are more known by their effects than by their immediate sensation'.[36]

When Stroud considers this suggestion, he points out that it commits Hume to the view that desires are to be conceived of as *the causes of actions.*[37] It might therefore be thought that Hume's suggestion should be of little interest to us. For I have argued that the only argument for the Humean theory, if there is to be one at all, will be that it alone is able to make sense of reason explanation as a species of teleological explanation, and that one may accept that reason explanations are teleological without accepting that reason explanations are causal (see section 4). Yet if we accept this conception of desire we immediately lock ourselves into a causal conception.[38]

However, though this makes acceptance of Hume's suggestion as it stands inappropriate, it seems to me that we would be wrong to abandon Hume's suggestion altogether. For if we are less interested in *Hume*'s view than in a *Humean* view then it seems to me that we can find in Hume's suggestion about the epistemology appropriate for the calm passions, the inspiration for a somewhat different conception of desires; a conception that allows us to remain neutral about whether desires are causes.

According to this alternative conception, desires are states that have a certain *functional role*. That is, according to this conception, we should think of the desire to ϕ as that state of a subject that grounds all sorts of his dispositions: like the disposition to ϕ in conditions C, the disposition to ϕ in conditions C', and so on (where, in order for conditions C and C' to obtain, the subject must have, *inter alia*, certain beliefs). For Hume's suggestion about how the calm passions are known may then be translated into the thought that the epistemology of desire is simply the epistemology of dispositional states—that is, the epistemology of such counterfactuals. This does not commit us, *as Humeans*, to the thesis that desires are to be conceived of as the causes of actions. For it is a substantial philosophical thesis to move from the claim that desires are dispositions to the claim that desires are causes.

A dispositional conception of desires enables us to solve many of the problems that we have confronted so far. For instance, a dispositional conception is precisely an account of what a desire is that explains how it can be that desires have propositional content, for the propositional content of a desire may then simply be determined by its functional role. (I say that it may 'simply' be determined by its functional role. But of course, there need be nothing simple about the functional theory that determines content.)

---

[36] *Treatise*, p. 417.   [37] *Hume*, p. 165.

[38] Perhaps this link between Hume's own conception of desire and a causal conception of reason explanations explains why McDowell thinks that the Humean theory finds support from a causal conception (see section 4).

A dispositional conception of desires also meets the constraint on the epistemology of desire argued for earlier; that the epistemology of desire allows that subjects may be fallible about the desires that they have.[39] For, given just the assumption that desires are dispositions to act in certain ways under certain conditions, it is implausible to suggest quite generally that if the counterfactuals that are thus true of a subject who desires to ϕ are true of him then he believes that they are, and it is likewise implausible to suggest quite generally that if a subject believes that such counterfactuals are true of him, then such counterfactuals are true of him.[40] Furthermore, a dispositional conception of desires is consistent both with the claim that certain desires have phenomenological content essentially and with the claim that certain desires lack phenomenological content altogether. For, according to this conception, desires have phenomenological content just to the extent that the having of certain feelings is *one* of the things that they are dispositions to produce under certain conditions. Some desires may be dispositions to have certain feelings under all conditions: these have phenomenological content essentially. Other desires, though they are dispositions to behave in certain ways, may not be dispositions to have certain feelings at all: these lack phenomenological content altogether.

We are also able, given a dispositional conception of desires to see why Platts is right that, in myriad ways, desires 'involve elements of belief'. For if the desire to ϕ is a certain sort of complex dispositional state of the kind described then desiring to ϕ may 'involve' elements of belief in each of the following ways: the obtaining of the conditions in which the subject ϕs may require that he has certain beliefs; the truth of the counterfactual 'Were the subject in conditions C he would ϕ' may require that the subject has certain other beliefs due to holistic constraints on desire attribution; and so on. Indeed, if we take Platts's own claims about the phenomenology of desire quite seriously, then we might suggest that desires involve beliefs in other more direct ways. For, if we agree with Platts that oftentimes when we act our only awareness of the desires we have comes via our beliefs concerning the desirability of various options then we might think that this too ought to be reflected in the kind of disposition a desire is. Thus, we might say, the desire to ϕ is also, *inter alia*, a disposition to believe, under certain

---

[39] Here I am grateful to Frank Jackson.

[40] Thus, I contend that a subject's false belief that he desires to ϕ is not a state that is potentially explanatory of his behaviour. Everyday experience supports this contention. Reflect on occasions when you stand at the edge of a cold swimming pool thinking that you desire to jump in. On some such occasions your body is totally unresponsive to the desires that you profess to have. As you stand there motionless you sometimes come to the conclusion that, contrary to what you thought, you didn't really want to go swimming after all. Thus, just as we would expect if this contention were true, there are cases in which a subject believes that he desires to ϕ right up until the time that he is supposed to act only to discover that he in fact has no such desire when his body fails to respond to his desire. Of course, we can construct cases in which it might *appear* that an agent's false beliefs about what he wants motivate him. The example of John the musician may perhaps be such a case. But I should claim that in such cases, as in John's, we will find that the appearance is misleading, and that there is in fact some other desire that does the motivating.

conditions, that ϕ-ing is *prima facie* desirable (= 'is desired by me'); or that there is a reason to ϕ; and so on.

Finally, a dispositional conception enables us to see why, despite the fact that in these many ways desires may involve elements of belief, we may properly say of one who has a desire that he is in a state *with which the world must fit*. Moreover, and for the Humean's particular purposes perhaps more importantly, a dispositional conception of desires enables us to cash the metaphor characterizing beliefs and desires in terms of their direction of fit, and therefore draws support from it. For the difference between beliefs and desires in terms of direction of fit comes down to a difference between the counterfactual dependence of a belief and a desire that p, on a perception that *not p*: roughly, a belief that p is a state that tends to go of existence in the presence of a perception that *not p*, whereas a desire that p is a state that tends to endure, disposing the subject in that state to bring it about that p. Thus, we may say, attributions of beliefs and desires require that different *kinds* of counterfactuals are true of the subject to whom they are attributed. We may say that this is what a difference in their directions of fit *is*.

These are important results. For they serve to make a dispositional conception of desire attractive *period*, quite independent of the theory of motivation that one happens to favour. Moreover, they license us to talk unashamedly of desires as states with which the world must fit, for such talk, though metaphorical, captures the feature that distinguishes desires from beliefs; that is, such talk, though metaphorical, aptly describes the kind of dispositional state that a desire is.

The Humean's reasons for believing P1—the principle that a motivating reason is constituted by the presence of a desire and a means–end belief— may now be stated rather simply. Given that, as we have seen, all theorists should accept a dispositional conception of desires, and given that this conception licenses us to talk of desires as states with which the world must fit, the Humean's reasons are also, I think, both intuitive and compelling.

7. *Desires, directions of fit, goals and motivating reasons*

What is it for someone to have a motivating reason? The Humean replies as follows. We understand what it is for someone to have a motivating reason at a time by thinking of him as, *inter alia*, having a goal at that time; the '*alia*' here includes having a conception of the means to attain that goal. That is, having a motivating reason just *is*, *inter alia*, having a goal. But what kind of state is the having of a goal? It is a state with which *direction of fit*? Clearly, the having of a goal is a state *with which the world must fit*, rather than *vice versa*. Thus having a goal is being in a state with the direction of fit of a desire. But since all that there is to being a desire is being a state with the appropriate direction of fit, it follows that having a goal just *is* desiring. In

short, then, the Humean believes P1 because P1 is entailed by the following three premises:

(1) Having a motivating reason *is, inter alia,* having a goal

(2) Having a goal *is* being in a state with which the world must fit

and

(3) Being in a state with which the world must fit *is* desiring.

Simple though it is, this argument is, I think, really quite powerful. After all, which premise in the argument could plausibly be denied? Let's consider them in turn.

Given just the assumption that reason explanations are teleological explanations (see section 4), (1) seems unassailable; indeed it has the status of a conceptual truth. For we understand what it is for someone to have a motivating reason in part precisely by thinking of him as having some goal.[41] (2) is likewise unassailable. For learning that the world is not as the content of your goal specifies is not enough for giving up that goal, but rather puts pressure on you to change the world. The most vulnerable premise is perhaps (3), the claim that being in a state with which the world must fit is desiring. I can imagine two sorts of objection to this premise. But neither objection goes very far.

First, according to Platts, Anscombe claims only that desire is 'a prime exemplar' of those states with which the world must fit. But, he might say, there are other states that have this direction of fit as well: hopes, wishes, and the like. Therefore, given (1) and (2), we should surely say that such states may constitute the having of goals as well. But, *ex hypothesi,* hopes and wishes are not desires.

However, an attack of this kind on the Humean's argument is clearly not an attack on the *spirit* of his argument, it is rather an attack on the *details* of his argument. The Humean may therefore concede the details to the objector. That is, if *desire* is not a suitably broad category of mental state to encompass all of those states with the appropriate direction of fit, then the Humean may simply define the term 'pro-attitude' to mean 'psychological state with which the world must fit', and then claim that motivating reasons are constituted, *inter alia,* by pro-attitudes.[42]

A second objection to (3) tackles the assumption that there are only states with one or the other direction of fit. Thus, it might be asked, why couldn't there be a state with *both* directions of fit; a state which is both such that the world must fit with it, and such that it must fit the world? If such a state were possible then, it might be said, it could constitute the having of a goal.

---

[41] See section 8 (i) for a discussion of (1) in relation to Nagel's views.

[42] Compare Davidson on the difference between desires and pro-attitudes in 'Actions, Reasons and Causes', p. 4.

But it would not be a desire, nor even a pro-attitude; for desires and pro-attitudes have only one direction of fit.[43]

However, though it may sound like a coherent possibility that there should be such a state, it really isn't. For, as we have understood the concept of direction of fit, the direction of fit of a state with the content that p is determined, *inter alia*, by its counterfactual dependence on a perception with the content that *not p*. A state with both directions of fit would therefore have to be such that *both*, in the presence of such a perception it tends to go out of existence, *and*, in the presence of such a perception, it tends to endure, disposing the subject that has it to bring it about that p. Taken quite literally, then, the idea that there may be a state with both directions of fit is just plain incoherent.

Of course, a more subtle objector might find fault with this reply. He might say that the reply works only if we take the suggestion that there is a state with both directions of fit quite literally. But, he might well ask, why take it so literally?

Indeed, he might go on the offensive. For he might suggest that our resistance to the suggestion shows the extent to which we are in the grip of what might be called an 'austere' psychological theory; a theory which, as far as the explanation of action goes, both makes use of and makes do with the concepts of belief and desire: states having the one or the other direction of fit, as that has been defined here. The objector may well admit that an austere theory can explain some of the phenomena. But he might insist that we recognize that it cannot explain all of the phenomena; that there are certain goings on that we can explain only if we enrich our psychological theory with the concept of a state that has, in a more relaxed sense, *both* directions of fit. He might cite the example of a moral 'quasi-belief' that x is good ('quasi-belief' because, as we shall see, it is no ordinary belief). For, he might point out, since a subject who has such a quasi-belief tends to go out of this state when presented with a perception that x is not good, this makes it appropriate to describe a moral quasi-belief as being such that it must fit the world. But since a subject's having the moral quasi-belief that x is good disposes him to promote x, this makes it appropriate to describe such a quasi-belief as being, in a more relaxed sense, such that the world must fit with it. Indeed, he might go on to insist that since the factor that determines the kinds of concept our psychological theories can make use of is the evidence that needs to be explained by our theories, so the example just given shows that we positively have reason to enrich our austere psychological theory with the concept of a quasi-belief: a state that is both belief-like and desire-like though identical with neither. For the evidence—our moral practices—can only be explained by the richer theory.

This more subtle objection needs careful handling. I do not know whether the richer theory is really coherent—no surprise, since to my

---

[43] David McNaughton put this objection to me.

knowledge no-one has actually attempted to formulate such a theory. But I do not think that we need to follow the objection that far down the line in order to find fault with it. For, as I see it, the problem with the objection is that it requires that we *revise* our psychological theories without proper warrant. If I have correctly described the objection, its success depends entirely on the claim that there is evidence that cannot be explained by an austere psychological theory. But the evidence the objector cites can be easily accommodated by the resources of an austere theory; that is, within the accepted framework of beliefs and desires.

In order to see that this is so, consider the following parody of the argument just given: 'There is evidence for the existence of state that is belief-like and desire-like but identical with neither. Consider, for instance, the "quasi-belief" that ϕ-ing is *prima facie* desirable ("quasi-belief" because, as we shall see, it is no ordinary belief). This state is appropriately described as having both directions of fit because, first, a subject tends to go out of this state if he is presented with a perception with the content that ϕ-ing is not *prima facie* desirable, and, second, because a subject's being in such a state disposes him to ϕ.' But this argument is hopeless. For, within the confines of our austere psychological theory, we may say that there are beliefs that a subject can have only if he has certain desires. Thus, we may say, a subject's quasi-belief that ϕ-ing is *prima facie* desirable is best thought of as being such a state. It is a genuine belief because it is a state that must fit the world; that is (since 'is *prima facie* desirable' = 'is desired by me') because its truth requires that ϕ-ing has the property of being desired by him. But it is also a belief the condition for having which is that a subject desires to ϕ (*modulo* fallibility about one's desires). We can thus explain why one who believes that ϕ-ing is *prima facie* desirable is generally disposed to ϕ by noting that the normal condition for having such a belief is desiring to ϕ, and desiring to ϕ is, *inter alia*, a disposition to ϕ.[44]

We therefore do not need to introduce a state of some further, mysterious,

---

[44] Does the 'normal' provide a problem here? I think not. The argument succeeds just in case it shows that there is a necessary connection of a certain kind between having the belief that ϕ-ing is *prima facie* desirable and being disposed to ϕ, a connection of much the same kind as that which exists between the belief that ϕ-ing is good and the disposition to ϕ. The 'normal' merely allows that it is a remote possibility that beliefs about desirability and desire come apart; a possibility that must be admitted because we must admit that subjects have only fallible access to their desires. But in order for this to provide a problem the objector would have to insist that there is no remote possibility that a subject who believes that ϕ-ing is good, be not disposed to ϕ. Yet what could the evidence for this claim be? Indeed, as far as evidence one way or the other is concerned, the evidence seems to point in just the opposite direction: see, for instance, Michael Stocker, 'Desiring the Bad' in *The Journal of Philosophy*, 1979, in which he reminds us that, in certain fits of depression, or self-deception, or in certain conditions of physical tiredness, one may believe that a certain course of action is good and yet be totally indifferent to it. I would myself resist the externalist conclusions that some would have us draw by consideration of such examples; that is, I resist the idea that the connection between moral judgement and motivation is wholly contingent, requiring some wholly added on desire to be moral. By all means, I say, let's give the internalist in ethics his due. But his due does not require any more than that we admit that there is a necessary connection of sorts between making a moral judgement and being disposed to act; his due requires only that we admit that, under certain conditions, moral judgement entails a disposition to act. But that we have admitted.

58   *Michael Smith*

hybrid kind, over and above beliefs and desires, in order to explain why beliefs about the desirability of certain courses of action are, in a certain respect, practical. Nor, if this is right, do I see why we need to introduce a state of some further, mysterious, hybrid kind in order to explain why moral beliefs are, in a certain respect, practical. Rather, we should think of moral properties on the model of the property of being *prima facie* desirable. For we may then think of moral quasi-beliefs as being genuine *beliefs* about the properties that persons, actions, states of affairs, and the like have. But, since they have these properties in virtue of standing in certain relations to the desires that the subject has, they are beliefs that the subject can have only if he has certain *desires*.[45]

8. *Nagel, McDowell and Platts again*

If some version of the argument given in the last section is correct then we should be able to diagnose the flaws in the as yet unconsidered objections of Nagel, McDowell and Platts to the Humean theory; and, indeed, we should be able to diagnose the flaws in the theories of motivation with which they would replace the Humean theory. I want to close with some necessarily brief remarks aimed at showing that this is indeed the case.

(i) Early on in *The Possibility of Altruism* Tom Nagel puts forward an objection to the Humean theory that seems aimed not so much at *refuting* the theory, as at *deflating* it, thereby opening up room for his own non-Humean view:

The assumption that a motivating desire underlies every intentional action depends, I believe, on a confusion between two sorts of desires, motivated and unmotivated . . . The claim that a desire underlies every act is true only if desires are taken to include motivated and unmotivated desires, and it is true only in the sense that *whatever* may be the motivation for someone's intentional pursuit of a goal, it becomes in virtue of his pursuit *ipso facto* appropriate to ascribe to him a desire for that goal. But if the desire is a motivated one, the explanation of it will be the same as the explanation of his pursuit, and it is by no means obvious that a desire must enter into this further explanation. Although it will no doubt be generally admitted that some desires are motivated, the issue is whether another desire always lies behind the motivated one, or whether sometimes the motivation of the initial desire involves no reference to another, unmotivated desire.[46]

But there is confusion here only if the idea of a desire motivated by a state that is not a desire is itself plausible. Is it plausible? The Humean thinks not. He argues as follows.

---

[45] I have defended this view in my 'Should We Believe in Emotivism?' in *Fact, Science and Morality: Essays on A. J. Ayer's Language, Truth and Logic*, edited by Crispin Wright and Graham Macdonald, Blackwells, Oxford, 1986. See also my comments on McDowell in section 8 (iii).

[46] *The Possibility of Altruism*, p. 29.

A motivated desire is a desire had for a reason; that is, a desire the having of which furthers some goal that the agent has. The agent's having this goal *is*, in turn, *inter alia*, the state that constitutes the motivating reason that he has for having the desire (from (1)). But if the state that motivates the desire is itself a reason, and the having of this reason is itself constituted by his having a goal, then, given that the having of a goal is a state with which the world must fit rather than *vice versa* (from (2)), so it follows (from (3)) that the state that motivates the desire must itself be a desire. Thus, the Humean will say, the idea that there may be a state that motivates a desire, but which is not itself a desire, is simply implausible.[47]

The same point can be made in another way, by considering how, according to Nagel's own preferred theory of motivation, a state that is not a desire may yet motivate a desire. Suppose a subject now accepts the judgement 'At t I have (tenselessly: i.e. have or will have) reason to speak Italian'. This judgement may properly be thought of as the expression of a *belief* that the subject presently has. In Nagel's view, this belief may motivate a subject to promote his speaking Italian at t quite independently of the relation he believes *t* stands in to *now*.[48] Here, then, we have an example of a belief that, according to Nagel's theory, may suffice to explain a subject's action. And since whenever there is something sufficient to explain motivation there is enough to warrant the ascription of a desire, so, *a fortiori*, according to Nagel, that belief may also explain his having a desire; the desire to promote his speaking Italian at t. But, as is perhaps already evident, the Humean has a principled objection to Nagel's theory of motivation. For consider Nagel's theory in the light of (1)—the claim that having a motivating reason *is*, *inter alia*, having a goal. Does the subject who now believes that he has at t (tenselessly) reason to speak Italian necessarily now have a goal that he speaks Italian at t? Evidently not. The subject may indeed now believe that at t he has (tenselessly) a goal that he speaks Italian. But this belief cannot constitute his having a goal *now* that at t he speaks Italian, for it is a state with the wrong direction of fit (from (2)). Nor does the truth of this belief require that he has as a goal *now* that he speaks Italian at t. Rather, its truth requires that *at t* he has a goal that he speaks Italian.

The Humean will therefore say this about Nagel's theory of motivation, and hence about the theory according to which it is possible for a desire to be motivated by a state that is not itself a desire. Either this theory requires a conception of motivating reasons that is inconsistent with (1)—a claim we should have thought to be a conceptual truth about the connection between having a motivating reason and having a goal—or it requires a conception of belief that permits tenseless beliefs to be such that the world must fit with

---

[47] The objection here is that the idea that there is such a state is implausible. If we had some argument to the effect that the very concept of a state having 'both directions of fit' (see section 7) is incoherent, then we would be able to make a correspondingly stronger objection to Nagel's argument.

[48] *The Possibility of Altruism*, pp. 68-9.

60   *Michael Smith*

them, that is, a conception inconsistent with (3)—a claim we should have thought to be a conceptual truth about the nature of desire.

This is a pleasant result. For it is on the basis of the distinction between motivated and unmotivated desires, and the alleged possibility that a desire may be motivated though not by another desire that Nagel, and McDowell following him, think that they can concede P2 to the Humean—the claim that motivation requires the *presence* of a desire and means-end belief— without thereby accepting P1—the claim that motivating reasons are *constituted* by desires and means-end beliefs. But, if the argument given here has been correct, it emerges that P2 is not a principle that we have any reason to believe in its own right. Rather, properly understood, our only reason for believing P2 is that it is entailed by P1.

(ii) As I said earlier, Mark Platts in fact considers and rejects, a defence of the Humean theory based on a conception of desires as states with which the world must fit (see section 5). But why does he reject it? Platts rightly points out that we should demand of the Humean an 'argument for the claim that any full specification of a reason for action must make reference to a mental state of the second, non-cognitive kind *vis-à-vis* direction of fit with the world'.[49] But he fails even to put a response to this demand in the Humean's mouth. Rather, he asks rhetorically, 'Why should it not just be a brute fact about moral facts that, without any such further element entering, their clear perception does provide sufficient grounding for action?'[50] But the answer to this can now be seen to be relatively simple.

Given that reason explanations are teleological, a subject's clear perception of some moral fact could provide sufficient grounding for action only if (from (1)) it constituted his having some goal. But that would require in turn (from (2)) that the perception be a state with which the world must fit. However, a perception is not a state with which the world must fit. Thus we have reason to reject Platts's suggestion. This is not, of course, to deny that the 'clear perception' of some moral fact may be something that a subject can have only if he has certain desires. This is parallel to the way in which the clear perception of the desirability of some state of affairs is something that a subject can have, in normal circumstances, only if he has certain desires. But then, though a subject who has such a clear perception may be disposed to act in certain ways, the state that grounds this disposition will be a desire, not a clear moral perception. I am therefore unimpressed by Platts's own reasons for rejecting a defence of the Humean theory based on direction of fit considerations.

(iii) In short, this is my objection to John McDowell's view that the virtuous agent may be motivated by his conception of a situation in which he perceives some moral requirement—something that McDowell claims is

[49] *Ways of Meaning*, p. 258.   [50] Ibid.

properly thought of as a cognitive state.[51] McDowell simply overlooks the possibility that, though the virtuous agent's conceptions are cognitive states, and though his having those conceptions suffices for his being in a state that motivates him, none the less the state that motivates him is a desire. This possibility is opened up once we realise that the Humean may admit that there are cognitive states that a subject can be in only if he is in some non-cognitive state.

(Nor need this be interpreted as the simple-minded idea that for each virtue an agent has, he has a corresponding desire, and that the condition for his having the conceptions associated with having that virtue is his having that desire.[52] Rather, we may think that having a virtue requires being disposed to have different sorts of desires in different sorts of situations. Taking this view allows us to hold that, though having certain desires is the condition for having the conceptions that a particular virtue makes possible, there is no straightforward mapping of desires onto virtues.)

9. *Conclusion*

It is, I hope, beginning to look as though the Humean theory is more plausible than many people have thought. The argument I have given for the theory has been really quite simple. However, it seems to have been overlooked by non-Humean theorists of motivation. Some have done so because they fail to distinguish motivating reasons from normative reasons. Others have done so because they hold a weak phenomenological, and hence inadequate, conception of desire. Most have done so because they have overlooked the implications of the fact that having a motivating reason is, *inter alia*, having a goal. However, once we keep it firmly before our minds that the Humean's is a theory of motivating reasons and equip ourselves with an adequate conception of desire, we see that only the Humean's claim that motivating reasons are constituted, *inter alia*, by desires is able to make proper sense of reason explanations as teleological explanations. For only an agent's desires may constitute his having certain goals. So, at any rate, I have argued.[53]

Department of Philosophy   MICHAEL SMITH
Princeton University
Princeton, N.J. 08544
U.S.A.

[51] 'Are Moral Requirements Hypothetical Imperatives?', p. 18; 'Virtue and Reason', pp. 335-6, 345-7.   [52] 'Non-cognitivism and Rule Following', pp. 144-5.
[53] I am grateful to the following people for comments on an earlier version of this paper: Simon Blackburn, Jonathan Dancy, Gilbert Harman, Frank Jackson, Mark Johnston, Lloyd Humberstone, David McNaughton, Michaelis Michael, Nathan Tawil, and Jay Wallace.

[2]

Practical Tortoise Raising

SIMON BLACKBURN

In 1895 Lewis Carroll wrote his famous *Mind* article "What the Tortoise said to Achilles". The problem he raised can succinctly be put like this: can logic make the mind move? Or, less enigmatically, how do we describe what is wrong with the tortoise's argument that, however many premises Achilles has him accept, he always has space to refrain from drawing the conclusion?

In this paper I am not so much concerned with movements of the mind, as movements of the will. But my question bears a similarity to that of the tortoise. I want to ask whether the will is under the control of fact and reason, combined. I shall try to show that there is always something else, something that is not under the control of fact and reason, which has to be given as a brute extra, if deliberation is ever to end by determining the will. This is, of course, a Humean conclusion, and the only novelty comes in the way I wish to argue for it. I believe that many philosophers think, erroneously, that Hume relies on a naive and outdated conception of facts, or on an even more naive and outdated conception of reason, in order to put passion on their throne. My tortoise defends Hume: what we do with our premises is not itself construed as acceptance of a premise.

As it stands the project is only described metaphorically. Presumably everything, including movement of the will, is under the control of facts in some sense, for even if they are only facts about our physiology or chemistry, still, they make us move. I am interested only in cognitive control, or control by the apprehension of fact and reason.

Day 1

Achilles, then, had overtaken the tortoise and was sitting comfortably on its back. "You see", he said, "the distances were constantly diminishing, and so—".

"But if they had been constantly increasing?", the tortoise interrupted, "how then? ... Well now, would you like to hear of a race-course, that most people fancy they can get to the end of in two or three steps, while it

really consists of an infinite number of distances, each one longer than the previous one? ... let us take a little bit of an argument for acting."

(P)   I would prefer eating lettuce to eating souvlaki.

(B)   The moment of decision is at hand.

(Z)   Let me choose to eat lettuce rather than souvlaki!

"Well", continued the tortoise, "there is no question of accepting (Z) as true, but there may be a question of accepting it. Let us agree that accepting (Z) amounts to actually doing whatever is involved in choosing lettuce rather than souvlaki. We accept (Z) only if the will is determined, and an intention is formed. Are we to suppose that if we accept (P) and (B), then we must accept (Z)?"

"Wait a minute", said Achilles, "I don't want to rush you. It occurs to me that some philosophers make a distinction between what you prefer and what you think you ought to prefer, or would prefer if you were ideally placed, for a tortoise. Perhaps this affects the issue."

"If you like", said the tortoise. "I too hate this modern fad for rushing past anything like that. Let us put it in."

(P)   I would prefer eating lettuce to eating souvlaki.

(M)   I think it is right to prefer lettuce to souvlaki.

(B)   The moment of decision is at hand,

(Z)   Let me choose to eat lettuce rather than souvlaki!

"That's better!" said Achilles. "That certainly wraps it up for (Z). Surely you must accept (Z) if all those are true!"

"I don't quite know" said the tortoise sadly. "Sometimes, well, I am not sure how important rightness is. I certainly get these urges to do what I think is wrong, don't you know. I am really quite good at what you Greeks keep calling *akrasia*; in fact I rather enjoy it."

"Good heavens", replied Achilles sternly yet compassionately. "If there is one thing modern moral philosophy will tell you, it is that any such behaviour is quite irrational. The norms of reason are foundations for the norms of ethics."

"And we don't want to be unreasonable, do we?" said the tortoise. "In fact, we had better add it, just to make sure."

(RM)   I think it is rational to do what I think is right

"There we are", announced Achilles in triumph. "Reason prevails!"

"Well, that is certainly a change" said the tortoise, "and yet sometimes, well, I am not sure how important rationality is. I certainly get these urges to act against reason, don't you know. I am really quite good at that kind of *akrasia*; in fact I rather enjoy it."

"Holy Apollo!" exclaimed Achilles. "Do you mean you have been reading the Romantics, so many millennia before their time? Are you in favour

of short-termism and spontaneity, and against prudence and economics? Or is it something else?"

"I don't know" said the tortoise, "but perhaps you can explain to me: *must* I be rational?"

"Oh certainly" said Achilles, "you must if ... well, if you want to be rational, you know."

"I love hypothetical imperatives", said the tortoise. "But I am not sure this one is going to help. Still, we could make sure that rationality and ethics pull together, if you like", he conceded helpfully.

(MR)   I think it right to do what I think is rational

"Hmmm" said Achilles. "I hadn't expected to put that in, but it is terribly decent of you to let me. And now at last we are home and dry!"

"Only", said the tortoise apologetically, "I get so terribly confused. We had to add (M) and I can't help wondering that although I am sure it is right to do what is rational, these fits of *akrasia* still afflict me so chronically. I must have been badly brought up" he added bashfully.

Achilles frowned as he replaced his pencil with a new one. "I think that is probably a bit morbid" he said. "Surely in general you prefer to do what is right and rational?" "Perhaps we should add it", encouraged the tortoise.

(P′)   I prefer to do what I think it right and rational to do.

"And now" said Achilles in triumph, "We really are getting somewhere. The last time I talked with you, a century ago, you made me keep adding different premises! But now there is simply nothing more to add!" And he did a little dance.

"I love the way you move yourself" said the tortoise, sitting comfortably. "All I admit is that I prefer to do what is right and rational. But then, after all, I preferred lettuce to souvlaki. And we had to add a bit to that, didn't we?" he laughed, modestly.

"Sacred Zeno!" expostulated Achilles. "You are not going to make me add another round are you! I can see it coming: you want me to add that it is right to prefer to do what you think it is right and rational to do, and so on and so on. You really are the most stubborn animal."

"Well, I am a bit careful" confessed the tortoise. "And I don't really know that I am all that confident that it is right and rational to prefer to do what I think it is right and rational to do. After all, many people are wrong and stupid in preferring to do what they think it is right and rational to do. I wouldn't want to act while I am worried in case I am like them!"

But great Achilles had flown to the libraries to collect some volumes on The Theory of Rational Choice. Munching some lettuce, the tortoise awaited his return.

Day II

"You know" resumed Achilles, "this whole business is off on the wrong foot. We have been talking as if there is a gap between preference and actual choice. Whereas I now read that in the best circles the thing is to believe in the theory of revealed preference. Which means we read your preference back from your choice. It is not an antecedent state whose apprehension determines choices—I admit that yesterday's conversation made that idea puzzling—but simply a logical construct from the choices you make!"

"Pardon me" said the tortoise. "I must have misunderstood something. Don't these economists and game theorists get paid for giving advice— advice about what to do?"

"Absolutely", said Achilles. "They are very rich and regarded as very good at it."

"Tell me more", said the tortoise admiringly.

"Well" responded Achilles putting on his lecturer's gown, "it seems to go like this.

"The reasoning behind talking of revealed preference comes in two parts.[1] In the bad old days, it goes, it was thought that 'utility' will be a Benthamite, empirical quantity which happened to be the object of desire, or ought to be the object of desire. But utilities so conceived prove both empirically and philosophically bogus, as indeed Bentham might have learned from Bishop Butler (1953, especially Sermons I and XI). It is nei- ther true nor useful as an approximation that people or tortoises act so as to maximize the intensity or duration of some state of themselves. They do not even always act with their own interests in mind, where these inter- ests are construed as states of themselves. Rather, we see them as having an interest in some object when that object figures in their decision making. But objects here include states that are not states of the subject: the survival of the whales, or the relief of the famine, or the death of the blasphemer, or the success of a friend. Indeed, notoriously, unless this is so the life resulting is apt to be unenviable and the selfishness is self-defeating. So let us instead reverse the equation: utilities are no longer empirically given, but are simply constructs from mathematically tractable ways of handling preferences. Given very weak assumptions, an agent with an ordering of preferences over each of some set of options can be represented as if she had attached measurable 'values', called utilities, to those options. The pro- vision of a scale is similar in principle to that of providing numerical mea-

---

[1] A forceful recent presentation by a leading practitioner is Binmore (1994, Vol. 1). See also Kreps (1990, p. 26), and Dawes (1988, p. 154 ff).

sures for weights, given only the results from a balance. A balance is an empirical determination of when one object weighs at least as much as another. The results of tests for whether one object is at least as heavy as another can be presented numerically, with the numbers representing 'weights' of the objects in the set. An element has at least as great a weight as another if and only if the other does not outweigh it, which is to tip the balance against it.[2]

"So if we have pairwise preferences across choices in a set, we can represent their expected utilities numerically. But what corresponds to the empirical results from the balance, telling us when choice *a* is preferred to choice *b*? The orthodox answer amongst economists and game theorists to accept the theory of revealed preferences. This was initially defended in the work of the economist Samuelson (1947), and holds that preferences themselves are not antecedent psychological states that happen to control (most) decisions. Rather, true preferences are those that are revealed by decisions. It is, after all, a truism that to know what you or anyone else wants, see what you or anyone else chooses, or would choose given suitable options. To know that you prefer oil to butter, you see whether you choose it, at least when nothing further hangs on the decision. The theory of revealed preferences is perhaps less popular among philosophers than economists. But we shall see below good reason for accepting it, for there is really no other candidate for the necessary empirical test. Putting the two foundation stones together then, we have:

> (*Util*) A utility function is defined such that the expected utility of *a* is at least as great as *b* if and only if *a* is weakly preferred to *b* (i.e. preferred to *b*, or at least as much as *b*). Such a function can be defined over a set of options if preference satisfies two consistency conditions: for all outcomes *a*, *b* either *a* is weakly preferred to *b*, or *b* to *a* (totality), and if *a* is weakly preferred to *b*, and *b* to *c*, then *a* is weakly preferred to *c* (transitivity).
>
> (*Revpref*) Choice behaviour is primitive. If a player makes choices, then he is making choices as though he were equipped with a preference relation which has that choice preferred to others. An eligible agent is always interpretable as though he were seeking to further a preference.

"In a nutshell, the first part of the approach makes utilities 'logical constructions' out of preferences, while the second makes preferences logical constructions out of actual choices.

"To whom do *Util* and *Revpref* apply? To anyone with consistent, transitive preferences over a set of options. We may call such persons *eligible* persons (it is vital not to confuse the issue by calling them rational, as is frequently done). An ineligible person would be someone who cannot be

---

[2] The classic presentation is by von Neumann and Morgenstern (1944).

700   *Simon Blackburn*

interpreted in terms of utilities, just as a balance that cannot weigh some element in a set, or that weighs $a > b$, and $b > c$, but $c > a$, cannot deliver a set of weights defined over the set. It is of the utmost importance, then, to realize that there are not two sorts of players in a prisoners' dilemma, or other game theoretic structures, the eligible ones and the ineligible ones. 'Ineligible' refers not to a kind of player, but to someone who *cannot be interpreted* as playing at all. An ineligible player is like someone who approaches chess by knocking over the board. It is. however. often a matter of judgment whether someone who appears to be ineligible through having intransitive preferences is so really, or is best interpreted as having redefined the options in front of her.

"Of course, neither *Util* nor *Revpref* have gone uncriticized. Amartya Sen, for example, introduces notions of sympathy (having your welfare affected by the position of others) and an individual's commitments (conceived of as standing outside, and even in opposition to their own welfare) as independent pressures on action.[3] He points out that preference, in the economics literature, has two liaisons: one is with choice, but the other is with welfare. That is, increased preference satisfaction is supposed to increase welfare, and he denies that a notion of preference based on *Revpref* can fulfill this second condition. For people may behave as if they had certain preferences (those are the preferences we would read back from their behaviour) when their welfare, or even their expected welfare, would be better served if they behaved differently. Sen also believes that this undermines the authority of an approach based on *Util*. If it does so, it also undermines *Revpref*, since if because of sympathy or commitment an agent acts against his preferences (what he would really like to do, if only the situation allowed it), then of course his action will not be revealing those preferences.

"The orthodox game theorists' response is that their framework is quite elastic enough to encompass whatever motivations we believe to exist. As I have already sketched, there is no need to deny that a player may care about other things than their own interests, real or perceived, or their own welfare as opposed to that of others. In the apt phrase of David Gauthier, 'it is not interests in the self, that take oneself as object, but interests of the self, held by oneself as subject, that provide the basis for rational choice and action'. Choice is the upshot of *whatever* the player cares about, and as I have sketched, utility derives from choice.[4] So it is wrong to criticize either axiom by reminding ourselves of the heterogeneous nature of

---

[3] Sen (1982) especially the essays collected in Part I.

[4] It is very easy to forget this. Binmore, for example, describes *homo economicus* as someone whose "concern is with his own self-interest, *broadly conceived*" (p. 19). But this is wrong: *homo economicus* need not be concerned with himself at all, under any conception of his own interests.

desire. Rather, we must simply be careful to build any apparently 'exogenous' or external independent desires into the payoffs represented in the choice situation.

"The same caveats apply if we start to contrast preference with principle or with conscience. There is certainly a vernacular distinction here, for we talk of being obliged to do what we do not prefer to do. But the concepts defined by our two axioms do not match this distinction, and are not refuted by it. Rather, preference, revealed by choice, may include the preference for acting on any specific principle: the preference to keep a promise, or keep a vow to God, or to avoid the gaze of the man within, or the preference to do one's bit, the preference for being the man who bought the Brooklyn bridge, rather than the man who sold it, or even the preference to try to live up to our better selves. The better way to describe the 'conflict' between a narrow sense of preference and what happens when principle is introduced is to say that sometimes we are obliged to do what we would not *otherwise have* preferred to do; but this leaves it open that now, in the presence of the obligation, our preference is actually that we conform to the requirements of obligation or duty. The counterfactual preference that we would have had, had we not made the promise or felt obliged to cooperate, or whatever it is, is not our all-things-considered preference."

"Splendid, absolutely splendid" interrupted the tortoise, a little sharply. "But now tell me how this translates into advice, for this is what we were hoping to find."

"Well" said Achilles, confidently "consider the familiar prisoner's dilemma.

		A	
		Hawk	Dove
B	Hawk	1,1	0,3
	Dove	3,0	2,2

"Each player acts independently, causally, of the other, and each knows the other's utilities. Now, looking at this the game theorist can advise you to be a hawk. For whatever your opponent does, you do better by playing hawk. Yet this advice has been contested, and indeed some people think it is rational to play dove."

"Well, well", said the tortoise. "If the advice has been contested, then it must be significant advice! But tell me, to whom does it apply exactly?"

"As we have explained", said Achilles huffily "to anyone eligible, and who is presented with the game."

702 *Simon Blackburn*

"Timeo Danaos et dona ferentis" said the tortoise, smugly. "Tell me, what would happen if I didn't follow the advice to choose hawk? Wouldn't I reveal a preference for being a dove?"

"Well, yes" admitted Achilles, somewhat impatiently.

"And if that is so" continued the tortoise imperturbably "how does it happen that these little figures you have in the boxes, are the *right* ones? I mean, I can see how they might represent money, or years in prison or something, but the game theorist is surely not telling me that it is rational to care only about money, or years in prison. I thought these figures represented the sum total of my preferences. But since these are revealed by choice, if I play dove, then they cannot be right."

"Explain to me" said Achilles, tottering slightly.

Here, the tortoise paused to put on the lecturer's gown. "Suppose a player makes the dove choice. Then he preferred one or both of the options in which he acts as a dove to the others; by *Revpref* we must construct a utility function in accordance with that preference, and hence he was not actually in a prisoners' dilemma. In the terms often used, his decision problem cannot have been accurately 'modelled' by presenting him as if he were in a prisoners' dilemma. For a prisoners' dilemma is defined so that the hawkish utilities outrank the doveish ones, and that in turn simply means that the hawkish options are the ones that get chosen. The conclusion ought to read that it is a tautology that an eligible player will necessarily choose hawk in the prisoners' dilemma."

"Aha" said Achilles, "it is not quite as simple as that. For in such strategic problems, we have to consider the other player's likely choice. Imagine, if you will, the poor agent lurching towards a choice, and knowing that on the other side of a mirror, as it were, but quite independently, his twin is doing the same. It will be better all round if they plump for dove, in spite of the way that such a choice is dominated. Mightn't they each do so?"

"Oh well" replied the tortoise, "If they know that it is a real twin, who will magically do exactly the same as they do, then the options are restricted to the symmetric ones, and playing dove dominates. But in real sitiations they don't know this, and they might do *anything*. If they have a minute to chose, then recalling what their twin is doing they might change their mind once in the first thirty seconds, again in the next fifteen seconds, again in half the remaining time, and so on. It would be like one of those lamps going on and off ever more quickly. I seem to remember you once modelled your running on just such a contraption" he said, nostalgically remembering his first foray into philosophy, more than two thousand years ago. "Heaven knows where they end. All I am saying is that if they do go haywire, as well they might, and plump for dove, then if anything

they reveal different preferences, and hence expected utilities, from the ones on show."

"For example", continued the tortoise, "when on p. 27 of his book Binmore stresses that 'it is *tautological* that *homo economicus* maximizes all the time', we might think that this is peculiar to that kind of *homo,* or equally to *testudo economicus,* whom we then may or may not want to imitate. Whereas in the light of *Util* and *Revpref,* it is tautological that any eligible agent maximizes all the time. In interpreting this it is well to remember the extremely weak imposition that consistency involves: only that you have transitive preferences over the entire set of options in play. In particular, consistency does not entail any particular attitude towards risk, or towards other people, or action on principle. Nor does it entail constancy, or consistency over time, which means making the same choice on later occasions as you made on earlier ones.[5]

"More importantly, it is to be remembered that inconsistent players are of no interest. For if a player is genuinely inconsistent, in any way that matters to the game, then we will be unable to construct a function from preferences to utilities. In such a case we cannot say what the utilities of the agent are under different choices, and the interpretation of him as in a prisoners' dilemma, or any other kind of specific decision theoretic problem, collapses. So in fact the tautology applies across the board: it is tautological than any player *who can be interpreted as being in a prisoner's dilemma,* chooses the dominant strategy. There exists no theory about non-eligible players, so the restriction to eligible players is insignificant."

"Surely the game theorists know all this?" queried Achilles.

"Well" said the tortoise, shaking his head mournfully, "they tend to be forthright about the official framework in some places, but more coy when they are offering all that richly-paid advice. For example, Binmore frequently describes himself as arguing against those who think that strongly dominated choices are rational (p. 174); he sometimes describes his opponents as supposing that 'out of equilibrium play can be sustained in the long run' (p. 175), and by contrast presents himself as the realistic, Hobbesian man who is hard-headed enough to know that eventually if we can get more for ourselves, we will be tempted to do so. Theorists such as Gauthier and McLennan, who think it is sometimes rational to choose the dominated strategy, are particular targets."

"But isn't that as it should be?", said Achilles, fumbling a little.

"Well, I think it should be clear" replied the tortoise, "that these attitudes are thoroughly incoherent. It is not that out of equilibrium play can-

---

[5] Why should it? Preferring butter today and oil tomorrow may be the key to a healthy diet. Change of preference is often good strategy, in poker, or in real and metaphorical battles. Some men find fickle inconstant women especially charming, in which case these are genetically successful traits.

not be sustained in the long run, or needs psychologies that we have not got, or is the private preserve of benighted and irrational bleeding-heart Kantians, but that it *cannot happen at all*. In out of equilibrium play in the prisoners' dilemma, an agent chooses what she recognizes as the dominated strategy. But by *Util* and *Revpref* this is impossible: if an agent chooses a strategy, then this shows that (if utilities and probabilities can be attached at all) the expected utility attached to it is higher than that attaching to any other strategy over which it was chosen."

"Hmmm", said Achilles. "And yet, hasn't the enterprise of bringing rational weight to bear against selfishness made the prisoners' dilemma the central parable of modern political theory? How can that be so if you are right?"

"Oh, it has nothing to do with rationality" said the tortoise. "Or even being good. The same point applies even if you want to be *bad*", and he shuddered slightly, which is hard for a tortoise.

"Explain", said Achilles wonderingly.

"Well, take blackmail" said the tortoise. "We can think of it in extended form in terms of a sequence of plays, one in succession by each of two players, Adam and Eve. At each node the player has to play one of two options, hawk or dove. We are assuming as usual that each of Adam and Eve's payoffs is known to themselves, and to the other.

Blackmail

(Adam's payoff is represented first)

t_1	A		t_2	E
Dove	1,2		Dove	2,1
Hawk	●		Hawk	0,0

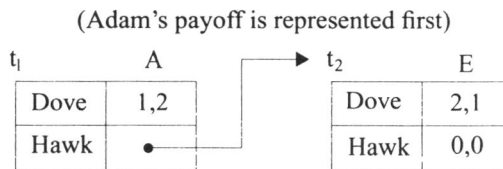

"The story is that before the game starts Eve has committed an indiscretion. If Adam does nothing (doveish) he has 1 unit of utility, and Eve 2. If he blackmails Eve (hawkish) and she submits (doveish) he takes 1 of Eve's units. But if she does not submit (hawkish) she blows the gaff on him, revealing him as a blackmailer, but also revealing her own indiscretion, leaving them both worse off, in the 0,0 finale.

"Orthodox decision theory has us reason as follows. In Blackmail, eligible Eve will not play the final hawkish option. For doing so represents simple loss. Eligible Adam knows that this is so. Hence he plays hawk, and since she then plays dove, his blackmail is successful.

"Suppose now that Adam knows *in advance* that this is the matrix. Then he knows in advance that eligible Eve will not choose to be a hawk when

it comes to her turn. For it would be a contradiction (by *Util* and *Revpref*) for Eve to choose 0 when she can have 1. So eligible Eve will play dove, and eligible Adam will play hawk. For, once more, it would be a contradiction for Adam to play dove when he could play hawk, leaving him with 1 instead of 2. So Adam does not face a choice: once he knows the matrix, he knows what is going to happen.

"Now remember that expert game theorists endorse both *Util* and *Revpref*, and Binmore, for example, implies that all the rest of their kind do so as well.[6] He believes that the 'advantages of the methodology in clarifying the underlying logic are overwhelming'. What this means is that the game theorist takes care of any facts about psychologies at the *modelling* stage (see esp. p. 162). We have successfully modelled a set of players only when they have no interests (nothing they care about) that are unrepresented in the game's payoff structure. Often persons with other elements in their psychologies will not be in such games when others are.

"So what Eve needs to be is someone who is *not* modelled correctly as being in this game even when other, nicer, people, would be. In short, she needs to present herself as being vengeful and proud, disinclined to submit to blackmail, preferring her own financial ruin and that of Adam to the feeling of having been done down by him. Should she know she will face such situations regularly, she needs to cultivate a nice public vicious streak, so that her threat to expose them both is all too credible. Of course, if she hasn't done that in advance, or had it done for her in school, she will be a plausible target for blackmail, poor thing."

"Good lord, or rather Zeus" said Achilles, correcting himself quickly. "I suppose philosophers like Gauthier would have to say that it is rational to be vicious." And he shuddered in his turn. "Let me try to sort it out. It certainly qualifies what we might have thought was meant by calling a strategy rational, or indeed calling the situation a game that calls for choices and strategies. We might have thought that if we talk of a game, and someone tells us that a particular strategy is rational, then we can interpret that as tantamount to giving us permission to follow it, or if it is uniquely rational, telling us to follow it. You do not in deliberation draw up two lists; one of what to do in given circumstances, and the other of

---

[6] Actually, I think he is wrong about this, at least as far as the founding fathers are concerned. Von Neumann and Morgenstern, for instance, write that "we shall therefore assume that the aim of all participants in the economic system is money, or equivalently a single monetary commodity ..." (1944, 2.2.1). Harsanyi (1977) contrasts the pursuit of "self interest and individual values" with the "rational pursuit of the interests of society as a whole", and sees games as modelling the former interest. The point is that in such approaches, an empirically given aim or type of aim is contrasted with others of a person's overall inclinations or concerns. Of course, any resultant advice is then hypothetical in form: if you want to maximize only these specific concerns, act as follows.

what it is rational to do in the same circumstances.[7] But in game theory as it is now being conceived, nothing can be translated into advice. For suppose we are 'advised' to follow the dominant strategy. This is null advice, equivalent to: behave so that a tautology is true of you. So if we don't follow the advice, then our choice reveals that it wasn't that game. But if it wasn't that game then the advice was inapplicable, and if the advice was inapplicable, then there was no point in following it in any event, for the game theorist had failed to model the situation properly. As Wittgenstein might have said, anything could accord with the advice, and that means that no advice was given. The economists' slogan 'Maximize!' turns out not to be an injunction at all, for nothing could count as failing to follow it.[8] So the promise that we can learn something about rationality by these means collapses. Or, if we prefer it, the idea that the notion of rationality gains any purchase here is refuted. It is inevitable that so-called counter-theoretical actions do not reveal the irrationality of the players, but the inadequacy of this application of the theory."

"You always did catch up fast" said the tortoise admiringly, "And it also suggests that the question is not so much one of whether it is rational for Eve to be vicious, as whether she has been educated so that she and her peers thrive in the situations in which they will be put. Some have, some haven't", he added sententiously, and sat down, which is also quite difficult for a tortoise, and ate some more lettuce.

Day III

"Look" said Achilles, forlornly contemplating his bonfire of books on The Theory of Rational Choice, "decision making is at least under the control of fact and reason in another way. There will come after us one greater than us, who will show that it is a dictate of pure practical reason that we treat every person as an end in themselves. And his name shall be called Immanuel. But let's not start on that", he added hurriedly.

"And every tortoise", I hope added the tortoise.

"If they are rational", assured Achilles, muttering something under his breath.

"Tell me", said the tortoise, "it sounds nice and impartial. *Must* I be impartial?" he asked, innocently.

---

[7] Unless "rational" is being used in an irrelevant, restricted sense in which what is rational contrasts with spontaneous or emotionally satisfying.

[8] Gauthier (1987, p. 27) points out the futility of this injunction on similar grounds. But his own views are not disentangled from the problem.

"Absolutely", said Achilles piously. "Even Hume, whom you somewhat resemble, realizes that we have to take up a common point of view. In a conversation with anyone else about what to do, there is a point where we must cease speaking the language of self-love, and correct our sentiments by invoking common standards, whereby we judge things and persons as they affect those surrounding them."

"And the penalty if we don't?" asked the tortoise.

"Well, practical reasoning could not go forward" said Achilles, "and we would lose the benefits of cooperation, or of putting the first person plural in place of the first person singular (Postema 1995). We couldn't even row boats together."

"We wouldn't want that", said the tortoise sociably. "But I remember a couple of days ago we thrashed out wants and preferences, and I am afraid I remained unmoved, if you remember. So what is new?"

"Kant improves upon Hume" said Achilles enthusiastically. "He shows how pure practical reason dictates respect for the law. For impartiality, fairness, and all that. All sorts of good things" he finished lamely.

"It sounds appetizing" agreed the tortoise, "but tell me about this dictation and this respect. What is my awful fate if I find this respect is not actually dictated?"

"Well if you don't respect the law" said Achilles, "you will not be free, not an autonomous self-governing tortoise."

"And I expect at least you are going to tell me that I wouldn't want to be anything else" chimed in the tortoise, "but that is not going to get us much further, is it? Presumably you really would like to tell me that it is contrary to reason not to respect the law, thereby achieving freedom and self-respect. And I doubt if I am going to believe you. For I fear that Kant will one day tell us that

> The real morality of actions, their merit or guilt, even that of our own conduct, thus remains entirely hidden from us. Our imputations can refer only to the empirical character. How much of this character is ascribable to the pure effect of freedom, how much to mere nature, that is, to faults of temperament for which there is no responsibility, or to its happy constitution, can never be determined … . (*Critique of Pure Reason*, A551/B579)

"And I am afraid my own self-respect as a just and caring tortoise is not beholden to any such murky transcendental facts. And", he added dropping his voice a little, "I rather doubt whether your self-respect as a hero is, either."

"But you *are* a just and fair and compassionate tortoise", reminded Achilles.

"You're too kind", said the tortoise blushing modestly. "But it is true. You will know how Adam Smith writes that

> The jurisdiction of the man within, is founded altogether in the desire of praise-worthiness, and in the aversion to blame-worthiness; in the desire of possessing those qualities, and performing those actions, which we love and admire in other people; and in the dread of possessing those qualities, and performing those actions, which we hate and despise in other people. (1759, *III*. 2, p. 33)

"Well, the same goes for the tortoise within", he added helpfully.

"But it is not *rational*" wailed Achilles, beating his head on the tortoise's shell.

"Just as well", said the tortoise, "given where *that* leaves us. And it is lucky my shell is so solid."

Day IV

"Listen", began Achilles, his locks disheveled by what appeared to have been a sleepless night. "At least you respect means-ends reasoning, do you not? And quite possibly there exists an argument that if you do that then you cannot remain unmoved in other ways. Once you have some musts then you have to allow others."

"Respect means-ends reasoning?", queried the tortoise, "Explain to me what you mean."

"Well, suppose you want some of that lettuce across the road. And you apprehend that the only way to get it is to cross the road, since lettuce is even less likely to move than you are. In other words, you know that if you want the lettuce, you must cross the road. So it follows that you conceive yourself under a necessity to cross the road. There would then be a kind of inconsistency in not crossing the road."

"I think I only know one kind of inconsistency", said the tortoise. "The kind that goes p & $\neg p$. Do you mean I am contradicting myself? It doesn't feel as if I am."

"But don't you agree that if you want the lettuce you must cross the road? And you want the lettuce (and the moment of decision is at hand) ... so you must cross the road."

"By modus ponens" said the tortoise, a nasty glint coming into his eye.

"Grrr", said Achilles warningly.

"All right", said the tortoise backing off relatively hastily, "but it isn't even modus ponens is it? I mean, if I want a million pounds I must buy a lottery ticket, and I do want a million pounds, but I don't see that I must buy a lottery ticket. It is one of those off-colour conditionals where musts

and oughts make the conclusion non-detachable. And in fact, I am not going to buy a lottery ticket" he concluded with a flourish.

"Aha", replied Achilles, "that must mean you want something else more, such as avoiding lotteries or sitting still."

"I rather think we are back in the world of *Revpref*" said the tortoise. "Of course I recognize that if I am to get what I want, I must adopt the only means available. If I am to get the lettuce I must cross the road, and wanting the lettuce as I do I expect in time to cross the road. If I don't do so, we might agree that I really didn't want the lettuce all that much, or perhaps that I wanted something else more. Maybe I just didn't want to cross the road. No harm in that" he concluded smugly.

"You make it sound a kind of accident if you choose the means to the end" complained Achilles. "Whereas I am trying to show that reason enjoins the choice! To coin a phrase, it is an a priori principle constitutive of practical rationality!"

"Not an accident, and not that, whatever it is" said the tortoise. "Naturally some difficult radical interpretation has to be done. If I prefer lettuce to starvation, and recognize crossing the road as the only means to lettuce, yet act as if I prefer the joint outcome <starvation, sit still> to <lettuce, cross the road> then we will cast around for other objects of concern to explain my choice. And equally obviously tortoises of a race that does not choose necessary means to ends will fail to achieve their ends; assuming their ends include satisfying their needs, then they will doubtless die out rather rapidly. I expect that is why I may be about to cross the road. On the other hand, tortoises who rush around buying lottery tickets may not do all that well either. The race is not always to the swift" he mused.

"But wouldn't you call a fellow tortoise who persistently failed to adapt means to ends unreasonable? Don't there have to be authoritative, instrumental norms?" fumed Achilles.[9]

"Oh, I call lots of people unreasonable", said the tortoise, "people who get angry too quickly or eat too much so that they can get sick and lose weight, or who enter dwarf-throwing competitions. It doesn't signify very much except that their behaviour doesn't make sense to me, or even that I disapprove of them. But as for norms, yes, indeed I am glad I am not the kind of tortoise who constantly fails to adapt means to ends. I am not sure I am ever going to meet any who do so fail, both because it is so hard to identify them, and because we agreed that they will have died out pretty quickly. But if I did, well I am sure they would really arouse my pas-

---

[9] This way of putting it is that of Jean Hampton (1995, p. 66). In the same issue Elijah Milgram (1995) thinks that Hume was, implausibly, a sceptic about practical reasoning. The tortoise suggests that we have no coherent concept of anything of which Hume was implausibly sceptical.

sions—good-for-nothing, useless animals, every last tortoise of them" he said with a frown.

"At least I can agree to that" replied Achilles, sadly.

"Why so sad?", asked the tortoise, caringly.

"Nothing", said Achilles, "It is just that I thought I had a different thought, and now I think I didn't."

Day V

"But look", said Achilles, "you have resisted all the arguments I could muster. And yet I notice that this pile of lettuce has steadily shrunk. So what is going on?"

"Oh, didn't I tell you?" said the tortoise, pausing surprised in mid-mouthful. "I have an absolute passion for the stuff. In fact, I scarcely ever resist it. Would you like some too?"[10]

Department of Philosophy   SIMON BLACKBURN
University of North Carolina
Chapel Hill, North Carolina 27599
USA
e-mail ublack@gibbs.oit.unc.edu

REFERENCES

Binmore, Ken 1994: *Game Theory and the Social Contract*. Cambridge, Massachusetts: MIT Press.

Butler, Joseph 1953: *Fifteen Sermons*. London: G. Bell & Sons.

Carroll, Lewis 1895: "What the Tortoise Said to Achilles". *Mind*, 4, pp. 278–80.

Dawes, Robyn M. 1988: *Rational Choice in an Uncertain World*. Orlando: Harcourt Brace.

Gauthier, David 1986: *Morals by Agreement*. Oxford: Oxford University Press.

Hampton, Jean 1995: "Does Hume Have an Instrumental Conception of Practical Reason?". *Hume Studies*, 21, pp. 57–74.

Harsanyi, John 1977: *Rational Behaviour and Bargaining Equilibrium in Games and Social Situations*. Cambridge: Cambridge University Press.

[10] This paper was read at a conference in Glasgow University commemorating the centenary of Carroll's paper. I am grateful to Nick Zangwill and Jim Edwards for the invitation, and to Pat Shaw, James Dreier, Gilbert Harman, and others in the audience for valuable commentary.

Kreps, David M. 1990: *Game Theory and Economic Modelling*. Oxford: Oxford University Press.

Milgram, Elijah 1995: "Was Hume a Humean?". *Hume Studies*, 21, pp. 75–93.

Postema, J. 1995: "Morality in the First Person Plural". *Law and Philosophy*, 14, p. 35.

Samuelson, P. A. 1947: *Foundations of Economic Analysis*. Cambridge, Massachusetts: Harvard University Press.

Sen, Amartya 1982: *Choice, Welfare and Measurement*. Cambridge, Massachusetts: MIT Press.

Smith, Adam 1759: *The Theory of Moral Sentiments*. Reprinted 1976, Oxford: Clarendon Press.

von Neumann, J. and Morgenstern, O. 1944: *The Theory of Games and Economic Behaviour*. Princeton: Princeton University Press.

[3]

MOTIVATIONAL INTERNALISM:
THE POWERS AND LIMITS OF PRACTICAL REASONING

ALFRED R. MELE

It is commonly supposed that when we act on the basis of practical reasoning, the reasoning plays a role in our being motivated to act as we do. But what is the role? And how is it, more specifically, that reasoning issuing in a judgment in favor of *A*-ing provides us with motivation to *A*? In particular, does the production of motivation to *A* by practical reasoning depend in some interesting way upon motivation that is already present in the agent?

Externalism about the motivational capacity of practical reasoning — or *motivational externalism,* for short — asserts that practical reasoning is capable of producing motivation that is not derivative from motivation already present in the agent (or what I shall call *antecedent motivation),* and that reasoning can motivate in virtue of its issuing in a pertinent evaluative belief. *Motivational internalism* denies this. Since both views can take a variety of forms, these formulations of the positions are rough sketches at best; but they will serve as a useful point of departure.

My aim in this paper is to articulate and defend a version of motivational internalism. The simplest version is a crude instrumentalism according to which reasoning can generate motivation in us only by identifying means to ends that we already desire. The view advanced here is much less restrictive.

Motivational internalism is a popular view, both in the philosophy of action and in moral philosophy. So why trouble readers with a paper on the topic, unless one is going to *attack* the view? There are at least two good reasons. First, the most credible version of the position should be isolated, and the best grounds for it identified. Second, because motivational internalism has encountered considerable resistance on normative grounds, it is well worth showing, as I attempt to do, that a plausible version does not have the normative consequences that are often claimed for the thesis — by opponents and proponents alike.

417

ALFRED R. MELE

1. MOTIVATIONAL INTERNALISM

Recent discussions of the internalist/externalist controversy about motivation typically focus on the nature of moral judgments or moral reasons.[1] Thus, for example, William Frankena, in his justly influential paper, "Obligation and Motivation in Recent Moral Philosophy," says that the dispute between internalists and externalists is over the question "whether motivation is somehow to be 'built into' judgments of moral obligation."[2] However, some motivational internalists understand their view more broadly. Aristotle and Hume propound versions of the thesis when they claim, respectively, that "intellect itself... moves nothing, but only the intellect which aims at an end and is practical" and that "reason is ... the slave of the passions, and can never pretend to any other office than to serve and obey them."[3] And they are not speaking about moral motivation exclusively, but about motivation in general. Moreover, there is a difference between the composition of a judgment and its causal history: internalists and externalists do not battle over the former alone.

To hold that judgments of a certain kind have a "built in" motivational component is not necessarily to take a stand on how those judgments, or their motivational components, are produced. One who maintains that judgments of moral obligation, for example, have built in motivation might either accept or reject motivational internalism. One might claim that even when certain internally motivational judgments are arrived at on the basis of reasoning, their motivational component is wholly nonderivative from antecedent motivation. Thus, we must distinguish between the view that judgments of a certain sort have built in or internal motivation and internalism about the production of motivation by reasoning. By 'motivational internalism' I mean only the latter.

We must also distinguish *motivational* internalism from what I shall call *normative* internalism. The former is a thesis about the motivational capacities of reasoning, whereas the latter is a thesis about the conditions under which normative claims such as the following are warranted: 'There is *reason* for S to A'; 'A-ing is the *rational* thing for S to do.' The normative internalist contends, in Bernard Williams's words, that the truth of sentences such as these "implies very roughly, that [S] has some motive which will be served or furthred by his [A]-ing...".[4] The motivational internalist is concerned instead with a *causal* question — roughly, whether reasoning that purports to show that there is some reason for S to A can generate in S motivation to A without the assistance of antecedent motivation.

MOTIVATIONAL INTERNALISM

The latter distinction has some ties (as we shall see in more detail in Sec. 4) to a familiar distinction between *motivational* and *justificatory* reasons for action.[5] Although it is a defining feature of motivational reasons for action that they have motivational force, this is arguably false of justificatory reasons for action.[6] Suppose that Green, upon Brown's telling him that he should do *A*, asks Brown why he should do it. On the face of it, Brown may intelligibly say that Green should do *A* because (for the reason that) it is the charitable thing to do, even though he is confident that Green is not at all motivated by considerations of charity, nor by anything else that could motivate him to be charitable. (Brown may offer him a motivational reason as well: "If you don't do *A*, I will break your neck.")[7] Justificatory reasons *can* be motivational, of course: A reason that provides an agent with some justification for *A*-ing may have some motivational force. But that they' *must* be motivational should not be granted in the absence of supporting argument. The *normative* internalist insists that justificatory reasons for action, if they are to be *reasons* for action, must have motivational force. The *motivational* internalist, as we shall see later, is not committed to this view.

The literature does not uniformly treat one kind of internalism as logically prior to the other. Williams, in "Internal and External Reasons," attempts to motivate acceptance of normative internalism on the basis of an argument for motivational internalism. Christine Korsgaard, in "Skepticism About Practical Reason," investigates arguments *from* normative internalism to a motivational counterpart. I shall advance an independent argument for motivational internalism and argue that the view does not entail normative internalism.

The antecedence of 'antecedent motivation,' again, is *temporal*. For the motivational internalist, the production of new motivation by reasoning involves motivation that is already in place — motivation present in what might be called, following Williams, the agent's antecedent *motivational set*. Williams claims, without explanation, that 'desire' "can be used, formally, for all elements in [the set]," including "dispositions of evaluation, patterns of emotional reaction, personal loyalties, and various projects... embodying commitments of the agent."[8] This point merits attention. If we are to adjudicate the dispute between motivational internalists and motivational externalists, we must have a firm grip on what counts as motivation.

First, there is a familiar distinction between *occurrent* and *latent* desires or wants.[9] Many cigarette smokers are strongly disposed to have an urge or desire to smoke when they see someone else smoking. This

ALFRED R. MELE

disposition is a latent desire. The activation of the disposition yields an occurrent desire to smoke — a desire to smoke that plays a role in the agent's psychological economy at a particular time. Second, there is a very broad use of 'desire' and 'want', quite common in the philosophy of action, according to which to have an occurrent want or desire to perform, possess, promote, etc., X is simply to be in a motivational state whose object is one's performing, possessing, promoting, etc., X. Desires or wants, in this sense, need not have a positive affective tone, nor any feel at all. If this violates ordinary usage of the terms, the blurred subtleties can be reintroduced by distinguishing among types of desire or want in the broad sense at issue — for example, felt urges and nonaffective motivational states.

Williams is evidently using 'desire' in the familiar broad sense. I shall follow him in this. And I shall include latent desires among the constituents of motivational sets. A motivational set, as I shall use the term, is composed *only* of items constituted partly or wholly of occurrent or latent wants, in the broad sense of the term identified. (Certainly, at least some dispositions of evaluation, emotions, etc., are so constituted.)

Motivational internalism has ties to a conceptual thesis bound up closely with a very old and influential distinction between cognition and conation or motivation. Let us say that a psychological event or state is *purely cognitive* only if it has no motivational force (occurrent or dispositional) of its own. The conceptual thesis can than be formulated as follows: No purely cognitive event or state is causally sufficient for the production of motivation. This is not to *say*, of course, that there are any purely cognitive events or states. But if there are none, motivational internalism will be very hard to reject. For in that case, all cognitive elements involved in reasoning will have motivational force, and therefore any belief arrived at by reasoning will be arrived at on the basis of something with antecedent motivational force — that is, motivational force antecedent to the acquisition of the concluding belief.[10] Motivational externalists could claim that the motivational aspect of the reasoning is irrelevant to the concluding belief's having motivational force and attempt to find a non-motivational explanation of the generation of this force; but, as we shall see, this is a difficult line to take.

If pure cognition alone is never sufficient to generate motivation, what is? Motivational internalism identifies another item that it holds to be centrally involved specifically in the generation of motivation by reasoning, namely, motivation antecedent to the reasoning's cognitive conclusion.

420

MOTIVATIONAL INTERNALISM

In ascertaining how antecedent motivation is supposed to be involved, a bit of technical terminology will prove useful. Let us say that the *positive motivational base* of a particular motivational item (e.g., of a desire to do *A*) is the collection of all motivations of the agent that make a positive contribution to the motivational strength of the item in question. Thus, for example, when I lit a match a few moments ago, the positive motivational base of my desire to light the match included my desire to smoke a cigarette.[11] One desire may contribute causally to the acquisition of another without being in its positive motivational base. In deliberating with a view to the achievement of a desired object, *O, S* may discover that his *A*-ing is a necessary means to his achieving *O*, with the consequence that he desires to *A*. This latter desire may figure in the etiology of the further desire by prompting means/end reasoning that issues in a desire to do *B*, an action that the agent thinks will promote his chances of *A*-ing. Although *S*'s desire to *A* is a causal antecedent of his desire to *B*, it need not contribute to the *strength* of his desire to *B*. The strength of the latter desire may derive wholly from the strength of *S*'s desire for *O*.

Many motivational items have both positive and negative motivational bases. The *negative motivational base* of a motivational item is the collection of all motivations of the agent that make a negative contribution to the strength of that item. Thus, my desire to honor a promise that I made to my children to smoke no more than two cigarettes per day is in the negative motivational base of my occurrent desire to smoke another cigarette, if the former desire renders the latter weaker than it would otherwise have been.

The positive and negative motivational bases of a motivational item constitute its *total motivational base*. The total motivational base of a motivational item does not always deterime the motivational strength of that item. An impressive body of experimental data indicates that cognitive factors often have a pronounced influence on motivational strength. For example, the manner in which one represents a desired object to oneself can have a marked effect on delay of gratification.[12] A plausible formulation of motivational internalism must accommodate this point about cognition.

Another requirement on a plausible motivational internalism is that it not entail that antecedent motivation *must* be involved in the generation of motivation by reasoning. Perhaps, in some possible world, other things occasionally do the work of antecedent motivation — for example, divine intervention. Rather, the idea is this:

ALFRED R. MELE

MI. Actual human beings and the real world are such that the
capacity of justificatory reasoning to generate in a human being,
S, a motivational item whose object is *S*'s *A*-ing and to do this in
virtue of that reasoning's providing *S* with what she takes to be
justification for *A*-ing rests (at least in part) upon *S*'s already
having motivation capable of providing a partial (or complete)
positive motivational base for the generated motivational item.

(I shall use, as a convenient bit of shorthand, *'non-accidentally* to
produce in *S* motivation to *A*' for the clause between 'reasoning' and
'rests' in *MI.*)

It can be agreed on all sides that intentional action is motivated
action. Motivational externalism and motivational internalism are
distinguished by their respective claims about the capacity of
justificatory reasoning to generate motivation.

2. MOTIVATIONAL INTERNALISM: SOME UNSUCCESSFUL ARGUMENTS

The present section addresses some unsuccessful arguments for
motivational internalism. My aim, in part, is to eliminate from
contention familiar but specious or tendentious gronds for accepting
the view. In the following section I shall contend that the plausibility of
motivational internalism rests on the role that it plays in a general
theory of action-explanation.

The arguments to be examined here are introduced by way of a single
claim of Bernard Williams's in his much-discussed paper, "Internal and
External Reasons." Williams attributes the following position to the
motivational externalist: In some cases, (1) an agent acquires motivation
because, on the basis of correct deliberation, he comes to believe a
certain "external reasons statement," and (2) this motivation is acquired
independently of any antecedent motivation (p. 24). He rejects this
view on the grounds that "*ex hypothesi,* there is no motivation for the
agent to deliberate *from,* to reach his new motivation" (ibid.).

It will prove instructive to consider various strategies for supporting
Williams's claim, *WC,* that in the absence of motivation for the agent to
deliberate from, he cannot acquire the "new motivation" at issue — that
is, motivation resulting from the agent's believing, on the basis of
correct deliberation, a certain external reasons statement. Aristotle
held that deliberation is, *essentially,* reasoning with a view to the
achievement of a desired end, and Williams may be following him in
this.[13] Or he may have in mind a more complex line about deliberation

MOTIVATIONAL INTERNALISM

— perhaps that the nature of deliberation (as opposed, say, to purely theoretical reasoning) is such that deliberation cannot provide justification for an agent's performing an action, *A*, independently of his having some motivation that both prompts his deliberation and speaks in favor of his *A*-ing.

To be sure, all intentional activities, including intentional reasoning, are motivated activities. Thus, instances of intentional reasoning must be prompted by some motive or desire, broadly construed. But it does not follow from this alone that motivation generated by a bit of intentional reasoning must be derived, in the pertinent sense, from the motivation that prompted the reasoning. A student for whom morality is a purely academic matter, who cares not a whit whether his behavior is morally proper, may be motivated to reason about what it would be morally best to do in a particular situation by a desire to write a good paper on the topic. Although motivational externalists might claim that this reasoning can non-accidentally result in motivation to do the action deemed best, they would quite properly deny that motivation to perform this action has the student's desire *to write a good paper* as a partial motivational base.

If it is replied that the student's reasoning is theoretical and not practical or deliberative, on the grounds that it is addressed to a theoretical and not a practical question, motivational externalists have a straightforward response: Theoretical reasoning about the right or the good can generate motivation that is not derivative from antecedent motivation. To show that they are wrong about this some distinct argument is needed. Of course, Williams attributes to his opponents the view that *deliberation* generates the new, external motivation. But they may be operating with a less restrictive notion that includes theoretical reasoning about practical matters, or they may just make Williams a present of the word.

This brings us to the possibility of defending *WC* on the basis of considerations about justification that do not rest on a particular conception of deliberation. Williams may be thinking that no (hypothetical) intentional action is to any degree *justified* (or rational) unless it is supported by the agent's antecedent motivational set — a *normative* internalist thesis. From this it would follow that *no* reasoning, deliberative or otherwise, could produce justification for the performance of an action that is not supported by antecedent motivation.

A salient problem with this line of argument is that motivational externalists (but not *normative* externalists) can grant that any

423

ALFRED R. MELE

(hypothetical or prospective) action depends for its being justified (or rational) upon supporting motivation antecedent to the *performance of the action.* They can simply contend that in some cases the required motivation is produced by justificatory reasoning whose conclusion in no way derives its motivational force from motivation that is already present. It is also worth noting that Williams's argument for the *normative* internalist thesis identified in the preceding paragraph rests on the alleged truth of motivational internalism (pp. 26f.). So he cannot, without vicious circularity, use that thesis to establish the truth of motivational internalism.

One might want to contend, in support of *WC* and partly on the basis of an alleged connection between an agent's being justified (or rational) in *A*-ing and his having motivation to *A*, that the *production* of motivation by justificatory reasoning depends upon the existence in the agent of motivation to which the reasoning can appeal. But such an argument, if successful, would support *MI* directly: No detour through *WC* is required. In any event, in the absence of a compelling argument for *normative* internalism, motivational internalists should leave open the possibility that *A* may be the rational thing for an agent to do even in the absence of motivation that supports his *A*-ing, and they should focus their critical efforts on the idea that reasoning can "externally generate" motivation in such cases.

3. MOTIVATIONAL INTERNALISM VERSUS MOTIVATIONAL EXTERNALISM

Motivational internalists are in a position in offer a relatively straightforward account of the generation of motivation by reasoning. The strength of their view lies here. This strength and the corresponding weakness of motivational externalism ought to be emphasized in a defense of motivational internalism. The simplest internalistic model is an instrumentalist one: Reasoning generates motivation by identifying means to a desired end or by locating something that the reasoner wants, with the result that antecedent motivation is directed toward a certain (sort of) action or object (cf. Hume's *Treatise,* p. 459). This model, as we shall see, is *too* simple; but the necessary revisions can be made with a little effort.

Motivational *externalists* also owe us some explanation of the manner in which reasoning generates motivation — especially when reasoning is alleged to do so independently of antecedent motivation. If motivational externalists are unable to provide such an explanation, or even a sketch of one, their opponents have won a major battle.

424

MOTIVATIONAL INTERNALISM

Motivational externalism's contribution to this battle is the focus of the present section.

In assessing motivational externalism we must distinguish between two claims:

> (i) Justificatory reasoning can non-accidentally generate a motivational belief in *S* without any of *S*'s antecedent motivations entering into the justification offered for the belief.
>
> (ii) Justificatory reasoning can non-accidentally generate a motivational belief in *S* without that belief's deriving its motivational force (even in part) from any of *S*'s antecedent motivations.

The following case illustrates a crucial difference between (i) and (ii). Suppose that Sarah is presented with, and convinced by, the following argument, and that her concluding belief has motivational force.

> 1. The great majority of people believe that *X* is good.
> 2. Whatever the great majority of people believe is probably true.
> ∴ 3. *X* is probably good.

Perhaps Sarah's believing (3) can have motivational force even though her believing (1) and her believing (2) do not. Perhaps although Sarah is not at all motivated by her belief about what the majority take to be good, nor by her belief that majority opinion establishes probable truth, once she comes to believe that *X* is probably good she is motivated to pursue it. If so, Sarah confirms (i). But she may confirm (i) without confirming (ii); for although none of Sarah's antecedent motivations enters into the justification offered for the conclusion, her concluding belief might still derive its motivational force from antecedent motivation of hers. It may well be the case, for example, that Sarah's concluding belief derives its motivational force from an antecedent motivational interest in goodness.

Proponents of the version of motivational internalism that I am advocating (*MI*) can readily grant (i); for they do not insist that some appeal to antecedent motivation must be involved in assent to the *premises* of a justificatory, motivation-producing argument, but only that justificatory reasoning cannot non-accidentally generate a motivational item whose force is wholly non-derivative from some antecedent motivation or other of the agent. The fact that the motivational force of the conclusion of a particular bit of reasoning is not derivative from motivation associated with the premises of that reasoning is quite compatible with its being derivative from *other*

ALFRED R. MELE

antecedent motivation. Claim (ii) is the central point of contenton. Motivational externalists owe us some explanation of its (alleged) truth.

It is not easy to see what form this explanation should take. Suppose that, on the basis of justificatory reasoning, S believes that A is B (e.g., that A is good, or morally right, or likely to contribute to Fred's well-being). How can S be motivated by this belief if she is not already motivated to some degree to pursue, promote, etc., what she takes to be B? If S is not antecedently motivated to promote Fred's well-being, how can her belief that her A-ing would help Fred provide her with motivation to A?

Some answers are beside the point. Perhaps someone's forming a belief on the basis of justificatory reasoning can trigger a post-hypnotic suggestion to be motivated in accordance with one's acceptance of the conclusion of the first convincing practical argument offered to one by Brown on Tuesday.[14] Perhaps, in some possible world, an internal biological mechanism occasionally brings it about, entirely independently of the agent's antecedent motivations, that she is motivated to do an action of type A when she comes to believe that A is B on the basis of reasoning. Or, one might suppose, the juxtaposition of thoughts of A and B in an agent's consciousness may directly result in her being motivated to do A even though she has no antecedent motivation concerning either of A and B. But these possibilities are not enough for motivational externalists. Their concern, presumably, is not with highly artificial cases, but rather with cases in which human beings *in quite ordinary circumstances* are "externally motivated" by justificatory reasoning. What externalists must explain, given the empirical nature of their thesis, is how there can be cases of the *latter* sort in which agents are motivated precisely in virtue of their coming to see the truth of an external reasons statement.[15]

More can be said about the preceding hypotheses, but it should be kept brief. An effective post-hypnotic suggestion to A under conditions C is plausibly regarded as creating a latent desire to A under C. Further, on the juxtaposition hypothesis, it is not in virtue of the apprehension of truth that the agent is motivated to do A; rather, it is the juxtaposition of thoughts of A and B that does the trick. And given that motivational externalism (like motivational internalism) is an empirical thesis, proponents of this view cannot take much comfort in the mere possibility of the above-mentioned biological mechanism.

One might suggest that, in the case of a motivational belief that A is B, motivation for B need not be present prior to S's acquiring the belief

MOTIVATIONAL INTERNALISM

and that the motivation may itself be non-accidentally generated, independently of antecedent motivation, by the justificatory reasoning that prompted the belief. But this simply pushes the original problem up another level. How is the motivation for B generated by the reasoning?[16]

Now, owing to a significant similarity between B and C, one who has no antecedent motivational interest in B might nevertheless be motivated to pursue B as a partial result of acquring the belief that A is B. Suppose that we try to convince S to A by demonstrating to her that her A-ing would help Fred, and suppose that she has no antecedent motivational interest in helping Fred in particular nor people in general. Suppose, however, that in showing her how her A-ing would help Fred (which is part of demonstrating to her that her A-ing would help Fred), we cause S to see Fred's plight as significantly like that of her beloved brother, with the result that S's belief that her A-ing would help Fred motivates her to A. S's motivation to A might not derive from any antecedent motivation to help Fred: We may suppose that she is not motivated to help him prior to forming the belief that A-ing would help. But, of course, the motivational externalist cannot infer from this that the motivation is wholly nonderivative from antecedent motivation. Indeed, it certainly looks as though her "new" motivation has a positive motivational base consisting, in part at least, of some motivation concerning her brother.

Consider the following externalistic move. Granted, a person cannot (under normal conditions) be motivated by justificatory reasoning in a particular case unless she has the *capacity to be motivated* by that bit of reasoning. But this capacity need not involve motivation, either dispositional or occurrent, that the agent has at the time. Consequently, motivation produced (under normal conditions) by practical reasoning need not be derivative, even in part, from antecedent motivation.

In what might the alleged motivational capacity consist in a particular case, if it does not involve items in the agent's motivational set? Stephen Darwall maintains that "a person's motivational capacities, in the broadest sense, are not constituted simply by his desires but also by capacities of imagination, sensitivity, and so on."[17] However, motivational externalists can effectively use the "capacity" argument only if they can at least *sketch* a plausible account of how it is that justificatory reasoning, with the assistance of certain capacities, non-accidentally generates motivational items whose motivational force is wholly non-derivative from antecedent motivation. Moreover, they owe us (and themselves) an account of the capacities in question that is

427

ALFRED R. MELE

detailed enough to support the claim that they do not involve anteceden
motivation.

Though the extended example that Darwall offers of the generation
of motivation by a desire-independent process features perceptual
experience rather than justificatory reasoning, brief consideration of
the case will prove instructive. Darwall's heroine, Roberta, first "sees a
film that vividly presents the plight of textile workers in the southern
United States," and then attends a discussion about what might be done
to alleviate the situation.[18] Even though she had no prior general desire
to relieve suffering, she is "shocked and dismayed by the suffering she
sees," and she "decides" — and desires — to help these unfortunate
people by promoting a boycott.

Darwall contends that Roberta "may have had no desire prior to
viewing the film that explains her decision to join the boycott." But this
strikes me as quite implausible. Suppose that Roberta had no antecedent
latent desire to relieve any suffering whatever — either her own or that
of loved ones. What would explain her being "*shocked* and *dismayed* by
the suffering she sees"? How could she have the feelings about suffering,
or the appreciation of it, necessary for a depiction of suffering to be
shocking and dismaying to her? Darwall may appreciate the force of the
question; for he mentions the possibility of Roberta's having been
moved in the past by the suffering of family, friends, and pets, and he
says only that Roberta has no *general desire* to relieve suffering — that
is, no desire to relieve suffering in general. This is consonant with the
very likely hypothesis that the film helped Roberta to feel about the
suffering of the textile workers and their families something akin to
what she already is disposed to feel about her own occasional suffering,
or the occasional suffering of loved ones and friends. This is not to say
that she desires to aid the textile workers as a means to satisfying some
more general desire or hers concerning suffering. Rather, the point is
that a very plausible etiology of her desire to help these people does
include pertinent antecedent motivation of hers — and in such a way as
to locate the antecedent motivation in the positive motivational base of
the desire. And, again, it is difficult to see how the desire to assist the
workers could have been generated by the documentary in the absence
of antecedent motivation concerning, for example, her own suffering or
the suffering of people close to her.

My aim thus far has been to articulate a promising version of
motivational internalism and to display its plausibility. The structure of
my argument for *MI* as against externalist competitors is quite simple
MI is part of a general theory of the etiology of intentional behavior

428

MOTIVATIONAL INTERNALISM

that seems capable of explaining how reasoning generates motivation. Conversely, it seems quite mysterious how, under ordinary circumstances and independently of appropriate antecedent motivation, a human being may acquire motivation to do *A* simply in virtue of her acquiring a belief that *A* is *B*. Motivational externalism smacks of creation *ex nihilo*.[19]

One might think that, mysterious or not, motivational externalism is something that we must learn to live with. Some might see no alternative, if they want, with Nagel, "some guarantee that reasons will provide a motive" and are convinced that there are external reasons.[20] Discussion of these matters is reserved for Section 4.

I condlude this section with a brief comment on an objection to the line that I have been pressing. Thomas Reid, in his *Essays on the Active Powers of Man*, contends that Hume's view on the relationship of reason to motivation can be defended only "by a gross and palpable abuse of words."[21] Reid's claim is that Hume helps himself to a victory by inventing a distinction between passion and reason that, contrary to ordinary usage, entails that everything motivational falls on the side of passion and passion alone. One may want to charge me with having done the same. Notice, however, that if sense can be given to the idea that reason has its own reservoir of motivation, *MI* does not commit one to insisting that reasoning can non-accidentally motivate only if it benefits from the existence of some reason-extrinsic (i.e., purely "passional" or "non-rational") motivation. *MI* does not specify the *sort* of motivation that justificatory reasoning relies upon when it generates motivation in virtue of its producing a belief. It insists only that (in human beings as they actually are) there is *some* antecedent motivational base for the generated motivation.

4. IMPLICATIONS OF MOTIVATIONAL INTERNALISM?

It is time now to inquire about implications of the version of motivational internalism that I have been defending. In the present section I ask first to what extent my position limits the powers of practical reasoning. In particular, does the motivational thesis that I have defended warrant Hume's contention (*Treatise,* p. 415) that "reason is, and ought to be, the slave of the passions, and can never pretend to any other office than to serve and obey them"? Toward the end of the section, I address the question whether motivational internalism entails normative internalism. My aim is to undercut familiar normatively based objections to motivational internalism by

429

ALFRED R. MELE

showing that the view does not have normative implications often
claimed for it.

We may begin by noting that not all practical reasoning is concerned
with identifying means to ends.[22] For example, an agent may engage in
practical reasoning about what would *constitute* his achieving a certain
desired end. Someone who wants to have the most impressive garden
on the block may need to reason not only about means to this end but
also about the qualities that his garden must have if it is to be the best on
the block. This point is compatible with Hume's master/slave metaphor
only if the latter can be so interpreted as to allow reason(ing) (on some
occasions) to decide what its master is commanding (when, e.g., it
commands that *S* have the most impressive garden on the block).

Moreover, the metaphor must be so interpreted that it permits
reason(ing) to make some decisions without having to appeal to a
higher master. Consider the following example. Theresa, a young
woman who is about to graduate from high school, has a burning desire
to do something important with her life. She wants this, not as a means
to a further goal, but simply as an end. However, because she has no
clear idea exactly what would constitute her goal, Theresa's desire gives
her little direction. Undaunted, she sets out to determine what it would
be to live an important life. She starts by examining the sorts of life that,
in her opinion, many people think to be important. Some of the
life-types, she decides, are not all that they are cracked up to be. For
example, any life dominated by a concern to make money is, she thinks,
irrational, since money has no intrinsic value. On the basis of various
items in her motivational set, she eliminates several other candidates:
She will commit herself to no type of life that is incompatible with her
being honest, bearing and raising at least one child, and so on. But she is
still left with a number of candidates and with a crucial question: If
these lives are important, what makes them so? She decides that she had
wrongly been thinking that a necessary condition of doing something
important with one's life is that one is thought by many to be an
important person; and she gradually comes to believe that truly
important lives have at least this in common: They are led by loving,
unselfish, autonomous individuals who are dedicated to the achievement
of a lofty goal or goals and possessed of strong moral character, and
who, in pursuing their goals, make a significant contribution to the
amelioration of the human condition. *This* is the kind of person she
now wants to be; these are the traits that she wants to exhibit. And after
further reflection she decides that, given her various talents, *she* can
best live an "important life" in the political realm.

430

MOTIVATIONAL INTERNALISM

Theresa's reflection and conclusions were undoubtedly influenced by items in her antecedent motivational set, but the process by which she reached her conclusions was not one of *discovering* some item in this set. Rather, through reflection, she developed a new, more detailed conception of a certain goal; and the newly acquired goal — living an important life, under the developed conception — supplanted the old one. (Notice that the content of what I have called the new goal is not that of Theresa's former desire to live an important life. For this reason, it is properly counted as a new goal.)

It is worth noting in passing that the case of Theresa gives some sense to the idea, embraced by Reid and others, of a motivational reservoir possessed by reason.[23] While reason has no special claim to instrumental desires that reasoning helps to generate, there may be some point in distinguishing reasoned from unreasoned desires for *ends*.

In any case, Hume's "slave" metaphor (whatever his own substantive position may have been) plainly cannot accommodate the observations made in the last few paragraphs. Slaves who are free to reject one master in favor of another and to fashion their own masters are not slaves at all (provided that they retain this freedom even after the "master" is chosen or fashioned). The version of motivational internalism that I have defended does not relegate reason (nor reason*ing*) to a subordinate role in directing an agent's behavior.

I have thus far been concerned with a non-normative question: What sense is properly given to the claim that reasoning cannot generate motivation independently of antecedent motivation? On what interpretation(s) of the claim is it most plausible? However, this question is sometimes thought to have an important bearing upon such normative questions as whether it can be *rational* for S to A if she has no antecedent motivation that supports her A-ing, and whether there can be *good reason* for S to A if nothing in S's motivational set supports her A-ing.[24]

The purpose of the remainder of this section is to show that the version of motivational internalism that I have been developing does not, by itself, entail normative internalism. From

> *MI.* Actual human beings and the real world are such that the capacity of justificatory reasoning to generate in a human being, S, a motivational item whose object is S's A-ing and to do this in virtue of that reasoning's providing S with what she takes to be justification for A-ing rests (at least in part) upon S's already having motivation capable of providing a partial (or complete) positive motivational base for the generated motivational item

431

ALFRED R. MELE

it does not follow, at least directly, that

> *NI.* There is good reason for S to A (and it is rational for her to do so) only if some member of S's antecedent motivational set would be served or furthered by her A-ing.

The following thesis goes some of the way toward filling the gap:

> *R.* There is good reason for S to A (and it is rational for her to do so) only if justificatory reasoning in support of her A-ing can, given S's antecedent motivational set, produce in her motivation to do A in virtue of its providing her with what she takes to be justification for A-ing.[25]

But the proponent of R must come to grips with what is, at least *prima facie,* an important distinction — namely, the distinction introduced earlier between motivational and justificatory reasons for action.

The relevance of this distinction is plain. R postulates a tight connection between what there is good reason for an agent to do and the agent's antecedent motivational set. However, the distinction between motivational and justificatory reasons points the way to a kind of reason-for-S-to-A that is in no way grounded in S's antecedent motivational set. The alleged existence of such reasons — "external reasons" — lies at the heart of the dispute between normative internalists and normative externalists.[26] Suppose that there are such reasons. And suppose that, in some cases, the rational course of action is dictated by such reasons. Then there may be cases in which there is good reason for S to A, even though S's antecedent motivational set is such that justificatory reasoning in support of her A-ing cannot do what R requires it to do. The crucial point, for present purposes, is that motivational internalists need not take a stand on these matters. *MI* is neutral on the question of the existence of external reasons. Normative externalists who accept *MI* may direct their attack at R.

Rachel Cohon has suggested that the task of "the defender of external reasons" is to find "some rational way in which an agent can come to be moved to act on an external reason."[27] Her claim here is that an external reasons theorist must identify a way in which an agent can be rationally moved to act on (or for) a reason that is not part of S's antecedent motivational set and in no way derives its motivational force from that set. A few lines later, intending to make the same point, she says that "external reasons theorists ... must find considerations that can obtain regardless of the agent's desires, aims, or sentiments, that would move the agent to action if she were well informed and thinking rationally."[28]

432

MOTIVATIONAL INTERNALISM

Part of what I have just been suggesting, in effect, is that the task described in the latter passage is not the one described in the former. Even if *no* agent's believing an external reasons statement can motivate her in the way — whatever it may be — that motivational externalists want to claim such beliefs can motivate, it does not follow that *there are no* external reasons. Nor does it follow that normative externalists cannot find considerations of the sort that, in the second passage, Cohon says they must find. It is open to normative externalists to argue that, precisely because certain agents lack certain antecedent motivations (e.g., a desire to be fair), they cannot reason rationally about some matters. Perhaps, because of the subject matter, rational reasoning about certain questions must be *impartial* reasoning; and some agents may be incapable of reasoning impartially about certain issues in the absence of a desire to be fair. Its being true that there is *no* "rational way in which [any] agent can come to be moved to act on an external reason" is quite compatible with its also being true that considerations *C,* which, as it happens, in no way rest upon a particular *S*'s antecedent motivational set, "would move [*S*] to action if she were well informed and thinking rationally." For it may be that rational (or wellinformed) thinking about the matter at hand depends upon one's having antecedent motivation of a sort that would render *C* motivational. Thus, it may be true that if *S* were well informed and thinking rationally, she would be moved by *C* — even though, given her antecedent motivational set, *C* cannot move her in the way that motivational externalists claim external reasons are capable of moving agents.

It is sometimes held that if *N* is to be a reason for *A*-ing relative to an agent, *S, N* must be capable of being a reason *for which S A*-s — that is, a reason that would help *explain S*'s *A*-ing. This view entails that statements, propositions, and the like cannot be reasons for action, since such things themselves would not help explain (in the requisite way) an agent's action. Rather, *S*'s having some sort of *attitude* toward these things would do the explanatory work at issue. But normative externalists can resist this view and make a case for an alternative conception of the connection between reasons *for which* agents act and the reasons that *there are* for agents to act.

Do *moral* reasons have a special motivational status? Must moral reasons be motivational because, say, morality is essentially practical or *action-guiding?* Would a morality be less than practical if it offered reasons for a particular agent to *A* that, given her antecedent motivational set, could not motivate her? I do not see why. The

433

ALFRED R. MELE

prescription of an essentially practical morality for such an agent may be moral education. And, as we all know, moral education is not accomplished only, nor even primarily, through justificatory reasoning. An agent's motivational set can be modified and enriched in other ways (e.g., through operant conditioning).

I do not wish to champion normative externalism. Rather, my point in the last few paragraphs is that if *MI* does support *NI*, it does so only in conjunction with something like *R* — a controversial principle that is not itself entailed by *MI*. Normative internalists cannot establish their position simply by appealing to motivational internalism. There is more to be done; and what reamins does not promise to be easy. Normative *externalists* need not seek to preserve their view by attacking *MI*. Again, they can focus their attack on *R* and its ilk.

My primary purpose in this papar has been to explain what sense ought to be given to the Humean/Aristotelian contention that reasoning cannot generate motivation independently of antecedent motivation, and to make a case for the view on the basis of its strengths and motivational externalism's weaknesses. The underlying idea, I have argued, is quite plausible. But, properly interpreted, it does not (by itself) have the normative implications that are sometimes claimed for it. Nor does it commit one to understanding reason(ing) as a mere instrument, or slave, of the passions.[29]

DAVIDSON COLLEGE
DAVIDSON, NORTH CAROLINA 28036
USA

NOTES

[1] See, e.g., Kurt Baier, "The Social Source of Reason" *Proceedings of the American Philosophical Association* 51 (1978); David Brink, "Externalist Moral Realism," *Southern Journal of Philosophy* 24 (1986); Stephen Darwall, *Impartial Reason* (Ithaca: Cornell University Press, 1983), Ch. 5; W.D. Falk, "'Ought' and Motivation," *Proceedings of the Aristotelian Society* 48 (1947/48); William Frankena, "Obligation and Motivation in Recent Moral Philosophy," in A. Melden, ed., *Essays in Moral Philosophy* (Seattle: University of Washington Press, 1958); Christine Korsgaard, "Skepticism About Practical Reason," *Journal of Philosophy* 83 (1986); Thomas Nagel, *The Possibility of Altruism* (Oxford: Oxford University Press, 1970), Ch. 2; Thomas Nagel, "Value," in S. McMurrin,

MOTIVATIONAL INTERNALISM

ed., *The Tanner Lectures on Human Values,* vol. 1 (Salt Lake City: University of Utah Press, 1980); Bernard Williams, "Internal and External Reasons," in R. Harrison, ed., *Rational Action: Studies in Philosophy and Social Science* (Cambridge: Cambridge University Press, 1979), reprinted in Williams, *Moral Luck* (Cambridge: Cambridge University Press, 1981).

2   Frankena, p. 41.

3   Aristotle, *Nicomachean Ethics* VI. 2 1139a35f.; in W. Ross, ed., *Works of Aristotle,* Vol. 9 (London: Oxford University Press, 1915); David Hume, *A Treatise of Human Nature,* ed., L.A. Selby-Bigge (Oxford: Oxford University Press, 1888), p. 415. For a defense of the suggested reading of Aristotle, see my "Aristotle on the Roles of Reason in Motivation and Justification," *Archiv für Geschichte der Philosophie* 66 (1984).

4   Williams, p. 17.

5   See, e.g., Hutcheson's and Frankena's distinction between "exciting" and "justifying" reasons. Francis Hutcheson, "Illustrations on the Moral Sense," in L. Selby-Bigge, ed., *British Moralists* (Oxford: Clarendon Press, 1897), pp. 403ff. Frankena, p. 44.

6   For a recent argument to this effect, see Brink.

7   That Green will have his neck broken if he does not do *A* may be a reason for him to do *A,* the charitable action; but it is not a reason for him to *be* charitable, nor to act from charitable motives.

8   "Internal and External Reasons," p. 20.

9   See, for example, William Alston, "Motives and Motivation," in P. Edwards, ed., *The Encyclopedia of Philosophy* (New York: Macmillan, 1967), and Alvin Goldman, *A Theory of Human Action* (Englewood Cliffs: Prentice-Hall, 1970), Ch. 4. The terminology varies.

10   For an explication and defense of the notion of motivational strength, see my *Irrationality: An Essay on Akrasia, Self-Deception, and Self-Control* (New York: Oxford University Press, 1987), pp. 11–15.

11   An *intrinsic* desire to *A* — that is, a desire whose object (one's *A*-ing) is desired as an *end* — is at least partially constitutive of its own motivational base. On this point, see my *Irrationality,* pp. 67f.

12   See, for example, Walter Mischel and Bert Moore, "The Role of Ideation in Voluntary Delay for Symbolically Presented Rewards," *Cognitive Therapy and Research* 4 (1980): 211–221; Walter Mischel and Harriet Mischel, "Self-Control and the Self," in T. Mischel, ed., *The Self: Psychological and Philosophical Issues* (Oxford: Basil Blackwell, 1977), pp. 31–64. For a discussion of the philosophical significance of recent experimental work on delay of gratification, see my *Irrationality,* pp. 89–95.

13   See, for example, *Nicomachean Ethics,* III. 3 and VI. 2.

14   Cf. Rachel Cohon, "Are External Reasons Impossible?" *Ethics* 96 (1986), p. 549.

15   Cf. Williams's description of externalism in "Internal and External Reasons," p. 24.

16   E.J. Bond claims that *S*'s desiring *X* is a necessary causal consequence of *S*'s acquiring a true belief that *X* is a value; and, for Bond, "all value is *necessarily*

ALFRED R. MELE

objective, in the sense that it is never a function of desire." See his *Reason and Value* (Cambridge: Cambridge University Press, 1983), pp. 69, 84. However, as Jan Narveson observes in his review of Bond's book (*Dialogue* 23 [1984], p. 329), Bond offers no explanation of the motivation-independent generation of a desire by the belief that something is good.

17   Darwall, p. 39.

18   Darwall, pp. 39f.

19   Christine Korsgaard argues that Hume's "skepticism about the scope of reason as a motive ... is entirely dependent upon his ... skepticism about what reason has to *say* about choice and action" (p. 7). It is worth noting that my argument against motivational externalism does not depend upon presuppositions about the propositional content of reason's pronouncements. What is problematic about motivational externalism is the supposed generation of motivation by justificatory reasoning alone — whatever the propositional content of its conclusions may be.

20   *The Possibility of Altruism,* p. 28.

21   Thomas Reid, *Essays on the Active Powers of Man* (Edinburgh: J. Bell, 1788), p. 212.

22   Cf. Williams, p. 20.

23   Reid, Essay 3, Ch. 2. The idea is at least as old as Plato. See, e.g., *Phaedrus* 237d9–238a2. Aristotle's notion of wish (*boulesis*), the only form of desire located in the "rational part of the soul" (e.g., *De Anima* 432b5), is particularly well-suited to the case of Theresa. On this last point, see my "Aristotle's Wish," *Journal of the History of Philosophy* 22 (1984).

24   See, e.g., Williams, pp. 26f.

25   Williams plainly is attracted to *R,* or something very similar. He contends at one point that an "external reasons statement itself might be taken as roughly equivalent to, or at least as entailing, the claim that if the agent rationally deliberated, then, whatever motivations he originally had, he would come to be motivated to *X*" (p. 24); and he asks a bit later (pp. 24f.): "*What* is it that one comes to believe when he comes to believe that there is reason for him to *X*, if it is not the proposition, or something that entails the proposition, that if he deliberated rationally, he would be motivated to act appropriately?"

26   Cf. Darwall, p. 51.

27   Cohon, p. 556

28   Cohon, p. 556

29   A distant ancestor of this paper was written for a 1984 NEH institute on human action directed by Robert Audi at the University of Nebraska. Another was composed during my tenure of a 1985/86 NEH Fellowship for College Teachers. Thanks are due to the NEH for its support and to Robert Audi, Joe Beatty, Richard Brandt, Irwin Goldstein, John Heil, Brad Hooker, David McNaughton, M.P. Smith, Lance Stell, and Art Walker for their comments on earlier drafts.

[4]

*—*The Presidential Address*

WHY THERE IS REALLY NO SUCH THING AS THE THEORY OF MOTIVATION

by Jonathan Dancy

One of the very many distinctions influential in moral theory is that between motivating and justifying reasons. According to this distinction there is a difference between the reasons why an action is or was right and the reasons why the agent did the action. As a distinction, this is quite uncontentious. It is perfectly obvious that the reasons why an agent did the action may not be reasons why it is right, either because it was not right or because, though it was right, the reasons why it was right were not the reasons why the agent did it. Contention comes in when we try to give an account of the two sides of the distinction, to back up and make theoretical sense of the difference. The theoretical account that I want to reject is one that is becoming increasingly common in the literature of moral theory. This account takes justifying reasons to be facts about the world, and motivating reasons to be combinations of beliefs and desires. The most striking feature of this account is that no justifying reason can be a motivating reason and no motivating reason a justifying one. The two classes of reason come to be seen as mutually exclusive.

I will eventually come to look at the arguments underlying this account. For the moment I want to elaborate on the importance attributed to the distinction, so understood. One use to which it has been put is in the attempt to undermine internalism in the theory of moral judgement. William Frankena, who is responsible for the account in its present form, argued that the internalist claim that moral facts are capable of motivating in their own right succumbs

*Meeting of the Aristotelian Society, held in the Senior Common Room, Birkbeck College, London, on Monday, 17th October, 1994 at 8.15 p.m.

2   JONATHAN DANCY

to the motivating/justifying distinction.[1] A moral fact is a justifying
reason for action, and thoughts about what is capable of motivating
in its own right belong not in the theory of justifying reasons but in
that of motivating ones. It is a simple mistake to suppose that the
commitment to moral facts as justifying reasons carries with it a
commitment to any view about motivation. This mistake is covered
up by the use of phrases like 'the moral fact is in and of itself a
reason for acting', read as a remark about motivation.

More subtle, perhaps, is David Brink's appeal to the distinction in
his attack on internalism.[2] He uses it to divide internalism into two
halves—internalism about motivation and internalism about reasons.
Brink argues, not as Frankena does that the motivating/justifying
distinction is itself sufficient to disprove internalist claims, but that
once we recognise the distinction, we can disentangle matters well
enough to see that internalism about motivation is false for moral
judgements, and internalism about reasons is false for moral facts.
Motive internalism is false because it is at least possible for an agent
to be totally indifferent to what she allows to be morally relevant
considerations, since she lacks the necessary desires. Internalism
about reasons is false because it is not incoherent to admit that one
has a moral obligation to act but to ask whether this gives one any
reason to act.

A second use of the distinction, with which I will be more concerned, is to defend some form of Humeanism in the theory of
motivation.[3] The suggestion here is that attempts to deny the truth of
Humean belief/desire theory appeal to considerations that properly
belong to the theory of justifying reasons, and that are improperly
transferred to the theory of motivation. We make a mistake if, having
accepted that there are facts about what is right and wrong (thus
becoming realists in the theory of justifying reasons), we then
suppose that this gives us ground for a purely cognitive theory of
motivation (i.e. a non-Humean one). The common suggestion is that
this is what protagonists of cognitive theories of motivation have

---

1   W. Frankena, 'Obligation and Motivation', in A. I. Melden ed. *Essays in Moral Philo-
    sophy* (Seattle: University of Washington Press, 1958), at pp. 43–5.

2   D. Brink *Moral Realism and the Foundations of Ethics* (Cambridge: Cambridge Uni-
    versity Press, 1989), ch. 3.

3   See M. Smith *The Moral Problem*, (Oxford: Blackwell, 1984), esp. ch. 4.2. I am very
    grateful to Michael Smith for his repeated attempts to explain his view to me.

done, and that it is necessarily an error because the theory of motivation is quite distinct from the theory of justifying reasons. So different are these theories supposed to be that we even read that the word 'reason' is ambiguous, and that this ambiguity is offered as the explanation of why people find it so easy to slide from thoughts about one sort of reason to thoughts about the other.

The mistake that we cognitivists have made, supposedly, is to notice that Hume was wrong about justifying reasons, and to suppose that in order to show this we have to show that he was wrong about motivating ones, or that since he is wrong in the one area he must also be wrong in the other. The distinction is thus used as part of the defence of Humeanism in the theory of motivation. It is also used, similarly, to reconcile a broadly Humean theory of motivation with some form of realism about values. It has been common to see some form of subjectivism or projectivism supported by remarks in the theory of motivation. But this is a mistake. Nothing in the theory of motivation could have such consequences, because of the sheer ambiguity in the notion of a reason.

At its most extreme, therefore, the role of the distinction is to create a limited area for Hume to have been right about. To the extent, then, that we set our face against admitting the truth of Humeanism in the theory of motivation, to that extent we are probably going to feel that there is no such thing as the theory of motivation, so conceived, at all. And that will be the position that this paper is trying to defend, though not only for this reason.

It might seem miraculous that so much can be extracted from the little distinction with which we started, between the reasons why an action was right and the agent's reasons for doing it. It is not so much the distinction itself which is the culprit, however, as the account of it that sees motivating reasons as complexes of beliefs and desires, i.e. as complexes of psychological states of whatever sort, and sees justifying reasons as truths. It is this account, which puts into form the attempt to combine value realism with Humean philosophical psychology, that leads to the results I have outlined above.

I

Let us start by taking it as a maxim in the theory of practical reason in general that reasons must be at least potentially explanatory of

actions. A reason must be something for which someone could have acted, and in any case where someone does act for that reason, the reason contributes to the explanation of her action.

This maxim is already in conflict with the account of the distinction between motivating and justifying reasons that I outlined above. For the maxim appears to say that justifying reasons must be capable of being motivating ones, and this is directly denied by the claim that motivating reasons are beliefs and desires, while justifying reasons are truths. The categorial difference between truth and psychological state means that no one thing could be a reason of both sorts.

One would suppose, therefore, that protagonists of the account would deny the maxim—or, more probably, admit it of motivating reasons but deny it of justifying ones. In fact, however, some do and some don't. Michael Smith is one of those who don't. Almost the only thing that reasons of the two sorts have in common, according to him, is that they are potentially capable of rendering actions intelligible. But it is hard to see how this can be true within the constraints that he accepts. According to his picture, it is complexes of beliefs and desires that explain the occurrence of actions, and truths do not contribute to this at all. They *do* contribute, of course, to the explanation of why the action was right; but the maxim does not concern itself with that sort of explanation at all. So it seems that justifying reasons fall foul of the maxim.

There is one move that could be made in reply to this complaint, which is that not all talk of 'rendering an action intelligible' is talk of explaining the action. The idea might be that the notion of rendering intelligible is itself ambiguous between justifying an action and explaining it. But to make sense of this we have to ask what the difference between rendering intelligible and explaining is supposed to be. To this question we will not find any very satisfactory answer.

One suggestion that Smith has made to me in correspondence is as follows. Suppose that someone returns a wallet that she found in the street to its owner. Without having the slightest idea why she did this, we already think that it is an intelligible thing to do. And the reason why we think of it as intelligible is that it is right. So justifying reasons necessarily render intelligible the actions they justify. But they do not thereby *explain* them.

IS THERE A THEORY OF MOTIVATION?   5

There are two things wrong with this attempt as it stands. The first is the idea that if an action is right, it is at least intelligible, whatever the agent's reasons for doing it. This idea of a sort of intelligibility which prescinds from the agent's reasons leaves us with too little to work on. One is tempted to say that if we do not take into account the reasons why the agent did it, we are not yet in a position to ask the question whether the action is intelligible. There is no such thing as an intelligibility that can be established in this way, irrespective of reasons.[4] What we do get from the thought that the action was right is that it is at least intelligible that someone should have done the action, provided that they did it for the reasons that in fact make it right, and understanding them as such. But this does nothing to show that justifying reasons render actions intelligible. What in this case renders the relevant action intelligible is the beliefs and desires that led to it and explain it—the motivating reasons.

The second difficulty is that unjustified, wrong actions are as intelligible, and for the same reasons, as justified ones. If someone finds a wallet, the action of returning it to its owner is no more intelligible than that of keeping quiet. If we had to list in advance, that is, all the intelligible actions which the finder of the wallet might do, prominent among them might be keeping the money for himself.

One might suggest now that there are good reasons for keeping the money, even if they are not good moral reasons. The action of keeping the money is as well grounded in reasons (e.g. in the fact that he has a good use for the money) as is that of handing it back. Just as justifying theoretical reasons do not show the beliefs which they justify to be true, but only reasonable, so justifying practical reasons do not show the actions they justify to be right, but only rational. The idea that wrong, unjustified actions are as intelligible as right ones, taken as an objection to Smith, turns out to be a mistake based on an equivocation between 'justified' as 'right' and 'justified' as 'rational'; in the second sense, wrong actions are as justified, and hence as intelligible, as right ones are.

---

4   It may be possible to establish a reason-free intelligibility in another way; Freud springs to mind.

6   JONATHAN DANCY

Smith however rejects this line of defence. I can think of two
reasons one might have for doing that. The first is that though there
are reasons for doing the wrong thing, the balance of reasons always
favours the right one. I don't accept this in general. I think that there
can sometimes be more reason to do the wrong thing. The second
is that he takes all justifying reasons to be *normative* truths. Again,
I don't accept this. According to me, some are normative truths and
some are not. For instance, the distress I will cause her if I plough
on is a reason for me to stop, and the truth that I will distress her is
not a normative truth. So I don't accept Smith's view that it is
morally right actions that are specially intelligible, rather than more
generally the ones for which there is most reason.

The reason he gives for his claim that right actions are antecedently intelligible in a way that wrong actions are not is an appeal
to the theory of interpretation. Just as in the interpretation of
utterance there is a preference for attributing true beliefs to the
Other rather than false ones, so in the interpretation of action there
will be a preference for attributing true *normative* beliefs to agents.
And if there is this preference, there will be an associated preference
for attributing consonant motivation to them. This gives us an
antecedent preference for seeing our agents as doing right actions
rather than wrong ones, since we should always prefer an interpretation which has the agent rightly believing that the balance of
reasons favours her action. We can redescribe this preference by
saying that justified, right actions enjoy a greater degree of antecedent intelligibility.

Whether this approach is sound depends on the reason for
believing that in radical interpretation we must understand the Other
as largely believing the truth. As I understand it, the argument is that
we have no alternative to identifying the truth conditions of the
Other's utterances with the events which cause them. The circumstances of radical interpretation mean that the Other will always be
interpreted as believing the true if this is possible. Now if this is the
argument, it seems to me that there are several significant differences between the situation of radical interpretation and the
situation we find ourselves in when we are attempting to assign
normative beliefs to other agents. Quite apart from the fact that the
situation is not the radical one, the beliefs we are here dealing with
are not concerned with our immediate surroundings, nor are the

contents of those beliefs 'occasion sentences', in any recognisable sense of Quine's phrase. What is more, the reason for attributing true beliefs to the Other does not extend to require us to attribute desires consonant to those beliefs. The reason for doing that is quite different, namely the sense that if we do it we end up with less to explain than if we don't.

So I do not accept the reason Smith gives for holding that right actions are antecedently intelligible in a way that wrong ones are not. But even if what he says about the requirements of radical interpretation were true, it would not have the consequences he claims. It is not that wrong actions would be antecedently unintelligible in some way, but only that the attribution of right ones, so far as one can, would be the only possible interpretational strategy. At the end of the day, intelligible wrong actions are intelligible in just the same sense as right ones are.

The same result holds even if we do not claim greater antecedent intelligibility for *morally right* actions, as Smith does, but for the actions for which there is the most reason. (This might include some wrong actions.) Suppose that the requirements of radical interpretation force us to attribute to our agents, so far as we can, the true belief that there is more reason to do what they are doing than to do anything else. This would not have the consequence that actions of which such beliefs are true are intelligible in a different sense from those of which the belief is false. As long as there is sufficient reason for the action, it is intelligible in just the same sense as would have been the action for which there is more reason.

There remains something that has not yet come to light. I try to tease it out by offering a picture of the situation which is different from Smith's, but which accepts the need to attribute true beliefs wherever possible. According to this picture we first establish a list of actions which the person engaged in a certain set of bodily movements might *intelligibly* be doing. This list evinces no preference for the right over the wrong. Then we attempt to attribute suitable beliefs and desires to the agent for each of the most plausible candidates on the list. *At this stage* there is a preference for true beliefs, and possibly for consonant motivation. It is not, therefore, that right actions are more intelligible than wrong ones. The preference for the right appears at another, later point.

8   JONATHAN DANCY

This picture is inadequate, in a way that cannot be brought out
by appeals to the theory of interpretation. The list of intelligible
actions *does* exhibit some preference for the right over the wrong,
in the following sense. If an action is right for reasons A–D, and if
an agent does that action for reasons A–D, understanding them as
such, her doing so would therefore be intelligible. By contrast, if
the action is wrong for reasons A–D, and the agent does the action
for those reasons, understanding them as such, her doing so is *not
yet* intelligible. To make it intelligible, we have to provide further
elements.

What this means, however, is just that if the action is right for
reasons A–D, an explanation of the action which appeals to the
agent's beliefs in A–D is a good explanation. In other cases it is not.
This does nothing to introduce a sense of 'render intelligible' that
is not to do with explanation. It only concerns itself with the
question which explanations are good ones. Smith is promoting a
picture with three elements:

1. justifying reasons, being facts, are categorially different from
   motivating ones, which are beliefs and desires;

2. both sorts of reasons render actions intelligible;

3. motivating reasons render actions intelligible in quite a different sense from that in which justifying reasons do.

But this picture turns out to be ungrounded. The sense of intelligibility at issue is the same both times.

Doesn't this just show that justifying reasons do serve to explain
actions, thus undermining my earlier argument that on Smith's
picture justifying reasons cannot be motivating ones? No. What has
been admitted is that normative truths about what is a reason for
what and what is a better reason than what are relevant to the
question whether a putative belief–desire explanation of an action
is a good one. But no sense whatever has been given to the idea that
a truth can motivate—that the truth figures *in* the explanation. And
this is what we would need if we were to show that justifying
reasons can be motivating ones.

IS THERE A THEORY OF MOTIVATION? 9

II

So it seems that the account of the distinction between motivating and justifying reasons does indeed fall foul of the maxim. Now this should not be news, exactly. For it is what I see as the main message of Bernard Williams' notorious paper 'Internal and external reasons'. Williams there suggests that external reasons always collapse into internal ones. conceived of as sub-Humean packages of beliefs and desires. The pressure which he applies to the notion of an external reason comes largely from the maxim. He urges that as soon as an external reason becomes capable of motivating an agent, the agent is one about whom a true internal reasons statement could be made.[5] External reasons cannot both remain external and satisfy the maxim.

This is just another way of making the point I have already made, against the protagonists of the radical account of the motivating/ justifying distinction. That point is that once we admit a Humean (or sub-Humean) account of motivating reasons, there can be no other reasons than these. At best. justifying reasons will be a subclass of motivating ones. In this sense, Williams argues that the theory of motivation (a theory which has an inbuilt tendency towards Humean answers) expands to cover the whole of the territory covered by the theory of practical reasons. The general form of this position is that with Humean reasons in place, we need no other sort of reasons than Humean ones. Or, more strongly, that with Humean reasons in place, there is *no space left* for any other sort of reason.

The most promising reply to this is that there is no reason why there should not be more than one style of explanation of the same event, without either competing with the other. Dan Dennett has made us used to the idea that the behaviour of a chess-playing computer can be explained in three different ways. So why shouldn't human actions be explained not only in the Humean way, but also in a quite different way that appeals to justifying reasons? The answer to this is that this might perhaps be possible if the second way was *quite different* from the first, as it would be if the first was,

5 Bernard Williams 'Internal and external reasons', reprinted in his *Moral Luck* (Cambridge: Cambridge University Press. 1981), p. 107.

as we might put it, brutely causal and the second were quite other—rational and normative. But that is not how things are in our case. Humean explanation is not presented as brutely causal, but causal and rational at once, since it is supposed to be a sort of causal explanation that is subject to normative rational constraints. That being so, it is necessarily incompatible with the co-existence of another style of rational explanation.

My own view, then, is that the structure of Williams' position is sound, and, what is more, that it is sound no matter how we tinker with the details of what I have so far been calling 'Humean theory of motivation'. It is common enough to see references to thinkers who reject the Humean picture of the way in which belief and desire combine in motivation. The vast majority, of course, accept that picture. But most of those who dispute it merely tinker with the details. The best known anti-Humean suggestions are those stemming from Nagel and McDowell. But all that these two do, at least on the surface, is to suggest that on some occasions beliefs can play a role other than that which Humeanism traditionally allows them: moral and some prudential beliefs can lead desires rather than follow them. Nagel and McDowell do not follow this up by considering what sort of things beliefs capable of functioning in this way must be, nor by asking whether this comparatively slight deviation from the Humean norm—a deviation, what is more, which is explicitly supposed to leave intact the Humean form of explanation for the vast majority of actions[6]—gives us anything like a different picture of how action-explanation functions. The most trenchant anti-Humean position that I know is the one which I adopted myself in my *Moral Reasons*,[7] where I argued that beliefs are capable of motivation without the sort of support from desires that Humeanism normally supposes necessary. But even this story is essentially playing the Humean game. The style of action-explanation that is being debated here is still the Humean style, and it is merely the players whose interrelations are being reassessed. If I announce that beliefs are not inert, secondary motivators, but meaty primary ones, all I have done is to tinker with the details.

6   Which is why I think of it as a hybrid theory that claims that Hume is sometimes right and sometimes wrong.

7   Oxford: Blackwell, 1993.

IS THERE A THEORY OF MOTIVATION?   11

It is impossible, therefore, both to accept the maxim and to run the distinction between motivating and justifying reasons in the ways that sees the former as any sort of complex of beliefs and/or desires and the latter as facts, normative or otherwise. Those who accept the distinction in this form do better, therefore, to deny the maxim. This is what David Brink does,[8] and he marks his denial by talking, not of the motivating/justifying distinction, but of the explanatory/justifying one—thus distancing himself from any attempt to say that justifying reasons explain. In Brink's view, justifying reasons explain why an action was right, and why a fully rational person would have done it, but they never explain actions done by ordinary mortals.

If the distinction is between explanatory and justifying reasons rather than between motivating and justifying reasons, we cannot accuse its proponents of flouting the maxim. For it is explicit that the maxim applies only to explanatory reasons. This puts pressure on us to say why the maxim is true for all practical reasons. Here is Smith's reason for thinking it true:

> Motivating and normative reasons do have something in common in virtue of which they both count as reasons. For citing either would allow us to render an agent's action intelligible. This is essential. For there is an *a priori* connection between citing an agent's reasons for acting in a certain way and making her acting in that way intelligible: that is, specifying what there is to be said for acting in the way in question.[9]

Now I think that this would leave Brink unmoved, since he would merely say that the notion of 'an agent's reasons' refers here only to explaining (motivating) reasons, and has no need also to refer to justifying ones. So what can we put in its place? Why should it be true that 'if there are reasons for action, it must be that people sometimes act for those reasons, and if they do, their reasons must figure in some correct explanation of their action'?[10] The best I can do is to resort to rhetoric. How could there be this complex structure of reasons favouring and disfavouring actions, if humans were incapable of registering the fact? And how could it be possible *in*

---

8 op. cit., pp. 39–40.

9 Smith, *op. cit.*, *ibid.*.

10 This way of putting the maxim is taken from Williams' *op. cit.*, p. 102.

general for people to recognise the fact and not to take it into account in practical deliberation? Is there any difference here between practical and theoretical deliberation? Suppose that there are reasons for and against different beliefs, as there are for and against different actions. Again it seems inconceivable that there should be this structure on the theoretical side unless humans were capable of recognising it, at least to some extent. And surely it is inconceivable that we should do other than take the things we recognise to be relevant to the question what to believe.

In my view, then, we have to accept that justifying reasons are capable of explaining actions. This returns us to the position we were in before. All available positions admit in some sense that Hume was right about something. And we have seen that once we admit this, whatever the details of our Humean theory of motivation, we end up with no room for other reasons than our Humean ones. So is there no other possibility? There had better be, if we are to remain realists about reasons, and suppose that there are matters of fact which constitute reasons for action. To the extent that we suppose that the fact that an action is wrong is a reason not to do it, or that her need for help is a reason for us to provide it, to that extent we appear to be expressing a realist perspective on reasons, and nailing ourselves to the mast of justifying or external reasons. How can we do this without falling foul of the constraints already identified? The most obvious manoeuvre is to abandon the attempt to add justifying reasons to Humean motivating ones, and to try to move in the reverse direction, understanding motivating reasons in some non-Humean way, in terms of what we have already laid down about justifying ones. This approach is the one which seems to bear the most promise of avoiding the trap we have identified, of so understanding the motivating ones that we leave no room for justifying ones at all.

Even the expressions I used in outlining this strategy need to be treated with care, of course, since the motivating/justifying distinction is itself in question. It would be best to start in a non-contentious way, trying to understand reasons in favour of acting, and then writing an account of reasons why someone acted within the constraints of the picture we have begun to develop. There is nothing prejudicial about *this* procedure. It remains to be seen whether it is possible, and that is what the rest of this paper is

concerned with. One possibility, however, is that at the end of the day we will find in our account no recognisable successor of the theory of motivation at all. The very idea that there is room for such a theory will turn out to be a Humean implant, which we had previously failed to notice as such.

III

What we are after, then, is a realist account of reasons in favour of an action. But our account must respect certain constraints. One of those constraints has already been identified; it is the maxim that anything that is a reason must be capable of explaining an action. Justifying reasons must be capable of being motivating reasons. The second constraint is the realist nature of the story we are eventually going to tell about reasons why agents act. This realist story is that justifying reasons are facts—often normative facts. For instance, the reason why her action was right was that it promoted something which is a good. However, we must also admit and somehow capture the fact that no state of the world can motivate unless it is recognised by the agent. This gives us three constraints:

1. A reason must be capable of explaining an action.(Justifying reasons must be capable of also being motivating ones).

2. Justifying reasons are facts or states of affairs—largely, but not exclusively, normative ones.

3. States of the world and facts cannot motivate unless recognised by the agent.

There is a fourth constraint to be added to these. This is that:

4. The distinction between true and false beliefs on the agent's part cannot affect the *form* of the explanation which will be appropriate to his actions.[11]

It is the last two constraints that raise the real difficulties. They form a large part of the pressure in favour of taking complexes of beliefs and desires (of whatever sort) as the sole possible explainers of actions. This works in the following way. Let us suppose, in line with the first two constraints, that justifying reasons are largely

11 This constraint is also operative in Williams *op. cit.*; see again p. 102.

normative facts, and that these normative facts are capable of
motivating. We have to allow, however, that false conceptions of
the normative are also capable of motivating. People can be led to
act by taking an action which is in fact wrong to be right. The fourth
constraint prevents us from saying that where our normative beliefs
are true, the *facts* believed are what motivate, and when they are
false, the motivation stems from the false *beliefs*. The third
constraint ensures that even in the favourable case, there is a belief
in play; for recognition of the fact amounts to no more than true
belief. Since we cannot appeal to facts on both sides, then, and since
we must find an explanation of the same form each time, we are
reduced to explaining by appeal to beliefs both times, i.e. to the
familiar Humean form of motivation.

   This form of the argument from illusion is the argument that takes
us from the apparently innocuous distinction between two sorts of
reasons—reasons in favour of acting and reasons why the action
took place—to the full-blown distinction between reasons as
motivating beliefs and desires and reasons as normative facts. We
have been forced to abandon the first constraint in the attempt to
satisfy the other three.

   There is a second, quite distinct form of pressure leading to the
same conclusion. This pressure arises when we try to understand
explanation by reasons as causal explanation, without adopting
anything very unusual in the way of a theory of causation. If
anything that motivates must be a cause, it is clear that justifying
reasons cannot motivate—cannot be anyone's reason for acting—if
we conceive of justifying reasons as facts. For facts are causally
impotent, especially if they are normative.

   I say that we are committed to this view so long as we do not play
clever with the theory of causation. There are moves in the theory
of causation which would undermine the supposed causal impotence of facts, notably ones that deny the causal primacy of events.
And there are others, some of which are owed to Hume, that amount
to denying the appeal of any notion of causal impotence. But I am
not tempted to make this move here. The real question is whether
we are committed to understanding explanation by reasons as
causal explanation.

   The point at the moment is only that once one insists on seeing
reasons-explanation as causal, one needs to see one's reasons as

IS THERE A THEORY OF MOTIVATION?   15

capable of being causes, and facts—especially normative facts—
appear to many to be incapable of playing this role. Normative
beliefs (and desires, of course), however, can play it as well as any
other beliefs. So we have this second, causal pressure to make all
our reasons-explanations Humean.

The two forms of pressure come together when we notice that in
cases where our normative beliefs are false, there are no normative
facts to do the causing, even if we did manage to attain a conception
of facts as causally potent.

The situation then is that we seem unable to respect all four
constraints at once. We can only respect the third and the fourth
constraint by abandoning the realist picture of justifying reasons as
normative facts.

IV

There is however a possibility which we have not so far considered.
Our realism amounted to the claim that people can be motivated by
how things are (either normatively or non-normatively). We assumed
that this had to mean that we can be motivated by normative facts—by
the truths we recognise rather than by our recognising them. But that
might not be quite correct. What is required might be something less
than that. To comply with our realism, what motivates must be
capable of being believed and capable of being true, but need not be
considered as something incapable of being false. We could, that is,
respect the fourth constraint without being reduced to seeing beliefs
as the common explainers. For between beliefs on the one hand,
conceived as psychological states, and normative truths, facts or
states of affairs (all of which are incapable of falsehood) lie such
things as *what is believed*. What motivates agents to action, I propose,
and what justifies their actions in favourable cases, is *what they
believe*, not their believing it. The belief may perhaps give their
reason, or reveal what the reason was, but it will not actually *be* that
reason.

Let us try, then, to give an account of reasons for action in terms
of what is believed rather than speaking directly in terms of truths.
This will mean yielding in a way to one form of pressure applied
by the third constraint. That constraint pulls us towards the
suggestion that belief is what is doing the motivating, so that truth

adds nothing. That suggestion is correct if it means that the truth of what explains the action adds nothing to the explanation, being all concerned with the question of justification, but false if it means that the thing which is capable of both truth and falsehood adds nothing. For how could what the agent believes fail to add to the explanation?

This position is capable of respecting all four constraints. Justifying reasons are capable of explaining actions, though of course they can only do so when actually believed. For them to do so, the first requirement is that what explains the action was a true conception of how things are, either normatively or non-normatively—using the term 'conception' as a synonym for 'what is believed'. In such a case a justifying reason is a motivating reason and the motivating reason a justifying one, i.e. one which succeeds in showing that the action was right. In unfavourable cases the action will still be explained as well as in a favourable case, though now not justified. But it is still the case that that which explains is the right sort of thing to do some justifying, and would have justified had it been true. Finally, the true/false distinction has turned out not to affect the form of the relevant explanation at all.

In this way, then, one satisfies all the constraints by making adjustments at both ends—at the motivating end and at the justifying end. At the motivating end we have abandoned the view that beliefs and desires are motivating reasons for action. Instead, we have announced that it is what is believed that motivates. At the justifying end we have drawn back to some extent from the claim that justifying reasons are facts—only to some extent, however, because it remains the case that when what you believe is true, it is a fact. In such cases what you believe both explains and justifies what you did. We have drawn back more severely from the claim that justifying reasons are states of affairs or parts of the world. Or rather, we can only make this further claim if we adopt either the metaphysical view that facts are parts or constituents of the world, or the externalist claim that what is believed can *be* a state of affairs. Nothing in what I have said, however, prevents that claim. For it would be wrong to think that if we make either of those moves, we are again in conflict with the fourth constraint. The fourth constraint speaks only about the *form* of the relevant explanation, and we have (comparatively trivially) been able to satisfy that constraint by

announcing that whether the beliefs are true or false, it is not the belief that motivates but what is believed. Nothing that I have said, however, does much to establish either the metaphysical claim that facts are part of the world, or the externalist claim that what is believed can be a state of affairs. At least I hope not, for I would like to be able to propound the view that it is what is believed that both motivates and justifies without needing yet to offer a substantial theory of what these peculiar objects are.

The real hackles that my account will raise are causal hackles. We noticed that truth is causally impotent. So surely is what is believed (most obviously when the belief is false). If it is genuinely what is believed that is doing the explaining and not the belief, how can any explanation that appeals to reasons be shown to be causal? The answer is that it cannot. Explanation by motivating reasons is one thing and causal explanation another. This is the price of saying that there are such things as justifying reasons. Whether it is possible that actions should be able to be explained in a brutely causal way as well as by appeal to reasons, and what the elements of such a causal explanation might be, I am doubtful. But I will not argue against the possibility here. If I did, my general line would be that it is not obvious what, other than rationality constraints, could prevent situations arising in which wholly unsuitable beliefs and desires are the ones that actually caused the action. On a brutely causal account, where the players are still supposed to be beliefs and desires (and not neural changes, for instance), what will rule out the possibility of my taking the bus being caused by the belief that it might have been called Henry and my desire to have worked harder when I was a student? Of course, the action is not *rationalised* by these two causes. But in my view it makes no sense to admit this and then still insist that they might have caused it none the less. So the notion of a brutely causal explanation of action seems to me to make no sense. We might have a brutely causal explanation of a bodily movement, but that is another matter.

We have perhaps become recently inured to talk of reasons as causes, partly because of remarks by Donald Davidson. But at best he only succeeded in dealing with one of the reasons for refusing to think of reasons as causes—the one that concerns our ability to provide independent specifications of cause and effect. There is another reason for denying that reasons are causes. This is that there

is no possible metaphysical distinction between the action and the reasons for it, for if we subtract the reasons from the action, there is not enough left to be an action at all. We would only have something like a bodily movement, or the initiation of a change. So we can make no real sense of the idea that one and the same action could have been done for different reasons, though we can of course understand well enough the claim that one and the same action-description can be instantiated in different actions, each with its own reasons.

V

Is there then such a thing as the theory of motivation? I suggested earlier that the very concept of a theory of motivation is a Humean concept. This is not because it is a causal concept; the theory of motivation can be conceived teleologically rather than causally. It is because the theory of motivation is one within which only broadly Humean answers are possible, once we distinguish between motivating and justifying reasons in the sort of way that I have tried to dismantle. To suggest, by contrast, that the agent can be motivated by what he believes is to abandon the theory of motivation, so understood, completely, and to put in its place the basis of a more homogeneous and explicitly normative theory of practical reason.

The reasons that explain our acting must indeed be psychologically real, as Michael Smith puts it, but they need not for that reason be psychological states. They can instead be what we believe, which is surely psychologically real in the sense of being psychologically present to us.[12]

Philosophy Department,
University of Keele,
Keele, Staffs ST5 5BG

12 I am grateful to David McNaughton and to Bernard Williams for advice about this paper, and to Derek Parfit for forceful discussion.

[5]

Taking Plans Seriously

We are planning creatures.[1] We frequently settle in advance on more
or less complex plans concerning the future, and then these plans
guide our later conduct. My plan for today includes beginning the
day by preparing my lecture for my afternoon class, turning to some
work on this paper, meeting Howard at the Faculty Club for lunch,
giving my lecture, talking with John if he is in his office and, finally,
picking up a manuscript at the computer center on the way home. As
the day proceeds I execute my plan though, of course, I also must
make further decisions (which route should I take to the computer
center?) and could always reconsider my plan.

In this paper I try to sketch answers to two questions. First, what
is involved in having such garden-variety plans? Second, what are
the general outlines of a theory of practical rationality that takes
such plans seriously?

1. Plans: Why We Bother and What They Are

I have spoken of my plan for the day. But this is ambiguous. On the
one hand, I could mean an appropriate abstract structure—some sort
of partial function from circumstances to actions, perhaps. On the
other hand I could mean an appropriate state of mind, one naturally
describable in terms of such structures. A more careful usage might
reserve "plan" for the former and "having a plan" for the latter; but
this is frequently stylistically awkward. In this paper I will use
"plan" to mean "having a plan"—that is, a state of mind. Thus,
plans are in the same category as though (for reasons that will
emerge) different from desires and beliefs.

I want to know what is involved in having a plan of the garden-
variety sort just described, and how such plans figure in a plausible
conception of practical rationality. To do this I think we need to ask
yet another question: Why, anyway, do we bother with such plans
for the future?[2] Why don't we just cross our bridges when we come
to them?

Part of the answer is that we thereby avoid the need for deliberation at the time of action. If I have settled on no relevant plan I will
have to figure out what to do when I come to the bridge. But if I
have settled on a plan to cross, and the situation at the bridge is at
least roughly as I expected it to be, such deliberation will not be
necessary. This can be quite useful in cases in which there will be
limited opportunity for reflection when I get there.

But this is not the only or even the most important reason why we
bother with such plans. We settle on such plans as a way of
coordinating various activities. Plans facilitate coordination both of
my own activities over time, and of my activities with yours. The
ability to settle on such plans thereby enables us to achieve complex
personal and social goals we would not otherwise be able to
achieve.

For example, my plan for today enables me to coordinate various
activities—including lecture-writing, paper-writing, and other
errands—so as to achieve a complex mix of goals. And it is because
both Howard and I are planning to meet each other for lunch that we
are able to coordinate our otherwise disparate activities so as to
achieve a common goal.

But how does this work? Just by *deciding* or *settling* at the
beginning of the day on a plan for the rest of the day I do not ensure
coordination. Such coordination requires, at the least, that there be
some influence on my (and Howard's) later conduct. And my decision, at the beginning of the day, does not reach its ghostly hand
over time to influence what I do later. Rather, it sets up a new
state—a kind of decision "trace"—which somehow has the needed
influence. This is the state of having a plan.[3] We make progress in
understanding what it is to have a plan by reflecting on those
features of this state which enable it to support such coordination.

Consider Howard and me. My plan to meet him at the Faculty
Club is based on my expectation that he will be there, an expectation
in turn based on my knowledge of his plan to be there. Howard's
plan is in turn based on his expectation that I will be there, an
expectation based on his knowledge of my plan. Now, how is it that
my knowledge of Howard's plan to go to the Faculty Club at lunch
time can support a reasonable expectation that he will?

A natural conjecture here is that this is in part because Howard's
plan tends to motivate him to act as planned. It is a *pro-attitude* in at
least the very general sense in which desires, inclinations, goals,
and valuations are, and ordinary beliefs are not. Pro-attitudes in this

Taking Plans Seriously 273

very general sense play a motivational role: in concert with our beliefs they can move us to act. Thus, in knowing Howard's plan I know of a state that will tend to lead to his going to the Faculty Club at lunch time.

But this is not enough to support the kind of expectation that underlies such garden-variety cases of interpersonal coordination. Here we need to distinguish between two kinds of pro-attitudes. Suppose I desire a milkshake for lunch, recognize that the occasion is here, and am guilty of no irrationality. Still, I might not drink a milkshake; for my desire for a milkshake still needs to be weighed against conflicting desires—say, my desire to lose weight. Even though my desire for a milkshake *influences* what I do at lunch time, in the normal course of events I still might not drink one.

Let us say that my desire is merely a conduct-*influencing* pro-attitude. Now, the motivational role of *plans* seems different; plans seem not to be *merely* conduct-influencers. Suppose that this morning I settled on a plan that included my having a milkshake at lunch. Lunch-time arrives, my plan remains, and nothing unexpected happens. In such a case I do not need yet again to tote up the pros and cons concerning milkshake drinking. Rather, in the normal course of events I will simply proceed to execute this part of my plan and order a milkshake. My plan will not merely influence my conduct, it will *control* it: it is a conduct-*controlling* pro-attitude.

This difference in motivational roles helps explain how plans facilitate coordination. If I only knew that Howard had a conduct-influencing pro-attitude in favor of lunch at the Faculty Club I would have a much harder time determining whether I could reasonably expect him to be there. I would have to know much more about Howard's psychology: what his other goals and desires were, how they ranked in importance, how he tended to weigh up conflicting considerations, and so on. Interpersonal coordination would be rather difficult.

But in fact I know more than this, and this is why such coordination can work so smoothly. I know that in the normal course of events Howard's plan to lunch at the Faculty Club will *control* his conduct at lunch time, so long as he does not change his mind. If he continues to have this plan and recognizes the occasion he will at least try to go there, without having to weigh this plan against other desires, goals, and whatnot. Howard has a conduct-controlling pro-attitude in favor of going to the Faculty Club, not merely a conduct-influencing one; and this helps support the expectations needed for coordination.

Plans are conduct-controlling pro-attitudes, and that is partly why they are able to play the role they do in interpersonal coordination. But this is still not the whole story. None of this would work if plans did not have a certain *stability*. I need to know that Howard's plan can be expected to stay around until lunch time. Of course, there is no reason to suppose that his plan is absolutely immune to change if something unexpected happens. But my reasonable expectation that he will be at the Faculty Club does not need such a supposition of rigidity. It just needs the supposition (roughly) that the plan will be stable within most of the sorts of variations in Howard's beliefs, desires and circumstances that are realistically possible between now and lunch.

What is it for a plan to be stable, in the sense that is relevant here? First, in the normal course of events it will not vary in response to ordinary, nonrational bodily processes, unlike my desires to eat and drink. Second, and most important, having a plan will involve a strong disposition *not to reconsider* it except in the face of a significant problem—as we might say, following John Dewey, except in the face of a "problematic situation." (Of course, Howard may fill in his plan, or make adjustments in its sub-plans, without reconsidering it.)

This associated disposition not to reconsider one's prior plan will play a significant role in later discussion, so let me say a bit more about it right away. Reconsidering a plan is something one *does*. It is not merely for the thought of acting differently to occur. Typically, to reconsider a plan is to reason with the aim of seeing whether some other plan would be better. In contrast, when I do *not* reconsider a plan of mine that is not normally an action of mine at all; normally it is just the absence of an action of reconsidering. Of course, there will be some cases in which I explicitly decide not to reconsider my plan, and intentionally refrain from reconsidering it. But normally not reconsidering does not involve intentionally refraining from reconsidering. Stability involves primarily a disposition not to reconsider, and only secondarily a disposition intentionally to refrain from reconsidering.

Plans, then, support interpersonal coordination, of the sort Howard and I are attempting, in part because they are relatively stable, conduct-controlling pro-attitudes. What about *intra*personal coordination? My plan for the day, I have said, facilitates the coordination of a complicated array of my activities over time. How?

In a way analogous to the interpersonal case. I begin the day by working on my lecture in part because of my expectation that I will

get to work on this paper later in the day. Otherwise I would feel compelled to work on this paper right away, given the pressing deadline and my ability to give an acceptable lecture without any preparation. My plan grounds this expectation. It does this despite my known proclivity to get caught up in lecture preparations. It grounds this expectation in part because it is a conduct-controlling pro-attitude, and so normally need not be weighed against conflicting considerations when the time to turn to this paper arrives. (If it did need to be weighed in this way I might be considerably less confident that I *will* turn to this paper, knowing my tendency to be overly impressed with the importance of detailed lecture-preparations when I am in their midst.) It grounds this expectation also because it is a relatively stable state. I am disinclined to reconsider it in the light of minor variations in my situation— including variations in the degree to which I am attracted to working on the lecture.[4]

It is at least in part because plans are relatively stable, conduct-controlling pro-attitudes that they are so *useful* to us in facilitating both interpersonal and intrapersonal coordination. The ability to have such plans is, for us, a kind of "universal means," useful in our pursuit of a wide variety of different ends.

2. Plans and Intelligent Activity

What would a theory of practical rationality look like if it took such plans, and their coordinating role, seriously? Part of the answer would consist of an account of constraints of consistency and coherence that are applicable to a person's plans both in isolation and together with his beliefs. Here I will draw on my earlier discussion of these matters.[5]

To serve their coordinating role well my plans will need, other things equal, to be both *consistent with each other* and *consistent with my beliefs*. It should be possible for my plans taken together to be successfully executed in a world in which my beliefs are true. Further, other things equal, my plans should also be *means-end coherent*. They should be filled in with appropriate sub-plans concerning how I am to do what I plan to do, sub-plans at least as extensive as I believe is now required to do what I plan. For example, at some point my plan may need to be filled in to include a sub-plan concerning my route home at the day's end.

The demand for means-end coherence is connected with the characteristic *incompleteness* of plans. Consider three ways in

which the plans people like us normally have are *partial*. First, they do not specify what to do in *every* conceivable circumstance. My plan for the day does not tell me what to do in the event of an earthquake; though I might have another "stand by" plan for dealing with such an untoward eventuality. Second, plans will not normally specify what to do down to the most detailed, physical level. My plans will typically be at a level of abstraction appropriate to my habits and skills. I may need a detailed plan for shooting a jumpshot, a plan that specifies which foot to jump off from, when to break my wrist, and so on. In contrast, Dr. J's plan may be just to shoot a jump shot and then to steal the ball on the in-bounds play. Third, when initially formulated a plan may only provide a relatively general specification of some later conduct, a specification the agent knows will need to be filled in prior to the time of action. My initial plan may only tell me to stop at the computer center on the way home. But I know I will need later to settle on a specific route.

The demand for means-end coherence arises from this third way in which plans are partial. It is not a demand to complete my plans with respect to every conceivable circumstance or physical movement I might make. It is only a demand to fill in my plans with specifications of how I am to do what I am planning to do, specifications that are only as detailed as is, on my view, needed for me successfully to execute my plan. Nor is it a demand that these specifications be filled in all at once. They need only be provided at appropriate later stages in the on-going construction of my plan. I can leave until later the choice of a specific route home.

My view, then, is that there is a pragmatic rationale, rooted in the coordinating role of plans, for demands for consistency and means-end coherence on those plans. In being subject to these demands, plans differ from ordinary desires. I might desire to have a milkshake for lunch, and desire to run four miles after lunch (which is not to say that I desire to have a milkshake and to run) all the time knowing that if I do the former I will not be able to do the latter. Yet there need be no irrationality here. It is just a conflict of a sort that occurs countless times in the life of a reasonable person. If, however, my *plans* include both actions then I *am* guilty of a criticizable form of inconsistency. Again, simply desiring to stop at the computer center on the way home places me under no rational requirement to settle on some means to doing so, in the way in which planning to stop there would.

Let us turn now to action. How should we think of rationality in action if we are going to take plans seriously?

On one dominant tradition, inspired by Hume, rationality in action is a matter of fit between the action and the agent's desires and beliefs, values and expectations, utilities and probabilities, or some similar conative-cognitive pair. Strict Humeans confine themselves to the agent's desires and beliefs at the time of action. Others see as also relevant what desires and beliefs the agent will have, or would have under certain conditions (for example, certain kinds of reflection).

Such approaches involve a *two-parameter* conception of practical reason. But our discussion of plans should make us skeptical that such a two-parameter conception will provide a complete picture. After all, my *plans* seem somehow relevant to whether I am acting reasonably when I am executing them. Yet having a plan seems an importantly different sort of state than having a desire or a belief. Plans are conduct-*controlling* attitudes, not merely conduct- *influencing* ones, as ordinary desires. Plans are subject to consistency and coherence constraints to which ordinary desires are not subject. And, as pro-attitudes, plans differ significantly from beliefs in their motivational role.[6]

The very idea that we have plans that are—and reasonably so— both *partial* and relatively *stable* will force us to complicate our account of rationality in action. You can see this in two ways. Consider, first, stability. To be stable is, in part, to resist reconsideration. So we will want to know when such resistance to reconsideration, and the conduct in which it issues, is reasonable. Now add partiality. A partial plan will need to be filled in later, prior to action. Given that the plan is relatively stable, the practical reasoning aimed at filling it in will take its main outlines for granted. This means that options will be seen as relevant only if they are compatible with those main outlines. We will want a theory of rationality in action somehow to illuminate the structure of such reasoning and the appropriate standards of reasonableness.

To make progress here let us reflect further on the role of deliberation and plans in intelligent activity. "Deliberation," Dewey teaches us, "has its beginnings in troubled activity."[7] The implicit contrast here is between smooth, on-going activity in which no further deliberation is called for, and cases in which deliberation is needed to "resolve entanglements in existing activity."[8] The phenomenon of plan-execution provides us with a special case of this general contrast.

On the one hand, there are cases in which the agent is engaged in an on-going activity involving the execution of a prior plan. He

recognizes no problem for his plan; he runs into no "entanglements." He simply proceeds to execute it without further reconsideration of its merits. This is a case of *non-deliberative plan-
execution.* On the other hand, there are cases in which the agent
deliberatively weighs the pros and cons in favor of and against
several conflicting options that present themselves for choice. He
deliberates because he has run into some "entanglement" in executing some plan, or because he has been presented with a choice of a
sort not anticipated in any such plan. This is a case of *deliberative
decision.*

When we come to assess the agent's conduct in such cases we will
need to ask slightly different questions. To keep track of these
differences let us say that deliberative decisions are more or less
rational, while in nondeliberatively executing a prior plan one is
acting more or less *reasonably.* Thus, as I am using these terms,
"rational" and "reasonable" are terms of assessment that apply to
different objects: the former to deliberative decisions, the latter to
cases of nondeliberative plan execution.[9]

Having said this, an important complexity should be noted immediately. Cases of "pure" deliberative decision or nondeliberative
plan-execution are clearly atypical extremes. Most real cases of
intelligent activity are a *hybrid,* involving elements of both.

This is because plans will typically have both a *hierarchical* and a
linear structure. More general plans will embed more specific plans;
as when my day's plan embeds a specific plan for getting to the
computer center. And more extensive plans will organize various less
extensive sub-plans either in sequence or meshed in some more or
less complicated way. This is what my plan for the day does with my
sub-plans concerning writing this paper and giving my lecture.
Suppose, then, I am nondeliberatively executing a plan at a certain
level of generality and extensiveness. I still might, at the same time,
be deliberatively weighing the pros and cons concerning various
ways of resolving a problem that has arisen at a more specific or
more limited level. I might be faced with a problem with the writing
of my lecture that requires some deliberative decision even while
nondeliberatively executing my more general and more extensive
plan for the day.

Indeed, it seems that most cases of deliberative decision are like
this: they take place within the framework of the nondeliberative
execution of a plan at a more general and/or more extensive level.
This plan provides a background framework for the deliberative

weighing of pros and cons. It does not merely influence one's decision between options, in the way that ordinary desires do. Rather, the background plan constrains what options are *relevant* options. Thus, I deliberate between different ways of presenting the Prisoner's Dilemma to my afternoon class; I do not consider putting down my lecture notes and going for a four-mile run. So long as I do not reconsider my more general plan I treat it as providing a fixed framework within which my more specific sub-plans are to be fit.

Of course, I *might* reconsider my more general plan for the day, and actually consider whether to run instead. Given a plan at any level of generality or extensiveness that one is nondeliberatively executing, it is always possible to reconsider and bring that plan into question. But we would cease to be planning creatures if we constantly reconsidered all our plans—if we always started from scratch. Typically we will be nondeliberatively executing some plans even while deliberating among various options, options duly constrained by the plans being executed.

This means that even cases of deliberative weighing will typically raise two sorts of questions: Was the agent's deliberative decision rational? And at the level at which the agent was nondeliberatively executing a plan, did his conduct satisfy plausible standards of reasonableness? A conception of rationality in action will need to address both such questions.

Within the Humean tradition cited above, it is common to see the rationality of a deliberative decision between several options presented for choice as a matter of the fit between those options and the agent's desires and beliefs. For example, it is common to suppose that a rational decision will favor that option with highest "expected utility." Now, I do not want to try to settle here on the merits of this conception. Rather, I want to point out that even if it were accepted as a conception of rational deliberative decision, we would still need a more elaborate framework for a full theory of rationality in action. This is because we would still be in need of an account of reasonable plan execution. I want now to try to sketch the outlines of such an account.

3. Reasonable Stability

We have noted that for plans to play their characteristic role in coordination they need to have a certain stability. We need to say something more about what such stability involves and about when the stability of a plan is more or less reasonable.[10]

The stability of my plan for the day is largely a matter of my associated disposition not to reconsider it. This disposition may be rather minimal: I might be inclined to reconsider my plan given only a slight divergence between the way the world is when I come to act and the way I expected it to be when I first settled on my plan. Or the disposition might involve substantial rigidity, as when I would only reconsider it in the face of some extreme divergence from my expectations—an earthquake, for example.

A plan might be stable in some respects and not in others. Perhaps my discovery that there is a special lecture today at lunch time would not trigger reconsideration of my plan, whereas my discovery that this paper is due a month later than I had thought would. In contrast, things might be the other way round for you. My plan might be unstable in a respect in which yours is relatively stable, and vice versa.

The stability of my plan may be rooted in a further, "second-order" plan, but it need not. I may actually plan to reconsider my day's plan if I learn of a change in the deadline. But I need not have such a further plan in order to be *disposed* to reconsider in such circumstances.

The stability of a plan is generally a long-term feature of that plan: I do not constantly adjust the stability of my plans. To do that would undermine the point of having plans, for I would then be constantly reconsidering their merits. Further, I normally do not *decide* how stable my plan is to be. Generally, I do not, having settled on a plan, begin to reason yet again about how stable my plan should be (though in special cases I might). Rather, the stability of my plan is largely determined by general, underlying dispositions of mine.

The stability of my plans will generally not be an isolated feature of those plans, but will be linked with other features of my psychology. For example, if I am the sort of person who is constantly on the alert for dangers in my environment, my plans are likely to have a kind of instability they would not have if I were a person too engrossed in my projects to be very senstive to such dangers.[11] I might be more likely than most to reconsider my planned route home upon hearing of a smog alert in the area. Frequently, the extent of stability of my plans will be connected with underlying tendencies to *take notice* of certain sorts of things and not others—to see certain features of my environment as *salient*. I may be more likely to take notice of certain kinds of hazards than you, and this fact may

well be tied to a certain kind of instability that my plans have and
yours do not.

In light of this discussion, what can we say about when a plan is
appropriately stable? *not stable enough* in certain respects? *too
stable* in other respects? Most generally, what can we say about
when the stability of a plan is *reasonable?* Here I do not have as
much an answer as the sketch of an answer—an answer that is
broadly consequentialist in structure.

Return for a moment to rational deliberative decision. As noted,
we might see this, in the Humean tradition, as a matter of fit with
relevent desires and beliefs. Or, taking a somewhat different tack,
we might see the rationality of such a decision as a matter of its
expected impact on the agent's overall good. I will not try to resolve
such differences here. What I do want to point out is that such
conceptions share a certain structure. They assess the rationality of a
deliberative decision by appeal to its expected impact on some
central *goal:* desire-satisfaction, the agent's overall good, or perhaps
something else.

Given such a goal, we may proceed in an analogous way in
assessing plan stability. Suppose that I have a plan that is stable in
certain ways. We can consider the general disposition to have one's
plans of this sort be stable in such ways. We can then ask about the
expected impact on the goal we have singled out, of my having this
general disposition. The better this expected impact the more
reasonable is the stability of my plan. The stability of my plan is
reasonable *simpliciter* when this expected impact exceeds an appropriate threshold.

The expected impact of such a disposition towards stability will
itself depend on a variety of factors. It will depend on what
psychological traits are involved in such plan-stability. It will depend on what sort of plan is in question: for example, how general
the plan is. It will depend on general facts about my social and
environmental circumstances. And, finally, it will depend on general
facts about my particular psychology that may vary even while the
disposition towards such stability remains fixed. For example, it
will depend on the extent of my general abilities to reason carefully
and quickly in the face of the unexpected.

Note that it is not only the impact on my *actions* that matters. This
will, of course, be one of the main considerations relevant to our
assessment of the stability of my plan. But there are other ways in
which stability, and its associated psychological traits, can have a

relevant impact. Suppose, for example, that the goal in terms of which we are assessing stability is the agent's long-term good. And suppose I have a high sensitivity to certain kinds of environmental hazards, a sensitivity associated with certain kinds of plan instability. Now, these kinds of instability may in fact conduce to certain kinds of useful preventive activity. But they may also conduce to a kind of apprehensive and fearful consciousness that will undermine my good. And that impact also is relevant to the assessment of such instabilities.

Another point to notice is that there will, in general, be a kind of social pressure towards increased stability. This is because the stability of my plans is one of the things that makes me a reliable partner in various schemes of inter-personal coordination—schemes that are to everyone's advantage.

So we have the following picture. A conception of rational deliberative decision can be expected to cite a central goal in terms of which such decisions are to be assessed. Given such a goal we may proceed to assess plan stability in a similarly consequentialist vein. This means that conceptions of rational deliberative decision can be *paired,* in a natural way, with conceptions of reasonable plan stability.

4. Reasonable Plan Execution

With this treatment of reasonable stability in hand, let us return to our question of when an agent acts reasonably in nondeliberatively executing a prior plan. Recall that this phenomenon is not limited to cases in which there is no deliberation between alternative options. In many cases such deliberation will take place within the context of the nondeliberative execution of a more general plan. In such cases the options seen as relevant will be constrained by the more general plan. Once in the classroom, I might stop my lecture for a moment and try to figure out which of several ways of making a certain point will work best. But, unless I reconsider my more general plan, I will not stop to determine whether it would be better to stop the lecture in the middle and head over to the gym. What we want to know is when such nondeliberative execution of my more general plan, even when accompanied by deliberation at a less general level, is reasonable.

My strategy will be to construct an answer in terms of two ideas that have already received some discussion: reasonable plan stability and rational deliberative decision. I will assume we have some

conception of when a deliberative decision, between several options presented for choice, is rational. This conception will be paired with a corresponding conception of reasonable plan stability. Given these two conceptions, what is it for my activity in nondeliberatively executing my plan to be reasonable?

My plans are constructed over time in different stages. We may suppose that at each stage in the construction of a plan I make a deliberative decision between different options, options themselves constrained by the structure of my plan as so far formed. Now let us consider a particular present plan of mine and suppose that the following conditions are satisfied. First, at each stage in the construction of my plan my deliberative decision, in favor of one element rather than others, was rational. Second, I have, until now, been successfully executing the earlier components of this plan. Third, my present plan, as so far formed, both satisfies our requirements of consistency and means-end coherence and is stable in various ways. Fourth, this stability is reasonable. Fifth, and finally, my present situation does not involve the sort of problem or "entanglement" that triggers reconsideration of my plan, given the ways in which it is stable. Given these conditions, I proceed nondeliberatively to execute part of my plan. What can we say about the reasonableness of my conduct in such a case?

It seems to me that, at least on one commonsense form of assessment, I am acting in a way that is not subject to a serious form of rational criticism: I am acting *reasonably* in so executing my plan. After all, I am engaged in the kind of plan-execution characteristic of the sort of planning creature I am—the sort of plan-execution the capacity for which we have seen to be so useful. And each element in my activity passes muster: my plan is the product of a sequence of rational deliberative decisions; it is now consistent, coherent and reasonably stable; and it is because of that stability that it is now being executed without further reconsideration.

I think, then, that we have here plausible sufficient conditions for reasonable, nondeliberative plan execution. A full account would provide plausible necessary conditions as well. But here I am content with a partial account that provides only sufficient conditions.

While only partial, this view of reasonable plan execution has several important consequences. First, my nondeliberative execution of my plan may be reasonable even though, as it happens, in this particular case it would have been better if I had reconsidered.

(By "better" I mean better in terms of the expected impact on the goal by reference to which deliberative decisions are to be assessed—desire-satisfaction, perhaps.) This may be so even taking into account the inconvenience and other costs associated with reconsideration.

For example, suppose it is true that if upon hearing of the special lecture I had stopped and reconsidered my plan to meet Howard, then I would have seen that I could persuade Howard to meet me there. This option would have been slightly better, even taking into account the costs of reconsideration, than my proceeding non-deliberatively with my original plan. Nevertheless, my disposition not to reconsider my original plan in the face of this new information about the lecture might well be a kind of stability that is quite reasonable for me. After all, a general tendency to reconsider my plans in such cases, in which only marginal improvements are likely, will have obvious disadvantages. We are not very good at detecting slight differences in the pros and cons of various options, so reconsideration in such cases will many times just lead to inefficient delay. And the more inclined we are in favor of such reconsideration, the more difficult will be various forms of coordination. So it may well be that I act reasonably in proceeding nondeliberatively with my plan to meet Howard at the Faculty Club. If my plan had been considerably less stable I would have reconsidered; and on this particular occasion that would have been fortunate. But then my plan may well have been unreasonably unstable.

A second corollary is that two people, Smith and Jones, can be quite similar in their desires, beliefs and plans, and yet still differ in ways important to a theory of rational conduct. This is because their plans can still differ in stability, or be similar in stability but this stability be reasonable for one person but not for the other. Suppose, first, that Smith's plan is stable in ways in which Jones's is not. Given differences in their abilities, however, both plans are *reasonably* stable. (Perhaps Jones is just better at reasoning quickly in the face of the unexpected: he is a better improviser.) Jones might then reconsider his plan in a situation in which Smith would not. Jones might proceed rationally to diverge form his prior plan, while Smith would have proceeded to act reasonably in nondeliberatively execut-ing that plan. So Smith and Jones would act differently and yet the former act reasonably and the latter rationally. Same beliefs, desires, and plans. Different actions. Yet both act in ways that are not criticizable by our theory.

Again, Smith's and Jones's plans may be quite similar in their stability yet, because of differences in their abilities, Smith's plan might be reasonably stable while Jones's is not. So, when they both proceed nondeliberatively to execute their plan it may be well that Smith acts reasonably while Jones does not. Same desires, beliefs, and plans. Same action. Yet one acts reasonably and the other does not.

The reasonableness of an agent's activity will depend, then, on his plans, the stability of these plans, and on the reasonableness of this stability. (Of course, it will depend on other things as well.) A theory of rationality in action that ignores this role of plans and their stability will be importantly incomplete.

5. Intentions and Plans

I began this paper by asserting that we are planning creatures. I have been arguing that we need to take this fact seriously in our accounts of the motivation and assessment of intelligent activity. This argument applies both to commonsense and to scientific psychology. Both a plausible reconstruction of the former, and a reasonable candidate for the latter will, it seems to me, need to include something like plans among the states that play a motivational role.[12] (This is not, of course, to say that *all* intentional activity is motivated by prior plans.) Such plans are importantly different sorts of states than ordinary desires and beliefs. And facts about them and their stability will play a basic role in an acceptable theory of practical rationality.

I conclude with a brief remark about intention. Anscombe begins her justly famous monograph[13] by distinguishing between intending to do something and doing something intentionally. She then proceeds to treat the latter as basic for the theory of action, and leaves us without a clear treatment of the former. Many treatments of intention in the wake of Anscombe's monograph have more or less gone along with this theoretical decision and treated intentional action as the basic case for our understanding of intention.[14] Once we take plans seriously, however, a different strategy recommends itself. Rather than try to understand intending to act in terms of the purportedly more basic phenomenon of intentional action, we turn to the phenomenon of future-directed plans. We understand what it is to intend to do something in large part in terms of such plans; for future intentions are, at least typically, elements in such larger plans. This is to follow the strategy of *the methodological priority of future*

286   **Social Theory and Practice**

intentions and plans. I conjecture that in this way we will gain a better understanding of the distinctive role intentions play in our lives.[15]

Notes

1. I want to thank Allan Gibbard for extremely helpful conversations on some of the topics of this paper, and for allowing me to see an as-yet unpublished paper of his on related issues. I also want to thank Patrick Suppes for providing detailed comments on an earlier draft that were immensely useful. I am also indebted to Robert Audi, Arnold Davidson, and Adrian Piper for many helpful comments. Initial work on this paper was supported by a summer research grant from the National Endowment for the Humanities.

2. I do not mean to be asking here about our specific reasons for settling on a prior plan in a particular case. My concern is, rather, with the general role such plans play in our lives.

3. Thus plans provide the connection between decision and future action decided upon, just as a "memory trace" may be thought to provide the connection between remembering and the past event remembered. Concerning the notion of a "memory trace" see C. B. Martin and M. Deutscher, "Remembering," *Philosophical Review* 75 (1966): 161–96.

4. Though plans normally support expectations of their successful execution as part of their contribution to coordination, there may still be cases in which I plan to *A* but do not believe I will. Though I will not pursue the point in this paper, I suspect that we have here a basis for a resolution of debates concerning the possibility of intending to *A* without believing I will. For conflicting views on this matter see Donald Davidson, "Intending," in *Essays on Actions and Events* (New York: Oxford University Press, 1980), pp. 83–102; and Paul Grice, "Intention and Uncertainty," *Proceedings of the British Academy* 57 (1971): 263–79.

5. In "Intention and Means-End Reasoning," *Philosophical Review* 90 (1981): 252–65 esp. pp. 259–60.

6. As indicated below, I see future intentions as, at least typically, elements in such plans. So what I am saying here amounts to a rejection of the sort of reductive approaches to intention offered by Audi, Beardsley, and Churchland. These philosophers try to analyze an intention to *A* as a complex of desires and beliefs. My remarks in this paragraph suggest some reasons for being wary of such attempts. But in the end I think the main argument for seeing plans—and so, intentions—as distinctive psychological phenomena lies in the theoretical usefulness of this approach. I take the present paper to be part of

Taking Plans Seriously **287**

an argument for such utility. See Robert Audi, "Intending," *Journal of Philosophy* 70 (1973): 387–403; Monroe Beardsley, "Intending," in *Values and Morals: Essays in Honor of William Frankena, Charles Stevenson, and Richard Brandt,* ed. Alvin Goldman and Jaegwon Kim (Dordrecht, Holland: Reidel, 1978), pp. 163–84; and Paul Churchland, "The Logical Character of Action-Explanations," *Philosophical Review* 79 (1970): 214–36.

7. John Dewey, *Human Nature and Conduct* (New York: Random House, 1957), p. 187.
8. Ibid.
9. I will be extending the scope of "reasonable" somewhat in the discussion to follow.
10. Here I am extending the scope of "reasonable" in the obvious way.
11. This example is derived from an example of Allan Gibbard's.
12. Atkinson and Birch seem inclined toward a similar conclusion in reflecting on the limitations of their theory when they write: "One reader of an early draft . . . was concerned with how the *planning* and *scheduling* of activities, which distinguishes human from animal behavior, is to be taken into account. And so are we. At this writing, we consider planning a covert conceptual activity of considerable motivational significance, although we have not, as yet, encompassed the topic in any systematic way." *The Dynamics of Action* (New York: John Wiley and Sons, 1970), p. 95n.
13. G. E. M. Anscombe, *Intention* (Ithaca: Cornell University Press, 1963).
14. This is even true of Davidson's work in the theory of action, even though he famously *dis*agrees with Anscombe on the issue of whether reasons are causes. See my "Davidson's Theory of Intention," forthcoming in a Festschrift in honor of Donald Davidson, edited by Merrill Hintikka and Bruce Vermazen (Oxford: Oxford University Press, 1984).
15. I expand on this point in "Two Faces of Intention," forthcoming.

Michael Bratman
Department of Philosophy
Stanford University

Part II
Reasons and Desires

[6]

How to Argue about Practical Reason

R. JAY WALLACE

This is the sixth of our commissioned 'State of the Art' series

What are the comparative roles of reason and the passions in explaining human motivation and behaviour? Accounts of practical reason divide on this central question, with proponents of different views falling into rationalist and Humean camps. By 'rationalist' accounts of practical reason, I mean accounts which make the characteristically Kantian claim that pure reason can be practical in its issue. To reject this view is to take the Humean position that reasoning or ratiocination is not by itself capable of giving rise to a motivation to act. This alternative position is most famously expressed in Hume's polemical assertion that 'reason is, and ought only to be the slave of the passions' in influencing the will or moving us to act.[1]

To fix terms, let us say that a process of thought is an instance of reasoning or ratiocination just in case it is governed by the principles or norms of rationality. To say that a principle or norm *governs* a process of thought is in turn to make an explanatory claim: it is to say, not just that the process of thought is in accordance with the rational principle or norm, but that the process of thought occurs *because* the person believes it to be in accordance with the principle or norm. Thus, if we say that it is a principle or norm of rationality that people should not hold inconsistent sets of beliefs, this does not just mean that they revise those sets of beliefs which they know to be inconsistent, but that they revise them *because* they know those sets of beliefs to be inconsistent.

In these terms, the dispute between the Humean and the rationalist is a dispute about the capacity of rational principles or norms to contribute to explanations of motivation. The rationalist holds that such rational principles have a *primary* role to play in the explanation of motivation, that the psychological processes which originally give rise to motivation can be processes which are governed—in the sense I have specified—by the principles or norms of reason. By contrast, the Humean maintains that such rational principles never have a primary role to play in the explanation of motivation or the fixing of our ends. Rather, the explanatory contribution they make is exclusively secondary, accounting for the extension of motivational influence (for example, along means/end lines), but never explaining the original formation of motivation.

---

[1] See Hume, *A Treatise of Human Nature*, ed. Selby-Bigge, Second Edition, Oxford, Clarendon Press, 1978, p. 415.

Mind, Vol. 99 . 395 . July 1990

356   *R. Jay Wallace*

The significance of this dispute about practical reason lies in its connection with central issues in moral philosophy, concerning the nature and scope of moral requirements. It is a common thought that moral requirements, if they are to provide reasons for action, must be capable of guiding behaviour, leading those who are aware of the requirements to be motivated in accordance with them. (This is, presumably, one thing that is meant by the multiply ambiguous word 'internalism'.) If we combine this internalist position with the Humean picture of practical reason, however, it seems to follow that moral requirements can only provide an agent with reason to act if they are appropriately related to the agent's antecedent desires; for all motivation and behaviour, on the Humean view, must be explained by reference to the agent's given, prior desires. The resulting account represents moral behaviour as dependent on the agent's existing dispositions, in a way that could restrict the scope of moral reasons (since the required prior desires may not be universally distributed). A Kantian approach to practical reason, by contrast, suggests a different picture of the psychological bases of moral behaviour, and a straightforward development of the idea that moral requirements are universal or inescapable in their scope. It does this by opening up the possibility that there are processes of pure reasoning or ratiocination which can explain moral behaviour by themselves, and which could equally lead all agents, regardless of their background desires, to be motivated to act on moral requirements.

All of this should be familiar to students of the history of philosophical ethics since Hume. Indeed, so familiar has it become that one might reasonably be sceptical whether there is anything to be contributed on the topic which has not already been said. In the event, however, such scepticism has not deterred contemporary philosophers from entering the fray, and recent years have seen a flurry of philosophical discussions purporting to defend or refute the different approaches to practical reason. My aim in this essay is to sort through these recent discussions, with an eye to reaching a clear assessment of the current state of argument between the opposing camps. I hope to show that recent work has in fact helped to advance the old debate between Humeans and rationalists. For one thing, it has become increasingly clear that the appeal of the Humean position is linked to the teleological character of intentional action, consideration of which suggests an a priori argument for the Humean claim that action must be explained ultimately in terms of desires. Rationalists have generally not paid sufficient attention to these teleological considerations and the a priori arguments they suggest, and this has made their pronouncements about the possibility of pure practical reason vulnerable. Or so I will suggest.

My own view is that the rationalist position can, in the end, be sustained against the challenge of these Humean arguments. To see why, however, it will be necessary to get clear about what is really at stake in the debate

about practical reason. A further aim of my discussion will accordingly be to sharpen our understanding of the issue that divides Humeans and rationalists. Here, I think it will be helpful to turn to the somewhat less recent work of Thomas Nagel, which contains important suggestions about how the issue dividing Humeans and rationalists should be conceived. This is, or ought to be, familiar territory—Nagel's work has hardly wanted for readers. But the issues are complicated, and Nagel himself has neither explained nor developed his proposals adequately. Hence, despite the influence his work has enjoyed, its significance for the debate about practical reason remains rather poorly understood. A clearer account of what is at stake in the debate, which draws on and develops Nagel's suggestions, should help to reveal the inadequacy of recent arguments for the Humean view, and lead to an improved understanding of how we should be thinking, and arguing, about practical reason.

1. Rationalist accounts of practical reason claim that principles or norms of reason can play a primary role in the explanation of action and motivation. In an incisive recent discussion, Christine Korsgaard has distinguished two kinds of scepticism about this rationalist position.[2] *Content* scepticism, as she describes it, is doubt about whether specific principles or norms of rationality are sufficient, by themselves, to guide practical reflection and to explain motivation and action. *Motivational* scepticism, by contrast, is not directed at specific proposals about the content of rational principles and norms. Rather, it purports to offer general grounds for doubting whether there could be such a thing as pure practical reason, grounds which are antecedent to consideration of rationalist proposals about the norms or principles of reason, and which turn on the alleged incapacity of reason to give rise to motivation.

Korsgaard herself rejects motivational scepticism. She says: 'motivational considerations do not provide any reason, in advance of specific proposals, for scepticism about practical reason'.[3] In support of this conclusion, Korsgaard suggests that motivational scepticism typically rests on a misinterpretation of the internalist requirement on practical reasons.[4] Humeans, she contends, often construe internalism as the requirement that rational considerations (or reasons) necessarily succeed in motivating us. So construed, internalism would lead fairly directly to motivational scepticism, since it is doubtful that there are any rational considerations which *necessarily* succeed in motivating us, independently of our desires. Korsgaard argues, however, that this is a misinterpretation of internalism, which does not require that reasons necessarily succeed in motivating us, but only that they 'succeed in motivating us insofar as we are rational'.[5] This,

---

[2] Christine Korsgaard, 'Skepticism about Practical Reason', *The Journal of Philosophy*, 1986.
[3] 'Skepticism about Practical Reason', p. 25. [4] 'Skepticism about Practical Reason', p. 15.
[5] 'Skepticism about Practical Reason', p. 15.

358   *R. Jay Wallace*

however, is a fairly trivial condition on reasons, which does not place any a priori constraints on the possible norms of practical rationality. Whether a candidate principle could motivate rational agents depends on what it is to be rational, and that in turn depends on what the norms or principles of reason are. Hence, Korsgaard concludes, 'motivational scepticism must always be based on content scepticism';[6] it has no independent force.

This conclusion, if correct, would already be a kind of victory for the rationalist approach. Motivational scepticism, as Korsgaard describes it, purports to offer a general argument against the very possibility of a principle or norm of pure practical reason. But if there is no such argument, then it is already possible that pure reason might be practical in its issue, and this, in its weakest form, *is* the rationalist position. A more substantial victory for the rationalist, however, would require specification of the norms or principles of practical reason. Here, as Korsgaard notes, the internalist requirement entails that rationalist proposals about the norms or principles of practical reason will have psychological implications, telling us something about what it would be like to be rational.[7] Some proponents of the rationalist approach, notably including Thomas Nagel, have seen in these psychological implications of internalism a fertile source of arguments in favour of specific rationalist proposals. Focusing on the case of prudence, Nagel argues that this class of motivations can better be explained in terms of principles or norms of reason than on the Humean assumption that motivation always has desire at its source.[8] His strategy is to show that the psychological implications of rationalist accounts, for the motivation of ideally rational agents, are more plausible than those of alternative, Humean accounts.

If we are to conceive the debate in this way, however, it must indeed be the case that there is no reason for questioning the very possibility of a rationalist explanation of motivation. On this point, Korsgaard's own argument seems to me too swift. She takes it that internalism will be seen as innocuous, for the rationalist, once it is correctly interpreted as a thesis about the motivations of the fully rational agent. But rationalism is not simply a stipulative claim, about the motivations that the fully rational agent will happen to have; it also makes an explanatory claim, to the effect that the rational agent's motivations can be explained in terms of norms or principles of correct reasoning. As I show in what follows, there is

---

[6] 'Skepticism about Practical Reason', p. 6.   [7] 'Scepticism about Practical Reason', pp. 23–5.

[8] Thomas Nagel, *The Possibility of Altruism*, Princeton, Princeton University Press, 1978, chs. VI–VIII. Nagel's discussion of prudence is guardedly endorsed by Philippa Foot, in 'Reasons for Action and Desires', in her *Virtues and Vices*, Oxford, Basil Blackwell, 1978; and there is a similar account of the rationality of prudence in Martin Hollis, *The Cunning of Reason*, Cambridge, Cambridge University Press, 1987, ch. 6. Derek Parfit offers some powerful objections to accounts of this sort in his discussion of the self-interest theory of practical rationality, in *Reasons and Persons*, Oxford, Oxford University Press, 1984, part two. See also Richard Kraut, 'Prudence and the Desire Theory of Reasons', *The Philosophical Review*, 1972; and Janet Broughton, 'The Possibility of Prudence', *Philosophical Studies*, 1983.

something about the teleological character of motivation that has seemed to rule out the possibility of such explanations in principle, and so to provide an a priori argument for motivational scepticism about the rationalist approach. It is this argument, and not simply a misunderstanding of the internalist requirement, that accounts for the persistence of Humean scepticism about the very possibility of pure practical reason. Only once this argument is understood, and conclusively laid to rest, can we proceed to assess the plausibility of specific rationalist proposals about the content of the principles or norms of reason.

2. The a priori argument I want to consider may be called the teleological argument, because it takes as its starting point the essentially teleological character of both motivation and intentional action. In saying that these are teleological phenomena, I mean that the person who acts intentionally, or who is motivated so to act, is in a goal-directed state. Any psychological explanation of these phenomena must account for the fact that to act intentionally, or to be motivated so to act, is necessarily to be in a goal-directed state. The teleological argument aims to show that conformity to rational principles cannot alone account for this fact.

The argument—which has been given its clearest and most vigorous statement in a recent discussion by Michael Smith[9]—proceeds as follows. To be in a goal-directed state, it is claimed, is to be in a distinctive kind of psychological condition. Specifically, it is to be in a state whose content is not meant to match or represent the way things are in the world, but which is such that the world is to be made to match or fit the content of the state.[10] This reflects itself in the fact that people who are in a goal-directed state will not, in general, give up the goal, upon learning that it has not been realized in the world, but will instead take steps to change the world so that the goal can be realized. The question arises, however, as to what it is to be in a psychological state which has this peculiar direction of fit *vis-à-vis* the world; and a plausible answer to this question must hold that,

[9] See Michael Smith, 'The Humean Theory of Motivation', *Mind*, 1987. Smith's article makes the significant contribution (which I have followed) of formulating the argument in terms of claims about the 'direction of fit' of psychological states, *vis-à-vis* the world. I suspect that similar considerations, less cogently expressed, have historically tended to move proponents of the Humean approach. They also seem to lie behind the common thesis that intention entails desire; for a recent discussion of this idea, see Robert Audi, 'Intending, Intentional Action, and Desire', in Joel Marks (ed.), *The Ways of Desire*, Chicago, Precedent Publishing, 1986.

[10] On the idea that psychological states may be differentiated according to their 'direction of fit' with the world, see, for example, G. E. M. Anscombe, *Intention*, Ithaca, Cornell University Press, 1963, sections 36, 40; Bernard Williams, 'Consistency and Realism', in his *Problems of the Self*, Cambridge, Cambridge University Press, 1973, pp. 203–5; John Searle, *Intentionality*, Cambridge, Cambridge University Press, 1983, pp. 7–9; and Richard Wollheim, *The Thread of Life*, Cambridge, Harvard University Press, 1984, pp. 52–3. Talk about 'direction of fit' applies literally to propositions; its application to psychological states may seem metaphorical or otherwise problematic. For attempts to explain and to defend talk about the 'direction of fit' of propositional attitudes, see Andrew Woodfield, 'Desire, Intentional Content and Teleological Explanation', *Proceedings of the Aristotelian Society*, 1981–2, pp. 82–6; and Smith, 'The Humean Theory of Motivation', section 6.

360   *R. Jay Wallace*

whatever else is involved in being in a goal-directed state, it cannot simply
be a matter of having a certain belief or set of beliefs. Beliefs are precisely
those psychological states which aim to match or represent the world, and
their direction of fit is therefore just the converse of that which
characterizes goal-directed states. Some other kind of state must thus be
present, whenever one acts intentionally or is motivated so to act.
Moreover, it is plausible to suppose that these further goal-directed states
will characteristically be constituted by desires; for there is a general
conception of desires according to which they are the psychological states
one is in whenever one is in a state such that the world must be made to fit
the content of the state (rather than vice-versa).[11]

   This argument, which looks fairly strong as far as it goes, establishes
that beliefs alone cannot account for motivations to action, but that desires
must also be present whenever an agent is so motivated. The Humean,
however, wishes to draw the stronger—or at any rate, different—conclusion that we cannot account adequately for motivation and intentional
action solely in terms of the following of rational principles or norms, and
to reach this conclusion on the basis of the teleological argument it is
necessary to make some further assumptions.[12] The most important such
assumption is the following: that rational principles will only be capable of
contributing to the explanation of motivation to the extent that desires are
not implicated in motivation. This assumption seems to be part of a
broader picture of rationality, according to which reasoning and
ratiocination are associated exclusively with the cognitive side of human
psychology—that is, with beliefs and relations among one's beliefs—and
contrasted with such non-rational states as desires and emotions (what
Hume refers to collectively as 'the passions'). Hume himself endorses
some version of this picture in the *Treatise*.[13] He distinguishes between

[11] The conception in question is dispositional (but non-behaviourist). See, for example, the
dispositional conceptions of desire sketched by Richard B. Brandt and Jaegwon Kim, in 'Wants as
Explanations of Actions', *The Journal of Philosophy*, 1963; and by William P. Alston, in 'Motives and
Motivation', in Paul Edwards (ed.), *The Encyclopedia of Philosophy*, New York, Macmillan and Free
Press, 1967. Apparent counter-examples to the claim that goal-directed states are always realized by
desires—such as hopes and wishes—are plausibly understood as involving an element of desiring; on
this point, see Wayne Davis, 'Two Senses of Desire', in Joel Marks (ed.), *The Ways of Desire*, p. 64.
Some philosophers, such as Brandt and Kim, find it more felicitous to use the term 'want' to refer to
the general, dispositional conception of desire, reserving the term 'desire' for appetitive states which
have a distinctive phenomenology; but nothing significant hangs on this terminological issue.

[12] This gets obscured in Smith's discussion, because he is content for the most part to represent the
Humean view as the claim that explanatory reasons for action are partly constituted by desires. This
formulation, however, does not bring out adequately the central point at issue between the Humean
and the rationalist, which is the extent to which rational processes of thought—those which are
governed by rational principles or norms—can contribute to the explanation of motivation.

[13] Book II, part iii, section iii (p. 415). I assume here that when Hume describes the passions as
original existences, he is not necessarily denying that they have propositional content, but only denying
that their content is 'representational'—such as aims to fit the way the world is. For discussion of this
and other possible interpretations, see Mark Platts, 'Hume and Morality as a Matter of Fact', *Mind*,
1988, sections 6–9.

the passions, as 'original existences', and those states of the understanding which admit of truth and falsity, suggesting that the latter states are alone the province of rationality. But this picture, when combined with the teleological argument, appears to make the Humean conclusion irresistible: if desires are necessarily present on occasions of motivation, and if desires are not themselves rational psychological states, what scope can there possibly be for the rational explanation of motivation and intentional action?

This, in outline, is the teleological argument for the Humean position. If sound, it would constitute an a priori argument against the very possibility of a rationalist account of practical reason, for it would show that rational principles or norms cannot contribute to the primary explanation of motivations, in the way the rationalist supposes. Motivation, being a teleological phenomenon, requires the presence of desire, and desires are simply beyond the range of explanation in terms of rational principles or norms.[14]

3. If we are to leave open the possibility of a rationalist account of practical reason, some response to the teleological argument will have to be made. In fact I think there are two strategies that might be followed in responding to the teleological argument. One strategy would be to question the conception of desire that figures in the argument. In particular, we might challenge the Humean assumption that to be in a teleological or goal-directed state is necessarily to be in a state of desire. Though some have followed this strategy, it does not seem a very promising line to take, because the conception of desire underlying the teleological argument is independently more plausible than the alternative accounts that have been proposed.[15] For this reason, I think that a different strategy will have to be pursued.

The immediate conclusion of the teleological argument, it should be recalled, is that a person cannot simply be in a state of belief, on an occasion when he acts intentionally or is motivated to act intentionally; some state of wanting or desiring is additionally required. As I said earlier

---

[14] This teleological aspect of action-explanations is entirely left out of account in the argument which Richard Warner gives for the coherence of a rationalist account of motivation, in *Freedom, Enjoyment and Happiness*, Ithaca, Cornell University Press, 1987, pp. 42–5. Warner describes a thought experiment in which we are to imagine a creature which takes thoughts as inputs and produces behaviour as output; the coherence of the description is then taken to show that a rationalist account is at least possible. But the description is coherent only if we interpret the creature's behaviour as mere bodily movement rather than as intentional action. The point of the teleological argument is that it is *not* coherent to suppose that intentional action could take place in the absence of a state of desire.

[15] The alternative accounts treat desires—or at any rate, 'genuine' desires, as opposed to mere formal desires—as states that have a distinctive phenomenology: see, for example, Mark Platts, *Ways of Meaning*, London, Routledge and Kegan Paul, 1979, ch. 10; and Don Locke, 'Beliefs, Desires and Reasons for Action', *American Philosophical Quarterly*, 1982. Smith effectively criticizes the idea that all genuine desires are states with a distinctive phenomenology, in 'The Humean Theory of Motivation', section 5. See also Alston, 'Motives and Motivation', pp. 402–3.

362   *R. Jay Wallace*

however this conclusion by itself is not yet damaging to the rationalist, or supportive of a Humean account of practical reason. To derive a Humean moral from the teleological argument, it is necessary to make the further assumption that the presence of desire precludes the rational explanation of motivation; that because the desires involved in motivation are themselves non-rational states, there is no scope for distinctively rational principles to enter into the explanation of motivation. The second and more promising strategy for challenging the Humean is to question this crucial assumption.

To understand the problem with this assumption, however, it will be necessary to provide a clearer account of what the debate between the Humean and the rationalist is all about. Now I suspect—though I am not certain about this—that the key to a proper understanding of the debate is to be found in chapter V of Thomas Nagel's book, *The Possibility of Altruism*. I say I am unsure about this, because Nagel's account of the debate turns on distinctions and concepts that are not adequately explained; certainly, his discussion has not prevented his readers from continuing to misunderstand the issue that divides Humeans and rationalists. In what follows I shall develop an interpretation of that issue which is at least broadly inspired by Nagel's discussion, with the aim of making more perspicuous than Nagel himself succeeded in doing the flaw in the Humean appropriation of the teleological argument.

Nagel starts by accepting the immediate conclusion of the teleological argument, and the associated conception of desires as states that realize one's having of an aim or goal. He says, for instance, that '*whatever* may be the motivation for someone's intentional pursuit of a goal, it becomes in virtue of his pursuit *ipso facto* appropriate to ascribe to him a desire for the goal'.[16] Desires, then, must always be present on occasions of motivation and intentional action. But a further issue arises, concerning the explanatory role of desires in accounting for motivation, and the resolution of this issue is absolutely crucial to the Humean interpretation of the teleological argument. Nagel raises this further issue by drawing a distinction between two broad categories of desires, which he calls 'motivated' and 'unmotivated'.[17] He explains the distinction in the following terms. Unmotivated desires are desires which simply assail us or come over us (Nagel cites as examples the appetites and certain emotions); whereas motivated desires

[16]   *The Possibility of Altruism*, p. 29.

[17]   *The Possibility of Altruism*, p. 29. Various historical precedents for this distinction have been cited. Nagel himself now claims that it has affinities with the Kantian distinction between inclination and interest; see his *The View from Nowhere*, New York, Oxford University Press, 1986, p. 151 (n. 3). N. J. H. Dent suggests a different parallel between Nagel's distinction and the distinction in Aristotle and Aquinas between 'deliberated appetites' and 'sense appetites', in *The Moral Psychology of the Virtues*, Cambridge, Cambridge University Press, 1984, ch. 4. I am myself doubtful how close Nagel's distinction really is to either of these antecedents—the category of motivated desires is much more encompassing than the earlier counterparts, at least on the interpretation of it I shall go on to offer.

are *'arrived at* by decision and after deliberation'.[18] Desires of both types are presumably susceptible of explanation—we can, for instance, explain the onset of an unmotivated desire to eat by citing the physiological factors associated with a lack of food. But only motivated desires admit of what Nagel calls 'rational or motivational explanation'.[19]

Now this account of the difference between motivated and unmotivated desires is not very helpful. It suggests that motivated desires will always be formed after a prior episode of deliberation, and that all unmotivated desires are like bouts of animal lust in 'assailing' the agent unfortunate enough to be in their grip; but I do not think this can have been the kind of distinction that Nagel was trying to draw. For one thing, Nagel's distinction looked like offering a comprehensive typology of desires; but a great many of the desires that we ascribe to people are neither states that simply assail the person who has them, nor states that the person goes into following an episode ofdeliberation. Consider, for instance, the important class of long-term or dispositional desires that are formed as a result of moral education, and help to constitute a person's overall character: these can hardly be said to 'assail' the person who has them, like lust or thirst, but at the same time they are not arrived at by decision and after deliberation, either.

More promising, in my view, is Nagel's suggestion that what marks the difference between motivated and unmotivated desires is the kind of explanation to which each is susceptible; in particular, the idea that motivated desires are distinctive in admitting of what he calls 'rational or motivational explanation'. So far, however, this idea is merely a suggestion, for Nagel's own discussion does nothing to clarify the important notion of rational or motivational explanation. Moreover, without a precise explanation of this notion, the significance of the distinction between motivated and unmotivated desires is apt to remain obscure—a point which I shall have occasion to illustrate, later in my discussion. Let me now offer my own account of the notion of rational or motivational explanation, and say in terms of it what is significant about the distinction between motivated and unmotivated desires.[20]

---

[18] *The Possibility of Altruism*, p.29.   [19] *The Possibility of Altruism*, p. 29.

[20] There is, in fact, a variety of ways of distinguishing between different kinds of desires, many of which are close to being coextensive with the distinction between motivated and unmotivated desires, as I shall construe it. Consider, for example, Stuart Hampshire's distinction between desires which are, and desires which are not, mediated by descriptions or conceptions, in *Freedom of the Individual*, Expanded Edition, Princeton, Princeton University Press, 1975, ch. 2; Stephen Schiffer's distinction between reason-providing and reason-following desires, in 'A Paradox of Desire', *American Philosophical Quarterly*, 1976; and the distinction Wayne Davis draws between volitive and appetitive desires, in 'Two Senses of Desire'. The near coextensiveness of these various distinctions may make it tempting to suppose that they are all, at bottom, different ways of marking the same basic difference between kinds of desires; but I suspect that this is not in fact the case. At any rate, my discussion in the text is meant only to give a sharper interpretation of a single distinction which is especially important for the debate about practical reason, that between what Nagel has called motivated and unmotivated desires.

The basic idea, I would suggest, is that when a person has a motivated desire, it will always be possible to explain that desire in a way that shows it to be *rationalized* by other propositional attitudes that the person has. That is, psychological explanation of motivated desires is not restricted to causal claims, about the states or conditions that trigger the onset of the desire. Rather, motivated desires also (and *necessarily*) admit of a different kind of psychological explanation, in which the propositional content of the desire is shown to be rationalized or justified by the content of other of the person's attitudes.[21] Of course, it is possible for one propositional attitude to be rationalized by other attitudes of the agent's, without the rationalizing attitudes *explaining* the formation of the state that is rationalized; a rationalizing explanation requires, more strongly, that the person should be in the rationalizing state *because* he has certain other attitudes that rationalize that state. But it is plausible to think that motivated desires can be explained in this distinctive, rationalizing way. Thus—to take Nagel's own simple example—if Wotan's desire to shop for groceries is a motivated desire, then there will be an explanation of it that reveals it to be rationalized by other propositional attitudes that Wotan has: for example, a desire to eat something, a belief that there is nothing at home to eat, plus various other beliefs of Wotan's (about grocery stores, shopping, etc.). It is because Wotan has these rationalizing attitudes that he forms the motivated desire to shop; but at the same time those rationalizing attitudes provide *reasons* for Wotan's motivated desire.[22]

To put the point this way, however, is potentially misleading. Rationalizing explanations, as I have introduced the notion, explain propositional attitudes in terms of other attitudes whose content rationalizes the state which is to be explained, where rationalization is construed as the provision of reasons or justifications. Strictly speaking, however, the *contents* of desires never provide reasons or justifications for other propositional attitudes; nor do they themselves appear directly susceptible of rationalizing explanation. For example, the propositional content of Wotan's desire to shop for groceries—that is, 'that he (Wotan) shop for groceries'—simply seems to have the wrong form either to justify, or be justified by, other propositions; read literally, it is not even in the indicative mood.[23]

It would be a mistake to conclude from this, however, that desires

[21] I do not mean to suggest that rationalizing explanations may not also be cause-giving explanations. For a useful recent discussion of this point, and of the nature of rationalizing explanation more generally, see Philip Pettit, 'Broad-Minded Explanation and Psychology', in Philip Pettit and John McDowell (eds), *Subject, Thought, and Context*, Oxford, Clarendon Press, 1986.

[22] There is an obvious analogy here with the case of beliefs. Many of a person's beliefs are held for reasons, where the reasons are other propositional attitudes which both rationalize the belief and explain the holding of it.

[23] Michael Smith made me see this point. It raises a potential problem for all accounts which hold that some desires are held for reasons, such as those of Stephen Schiffer, in 'A Paradox of Desire', and Wayne Davis, in 'Two Senses of Desire'.

cannot enter into rationalizing explanations at all. To see how they can, we need only note that desires are characteristically associated with evaluative beliefs. Thus, if Wotan wants to shop for groceries, it will—in the normal case, at least[24]—be legitimate to ascribe to him an evaluative belief, to the effect that shopping for groceries is (prima facie) desirable.[25] The content of this evaluative belief, however, can straightforwardly enter into relations of rationalization and justification with other contents of propositional attitudes. For example, we might deploy the schema of the practical syllogism to explain the belief that shopping for groceries is (prima facie) desirable in terms of the following, further propositional attitudes: the evaluative belief that eating is (prima facie) desirable; and the belief that in order to eat it is necessary to go shopping for groceries.[26] The content of these propositional attitudes justifies or provides a reason for the conclusion that shopping for groceries is (prima facie) desirable. And, a person might have reached this conclusion *because* that person holds these further, rationalizing beliefs.

Evaluative beliefs can in this way straightforwardly enter into relations of rationalizing explanation. If this much can be admitted, however, then we have a way of drawing the distinction between motivated and unmotivated desires in terms of the notion of rationalizing explanation. We may say, to start with, that motivated desires are desires whose associated evaluative beliefs admit of a rationalizing explanation. Furthermore, when the evaluative belief associated with a desire admits of a rationalizing explanation in this way, the factors which justify and support the belief can equally be said to justify and support the desire associated with the belief; so that the reasons for the belief may be considered reasons for acquiring the desire as well. To give a a rationalizing *explanation* of the desire in terms of these reasons, it need only be supposed in addition that the desire has been formed *because* the agent has endorsed the evaluative

[24] The abnormal cases are those in which one desires something which one does not value at all, not even instrumentally. Such cases are discussed by Harry Frankfurt, in 'Freedom of the Will and the Concept of a Person', *The Journal of Philosophy*, 1971; and Gary Watson, 'Free Agency', *The Journal of Philosophy*, 1975. See also Frankfurt's more recent discussion 'Identification and Wholeheartedness', in Ferdinand Schoeman (ed.), *Responsibility, Character, and the Emotions: New Essays in Moral Psychology*, New York, Cambridge University Press, 1987. For present purposes it is enough to acknowledge that such desires exist, and to observe that they cannot, strictly speaking, provide material for practical reasoning or deliberation. (Reasoning or deliberation involving such desires requires the *pretence* that their objects satisfy some evaluative predicate or other.)

[25] The predicate 'is (prima facie) desirable' is meant only as an example; it should be construed as ranging over both instrumental and intrinsic kinds of desirability. Similar points might be made, with appropriate modifications, in terms of other specific evaluative predicates; or in terms of 'ought'-judgements, or judgements about reasons for action.

[26] That these apparently simple syllogistic explanations mask the complexity of even instrumental reasoning is a point made by Jaakko Hintikka, in 'Theoretical Reason—An Ambiguous Legacy', in Stephan Körner (ed.), *Practical Reason*, Oxford, Basil Blackwell, 1974; see also David Wiggins, 'Deliberation and Practical Reason', in Amélie Oksenberg Rorty (ed.), *Essays on Aristotle's Ethics*, Berkeley, University of California Press, 1980. The point does not seem to me to detract from the usefulness of the practical syllogism, as a framework for certain kinds of rationalizing explanations.

judgement and the reasons that directly support it. This would often seem to be a plausible assumption to make.

A distinction can thus be drawn between two broad classes of desires—the motivated and the unmotivated—in terms of whether the evaluative beliefs associated with the desires admit of a distinctively rationalizing explanation. Moreover, it should be clear that this distinction has some relevance to the Humean appropriation of the teleological argument. The Humean concludes, from the fact that desires are always present on occasions of motivation, that motivation cannot be explained rationally, assuming that the presence of desires necessarily limits the scope for explanation in terms of rational principles or norms. But Nagel's distinction, at least on the interpretation of it I have offered, calls this assumption into question. Many of the desires that figure in motivation are themselves motivated propositional attitudes—in my terms, states which admit of a further rationalizing explanation, via their associated evaluative beliefs. Their presence on occasions of motivation therefore does not necessarily preclude the purely rational explanation of motivation. For all that the teleological argument shows, the rationalizing explanation of motivated desires may sometimes rely solely on the agent's beliefs, together with rational principles or norms, and in such cases it would be possible to give a purely rational explanation of both motivation and the desires necessarily implicated in it.

4. It will be well to pause over the distinction between motivated and unmotivated desires, to get clearer about its implications for the debate between the Humean and the rationalist. On the interpretation I have urged, a motivated desire is one whose associated evaluative belief admits of a rationalizing explanation, where the desire is formed *because* the agent has arrived at the evaluative belief. A crucial assumption here is that the rational explanation for an evaluative belief may account for the formation of the motivated desire as well, so that the reasons which explain the belief will equally be reasons for the motivated desire. To say this, it seems, is to admit that it is an independent principle or norm of rationality that one should desire in accordance with one's evaluative beliefs, where this means that one should desire those ends and activities one takes to be desirable, to the extent one takes them to be desirable. Only on this assumption are we entitled to maintain that the rational explanations and justifications of evaluative beliefs may extend as well to the motivated desires associated with them.

This would seem to be a plausible minimal assumption to make about the content of the principles or norms of practical reason, since we do in fact try to adjust our desires to our evaluative beliefs, and take ourselves to be subject to rational criticism when we fail. Officially, of course, Hume himself would deny that this is a legitimate assumption, since he is on

record as holding that rational criticism is restricted to the theoretical sphere of beliefs and the relations between them. But as Nagel and Korsgaard have persuasively suggested, Hume's own discussion of practical reason appears to take for granted some irreducible principles of practical rationality, such as the principle that one should adjust one's desires to one's evaluative beliefs.[27] Thus, Hume notes that people who cease to believe that a certain action or object is a means to some valued end will immediately desist from desiring that action or object.[28] But how are we to understand this tendency? Behind it, there seems to lie the assumption (or something equivalent to it) that it is rational to adjust one's desires at least to one's beliefs about what is instrumentally valuable; plus the assumption that people are, in this respect, characteristically rational. Hume himself thus seems poorly placed to reject out of hand the principle that rational agents adjust their desires to their evaluative beliefs.

This has important implications for the debate about practical reason. It shows that if we are to make sense of the notion of a motivated desire—a desire, that is, which is explicable in terms of the agent's reasons—then we must deny the most extreme Humean claim that there are no irreducible principles or norms of practical reason, only principles or norms of theoretical rationality. To deny this claim, however, is not yet to settle the issue between the Humean and the rationalist. That issue concerns the possibility of explaining motivation and intentional action in purely rational terms. But for all that has been established so far, it might be that the irreducible principles of practical reason are exclusively principles of instrumental or derivative rationality, accounting for the rational extension of motivational influence, but not capable of explaining the original formation of motivation or the original fixing of an agent's ends.

Rationalists, of course, deny this. They maintain that the principles or norms of practical reason are such that reasoning in accordance with them can explain, not just the extension of given motivations, but the original formation of motivation and the fixing of one's ends. If I am right, explanations of this sort would have to be capable of yielding explanations of an agent's motivated desires, since, by the teleological argument, desires are invariably present on occasions of motivation. What would a distinctively rationalist explanation of motivated desires look like?

For purposes of illustration, we may consider two possibilities. The rationalizing explanation of desires, I have suggested, will proceed via the rationalizing explanation of their associated evaluative beliefs. One way we might provide these explanations is to deploy the schema of the practical syllogism, relating specific evaluative conclusions to more general evaluative premises, by way of intervening factual beliefs, until we arrive at

[27] Nagel, *The Possibility of Altruism*, pp. 33–4; Korsgaard, 'Skepticism about Practical Reason', section III.
[28] Hume, *A Treatise of Human Nature*, p. 416.

368   *R. Jay Wallace*

basic principles about what is intrinsically valuable. The rationalist might
then attempt to establish that these basic evaluative principles can
themselves be given a rational justification, one which shows them to be
valid independently of considerations about the desires that particular
agents may happen to have.

Consider, for example, Nagel's argument in part III of *The Possibility of
Altruism*.[29] We might reconstruct Nagel's rationalist position, in accordance with the model I have just sketched, in the following terms. Suppose
someone has a desire to perform a specific action of type *R*, and an
associated evaluative belief that doing that action is (prima facie) desirable
(where '*R*' = an act of relieving someone's pain). On one reading of Nagel's
account, the rationalizing explanation of this evaluative belief may relate it
to a basic evaluative principle that the agent accepts, to the effect that *any*
action which would relieve someone's pain is (prima facie) desirable. This
basic evaluative principle may then in turn be given a rational justification,
on the reading of Nagel's argument now under consideration, in so far as
rejection of the principle would commit one to the constitutively irrational
doctrine of solipsism.[30] But if such a justification can successfully be
carried through, then the rational considerations which figure in it could
be invoked to explain, not just the basic evaluative principles and the
specific evaluations derived from them, but also an agent's desires in
accordance with these (basic and derived) evaluations. For we are
assuming that it is an independent principle of rationality that one should
desire in accordance with one's evaluative beliefs.

This is not, however, the only way that a rationalist explanation of
motivated desires might be developed. A second possibility is that the
rationalizing explanation of specific evaluative beliefs may depart from the
schema of the practical syllogism; so that we are sometimes able to explain
a specific evaluation rationally by relating it *directly* to further beliefs that
the agent holds, together with background principles of rational reflection.
To return to the example of Nagel's argument, this model suggests a
different way of explaining the specific evaluative belief that it is (prima
facie) desirable to perform a particular action of type *R* (where '*R*' = an act
of relieving someone's pain). In particular, we might rationally explain the

---

[29] What follows is based only very loosely on Nagel's complicated discussion, but I hope the
parallels will be apparent. It should be stressed, too, that I am not trying to argue for Nagel's position,
but only trying to see what a rationalist position might look like, by considering how Nagel's claims
might variously be formulated.
[30] Nicholas Sturgeon seems to interpret Nagel this way, as trying to provide a *justification* for a
basic evaluative principle in favour of altruistic motivation, in 'Altruism, Solipsism, and the
Objectivity of Reasons', *The Philosophical Review*, 1974 (especially pp. 375, 393–4). Aristotle's ethical
theory is sometimes interpreted as an attempt to provide a similar rational justification for such basic
evaluative principles (fixing the ends of action). See, for example, T. H. Irwin, 'Aristotle on Reason,
Desire, and Virtue', *The Journal of Philosophy*, 1975, especially pp. 574–6; and Norman O. Dahl,
Practical Reason, Aristotle, and Weakness of the Will, Minneapolis, University of Minnesota Press,
1984, Part One.

belief by relating it, simply, to the agents belief that the action is of type R; for on a second interpretation of Nagel's argument, background principles of rationality license a *direct* inference from the belief that an act would relieve someone's pain to the evaluative conclusion that the act is (prima facie) desirable.[31] Furthermore, this rationalizing explanation of the evaluative belief may carry over to the desire which is associated with it, since (again) we are assuming the rational requirement that one should desire in accordance with one's evaluative beliefs.

We have, then, two models for explaining motivated desires in accordance with the rationalist claim that pure reasoning can be practical in its issue. What, on the other side, would a Humean position look like? Here, the simplest approach would be to deploy the schema of the practical syllogism to explain specific evaluative beliefs. That is, we should suppose that, when specific evaluative beliefs admit of a rationalizing explanation, the explanation offered will relate the beliefs to more general evaluative premisses, by way of factual beliefs, until basic principles are reached about what is intrinsically desirable. So far, the Humean approach would follow the first model for a rationalist account which I sketched above. Unlike the rationalist, however, the Humean must deny that the basic evaluative principles with which syllogistic explanations terminate can be given an independent rational justification. Rather, the Humean will suppose that these basic evaluative principles are fixed by the agent's intrinsic desires, desires which cannot themselves be given a further, rationalizing explanation.[32] Only if we make this assumption will it be the case—as the Humean claims—that practical reason is restricted to accounting for the extension of motivational influence from fixed, antecedent ends.

To put the issue in these terms is to admit that, even on a Humean account, rational explanations of motivation can be given exclusively in terms of the agent's (evaluative) beliefs. For on the kind of Humean position I have sketched, the rational explanation of motivation terminates with citation of the agent's basic principles or beliefs about what is

[31] An interpretation on these lines seems the more proper way of reading Nagel's argument. The burden of the argument is not to provide a rational justification for some basic evaluative premiss, such as figures in the first model of the rationalist position which I sketched. Rather, it is to provide an *interpretation* of the inference patterns characteristic of moral reflection, showing those inference patterns to be rational by displaying their connections with broader patterns of inference that are paradigmatically rational. See Nagel's remarks about the 'method of interpretation', in *The Possibility of Altruism*, pp. 4, 18–23.

[32] The most straightforward way to develop this claim would be to say (with Hobbes) that a person's basic values are, simply, those things which the person desires for their own sakes. A more plausible proposal would allow room for discrepancies between a person's actual, first-order desires and the person's values, treating values (for instance) as some function of the agent's second-order desires (cf. Frankfurt, 'Freedom of the Will and the Concept of a Person' and 'Identification and Wholeheartedness').

Note too that it will often be possible to provide *non*-rationalizing explanations of an agent's intrinsic desires. For instance, in some cases they might be taken to result from a process of Aristotelian habituation or training.

370   *R. Jay Wallace*

intrinsically valuable. It is true that, on the Humean acount, these basic
beliefs will in turn be fixed by the agent's intrinsic desires; but those
desires do not *rationalize* or *rationally* explain the basic evaluative beliefs.
To think that they do is to suppose that it is a basic principle of practical
rationality that one should adjust one's evaluative beliefs to one's (intrinsic) desires. But in fact rationality does not require that we adjust our
evaluative beliefs to our desires in this way (it can be perfectly rational to
hold that one's intrinsic desires sometimes aim at objects or activities
which are not valuable at all). Still, even if intrinsic desires do not
rationally explain an agent's basic evaluative beliefs, on the Humean view,
there is a looser but more important sense in which they determine the
starting points for practical reasoning and deliberation. So long as basic
evaluations are fixed by an agent's intrinsic desires, rational criticism of the
agent's ends will not be a possibility, and practical reason will be restricted
to accounting for the extension of motivational influence from given,
antecedent ends.[33]

   This discussion may be summarized by saying that Humeans are
committed to a distinctive thesis about the form taken by rationalizing
explanations of desires. In particular, they are committed to the view that
rationalizing explanations of desires must terminate, at some point, with
the citation of a basic evaluative belief of the agent's which cannot itself be
justified or explained in rational terms. An agent's particular evaluative
beliefs and motivated desires may be explained, in the first instance, by
being related to basic evaluative principles that the agent holds; but on the
Humean view these basic principles are always fixed or determined by the
agent's intrinsic desires, and so beyond range of rational justification or
explanation. This thesis about the form taken by rationalizing explanations
of desires might be called the 'desire-out, desire-in' principle, since it
maintains that processes of thought which give rise to a desire (as 'output')
can always be traced back to a further desire (as 'input'), one which fixes
the basic evaluative principles from which the rational explanation of
motivation begins. An adequate defence of the Humean position must
provide a reason for accepting this distinctive thesis about the form taken
by rationalizing explanations of desires.

   Once the issue is seen in this way, however, it becomes apparent that the
teleological argument by itself has no direct bearing on the dispute

---

[33] This point seems to be neglected by Don Locke, in 'Beliefs, Desires and Reasons for Action'.
Locke argues against the Humean approach by insisting that rational explanations of motivation can be
given exclusively in terms of an agent's evaluative beliefs (in particular, he suggests explanations in
terms of what he calls 'sufficient reason' beliefs: see 'Beliefs, Desires and Reasons for Action', pp.
246–7; also Locke's 'Reasons, Wants, and Causes', *American Philosophical Quarterly*, 1974, pp.
170–2). But Locke admits that these sufficient reason beliefs may simply 'derive from' the agent's
desires ('Beliefs, Desires and Reasons for Action', p. 247). In the terms I have proposed, however, this
is not an admission which it is open to an anti-Humean to make, since the distinctive Humean claim is
precisely the claim that the evaluative beliefs in terms of which we explain desires are themselves
'derived from' or fixed by the agent's desires.

between the Humean and the rationalist. That argument establishes only that desires must be present on occasions of motivation. It leaves it an open question whether the present desires are themselves motivated or unmotivated; and, still more significantly, it says nothing at all about the form that must be taken by rationalizing explanations of motivated desires. An a priori argument for the Humean account would have to be a defence of the desire-out, desire-in principle, and the teleological argument sketched earlier does not by itself provide a defence of that crucial principle.

I would suggest, then, that the significance of the distinction between motivated and unmotivated desires is that it sharpens our conception of the debate between the Humean and the rationalist. Interpreting this distinction as I have done, we see that the real burden on the Humean is to defend a claim about the rationalizing explanation of desires, the claim I have called the desire-out, desire-in principle. It is because the teleological argument by itself lends no support to this crucial principle that it fails to settle the issue between the Humean and the rationalist.

5. Of course, the failure of one attempted a priori argument for the Humean position does not rule out other strategies that might be pursued in support of the Humean approach. In this section I wish to consider, briefly, three further arguments that purport to offer general support for a broadly Humean account. The interpretation of the debate I have developed in the preceding sections should help us to see why none of these further arguments succeed.

An assumption commonly made about rationalist accounts is that they end up identifying desires and beliefs, saying that there are certain beliefs which are desires, or which serve as desires, or which are necessarily connected with desires.[34] But the idea that desires might be identified with beliefs in this way has recently come under attack, on grounds that it is incompatible with the accounts of belief and desire provided by decision theory.[35] The idea, roughly, is that on decision-theoretic accounts, beliefs and desires should evolve in different ways, when new information is added to an existing set of attitudes, thus precluding the identification of desires with beliefs. If this is right,[36] it should provide a general reason for

[34] See, for example, Warner, *Freedom, Enjoyment and Happiness*, ch. 1, where it is suggested that, on a rationalist view, certain thoughts may 'serve as' desires; and Philip Pettit, 'Humeans, Anti-Humeans, and Motivation', *Mind*, 1987, who proposes a version of rationalism on which the presence of desires is sometimes entailed by the presence of beliefs.

[35] See David Lewis, 'Desire as Belief', *Mind*, 1988, where the argument is presented using Bayesian decision theory; and John Collins, 'Belief, Desire, and Revision', *Mind*, 1988, who reaches a similar conclusion using non-quantitative decision theory.

[36] For some doubts, see Huw Price, 'Defending Desire-as-Belief', *Mind*, 1989. A better objection, found in very recent work by John Collins, challenges the argument's premiss that rational belief-revision is always by conditionalization (or its non-quantitative analogue). Collins now thinks that there are independent reasons for holding that belief revision follows two, distinct methods:

anyone who accepts decision theory to resist the identification of desires with beliefs.[37] It is doubtful, however, whether this result has any direct bearing on the debate between the Humean and the rationalist, as I have reconstructed it. For on neither of the models of a rationalist account which I have sketched is the rationalist committed to identifying desires and beliefs, or to holding that they are necessarily connected. What the rationalist does maintain is that certain kinds of desires can be given a rational explanation, in terms of an agent's beliefs (together with principles or norms of practical rationality). This would establish, perhaps, a *rational* connection between certain beliefs and certain desires. But to conclude, on this basis, that the beliefs and desires in question are identical, or necessarily connected, is to confuse the rational connections of explanation and justification with laws of psychological necessity. People are irrational, much of the time, and for this reason alone no rationalist account should identify beliefs with desires, or hold that they are necessarily connected.[38]

Still, the rationalist must establish the claim that there is at least a rational connection between beliefs and desires, and attempts to make out such a connection might appear to run into a different kind of problem. To see this, observe that the two models for a rationalist account which I sketched above both apparently license an inference from *factual* premisses to an *evaluative* conclusion. On the first model, this occurs at the point at which a rational justification is provided for basic evaluative principles; on the second model, it occurs in the allegedly rational inference from specific factual beliefs to specific evaluative conclusions. Noticing this feature of rationalist accounts, Mark Platts has recently suggested that the force of Hume's own argument against the rationalist rests on his famous strictures against deducing 'ought'-conclusions from 'is'-premisses.[39] For the ban

conditionalization, which is appropriate for genuine updating of belief; and the merely *hypothetical* revision implicit in the decision theoretic definition of expected value, which has quite different formal properties. The theorems proved in the papers by Collins's and Lewis (see n. 35 above) give us further reasons for acknowledging these two distinct methods of belief revision; but they do not rule out the possibility that beliefs and intrinsic desires are necessarily connected. Collins' new position is developed in his paper 'Updating and Supposing', read at the A.A.P. Conference in Canberra in July 1989.

[37] Stephen Darwall has argued from decision theory to the opposite conclusion that the Humean approach must be wrong, in *Impartial Reason*, Ithaca, Cornell University Press, 1983, ch. 6. He maintains that we can only make sense of the decision-theoretic requirement of transitivity of individual preferences on the assumption that an agent's preferences are criticizable in terms of reasons. Even if this is correct, however, it does not yet establish that the terms for criticism of desires conform to a rationalist rather then a Humean pattern: the basic values which lie behind an agent's preferences, and render them commensurable, may themselves merely reflect the agent's intrinsic desires.

[38] This is the moral of Korsgaard's discussion of internalism, in 'Skepticism about Practical Reason'. See also Nagel, *The Possibility of Altruism*, pp. 20–2, 65–7; Michael Smith, 'On Humeans, Anti-Humeans, and Motivation: A Reply to Pettit', *Mind*, 1988, pp. 591–2; and Michael Smith, *The Moral Problem*, Oxford, University D. Phil., 1989, ch. 6, section 4.

[39] Platts, 'Hume and Morality as a Matter of Fact', pp. 201–3. It should be stressed that Platts offers this as an interpretation of Hume, not as an argument he himself endorses. In discussing Platts's suggestion, I shall put aside the question of whether Hume's intent in the is-ought passage was really to propose a strict ban on deriving 'oughts' from 'is'-premisses.

on such inferences, if it could be sustained, and extended to all inferences from factual premisses to evaluative conclusions, would indeed seem to rule out the rationalist explanation of motivated desires.

As an interpretation of Hume, however, this seems to me to get things the wrong way around: coming long after the Hume's discussion of the influencing motives of the will,[40] and lacking any independent support, the is-ought considerations appear simply to reflect Hume's basic anti-rationalist convictions, not to provide an argument for them. The point, moreover, is a general one. *Any* argument against rationalist accounts which merely invokes the alleged gap between is and ought (or between facts and values) seems bound to fail, because Humean strictures against deriving 'oughts' from 'is'-premisses are not independent of Humean accounts of practical reason. An argument for accepting the ban on deriving 'oughts' from 'is'-premisses would already *itself* be an argument for rejecting the rationalist approach to practical reason. But then the Humean needs to show us what that argument is; it is no use simply invoking the is-ought strictures, as if they had the status of an independent and established conclusion in the context of the debate between the Humean and the rationalist.

A third general argument against the rationalist approach has recently been suggested by Michael Smith.[41] Like the argument I presented in section 2 above, this argument turns on the teleological character of reason explanations. The apparent aim of Smith's new argument, however, is to show, not just that desires must be present on occasions of motivation, but that the explanation of motivated desires must conform to the principle of desire-out, desire-in. As we have seen, this is precisely what a general argument for the Humean account must establish.

Smith's own presentation of his position is succinct enough to be quoted virtually in its entirety:

A motivated desire is a desire had for a reason; that is, a desire the having of which furthers some goal that the agent has. The agent's having this goal *is*, in turn, *inter alia*, the state that constitutes the motivating reason that he has for having the desire.... But if the state that motivates the desire is itself a reason, and the having of this reason is itself constituted by his having a goal, then, given that the having of a goal is a state with which the world must fit rather than *vice versa* ..., so it follows ... that the state that motivates the desire must itself be a desire. Thus, the Humean will say, the idea that there may be a state that motivates a desire, but which is not itself a desire, is simply implausible.[42]

---

[40] The is-ought passage is in book III, part i, section iii of the *Treatise*, a full fifty pages after the discussion of the influencing motives of the will, which appears in book II, part iii, section iii.

[41] See Smith, 'The Humean Theory of Motivation', pp. 58–60; the argument is repeated in Smith's book *The Moral Problem*, ch. 6, section 5. A different argument, which like Smith's assumes that the states which rationally explain a desire must themselves be motives, may be found in Joel Marks, 'The Difference between Motivation and Desire', in Marks (ed.), *The Ways of Desire*, pp. 136–42; my remarks about Smith's argument tell equally against the one that Marks offers.

[42] 'The Humean Theory of Motivation', p. 59.

The structure of this argument is extremely straightforward. A motivated desire, Smith notes, is one that is explicable in terms of reasons. But reason explanations are essentially teleological, attributing a goal to the person who has the reason; and to have a goal is already to be in a state of desire. Of course that further desire may itself be motivated by a reason, but simple iteration of Smith's teleological argument suffices to show that the chain of explanations must eventually terminate in an unmotivated desire. Hence it is not an open question whether explanations of desires themselves always terminate in a desire. On the contrary, teleological considerations concerning the nature of reason explanations suffice to establish the Humean principle of desire-out, desire-in.

So Smith argues; but his argument seeks to prove too much. It turns on the claim that reason explanations are necessarily teleological, in the sense that the psychological states which constitute one's reasons are always goal-directed states. But if this were true, then to have a reason for *believing* something would equally be to have some desire which enters into the explanation of the belief. This is clearly not the case, however, since rationalizing explanations of beliefs are ordinarily given exclusively in terms of further beliefs that the agent holds (together with principles or norms of theoretical rationality). Thus, when Smith confronts the rationalist with what is supposed to be a dilemma—that is, a choice between denying that to have a reason is necessarily to have a goal, and denying that desires are the states that realize one's having a goal[43]—the appropriate response is to grasp the first horn. Far from its being, as Smith suggests, a conceptual truth, the principle that 'to have a reason is to have a goal' is simply *false*, on the interpretation of it that is relevant to the dispute between the Humean and the rationalist. What the Humean needs to establish is something at once less general and more difficult: not that to have a reason which explains a propositional attitude is always to have a goal, but that it is to have a goal whenever the attitude to be explained is itself a goal-directed state. That is the desire-out, desire-in principle, and there is nothing in the considerations Smith adduces that would support this crucial claim.

In fairness, however, it should be mentioned that Smith's apparent misinterpretation of the rationalist position is one that is directly encouraged by Nagel's own presentation of that position. As I explained in section 3, Nagel attaches great significance to the distinction between motivated and unmotivated desires, without making it adequately clear what it is for a desire to be motivated. Taking the terminology of 'motivated' and 'unmotivated' states quite literally, Smith seems to have assumed that a motivated desire is one that is formed for something like an

---

[43] 'The Humean Theory of Motivation', pp. 59–60.

ulterior motive.[44] That is, he interprets motivated desires as states which are precisely *not* rationalized by other of the agent's propositional attitudes, but rather formed under pressure of some further aim or goal that the agent has (as in a case of wishful thinking). This is what leads him to suppose that explanation of motivated desires has to postulate some further, goal-directed state of desire. Once we are quite clear about what is at stake in the debate between the Humean and the rationalist, however, it also becomes clear that teleological considerations are not going to determine the outcome of the debate.

6. To this point, I have offered an interpretation of the debate between the Humean and the rationalist, and in light of this account I have tried to show why teleological and other considerations do not provide general grounds for preferring the Humean to the rationalist account. We are, I would submit, now in a much stronger position to accept Korsgaard's contention that motivational scepticism about the rationalist position cannot be sustained. Still further support for this conclusion may be provided by considering one additional and extremely influential discussion of practical reason, that found in Bernard Williams's paper 'Internal and External Reasons'.[45] Williams's discussion has widely been interpreted as an attempt to raise a quite general problem for rationalist accounts of practical reason, and while there is now some evidence that Williams himself does not share this interpretation,[46] it will be useful to take up his argument on the assumption that it does in fact aim to support the Humean account.

Williams's argument starts from what might be called an internalist view of practical reasons. That is, Williams assumes that a person's reasons for action must be deliberatively accessible to the person, in the sense that it must be possible for the person to become motivated by her reasons for action as a result of purely rational reflection.[47] Given this assumption,

---

[44] On this point, see pp. 251–2 of Smith's more recent paper 'Reason and Desire', *Proceedings of the Aristotelian Society*, 1987–8. See also Smith, *The Moral Problem*, ch. 8, section 4.

[45] Reprinted in his *Moral Luck*, Cambridge, Cambridge University Press, 1981.

[46] See his book *Ethics and the Limits of Philosophy*, Cambridge, Harvard University Press, 1985, pp. 223–4 (n. 19), where Williams attributes to Kant the denial 'that there can be an absolutely "external" reason for action, one that does not speak to any motivation the agent already has'. The clear implication here is that the internal reasons theory which Williams has defended is something to which *both* Humeans and (Kantian) rationalists are committed; so that the difference between Humeans and rationalists would become a difference about the content of the dispositions which are to be included in the subjective motivational sets of rational agents. (See also Korsgaard, 'Skepticism about Practical Reason', section vi, where a similar reading of the internal reasons model is offered as part of an argument against Williams's position in 'Internal and External Reasons'.) If this is Williams's present view, however, it is difficult to reconcile with the text of 'Internal and External Reasons', which connects the internal reasons theory much more closely with the Humean approach to practical reason.

[47] 'Internal and External Reasons', pp. 108–9. Actually Williams attributes this assumption to the 'external reasons' theorist, rather than endorsing it *in propria persona*; but it seems clear from the course of his argument that he takes the assumption to describe a genuine condition on practical reasons for action.

Williams goes on to distinguish two positions about the conditions under which one may have a given practical reason. On the first view—in Williams's slightly confusing terminology,[48] the 'internal reasons theory'—people may only have a given reason if they could come to be motivated to act on the reason by deliberating *from* some desire in their 'subjective motivational set'. On an 'external reasons theory', by contrast, one's reasons are not required to stand in this kind of deliberative relation to one's antecedent desires.

Williams correctly takes the decision between these two positions to depend crucially on the question of the possibilities for rational explanation of motivations—the question, that is, that divides Humean and rationalist accounts of practical reason. Given the general internalist assumption, the external reasons theorist must hold that agents can acquire the motivation to act on their reasons as a result of rational reflection. At the same time what is distinctive about this view is precisely the denial that one's reasons need be restricted by one's prior desires, as considerations one could come to be motivated on by deliberation *from* those prior desires. The external reasons theorist thus needs to defend a rationalist account of practical reason, to show that rational reflection can give rise to new motivations without taking the form of deliberation *from* prior desires in the agent's subjective motivational set. Once these requirements are clearly set out, however, Williams apparently finds the external reasons theory easy to dismiss. He says, simply: 'I see no reason to suppose that these conditions could possibly be met.'[49]

The real problem, however, is to see how, at this level of generality, any such statement about the prospects for an external reasons account could possibly be defended. Williams may be taking for granted here some version of the teleological argument, correctly assuming that the explanation of motivation requires the postulation of a desire on the part of the agent who is motivated, and inferring from this that practical deliberation must be deliberation *from* the desires in one's prior motivational set. But the inference is unsound, as we have seen: the desire implicated in motivation, by the teleological argument, may itself be a motivated desire, in which case it will constitute not the starting point for practical deliberation but its conclusion. General scepticism about the possibility of pure practical reason would have to be based on a defence of the desire-out, desire-in principle, in rationalizing explanations of desires. But Williams, in line with most proponents of the Humean view, provides no grounds for this crucial Humean principle.

---

[48] The terminology is confusing because both Williams's 'internal reasons theory' and his 'external reasons theory' are, in a more conventional sense, *internalist* accounts, postulating a necessary connection between agents' reasons for action and their motivational capacities.

[49] 'Internal and External Reasons', p. 109.

He does, it is true, at one point allege that there is a circularity in what he presumably takes to be the most plausible version of an external reasons theory.[50] This is an account according to which agents can come to be motivated in a certain way simply by coming to believe that they have reason to act in that way, where coming to believe such a thing is not necessarily a matter of deliberating *from* the motives in one's prior subjective motivational set. About this proposal, Williams demands to know in what the content of such a belief could possibly consist. Answering this question himself, he suggests that the content of the belief must consist in 'the proposition, or something that entails the proposition, that if [the agent] deliberated rationally, he would be motivated to act appropriately'.[51] But this answer, Williams observes, merely takes for granted the possibility of pure practical reason, without showing us how reasoning which does not start from the agent's prior desires can generate by itself a new motivation.

To see why this is a weak objection, consider the following analogy with a case of theoretical reasoning, or reasons for belief. Presumably, everyone would agree that an agent could come to draw a new theoretical conclusion by coming to believe that there is reason to draw that conclusion. But suppose we now ask the question that is the analogue of Williams's question in the practical case: namely, in what might the content of the belief possibly consist? Here, it appears, there are any number of answers that might be given, such as that the new conclusion is a logical consequence of other beliefs of the agent's which she is not prepared to give up. To follow Williams's treatment of the practical case, this propositional content may indeed *entail* (in conjunction with some minimal assumptions about theoretical rationality) that if the agent were to reason correctly, she would draw the new theoretical conclusion. But this does nothing to show that the original answer was circular, or question-begging, or otherwise uninformative.

Perhaps Williams was misled here by an ambiguity in his formulation of the rationalist position. It is, he says, the view that an agent can acquire a new motivation as a result of coming to believe that there is reason for him to act in a certain way. But the existential proposition that gives the content of this belief may be read in two different ways: either as the claim that there is some such reason for action or other, where the agent does not necessarily know what that reason is; or as the claim that there is a particular practical reason which the agent grasps and understands.[52] Naturally the first interpretation of the proposition would leave us

---

[50] 'Internal and External Reasons', pp. 109-10. Cf. Brad Hooker, 'Williams' Argument against External Reasons', *Analysis*, 1987, for a similar criticism of this part of Williams's discussion.

[51] 'Internal and External Reasons', p. 109.

[52] Williams himself, in a different context, notices precisely this ambiguity in existential claims about reasons; see p. 107 of 'Internal and External Reasons'.

unsatisfied about the possibility of a purely rational explanation of motivation and motivated desire, if it were indeed all the rationalist had to say about the matter. But as the analogy with belief shows, the interpretation to opt for would anyway be the second. That is, the rationalist should say that pure practical reason is possible, because agents can acquire both new motivations, and the motivated desires implicated in such motivations, by coming to grasp and understand the particular reasons that they have for acting in certain ways. Of course, for this to be a satisfying account we will need to be convinced that the motivated desires involved here really are explicable solely in terms of the agent's new beliefs, plus principles or norms of rationality; otherwise what is represented as 'coming to grasp and understand the particular reason for action that one has' will not be a genuine case of *pure* practical reflection. But again, Williams has said nothing that would rule out this form of explanation in principle.[53]

7. My topic in this essay has been a question about the explanation of motivation and action, the question, namely, whether we can explain motivation and action in distinctively rational terms. To provide explanations of this kind—particularly explanations of moral motivation and behaviour—has been a characteristic aspiration of Kantian approaches to moral philosophy, and I have urged that there is no reason to think that this aspiration would be impossible to satisfy. Some recent work, however, has suggested a different way of developing a Kantian (or at any rate, anti-Humean) approach to practical reason, one which is not committed to the possibility of explaining motivation and action in purely rational terms. This possibility requires brief consideration.

Even if, as I have argued, rational explanations of action could in principle be carried through, it might be that they would add nothing significant to the formulation of a Kantian position in ethics. This, in effect, has been suggested by Michael Smith.[54] Smith distinguishes between two ways of understanding the Kantian claim that moral requirements are, or are based on, norms or requirements of practical reason. 'Belief-rationalism', as he calls it, takes the norms or requirements of practical reason to be capable of explaining motivation and motivated desire, in line with my depiction of the rationalist position in this paper. What Smith calls 'desire-rationalism', by contrast, holds that explanations of motivation and desire conform to the the Humean principle of desire-out, desire-in. Unlike the Humean, however, Smith's desire-rationalist

[53] For further discussions of Williams's account, see Rachel Cohon, 'Are External Reasons Impossible?', *Ethics*, 1985–6; John McDowell, 'Might There be External Reasons?' (Abstract), *Proceeding and Addresses of the American Philosophical Association*, 1987; and Martin Hollis, *The Cunning of Reason*, ch. 6.

[54] See Smith, 'Reason and Desire', section 4; and *The Moral Problem*, ch. 8, section 4.

maintains that certain basic desires are intrinsically rational, in the sense that all rational agents must have those basic desires. On this view, the norms or requirements of reason tell us that certain intrinsic desires are rationally required, without being able to explain the formation of such desires.[55]

Having introduced these two rationalist positions, Smith proceeds to question the significance of the differences between them, and hence to raise a doubt about the importance of the aspiration to explain motivation in rational terms. He notes that both positions will be able to identify the same sorts of behaviour as irrational: where the belief-rationalist says (for instance) that the amoral person is failing to reason correctly, in accordance with norms or principles of rationality, the desire-rationalist will say that the person lacks a basic desire which is intrinsically rational.[56] The same conclusion holds for rational behaviour, on Smith's view. On the belief-rationalist account, the rational agent will have specific moral desires which can be explained rationally in terms of principles or norms of reason. But Smith argues that any agent who has such specific moral desires could equally be credited with a basic dispositional desire with moral content, which the desire-rationalist may characterize as intrinsically rational.[57]

This seems to me correct, as far as it goes, but Smith is wrong to conclude from it that the differences between his two forms of rationalism are insignificant.[58] Take the case of the fully rational agent. It is true that on both views, such an agent may be credited with the same standing or dispositional desires. But these desires will have very different explanatory roles in the two kinds of account. For the desire-rationalist, they fix the starting points for the rational explanation of any specific moral desires that the rational agent may have, since the desire-rationalist only admits explanations of desires that satisfy the Humean desire-out, desire-in principle. On a belief-rationalist account, by contrast, it is possible to explain specific intrinsically moral desires in purely rational terms; and these explanations may equally account for the dispositional or standing desires that we ascribe to rational agents in virtue of their specific moral desires.[59]

Thus, Smith's two kinds of rationalist position continue to differ in their implications for the rational explanation of motivation. Nor is this difference an insignificant one. Its importance is clearest in cases where a

[55] Smith suggests that the critical present aim theory discussed by Derek Parfit might be a version of desire-rationalism, in so far as it claims that certain desires are rationally required, certain others intrinsically irrational; see Parfit, *Reasons and Persons*, part two (especially section 46).
[56] Smith, 'Reason and Desire', pp. 253–4.
[57] Smith, *The Moral Problem*, ch. 8, section 4.
[58] Still less does it seem correct to say that belief-rationalism 'collapses into' desire-rationalism, as Smith suggests in *The Moral Problem*, ch. 8, section 4.
[59] I take it this is the possibility Nagel is suggesting, when he offers the following comparison with the beliefs involved in deductive inference (in *The Possibility of Altruism*, p. 31): 'If someone draws conclusions in accordance with a principle of logic such as *modus ponens*, it is appropriate to ascribe to him the belief that the principle is true; but that belief is explained by the *same* thing which explains his inferences in accordance with the principle.'

380   *R. Jay Wallace*

formerly amoral agent comes to acquire the desires and motivations characteristic of virtue. On both of the rationalist positions Smith describes, this transition will mark a change from irrationality to rationality. But if desire-rationalism is correct, the transition cannot itself be explained in rational terms; rather it must be described as something akin to a conversion—the acquisition of a new motivation which is constitutively rational, but which does not admit of a rational explanation. Belief rationalism, on the other hand, would enable us to see the transition from amoralism to virtue as a *reasoned* change in the agent's motivations, the result of a process of reasoning or reflection in accordance with the norms or principles of practical rationality. Thus belief-rationalism promises to offer terms for a rational discussion with the amoralist, terms which—in principle, at least—the amoralist might be persuaded by, leading to a reasoned adjustment of or addition to the amoralist's motivations.[60] There is no such possibility on the view that Smith calls desire-rationalism.

I conclude that the aspiration to explain motivation and behaviour in purely rational terms makes a distinctive contribution to the Kantian approach to ethics. Once this is granted, however, a further question arises, concerning the extent to which other characteristically Kantian or anti-Humean claims about practical reason can be made by a theory which renounces the aspiration to provide purely rational explanations of motivations. This question is posed, albeit in very different ways, by the recent work of John Rawls, T. M. Scanlon, and John McDowell.[61] These philosophers reject the Humean claim that practical reason is exclusively instrumental in its function, restricted to identifying means to the satisfaction of individual ends; and they reject equally the modern development of the instrumentalist approach, according to which practical reason is directed toward maximizing the joint satisfaction of sets of desires or preferences. Instead, Rawls, Scanlon, and McDowell all contend that there are non-instrumental patterns of practical reasoning in terms of which we can criticize actions and social institutions morally, and explain distinctively moral kinds of motivation and concern. And yet, none of these philosophers seems to suppose that the morally distinctive patterns of practical reasoning are equally accessible to all agents, regardless of those agents' antecedent desires.[62]

---

[60] It need not be supposed that such reasoned discourse with the amoralist would be an easy thing to bring off in practice; only that it would be possible.

[61] See John Rawls, 'Justice as Fairness: Political Not Metaphysical', *Philosophy and Public Affairs*, 1985; T. M. Scanlon, 'Contractualism and Utilitarianism', in Amartya Sen and Bernard Williams (eds), *Utilitarianism and Beyond*, Cambridge, Cambridge University Press, 1982; and John McDowell, 'Virtue and Reason', *The Monist*, 1979.

[62] On this point, see Rawls's remarks about the role of consensus in political justification, in 'Justice as Fairness: Political Not Metaphysical', pp. 229, 246–7; Scanlon's suggestion that the desire to be able to justify one's actions may be the basis of moral motivation, in 'Contractualism and Utilitarianism', pp. 116–8; and McDowell's denial that those who lack the desires characteristic of virtue need be irrational, in 'Are Moral Requirements Hypothetical Imperatives?', *The Aristotelian Society Supplementary Volume*, 1078, pp. 13, 24.

If this is right, it suggests that there may be considerable work for a Kantian or anti-Humean[63] approach to ethics, even if it renounces or suspends the aim of explaining motivation and action in purely rational terms. The work would consist in showing that there are patterns of reasoning *from* an agent's desires—to use Bernard Williams's expression[64] —which are not forms of instrumental or maximizing reasoning. This seems to me a fertile area for further research and discussion: questions arise, for instance, concerning the explanatory *role* that desire plays in forms of practical reasoning that are neither instrumental nor maximizing, but that nevertheless, in some sense, begin from an agent's desires. But however these questions are answered, the possibility that reasoning from one's desires need not take a maximizing or instrumental form is an important one. It does not undermine the aspiration to provide purely rational explanations of motivation, or show it to be misguided. But it suggests that rather less may hang on the satisfaction of the aspiration than some Kantians have supposed.

8. I have argued that Humeans have so far failed to give us good reasons for accepting motivational scepticism about the rationalist approach. To support this conclusion, it has been necessary to get clearer about what is at stake in the debate between Humeans and rationalists. Developing a suggestion of Thomas Nagel's, I have proposed that the issue turns on the form taken by rationalizing explanations of desires and motivations; in particular, the question is whether such explanations conform to the Humean principle of desire-out, desire-in. Once the question is correctly seen in this way, however, it becomes clear that recent arguments, purporting to offer general support for the Humean approach, do not succeed.

How are we to proceed beyond this point? One approach that suggests itself is to turn to phenomenology to settle the issue. The idea would be that, once we see that there is nothing to rule out or determine either kind of account on general or a priori grounds, we may appeal to the evidence of the moral life to see what kinds of explanations of motivation are actually accepted in practice. Evidence of this sort, however, seems to me of extremely limited value in the context of the debate between the rationalist and the Humean. The main reason for this is that the conception of desire with which the Humean operates is a dispositional rather than a phenome-

---

[63] Rawls's and Scanlon's accounts are broadly Kantian, whereas McDowell's is more directly inspired by his reading of Aristotle.

[64] See 'Internal and External Reasons', pp. 104–5, where Williams too contends that reasoning from the elements in one's subjective motivational set need not take an instrumental or maximizing form. I do not mean to suggest that Rawls, Scanlon, and McDowell would all agree with Williams's way of putting the point (see McDowell, 'Might There be External Reasons?', for some objections). Whether disagreements on this point are significant, however, will depend on how the notion of reasoning *from* one's desires is developed.

nological conception, a conception, that is, on which one may be in a state of desire without being aware that one is in such a state. But if desires are not phenomenological states, it is unclear how phenomenological or experiential evidence could possibly settle the issue of whether desires always serve as the ultimate source of our motivations.

Indeed, so long as the issue is joined in experiential terms alone, it is open to the Humean to confront the rationalist with a dilemma. The rationalist will want to say that certain motivations and motivated desires may be explained in terms of beliefs, because in moral experience it seems (for instance) as if the desire to perform a given action may be both justified and explained by the agent's belief that the action would be, say, helpful, or just. If this is an ordinary belief, however, then it should be equally open to an amoral agent to have the belief; and yet the belief that an action would be helpful or just will not give rise, in the amoralist, to the motivated desire to perform the action.[65] Pointing to this difference, the Humean will say that it can best be explained by supposing that the virtuous agent has, while the amoral agent lacks, a dispositional desire to perform actions that are helpful or just, where this dispositional desire is the real source of the virtuous person's motivations. Phenomenological evidence, in other words, seems rather to support the Humean approach than to confute it. The rationalist may try to avoid this outcome, perhaps, by denying that the beliefs which seem to explain motivations and motivated desires are ordinary beliefs, available equally to those who are not motivated by them.[66] But this conception of 'extraordinary' beliefs seems questionably coherent; and in any case, its invocation is completely *ad hoc* so long as the debate is being conducted on phenomenological or experiential grounds alone.

What the rationalist needs to establish is that it is *irrational* to have certain sorts of beliefs, but lack the corresponding desires and motivations. To show this, it is necessary to go beyond phenomenology, by specifying the relevant principles or norms of reason, or by offering a conception of rationality in terms of which the inferences in question can be shown to be

[65] Richard Warner offers an experiential argument against the Humean which allows for this possibility (namely, that the very same beliefs which motivate may sometimes fail to serve as motives), in *Freedom, Enjoyment and Happiness*, pp. 46–51. His anti-Humean position is different from the one I am considering in the text in holding, not that beliefs explain desires, but that they sometimes 'serve as' desires (see section 5 above, for a discussion of this proposal). I am supposing, however, that an experiential argument similar to Warner's could be mounted in support of the conclusion that beliefs may sometimes explain desires; and that both arguments would be subject to the same objection.

[66] See John McDowell, 'Are Moral Requirements Hypothetical Imperatives?', pp. 16–17, for this suggestion. The extraordinary character of the beliefs McDowell here takes to be explanatory of moral behaviour is revealed by his admission that ascription of the beliefs is independent of 'ordinary' tests for mastery of the language in which the content of the beliefs is expressed ('Are Moral Requirements Hypothetical Imperatives?', p. 22). Doubt about the coherence of this notion is suggested by Sabina Lovibond in *Realism and Imagination in Ethics*, Minneapolis, University of Minnesota Press, 1983, section 12. (I take it that in 'Virtue and Reason', referred to in section 7 above, McDowell offers further, non-experiential support for his anti-Humean conception of practical reason.)

rationally required. The real burden of the rationalist position is to find a way of defending such a conception of rationality or of the specific principles or norms of reason. One strategy, adverted to in section 1 above, would proceed by showing that a rationalist account of the principles or norms of reason yields a more plausible ideal of rational attainment than alternative, Humean accounts. Or, rationalists might try to establish that their conception of practical rationality develops or extends certain aspects of theoretical rationality (such as impersonality, consistency, or universality) that may be taken as paradigmatic.

Much work remains to be done, before we can definitively judge the outcome of these strategies (which are themselves rather poorly understood). At this point, I would only venture to say that the success of the rationalist strategies is likely to be affected by the increasing sophistication of accounts which deny that pure reason can be practical in its issue (or which at least remain non-committal on this question). Thus, to the extent that such accounts can be freed from an instrumental or maximizing conception of practical reason (see section 7 above), it will become correspondingly difficult to show that rationalist accounts provide a uniquely plausible ideal of rational attainment. Difficult, but not impossible: further progress with this debate is only going to be made once we give up the thought that there must be something wrong in principle with the attempt to explain motivation in rational terms, and begin assessing particular rationalist and Humean proposals on their merits.[67]

Department of Philosophy   R. JAY WALLACE
The University of Pennsylvania
Philadelphia, PA 19104-6385
USA

References

Alston, William P., 'Motives and Motivation', in Paul Edwards (ed.), *The Encyclopedia of Philosophy*, New York, Macmillan and Free Press, 1967.
Anscombe, G. E. M., *Intention*, Ithaca, Cornell University Press, 1963.
Audi, Robert, 'Intending, Intentional Action, and Desire', in Joel Marks (ed.), *The Ways of Desire*.
Brandt, Richard B. and Jaegwon Kim, 'Wants as Explanations of Actions', *The Journal of Philosophy*, 1963.
Broughton, Janet, 'The Possibility of Prudence', *Philosophical Studies*, 1983.
Cohon, Rachel, 'Are External Reasons Impossible?', *Ethics*, 1985–6.

[67] I have had helpful comments on predecessors of this paper from Simon Blackburn, John Collins, Samuel Freeman, Gilbert Harman, Sally Haslanger, Katharina Kaiser, Wolfgang Mann, and an audience at the University of Pennsylvania. I owe a special debt to Michael Smith, with whom I have had the benefit of many stimulating discussions about practical reason. Work on this paper was partially supported by a grant from the Research Council of the University of Pennsylvania.

384   R. Jay Wallace

Collins, John, 'Belief, Desire, and Revision', *Mind*, 1988.
——— 'Updating and Supposing', read at the A.A.P. Conference in Canberra in July 1989.
Dahl, Norman O., *Practical Reason, Aristotle, and Weakness of the Will*, Minneapolis, University of Minnesota Press, 1984.
Darwall, Stephen, *Impartial Reason*, Ithaca, Cornell University Press, 1983.
Davis, Wayne, 'Two Senses of Desire', in Joel Marks (ed.), *The Ways of Desire*.
Dent, N. J. H., *The Moral Psychology of the Virtues*, Cambridge, Cambridge University Press, 1984.
Foot, Philippa, 'Reasons for Action and Desires', in her *Virtues and Vices and Other Essays in Moral Philosophy*, Oxford, Basil Blackwell, 1978.
Frankfurt, Harry, 'Freedom of the Will and the Concept of a Person', *The Journal of Philosophy*, 1971.
——— 'Identification and Wholeheartedness', in Ferdinand Shoeman (ed.), *Responsibility, Character, and the Emotions: New Essays in Moral Psychology*, New York, Cambridge University Press, 1987.
Hampshire, Stuart, *Freedom of the Individual*, Expanded Edition, Princeton, Princeton University Press, 1975.
Hintikka, Jaakko, 'Theoretical Reason—An Ambiguous Legacy', in Stephan Körner (ed.), *Practical Reason*, Oxford, Basil Blackwell, 1974.
Hollis, Martin, *The Cunning of Reason*, Cambridge, Cambridge University Press, 1987.
Hooker, Brad, 'Williams' Argument against External Reasons', *Analysis*, 1987.
Hume, David, *A Treatise of Human Nature*, ed. Selby-Bigge, Second Edition, Oxford, Clarendon Press, 1978.
Irwin, T. H., 'Aristotle on Reason, Desire, and Virtue', *The Journal of Philosophy*, 1975.
Korsgaard, Christine, 'Skepticism about Practical Reason', *The Journal of Philosophy*, 1986.
Kraut, Richard, 'Prudence and the Desire Theory of Reasons', *The Philosophical Review*, 1972.
Lewis, David, 'Desire as Belief', *Mind*, 1988.
Locke, Don, 'Beliefs, Desires and Reasons for Action', *American Philosophical Quarterly*, 1982.
——— 'Reasons, Wants, and Causes', *American Philosophical Quarterly*, 1974.
Lovibond, Sabina, *Realism and Imagination in Ethics*, Minneapolis, University of Minnesota Press, 1983.
McDowell, John, 'Are Moral Requirements Hypothetical Imperatives?', *The Aristotelian Society Supplementary Volume*, 1978.
——— 'Might There be External Reasons?' (Abstract), *Proceedings and Addresses of the American Philosophical Association*, 1987.
——— 'Virtue and Reason', *The Monist*, 1979.
Marks, Joel, 'The Difference between Motivation and Desire', in Joel Marks (ed.), *The Ways of Desire*.
——— (ed.), *The Ways of Desire: New Essays in Philosophical Psychology on the Concept of Wanting*, Chicago, Precedent Publishing, 1986.
Nagel, Thomas, *The Possibility of Altruism*, Princeton, Princeton University Press, 1978.

How to Argue about Practical Reason 385

—— *The View from Nowhere*, New York, Oxford University Press, 1986.
Parfit, Derek, *Reasons and Persons*, Oxford, Clarendon Press, 1984.
Pettit, Philip, 'Broad-Minded Explanation and Psychology', in Philip Pettit and John McDowell (eds), *Subject, Thought, and Context*, Oxford, Clarendon Press, 1986.
—— 'Humeans, Anti-Humeans, and Motivation', *Mind*, 1987.
Platts, Mark, 'Hume and Morality as a Matter of Fact', *Mind*, 1988.
—— *Ways of Meaning*, London, Routledge and Kegan Paul, 1979.
Price, Huw, 'Defending Desire as Belief', *Mind*, 1989.
Rawls, John, 'Justice as Fairness: Political Not Metaphysical', *Philosophy and Public Affairs*, 1985.
Scanlon, T. M., 'Contractualism and Utilitarianism', in Amartya Sen and Bernard Williams, (eds), *Utilitarianism and Beyond*, Cambridge, Cambridge University Press, 1982.
Schiffer, Stephen, 'A Paradox of Desire', *American Philosophical Quarterly*, 1976.
Searle, John, *Intentionality*, Cambridge, Cambridge University Press, 1983.
Smith, Michael, 'The Humean Theory of Motivation', *Mind*, 1987.
—— *The Moral Problem*, Oxford University D. Phil., 1989.
—— 'On Humeans, Anti-Humeans, and Motivation: A Reply to Pettit', *Mind*, 1988.
—— 'Reason and Desire', *Proceedings of the Aristotelian Society*, 1987–8.
Sturgeon, Nicholas, 'Altruism, Solipsism, and the Objectivity of Reasons', *The Philosophical Review*, 1974.
Warner, Richard, *Freedom, Enjoyment and Happiness*, Ithaca, Cornell University Press, 1987.
Watson, Gary, 'Free Agency', *The Journal of Philosophy*, 1975.
Wiggins, David, 'Deliberation and Practical Reason', in Amélie Oksenberg Rorty (ed.), *Essays on Aristotle's Ethics*, Berkeley, University of California Press, 1980.
Williams, Bernard, 'Consistency and Realism', in his *Problems of the Self*, Cambridge, Cambridge University Press, 1973.
—— *Ethics and the Limits of Philosophy*, Cambridge, Harvard University Press, 1985.
—— 'Internal and External Reasons', in his *Moral Luck*, Cambridge, Cambridge University Press, 1981.
Wollheim, Richard, *The Thread of Life*, Cambridge, Harvard University Press, 1984.
Woodfield, Andrew, 'Desire, Intentional Content and Teleological Explanation', *Proceedings of the Aristotelian Society*, 1981–82.

[7]

NOÛS 30:2 (1996) 197–220

Williams' Argument Against External Reasons*

Elijah Millgram
Princeton University

In his agenda-setting paper, 'Internal and External Reasons', Bernard Williams has argued that there are only internal, and no external, reasons for action; in Williams' terminology, an 'internal reason' is one that 'display[s] a relativity . . . to the agent's subjective motivational set' (as Williams denotes it, his S), in contrast to an 'external reason', which does not.[1] Put more colloquially, the thought is roughly that someone's reason for doing something has to bottom out in what that person wants. Williams' arguments are of interest in part because they inherit the mantle of a familiar debate about the force of the demands morality makes on us: must those demands appeal to our sometimes selfish and variable wants, or does morality have an authority that is independent of our aims and desires?[2] And his arguments have a further claim on our attention as well. Experience shows that the internalist take on reasons can appear enormously compelling to a very wide range of the philosophically inclined, from freshmen in their first ethics class to seasoned professionals in their most tough-minded moods; but the considerations that so often make internalism seem inescapable tend to be unformed and largely mute. In Williams' arguments these motivations are articulated, in both senses of the word, and I here want to use the arguments to bring these usually implicit considerations into clear focus.

1

We can start by getting Williams' two arguments on the table. The point of the first is that reasons must be able to explain actions, but to explain actions, one must appeal to motivations; and an explanation that adduces motivations is an internal, and not an external, reasons explanation. The second argument is intended to improve on the first by emphasizing the normative as opposed to the simply explanatory aspect of reason attribu-

tions. The idea is that reasons for actions are to be understood through their role in practical deliberation; if someone has a reason for action then, if he were to deliberate, it would motivate him to act. But practical deliberation requires motivational fuel; so reasons for action must be internal rather than external. Here are the arguments; the first runs as follows:

1. 'If there are reasons for action, it must be that people sometimes act for those reasons, and if they do, their reasons must figure in some correct explanation of their action . . .' (102)[3]
2. 'no external reason statement could *by itself* offer an explanation of anyone's action . . . [because] nothing can explain an agent's (intentional) action except something that motivates him so to act' (106f).
3. An external reason statement can explain action only conjointly with some further element linking it and the action, but that further element must be an element of the agent's subjective motivational set; consequently, 'this agent . . . appears to be one about whom, now, an *internal* reason statement could truly be made' (107).
4. Consequently, would-be external reason explanations turn out, when they are successful, to be *internal* reason explanations; there are no external reasons.

Williams' second argument has this skeleton:

5. If an agent has an external reason to ϕ, then 'if the agent rationally deliberated . . . he would come to be motivated to ϕ' (109).
6. Practical deliberation proceeds from available motivation.
7. Where deliberation proceeds from an external reason 'there is no motivation for the agent to deliberate *from*' (109; by definition of external reasons).
8. Therefore, 'all external reason statements are false' (109).

Let's call the premise (1), which states that reasons explain actions, REA. And, while we're labeling premises, let's call (5), which says that reasons entail counterfactuals of a specified kind, REC. The starting points of the two arguments, REA and REC, are themselves connected by a further argument:

i. Reasons have to be able to explain action (REA; 106).
ii. The link between external reason and action would have to be '*A*'s believing an external reason about himself' (107).
iii. '[T]he external reasons theorist essentially wants, that the agent should acquire the motivation *because* he comes to believe the reason statement, and . . . because . . . he is considering the matter aright' (108f).
iv. '[T]he condition under which the agent appropriately comes to have the motivation [must be] . . . that he should deliberate correctly' (109).
5. Therefore, if an agent has an external reason to ϕ, then 'if the agent

rationally deliberated . . . he would come to be motivated to ϕ' (REC; 109).

John McDowell has criticized the transition from (iii) to (iv) on the grounds that conversion, or simply good upbringing, can substitute for deliberation in bringing one around to motivation that one has because one is considering the matter aright.[4] Later on in the paper, I will mention a class of cases that do the work of McDowell's examples without their bolt-from-the-blue quality. For now, the point to notice is that while REA and REC are quite close to one another in spirit, McDowell's objection shows that they are not in fact equivalent.

2

A number of very competent commentators have approached these arguments directly, but I want to take a more roundabout approach.[5] The arguments in front of us are conducted at an overly high level of generality, and so ought to prove too much. They seem to turn on what it takes to be a reason at all, specifically, on the idea that *being* a reason must be made out in terms of *giving* reasons, that is, in terms of the deliberation and explanations that invoke reasons. Reasons must be cognitively on-hand if they are to be given, so having them depends on having mental states of the appropriate kinds. These highly general considerations are too broad to effectively support a conclusion that is clearly, and correctly, meant to be restricted to reasons for action. There is evidently more (or less) going on in these arguments than meets the eye.

I will press this point by constructing analogues of Williams' core arguments applicable within the sphere of theoretical—as opposed to practical—reason. These will have as their conclusion that there are no external reasons for belief. (As a notational convenience, I will indicate reasons for a belief by the subscript '$_B$', and I will sometimes mark reasons for action with the subscript '$_A$'.) Since externalism is far more obviously false in the theoretical domain than in the practical, developing these analogues will have several payoffs. First, by determining why the arguments do not go through when beliefs are at issue, we will be able to isolate the further ingredient that is being relied upon when they are applied to reasons for action; an incidental bonus will be to highlight a number of pressure points in Williams' arguments. Second, we will equip ourselves to meet a demand that Williams quite legitimately makes. In challenging the external reasons theorist to say what the content of an external reason for action would be, Williams suggests that in dismissing external reasons, no real possibility is being excluded. By using external reasons for belief as a model, we will be able to come to a fairly concrete idea of what the content of an external reason for action might be like; this will allow us to

see what real possibility *is* being excluded. And third, once we have
isolated the further ingredient at work in the practical domain, we will
have shifted the focus of argument, away from the overly general plane
on which arguments for and against internalism tend to be conducted, and
to the relatively substantive question on which the debate over internalism really turns.

To proceed. An internal reason$_B$ statement is one that is falsified by the
absence of some appropriate element from C, the set of things of which the
agent is convinced or finds convincing.[6] The elements of C may be formally
called beliefs, but, as with Williams' S (105), a broader notion is intended;
one's C may include gut feelings, prejudices, working hypotheses, larger
theoretical commitments, and so on. C is of course not fixed: processes of
theoretical reasoning may add elements to, or subtract them from, one's C.
But all of these processes, insofar as they are processes of *reasoning*, are
controlled by, or are responsible to, elements of one's C.[7]

External reasons$_B$, by contrast, do not display this relativity to a reasoner's C. We can make this point by shifting perspectives within one of
Williams' examples.[8] A battered wife who does not leave her husband may
stay because she does not believe that he will keep on beating her, and she
does not think he will keep on beating her because, she tells us, he is not
really like that. Suppose one reason$_B$ for thinking that he will continue to
beat her is that he *is* like that. This reason$_B$ is external to someone who does
not find it convincing that he is like that. Someone who does not find it
convincing will not use his being like that as a premise or starting-point of
her reasoning, and, *a fortiori*, will not use it as a premise of reasoning the
conclusion of which is that he will continue to beat her. A statement may be
true, but it will not enter as a premise into one's reasoning, and will not
control one's deliberation, if one does not believe it. If a friend were to
claim that his being like that was a reason for her to believe that he will
continue to beat her, the friend would be invoking an external reason$_B$.

Now if when reasons$_B$ rationally determine belief they must figure in an
explanation of the belief they support, then there could be no external
reasons$_B$. Nothing can explain reasoned acquisition of belief except *convincing* reasons. A putative external reason$_B$ could explain belief only conjointly with some further element linking it and the conclusion (for example, a willingness to believe whatever a certain person tells one). But that
further element must be counted as belonging to the reasoner's C; such an
agent would be one about whom an *internal*, not merely an external, rea-
son$_B$ statement could truly be made. This is the doxastic analogue of Williams' first argument.

Again, suppose it is true that if an agent has an external reason to
believe that p, then if he rationally deliberated, he would come to find p
convincing.[9] Theoretical reasoning, we have pointed out, proceeds from

elements of one's *C*. Therefore, there could be no true external reason$_B$ statements, i.e., attributions of reasons$_B$ that do not appropriately invoke elements of one's *C*. This is the analogue of Williams' second argument.

There is a further parallel to one of Williams' subsidiary arguments. To the objection that one might be motivated to act when one thought that one had an external reason$_A$, Williams asks: what is the content of the proposition, that one has an external reason to ϕ, if not that, if one deliberated rationally, one would be motivated to act? Similarly, to the objection that one might be willing to find convincing what one had external reason$_B$ for, we can ask: what does the proposition that one has an external reason$_B$ to believe that *p* come to, if not that, were one rationally to deliberate, one would find *p* convincing?

As I have already suggested, one question we are going to have to answer is this. If the arguments I have just given are structurally identical to those Williams advances against external reasons$_A$, why aren't the objections to external reasons for action merely a special case of a fact about reasons generally? Later I will try to say why Williams takes the arguments he presents to be showing something specific to reasons for action. But before I get to that, I want to press and prod the newly constructed arguments a little; doing this will prepare us to see what is being excluded by Williams' original arguments, what is being presupposed by them, and what an external reason for action might look like, if there were such a thing.

3

How convincing do we find the doxastic analogues of REA and REC, the premises from which the arguments that there are no reasons$_B$ proceed? Let me begin by developing two candidate counterexamples to the claim that to have a reason to believe just amounts to, or at least entails that, were one rationally to deliberate, one would find the belief convincing.

Imagine a theory T_1 that explains and predicts one's cognitive abilities and disabilities, and suppose that T_1 is so complicated that, given one's .ognitive disabilities, one will never be able to understand the theory itself, and consequently will never be able to believe it. Let us suppose that T_1 applies to *me*, and that it allows me to grasp the evidence for it; a more inferentially capable being would be able to infer T_1 from this evidence. (If you want, you can suppose that the evidence I believe logically entails T_1.) In this case, I have reasons for T_1 (what, if not sufficient evidence, could amount to reason for T_1?), but it is not the case that, were I rationally to deliberate, I would come to believe T_1. If I *were* able to deliberate well enough to judge T_1's merits, T_1 would be *false* (and there would, presumably, be no evidence conclusively supporting it).[10]

Although T_1 resists a Williams-style attempt to cash the reasons for it out in terms of counterfactuals, the reasons for it are nonetheless internal, in the sense of being suitably linked to the agent's C. (The agent is unable to forge the link himself, but the burden is taken up by our grasp of the logical relations between the evidence for T_1 and T_1 itself.) So let us now consider a slightly more restrictive theory, T_2. Suppose that, according to T_2, I will never even believe the evidence for T_2; these are not reasons that are available to me, if T_2 is true. I do not find them convincing, which is to say, they are not elements of my C. So if they are reasons at all, they are external reasons. In any case, it is evidently as untrue of T_2 as it is of T_1 that if I were to deliberate rationally, I would come to believe it. If I were to believe the premises from which T_2 might be inferred, T_2 would be false. If the bodies of evidence for T_1 and T_2 are the reasons for believing T_1 and T_2, they are reasons for which REC (or, more precisely, its analogue REC_B) is false. And moreover, if the reasons for T_2 *are* reasons, they are external reasons, since they fail to display the appropriate relativity to my C. Internalism runs together two ideas: that a person's reasons are not independent of the uses he can make of them, and that a person's reasons are derivable from the mental states (here, beliefs or desires) he now has. Putting T_1 side by side with T_2 shows that these are *different* ideas.

We can imagine someone who understands either T_1 or T_2 and the reasons for believing them (maybe, if they are very complicated, God) saying of me: 'There are good reasons to believe $T_{1,2}$, although he cannot find them convincing.' It is important, however, that the plausibility of this pronouncement is not independent of my relation to the evidence. Under what circumstances are we willing to say that 'so-and-so has reasons$_B$', of someone who does not find them convincing?[11] It does not suffice that we know facts that so-and-so does not. If Joe thinks that Smith will win, but I and my co-conspirators have secretly fixed the computer to make Jones win, we are not entitled to say that Joe has (external) reasons to think Jones will win. But suppose the necessary facts are *available* to Joe: they are the common currency of the newspaper he reads, his bar buddies mention them on regular occasions, they are, we would say, staring him in the face; but, because of his faith in the Party, Joe refuses to believe them. In such circumstances, we would say that Joe has reasons, albeit reasons he does not acknowledge. From here it is only a step to T_2, evidence for which is widely available, but which Joe cannot believe (if T_2 is true), because the content of T_2 is, *inter alia*, that Joe cannot believe the evidence for T_2.

If we accept these cases as examples of reasons for belief, then both REA_B and REC_B (the doxastic analogues of REA and REC) are false: it is possible to have reasons for belief that cannot explain one's having the beliefs they are reasons for; and it is possible to have reasons for belief whose content cannot be made out in terms of counterfactual deliberation.

And if REA_B and REC_B are false, then the doxastic analogues of Williams' arguments are unsound, and fail to show that there can be no external reasons$_B$. I want to postpone considering whether cases like these *are* examples of external reasons$_B$ in favor of extending the analogy between the domains of reasons for belief and reasons for actions; I will do this by constructing analogous candidate counterexamples to the claim that having a reason$_A$ to ϕ entails that if one were rationally to deliberate, one would be motivated to ϕ.

As in our construction of the theories $T_{1,2}$, we can try to produce a reason that deliberation cannot transform into motivation by picking a reason such that one has it if and only if one is unable to deliberate in such a way as to bring it about that one acts from that reason. By way of example, consider an insensitive person named Archie. Because he is insensitive, his life is worse than it might be; his home is mean and loveless, his colleagues unpleasant to him, his (so-called) friends as insensitive as himself. He himself realizes that things are not going well (maybe he complains bitterly about not being invited to parties); but his insensitivity prevents him from seeing why. Archie's insensitivity is a reason to act: reason to avoid acquaintances in their hour of grief, for example (he only makes things worse). Maybe it is even a reason, in California at any rate, to take steps to make himself more sensitive. To simplify the example, let us think of Archie's insensitivity as unusual in the following way. It is not the kind of insensitivity that allows of minor amelioration. Becoming more sensitive, in Archie's case, requires becoming a *good deal* more sensitive.

Archie's insensitivity is a deliberative incapacity: it consists in being unable to appreciate certain reasons for action, these among them. Because he is insensitive, he cannot see that his own insensitivity gives him reasons for action. ('*Insensitivity*,' he sniffs, his voice dripping with contempt.) If he could reason in this way (e.g., 'I had better stay away from the funeral; if I go, I'll only make things worse') he would *ipso facto* be sensitive enough not to have these reasons. Archie has a reason for action which is not such that if he deliberated correctly it would motivate him to action. For if he *could* so deliberate, then he would no longer have this reason.

In such a case we may regard an agent as having a reason to ϕ, yet reject 'the claim that if the agent rationally deliberated, then . . . he would come to be motivated to ϕ'. For if the agent were able rationally to deliberate in the appropriate way, he would not have the reason that is the proposed ground of the motivation. That is, if we take the example as presented, we must take REC to be false, and the argument that proceeds from it to be unsound.[12] Should it be objected that we ought to consider what the agent *would* do *if* he were fully informed and deliberatively competent, we may remind ourselves that if the agent *were* fully informed and deliberatively

204 *NOÛS*

competent, he would not have reasons to act springing from deliberative incompetence, and so would not act on them.[13,14]

Before going on to the next case, notice that would-be counterexamples like this one are directed not only against REC, a fact I have been emphasizing, but against REA as well. I remarked earlier that McDowell takes issue with the transition from REA to REC, and I will in a little while consider a way of reinforcing his objection. But, and this is the point I want to bring forward now, we need not wait until the argument has progressed as far as this. Our proposed counterexample—and again, I am postponing the question, whether it is in fact a counterexample—suggests that one can deny that, whenever one has a reason for an action, the action could be performed for the reason, and the reason would then explain the action. For the reason proposed by the example is a reason only when it is unavailable to the agent, and thus, only when it fails to explain action.[15]

We need to deal with the objection that, even if the example shows the letter of Williams' attempted specification of the content of an external reason to be unsatisfactory, the spirit of his internalism has still not been adequately addressed. What is at issue is not just the counterfactual required by REC, but the 'relativity of the reason statement to the agent's subjective motivational set' (102, emphasis deleted). The reason given for Archie to avoid funerals, become more sensitive, and so on, is that he would be invited to more parties, and the desire to be invited to more parties is in his S. So this reason is still appropriately linked to Archie's S, even if he is unable, even counterfactually, to forge the link himself.

So let us specify Archie's affliction a little more tightly. (This is the analogue of moving from T_1 to T_2.) There are rewards to sensitivity that Archie is not now prepared to appreciate; for example, the flourishing of trust in his friendships, or the ability to respond sympathetically and effectively to others' concerns. The desires for these rewards are not elements of his S; when Edith, his wife, mentions some of these rewards to him, he responds with scorn and disgust. But were he to experience them, he himself would acknowledge the extent to which his life had improved. It is natural to say that Archie has reasons to change his ways, reasons which are not grounded in elements of his S and are consequently external reasons. As before, if these considerations *are* reasons, they are reasons of which neither REA nor REC are true, and they show the arguments proceeding from REA and REC to be unsound.[16]

4

Now at this point someone might again want to object that the proposed counterexamples are not in fact counterexamples, because the purported reasons are not *actually* reasons. But I want, once again, to defer this

objection, and instead to use the last of the Archie cases to address what I take to be the demand that most centrally informs Williams' objections to external reasons: that we be able to say what the *content* of an external reason statement is. If there are true external reason statements, there must be some difference between them and the kind of browbeating that Williams properly calls 'bluff' (111). To this end, we may contrast the second Archie case with Williams' example of a would-be external reason. (In the example, Owen Wingrave has no motivation to join the army, but his father insists that he has a reason to do so nonetheless, 'since all his male ancestors were soldiers, and family pride requires him to do the same' (106). It is, I think, a demerit of Williams' exposition that he picks a particularly implausible example of a would-be external reason, one of which we would be inclined to say that the agent *has* no reason, and then proceeds as if all external reasons had to be like *that*.)

While discussing the bearing of facts that the agent does not know on whether we should ascribe reasons$_A$ to him, Williams remarks that '[f]or it to be the case that he actually has such a reason . . . the relevance of the unknown fact to his actions has to be fairly close and immediate; otherwise one merely says that A would have reason to ϕ if he knew the fact' (103). This remark is on target, and applies not just to the auxiliary beliefs brought to bear in generating reasons for action. Some condition that would naturally be expressed using the phrase 'fairly close and immediate' needs to be made out with regard to external reasons as well. When we were discussing T_2, we described the facts not believed as 'staring the agent in the face'; not just any true fact counts as a reason$_B$, but facts like these do.

Can we find an appropriate kind of proximity between Archie and the reasons we have proposed for him? While these reasons do not proceed from Archie's S, they nevertheless appeal to his stake in aspects of his own well-being. Archie should treat people more nicely, even though he does not want to, because he will be better off if he does—despite the fact that he is now unable to appreciate the ways in which he would be better off as ways in which he would be *better* off. I do not of course insist that all external reasons$_A$ must look precisely like this, and when we explore the possibility further it will be clear that proximity need not always amount to self-interest. The question now is whether this kind of proximity will allow us a way of saying what the content of an external reason might be.

There is an objection to this proposal that I had better mention right away. An internalist might concede that being better off is a reason to act, but object that desires for well-being, happiness, and so on are necessarily, or at any rate usually, elements of an agent's S; and it is these elements that render plausible our taking the improvement in Archie's life to be a reason for him to take action. These are reasons, runs the objection, but they are

internal reasons; Archie's failure lies in his inability to see what means would most effectually obtain him these very general ends. Having mentioned the objection, I want to dispose of it without giving it anything like the treatment it deserves; the way of thinking about happiness and well-being that it expresses is too deeply confused to be cleared up here.[17] For now, we can say that the *available content* of such notions as well-being, happiness, and so on, is a matter of other, more determinate elements of the agent's *S*.[18] Archie's conception of happiness must be substantive to the extent that it is to play the requisite role in deliberation (i.e., a role that will underwrite explanation of action); and we have stated that it specifically excludes those elements that could underwrite the reasons in question.

Still, why is insisting that someone will be better off when he ϕs, when he does not want what he will get when he ϕs, not simply more browbeating and bluff? How can we give the claim that the agent has a stake in the matter content that is not exhausted by the elements of his *S*? Recall that we said that Archie, if he were to experience the benefits of sensitivity, would himself acknowledge that he had been mistaken. Just as reasons for belief are subject to correction by experience, so are reasons for action. They may be corrected by disappointment, on the one hand, and by unanticipated enjoyment, on the other. To change examples for a moment, one's *S* may contain only desires for luxury, and the most thorough deliberation proceeding from those desires may produce only action aimed at luxury; but luxury attained may prove empty and unsatisfying. The story is familiar enough, and it may prompt those with more experience to say that so-and-so has excellent reason to attend to things besides the pursuit of luxury— for although he does not now find these reasons motivating, he may yet come to regret his mistake. (He himself will of course admit the possibility of disappointment in general, but this is not necessarily to see, of any particular item that he is now pursuing, how it might be disappointing; and the inability, I will argue shortly, need not be blindness to some matter of *fact*.) That correction need not only be a matter of disappointment is recognized by the expression, 'Don't knock it till you've tried it.' Each of us is familiar with the surprise of discovering that one enjoys, or thrills to, or is intrigued by, or cherishes, something about which one had not realized that one could care.

I have been promising an improvement on McDowell's objection to the argument linking REA and REC, and I am now ready to make good on that promise. Consider the core of the doxastic analogue of the argument: if someone comes to believe something for a reason, he must come to believe because he is seeing the matter aright, and this entails that he come to believe because he is deliberating correctly. McDowell's objection was that one could come to believe because one was seeing the matter aright, yet without deliberating; and he adduced conversion and being well

brought up as ways in which this might happen. These examples have a bolt-from-the-blue quality to them; if you become converted to the right, as opposed to the wrong, way of seeing things, or if you are well, as opposed to poorly, brought up, that is just luck—*pure* luck. But in the doxastic case it is obvious that there is a much more straightforward, and far less arbitrary way in which one can, non-deliberatively, come to believe because one is seeing matters aright, and that is to literally *see* matters aright. (This is not, of course, to deny that luck may be involved in getting into a position from which one can see matters aright.)

What I want to suggest is that, just as reasoning can be practical as well as theoretical, so experience can be practical too. Using 'fact' and 'value' for the moment as contrasting terms, we can say that there may be no relevant *fact* about some upcoming situation of which I am unaware, and there may be no element of my S that I am unable to deploy deliberatively, but that does not mean that I can know what it will be *like* without living through it. One reason for this is that what something is like is, often enough and in large part, a matter of my evaluation of it; and it is this evaluative aspect of what it is like that makes what it is like not simply a further fact available to the internalist. (I do not mean to suggest that all there is to, or is to be learned from, practical experience is: what it is like.) Aristotle was right to think that experience is necessary to develop the powers of practical judgment; we cannot expect a child raised in a narrow and inactive life to grow up into a *phronimos*, into someone whose practical judgment we might trust, no matter how much book learning, no matter how much *factual information*, he has.

We now have a way to respond to Williams' rhetorical question regarding the content of an external reason statement: '*What* is it that one comes to believe when he comes to believe that there is reason for him to ϕ, if it is not the proposition, or something that entails the proposition, that if he deliberated rationally, he would be motivated to act appropriately' (109)? One possible answer now seems to be: if he underwent the tutelage of experience, he would be motivated to act appropriately. (Of course, we now know not to rely too strongly on the counterfactual formulation, so this way of putting the point should be thought of as a placeholder.) As the Alka-Seltzer ad had it: 'He said, "Try it; you'll like it." I almost died.'

I need to consider two objections to the point I have just made. One is a rejoinder to the effect that I *must*, in principle, be able to know what it will be like, and that if I do not, it is because I am unaware of some fact, or because I have not sufficiently exercised my imagination. I will discuss this objection a few bends down the road. The other objection, which I will tackle now, claims that if I am not unaware of some fact or other about the situation, then I must be unaware or ignorant of some element in my S. In particular, Williams explicitly states that one's S 'can contain such things as

dispositions of evaluation' (105). Suppose someone's habits will prove infinitely irritating when one moves in with them. Even if one is confident beforehand that this will not be the case, the disposition to find them infinitely irritating is nonetheless there, and is an element of one's *S*— albeit an element of which one was ignorant. Experience is merely bringing one face to face with what some other way of exploring the contents of one's soul—perhaps psychoanalysis, as it is popularly conceived—would have found to be antecedently there. So the reasons which are revealed by experience are tied to one's *S* and are in fact internal reasons.[19]

There are two reasons why this response is unsuccessful. The first has to do with the internalist's appeal to the explanatory dimension of reasons. Cases of this kind can be set up such that they can be handled in this way only by emptying the notion of a subjective motivational set of explanatory power, not to mention content. Suppose that before time t my heart was set on X, and after experiencing X at t I wish I had never laid eyes on X. Before t the only motivation that can contribute to the explanation of action is my desire for X; if I could retroactively ascribe to myself, prior to t, my fervent and univocal desire never to have laid eyes on X, both REA and REC would have to be abandoned. (Think about the lessons of experience that, necessarily, arrive too late to be the basis for action, for instance, what as an adult one finally understands about one's youth.)

The second reason that this response fails has to do with the need for a theory about reasoning to be able to distinguish between dispositionally (as opposed to occurrently) held attitudes, and attitudes that one does not hold but is disposed to adopt in other circumstances.[20] It *is* often the case that experience brings me face to face with a fact about myself, rather than a feature of my world; perhaps my irritation forces me to acknowledge a longstanding but unadmitted contempt for habits like his, rather than teaching me anything genuinely new about those habits, or about what living with them is like. The question is whether we have the option of uniformly interpreting the tutelage of experience in this way.

In the *Meno*, Plato's Socrates adopts a similar strategy with regard to the conclusions of geometrical reasoning: the slave boy is not arriving at new beliefs but rather simply discovering beliefs he already has. (Socrates endorses the unlikely upshot, that infants already believe the entire panoply of geometrical theorems; it is important to see that the objection we are considering would require similarly attributing an implausible complexity to the personalities of the inexperienced.) Plato's dialogue shows us that, just as response to experience can be construed as revealing a mental state that both explains the response and shares its content, so response to argument can be construed as revealing a mental state that both explains the response and has its content. (It is the attribution of the content to the preconscious state that allows us to think of it as an element of the agent's

S, rather than something along the lines of a physical disposition.) But *this* move, which replaces deliberation with discovery of one's already-present mental states, is not one which someone who has come this far with Williams can afford to make. The agent's *S* is a basis for practical reasoning, that is, for mental activity in which one arrives at (practical) conclusions that one had not previously accepted. Suppose I desire to drink some gin, and believe that this is gin. If I think about it, I may come to desire to drink this; and when I do, I may be genuinely changing my mind about what I want to do. If we do not want to be put in the position of insisting that I am not arriving at any new conclusion, but simply discovering a previously concealed desire to drink this, we must acknowledge that there is a difference, and a way to tell the difference, between dispositional beliefs and desires (that is, things I now think or want that are, however, not at the moment being actively considered) and beliefs and desires that I do not have, but am disposed to arrive at in certain circumstances. But once the difference is acknowledged, then we can bring it to bear on our practical responses to experience. Someone who agrees that arguments can proceed from already-endorsed premises to not-yet-endorsed conclusions is in no position to insist that experience cannot lead us from genuinely not caring about something, to caring about it, on the grounds that we must already *dispositionally* care about it.

5

We're now far enough along to face the following pair of problems. First, given the similarities between Williams' own arguments and their doxastic analogues, why does Williams take himself to be making a point specific to reasons for *action*? Second, given the pressure it's possible to put on REA and REC, and given the straightforwardness with which the analogy allows us to make out a possible content for external reason statements, why does Williams nonetheless conclude that there are only internal reasons? To address these problems, I want to turn back to Williams' introduction of what he calls 'the sub-Humean model'. Williams states there that 'any model for the internal interpretation must display a relativity of the reason statement to the agent's subjective motivational set' (102, italics deleted); I need to spell out a little further the notion of 'relativity' that Williams has in mind.

On the following page, Williams denies that '[a] member of *S*, *D*, will . . . give *A* a reason for ϕ-ing if . . . *A*'s belief in the relevance of ϕ-ing to the satisfaction of *D* is false' (103). This seems to imply that one has a reason to ϕ only if there is some element of one's *S* whose satisfaction will be served by one's ϕ-ing, and so suggests exploring the idea that the notion of relativity to one's *S* that we are examining is to be made out entirely in terms of *satisfac-*

tion of elements of one's *S*. I will call a reason whose force is to be made out entirely in terms of such satisfaction an *instrumental* reason. The question, then, is whether Williams' conception of practical reasoning is uniformly instrumental, that is, whether it allows only for reasons for action whose force can be made out in terms of such satisfaction.[21]

Since deliberation consists in the deployment of reasons, a survey of forms that can be taken by deliberation would be a good place to get an idea of what someone thinks reasons can look like, and Williams provides such a survey (104). He mentions 'practical reasoning . . . leading to the conclusion that one has reason to ϕ because ϕ-ing would be the most convenient, economical, pleasant etc. way of satisfying some element in *S*', 'thinking how the satisfaction of elements in *S* can be combined', 'where there is some irresoluble conflict among the elements of *S*, considering which one attaches most weight to' (in order, I take it, to determine which to actually try to satisfy), and 'finding constitutive solutions, such as deciding what would make for an entertaining evening, granted that one wants entertainment.' All of these are clearly in the service of satisfying elements of one's *S*. Williams also mentions the ability of imagination to produce and eliminate desires; I will return to that item shortly.[22] While it is doubtful that Williams intends the list to be exhaustive, the generally instrumental cast of its elements is highly suggestive.[23]

Notice that while these forms of reasoning serve the satisfaction of elements of one's *S*, they are not entirely controlled by them. When conflicts arise, one may have to choose if one is not, like Buridan's ass, to fail to satisfy any of the conflicting desires; but there may be nothing in those elements of one's *S* (or even in any elements of one's *S*) to univocally determine the choice. Sarah Broadie has pointed out that constitutive reasoning, in going from the less to the more determinate, outruns its premises; the conclusion may serve the satisfaction of a desire, but it is not fully controlled by it.[24] Williams himself states that his first form of deliberation is 'controlled by other elements in *S*', but 'not necessarily in a very clear or determinate way'. How can a wholly instrumental conception of reasons for action be squared with this kind of slackness in the reins?

Williams handles the difficulty by allowing that 'there are no fixed boundaries on the continuum from rational thought to inspiration and conversion' (110). We must interpret this kind of slack in deliberation as meaning that we have something like a mixture of, on the one hand, the fully rational deployment of reasons, and, on the other, the use of faculties that are not themselves responsible to considerations that might subject them to correction. This is not to say that we might be able to factor out somehow the rational and inspirational or imaginative contributions to a particular episode of deliberation; nor is it to suggest that it would be possible or desirable to eliminate the non-rational contribution. The point

is just that, on this picture, whatever there is to a reason for action that cannot be derived from the content of some desire makes our understanding of the process of derivation as *reasoning* blur.

It is not my purpose here to argue that the instrumentalist model of practical reasoning is mistaken. But since I do think that it is,[25] I will try to explain what it is that Williams has overlooked.

The notion that there is some pattern of argument that can be used to bring any rational agent around to (say) morally satisfactory motivations, no matter *what* the agent cares about, Williams rightly regards as implausible. So one's reasons must be *rooted* in one's motivations, and if the only available form of rootedness is, being directed toward their satisfaction, then all reasons must be internal.[26] What is being left out of account is the possibility that reasons may be rooted in an agent's subjective motivational set without being directed toward the satisfaction of elements of that set. Let me try to indicate by illustration what such a relation might come to.

Imagine someone brought up on the pleasures of light verse: the deft rhyme, the cleverly enjambed phrase, the incongruous image subtly played out. What we might call a strong appreciation for the accomplishments of lesser poems is firmly a component of his *S*. Now suppose he is directed to a passage such as, say, the second part of Yeats' 'A Dialogue of Self and Soul'. It is characteristic of such poems that appropriate reactions to them are complex and not easily summarized, but we may suppose that one component of his reaction amounts to, 'I had no idea a poem could be like *that*', and that his *S* now contains desires to read more poetry of this kind. (We do not now need to try to say what 'this kind' is, but it is important that the conceptual resources this would require can go beyond those available to him before his encounter with the 'Dialogue'. In such a case, it is especially implausible to insist that his former *S* contains the resources to account for his present reasons.) Now the augmentation of his *S* by these new elements is rooted in his previous *S*, but is not a matter of satisfying already present elements of it. His engagement by the poem required having been prepared, by his interest in verse and, to be sure, other things; it is not as though there is a way to make anybody, no matter what his concerns, have this reaction to the piece. But his desire to read and reread poems like the 'Dialogue' is not a way of satisfying any desires he already had. And, finally for now, it is fairly clear what the force of someone's advising him that he had reason to take a look at this poem might have been.

An instrumental view of reasons for action explains how one might invoke REA and REC without seeming to oneself to be committing the conditional fallacy. The conditional fallacy is committed when a definition is given in terms of a counterfactual, and the class being defined has in-

stances that involve the falsehood of the antecedent of the counterfactual.[27] Williams' formulation of what it takes to have a reason for action seems, I have argued, to commit this fallacy; having a reason for action cannot consist in the fact that if you were rationally to deliberate, you would be motivated, if some reasons for action come down to one's inability rationally to deliberate. However, if one were an instrumentalist, and especially if one were an instrumentalist with Williams' sensitivities to the actual workings of instrumental reasoning, one might quite reasonably think that there had been no fallacy committed.

In order to show up a counterfactual-based definition of this kind, one needs to be able to point out the antecedent-falsifying instance. In the case of internalism about reasons for belief, this was, we saw, easy enough: if you are blind or obtuse, you may be unable to see, or see the import of, the evidence for those very facts. But instrumentalism blocks the analogous move against internalism about reasons for action. Instrumentalism is an unsettlingly narrow view of what practical inferences are possible: we can see this by observing that no analogue of instrumentalism in the domain of belief would be remotely plausible; it is just too evident that we have beliefs learned from, and corrected by, experience, that is, that there are empirical patterns of theoretical inference. Because, on the instrumentalist view, all practical inference is directed toward the *satisfaction* of elements of one's S, and, ultimately, of elements of one's S that are not themselves derived from further satisfaction-demanding elements, there is no logical room for control of those elements from the outside. This upshot of the instrumentalist thesis tends to get expressed in something like the following picture. When someone falsely believes himself to have a reason to ϕ, he may be mistaken about the contribution of ϕ-ing to the satisfaction of elements of his S, he may be mistaken about factual presuppositions of elements of his S, and he may be mistaken about the relations in which elements of his S stand to one another. But once we have got past these errors, there is no room to correct elements of an S, just because there is no further way in which they can be wrong. On this picture, there is simply nothing for them to be wrong *about*. If truth is the formal object of belief, we can sum up this view with the claim that there is no real analogue of truth in the practical domain. Now a picture, of course, is only a picture. Just as we have no hold on the notion of truth other than our hold on the inferential patterns in which beliefs figure, so we have no hold on what might be the practical analogue of truth over and above our hold on the inferential patterns in which practical attitudes figure. So the picture is merely a dramatic reiteration of the instrumentalist thesis, rather than independent support for it.

The instrumentalist, then, is in a position to disregard T_2-type counterexamples; his exclusive interest in satisfaction makes the notion of an

outside source of correction unintelligible. But what about T_1-like cases? Can't the logical relations between means and end hold even when necessarily unappreciated?

Perhaps not. Williams' survey of the different forms instrumental reasoning can take makes clear his awareness of its logical *softness*. Typically, there are many available means to an end, and an instrumental reasoner must choose one. (If I want a copy of a certain book, I could go to the library, or to the local bookstore, or I could break into a colleague's office, or I could fly to England, where there are more bookstores . . .) Most of the options are, usually, just crazy, and it would be a mistake *of reasoning* to choose one of the just crazy options; but there is no clean way to say which of the options are and are not just crazy. There is nothing like the model-theoretic specification of validity for deductive reasoning; indeed no formally specifiable notion of validity seems to be available.[28] Instead, we end up relying on the practical intelligence of the reasoner to pick the right, or a reasonable, alternative out of the lot. But if we have no hold on the inference pattern independent of the dispositions of practically intelligent reasoners, then we are not in a position to pick out a case in which the inferential relations hold, but the dispositions fail.

Internalism, we saw, is not a plausible take on reasons for belief. Instrumentalism, I am suggesting, is the extra ingredient that makes internalism about reasons for action a reasonably held position. This is a controlling exegetical consideration, one which underwrites an instrumentalist reading at ambiguous moments in Williams' writing, and overrides what would be their author's likely surprise at having the label adhere to his own carefully nuanced views. But the point is not in the first place exegetical: the substantive issue at the core of the debate over internalism is the adequacy of the instrumentalist model of practical reasoning.

Internalism and instrumentalism are at first glance only indirectly related views. Internalism is a view having to do with what is required for something to be a reason, of any kind, at all; instrumentalism is a claim about what patterns practical inference can take—a claim about what belongs on the list of, broadly, valid rules of inference. But, as developing analogies between doxastic and orectic internalism has shown, the merely formal considerations adduced in support of internalism are insufficient: they are identical on both sides of the analogy, and internalism about belief is obviously false. Internalism about reasons for action must be motivated by some further doctrine that is being kept out of sight in the apparently very general arguments; if I am right in thinking that Williams is articulating the considerations that have made internalism broadly attractive, our discussion suggests is that it is only when internalism is considered against a background of instrumentalist presuppositions that it seems inevitable.

6

I want to conclude by asking what might make it seem plausible that one is necessarily infallible in the contents of one's *S*. The question is particularly pressing in the light of the examples we have been examining: if we learn from, which is to say, are corrected by, experience, and if correction makes sense only when we have room for being mistaken, then the infallibility to which the internalist or instrumentalist conception is committed must go by the board. But the ways in which we learn from experience are too common, and too important, to be overlooked. What does the internalist make of them?

The question is not, at this point, why someone might *want* to think that one cannot in this way learn from experience. (Instrumentalism has obvious and respectable philosophical attractions; for example, the legitimacy of instrumental reasoning is relatively uncontroversial.) Rather, I want to ask how one might suppose that one has the *liberty* to think that one cannot learn from experience, given the *prima facie* implausibility of this thought. After all, it is not only *hubris* to hold that life has nothing to teach us about what matters. It is a procrustean attitude to some very familiar, but quite messy, phenomena. On what basis am I willing to insist that when the maturing child no longer wants to become a fireman, this *must* be understood as a matter of learning facts, on the one hand, and change in his orectic system that is not a matter of correction by experience, on the other? When you discover to your astonishment that your ex-spouse means more to you than the job for which you left him or her, *need* it be the case that you had overlooked either some fact, or one of your desires? Our understanding of cases like these should be sufficiently tentative to make the internalist's willingness to insist on his construal of them, before examining the actual cases, surprising.[29]

Now while an internalist will find it very hard to deny that we do learn from experience, he can explain our doing so in the following way. Human beings are, as it happens, not very good at telling how complicated situations will (or won't) satisfy our complicated *S*s. For this reason, we may have anticipated the facts, yet be surprised at our reaction when we come face to face with them. But in principle, if we had pictured the anticipated situation very accurately, while giving our *S* a kind of reactive free rein, we would have been able to anticipate our own responses, and we would not be surprised by them. That is, we learn what matters from experience only because we have not sufficiently exercised our imaginations.

It is hard to be certain, but I suspect that some such notion of imagination is in play in "Internal and External Reasons". Williams writes that

the agent . . . may think he has reason to promote some development because he has not exercised his imagination enough about what it would be like if it

came about . . . he may come to have some more concrete sense of what would be involved, and lose his desire for it, just as, positively, the imagination can create new possibilities and new desires. (104f; cf. Williams, 1989, p. 4)

The suggestion seems to be that if only the facts were pictured clearly enough, and the bearing, not always obvious, and not always routinely discoverable, of the facts on the satisfaction of the elements of one's *S* were made clear, it would become evident what one really wanted; which is to say that the lessons that experience holds in store for one might be anticipated.

Now 'imagination' is one of those words in philosophy that are overused and underexamined, and which usually signal an appeal to black magic. Here I will make a few dogmatic remarks about what can be done with the notion. Imagination is just thought: to say, 'imagine what it would be like', is to say no more than, 'think about what it would be like'. Consequently, imagination cannot outrun the resources of thought. (In fact, the view of imagination that is congenial to the internalist, which we can call 'the simulator view', will concede that you can't imagine what something would be like if you are missing relevant information, perhaps some fact of which you are unaware.) What is important here is that the internalist's appeal to imagination, at a point in the argument where he is concerned to resist the idea that experience can teach us what matters, is question-begging. For it supposes that once the facts and my *S* are in, nothing further is required for the successful exercise of imagination. But if successfully thinking about what matters requires further premises obtainable only from experience, then imagination, which is simply thinking, requires these premises too.

Imagination is a human faculty, and there are accordingly limits to its capabilities. My most perfect imaginings may lead me to believe that one course of action is what I want; and I will only discover that it is not when it actually occurs. I may have a stake in things turning out one way rather than another, and yet have no way to find this out short of living through one of the options. In particular, I may have no way that proceeds from my current subjective motivational set through any deliberative process whatsoever. Learning, in our earlier example, what a poem can be amounts to change in motivation that, just because it is a child of experience, is not fully responsible to one's initial subjective motivational set. We can learn from experience, and this education is neither a substitute for the imaginative exploration of present desires, nor simply an arbitrary alteration of them.[30]

Let me return briefly to an objection that I have put off more than once, to the effect that the examples of external reasons that I have given are not really examples of reasons—or of external reasons—at all. If objections in this vein are to be anything more than mere counterassertion, the willing-

ness to dismiss the candidate counterexamples needs to be motivated. What I have tried to do is elicit and disarm the motivations most likely to give rise to the objection. Only one of these is still viable: the instrumentalist theory of practical reasoning. But because internalism and instrumentalism are, as it has turned out, so very tightly linked, in disarming the motivations for the objection, I have also inventoried, and given reason to reject, what I have found to be the most common conversationally adduced defences of instrumentalism: the appeals to imagination, to dispositional desires, and so on. The issue remaining from the debate over internalism turns out to be whether there are patterns of practical inference that are not directed toward the satisfaction of desire; if we have in fact in the course of the argument dismantled the reflexively invoked defences of instrumentalism, much of the clutter around *this* question has been cleared away.

Notes

*For comments on earlier drafts, I'm grateful to Alyssa Bernstein, Sarah Buss, Alice Crary, Garrett Deckel, Gilbert Harman, Wilfried Hinsch, Jenann Ismael, Lee Overton, Jim Pryor, Tim Scanlon, Seana Shiffrin, Bill Talbott and several anonymous reviewers.

[1]P. 102, italics deleted. References by page number alone will be to Williams, 1981; like Williams, I intend mentions of internal and external reasons to be paraphrasable by locutions mentioning reason-*statements*. Williams has restated and further developed the argument in Williams, 1989. Hieronymi, 1993, discusses tensions between these papers and the uses to which he elsewhere puts the views he develops in them.

[2]For a recent overview, see Brink, 1989, pp. 37–62; for an earlier survey, see Frankena, 1958/1976. Cf. also Darwall, 1983, esp. chs. 2–5. Note that different authors mean very different things by the terms 'internal', 'internalist', 'external', 'externalist', and their relatives. I will be following Williams' usage.

[3]We must construe the expression 'people sometimes act' modally; that is, we must read Williams as insisting that persons *could* act for the reason they have (for reasons of that type), even if in fact no one ever does. After all, it is easy enough to imagine that someone comes one day to have a reason for action that he has never had before and will never have again; Cathy and Larry's wedding is a reason for me to fly to San Francisco, and I do not expect them to marry one another more than once. On that occasion, however, the reason may not suffice for action; I have other commitments that do not allow me to fly to the West Coast. Charity requires us to take Williams as allowing for such cases—if we are sufficiently fine-grained in our characterizations of reasons, they will be frequent enough—which means taking his claim modally. There is further textual support for this interpretive point. (1) is introduced by Williams' remark that he will return to the issue of the 'explanatory dimension' of reasons (102). Later, he tells us 'to remember again the dimension of possible explanation'; and here he phrases the condition using an explicit modal: 'If something can be a reason for action, then it *could* be someone's reason for acting on a particular occasion . . .' (106, my emphasis). Equally worth emphasizing, I take it that the point is not that *one* person has a reason if some *other* person could act from it. Rather, it is that a person has a reason for action only if *that* person could act for that reason, and that if he did, the reason would figure in some correct explanation of his action. (Cf. Williams, 1989, p. 5.)

[4]McDowell, 1995.

[5]Discussion includes Hooker, 1987, McDowell, 1995, Robertson, 1986, Korsgaard, 1986, Hollis, 1987, ch. 6, Velleman, 1996, Smith, 1992, and Cohon, 1986.

[6]I will distinguish between these in order to have a way of representing the analogue of the distinction between motivation (which may be overridden by more powerful motivations) and all-out motivation—the resolution, as it were, of one's motivations that determines action.

According to this (somewhat strained) usage, to find something *convincing* need not involve thinking it *true*. I may think it only likely, or I may actually think it unlikely: even though I know the snake-oil salesman's apparent sincerity is a tool of his trade, and so am not *convinced* by it, it is *convincing*, that is, it exerts a cognitive pull on my opinions—and can do so even when I am sure he really is not sincere. To be *convinced* of something entails thinking it true.

I will ignore complications arising from the possibility of contradictory elements in one's *C*.

[7]There may be said to be internal reasons$_B$ of which one is unaware—typically, items entailed by elements of one's *C*. These do not provide us the precise analogue of Williams' example of someone who wants to drink gin, and fails to realize that this petrol is not gin (102), since this case invokes an explanation of action involving two elements, one of which *is* in one's *S*, and the other of which is *not* in one's *C*. The analogue for this might be a case in which one refrained from drawing conclusions from one's beliefs out of contempt for consistency, fear of the truth, or simple disinterest in the subject. Here we might say that the agent has internal reasons$_B$ for believing the conclusion, but lacks internal reasons$_A$ to draw it.

[8]Williams, 1989, p. 5.

[9]Which is not to say that other, stronger reasons to the contrary may prevent him from being *convinced*. There is an apparent disanalogy here between reasons$_A$ and reasons$_B$: often, if I have a better reason for believing p than $\sim p$, the evidence for $\sim p$ loses all of its plausibility. On the other hand, a desire for X may conflict with, and outweigh, a desire for Y, without the desire for Y losing its force. But the disanalogy is not as clear-cut as it might seem at first glance. For one thing, the pull of competing reasons$_B$ often remains even after I settle on one of the beliefs; for another, certain kinds of incompatibility between desires may result in one of the desires losing its motivational force entirely.

[10]I am *not* suggesting that we consider a case in which T_1 is true and I deliberate rationally about its truth; the point is that when T_1 is true, I cannot deliberate rationally, and the counterfactual ceases to provide a handle on the logical connections between T_1 and the evidence for it.

Perhaps, even if I cannot see that the evidence entails T_1, someone more clear-headed than myself might do so. To see why this is not a promising option, consider a theory so complicated that *no* individual could, even in principle, understand it; the recent development of complexity theory allows us to give quite precise content to this suggestion. For related discussion, see Cherniak, 1986.

[11]It might be thought that we, the ascribers, must find them convincing ourselves. But this is belied by cases in which we are considering red herrings we know to have been planted in our subject's way: we, who know them to be red herrings, are not convinced, and the subject, who is failing to draw the obvious conclusion, is not convinced either. Our claim that he has reasons amounts to something like: given the evidence available to him, he should draw the conclusion to which it points.

[12]It might here be pointed out on Williams' behalf that REC, i.e., (5), has the form $p \supset (q \supset r)$. The example chosen, in which the agent cannot rationally deliberate when he has the given reason, sets q false when p is true; but it thus does not falsify (5), because the falsity of q makes $q \supset r$ true, which in turn makes $p \supset (q \supset r)$ true. But this objection would be doubly incompatible with the role Williams intends (5) to play. (5) is 'taken as roughly equivalent to, or at least as entail[ed]' by 'the external reasons statement itself' (109), by way of specifying 'the content of the external type of [reasons] statement' (108). A vacuously true statement fails to provide content; this can be seen by noting that (5), so construed, would fail to distinguish between deliberatively impaired agents with and without external reasons. Moreover, this construal of (5) would render Williams' argument invalid, inasmuch as it would only warrant the much weaker alternative to (8),

9. All external reason statements unaccompanied by an appropriate deliberative incapacity are false.

[13]For another example that makes this point, see Lear, 1984, p. 143.

[14]Note that we had better not replace REC with a claim of the form: a reason for Archie to

act is one that a counterfactual deliberatively competent Archie would advise his deliberatively incompetent counterpart to act on. First, as in note 10, above, we can turn to deliberative incapacities that are inevitable. Second, consider *your* idealized counterpart: why would you want to take his advice? Even if he is in a position to figure out what *he* ought to do, why does this put him in a position to advise *you*? If the two of you share an *S*, and your own *S* is not particularly focussed on improving the predicaments of others, then he will be unlikely to notice the relevant features of your circumstances, or be able to think them through helpfully. And if his *S* differs from yours, then why, on an internalist's view of the matter, should you listen to what he tells you? (This latter option is by far the more realistic, inasmuch as one's *S* is in large part an upshot of one's deliberative history. Deliberatively incapacitated, you've been made a fool of all your life, and so want, more than anything, not to be laughed at. Your deliberatively competent counterpart, never having been teased, doesn't particularly mind being laughed at.) In short, the counterfactual counterpart's deliberation is a far cry from the *agent* so deliberating, or acting: recall that Williams' example of a father advising his son to enter the army on the basis of reasons not available to the latter's deliberative processes was used to introduce and illustrate the notion of *external* reasons.

¹⁵This is of course not to imply that having reasons for action might have *no* close connection to the possibility of acting for reasons; our having reasons on which we could not act is intelligible only against a background of having reasons on which we can.

¹⁶If the proposed counterexamples *are* counterexamples, then Williams has committed a fallacy, called 'the conditional fallacy' by Shope (1978); and I think it is evident that the doxastic analogues of Williams' arguments do commit this fallacy. I will return later to the question of why someone might think they had avoided this fallacy when it is reasons for action to which the arguments are applied.

There are interesting similarities between internalism and other more familiar forms of reductionism. (On this point, see Robertson, 1986, p. 133.) For instance, there is an antiphenomenalist analogue to the counterexamples we developed to REC: a physical state that prevented sensation could not be reduced to possibilities of sensation. Physical injury resulting in blindness could not be visually verified.

¹⁷Some preliminary discussion can be found in Millgram, 1993, sec. 6.

¹⁸For related criticism, see Robertson, 1986, pp. 129ff, on 'Platonic internalism'.

¹⁹A reaction of this kind is likely to be prompted by the thought that the tutelage of experience, especially when it is tutelage regarding one's self-interest, is amenable to an internalist construal. Invoking the analogy with theoretical reasoning is a helpful way of inducing hesitation: when the tutelage of experience consists in, say, astronomical observation, no-one is tempted by the thought that an internalist construal must be available. Why, we are asking, are the two cases supposed to be, at this point, disanalogous?

²⁰I do not mean to suggest that making the distinction is always easy; or that being able to make the distinction means having a *procedure* for making the distinction.

²¹The terminology is slightly non-standard; see note 23, below.

²²Commentators tend to regard Williams' conception of deliberation as quite generous. McDowell, for example, allows that Williams has 'a subtle and flexible conception of the materials available to the internal interpretation', specifically, an understanding of 'practical reasoning, conceived on . . . unrestrictive lines' (1995, sec. 2). More ambiguously, both Hooker, 1987 (working out a point he attributes to Robert Gay), and Robertson, 1986, p. 127, point out ways in which Williams' second argument trades on the manner in which 'the deliberative process . . . may be more or less ambitiously conceived' (110). If I am right, however, the conception of deliberation in play here is narrower than has been thought.

²³Because my use of 'instrumental' here is mildly unusual, let me preempt a couple of possible confusions. Constitutive reasoning is often contrasted with instrumental reasoning; when this contrast is drawn, instrumental deliberation is thought of as reasoning about causal connections (to get the ball into the outfield, I have to hit it with the bat), and constitutive deliberation, as a matter of determining the parts or elements or components of something (to win the game, we must score more runs than the opposing team, and avoid being disqualified by the way we do it). Both types of reasoning may be a matter of figuring out how to get something fairly definite that one already wants (e.g., winning the game), and when they are, they come under the heading of instrumental reasoning, as I am now using the term. Constitu-

tive reasoning, when it is not simply a matter of joint constraint satisfaction, or a listing of standard constituents, may also be non-instrumental (in my sense); that is, it may amount to figuring out what one wants in the first place, rather than what is involved in getting what one wants. (When it does, it is externalist reasoning; see Millgram, 1993, sec. 6.) Williams' example strongly suggests that it is the instrumental (in my sense) version of constitutive reasoning he has in mind: when we ask what would make an entertaining evening, we are normally trying to figure out what it would take to satisfy a fairly substantial desire (i.e., to find something that will count as satisfying an element of our respective *S*s), rather than trying to figure out what the content of the desire we are considering satisfying might be (i.e., rather than replacing a thin desire for entertainment with a substantially new, and much richer desire for what we now understand 'entertainment' to mean).

²⁴Broadie, 1987, pp. 238f.

²⁵For an argument that it is mistaken, see Millgram, forthcoming, ch. 2.

²⁶Notice that in this sense of 'rooted', even the conversions that McDowell considers are rooted in the agent's prior *S*. It is implausible that there is a conversion technique that will work on anyone, no matter what it is he cares about. And notice that the rootedness of practical reasons resembles that of reasons for belief: experience delivers external reasons for belief, but we should not expect any experience to bring one around to a particular belief *regardless* of what else one believes.

²⁷See note 16, above.

²⁸Cf. e.g., Searle, 1991.

²⁹It is still, at this point, *open* to the internalist to insist that such transformations of one's motivational set must be mere change (albeit change that creates new reasons for action). Though we can now say that this would be *mere* insistence—the internalist is, at this point, short both on argument and on convincing renderings of realistic examples—it would be nice to have an argument that decisively closes off the option. I advance an argument meant to do the job in Millgram, forthcoming.

³⁰I am not of course supposing that I have here laid out the means for distinguishing learning from mere change in goals, or of saying what the standard is against which satisfying desires that—one wants to say—one did not know enough to have counts as an *improvement* in one's circumstances.

References

Brink, David. (1989) *Moral Realism and the Foundations of Ethics*, Cambridge University Press, Cambridge.

Broadie, Sarah. (1987) "The Problem of Practical Intellect in Aristotle's Ethics," *Proceedings of the Boston Area Colloquium in Ancient Philosophy, Vol. III*, John Cleary (ed.), University Press of America, Lanham, 229–52.

Cherniak, Christopher. (1986) *Minimal Rationality*, MIT Press, Cambridge, Mass.

Cohon, Rachel. "Are External Reasons Impossible?" *Ethics, 96*, 545–556.

Darwall, Stephen. (1983) *Impartial Reason*, Cornell University Press, Ithaca.

Frankena, William. (1958/1976) "Obligation and Motivation in Recent Moral Philosophy," *Perspectives on Morality*, K. Goodpaster (ed.), University of Notre Dame Press, Notre Dame.

Hieronymi, Pamela. (1993) "Internal Reasons and the Integrity of Blame," unpublished manuscript.

Hollis, Martin. (1987) *The Cunning of Reason*, Cambridge University Press, Cambridge.

Hooker, Brad. (1987) "Williams' Argument Against External Reasons," *Analysis, 47(1)*, 42–44.

Korsgaard, Christine. (1986) "Skepticism about Practical Reasoning," *Journal of Philosophy, 83(1)*, 5–25.

Lear, Jonathan. (1984) "Moral Objectivity," *Objectivity and Cultural Divergence*, S. C. Brown (ed.), Cambridge University Press, Cambridge, 135–170.

McDowell, John. (1995) "Might There Be External Reasons?" *World, Mind and Ethics: Essays on the Ethical Philosophy of Bernard Williams*, J.E.J. Altham and Ross Harrison (eds.), Cambridge University Press, Cambridge, 68–85.

Millgram, Elijah. (1993) "Pleasure in Practical Reasoning," *The Monist, 76(3)*, 394–415.

Millgram, Elijah. (forthcoming) *Practical Induction*, Harvard University Press, Cambridge, Mass.

Robertson, John. (1986) "Internalism About Moral Reasons," *Pacific Philosophical Quarterly, 67*, 124–135.

Searle, John. (1991) "Desire, Deliberation, and Action," unpublished manuscript.

Shope, Robert. (1978) "The Conditional Fallacy in Contemporary Philosophy," *The Journal of Philosophy, 75(8)*, 124–135.

Smith, Michael. (1992) "Valuing: Desiring or Believing?" *Reduction, Explanation, and Realism*, D. Charles and K. Lennon (eds.), Clarendon Press, Oxford, 324–359.

Velleman, J. David. (1996) "The Possibility of Practical Reason," *Ethics*.

Williams, Bernard. (1981) "Internal and External Reasons," *Moral Luck*, Cambridge University Press, Cambridge.

Williams, Bernard. (1989) "Internal Reasons and the Obscurity of Blame," *Logos: Philosophic Issues in Christian Perspective, 10*, 1–11.

[8]

Philosophy and Phenomenological Research
Vol. LV, No. 1, March 1995

Internal Reasons

MICHAEL SMITH
Australian National University

Introduction

According to one popular version of the dispositional theory of value, the version I favour, there is an analytic connection between the desirability of an agent's acting in a certain way in certain circumstances and her having a desire to act in that way in those circumstances if she were fully rational (Rawls 1971: Chapter 7; Brandt 1979: Chapter 1; Smith 1989, 1992, 1994).[1] If claims about what we have reason to do are equivalent to, or are in some way entailed by, claims about what it is desirable for us to do—if our reasons follow in the wake of our values—then it follows that there is a plausible analytic connection between what we have reason to do in certain circumstances and what we would desire to do in those circumstances if we were fully rational.

The idea that there is such an analytic connection will hardly come as news. It amounts to no more and no less than an endorsement of the claim that all reasons are 'internal', as opposed to 'external', to use Bernard Williams's terms (Williams 1980). Or, to put things in the way Christine Korsgaard favours, it amounts to an endorsement of the 'internalism requirement' on reasons (Korsgaard 1986). But how exactly is the internalism requirement to be understood? What does it tell us about the nature of reasons? And where-in lies its appeal? My aim in this paper is to answer these questions.

The paper divides into three main sections. In the first I distinguish between two different models of the internalism requirement—the 'advice' model and the 'example' model—and I say why the requirement should be understood in terms of the advice model. In the second and longest section I spell out the requirement in some detail and I explain why, contrary to

---

[1]   Adherents of other versions of the dispositional theory may agree that desirability is a feature that elicits an appropriate response in subjects under conditions of full rationality, but disagree about whether that response is desire (Johnston 1989 appears to take this view), or they may instead agree that desirability is a feature that elicits desire in agents under the appropriate conditions, but disagree about whether those are conditions of full rationality (Lewis 1989 appears to take this view).

Bernard Williams, it is not especially allied to a relativistic conception of reasons—indeed I say why those of us who embrace the requirement should endorse a non-relative conception. And in the third section I use the advice model, understood in the way explained in the second section, to explain the appeal of the internalism requirement. As we will see, the internalism requirement helps us solve an otherwise troubling problem about the effectiveness of deliberation.

1. The advice model versus the example model

The internalism requirement tells us that the desirability of an agent's φ-ing in certain circumstances C depends on whether she would desire that she φs in C if she were fully rational. This idea can be made more precise as follows.

We are to imagine two possible worlds: the *evaluated* world in which we find the agent in the circumstances she faces, and the *evaluating* world in which we find the agent's fully rational self. In these terms, the internalism requirement tells us that the desirability of the agent's φ-ing in the evaluated world depends on whether her fully rational self in the evaluating world would desire that she φs in the evaluated world. Note what I have just said, for the precise formulation is important. The idea is that we are to imagine the agent's fully rational self in the evaluating world looking across at herself in the evaluated world (so to speak) and forming a desire about what her less than fully rational self is to do in the circumstances she faces in that evaluated world. We might imagine that the self in the evaluating world is giving the self in the evaluated world advice about what to do. Accordingly, this is what I call the 'advice' model of the requirement.

The advice model of the requirement contrasts with the example model. On this alternative way of thinking about the requirement, the idea is that the desirability of an agent's φ-ing in the evaluated world depends on whether her fully rational self in the evaluating world would desire to φ *in the evaluating world*. We are not to suppose that the agent's fully rational self is giving advice to herself in the evaluated world, but rather that the agent's fully rational self is setting up her own behaviour in her own world, the evaluating world, as an example to be followed by the self in the evaluated world. The issue of interpretation, then, turns on whether the internalism requirement tells us that in acting on reasons we follow the *advice*, or the *example*, of our fully rational selves.

I said that the details of the formulation are important, and the reason why is because the details are something about which those who accept the requirement may yet disagree. Consider, for example, Christine Korsgaard's own official formulation of the requirement. According to Korsgaard the internalism requirement is the claim that the considerations that constitute reasons must 'succeed in *motivating* us insofar as we are rational' (1986: 15,

emphasis is mine). But on the plausible assumption that a fully rational agent's desires will only succeed in motivating *her* if they are desires that concern the circumstances in which *she* finds *herself*, the idea, in our terms, must be that a consideration constitutes a reason in the evaluated world just in case, in the evaluating world, the agent's fully rational self would desire that she acts on that consideration *in the evaluating world*. Korsgaard thus seems to have in mind the example model of the internalism requirement, not the advice model.[2]

But the example model is plainly wrong. In order to see why consider the following case, a variation on an example of Gary Watson's (1975). Suppose I have just been defeated in a game of squash. The defeat has been so humiliating that, out of anger and frustration, I am consumed with a desire to smash my opponent in the face with my racket. But if I were fully rational, we will suppose, I wouldn't have any such desire at all. My desire to smash him in the face is wholly and solely the product of anger and frustration, something we can rightly imagine away when we imagine me in my cool and calm fully rational state. The consideration that would motivate me if I were fully rational is rather that I could show good sportsmanship by striding right over and shaking my opponent by the hand. In that case, does it follow that what I have reason to do *in my uncalm and uncool state* is stride right over and shake him by the hand?

In essence, this is what Korsgaard's formulation of the internalism requirement tells us, for she supposes that a consideration constitutes a reason just in case it would motivate the fully rational person, and this is what my fully rational self would be motivated to do. And yet this is surely quite wrong. Striding right over and shaking my opponent by the hand might be the last thing I have reason to do, especially if being in such close proximity to him, given my anger and frustration, is the sort of thing that would cause me to smash him in the face. Rather, we might plausibly suppose, what I have reason to do in my uncalm and uncool state is to smile politely and leave the scene as soon as possible. For this is something that I can get myself to do and it will allow me to control my feelings. Moreover—and importantly for the advice model—*this is exactly what my fully rational self would want my less than fully rational self to do in the circumstances that my less than fully rational self finds himself.* But, to repeat, it is not something I would be motivated to do if I were fully rational because it is not something that I would have any *need* to be motivated to do if I were fully rational.

---

2   Rawls (1971) and Brandt (1979) seem to have had in mind the example model of the internalism requirement as well. Contrast Peter Railton's account of a person's own good (1986) which is formulated in terms in terms of the advice model precisely to avoid problems like those I go on to describe in the text. For criticisms of Rawls's and Brandt's 'example' versions of the internalism requirement see Shope (1978) and Pettit and Smith (1993). (Here I am grateful to Stephen Darwall.)

The example model of the internalism requirement thus gives us the wrong answer in cases in which what we have reason to do is in part determined by the fact that we are irrational. For what an agent's fully rational self is motivated to do will depend on the circumstances in which she finds herself, and, by definition, these circumstances will never include her own irrationality. It therefore seems to me that we should reject the example model of the internalism requirement in favour of the advice model. What we have reason to do in the circumstances in which we find ourselves is fixed by the advice our fully rational selves would give us about what to do in these circumstances that we face.

2. The internalism requirement and the idea of being fully rational

The internalism requirement tells us that it is desirable for an agent to φ in certain circumstances C, and so she has a reason to φ in C, if and only if, if she were fully rational, she would desire that she φs in C. The content of our reasons is thus fixed by the advice we would give ourselves if we were fully rational. However, note that I haven't yet said anything about what being 'fully rational' means, and that we must do so if we are to understand what the internalism requirement tells us, substantively, about the reasons we have.

In his own similar analysis of internal reasons Bernard Williams suggests, in effect, that to be fully rational in the practical sphere an agent must satisfy the following three conditions:

    (i)   the agent must have no false beliefs

    (ii) the agent must have all relevant true beliefs

    (iii) the agent must deliberate correctly

His reason for insisting on the first two conditions is straightforward enough.

If our desire to do something is wholly dependent on false beliefs, then we ordinarily suppose that it isn't really desirable to do that thing. Suppose, for example, I desire to drink from a particular glass, but that my desire to do so depends on my belief that the glass contains gin and tonic when in fact it contains gin and petrol. Then we would ordinarily say that though I might think that it is desirable to drink from the glass, it isn't really desirable to do so. Why not? Because I would not desire that I do so if I were fully rational: that is, if, *inter alia*, I had no false beliefs—thus condition (i).

Similarly, in the case of condition (ii), if we fail to desire something, and if our failure to do so is wholly dependent on our failure to believe something that is true, then we ordinarily suppose that that thing may yet be desirable. Suppose, for example, that I do not desire to drink from a particular glass,

but that my failure to do so is to be explained by the fact that I am ignorant of the contents of the glass. In fact it contains the most delicious drink imagineable. Then we would ordinarily say that despite the fact that I do not desire to drink from the glass, doing so may yet be desirable. Why? Because I may well desire that I do so if I were fully rational: that is, if, *inter alia*, I had all relevant true beliefs.

But what about condition (iii)? Williams's idea here is that even if we fail to desire that we φ, φ-ing may still be desirable because we would desire that we φ if our other beliefs and desires interacted in the ways appropriate for the generation of new desires: that is, if we deliberated and did so correctly. For example, the means to an end is desirable, but we will in fact desire the means to our ends only if we reason in accordance with the means-ends principle, for only so does a desire for an end turn into a desire for the means.

Moreover, as Williams points out, means-ends reasoning is only one mode of rational deliberation among many. Another example is

> ...practical reasoning...leading to the conclusion that one has reason to φ because φ-ing would be the most convenient, economical, pleasant etc. way of satisfying some element in...[one's set of desires]...and this of course is controlled by other elements in...[one's set of desires]...if not necessarily in a very clear or determinate way....[And]...there are much wider possibilities for deliberation, such as: thinking how the satisfaction of elements in...[one's set of desires]...can be combined: e.g. by time-ordering; where there is some ir-resoluble conflict among the elements of...[one's set of desires]...considering which one attaches most weight to...; or, again, finding constitutive solutions, such as deciding what would make for an entertaining evening, granted that one wants entertainment. (1980: 104)

And he thinks that there are other, more radical, possibilities for deliberation as well.

> More subtly,...[an agent]...may think he has reason to promote some development because he has not exercised his imagination enough about what it would be like if it came about. In his unaided deliberative reason, or encouraged by the persuasions of others, he may come to have some more concrete sense of what would be involved, and lose his desire for it, just as positively, the imagination can create new possibilities and new desires. (1980: 104–5)

Thus, according to Williams, we must include the operation of the imagination in an account of what is involved in deliberating correctly as well.

Williams's conditions (i) through (iii) seem to me to constitute a fairly accurate spelling out of our idea of what it means to be practically rational. An agent who has defective beliefs or who deliberates badly is indeed the sort of agent we tend to think of as being practically irrational in some way. It seems to me that Williams's conditions do require supplementation and amendment, however. For one thing, I see no way in which the effects of anger and frustration could be precluded by conditions (i) through (iii) —unless some such constraint is supposed to be presupposed by condition (iii), the condition of correct deliberation. Yet, as we have seen, emotions can

cause us to desire to do what we have no reason to do (remember the effects
of that humiliating defeat I suffered in squash). Here, then, there is need for
supplementation. And for another—and this is the point on which I wish to
focus—it seems to me that Williams omits from his discussion of condition
(iii) an account of perhaps the most important form of deliberation. The
omission is serious as it leads him to overstate the role of the imagination in
deliberation. Here, then, as we will see, there is need for both supplementation and amendment.

Williams admits that deliberation can produce new and destroy old underived desires. As he puts it, an agent 'may think he has reason to promote
some development because he has not exercised his imagination enough
about what it would be like if it came about', just as, more 'positively, the
imagination can create new possibilities and new desires'. When the imagination does create and destroy desires in these ways Williams tells us that we
take its operations to be sanctioned by reason.

Williams is right, I think, that deliberation can both produce new and destroy old underived desires. But he is wrong that the only, or even the most
important, way in which this happens is via the exercise of the imagination.
By far the most important way in which we create new and destroy old underived desires when we deliberate is by trying to find out whether our desires
are, as a whole, *systematically justifiable*. And, if this is right, then that in
turn requires a significant qualification of Williams's claim that reason sanctions the operation of the imagination.

What do I mean when I say that we sometimes deliberate by trying to find
out whether our desires, as a whole, are systematically justifiable? I mean
just that we can try to decide whether or not some particular underived desire
that we have or might have is a desire to do something that is itself non-
derivatively desirable, and that we do this in a certain characteristic way:
namely, by trying to integrate the object of that desire into a more *coherent*
and *unified* desiderative profile and evaluative outlook. Rawls describes the
basics of this procedure of systematic justification in his discussion of how
we attempt to find a 'reflective equilibrium' among our specific and general
evaluative beliefs (Rawls 1951; Daniels 1979). I will restrict myself to saying a little about the way in which achieving reflective equilibrium may also
be a goal in the formation of underived desires.

Suppose we take a whole host of desires we have for specific and general
things, desires which are not in fact derived from any desire we have for
something more general. We can ask ourselves whether we wouldn't get a
more systematically justifiable set of desires by adding to this whole host of
specific and general desires another general desire, or a more general desire
still, a desire that, in turn, justifies and explains the more specific desires that
we have. And the answer might be that we would. If the new set of desires—
the set we imagine ourselves having if we add a more general desire to the

more specific desires we in fact have—exhibits more in the way of coherence and unity, then we may properly think that the new imaginary set of desires is rationally preferable to the old. For the coherence and unity of a set of desires is a virtue, a virtue that in turn makes for the rationality of the set as a whole. This is because exhibiting coherence and unity is partially constitutive of having a systematically justified, and so rationally preferable, set of desires, just as exhibiting coherence and unity is partially constitutive of having a systematically justified, and so rationally preferable, set of beliefs.

The idea here is straightforwardly analogous to what Rawls has to say about the conditions under which we might come to think that we should acquire a new belief in a general principle given our stock of rather specific evaluative beliefs. The thought there is that we might find that our specific value judgements would be more satisfyingly justified and explained by seeing them as all falling under a more general principle. The imaginary set of beliefs we get by adding the belief in the more general principle may exhibit more in the way of coherence and unity than our current stock of beliefs. Likewise, the idea here is that our imaginary set of desires may exhibit more in the way of coherence and unity than our current set of desires.

If we do come to believe that our more specific desires are better justified, and so explained, in this way, then note that that belief may itself cause us to have a new, underived, desire for that more general thing. And, if it does, then it seems entirely right and proper to suppose that this new desire has been arrived at by a rational method. Indeed, the acquisition of the new more general desire will seem rationally required in exactly the same way that the acquisition of the new belief that the object of the desire is desirable will seem rationally required. In fact, if the internalism requirement is right, the acquisition of a new evaluative belief will be the cognitive counterpart of the acquisition of the new desire. For, according to the requirement, an evaluative belief is simply a belief about what would be desired if we were fully rational, and the new desire is acquired precisely because it is believed to be required for us to be more rational.

Moreover, if this is agreed, then note that we can not only explain how we might come to have new underived desires as the result of such reflection, but that we can also explain how we might come to lose old underived desires as well. For, given the goal of having a systematically justifiable set of desires, it may well turn out that, as the attempt at systematic justification proceeds, certain desires that seemed otherwise unassailable have to be given up. Perhaps because we can see no way of integrating those desires into the set as a whole they will come to seem *ad hoc* and so unjustifiable to us. Our belief that such desires are *ad hoc* may then cause us to lose them. And, if so, then it will seem sensible to describe this as a loss that is itself mandated by reason; as again straightforwardly analogous to the loss of an unjustifiable, because *ad hoc*, belief.

As this procedure of systematic justification continues we can therefore well imagine wholesale shifts in our desiderative profile. Systematic reasoning creates new underived desires and destroys old. Since each such change seems rationally required, the new desiderative profile will seem not just different from the old, but better; more rational. Indeed, it will seem better and more rational in exactly the same way, and for the same reasons, that our new corresponding evaluative beliefs will seem better and more rational than our old ones.

To a first approximation, then, this is what I mean by saying that we can create new and destroy old underived desires by trying to come up with a set of desires that is systematically justifiable. But even this first approximation is enough to see why Williams's claims about the role of the imagination in deliberation requires significant qualification. For true though it is that the imagination can produce new and destroy old underived desires via vivid presentations of the facts, its operations are not guaranteed to produce and destroy desires that would themselves be sanctioned in an attempt at systematic justification of the kind just described. In fact quite the opposite is the case. For the imagination is liable to all sorts of distorting influences, influences that it is the role of systematic reasoning to sort out. Consider an example. Vividly imagining what it would be like to kill someone, I might find myself thoroughly averse to the prospect no matter what the imagined outcome. But, for all that, I might well find that the desire to kill someone, given certain outcomes, is one element in a systematically justifiable set of desires. Merely imagining a killing, no matter what the imagined circumstances, may cause in me a thoroughgoing aversion, but it will not justify such an aversion if considerations of overall coherence and unity demand that I have a desire to kill in certain sorts of circumstances, and such considerations may themselves override the effects of the imagination and cause me to have the desire I am justified in having.[3] The role played by attempts at systematic justification is thus what is crucially required for an understanding of how deliberation creates new and destroys old underived desires, not the role played by the imagination.

Let's recap. According to the internalism requirement, the desirability of an agent's ϕ-ing in certain circumstances C is fixed by whether or not she would desire that she ϕs in C if she were fully rational. The aim in this section is to spell out the idea of being fully rational. Taking our lead from Bernard Williams the suggestion so far is that an agent is fully rational just in case she has no false beliefs and all relevant true beliefs, and just in case she deliberates correctly in the light of these beliefs, and an agent is in turn understood to have deliberated correctly just in case her underived desires are

---

3   Mark Johnston (1989) pursues a similar line in his criticism of David Lewis's account
of the role of imaginative acquaintance in valuing (1989).

systematically justifiable: that is, to a first approximation, just in case her underived desires form a maximally coherent and unified desire set. Do we need to say more? Indeed we do, something we see clearly once we focus on a consequence Williams wants us to draw from his own similar analysis of reasons.

According to Williams, the internalism requirement supports a *relative* conception of reasons. He puts the point this way.

[T]he truth of the sentence…['A has a reason to φ']…implies, very roughly, that A has some motive which will be served or furthered by his φ-ing, and if this turns out not to be so the sentence is false: there is a condition relating to the agent's aims, and if this is not satisfied it is not true to say…that he has a reason to φ. (1980: 101)

And again later:

Basically, and by definition,…[an analysis of reasons]…must display a relativity of …[a]…reason statement to the agent's *subjective motivational set*…(1980: 102)

Now in fact it is initially quite difficult to see why Williams says any of this at all. For, as we have seen, what the internalism requirement suggests is that claims about an agent's reasons are claims about her *hypothetical* desires, not claims about her *actual* desires. The truth of the sentence 'A has a reason to φ' thus does not imply, not even 'very roughly', that A *has* some motive which will be served by his φ-ing; indeed A's *motives* are beside the point— that was the difference between the advice model and the example model. What the internalism requirement implies is rather that A has a reason to φ in certain circumstances C just in case he *would* desire that he φs in those circumstances if he were fully rational.

Williams might concede this. But, he might say, it doesn't show that he is wrong when he says that the requirement supports the relativity of an agent's reasons to her actual desires, it simply shows that the relativity of reasons requires more careful formulation. The crucial point, he might insist, is that the desires an agent would have if she were fully rational are themselves simply functions from her actual desires, where the relevant functions are those described in conditions (i) through (iii). An agent's reasons are thus relative to her actual desires, he might say, because under conditions of full rationality agents would all have different desires about what is to be done in the various circumstances they might face. Even if it is rational for each of us to change our actual desires by trying to come up with a set of desires that can be systematically justified, in the manner captured by conditions (i) through (iii), such changes will always fall short of making us have the same desires as our fellows; they will always reflect the antecedent fact that we have the actual desires that we have. The content of the maximally coherent and

unified desire set any particular agent could have will always reflect the content of that agent's actual desires.

As I see it, this is what Williams has in mind when he says that our reasons are all relative.[4] It explains why he rightly insists that he is defending a 'Humean' conception of reasons (1980: 102). For his conception of reasons, like Hume's own, is predicated on skepticism about the scope for reasoned change in our desires (Korsgaard 1986); predicated on denying that, through a process of rational deliberation—through attempting to give a systematic justification of our desires, for example—we could ever come to discover reasons that we all share. For what we have reason to do is given by the content of the desires we would have if we were fully rational, and these may differ in content from agent to agent.

Williams claims to derive this relative conception of reasons from the internalism requirement. But as a *derivation* this is hardly compelling. It goes through only if we assume that it is no part of our task, in trying to come up with a systematically justifiable set of desires, to come up with the same set of desires as our fellow rational creatures would come up with if they set themselves the same task. And this suggests, in turn, that there are therefore two quite distinct conceptions of *internal* reasons. There is a relativistic, Humean, conception of internal reasons—the conception embraced by Williams—and there is also a non-relativistic, anti-Humean or Kantian conception according to which, if we were to engage in a process of systematically justifying our desires we would all eventually reason ourselves towards the same conclusions as regards what is to be done. That is, according to the opposing conception, all possible rational creatures would desire alike as regards what is to be done in the various circumstances they might face because this is, *inter alia*, what defines them to be 'rational'. Part of the task of coming up with a maximally coherent and unified set of desires is coming up with a set that would be converged upon by other rational creatures who too are trying to come up with a maximally coherent and unified set of desires; each rational creature is to keep an eye out to her fellows, and to treat as an aberration to be explained, any divergence between the sets of desires they come up with through the process of systematic justification.[5, 6]

---

4   See especially Williams's discussion of the Owen Wingrave example (1980: 106–11).

5   Compare Philip Pettit on rule-following (1993, especially 96–97).

6   The claim is not that on the non-relative conception of reasons the existence of reasons-in-the-actual-world presupposes a convergence in the desires of fully rational creatures in the actual world. For this is itself a relative conception of reasons: reasons are *world*-relative. The non-relative conception really is *non*-relative. It claims that there is a convergence in the desires that all possible creatures would have, so long as those creatures are fully rational, whether those creatures exist in the actual world or not. Angels, ourselves in other possible worlds, the inhabitants of Mars—on the non-relative conception we are all of us supposed to desire the very same thing for the various circumstances we might face, at least insofar as we are rational.

The final question to ask, then, in spelling out our idea of 'full rationality', is whether Williams is right that our ordinary concept of a reason is
Humean or anti-Humean. Does our ordinary concept of a reason presuppose
skepticism about the scope for reasoned change in our desires? In other words,
does it presuppose that there will, or alternatively that there will not, be a
convergence in the desires that we would have under conditions of full rationality? If it presupposes that there will not be such a convergence then our
concept of a reason is indeed relative, just as Williams says. If it presupposes
instead that there will be such a convergence then our concept of a reason is,
by contrast, non-relative.

Let me emphasise that we are asking a conceptual question, not a substantive question. We are asking what we mean when we talk of people being
fully rational; whether it is part of what we mean by 'rational' that fully rational people converge in their desires, or whether this is no part of what we
mean by 'rational'. And note as well that no matter how we answer this question, we do not thereby beg any substantive questions. For example, even if
our concept of a reason is itself non-relative—even if our concept optimisti-
cally presupposes that we would all converge on the same desires under conditions of full rationality—the world might disappoint us. Entrenched and apparently rationally inexplicable differences in what we desire might make it
impossible to believe, substantively, that there are any such non-relative reasons (Smith 1991, 1993, 1994).

Let's, then, confront the conceptual question head on. Is our ordinary concept of a reason relative or non-relative? The relativity of a claim should manifest itself in the way we talk. Consider, for example, the schematic claim 'It
is desirable that p in circumstances C'. On the non-relative conception of internal reasons—at least if we abstract away from some complications to be
dealt with presently— this claim has a straightforward truth condition: it is
desirable that p in C just in case we would all desire that p in C if we were
fully rational. There is, then, a sense in which we can talk about rational
justification or desirability *simpliciter*. When you and I talk about the reasons
that there are for acting, we are therefore talking about the same thing. We are
talking about reasons *period*; about the common set of reasons that are appreciable by each of us.

On the relative conception, however, matters are quite different. For in order to give the truth condition of the schematic claim 'It is desirable that p in
C' we need first to know from whose perspective the truth of the claim is to
be assessed. For while 'It is desirable that p in C' as assessed from A's perspective is true if and only if A would desire that p in C if A were fully rational, 'It is desirable that p in C' as assessed from B's perspective is true if
and only if B would desire that p in C if B were fully rational, and so on and
so forth. There is thus no such thing as desirability or the considerations that
rationally justify *simpliciter*, but only desirability$_A$, desirability$_B$,...; consid-

erations that rationally-justify-from-A's-perspective, rationally-justify-from-B's-perspective,...and so on. If I say to you 'There is a reason for φ-ing', and you deny this, we are therefore potentially talking about quite different things: reasons$_{me}$ and reasons$_{you}$. The question to ask is therefore whether the way in which we talk about reasons for action and the considerations that rationally justify our actions reflects a relative or a non-relative conception of the truth conditions of reason claims.

One reason for thinking that it reflects the non-relative conception comes from the broader context in which the question is being asked. For it is important to remember that we have a whole range of normative concepts: truth, meaning, support, entailment, desirability, and so on. Between them these concepts allow us to ask all sorts of normative questions, questions about what we should and should not believe, say and do. But how many of these other normative concepts are plausibly thought to give rise to claims having relativised truth conditions? As I understand it, none of them do.

Consider our concept of support, by way of example. It seems quite implausible to suppose that the truth of claims about which propositions support which others is implicitly relative to the individual; that when A says 'p supports q' and B says 'p does not support q' they are potentially talking about quite different things: that A is talking about what supports$_A$ q and B is talking about what supports$_B$ q, for instance. For if this were the case then we should expect to find that we are sometimes able to dissolve apparent disagreements by finding that both parties are speaking truly. It should be permissable for B to say 'A said "p supports q" and what she said is true, but p does not support q'. However it is a striking feature of our talk about which propositions support which others that we *never* dissolve apparent disagreements in this way. Propositions have normative force *simpliciter*, not just normative-force-relative-to-this-individual or -relative-to-that. When one individual says 'p supports q' and the other says 'p does not support q' they thus express their disagreement about whether p supports q in a *non-relative* sense.

If our concept of desirability were implicitly relativised, then, it seems that this would mark a significant difference between this concept and our other normative concepts. We should expect to find that with claims about what is desirable, unlike claims about which propositions support which, we *are* able to dissolve apparent disagreements in the way just described. But do we find this?

It might be thought that we do. After all, aren't there all sorts of familiar cases in which we say things like 'That may be a reason for you, but it isn't for me', 'Desirable for you maybe, but not desirable for me', and the like? But though there are indeed such cases, it is important to note that the sort of relativity we signal when we say such things is quite different from the kind just described; quite different from the kind of relativity Williams has in mind. For, in the familiar cases, 'That may be a reason for you, but it isn't

for me' signals the fact that there is a relativity built in to the *considerations* that we use to rationally justify our choices. It does not signal the fact that *our concept of a reason* is itself relative to the individual; that there is no such thing as which considerations, relative or not, rationally justify our choices, but only which considerations rationally-justify-relative-to-this-person or rationally-justify-relative-to-that-person. Here, then, we come to the complications abstracted away from earlier.

Sometimes what we have in mind when we say 'That may be a reason for you, but it isn't for me' is that the considerations that rationally justify our choices are, to use Parfit's terms, *agent-relative*, rather than *agent-neutral* (Parfit 1984). Suppose you are standing on a beach. Two people are drowning to your left and one is drowning to your right. You can either swim left and save two, in which case the one on the right will drown, or you can swim right and save one, in which case the two on the left will drown. You decide to swim right and save the one and you justify your choice by saying 'The one on the right is my child, whereas the two on the left are perfect strangers to me'.

In one sense, of course, I may well say 'That may be a reason for you, but it isn't for me'. For if the three people drowning are all perfect strangers to me then, had I been standing on the beach instead of you, I would not have been able to justify the choice of swimming right and saving the one. But in another sense it seems that what is a reason for you may indeed be a reason for me. For if I had been standing on the beach instead of you, and if the one on the right had been my child—that is, if my circumstances had been in all crucial respects *the same* as your's—then surely I too would have been able to justify the choice of swimming right and saving the one by saying 'The one on the right is my child'. Indeed, if we think that a parent who fails to save her child in such circumstances fails to act on a reason available to her— as it seems to me that we do—then we are in fact obliged to say this; obliged to assume the non-relative conception of internal reasons.

What this sort of example shows is therefore that, even if reasons are non-relative in the crucial sense at issue here, among the considerations that may rationally justify our choices are both considerations that are properly given a *de dicto* formulation and considerations that are properly given a *de se* formulation (see also Lewis 1989). That is there are both *de dicto* and *de se* internal reasons. We can each express the content of the *de dicto* reason relevant in this case by using the words 'There is a reason to save people quite generally'. And we can each express the content of the *de se* reason by using the words 'There is a reason to save my child in particular'. In these terms what is a reason for you, in this case, is not a reason for me in the sense that, if it had been me standing on the beach rather than you, and if the same people had been drowning, then the only consideration that would have been relevant to my choice is the *de dicto* reason. The *de se* reason would not have been rel-

evant to my choice because the people who are in fact drowning are all perfect strangers to me. But in another sense what is a reason for you is indeed a reason for me. For if I had been standing on the beach and the one person on the right had been my child, as the one on the right is your child, then both the *de se* and the *de dicto* reason would have been relevant to my choice in just the way they are both relevant to your's.

I said that this sort of relativity is entirely different from the kind that Williams has in mind and it should now be plain why this is so. For, in terms of the analysis, even if some of the considerations that rationally justify our choices are relative because *de se*, the existence of such *de se* reasons may still require a convergence in the desires that we would all have if we were fully rational. That is, the existence of reasons with *de se* contents may still require that, under conditions of full rationality, we would each have desires whose contents we would express by using words like 'to help my children', 'to promote my welfare', and the like. The mere existence of *de se* reasons is thus quite different from the relativity Williams has in mind. For his claim is that reasons are relative in the sense of requiring no such convergence; that the fact that my act helps my child may constitute a reason$_{me}$ even though the fact that your act helps your child does not constitute a reason$_{you}$.

There is another familiar sort of relativity in our claims about the reasons we have as well, a sort that derives from the fact that what we have reason to do is relative to our circumstances, where our circumstances may include aspects of our own psychology. Suppose, for example, that you and I differ in our preferences for wine over beer. Preferring wine, as you do, you may tell me that there is a reason to go to the local wine bar after work for a drink, for they sell very good wine. But then, preferring beer, as I do, I may quite rightly reply 'That may be a reason for you to go to the wine bar, but it is not a reason for me'.

Now while this might initially look like the claim that our reasons are relative to our desires in something like the sense Williams has in mind, it again isn't really. For the crucial point in this case is that a relevant feature of your circumstances is your preference for wine, whereas a relevant feature of my circumstances is my preference for beer. That this is a relevant feature of our circumstances is manifest from the fact that I can quite happily agree with you that if I were in your circumstances—if I preferred wine to beer—then the fact that the local wine bar sells very good wine would constitute a reason for me to go there as well, just as it constitutes a reason for you.

This sort of relativity is thus completely different from the kind that Williams has in mind as well. For, in terms of the analysis, even if an agent's preferences may enter into a specification of the circumstances that she faces it might still be the case that whether or not she is rationally justified in taking her own preferences into account, and the way in which she is

justified in taking them into account, if she is, depends on whether fully rational agents would all converge on a desire which makes the preferences she in fact has relevant in that way to her choice. In this case, for example, it may be crucial that, under conditions of full rationality we would all converge on a desire to satisfy whatever preferences we might have (perhaps within limits) in deciding where to go for a drink after work.[7] The fact that in rationally justifying our choices our preferences may sometimes be a relevant feature of our circumstances thus does nothing to support Williams's view that our reasons are relative; does nothing to support the view that really there are only the considerations that rationally-justify-relative-to-this-person or rationally-justify-relative-to-that.

In order to find support for the sort of relativity Williams has in mind, we therefore need to look for cases in which it is permissable to make much more radically relativised claims about what there is reason to do. But in fact, as far as I can tell, we find no such claims. Suppose someone tells me that she has a reason to take a holiday and that I think I would have no reason to take a holiday in the circumstances she faces. Provided we have taken proper account of the *de se* considerations that might be relevant to her choice, and provided we have taken proper account of the way in which her preferences may constitute a relevant feature of her circumstances, it seems that I straightforwardly disagree with her about the rational justifiability of her taking a holiday in the circumstances she faces, a disagreement I can express by saying 'She thinks that there is a reason to take a holiday in her circumstances, but there is no such reason'. If she cites a consideration in support of her taking a holiday that I think fails to justify, then I do not conclude that it may justify-relative-to-her, though not justify-relative-to-me, I conclude that it fails to justify *simpliciter*.

The point is important, for it suggests that when we talk about reasons for action we quite generally take ourselves to be talking about a common subject matter: reasons *period*. We are thus potentially in agreement or disagreement with each other about what constitutes a reason and what doesn't. This is why, when we find ourselves in disagreement—as for example in the case of disagreement about whether or not there is a reason to take a holiday in certain circumstances—we always have the option of engaging in argument in the attempt to find out who is right and who is wrong. Other people's opinions about the reasons that there are thus constitute potential challenges to my own opinions. I have something to learn about myself and my own assessment of the reasons that there are by finding out about others and

---

7   Note that the preferences we have are not always a relevant feature of our circumstances. If I just so happen to prefer kicking the cat to leaving it sleep in peace, my fully rational self might want that I do not kick the cat despite my preference. For relevant discussion of this point, and the relevance of actual desires to the desirability or justifiability of our actions generally, see Pettit and Smith 1990, 1993, forthcoming.

their assessment. This is why books and films are so engaging. All of this is flat out inconsistent with the claim that our concept of a reason for action is quite generally relative to the individual; that it typically means reason$_{me}$ out of my mouth, reason$_{you}$ out of your's, reason$_{her}$ out of her's and so on. It suggests rather that our concept of a reason is stubbornly non-relative.

Indeed, it seems to me that we have no choice but to think this. For if reasons were indeed relative then mere reflection on that fact would itself suffice to undermine their normative significance. In order to see why, remember that on the relative conception it turns out that, for example, the desirability$_{me}$ of some consideration, p, is entirely dependent on the fact that *my* actual desires are such that, if *I* were to engage in a process of systematically justifying *my* desires, weeding out those that aren't justified and acquiring those that are, a desire that p would be one of the desires *I* would end up having. But what my actual desires are to begin with is, on this relative conception of internal reasons, an entirely *arbitrary* matter, one without any normative significance of its own. I might have had any old set of desires to begin with, even a set that delivered up the desire that not p after a process of systematic justification! The desirability$_{me}$ of the fact that p thus turns out to be an entirely arbitrary fact about p. But this is surely a *reductio*, as *arbitrariness* is precisely a feature of a consideration that tends to undermine any normative significance it might initially appear to have. Internal reasons on the relative conception are thus without normative significance (Darwall 1983, 218–39; Smith 1989; Darwall, Gibbard and Railton 1992). And if this is right then it follows that *relative* internal reasons are not *reasons* at all.

On the non-relative conception, by contrast, reflection on our concept of desirability reveals no such arbitrariness. For on that conception everyone is supposed able to reason themselves towards the same desires if they engage in a process of systematic justification of their desires, and they are supposed able to do so precisely because the task of systematic justification is *inter alia* a matter of finding desires that can be shared by their fellow rational creatures. Which desires *I* would end up with, after engaging in such a process, thus in no way depends on what *my* actual desires are to begin with, because reason itself determines the content of our fully rational desires, not the arbitrary fact that we have the actual desires that we have. On the non-relative conception, reflection on the concept of desirability thus leaves the normative significance of facts about what is desirable and undesirable perfectly intact.

This, then, is the final element in our account of what it means when the internalism requirement tells us that the desirability of an agent's φ-ing in certain circumstances C depends on whether or not she would desire that she φs in C if she were 'fully rational'. Fully rational agents *converge* in their desires about what is to be done in the various circumstances they might face. Of course, the mere fact that a convergence in the hypothetical desires of fully rational creatures is required for the truth of internal reason claims does noth-

ing to guarantee that such a convergence is forthcoming. In defending the non-relative *conception* of internal reasons we have said nothing to suggest that, *substantively*, there are any such reasons. But what we have said does suggest that, in order to discover whether there are any such reasons, and if so what they are, we have no alternative but to give the arguments and see where they lead. Substantive convergence is always assumed available, in so far as we converse and argue about the reasons that we have. But whether or not this assumption is true is always *sub judice*; something to be discovered by the outcome of those very conversations and arguments; something that will emerge when we see where our attempts to systematically justify our desires lead us.

3. The advice model and the appeal of the internalism re-quirement

So far I have argued that the internalism requirement on reasons is best understood in terms of the 'advice' model, rather than the 'example' model, and I have argued that reasons, understood in terms of the 'advice' model, are best thought of as being non-relative, rather than relative. The two points are related, of course. For I have argued that it is only if we think of reasons on the 'advice' model, and it is only if we think of reasons as being non-relative, that we can properly account for the normative significance of reason claims. However the most important question about the internalism requirement remains yet to be answered. Why exactly should we accept the internalism requirement in the first place? Why shouldn't we think, instead, that reasons have nothing to do, constitutively, with the desires of fully rational agents, as I have defined the idea of 'full rationality'? The answer is that the internalism requirement on reasons enables us to solve an otherwise disturbing puzzle about the role of deliberation in the production of action. Let me begin by explaining the puzzle.

Hume taught us that desires and means-end beliefs each play an essential role in the explanation of action (Smith 1987). Suppose, for example, that all we know about someone is that she believes that if she flicks a particular switch the light will go on and that if she refrains the light will stay off. Then, so far, we have no more reason to suppose that she will flick the switch than refrain. Whether she will flick or refrain must therefore depend on something else about her beyond her beliefs about the way the world is. And indeed it does. It depends on what she happens to desire. Does she desire the causal upshot of flicking the switch, the light's being on, or the causal upshot of refraining from doing so, the light's being off? If the former, then she will flick the switch; if the latter, then she will refrain. Desires are thus essential for the explanation of action. But so are beliefs as well. For if all we know about someone is that she desires the light to be on then, again, so far we have no more reason to suppose that she will flick the switch than that

she will refrain. For whether she will flick the switch or refrain depends on whether she believes the light's being on is the causal upshot of flicking or refraining. To sum up: beliefs alone are unable to motivate action, for beliefs can only motivate action in conjunction with a separate desire; but desires alone are also unable to motivate action, for desires can only motivate action in conjunction with a separate means-end belief.

Compelling though this Humean story of how we explain action is, it presents us with a disturbing puzzle about the role of deliberation in the production of action. For it seems undeniable that we sometimes deliberate in order to find out what we are rationally justified in doing: that is, we sometimes deliberate in order to form beliefs about what it is desirable to do. And it also seems undeniable that we sometimes act upon the outcome of those very deliberations: that is, we sometimes do what we do because we believe that doing so is desirable. But the Humean story about how we explain action seems to leave no room for these undeniable facts. For the belief that it is desirable to act in a certain way is not itself a desire, it is a belief, and so whether or not we happen to act in accordance with this belief, given the Humean story about how we explain actions, must depend entirely on whether we just so happen to have a desire to act in that way, or just so happen to have some other desire which can combine with this belief to yield a desire to act in that way.[8] On Hume's account of the matter it thus appears to be a massive fluke, an inexplicable miracle of nature, that our desires match our beliefs about what it is desirable to do to the extent that they do. For there is nothing in the nature of our evaluative beliefs to explain why this should be the case. What is needed is an extra desire, an extra desire we are not rationally required to have.

Here we see the real appeal of the internalism requirement. For it promises to explain how it can be that our beliefs about what we are rationally justified in doing play a proper causal role in the genesis of our actions, and it promises to do so while leaving Hume's story about the way in which actions are explained largely intact. In order to see why, consider again what the requirement tells us about the content of our evaluative beliefs, at least on the advice model.

When I believe that it would be desirable to ϕ in certain circumstances C, the internalism requirement tells us that my belief has the following content: that I would desire that I ϕ in C if I were fully rational. But now, if indeed I do believe this, and if I believe that I am in circumstances C, then surely the only rational thing for me to desire is to ϕ. For a psychology that includes

---

8   For example, it might be supposed that when we deliberate we *de facto* have a desire to do what we believe it is desirable to do. I will have more to say about this in footnote 10. The point here is simply that the Humean must regard it a happy accident that we all just so happen to have such a desire. For the Humean cannot agree that such a desire is itself required by reason.

both the belief that I would desire that I φ in C if I were fully rational—that is, the belief that I would have that desire if my desires formed a maximally coherent and unified set—*and* the desire that I φ in C is itself a more coherent and unified psychology than one that includes the belief that I would desire to φ in C if I were fully rational and yet *lacks* the desire to φ in C. Coherence and unity are thus on the side of a *match* between the content of our evaluative beliefs and our desires.

Here is another way of putting the same point. What would an agent's fully rational self want her less than fully rational self to desire in circumstances in which her less than fully rational self believes that she would desire to φ in C if she were fully rational? On the plausible assumption that the agent's fully rational self desires that the psychology of her less than fully rational self is as coherent as possible she will want her less than fully rational self to desire that she φs in C. It thus follows that it is desirable for an agent to desire that she φs in C in circumstances in which she believes that it is desirable that she φs in C. Agents thus quite generally have a reason to desire in accordance with their evaluative beliefs.[9]

But if this is right then it follows that in *rational* creatures at least—that is, in those who do not manifest the form of unreasonableness or irrationality just described, those who are sensitive to the facts about what they have reason to desire—we would therefore expect there to be a causal connection between believing that it is desirable to act in a certain way and desiring to act in that way. That is, given the internalist account of the content of our evaluative beliefs, we would expect a rational deliberator's evaluative beliefs to cause her to have matching desires in much the same way, and for much the same reason, as the rational thinker's beliefs that p and that p → q cause her to believe that q. For the psychological states of rational deliberators and thinkers connect with each other in just the way that they rationally should. In this way, then, the internalism requirement can thus underwrite not just the rationality of desiring in accordance with our evaluative beliefs, but also the effectiveness of our evaluative beliefs in bringing about these desires in those who are rational.[10]

---

9   It is, of course, consistent to claim both that: (i) it is desirable that an agent desires to φ in C *in circumstances in which she believes that it is desirable to φ in C*, and (ii) it is not desirable that an agent desires to φ *in circumstances C*. For whereas (i) tells us what an agent's fully rational self would want her less than fully rational self to desire in one set of circumstances, (ii) tells us what her fully rational self would want her less than fully rational self to desire in another, quite different, set of circumstances. The point is important, as it serves to explain why certain theories of reasons for action are properly thought to be *self-effacing* (Smith 1994, chapter 5 footnote 2).

10 Note that the externalist who tries to explain the effectiveness of deliberation by positing an extra desire to do what we believe desirable (see footnote 8) has an explanation that is inferior to the internalist's explanation just given in two respects. First, since the externalist claims that the extra desire to do what we believe desirable is itself rationally optional, he is committed not just to the view that it is a miracle of nature, a

Note that the explanation just given is simply unavailable if we reject the internalism requirement. For on an externalist conception of reasons, the reasons we have are not themselves defined in terms of what we would desire if our psychology exhibited maximal coherence and unity. Without inquiring further into what exactly the content of a reason claim on such a conception is we can therefore already see that there is no reason to expect that a psychology which pairs a belief that there is reason to φ in circumstances C with a desire to do something other than φ in C will exhibit less in the way of coherence and unity than a psychology that pairs that belief with the desire to φ in C. It thus appears that externalists will be unable to explain why it is rational to desire in accordance with our beliefs about the reasons that we have.

Note also that the explanation just given presupposes not just the internalism requirement, but the internalism requirement understood in terms of the advice model. For if we interpret the internalism requirement in terms of the example model, the argument just given simply fails to go through at the crucial point. Suppose, for instance, that you believe your fully rational self would desire to φ in the circumstances she faces; that this is the example she would set for you in her own world. Why should this have any effect at all on what you desire to do in the circumstances you face? If your circumstances are quite unlike her's, then you can quite rationally acknowledge her example, and be impressed by it, while still being left entirely unmoved. Coherence and unity do not argue in favour of acquiring a desire like her's because her example—marvelous though it is in the circumstances in which *she* finds *herself*—doesn't engage with the circumstances in which *you* find *yourself*. This is not the case if instead we interpret the requirement in terms of the advice model. For then what you have to believe is that your fully rational self would want your less than fully rational self to φ in the circumstances your less than fully rational self actually faces. Your fully rational self's advice engages with your predicament because it is precisely tailored to it. You may

massive fluke, that so many of us just so happen to have such a desire, but also to the view that if someone just so happened to lack such a desire, that would not itself suffice to show that that person was irrational. By contrast the internalist has a principled reason for insisting that someone who lacks a desire to φ while believing that φ-ing is desirable is *as such* irrational. Second, the externalist who posits a quite general desire to do what is desirable must think that if we end up desiring to, say, φ in C, as a result of coming to believe that it is desirable to φ in C, then the desire to φ in C must itself, of necessity, be an *instrumental* desire. The externalist must therefore hold that deliberation never produces a non-instrumental desire to do what we believe desirable, where this is read *de re* rather than *de dicto*. The only thing we desire to do non-instrumentally, when we deliberate, is what it is desirable to do, where this is read *de dicto* rather than *de re*. This seems to me to be an extremely implausible claim. Indeed, as I have argued elsewhere, it seems to constitute a *reductio* of externalism (1994: Chapter 3). The internalist, by contrast, has an explanation of how the belief that it is desirable to φ in C generates a desire to φ in C that is perfectly consistent with the claim that the resulting desire to φ in C is *non-instrumental* in character.

still say 'So what?', of course, but if you do you simply reveal that you are unable to accept good advice; you reveal the extent to which your psychology fails in terms of norms of coherence and unity that define a systematically justified psychology. You thus simply betray your own irrationality.

Here, then, we see the real appeal of the internalism requirement. It offers us an explanation of how and why our evaluative beliefs come to play a proper causal role in the production of our desires, an explanation that leaves the Humean's claim that intentional actions are themselves the product of desires and means-end beliefs perfectly intact. The crucial idea, to repeat, is that given the content of an agent's evaluative beliefs—that is, given the internalism requirement—the desires that the Humean rightly supposes play a causal role in the genesis of intentional actions will themselves be caused by the agent's evaluative beliefs to the extent that she is a rational deliberator. The Humean's account has thus been supplemented, not replaced.

Conclusion

My aim in this paper has been to answer three questions. How exactly is the internalism requirement on reasons to be understood? What does it tell us about the nature of reasons? And where-in lies its appeal?

As regards the first question, I have argued that the content of the internalism requirement is best captured by what I have called the 'advice' model rather than the 'example' model. According to the advice model, the desirability of an agent's ϕ-ing in certain circumstances C is fixed by whether or not her fully rational self would advise her less than fully rational self to ϕ in the circumstances that she, the less than fully rational self, faces: that is, in circumstances C. The idea is not that the desirability of an agent's ϕ-ing in C is fixed by the example her fully rational self would set for her less than fully rational self by her own behaviour in her own world. Thus, even though the requirement is concerned with the *desires* of a fully rational agent, it is crucially not concerned with the *motivations* of a fully rational agent.

As regards the second question, I have argued that the substantive content of the internalism requirement depends on the way in which we understand the key idea of having certain desires under conditions of 'full rationality'. My claim has been that it is part of our concept of 'full rationality' that fully rational agents are those who have a systematically justifiable set of desires, where this idea is to be cashed out in terms of having a psychology that is maximally coherent and unified, and where it is presupposed that the maximally coherent and unified set of desires any one particular fully rational agent would come up with is exactly the same as the maximally coherent and unified set of desires any other rational agent would come up with. The internalism requirement is thus best understood as offering us a non-relativistic, rather than a relativistic, conception of reasons.

Finally, as regards the third question, I have argued that, given our answers to the earlier two questions, the appeal of the internalism requirement
is easy to understand. For it allows us to see that though the Humean is right
that all *actions* are caused by desires, in rational deliberators at least, the *desires* that cause an agent's actions may themselves be caused by her evaluative beliefs. The internalism requirement thus enables us to assign a proper
causal role to an agent's beliefs about the rational justifiability of her actions
when she deliberates.

For all I have said it of course remains an open possibility that there are
no internal reasons—and hence that there are no reasons for action at all. After all, the mere fact that our concept of a reason presupposes that fully rational creatures would converge in their desires does nothing to show that such a
convergence is forthcoming. But that is no objection to what has been said
here. For my aim has not been to argue that there are any reasons, it has
rather been to articulate the conceptual framework in which debates about
what our reasons are, if there are any, can sensibly take place.[11]

REFERENCES

Brandt, Richard 1979: *A Theory of the Good and the Right*. Oxford University Press.

Daniels, Norman 1979: 'Wide Reflective Equilibrium and Theory Acceptance
in Ethics' *Journal of Philosophy*. 256–82.

Darwall, Stephen 1983: *Impartial Reason*. Cornell University Press.

_____ Allan Gibbard and Peter Railton 1992: 'Toward *Fin de siecle* Ethics:
Some Trends', *Philosophical Review*. 115–89.

Korsgaard, Christine 1986: 'Skepticism about Practical Reason', *Journal of
Philosophy*. 5–25.

Lewis, David 1989: 'Dispositional Theories of Value', *Proceedings of the
Aristotelian Society* Supplementary Volume. 113–37.

Johnston, Mark 1989: 'Dispositional Theories of Value', *Proceedings of the
Aristotelian Society* Supplementary Volume. 139–74.

Parfit, Derek 1984: *Reasons and Persons*. Oxford University Press.

Pettit, Philip 1993: *The Common Mind*. Oxford University Press.

_____ and Michael Smith 1990: 'Backgrounding Desire', *The Philosophical
Review*. 565–92.

[11]   An earlier version of this paper was presented at 'Internal and External Reasons', a
symposium held at the Pacific Division APA meetings in Los Angeles, April 1994. I
would like to thank Stephen Darwall for the many useful suggestions and observations
he made as commentator on that occasion, suggestions and observations that have
helped me greatly improve the paper. I also received useful advice from John Broome,
David Copp, Frank Jackson, Douglas Maclean, Kevin Mulligan, Philip Pettit, Denis
Robinson, Holly Smith, Galen Strawson, Anita Superson, Sigrun Svavarsdottir, David
Velleman and Susan Wolf. The second section of the paper draws on material that appears in Chapter Five of *The Moral Problem* (Basil Blackwell, 1994).

_____ and Michael Smith 1993: 'Brandt on Self-Control' in Brad Hooker, ed., *Rationality, Rules and Utility*. Westview Press.

_____ and Michael Smith forthcoming: 'Parfit's P' in Jonathan Dancy, ed., *Parfit and his Critics 2: Reasons*. Blackwell.

Railton, Peter 1986: 'Moral Realism', *The Philosophical Review*. 163–207.

Rawls, John 1951: 'Outline of a Decision Procedure for Ethics', *Philosophical Review*. 177–97.

_____ 1971: *A Theory of Justice*. Harvard University Press.

Shope, Robert K. 1978: 'Rawls, Brandt, and the Definition of Rational Desires', *Canadian Journal of Philosophy*. 329–40.

Smith, Michael 1987: 'The Humean Theory of Motivation', *Mind*. 36–61.

_____ 1989: 'Dispositional Theories of Value', *Proceedings of the Aristotelian Society* Supplementary Volume. 89–111.

_____ 1991: 'Realism' in Peter Singer, ed., *A Companion to Ethics*. Basil Blackwell. 399–410.

_____ 1992: 'Valuing: Desiring or Believing?' in David Charles and Kathleen Lennon, eds., *Reduction, Explanation, Realism*. Oxford University Press. 323–60.

_____ 1993: 'Objectivity and Moral Realism: On the Phenomenology of Moral Experience' in John Haldane and Crispin Wright, eds, *Reality, Representation and Projection*. Oxford University Press. 235–36.

_____ 1994: *The Moral Problem*. Basil Blackwell.

Watson, Gary 1975: 'Free Agency' reprinted in Gary Watson, ed., *Free Will*. Oxford University Press. 1982. 96–110.

Bernard Williams 1980: 'Internal and External Reasons' reprinted in his *Moral Luck*. Cambridge University Press. 1981.

[9]

The Possibility of Practical Reason*

J. David Velleman

Suppose that reasons for someone to do something must be considerations that would sway him toward doing it if he entertained them rationally.[1] And suppose that the only considerations capable of swaying someone toward an action are those which represent it as a way of attaining something he wants, or would want once apprised of its attainability.[2] These assumptions, taken together, seem to imply that

* I am grateful to Sonja Al-Sofi, Stephen Darwall, Jennifer Church, Paul Boghossian, Alfred Mele, Elijah Millgram, Derek Parfit, Peter Railton, Sigrun Svavarsdottir, Nicholas White, Bernard Williams, Stephen Yablo, and several anonymous referees for helpful discussions of the issues raised in this article. Earlier versions of the paper were presented to the philosophy departments at New York University, Stanford University, the University of Illinois at Urbana-Champaign, and the University of Houston; and to the philosophy faculty colloquium at the University of Michigan. Some of the material was also presented to Michael Bratman's 1993 National Endowment for the Humanities seminar on intention. I have benefited from comments received on all of these occasions, especially the comments of Frances Kamm, Fred Dretske, Rachel Cohon, Allan Gibbard, Sally Haslanger, David Hills, Tomis Kapitan, Jeff McMahan, Patrick Hays, and David Phillips. Finally, I received many helpful comments from participants in a graduate seminar taught at the University of Michigan in the winter of 1993. Work on this article was supported by the Edna Balz Lacy Faculty Fellowship at the Institute for the Humanities, University of Michigan.

1. This principle is meant to apply only to complete sets of reasons, not to reasons taken individually. That is, if a particular consideration counts as a reason only in the context of a larger set or series of considerations, then it need not be capable of swaying the agent unless it is considered in that context. The assumption that 'reasons' denotes complete sets of reasons will be in force throughout the following discussion. I shall also rely on the success-grammar of the word 'considerations': considerations are, by implication, true considerations—or, as I shall sometimes call them, facts.

2. The last clause is meant to account for cases like this: "It may be true of me that were the aroma of fresh apple pie to waft past my nose I would be moved to discover its source and perhaps to try to wangle a piece. It does not follow from this, however, that before I smell the pie I desire to eat it or to eat anything at all" (Stephen L. Darwall, *Impartial Reason* [Ithaca, N.Y.: Cornell University Press, 1983], p. 40). Here apple pie is something that the agent doesn't yet want but will want once he considers its attainability, and so considerations about how to obtain it are capable of influencing

Ethics 106 (July 1996): 694–726

the only considerations that can qualify as reasons for someone to act are considerations appealing to his antecedent inclinations[3]—that is, his desires or dispositions to desire.[4]

This conclusion amounts to an admission that reason really is, as Hume put it, the slave of the passions,[5] and Hume's conclusion is one that many philosophers hope to avoid. Some try to avoid the conclusion by rejecting one of the premises from which it appears to follow.[6] Others prefer to keep the premises while arguing that the conclusion doesn't actually follow from them.[7]

In my view, the question whether reasons do or do not depend on an agent's inclinations should simply be rejected, because it embodies a false dichotomy. This dichotomy has recently come to be formulated in terms introduced by Bernard Williams.[8] In Williams's terminology,

---

him in the requisite way. I take it that this mechanism is what David Hume regarded as the first of the two ways in which reason can influence action: "Reason . . . can have an influence on our conduct only after two ways: Either when it excites a passion by informing us of the existence of something which is a proper object of it; or when it discovers the connexion of causes and effects, so as to afford us means of exerting any passion" (*A Treatise of Human Nature*, ed. by L. A. Selby-Bigge [Oxford: Clarendon, 1978], p. 459).

3. Note that I am not using the word 'inclination' in its Kantian sense. I am using it as the generic term for conative or motivational states of all kinds.

4. The argument presented here is discussed at length in Darwall, *Impartial Reason*, esp. chaps. 2 and 5.

5. Hume, p. 415. I do not claim that the argument offered above for Hume's conclusion should necessarily be attributed to Hume.

6. The most frequent target has been the second assumption, which is sometimes called the Humean theory of motivation. See, e.g., Thomas Nagel, *The Possibility of Altruism* (Princeton, N.J.: Princeton University Press, 1970); John McDowell, "Are Moral Requirements Hypothetical Imperatives?" in *Proceedings of the Aristotelian Society*, suppl. ser., 52 (1978): 13–29; Darwall, *Impartial Reason*, chap. 5; Rachel Cohon, "Are External Reasons Impossible?" *Ethics* 96 (1986): 545–56. For arguments defending this assumption, see Michael Smith, "The Humean Theory of Motivation," *Mind* 96 (1987): 36–61; and Alfred Mele, "Motivational Internalism: The Powers and Limits of Practical Reasoning," *Philosophia* 19 (1989): 417–36. Arguments against the first assumption are rare, although some philosophers have argued against a related assumption applied to moral requirements rather than reasons for acting. See, e.g., William Frankena, "Obligation and Motivation in Recent Moral Philosophy," in *Essays on Moral Philosophy*, ed. A. I. Melden (Seattle: University of Washington Press, 1958), pp. 40–81; and David Brink, *Moral Realism and the Foundations of Ethics* (Cambridge: Cambridge University Press, 1989), chap. 3.

7. See Christine Korsgaard, "Skepticism about Practical Reason," *Journal of Philosophy* 83 (1986): 5–25.

8. Bernard Williams, "Internal and External Reasons," in *Moral Luck* (Cambridge: Cambridge University Press, 1981), pp. 101–13; "Internal Reasons and the Obscurity of Blame," in *Making Sense of Humanity and Other Philosophical Papers* (Cambridge: Cambridge University Press, 1995), pp. 35–45; "Replies," in *World, Mind, and Ethics; Essays on the Ethical Philosophy of Bernard Williams*, ed. J. E. J. Altham and Ross Harrison (Cambridge: Cambridge University Press, 1995), pp. 185–224.

696   *Ethics   July 1996*

"internal" reasons are those which count as reasons for someone only by virtue of his antecedent inclinations; "external" reasons are those which count as reasons for someone independently of his inclinations.[9] The Humean conclusion implies that all reasons are internal, in this sense, and it is therefore called internalism; its denial is called externalism.[10] My thesis is that we do not in fact have to choose between the two.

*   *   *

Christine Korsgaard has pointed out that the foregoing argument doesn't necessarily yield any constraint on what counts as a reason for acting.[11] It may instead yield a constraint on who counts as a rational agent.

9. Here I am choosing one of two possible readings that have occasioned considerable confusion in the literature. The confusion can be traced to the casual manner in which Williams introduces the term 'internal reason'. Williams carefully defines what he calls the "internal interpretation" of the statement "A has reason to ϕ." Interpreted internally, the statement implies that A has some motive that can be served by his ϕ-ing. Williams then says "I shall also for convenience refer sometimes to 'internal reasons' and 'external reasons'" ("Internal and External Reasons," p. 101). But Williams never explains how a scheme for interpreting reason-attributions can be transformed into a scheme for classifying reasons themselves.

Two different schemes of classification have suggested themselves to philosophers writing in this area. One scheme classifies as internal any reason that can engage one of the agent's motives so as to sway him toward doing that for which it is a reason. The other scheme classifies as internal only those reasons whose status as reasons depends on their capacity to engage the agent's motives in this way. An internal reason, on this latter scheme, is one that wouldn't be a reason if the agent didn't have a motive that it could engage. The difference between these schemes of classification can be illustrated by the case of an agent who has both a reason and a corresponding motive. According to the first scheme, this reason is definitely internal, since the agent has a motive corresponding to it. According to the second scheme, however, this reason could still be external, if it would remain a reason for the agent whether or not he had the motive.

Only the latter scheme captures the entailment that distinguishes Williams's "internal interpretation" of reason-attributions. For on the former scheme, the agent's having a reason doesn't require him to have a motive. If he lacks a corresponding motive, then his reason doesn't necessarily cease to be a reason, on this scheme; it simply ceases to be internal. Yet under the internal interpretation of reason-attributions, the agent must have the motive in order for it to be true that he has a reason at all. I therefore prefer the latter scheme of classification.

10. Note that this usage differs somewhat from that of other philosophers, for whom the term 'internalism' refers to our first premise, requiring reasons to have the capacity of exerting an influence.

11. Korsgaard, "Skepticism about Practical Reason." For other discussions of Williams, see Cohon, "Are External Reasons Impossible?" and Rachel Cohon, "Internalism about Reasons for Action," *Pacific Philosophical Quarterly* 74 (1993): 265–88; Martin Hollis, *The Cunning of Reason* (Cambridge: Cambridge University Press, 1987), chap. 6; Brad Hooker, "Williams' Argument against External Reasons," *Analysis* 47 (1987): 42–44; John McDowell, "Might There Be External Reasons?" in Altham and Harrison, eds., pp. 68–85; Elijah Millgram, "Williams' Argument against External Reasons," *Nous* 30 (1996): 197–220.

The first premise of our argument doesn't entail that if a consideration fails to influence someone, then it isn't a reason for him to act; it entails that if a consideration fails to influence someone, then either it isn't a reason for him to act or he hasn't entertained it rationally. The inclinations that would make an agent susceptible to the influence of some consideration may therefore be necessary—not to the consideration's being a reason for him—but rather to his being rational in entertaining that reason. And our premises may consequently imply that an agent's inclinations determine, not what he has reason for doing, but whether he is rational in his response to the reasons he has.

Korsgaard favors the latter conclusion over the former.[12] In denying the dependence of reasons on inclinations, she qualifies as an externalist, in Williams's terminology.[13]

Korsgaard's critique of Williams suggests a version of externalism that goes something like this.[14] Being a rational agent entails having

---

12. See also Michael Smith, "Reason and Desire," *Proceedings of the Aristotelian Society* 88 (1988): 243–58. Smith seems to think (pp. 248–52) that he and Korsgaard disagree, but I think that they don't. In particular, Smith believes that Korsgaard rejects the second premise, that considerations can influence an agent only in conjunction with his conative attitudes. But I don't interpret Korsgaard as rejecting this premise. Korsgaard never claims that a consideration, or belief, can move an agent without the help of a conation or motive; what she claims, I think, is that the desires and values mediating the influence of a consideration need not be ordinary motives, of the sort that are directed at the agent's ends, since they can instead constitute his virtue of rationality.

Williams responds to this argument but seems to misunderstand it. He seems to think that if all rational agents have, say, a motive for doing what's right, then the fact that an action is right will turn out to be an internal reason for them, after all: "If this is so, then the constraints of morality are part of everybody's [motivational set], and every correct moral reason *will be* an internal reason" ("Internal Reasons and the Obscurity of Blame," p. 37). But here Williams adopts a sense of the phrase 'internal reason' that fails to capture his own "internal interpretation" of reason-attributions, as I have explained in n. 9, above. In this sense, an internal reason is one with the capacity to engage an agent's motives, but not necessarily one whose very status as a reason depends upon that capacity.

I believe that Korsgaard is working with the alternative (and, to my mind, preferable) sense of 'internal reason', according to which an internal reason is one whose status as a reason depends on its capacity to engage the agent's motives. And what Korsgaard envisions is that reasons for behaving morally will qualify as reasons whether or not people have motives that such reasons can engage. Even if people happen to have the relevant motives, reasons for behaving morally will still be independent of them, in Korsgaard's view, and such reasons should be classified as external.

For a misinterpretation similar to Williams's, see John Rawls, *Political Liberalism* (New York: Columbia University Press, 1993), p. 85, n. 33.

13. I do not mean that Korsgaard would call herself an externalist, since she uses the term in a somewhat different sense. See n. 10 above.

14. I don't mean to claim that Korsgaard holds this version of externalism. Korsgaard's "Skepticism about Practical Reason" seems designed to be independent, in many respects, of her larger metaethical project. It therefore leaves open various versions of externalism that Korsgaard herself would not necessarily endorse. Indeed, I suspect that the version of externalism discussed here in the text corresponds to what Korsgaard

various motives, including a preference for one's own greater good[15] and an acceptance of moral principles.[16] A rational agent is influenced by a reason for doing something when, for example, he considers some respect in which doing it is morally required; and this consideration can influence him because an inclination to abide by moral requirements is partly constitutive of his rationality. If an agent lacks this inclination, its absence won't prevent him from having moral reasons for acting: moral requirements will still count as reasons for him to act. Rather, lacking an inclination to abide by moral requirements will render the agent irrational, by making him insensitive to this particular kind of reason.

THE EXTERNALIST'S BURDEN OF JUSTIFICATION

One liability of this model is that it must identify particular features of an action as constitutive of reasons for taking it, whether an agent cares about them or not, and it must then criticize an agent as irrational if he should fail to care about those features. The model thus incorporates specific normative judgments, to the effect that one ought to be inclined toward courses of action with the features in question.

What entitles the externalist to build these normative judgments into his model of practical reason? As Williams puts it, "Someone who claims the constraints of morality are themselves built into the notion of what it is to be a rational deliberator cannot get that conclusion for nothing."[17]

Korsgaard does not try to get this conclusion for nothing, however. On the contrary, she insists that the normative judgments built into her conception of practical reason will require an "ultimate justification," which the externalist hopes to provide.[18] Indeed, the possibility of such a justification is the centerpiece of her paper.

Korsgaard's quarrel with Williams, after all, is that he prematurely discounts the possibility of justifying externalism. In assuming that an agent's imperviousness to a consideration impugns its status as a reason, rather than the agent's rationality, Williams assumes that its status as a reason cannot be established independently. For if a consideration could be certified as a reason for someone irrespective of whether he's susceptible to it, then his lack of susceptibility would thereby come to impugn his rationality instead. Yet certifying something as a reason

rejects under the label "dogmatic rationalism" in "The Normativity of Instrumental Reason," in *Value and Practical Reason*, ed. Garrett Cullity and Berys Gaut (Oxford: Oxford University Press, in press).

15. Korsgaard, "Skepticism about Practical Reason," p. 18.
16. Ibid., p. 22.
17. Williams, "Internal Reasons and the Obscurity of Blame," p. 37.
18. Korsgaard, "Skepticism about Practical Reason," p. 22.

for someone irrespective of his susceptibilities would amount to
showing that it is an external reason, and hence that externalism is
true. When Williams presupposes the impossibility of such a showing, he is presupposing the impossibility of justifying externalism.
His case for internalism thus rests on antecedent skepticism about
the alternative.

So Korsgaard argues—cogently, I believe. Yet even if she is right
that the case for internalism rests on skepticism about externalism,
the question remains whether we aren't entitled to be skeptical. What
are the prospects for showing that something is a reason for someone
whether or not he has the inclinations to which it would appeal? How
will the externalist demonstrate that there are considerations by which
any agent ought to be moved?

                    *   *   *

One might think that an externalist could avoid this burden of justification by avoiding the identification of any particular considerations
as reasons, or of any particular inclinations as rational. But I doubt
whether this strategy can work.

The version of externalism outlined above incurs a burden of
justification because it judges an agent to be irrational unless he is
inclined to be swayed by particular, substantive features of actions,
whose value or importance may be open to question. All that externalism needs to say, however, is that the inclination responsible for
the influence of reasons is one that's essential for the agent's rationality.
Does this inclination have to be an inclination to be swayed by particular considerations, specified by their substance? Maybe it can be an
inclination to do whatever is supported by reasons as such, or whatever
is rational as such.

The inclination that's now being proposed isn't an inclination to
do things with any particular features, other than the feature of being
favored by reasons (whatever they may consist in) or the feature of
being rational (whatever that is). Hence the claim that this inclination
is essential to an agent's rationality doesn't call for any justification.
For how could rationality fail to require an inclination to do what's
rational, or what's favored by reasons?

                    *   *   *

Unfortunately, this version of externalism doesn't ultimately succeed
in shedding the burden of justification, since it doesn't avoid the need
to specify what counts as a reason or a rational action. To be sure, all
it requires of a rational agent is that he be inclined to act in accordance
with reasons or rationality as such. But in order for reasons to influence
an agent by way of this inclination, he must recognize them as reasons,

or as evidence of rationality, and so he needs some criterion of what counts as a reason or as a rational action. And until such a criterion is supplied, the proposed version of externalism will be nothing but the trivial assertion that rationality is a disposition to be influenced by reasons.

What's needed to save this version of externalism from triviality is a criterion specifying what it is about an action that makes it rational or constitutes a reason for taking it. And this criterion will once again require justification.

At this point, the externalist may attempt to repeat his earlier evasive maneuver. He is committed to the existence of a criterion by which an agent can recognize reasons or rational actions; but is he committed to its being a substantive criterion, which would have to be justified? Maybe an agent can recognize reasons or rational actions by their satisfying the generic concepts of what it is to be a reason or a rational action as such.[19]

Yet this strategy of continually postponing controversy is unlikely to help. Asking the agent to identify a rational action under the guise of rationality as such, or to identify a reason for acting under the guise of a reason as such, would be somewhat like asking him to hunt for something described only as "the quarry," or to play a game with an eye to something described only as "winning." It would be to assign him a task with a formal object but no substantive object—and hence with no object at all.

THE OBJECT OF PRACTICAL REASONING

The formal object of an enterprise is a goal stated solely in terms of, or in terms that depend on, the very concept of being the object of that enterprise.[20] Thus, for example, winning is the formal object of a competitive game, since "winning" just is the concept of succeeding in competition. Similarly, the formal object of a search or hunt is the quarry, and the formal object of a question is the answer.

Any enterprise that has a formal object must have a substantive object as well—that is, a goal that is not stated solely in terms that

19. I believe that Korsgaard proposes this very strategy ("Skepticism about Practical Reason," pp. 30–31). And I believe that there may be a way—a distinctively Kantian way—of making the strategy work. I discuss this Kantian version of the strategy briefly in n. 25, below. Note, then, that the present argument does not purport to prove that the strategy in question is unworkable. It's meant to justify doubts about the strategy, by showing just how difficult it will be to carry out.

20. I suspect that the argument offered in this section is related to the argument offered by Williams on pp. 109–10 of "Internal and External Reasons." Because I don't fully understand the relevant passage, however, I hesitate to attribute the argument to Williams.

depend on the concept of being the object of that enterprise.[21] In the case of a competitive game, there must be a substantive object of the game, something that constitutes winning but cannot simply consist in winning, so described. A game whose object was specifiable only as "winning" wouldn't have an object—that is, wouldn't have any object in particular. And if a game had no particular object, then there would be no such thing as winning it, and so it wouldn't be a fully constituted competitive game. Similarly, a hunt whose object was specifiable only as "the quarry" wouldn't be a fully constituted search, and the question "What is the answer?" isn't by itself a fully constituted question.

*   *   *

Since practical reasoning is an enterprise at which one can succeed or fail, it must have an object against which success or failure can be measured. What, then, is the object of practical reasoning?

One might suggest that practical reasoning has the object of figuring out what to do, or answering the question "What shall I do?" But this suggestion either misstates the object of practical reasoning or states it in merely formal terms.

The statement that practical reasoning has the object of figuring out what to do may simply mean that it has the object of arriving at something to do or of issuing in an action. So interpreted, however, the statement is mistaken, since issuing in an action—some action or other—is not the object of practical reasoning. Issuing in an action may be what makes reasoning practical, but the object of such reasoning is, not to issue in just any action, but to issue in some actions rather than others.

The object of practical reasoning must therefore be to arrive at a privileged action or an action in some privileged class. And when "figuring out what to do" is interpreted as expressing this object, it turns out to be a merely formal specification, since "what to do," so interpreted, simply means the correct or privileged thing to do, the thing whose discovery is being attempted. Hence there must be a further, substantive specification of the action or kind of action that practical reasoning aims to identify. A mode of reasoning whose goal was specified solely as "figuring out what to do" would be like a search

---

21. The distinction between the formal and substantive aims of practical reason is discussed by Derek Parfit in *Reasons and Persons* (Oxford: Clarendon, 1984), pp. 3, 9, 37. As David Gauthier has pointed out ("Rationality and the Rational Aim," in *Reading Parfit*, ed. Jonathan Dancy [in press]), Parfit is less than clear on the relation between these aims; in particular, Parfit doesn't appear to believe that the substantive aim of practical reason, as identified by a particular theory, is a specification of the formal aim. Like Gauthier, I prefer to use the phrase 'substantive aim' for that which specifies what it is to achieve the formal aim.

whose object was specified solely as "figuring out where to look," or a question whose object was specified solely as "figuring out how to reply."

Similar remarks apply to the notion that practical reasoning aims at figuring out the best thing to do.[22] This notion is correct if 'the best thing to do' means "the privileged action"—that is, the action that uniquely satisfies the standard of success for this very reasoning. But in that case, it merely expresses the formal object of the enterprise. There can be an enterprise of figuring out the best thing to do, in this sense, only if that enterprise also has a substantive standard of success, just as there can be an enterprise of figuring out the best way to reply only if there is a substantive question, and there can be an enterprise of figuring out the best place to look only if there is a substantive quarry.

Of course, 'the best thing to do' might be interpreted, alternatively, as already expressing a substantive value: it might mean, for example, "the action that's optimific," in the sense that it contributes most to the agent's welfare or to the welfare of everyone. But in that case, the notion that practical reasoning aims to figure out the best thing to do will once again express a value judgment that calls for justification.

*   *   *

What, then, about rational action or reasons for acting? Can the object of practical reasoning be to identify a rational thing to do, or a thing that one has reason for doing?

The concepts of rational action and reasons for acting are potentially confusing in that they can have both generic and specific uses. If we specify a substantive kind of action as the object of practical reasoning, then we can grant it the honorific "rational," so that the phrase 'rational action' names actions of the specified kind. Similarly, if we specify substantive features that practical reasoning looks for in an action, we can grant the honorific "reasons for acting" to those features. Practical reasoning will then turn out to aim at the rational thing to do, or at what there is reason for doing, but only because 'rational' and 'reasons' are names for substantive objects.

What cannot be the aim of practical reasoning is rational action merely as such—that is, action conceived as rational in the generic sense, rather than in a sense defined by a specific standard. The generic concept of rational action is just the concept of action that would issue from competent practical reasoning. Until there is something that

---

22. This notion is, for example, the basis of Donald Davidson's conception of practical reasoning. See his *Essays on Actions and Events* (Oxford: Clarendon, 1980). The problems mentioned here are discussed further in the text accompanying n. 45 below.

counts as competence in practical reasoning, nothing counts as a rational action in the generic sense. And competence in practical reasoning
can be defined only in relation to the object of the enterprise, since
competence is a disposition toward success. To be indicative of competent practical reasoning is to be indicative of practical reasoning that's
well suited to achieving its object. Defining the object of practical
reasoning as action that's rational in this sense would thus be to string
definitions in a circle, leaving the object of practical reasoning still
undefined. It would be like trying to teach someone a game by telling
him that the object was to make a competent showing; whereas what
counts as a competent showing always depends on the substantive
object of the game.[23]

Similarly, the sole aim of practical reasoning cannot be action
supported by reasons merely as such—that is, reasons conceived under
the generic concept expressing what it is to be a reason. The generic
concept of a reason for acting is the concept of something that warrants
or justifies action. And to justify something is to show or indicate it to
be just—that is, in accordance with a *jus*, or rule of correctness. Until
there is something that constitutes a correct conclusion or a correct
inference, there can be nothing that constitutes justifying a conclusion
or an inference, and so there can be nothing that constitutes a reason
for a conclusion or an inference, in the generic sense. So, too, until
there is something that constitutes correctness in actions, or in outcomes of practical reasoning, there can be nothing that satisfies the
generic concept of a justification for action, or a justification in practical reasoning; and so there can be nothing that satisfies the generic
concept of a reason for acting.

JUSTIFYING A SUBSTANTIVE CONCEPTION OF REASONS

This argument suggests that the externalist cannot indefinitely postpone giving substantive characterizations of rationality or reasons.
The externalist must at some point provide practical reasoning with
a substantive standard of success, which will either consist in or give
rise to a substantive account of the features that constitute reasons
for an action. The externalist will then have to justify his normative
judgment that an agent ought to be swayed by consideration of the
specified features.[24]

---

23. Of course, we could introduce a substantive conception of competent practical
reasoning—a substantively specified procedure, adherence to which constitutes good
reasoning. In that case, however, the definition of rational action as that which would
issue from competent practical reasoning will become a substantive concept, which once
again requires justification.

24. The notion that practical reasoning is framed by a criterion of success for
actions is discussed by David Gauthier in "Assure and Threaten," *Ethics* 104 (1994):

What's more, the requisite justification is unlikely to emerge from an analysis of concepts such as "reason" or "rational action." As we have seen, these are formal concepts that have no application except in relation to a substantive object or standard of success. Because these concepts implicitly require such a standard to be supplied, we can hardly expect to deduce it from them, any more than we should expect to deduce the object of a game from the mere concept of winning, or the object of a hunt from the mere concept of a quarry.[25]

I cannot prove that the task of justifying an externalist conception of reasons is impossible, but I think it's going to be awfully hard. I'm just a fainthearted externalist, I guess. Being fainthearted, however, I want to consider whether the benefits of externalism can be obtained without the burdens. I shall therefore turn to an alternative conception of practical reason, which straddles the line between internalism and externalism.

OUTLINE OF AN ALTERNATIVE VIEW

Suppose that we want to frame a conception of reasons that isn't relativized to the inclinations of particular agents. That is, we want to identify particular things that count as reasons for acting simpliciter and not merely as reasons for some agents rather than others, depending on their inclinations.

One way to frame such a conception is to name some features that an action can have and to say that they count as reasons for someone whether or not he is inclined to care about them. The problem with the resulting conception, as we have seen, is that it entails the normative judgment that one ought to be inclined to care about the specified features, on pain of irrationality, and this normative judgment requires justification.

The advantage of internalism is that it avoids these normative commitments.[26] It says that things count as reasons for someone only

---

690–721. I discuss Gauthier's treatment of this notion in my "Deciding How to Decide," in Cullity and Gaut, eds.

25. Kant's conception of practical reason, as I understand it, is an attempt to circumvent this problem, by using the concept of a reason, not to identify which features are reasons, but rather to identify which features aren't, and by replacing the rule of acting for reasons with a rule of not acting for nonreasons. On Kant's conception, as I understand it, the object of practical reasoning is to act on any consideration but one whose being a reason would entail a contradiction. It's like a hunt whose object is to locate anything but that which could not possibly be a quarry. Perhaps the generic concepts of a quarry or a reason can indeed serve this modest role.

26. I don't mean to imply that internalism avoids all normative commitments. In "Skepticism about Practical Reason," Korsgaard suggests that the instrumental principle of adopting the means to one's ends is a substantive norm; she defends this point at length in "The Normativity of Instrumental Reason." But even if internalism has to justify requiring us to care about the means to what we already care about, it avoids

if he is inclined to care about them, and so it leaves the normative question of whether to care about them entirely open. Yet if we try to leave this question open, by defining things as reasons only for those inclined to care about them, we'll end up with a definition that's relativized to the inclinations of particular agents—won't we?

Not necessarily. For suppose that all reasons for acting are features of a single kind, whose influence depends on a single inclination. And suppose that the inclination on which the influence of reasons depends is, not an inclination that distinguishes some agents from others, but rather an inclination that distinguishes agents from nonagents. In that case, to say that these features count as reasons only for those who are inclined to care about them will be to say that they count as reasons only for agents—which will be to say no less than that they are reasons for acting, period, since applying only to agents is already part of the concept of reasons for acting. The restriction on the application of reasons will drop away from our definition, since it restricts their application, not to some proper subset of agents, but rather to the set of all agents, which is simply the universe of application for reasons to act.

*   *   *

The foregoing paragraph is an outline for a conception of reasons for acting—a bare outline that needs filling in. The remainder of this article will be devoted to filling it in, at least to some extent, though not, I admit, to the extent that's needed. I shall begin by making a digression into the subject of theoretical reasoning. My hope is that we can understand reasons for acting by analogy with reasons for belief.[27]

The nature of reasons for belief, and the inclination that mediates their influence, are fairly clear. The object of theoretical reasoning is to arrive at true belief;[28] and since true belief needn't be defined in

---

the further and heavier burden of justifying any requirements to care about particular things.

27. The analogy between theoretical and practical reason is being pursued independently by my colleague Peter Railton, with somewhat different results. See his "What the Noncognitivist Helps Us to See the Naturalist Must Help Us to Explain," in *Reality, Representation, and Projection*, ed. John Haldane and Crispin Wright (New York: Oxford University Press, 1993), pp. 279–300, pp. 292 ff.; "A Kind of Nonsubjective Reason?" in *Essays in Honor of Kurt Baier*, ed. J. Schneewind (New York: Open Court, in press); and "On the Hypothetical and Non-hypothetical in Reasoning about Action," in Cullity and Gaut, eds. David Gauthier also discusses the analogy, but he ultimately rejects it ("Assure and Threaten," pp. 699–702).

28. Some may be inclined to think that the object of theoretical reasoning is not true belief but empirically adequate and explanatorily fruitful belief, or belief of some other kind. My argument doesn't depend on the outcome of this disagreement. What matters for my purposes is that theoretical reasoning aims at some outcome specified substantively (i.e., not in terms of its being the object of theoretical reasoning or belief).

terms of success in theoretical reasoning, it constitutes a substantive rather than formal standard of success.[29] Reasons for a particular belief are recognized by their perceived relevance to this substantive standard of success, as considerations that appear to guarantee or probabilify the truth of the belief.[30] And these considerations influence a person's beliefs by virtue of an inclination to believe what seems true. Here, then, are considerations of a single kind and a single inclination to mediate their influence.

Perhaps we should ask whether the absence of this inclination would undermine the existence of reasons for belief or would alternatively undermine the believer's claim to rationality.[31] The answer to this question would determine whether reasons for belief were internal or external reasons. If someone weren't inclined to believe what seemed true, would signs of truth in a proposition no longer count as reasons for him to believe it? Or would he no longer qualify as a rational believer?

                    *   *   *

Both, I think—which goes to show that the question incorporates a false dichotomy. I shall argue that the dichotomy should be replaced with a subtler account of theoretical reasoning, along the following lines.

If someone isn't inclined to believe what seems true on a topic, he is no longer subject to reasons for believing things about it; but he is no longer subject to reasons for belief about it, I shall argue, because he is no longer a believer about it at all, and a fortiori no longer a rational believer.[32] He isn't in the business of forming beliefs on the

29. The claim that truth isn't defined in terms of success in theoretical reasoning is potentially controversial. It must be rejected by those who hold a pragmatist conception of truth as the eventual deliverance of rational inquiry. In my view, however, the pragmatist conception renders theoretical reasoning vacuous, like a game whose only object is winning.

30. In the case of inductive reasoning, of course, we may have trouble saying what relevance reasons have to the truth of a belief. Nevertheless, such reasons count as reasons for a belief because they make it seem true, even if we cannot say how or why. (An alternative way of handling this case would be to point out that inductive reasons satisfy a substantive procedural criterion of correctness in inductive inference. See n. 23 above.)

31. Williams raises this question and seems to suggest that the absence of an inclination toward the truth would undermine the existence of reasons for belief ("Internal Reasons and the Obscurity of Blame," p. 37). This is, of course, the internalist answer to the question.

32. I believe that Korsgaard makes a similar point ("The Normativity of Instrumental Reason," p. 42). In passages such as this, where Korsgaard seems to be pursuing a strategy like the one I am developing here, I begin to doubt whether she really is an externalist, in Williams's sense of the term. My reasons for this doubt will be explained in the text, below, when I explain why I do not regard the present strategy as a version of externalism.

topic, to begin with, unless he is inclined to believe what seems true about it.

Thus, reasons for believing something apply only to those who are inclined to believe what seems true on the topic, and so they are like internal reasons; but to say that they are reasons only for those who are so inclined is just to say that they are reasons only for potential believers on the topic—which is to say no less than that they are reasons for believing, period. Reasons for belief can therefore be identified independently of the inclinations of individuals, and so they are like external reasons, too.

The foregoing paragraph is a bare outline for an account of theoretical reasoning, and this outline also needs filling in. In order to fill it in, I shall have to explore the sense in which being inclined toward the truth is essential to being a subject of belief. I therefore turn to a different thesis associated with the name of Bernard Williams, the thesis that belief is an attitude that "aims at the truth."[33]

THE CONSTITUTIVE AIM OF BELIEF

The grounds for this thesis emerge when we try to distinguish belief from the other propositional attitudes. One difference between belief and other attitudes is that it entails regarding its propositional object as true.

The difference between believing that *P* and desiring that *P*, for example, is that the former attitude treats *P* as a report of how things are, whereas the latter treats *P* as a mandate for how things are to become.[34] Desire takes its propositional object as representing *facienda*—things that aren't the case but are to be brought about. By contrast, belief takes its propositional object as representing *facta*—things that are the case and in virtue of which the proposition is true.[35]

33. Bernard Williams, "Deciding to Believe," in *Problems of the Self* (Cambridge: Cambridge University Press, 1973), 136–51.

34. This difference between belief and desire can be obscured by the fact that desiring that *P* entails desiring *P* to be true, just as believing that *P* entails believing it to be true. These locutions obscure the difference between belief and desire because they use the infinitive 'to be', which is required for indirect discourse, to replace what would be different moods of the copula in direct speech. In believing *P* to be true, one believes in its completed truth, as would be expressed by the indicative statement that *P* is true; whereas in desiring *P* to be true, one desires its to-be-completed truth, as would be expressed by the optative that it *be* true. Thus, although we can speak either of believing or of desiring *P* to be true, transposing these statements from *oratio obliqua* to *oratio recta* reveals an underlying difference in the relation that *P* is taken as bearing to the world.

35. The language used in this contrast should not be overinterpreted. To say that belief involves regarding a proposition as true, or that desire involves regarding it as to be made true, is simply to articulate our concepts of belief and desire as propositional attitudes. We express the fundamental similarity among these content-bearing mental

*   *   *

This conception of belief is correct as far as it goes, but it doesn't go far enough. It's incomplete because regarding a proposition as true is involved in many cognitive attitudes, including not only belief but also other attitudes from which belief must still be distinguished. Assuming a proposition—say, for the sake of argument—entails regarding it as a report rather than a mandate, as a truth rather than something to be made true. Even imagining that P entails regarding it as a completed rather than a to-be-completed truth. One hasn't imagined that P unless one has regarded P as reflecting how things are, and hence as true. Yet to assume that P or imagine that P is not to believe it, and so regarding a proposition as true must not be sufficient for belief.[36]

Of course, there is a sense in which things that are merely assumed or imagined are not regarded as really true. But the relevant sense is not that they aren't regarded as true at all; it's rather that they are regarded as true but not really—regarded as true, that is, but not seriously or in earnest. What distinguishes a proposition's being believed from its being assumed or imagined is the spirit in which it is regarded as true, whether tentatively or hypothetically, as in the case of assumption; fancifully, as in the case of imagination; or seriously, as in the case of belief.

*   *   *

What's the difference between seriously regarding a proposition as true and doing so in some other spirit? Here is the point at which belief is distinguished from other attitudes by its aim.

---

states by describing them as ways of regarding propositional contents, and we express the differences among them by differentiating among the ways in which those contents can be regarded. The resulting locutions should not be understood as positing any particular mental architecture, least of all an inner eye that squints at propositions or raises its eyebrow at them so as to regard them in different ways. Rather, these locutions simply translate our terms for propositional attitudes into a common vocabulary, in which their similarities and differences can be clearly expressed. To say that belief entails regarding a proposition as true is therefore not to commit ourselves to any particular theory about which physical, neurological, or otherwise subdoxastic states make up the mental state of belief. It commits us only to a view about what such states must amount to if they are to constitute belief—namely, that they must amount to the state of regarding a proposition as true. For recent discussions of this phenomenon, commonly called "direction of fit," see Lloyd Humberstone, "Direction of Fit," *Mind* 101 (1992): 59–83; and G. F. Schueler, "Pro-attitudes and Direction of Fit," *Mind* 100 (1991): 277–81. Note that I understand direction of fit somewhat differently from these and other authors. For a fuller treatment of the differences, see my "The Guise of the Good," *Nous* 26 (1992): 3–26; and n. 55 below.

36. For related discussions of the similarities and differences among these cognitive states, see Jennifer Church, "Judgment, Self-Consciousness, and Object Independence," *American Philosophical Quarterly* 27 (1990): 51–60; and Mark Leon, "Rationalising Belief," *Philosophical Papers* 21 (1992): 299–314.

The sense in which fantasies and assumptions aren't serious is
that they entail regarding a proposition as true—or accepting the
proposition, as I shall put it—without sensitivity to whether one is
thereby accepting the truth. We assume a proposition when we regard
it as true for the sake of thereby framing a possibility to be entertained
in argument or inquiry and when we can therefore be said to accept
it for polemical or heuristic purposes. We imagine a proposition when
we regard it as true for the sake of thereby stimulating or vicariously
satisfying our desires and when we can therefore be said to accept it
for recreational or motivational purposes. But we believe a proposition
when we regard it as true for the sake of thereby getting the truth
right with respect to that proposition: to believe something is to accept
it with the aim of doing so if and only if it really is true.

Thus, the purpose or aim with which a proposition is regarded
as true is partly constitutive of the resulting attitude toward the proposition. It determines whether the proposition is being accepted hypothetically, as in assumption; playfully, as in imagination; or seriously,
as in belief. These attitudes can therefore be conceived as having two
tiers. The first tier, which they share and by virtue of which they differ
as a group from the conative attitudes, is the attitude of regarding a
proposition as true—the attitude of bare acceptance. The second tier,
in which the various cognitive attitudes differ among themselves, encompasses the different aims with which a proposition can be accepted.[37]

To say that our attitude toward a proposition is partly constituted
by the aim or purpose with which we accept the proposition is not to
say that the aim is itself an attitude of ours, or that acceptance is an
action. This point cannot be overemphasized.[38] Acceptance is a mental

37. An example that can help to illustrate this conception of the propositional
attitudes appears in Bernard Williams's discussion of "Imagination and the Self" (in
Problems of the Self, pp. 29–31). Williams compares two men who imagine assassinating
the Prime Minister in the person of Lord Salisbury. One man imagines assassinating
the Prime Minister but falsely believes that Lord Salisbury occupies that position; the
other man, who knows that Lord Salisbury isn't Prime Minister, nevertheless imagines
him to be, while also imagining a similar assassination. "On the purely psychological
level," Williams remarks, "the same visualisings, the same images, could surely occur
in both cases. The difference lies rather in how the story is meant" (p. 31). According
to my account, "how the story is meant" should be understood in terms of the aim with
which it is regarded as true that Lord Salisbury is Prime Minister. Each subject includes
this identification in his "story," and thereby regards it as true. But one subject regards
it as true for the sake of correctly identifying the Prime Minister, whereas the other
regards it as true for the sake of his own entertainment.

38. The point will be lost on those who believe that any goal-directed movement,
mental or physical, automatically qualifies as an intentional action. I reject this view, as
will become clear on pp. 715 ff. My reasons for rejecting it are developed more fully
in my "Guise of the Good" and "What Happens When Someone Acts?" *Mind* 101
(1992): 461–81. In any case, the present account of belief will be misunderstood if
aims are assumed to be necessarily agential.

state whose aim may be emergent in the cognitive mechanisms by which that state is induced, sustained, and revised. For example, if our acceptance of a proposition is regulated by mechanisms performing their function of therein framing a possibility to be tested, then our acceptance may have a heuristic aim whether or not we have heuristic motives or take any action toward heuristic ends. Similarly, if our acceptance of a proposition is regulated by mechanisms performing their function of therein tracking the truth of the proposition, then it may have an epistemic aim whether or not we have or act on such an aim.[39] In short, our acceptance of a proposition may be aimed at the truth by our cognitive faculties rather than ourselves.

*   *   *

This possibility suggests that one can have beliefs—aimed, as required, at the truth—while also being indifferent, at another level, to the truth of those beliefs. There are two ways of being indifferent to the truth, of which only one is an obstacle to believing.

To begin with, I can accept a proposition in a manner indifferent to its truth, thereby forming an assumption or fantasy rather than a belief. I am not then proceeding with indifference to the truth of a belief; I'm proceeding with indifference to the truth of what I accept, thereby falling short of belief altogether.

In another sense, however, I can be indifferent to the truth of something conceived as a belief. I cannot believe something without accepting it seriously—in an attempt, by me or my cognitive faculties, to arrive at acceptance of the truth—but I can still have further, second-order goals with respect to this attempt. For example, I can try to ensure that an attempt to accept what's true with respect to a proposition will lead to acceptance of that proposition whether it's true or not. This second-order attempt, to manipulate the outcome of a first-order attempt to accept what's true, is precisely what I undertake when I try to get myself to hold a particular belief irrespective of its truth. And in this case I am indifferent to the truth specifically of a

---

39. As David Phillips has pointed out to me, the mechanisms whose function is to track the truth may employ assumptions or even fantasies along the way. Thus, whether a particular instance of acceptance is an hypothesis, fantasy, or belief cannot depend on the ultimate aim toward which it is directed. Rather, the nature of each acceptance must depend on its immediate aim, as I have tried to indicate with the words 'therein' and 'thereby': to assume that P is to accept P for the sake of thereby formulating a possibility to be tested, whereas to believe that P is to accept P for the sake of thereby accepting the truth with respect to P. (Peter Railton raises the same problem in his "Truth, Reason, and the Regulation of Belief," *Philosophical Issues* 5 [1994]: 71–93.)

belief, because my indifference is directed at the success of something conceived as an attempt at accepting the truth.[40]

*   *   *

I can thus fail to care about the truth of my beliefs. Yet if indicators of truth in a proposition are reasons for believing it, then indifference to the truth of my beliefs would seem to leave me insensitive to reasons, and hence irrational. My conception of theoretical reason would thus seem to resemble externalist conceptions of practical reason, in mandating a particular concern or inclination as required for rationality.

But this appearance is misleading. The conception of reasons for belief as indicators of truth doesn't imply that indifference to the truth of my beliefs would be irrational. Indifference to the truth of my beliefs would not in fact make me insensitive to the associated reasons for believing.

Of course, evidence for the truth of some belief may not sway me toward wanting or getting myself to hold that belief, if I'm indifferent to its truth. But we don't necessarily think that indicators of truth are reasons for such second-order measures as wanting or getting myself to hold beliefs. We identify them as reasons for *believing*, which are simply reasons for accepting something in the course of an attempt to arrive at acceptance of what's true. And insofar as I or my cognitive faculties attempt to arrive at the truth on a topic, that attempt will already make me potentially sensitive to indicators of the truth; whereas if no such attempt is in the works, the topic will be one on which I am not in the business of holding beliefs, in the first place.

What provides my sensitivity to reasons for believing, then, is not a second-order aim of having true beliefs but rather the first-order aim that makes my acceptance of something into a belief. And if this first-order aim is lacking from my approach to some topic, then I am not irrationally insensitive to reasons for belief about it; I am out of the business of having beliefs about it altogether, and so I am no longer subject to reasons for belief about it at all. Thus, my conception of theoretical reason doesn't condemn this form of indifference as irrational, either.

---

40. As Williams noted in "Deciding to Believe," this account of indifference to the truth of a belief explains the difficulty of acting on that indifference. In order to end up believing the proposition that I want to believe, I must accept it in the course of an attempt to accept what is true, not an attempt merely to accept this proposition. Indifference to the truth must not seep into my first-order attempt from my second-order attitude toward its success or failure. Some psychological partitioning is therefore necessary. On the difficulty of manipulating beliefs, see also Leon.

*   *   *

In identifying something as a reason to believe a proposition, we are implicitly identifying it as a reason for a potential believer, someone who is in a position to believe or disbelieve the proposition at issue. Now, someone can be in a position to form a belief even though he lacks an interest in the truth of that belief—the second-order interest in the success of this attempt at accepting what's true. But he is not prepared to believe or disbelieve a proposition if he isn't prepared for an attempt to accept what's true with respect to it. Thus, he is not a potential believer with respect to a proposition—and hence not subject to reasons for believing it—in the absence of an inclination that would cause him to be swayed by indicators of its truth.

So when we say that indicators of truth are reasons for belief, we aren't making a normative judgment about whether to be inclined toward the truth; we're saying that they're reasons for someone only if he is inclined toward the truth, since we're identifying them as reasons of a kind whose universe of application is the set of potential believers, who are constitutively truth inclined. The question whether to be inclined toward the truth on some topic—and hence whether to be subject to reasons for belief about it—is left entirely open.

*   *   *

In some sense, theoretical reasoning now seems to fit the model of internalism. Indicators of truth count as reasons for someone to believe only if he has a cognitive inclination that makes him susceptible to their influence. And reasons that apply to someone only if he's susceptible to their influence are supposed to be internal reasons.

At this point, however, the distinction between internal and external reasons is out of its depth, so to speak. Reasons for belief are dependent on a particular inclination, all right, but they're dependent on that inclination which makes one a believer. They don't depend on one's peculiar inclinations *as* a believer—on one's second-order attitudes toward or preferences among beliefs.

Indeed, the dependence of theoretical reasons on a cognitive inclination does not justify relativizing them to particular believers at all. The inclination on which these reasons depend is constitutive of belief itself, and to that extent they are reasons simply *for belief* rather than for any particular person to believe.[41] If something counts in a particular epistemic context as a reason to believe that *P*, then it counts in that

41. Of course, reasons for belief are also relative to an informational context, and insofar as different people are in possession of different information, they will be subject to different reasons. But if the informational context is held constant, the relativity of reasons to persons disappears.

context as a reason simply to believe that *P*, and not just for this or
that believer to do so, since all potential believers of *P* are alike in the
cognitive inclination that gives application to such a reason.

The question of whether reasons for belief are internal or external reasons thus presents a false dichotomy. Reasons for belief are
like internal reasons in that they exist and exert an influence only
in relation to a particular inclination; but they are like external
reasons in that the inclination on which they depend is embedded
in the attitude of belief, so that they can count as reasons for belief
per se, in abstraction from motivational differences among individual believers.

*   *   *

Maybe the way to understand the status of reasons for belief is to
consider an analogy between belief and another enterprise that's partly
constituted by a substantive aim. Consider reasons for sacrificing a
pawn in the game of chess.

Reasons for sacrificing a pawn depend for their existence on a
goal or aim, and in this respect they look like internal reasons. But
the goal on which reasons for this move depend is partly constitutive
of the move itself, because sacrificing a pawn is by definition a move
in the game of chess, which is partly defined by its object; and because
the move is by definition a sacrifice, which it can be only in relation
to the object of the game. Reasons for sacrificing a pawn therefore
exist in abstraction from the temperament of any particular player:
they are reasons simply for the move itself, and in this respect they
look like external reasons, too.

A player may have second-order aims with respect to his success
or failure in a particular game of chess. He may even have the goal
of losing a game—if his opponent is a sensitive eight-year-old, for
example. But in order to lose a game of chess, he must stay in the game,
by continuing to pursue its object, however insincerely or ineffectually.
And so long as he is pursuing that object, he will have the inclination
that answers to reasons for sacrificing a pawn.

A player can lose his susceptibility to those reasons only by giving
up the associated object—moving his pieces around aimlessly, for
example. In that case, he will in effect have quit the game: his opponent will say, not just "You're letting me win," but "You're not playing
any more." Once the player has quit the game of chess, however, he
has quit the only game in which pawns can be sacrificed, and his
resulting insensitivity to reasons for sacrificing a pawn will not make
him irrational. To someone who isn't playing chess, reasons for sacrificing a pawn simply don't apply.

In sum, reasons for sacrificing a pawn apply to anyone with the
capacity to do so, irrespective of his inclinations about how to exercise

that capacity. They apply to him only because he has an inclination that lends them an influence, of course, but the requisite inclination is the one that makes him a chess player, not one that determines his individual style of play.

APPLYING THE ANALOGY TO PRACTICAL REASONING

I think that practical reasoning occupies the same middle ground between internalism and externalism. That is, reasons for acting apply to someone only because he has an inclination that lends them an influence, but the requisite inclination is the one that makes him an agent, not one that determines his individual course of action.

This account of practical reason simply follows the structure of theoretical reason, as analyzed above. That analysis began with the claim that belief is distinguished from other cognitive states by a substantive goal, and then it claimed that an inclination toward this goal creates the susceptibility necessary to the application of reasons for believing. Perhaps, then, action can be distinguished from other forms of behavior by a substantive goal, and an inclination toward this goal can create the susceptibility necessary to the application of reasons for acting. In that case, reasons for acting would be considerations relevant to the constitutive aim of action, just as reasons for believing are indicators of truth, which is the constitutive aim of belief. And anyone who wasn't susceptible to reasons for acting, because he had no inclination toward the relevant aim, wouldn't be in a position to act, anyway, and therefore wouldn't be subject to reasons for acting; just as anyone who has no inclination toward the truth isn't in a position to believe and isn't subject to reasons for belief.

The account rests, of course, on the initial claim that behaviors qualify as actions by virtue of having a particular aim. Let me say a word about the philosophical point of such a claim.

The point of specifying which behaviors qualify as actions is not, I think, to delineate the extension of 'action' or 'to act' as used in ordinary language. These terms are used quite loosely, in application not only to paradigm cases of action, in which human agency is exercised to its fullest, but also to marginal cases, in which agency is exercised only partially or imperfectly. The fundamental question in the philosophy of action is not how imperfect an exercise of agency can be while still qualifying as an action. The question is the nature of agency itself, and agency, like any capacity, fully reveals its nature only when fully exercised. We therefore want to know what makes for a paradigm case of action, a full-blooded action, an action par excellence.

I claim that what makes for an action, in this sense, is a constitutive aim. This claim sounds odd, to say the least. We may think that a full-

blooded action must have some goal or other;[42] but we tend to think
that its status as an action doesn't depend on what goal it has. Action,
we tend to think, is just behavior aimed at some goal, any goal.

*   *   *

In my opinion, however, we are mistaken in assuming that behavior
approaches full-blooded action by having a goal of the sort that varies
from one action to another. Simply being goal directed is not a mark
of action.

Consider a case of unintentional behavior. An old friend unexpectedly walks into your office, and surprise lights up your face: your
eyes widen, a smile flashes, an exclamation escapes your lips. These
reactions just happen to you, and they may even hit you with an
aftershock of surprise. Now suppose, instead, that you encounter your
friend on the quad, recognizing him as he approaches. You are moved
to the same reactions, but you now have a chance to modulate them
or compose them into an intentional expression of surprise.

Take another case of unintentional behavior. Say, a child accidentally brushes a glass off of the table, and your hand shoots out to catch
it. Everything happens so fast that you see your hand catching the
glass before you fully realize that the glass is falling. Now suppose,
finally, that another child—an older and sassier child—hefts the glass
with a smirk and calls, "Here, catch!" You then undertake the same
behavior, but as a fully intentional action.

The first instance in which you catch the glass is an instance of
behavior directed at a goal, but it isn't a full-blooded exercise of your
agency. Unlike your reflexive expression of surprise, which springs
out of the emotion of surprise but not *toward* any purpose or goal,
the reflexive extension of your hand is aimed at something—namely,
preventing the glass from smashing on the floor.[43] Despite being goal
directed, however, this behavior still lacks some element that's necessary to full-blooded action. So what makes for action is not simply
being goal directed.

*   *   *

The question is what's missing from this goal-directed behavior. In my
view, what's missing is some additional goal that every action shares, no
matter what its other, contingent goals may be.

42. See, e.g., Jay Wallace, "How to Argue about Practical Reason," *Mind* 99 (1990):
355–85, p. 359: "To act intentionally . . . is necessarily to be in a goal-directed state";
see also Smith, "The Humean Theory of Motivation."
43. The idea that some actions spring out of motives without being directed toward
any ends or goals is defended by Michael Stocker, "Values and Purposes: The Limits
of Teleology and the Ends of Friendship," *Journal of Philosophy* 78 (1981): 747–65.

There is an ancient thesis along these lines, to the effect that action, no matter where it aims, must thereby aim at the good.[44] This thesis identifies a constitutive goal of action—the good—and it thus implements the strategy of analysis that I favor. But in this implementation, the strategy fails to achieve its purpose, since it doesn't avoid the twin pitfalls of internalism and externalism.[45]

The thesis that action constitutively aims at the good can be interpreted in at least two ways. It may simply mean that an action must aim at something, which consequently counts as good in the sense of being that whose attainment will make the action a success. But this sense of the word 'good' is a formal sense, denoting whatever is the aim of an action. It identifies no particular thing at which every action must aim, and hence no particular kind of consideration as capable of influencing anyone insofar as he is an agent. If the thesis uses this formal sense of the word 'good', then the considerations that it classifies as reasons will vary along with the good being aimed at. Reasons will then depend for their application on one's inclinations as an agent, as they do under internalism.

In order to avoid this consequence of internalism, the ancient thesis would have to identify a substantive goal for action, by saying that every action aims at something conceived as good in a sense independent of its being the aim. But when the thesis uses a substantive sense of the word 'good' in this manner, it characterizes action as necessarily well-intentioned, thus ruling out various kinds of perversity. To those who believe, as I do, that behavior can still qualify as action even if its end-in-view is conceived as bad, the thesis will now appear to be burdened with controversial normative commitments, like the version of externalism considered above.[46]

*   *   *

The ancient thesis goes wrong, I think, in treating the constitutive aim of action as something shared or jointly promoted by all of an agent's other ends-in-view, as if it were an ultimate or all-encompassing end. If action is to be constituted by an aim, however, that aim cannot be an end at all.

44. This view is echoed by Donald Davidson in "How Is Weakness of the Will Possible?" in *Essays on Actions and Events*, pp. 21–42, p. 22.

45. This problem was foreshadowed in the text accompanying n. 22, above.

46. In adopting an evil end, the perverse agent may of course be said to make evil his good, as Satan does in *Paradise Lost* (bk. 4, line 110). But Satan makes evil his good only in the formal sense that its attainment will be the criterion of his success. The fact that even Satan's actions aim at the good in this formal sense doesn't help us to identify a substantive aim that constitutes them as actions. G. E. M. Anscombe discusses this passage (*Intention* [Ithaca, N.Y.: Cornell University Press, 1963], p. 75), and I have elsewhere criticized her discussion ("Guise of the Good," pp. 18 ff.).

An end is something conceived by an agent as a potential object of his actions. It is therefore something that one cannot have unless one already is an agent, in a position to act, and so it cannot be something that one must already have in order to occupy that position. If action is to be constituted by an aim, that aim must be, so to speak, subactional or subagential—something that a subject of mere behavior can have, and by having which he can become an agent, as his behavior becomes an action.

This subactional aim can be discerned, I think, in our contrasting pairs of behaviors. It is that which the unintentional behaviors are missing in comparison with the corresponding full-blooded actions.

*   *   *

Intuitively speaking, what these behaviors lack is that, while directed *at* various things, they are not directed *by* you. When the glass is brushed off the table, for example, behavior aimed at arresting its fall is initiated and completed before you know it, and so you have no chance to take control of that behavior. In the intentional instance, the same goal-directed behavior occurs, but it occurs under your control.

The kind of control at issue here is not the sensorimotor process that adjusts ongoing behavior in light of perceived progress toward a desired outcome. That process of real-time adjustment is simply eye-hand coordination, which occurs in both the intentional and the reflexive cases. What's missing from the reflexive case is conscious direction on your part, which is something other than eye-hand coordination. When goal-directed behavior proceeds under this conscious control, it becomes a full-blooded action, rather than a well-coordinated reflex.[47] And behavior that isn't directed at a goal can become an action in the same fashion. The smile that springs spontaneously from your emotion of surprise isn't aimed at any result, but it, too, can be transformed into a full-blooded action if it is brought under your conscious control.

Now, if an action comprises behavior of which you take control, then taking control of your behavior cannot itself be an action; otherwise, a vicious regress will ensue. Yet controlling your behavior is indeed an activity: it's something that you do. The reason why the falling glass leaves you no time to perform a full-blooded action is that, although it leaves you time to stick out your hand, it doesn't leave you time to do something else that's essential to a full-blooded

47. I do not mean that every part or aspect of the behavior must come under your conscious control in order for the behavior to constitute a full-blooded action. How you execute the catch may still be left to those reflexes which make up your skill as a catcher; that you execute a catch, however, must come under your control, or the catch won't be an action in the fullest sense.

action—that is, to exercise conscious control of your catch. Hence when you catch the glass intentionally, you must be doing two things: extending your hand in order to avert a mishap and exercising control over that behavior.

Let me reiterate that I am using the noun 'activity' and the verb 'to do' in senses that do not imply the performance of a full-blooded action. To suggest that an action comprises behavior on which you perform the action of exercising control would be absurd. But you do many things that aren't actions—such as when you reflexively stick out your hand to catch a falling glass or smile out of surprise. And exercising conscious control over your behavior is indeed something that you do, in this thin sense of the verb.

I therefore suggest that our ordinary concept of a full-blooded action is in fact the concept of two, hierarchically related activities. Action is like the corporate enterprise of work performed under management: it's behavior executed under conscious control. And just as the corporate enterprise includes both a basic work activity and the higher-order activity of managing that work (neither of which is itself a corporate enterprise), so full-blooded action comprises both a basic activity and the higher-order activity of controlling it (neither of which is itself an action).

*   *   *

This analysis of action suggests how action might have a constitutive goal. According to the analysis, various actions involve various behaviors—directed, in many cases, at various goals—but they also share an additional, higher-order activity, the activity of consciously directing these behaviors. This activity is constitutive of action, in the sense that its addition is what makes a full-blooded action out of a merely reflexive or unintentional movement. If this higher-order activity entails the pursuit of a goal, then there may indeed be a constitutive goal of action.[48]

What I have in mind here is not an ulterior goal or aim toward which behavior is consciously directed, as a corporation's work activity might be managed toward the end of maximizing profits. The executive officers can still manage the work of a corporation without having the goal of profit maximization, in particular, and so this goal is not itself essential to work's being performed under management. Similarly, a goal toward which behavior is consciously directed may not be

---

48. I have elsewhere presented an independent argument for this thesis ("What Happens When Someone Acts?"). The idea that practical reason has motives of its own, directed at the control of one's behavior, is contained in the theory of motivation attributed to Plato by John Cooper, "Plato's Theory of Human Motivation," *History of Philosophy Quarterly* 1 (1984): 3–21.

essential to the behavior's being consciously directed, insofar as behavior might be consciously directed at other goals or no goal in particular.

What I have in mind is a goal that must be pursued if behavior is to be consciously directed at all. This goal will not be one of the agent's ends-in-view, nor will it be something on which those ends converge. Rather, it will be something whose pursuit is ancillary to theirs—something whose pursuit transforms them, from outcomes sought unconsciously or reflexively, into ends at which action is consciously directed.

THE CONSTITUTIVE GOAL OF ACTION

What is this goal? A hint lies in the fact that consciously controlling one's behavior is not something that one can do without aiming to.[49] Maybe, then, the aim without which there is no conscious control of behavior is simply the aim of being in conscious control of one's behavior. If so, then the constitutive aim of action will turn out, in Kantian fashion, to be autonomy.[50] And considerations will turn out to qualify as reasons—also in Kantian fashion—by virtue of their relevance to our autonomy rather than their relevance to our interests or our good.[51]

These remarks are merely suggestive at best, and this is not the place to develop them into a full account of autonomy or its role as the constitutive goal of action.[52] I can only sketch how they might be developed.

*   *   *

My sketch begins with the conception of autonomy as conscious control over one's behavior. Consciously controlling one's behavior in-

---

49. Bernard Williams has pointed out to me that one can consciously control one's behavior while aiming not to—as, for example, when one unsuccessfully tries to let one's reflexes or instincts take over. But this point strikes me as compatible with my claim that one cannot consciously control one's behavior without aiming to. Trying not to control one's behavior involves a second-order goal, of relaxing one's first-order efforts at control. If one continues to control one's behavior while trying not to, the reason is that one continues to aim at controlling it while trying not to persist in that aim. (Remember that the aims under discussion here may be subagential. See pp. 716–17, above).

50. Thanks to Chris Korsgaard for publicly daring me to express this thought.

51. Stephen Darwall has proposed a similar conception of reasons, under the name 'autonomist internalism' ("Autonomist Internalism and the Justification of Morals," *Nous* 24 [1990]: 257–68). Of course, considerations may be relevant to our autonomy because of their relevance to our interests. The point is that their relevance to autonomy will be what makes them reasons for acting.

52. See my *Practical Reflection* (Princeton, N.J.: Princeton University Press, 1989); and "The Story of Rational Action," *Philosophical Topics* 21 (1993): 229–54.

volves two elements: being conscious of one's behavior and controlling it. How are these elements connected?

One possibility is that they aren't connected at all. Conscious control might just be the sum of two independent elements, control over what one is doing and consciousness of what one is doing. Another possibility is that exercising control over one's behavior is what brings it to consciousness. One might control what one is doing and thereby become conscious of that behavior.

The problem with these possibilities is that they would leave an agent's knowledge of his behavior dependent on the usual inbound channels, such as perception of the behavior itself or introspection on the process by which it is directed. And as many philosophers have noted, an agent's knowledge of his behavior is not receptive knowledge: an agent knows what he is doing, as they say, without observation.[53]

The work of these philosophers points to a third possibility for the relation between self-control and self-awareness. Maybe consciousness of what one is doing is that by which one exerts control. Consciously controlling one's behavior would then be—not just controlling it and also, or thereby, becoming conscious of it—but rather having a *controlling consciousness* of one's behavior, a guiding awareness of what one is doing. This possibility would account not only for an agent's self-control but also for the quality of his self-awareness, since his knowledge of what he was doing would be, so to speak, directive rather than receptive knowledge.[54]

*   *   *

But how can knowledge be directive? For the answer, let me return to my earlier account of cognition. (I'll give the answer in this section and then illustrate it in the next.)

Consciousness or knowledge must be a cognitive state, and so it must involve regarding propositions as true rather than as to be made

53. See Anscombe, *Intention;* Stuart Hampshire, *Freedom of the Individual* (Princeton, N.J.: Princeton University Press, 1975), chap. 3; Brian O'Shaughnessy, *The Will: A Dual Aspect Theory* (Cambridge: Cambridge University Press, 1980), chap. 8. See also Ludwig Wittgenstein, *Philosophical Investigations*, trans. G. E. M. Anscombe (Oxford: Blackwell, 1967), secs. 627 ff.

54. Compare the ancient and medieval notion of "practical knowledge," which is "the cause of what it understands" (Aquinas, *Summa Theologica*, Ia IIae, Q3, art. 5, obj. 1). Anscombe discusses this notion in the last two paragraphs of her paper "Thought and Action in Aristotle" (in *New Essays on Plato and Aristotle*, ed. by R. Bambrough [London: Routledge & Kegan Paul, 1965], 143–58), thereby picking up a theme that was left undeveloped in *Intention*, pp. 1–5, 56–58, 87. See also David Pears, *Motivated Irrationality* (Oxford: Clarendon, 1984), chap. 8; and Arthur Danto, "Action, Knowledge, and Representation," in *Action Theory*, ed. by Myles Brand and Douglas Walton (Dordrecht: Reidel, 1976), pp. 11–25.

true. It must also be a serious cognitive state, regarding propositions as true in an attempt thereby to get the truth right. Indeed, the success that's implied in the concept of consciousness or knowledge is success in this very attempt, to regard as true what really is true.

But there are two ways of attempting to regard as true, or accept, what really is true. One way is to accept a proposition in response to its being true; the other is to accept a proposition in such a way as to make it true. Note that the latter method does not entail regarding the proposition as *to be made* true. It entails attempting to make the proposition true by regarding it as such, but attempting to make a proposition true by regarding it as true is quite different from regarding it as to be made true. The proposition is regarded as fact, not *faciendum*, and so it is accepted, in a cognitive rather than conative attitude. What's more, the proposition is accepted seriously, not hypothetically or frivolously. For in attempting to accept something so as to make it true, one attempts to reach the position of accepting a genuine truth, no less than when one attempts to accept something in response to its being true. In either case, one's acceptance aims at correspondence between what's regarded as true and what is true, and so it is a serious cognitive attitude, whose success deserves to be called knowledge.[55]

How can one regard a proposition as true in such a way as to make it true? Well, when one accepts a proposition in response to its truth, one registers the influence of evidence and other reasons for belief, thereby manifesting an inclination to conform one's acceptance to the facts. Accepting a proposition in such a way as to make it true would simply require a converse inclination, to conform the facts to

---

55. Here I am expanding on two themes that I have discussed elsewhere. First, I am expanding an earlier critique of the traditional notion of direction of fit (in my "Guise of the Good"). In my view, this notion conflates two different distinctions. One is the distinction between the cognitive and the conative—the distinction between accepting, or regarding as true and approving, or regarding as to be made true. The other is a distinction between the receptive and the directive, which are two different ways of attempting to accept what's true—namely, by accepting so as to reflect the truth, and by accepting so as to create the truth. If these distinctions are conflated under the heading 'direction of fit', then one and the same mental state can appear to have two different directions of fit, since a subject can attempt to accept what's true by accepting something so as to make it true. The resulting state is cognitive rather than conative, but directive rather than receptive: it's directive cognition. I would claim that this state of directive cognition is the state of intending to act. This is the second theme on which I am currently expanding. In the past, I have said that an intention is a self-fulfilling and self-referring belief (*Practical Reflection*, chap. 4; see also "How to Share an Intention," *Philosophy and Phenomenological Research* 57 [1997]). The present discussion explains why I call it a belief, but also why I can dispense with that label. What matters is that intention is a state of directive cognition, not whether that state should be called belief.

722   *Ethics   July 1996*

one's acceptance. And one can indeed be inclined to conform the facts to one's acceptance, if the proposition accepted is about one's own behavior. One need only be inclined to do what one accepts that one will do. If one has this inclination, then accepting that one will do something can be a way of making this proposition true, and it can therefore be an attempt at accepting the truth.

*   *   *

This admittedly convoluted proposal can be applied to the contrast between your reflexively and intentionally catching that glass. In both cases, your desire to save the glass causes your hand to extend. In both cases, you're aware of this causal sequence, since you're aware of extending your hand in order to save the glass. But in only one of the cases is your knowledge directive, or your behavior autonomous.

When you extend your hand reflexively, you react before you know it, but then you observe your reaction. Extending your hand in order to save the glass causes you to accept the proposition that you're doing so. When you react intentionally, however, acceptance precedes behavior: you accept that you'll extend your hand to save the glass, and this acceptance is what prompts you to do so.

In the latter case as well as the former, your acceptance is an attempt to accept something true. You're not just hypothesizing or fantasizing that you'll extend your hand: you're seriously regarding it as true that you will extend it. Of course, your acceptance of this proposition is not an attempt to accept something that's true anteced-ently; it's an attempt to accept something whose truth will follow as a result. But it is not therefore less serious as an attempt to accept a truth. If the proposition accepted comes true, then its acceptance is a cognitive success—an instance of directive knowledge.

In sum, instead of reacting before you know it, you react after and because you know it, and that's what makes your behavior an autonomous action. You act autonomously because you extend your hand in, and out of, a knowledge of what you're doing.

*   *   *

But why would your extending a hand to save the glass result from your accepting that you would do so?

Suppose that you have an inclination toward being in conscious control of your next move. This inclination will inhibit you from doing anything out of other motives until you've accepted that you're going to—precisely so that you'll do it only after and because you know it, and hence under conscious control. Once you accept that you're going to do something, however, the inclination toward being in conscious

control will reinforce your other motives for doing it, since doing what you've accepted you'll do is what puts consciousness in control. Your inclination toward conscious control is thus converted, from an inhibition against doing something into a motive in favor of doing it, by your accepting that you'll do it. Accepting that you'll extend your hand to save the glass can therefore prompt you to do so.

Here, then, is how autonomy can serve as the constitutive goal of action. The goal-directed movement of your hand comes under your conscious control because it is prompted by your accepting that you will perform such a movement. And it is prompted by that acceptance because of your inclination toward conscious control of what you're doing—which is just an inclination toward autonomy. Your movement thus becomes autonomous precisely by manifesting your inclination toward autonomy; and in becoming autonomous, it becomes a full-blooded action. A full-blooded action is therefore behavior that manifests your inclination toward autonomy, just as a belief is a cognitive attitude that manifests your inclination toward the truth.

*   *   *

My view is that your inclination toward the constitutive goal of action also mediates the influence of your reasons for acting, just as your inclination toward the truth mediates the influence of your reasons for belief. Your reasons for acting can be displayed as the premises of a practical inference:

> I want to save that glass.
> I could save the glass by extending my hand.
> So I'll extend my hand.

Since the premises of this inference are about how to fulfill a desire of yours, they sound like reasons that Williams would call internal. But in my view, they don't influence you in quite the way that internal reasons are supposed to.

Here is how internal reasons are supposed to work. The first premise of your inference is about a desire of yours: "I want to save that glass." The second premise is about the means to the object of that desire: "I could save the glass by extending my hand." The desire mentioned in the first premise and the belief expressed in the second combine to motivate the action mentioned in your conclusion: "So I'll extend my hand." According to the internalist tradition, this process of motivation is the very process whereby reasons for acting exert their influence as reasons.

This conception of how reasons exert their influence encourages a particular reading of the statements displayed above. Since the influence of reasons is conceived as the motivational influence of desire and belief,

and since the second premise expresses the operative belief, the first premise is read as expressing the associated desire.[56] Similarly, the conclusion is sometimes read as expressing—or standing in for—the action itself, which is said to be the real conclusion of your inference.[57] The three displayed statements are thus interpreted as expressions of your reasons and of the action that they influence you to perform.

I don't dispute the traditional account of how desire and belief motivate behavior. My quarrel is with the claim that when desire and belief motivate behavior, they exert the influence of reasons.[58] You extend your hand, I agree, out of a desire for something and a belief about how to attain it. But you can extend your hand out of a desire and belief even when you do so reflexively, without knowing what you're doing or why, and hence without the benefit of practical reasoning.

In my view, extending your hand out of a desire and belief is the underlying behavior over which you may or may not exercise conscious control—the underlying work that may or may not come under your executive management. And practical reasoning is the process by which you exercise conscious control over this activity in some cases but not others. If you extend your hand without any guiding knowledge of what you're doing, then even though your behavior is motivated by a desire and belief, it isn't under your conscious control, and so it isn't a full-blooded action. Your behavior amounts to a full-blooded action only when it is performed in, and out of, a knowledge of what you're doing—or, as I have said, after and because you know it.[59]

*   *   *

This view of practical reasoning encourages a different interpretation of the statements displayed above. The first premise expresses a desire-

56. See Davidson, "Intending," in *Essays on Actions and Events*, pp. 83–102, p. 86. Because Davidson thinks that this premise should express your desire, he would reformulate it, from "I want to save that glass" to "Saving that glass would be desirable."

57. Davidson, "How Is Weakness of the Will Possible?" p. 32; and "Intending," pp. 98–99.

58. This quarrel is a continuation of my "Guise of the Good" and "What Happens When Someone Acts?"

59. Note that in my account, your autonomy isn't an ability to control the motions of your hand; it's an ability to control your behavior, which is bodily motion psychologically understood, in terms of its motivation. Even a robot can control whether its hand moves. It takes an autonomous agent to control whether he moves his hand out of a desire to save a glass. The object of autonomous control is thus the entire behavior, comprising motivation as well as movement. The same point can be put in (somewhat) Kantian terms, as follows. Acting autonomously isn't just moving in accordance with one's idea of a movement; it's acting in accordance with one's idea of a law—in this case, the law of motivation.

based reason, in my view, but the reason expressed is not the desire itself. The reason expressed by "I want to save that glass" is your recognition of the desire.

This recognition is a reason because, together with the belief expressed in your second premise, it forms a potentially guiding awareness of what you would be doing in extending your hand. The awareness that you want to save the glass, and that extending your hand would save it, puts you in a position to frame a piece of directive knowledge—"I'm extending my hand in order to save the glass"—a proposition that you can now make true by accepting it. Your awareness of the desire thus presents the behavior of extending your hand in a form prepared for your conscious control, as a potential object of your directive grasp. It presents the behavior, if you will, as fit for (en)action, given the constitutive aim of action, just as theoretical reasons present a proposition as fit for belief, given the constitutive aim of belief.

This view of practical reasoning requires far more elaboration and defense than I can offer here. Its only relevance to this article is that it implements the compromise that I favor between internalism and externalism. For according to this view, even desire-based reasons for acting derive their influence from an inclination other than the desires on which they are based.

*   *   *

The reasons displayed above are desire based in the sense that they mention your desire to save the glass and the means to fulfilling that desire. Yet their influence as reasons is not mediated by the desire that they mention.

Your desire to save the glass does exert a motivational influence in this example. But its influence as a motive contributes to the underlying activity of extending your hand in order to save the glass—the activity that comes under the control of your practical reasoning. And the contribution of your reasons to the control of this activity is distinct from the contribution of your motives to the activity itself.

What exerts the influence of a reason in this example is the recognition that you want to save the glass. And this recognition doesn't influence you by engaging your desire to save the glass. Wanting to save the glass is a motive that can be engaged by considerations about how to save it, not by the recognition that you want to. The recognition that you want to save the glass engages a different inclination, your inclination toward autonomy—toward behaving in, and out of, a knowledge of what you're doing. And it thereby exerts a rational influence distinct from the motivational influence of the desire that it's about.

*　　*　　*

Now, if desire-based reasons derive their influence from something other than the desires on which they are based, then perhaps the same influence is available to considerations that aren't based on desires at all. Perhaps considerations that aren't about your inclinations can still provide potentially directive knowledge.

Such considerations would still have the influence of reasons, by virtue of their capacity to engage your inclination toward autonomy. But they wouldn't depend for their influence on the inclinations that differentiate you from any other agent, and they wouldn't be about such inclinations, either. They might therefore be reasons that Williams would call external.

My thesis, in any case, is that reasons for acting shouldn't be classified as external or internal, since they don't conform to the assumptions underwriting the use of these terms. A reason applies only to those whom it can influence, but its application is not therefore limited to agents of a particular temperament. The inclination that makes one susceptible to a reason for acting is just the inclination that makes one an agent.

.

[10]

REASONS AND MOTIVATION

Derek Parfit and John Broome

I—Derek Parfit

As rational beings, we can ask:

What do we have most reason to want, and do?

What is it most rational for us to want, and do?

These questions differ in only one way. While reasons are provided by the facts, the rationality of our desires and acts depends instead on what we believe, or—given the evidence, ought rationally to believe. When we believe the relevant facts, these questions have the same answers. In other cases, it can be rational to want, or do, what we have no reason to want, or do. Thus, if I believe falsely that my hotel is on fire, it may be rational for me to jump into the canal; but I may have no reason to jump. Since beliefs aim at truth, and to be rational is to respond to reasons, it is the first question that is fundamental.

This question is about *normative* reasons. When we have such a reason, and we act for that reason, it becomes our *motivating* reason. But we can have either kind of reason without having the other. Thus, if I jump into the canal, my motivating reason was provided by my belief; but I had no normative reason to jump. I merely thought I did. And, if I failed to notice that the canal was frozen, I had a reason not to jump that, because it was unknown to me, did not motivate me.

Though we can have normative reasons without being motivated, and vice versa, such reasons are closely related to our motivation. There are, however, very different views about what this relation is. This disagreement raises wider questions about what normative reasons *are*, and about *which* reasons there are. After sketching some of these views, I shall discuss some arguments by Williams, and then say where, in my opinion, the truth lies.[1]

1. Given the size of this territory, my map will have to be rough. I must make some claims which, unless further qualified, could not have a hope of being true. In writing this paper, I have been helped by several people, especially Bernard Williams, Jonathan Dancy, John Broome, Jeff McMahan, Ingmar Persson, Roger Crisp, Julian Savulescu, Brad Hooker, Jerry Cohen, Susan Hurley, Tim Scanlon, Jonathan Bennett, Philippa Foot, David McNaughton, Sigrun Svavarsdottir, Mary Coleman, Ken O'Day and Sophia Reibetanz.

I

Following Williams, we can distinguish two kinds of theory.[2]
According to

> *Internalism about reasons*: All normative reasons are in this
> sense *internal*: for it to be true that
>
> > (R) we have a reason to do something,
>
> it must be true that either
>
> > (D) doing this thing might help to fulfil one of our
> > present intrinsic desires,
>
> or
>
> > (M) if we knew the relevant facts, and deliberated
> > rationally, we would be motivated to do this thing.

Our desire for something is *intrinsic* if we want this thing for its
own sake. Facts are *relevant* if our knowledge of them might affect
our motivation. We can be *motivated* to do something without being
moved to do it. But, for us to be motivated, it must be true that,
given the opportunity, and in the absence of contrary or competing
motivations, we would do this thing.

Many Internalists believe that, if either (D) or (M) is true, that is
not only necessary but also sufficient for the having of a reason.
Though my remarks will often apply to this simpler view, I shall not
say when that is so. Similarly, though (D) could be true while (M)
is false, and vice versa, I shall here, like Williams, set (D) aside.

According to *Externalists*, at least some reasons for acting are
not internal, since they do not require the truth of (M). Suppose
that I have borrowed money from some poor person. This fact,
some Externalists would claim, gives me a reason to return this
money. In calling this reason *external*, they would not mean that I
am not motivated to return this money. They would mean that I
have this reason whatever my motivational state.

Consider next one of Williams's examples. Suppose that, by
taking a certain medicine, someone could protect his health against

---

2. Williams drew this distinction in his 'Internal and External Reasons', henceforth *IER*,
reprinted in his *Moral Luck* (Cambridge University Press, 1982). He returned to it in 'Internal
Reasons and the Obscurity of Blame', henceforth *IROB*, in *Making Sense of Humanity*
(Cambridge University Press, 1995); and again in *World, Mind, and Ethics*, henceforth *WME*,
edited by J.E.J. Altham and Ross Harrison (Cambridge University Press, 1995) pp. 186–194
and 214–16.

REASONS AND MOTIVATION 101

some illness in the further future. According to Internalists, if this person did not care about his further future, and his indifference would survive any amount of informed and rational deliberation, he would have no reason to take this medicine.[3] Most Externalists would disagree. On their view, we all have reasons to protect our health, and to prevent our own future suffering, and these reasons do not depend on whether, after informed and rational deliberation, we would care about these things.

There is now a complication. Many Externalists would claim that, if we knew the relevant facts and were fully rational, we would be motivated to do whatever we had reason to do. This claim is not, as it may seem, a concession to Internalism. According to these Externalists, if

(R) we have a reason to do something,

that entails that

(E) if we knew the relevant facts, and were fully *substantively* rational, we would be motivated to do this thing.

To be substantively rational, we must care about certain things, such as our own well-being. If Williams's imagined person were fully rational, these Externalists would claim, he would be motivated to take the medicine that he knows he needs. That could be true even if, because he is not fully substantively rational, no amount of informed deliberation would in fact motivate him.

Internalists hold a different view. On their view, more fully stated, for it to be true that

(R) we have a reason to do something,

it must be true that

(M) if we knew the relevant facts, and deliberated in a way that was *procedurally* rational, we would be motivated to do this thing.

To be procedurally rational, we must deliberate in certain ways, but we are not required to have any particular desires or aims, such as concern about our own well-being. If Internalists allowed such further requirements, then, as Williams writes, 'there would be no

3. Williams discusses this example in *IER*, pages 105–6. (To make the case more plausible, I have added the reference to the further future.)

significant difference between the internalist and externalist accounts', since Internalism would allow 'anything the externalist could want'.[4]

Given the difference between (E) and (M), the distinction between these views is deep. Most Internalists describe deliberation in partly normative terms. But, since their conception of rationality is procedural, it is an empirical, psychological question whether claims like (M) are true.[5] Thus we might be unable to predict whether, if Williams's imagined person were procedurally rational, he would be motivated to take the medicine that he knows he needs.[6] When Externalists appeal to (E), their claim is not empirical. It is a normative question whether, if this person failed to be motivated, that would make him less than fully rational.

There is a related difference in the way the inferences run. According to Internalists, if (R) is true, that is *because* (M) is true. The psychological fact described in (M) is, or is part of, what makes (R) true. According to Externalists, (E) is merely a consequence of (R). What gives us reasons for acting are not facts about our own motivation, but facts about our own or other people's well-being, or facts about other things that are worth achieving, or—some would add—moral requirements. Internalists derive conclusions about reasons from psychological claims about the motivation that, under certain conditions, we would in fact have. Externalists derive, from normative claims about what is worth achieving, conclusions about reasons, and about the motivation that we ought to have.

If we turn to morality, there is a similar pair of views. According to

> *Moral Internalism*: We cannot have a duty to act in some way unless (M) is true.

This view restricts the range of those to whom moral claims apply. According to Moral Internalists, if informed and rational deliberation would not lead us to be motivated to do something, it cannot be our duty to do this thing. Those who were sufficiently ruthless, or amoral, would have no duties—and, some Internalists conclude,

---

4. *IROB*, p. 36.

5. More precisely, while it is a normative question which kinds of deliberation are procedrally rational, it is an empirical question whether, if we deliberated in such a way, we would be motivated to act.

6. As Williams writes: 'I take it that insofar as there are determinately recognisable needs, there can be an agent who lacks any interest in getting what he needs. I take it, further, that lack of interest can remain after deliberation' (IER, p. 105).

could not be held to be acting wrongly. *Moral Externalists* reject these claims. On the simplest version of their view, moral requirements apply to all of us, whether or not (M) is true.

We should also consider a view, not about the motivational implications of reasons or morality, but about moral reasons. According to

> *Moral Rationalism*: Moral requirements always give, to those to whom they apply, reasons for acting.

According to those who reject Moral Rationalism, people who do not care about morality might have a duty to act in some way without having any reason to do so.

The relation between these views can be shown as follows:

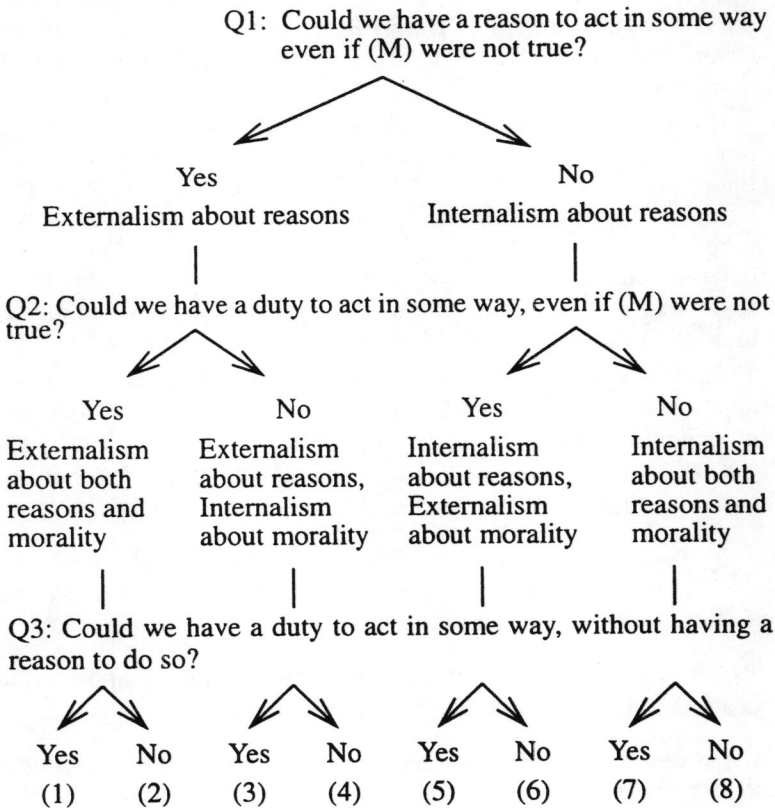

Q1: Could we have a reason to act in some way
even if (M) were not true?

Yes   No
Externalism about reasons   Internalism about reasons

Q2: Could we have a duty to act in some way, even if (M) were not true?

Yes   No   Yes   No

Externalism   Externalism   Internalism   Internalism
about both   about reasons,   about reasons,   about both
reasons and   Internalism   Externalism   reasons and
morality   about morality   about morality   morality

Q3: Could we have a duty to act in some way, without having a reason to do so?

Yes   No   Yes   No   Yes   No   Yes   No

(1)   (2)   (3)   (4)   (5)   (6)   (7)   (8)

104   I—DEREK PARFIT

If we are Externalists about both reasons and morality, we may believe that we always have a moral reason to do our duty. This is view (2), or Externalist Moral Rationalism. On a stronger version of this view, if some act is our duty, that makes it what we have most reason to do.

Though Double Externalists can be Moral Rationalists, they do not have to be. According to some writers, for example, though self-interest provides external reasons, morality does not. Such people accept view (1).[7]

If we are Double Internalists, we are likely to be Moral Rationalists, accepting (8) rather than (7). On this view, we cannot have a duty to act in some way unless (M) is true, and we are likely to believe that (M)'s truth would, in such cases, give us a reason for acting. We would then conclude that we always have a reason to do our duty. This version of Moral Rationalism is weaker than the Externalist version, since it restricts morality to those who have moral motivation.

Even if we are Internalists about reasons, we may believe that moral requirements apply to everyone. We shall then combine Internalism about reasons with Externalism about morality. On this view, we cannot be Moral Rationalists. We preserve morality's scope at the cost of denying its reason-giving force. Though we believe that people can have duties whatever their motivational state, we must admit that, on our view, people may have no reason to do their duty. Since this view implies (5), (6) is untenable.

The remaining views are (3) and (4), which combine Externalism about reasons with Internalism about morality. Though not incoherent, these views are too implausible to be worth discussing.

Consider now, not our *having* some reason for acting, but our *believing* that we have some reason. According to

> *Belief Internalism*: Beliefs about reasons necessarily involve motivation. We cannot believe that we have a reason to do something without being motivated to do this thing.

Belief Externalists reject this claim. More commonly appealed to is another, more restricted view. According to

---

7. This view was suggested, for example, in Philippa Foot's 'Morality as a System of Hypothetical Imperatives'.

Moral Belief Internalism: Moral beliefs necessarily involve motivation. We cannot believe some act to be our duty without being motivated to do it.

On a stronger version of this view, we cannot have a moral belief without being moved, if the opportunity arises, to act upon it.[8]

Consider next some views about motivation. According to

the Humean theory: No belief could motivate us unless it is combined with some independent desire.

Such a desire is *independent* when it is not itself produced by our having this belief.

As Nagel and others claim, we can reject this theory.[9] When we come to have some belief—such as the belief that some aim is worth achieving—that might cause us to have some wholly new desire. Such a belief could not all by itself cause us to have this desire, since we would have to be *such that*, if we came to have this belief, that would cause us to have this desire. But this disposition may not itself be a desire. On a variant of this anti-Humean view, whenever a belief moves us to act, we can be truly said to have wanted to act as we did; but this desire may not be a distinct mental state, since it may consist in our being moved by this belief. In either of these ways, reason might have the power that Hume denied. By giving us such beliefs, reason might motivate us without the help of any independent desire.

Humeans might retreat to the view that, for beliefs to motivate us, they must be combined with desires, even if these beliefs themselves produce these desires. But, with this revision, the Humean theory would lose most of its significance. According to Hume, reason is, and must be, wholly inert or inactive, as must be anything that reason alone could produce.[10] We could not claim that reason cannot be active on the ground that, though it might

8. In drawing these distinctions, I follow Stephen Darwall, *Impartial Reason* (Cornell University Press, 1983) p. 54.

9. *The Possibility of Altruism*, Oxford University Press, 1970, Chapter V. Of the other authors who challenge this theory, I have learnt most from Jonathan Dancy, *Moral Reasons* (Blackwell, 1993) Chapters 1 to 3, and 'Why there is really no such thing as the Theory of Motivation', *Proceedings of the Aristotelian Society*, 1995, pp. 1–18; and Francis Snare, *Morals, Motivation, and Convention* (Cambridge University Press, 1991) Chapters 1 to 5.

10. In Hume's words, 'an active principle can never be founded on an inactive', *A Treatise of Human Nature*, edited by L. A. Selby-Bigge, (Oxford University Press), p. 457.

motivate us, it could do that only by producing some new desire. That would be like claiming that some bomb cannot be destructive because, though it might destroy us, it could do that only by producing some explosion.

Consider finally two Humean arguments. According to some non-cognitivists:

> (A) If we have some moral conviction, we must be motivated to act upon it.
>
> (B) If moral convictions were beliefs, (A) could not be true.

Therefore

> (C) Moral convictions cannot be beliefs.

In defending (B), these non-cognitivists appeal to the Humean theory. They might say: 'If moral convictions were beliefs, they could not motivate us without the help of some independent desire, so it would be conceivable that we might have some moral conviction without being motivated to act upon it. Since that is inconceivable, moral convictions must themselves be desires, or pro-attitudes.'

If we are cognitivists about morality, and wish to deny (B), it would not be enough to show that we can reject the Humean theory. Even if moral beliefs *could* motivate us without the help of some independent desire, that would not explain how such beliefs *necessarily* involve motivation. To reject (B), we might appeal to

the Platonic theory: Moral knowledge necessarily motivates.

Or we might claim that, unless we cared about morality, we would not be able to have moral beliefs. But, for cognitivists, both claims are hard to defend and explain.[11]

We may find it easier to question (A), or Moral Belief Internalism. Or we might try to show that, in the sense in which (A) is true, it does not support non-cognitivism. Thus we might claim that, while moral beliefs are not called 'convictions' or 'sincere' unless they involve motivation, those who lack such

---

11. We would also need to extend the Platonic theory so that it covered even false moral beliefs.

motivation might still know that their acts were wrong. Such knowledge may imply belief in the sense that cognitivism requires. According to another Humean argument:

> (D) When moral convictions motivate us, they can do that without the help of any independent desire.

> (E) No belief could have this property.

Therefore

> (C) Moral convictions cannot be beliefs, but must themselves be desires.

This argument is weaker. Unlike (A), (D) has little intuitive appeal.[12] And, to deny (E), it *is* enough to reject the Humean theory.

My description of these views differs from those that are sometimes given. Several writers, for example, conflate my four versions of Internalism. That leads them to overlook important possibilities. Consider next what Korsgaard calls

> *the internalism requirement*: 'Practical reason claims, if they are really to present us with reasons for action, must be capable of motivating rational persons.'[13]

My Externalists could accept this requirement. Some would make the stronger claim that, if we believe that we have a reason to do something, and we are fully practically rational, we *must* be motivated to do this thing.

Korsgaard also says that, according to externalists, an act's rightness is not a reason for doing it.[14] Several other writers make such claims.[15] This use of 'externalist' conflicts with mine. It is my Double Externalists who can most easily be Moral Rationalists, since they can regard morality as always giving everyone reasons for acting. Why do these writers claim that, if we are externalists, we shall deny that an act's rightness is a reason for doing it? They may assume that, even if we are Externalists about morality, or

---

12. Though it might be claimed that (D) is implied by (A).

13. 'Skepticism about Practical Reason', *The Journal of Philosophy*, Volume 83, No 1 (January 1986) reprinted in Christine Korsgaard, *Creating the Kingdom of Ends* (Cambridge University Press, 1996), p. 317.

14. *Creating the Kingdom of Ends*, p. 43.

15. See, for example, David Brink, *Moral Realism and the Foundations of Ethics* (Cambridge University Press, 1989) pp. 37–43, and Michael Smith, *The Moral Problem* (Blackwell, 1994) pp. 62–3.

108   I—DEREK PARFIT

moral beliefs, we must be Internalists about reasons.[16] Or they may
conflate normative reasons and motivating states.[17]

We can now draw some more distinctions. According to
Internalists, for it to be true that

> (R) We have a reason to do something,

it is necessary—and, some add, sufficient—that

> (M) if we deliberated on the facts in a procedurally rational
> way, we would be motivated to do this thing.

This view can take at least three forms:

> *Analytically Reductive:* When we assert (R), what we mean
> is (M).

> *Non-Analytically Reductive:* Though these claims do not
> mean the same, when (R) is true, that normative fact is the
> same as, or consists in, the fact reported by (M).

> *Non-Reductive:* The facts reported by (R) and (M) are very
> different. While (M) is psychological, (R) is an irreducibly
> normative truth.

Reductive Internalism is a form of naturalism. Non-Reductive
Internalism is a form of non-reductive normative realism.

There is another form of Internalism that is, in a weak sense,
non-reductive. According to some non-cognitivists, since (R) is a
normative claim, it cannot be, in a strong sense, true. If we claim
that (R) requires (M), we are expressing some kind of attitude.[18]

Similar remarks apply to Externalism. Thus, according to most
Externalists,

16. Thus David McNaughton writes that, according to externalists, 'someone who has no
concern for human welfare may still recognize that inflicting unnecessary suffering on others
is morally wrong. But that recognition is held not to be in itself sufficient to give him a reason
to desist from causing such suffering. If he lacks the appropriate desires then he has no reason
to act in accordance with moral requirements', (*Moral Vision* (Blackwell, 1988) pp. 48–9).
My Externalists can deny that reasons presuppose desires.

17. Thus McNaughton also writes that externalism regards 'moral questions as factual ones
but distances them from *motivation* in its claim that moral commitments do not, in
themselves, provide the agent with *reason* to act'; in contrast, on 'an internalist account of
moral *motivation*', there are facts awareness of which 'will supply the observer with *reason*
to act' (*op. cit.,* pp. 49 and 105, my italics).

18. Cf. Allan Gibbard, *Wise Choices, Apt Feelings* (Oxford University Press, 1990). I must
here ignore such views.

(P) We have a prudential reason to act in some way

if and only if

(S) this way of acting would promote our own well-being.

(P) and (S) might mean the same, or report the same fact in two different ways, or report two very different facts, or this Externalist view might consist in the holding of some attitude.

That completes my proposed taxonomy. I shall now begin to suggest why, as I believe, we should be non-reductive normative realists, and should regard all reasons as external.

II

In the articles that have done most to clarify and to show the importance of these questions, Williams argues that there are no external reasons.

Williams's main objection is that Externalists have not explained what such reasons could be. He considers someone who maltreats his wife, and whose attitudes and acts would not be altered by informed and rational deliberation. If we are Externalists, we might claim that, despite this man's motivational state, his wife's unhappiness gives him reasons to treat her better. In rejecting this claim, Williams asks:

> what is the difference supposed to be between saying that the agent has a reason to act more considerately, and saying one of the many other things we can say to people whose behaviour does not accord with what we think it should be? As, for instance, that it would be better if they acted otherwise?[19]

We might answer: 'The difference is that, if we merely said that it would be better if this man acted more considerately, we would not be claiming that, as we believe and you deny, he has reasons to do so.'

Williams's ground for rejecting this claim is that he finds it 'quite obscure' what it could mean. As he writes elsewhere, Externalists do not 'offer any *content* for external reasons statements'.[20]

19. *IROB*, pp. 39–40.
20. *WME*, p. 191, my italics.

110   I—DEREK PARFIT

Williams may here be assuming Analytical Internalism.[21] On this
view, in claiming that

> (1) this man has reasons to treat his wife better,

we would mean that

> (2) if he deliberated rationally on the facts, he would be
>   motivated to treat her better.

If (1) meant (2), and we knew that (2) was false, it would indeed be
obscure what, in claiming (1), we could mean. *Non*-Analytical
Internalists would not find our claim so obscure. Such Internalists
believe that, though (1) is true only if (2) is true, these claims have
different meanings. These Internalists would understand—though
they would reject—the view that, despite this man's motivational
state, he has reasons to treat his wife better.

Discussing another, similar example, Williams asks:

> What is gained, except perhaps rhetorically, by claiming that A has
> a reason to do a certain thing, when all one has left to say is that
> this is what... a decent person... would do?[22]

This question seems to assume that, if our claim about A does not
have the sense described by Analytical Internalists, there is nothing
distinctive left for it to mean. We couldn't mean that, despite A's
motivational state, A has a reason to do this thing. If we could mean
that, there would be a simple answer to Williams's question. We
might be saying something that was both distinctive and true.

Williams continues:

> it would make a difference to ethics if certain kinds of *internal*
> reason were very generally to hand... But what difference would
> external reasons make?... Should we suppose that, if genuine
> external reasons were to be had, morality might get some leverage
> on a squeamish Jim or priggish George, or even on the fanatical
> Nazi?... I cannot see what leverage it would secure: what would
> these external reasons do to these people, or for our relations to
> them?

21. As he seems to do elsewhere. Thus he writes: 'I think the sense of a statement of the
form "A has a reason to *phi*" is given by the internalist model' (*IROB*, p. 40). See also *IER*,
pp. 109–10, and *IROB*, p. 36. In his most recent discussion, however, on *MWE*, p. 188,
Williams rejects Analytical Internalism.

22. *WME*, p. 215.

These remarks assume that, for external reasons to make a difference to ethics, such reasons would have to get *leverage* on people, by motivating them to act differently. This conception of ethics is, I believe, too utilitarian. When we believe that other people have reasons for caring, or for acting, we do not have these beliefs as a way of affecting those people. Our aim is, not influence, but truth. Similar remarks apply to morality. Someone might say:

> What difference would it make if it were true that the Nazis acted wrongly? What leverage would that moral fact have secured? What would the wrongness of their acts have done to them?

Even if moral truths cannot affect people, they can still be truths. People can be acting wrongly, though the wrongness of their acts does not do anything to them.

After asking what external reasons would do to such people, Williams writes:

> Unless we are given an answer to that question, I, for one, find it hard to resist Nietzsche's plausible interpretation, that the desire of philosophy to find a way in which morality can be guaranteed to get beyond merely *designating* the vile and recalcitrant, to trans-fixing them or getting inside them, is only a fantasy of *ressentiment*, a magical project to make a wish and its words into a coercive power.[23]

Williams has a real target here. Many philosophers have hoped to find moral arguments, or truths, that could not fail to motivate us. Williams, realistically, rejects that hope.

Note however that, in making these remarks, Williams assumes that claims about reasons could achieve only two things. If such claims cannot get inside people, by inducing them to act differently, they can only designate these people. On the first alternative, these claims would have motivating force. On the second, they would be merely classificatory, since their meaning would be only that, if these people were not so vile, or were in some other way different, they *would* act differently. As before, however, there is a third possibility. Even when such claims do not have motivating force, they could be more than merely classificatory.

23. *WME*, p. 216.

They could have *normative* force. Perhaps these people *should* act differently.

We should remember next that Externalists need not be Moral Rationalists. Some Externalists would agree with Williams that those who act wrongly may have no reason to act differently. These people are Externalists in their beliefs about prudential reasons. Return to Williams's imagined person who needs some medicine to protect his health, and whose failure to care about his future would survive any amount of informed and procedurally rational deliberation. Such a person, Williams writes, would have no reason to take this medicine.[24] He might ask:

> What would be gained by claiming that this person has such a reason? What would that add to the claim that, if he were prudent, he would take this medicine?

This claim would add what Williams denies. This person, these Externalists believe, ought rationally to take this medicine. He has reasons to care about his future; and, since these are reasons for caring, this person's failure to care does not undermine these reasons. Such claims, I believe, make sense, and might be true.

Williams suggests several arguments against their sense and truth. According to one such argument:

(A) Normative reasons must be able to be motivating reasons. It must be possible that we should act *for these reasons*.

(B) Motivating reasons must be internal, since our acts must be in part explained by our desires, or other motivating states.

Therefore

(C) Normative reasons must be internal.[25]

If we reject the Humean theory of motivation, we might question (B). Some of our acts, we might claim, are fully explained by our beliefs.

---

24. *IER*, 105–6.

25. This argument, which Williams may not intend, is suggested by remarks in *IER*, pp. 102 and 106–7, and in *IROB*, p. 39.

We can also claim, that in the sense in which (A) is true, it does not support (C). Suppose that, unlike Williams's imagined person, I care about my future. As Internalists would then agree, if it is true that

(3) I need some medicine to protect my health,

this fact would give me a reason to take this medicine. For (3) to give me such a reason, it must be possible, as (A) claims, that I should act for this reason. That condition would be met if, when asked why I took this medicine, I could truly answer, 'Because I need it to protect my health'. The normative reason provided by (3) could then be said to *be* my motivating reason. But, though these reasons would be in that sense the same, they would still differ in at least two ways. First, for (3) to have given me my motivating reason, I must have believed (3). But, even if I had not had this belief, (3)'s truth would have given me a normative reason to take this medicine. We can have reasons of which we are unaware.[26] Second, I would have had this same motivating reason even if my belief had been false.[27] But, if (3) had been false, I would have had no normative reason to take this medicine: I would have merely thought I did. So, while motivating reasons require that we have some belief, whether or not this belief is true, normative reasons are provided by some truth, whether or not we believe it.

Return now to the argument sketched above. Perhaps, for (3) to have given me my motivating reason, I must have wanted to protect my health, or had some other relevant desire. That might make this reason internal. But that would not show that my normative reason must have been internal. As we have just seen, normative and motivating reasons are not identical. Though motivating reasons require that we have some belief, that is not true of the corresponding normative reasons. Since an appeal to (A) could not show that, to have some normative reason, we must have some belief, it cannot show that, to have some normative reason, we must have some desire, or other motivating state. Externalists are free to claim that, even if I had not cared about my health, and my indifference would have survived procedurally rational deliber-

26. As Williams would agree. See, for example, *IER*, pp. 102–3.
27. As Williams writes: 'The difference between false and true beliefs on the agent's part cannot alter the *form* of the explanation which will be appropriate to his action' (*IER*, p. 102).

ation, I would have had a normative reason to take the medicine that I need.[28]

Consider next someone who has no internal reason to act in some way. Let us call this person *Jack*, and this way of acting *X*. Suppose we claim that

>   (4) Jack has some external reason to do X.

Williams writes that, if Jack comes to believe (4), 'he will be motivated to act; so coming to believe it must, essentially, involve acquiring a new motivation. How can that be?'[29] These remarks suggest that, if we are Externalists, we cannot explain the truth of Belief Internalism.

There is, I believe, nothing to explain. Belief Internalism is most clearly false when applied to people who accept Reductive Internalism. Suppose that such a person comes to believe that

>   (5) if he knew certain facts, and deliberated rationally, he would be motivated to act in some way.

As a Reductive Internalist, this person may conclude that he has a reason to act in this way. But, because he doesn't yet know these facts, he might not be motivated to do so. People often try to avoid

---

28. It may be objected that, if I had not cared about my health, and my indifference would have survived such deliberation, it would *not* have been possible, as (A) requires, that I should have acted for this reason. But, in the sense in which (A) is uncontroversial, it means only that, if certain facts are claimed to provide normative reasons, it must be true that '*people sometimes* act for these reasons' (*IER*, p. 102, my italics). The kind of reason that (3) provides meets that requirement. People sometimes take medicine that they know they need. This last objection takes (A) to mean that, for it to be true that some particular person has some normative reason, it must be possible that, on *this* occasion, and *without* any further change in this person's motivational state, *this* person should act for this reason. So interpreted, (A) could not support an argument for Internalism, since it would merely restate this view.

Much more needs to be said about motivating reasons. Such reasons can be acceptably regarded in two ways. On the *psychological account*, motivating reasons are beliefs and/or desires, when these explain our decisions and our acts. On the *non-psychological account*, motivating reasons are *what* we believe and/or *what* we want. Thus, when asked, 'Why did he jump?', we might truly claim: 'Because the hotel was on fire', or 'Because he believed the hotel was on fire', or 'To save his life', or 'Because he wanted to save his life'.

Since both accounts are acceptable, we should accept both, and should thus conclude that there are two kinds of motivating reason: one kind are mental states, the other are the contents or objects of these states. These two kinds of reason always go together. For some purposes, especially normative discussion, the non-psychological account is more natural; for others, such as causal explanation, we must appeal to the psychological account. The acceptability of both accounts can, however, cause confusion. On one account, motivating reasons are the true or apparent normative reasons belief in which explain our decisions and our acts. On the other account, motivating reasons are motivating states. Since *motivating* reasons can thus be regarded *both* as normative reasons *and* as motivating states, that may suggest that *normative* reasons are motivating states. That, I believe, is a grave mistake.

29. *IER*, p. 108.

learning certain facts because they want to avoid the motivation which, as they predict, that knowledge would arouse in them.

Externalists need not claim that, if Jack came to believe (4), that would guarantee that he would be motivated to do X. But they might claim that, if Jack were rational, his coming to have this belief would motivate him. For that to be so, Williams writes, (4) 'will have to be taken as roughly equivalent to, or at least as entailing', the claim that

> (6) if Jack 'rationally deliberated, then, whatever moti-
> vations he originally had, he would come to be
> motivated' to do X.

But, if (4) entails (6), Williams continues,

> it is very plausible to suppose that all external reason statements
> are false. For, *ex hypothesi*, there is no motivation for the agent to
> deliberate *from*, to reach this new motivation.

If Jack did become motivated to do X, as a result of such deliberation, Jack's new motivation would have to have been reached *from* some earlier motivation. But 'in that case', Williams objects, 'an *internal* reason statement would have been true'.[30]

If we are Externalists, we could give three replies. First, this objection seems to assume the Humean theory. As I have said, we can reject this theory. When Jack comes to believe (4), that might produce in him some wholly new desire.[31] For that to happen, Jack would have to be such that, if he came to believe (4), he would develop this new desire; but that disposition may not itself be a desire, or other motivating state. Since Jack would not be deliberating *from* some earlier motivation, it is doubtful whether, before he developed this desire, he would have had an internal reason to do X.

Second, even if Jack would have had such a reason, that would not show it to be false that

> (4) Jack has some external reason to do X.

(4) does not imply that Jack has no internal reason to do X. (4) means that Jack has a reason to do X that is not provided by, and

---

30. *IER*, p. 109, my italics.

31. Williams himself writes that 'reason, that is to say, rational processes, can give rise to new motivations' (*IER*, p. 108). The argument that we are now discussing must, however, assume that Jack could not rationally become motivated to do X except by deliberating from some earlier motivation. Without that assumption, (4) might both entail (6) and be true.

does not require, the motivational fact—(M)—to which Internalists appeal. Jack may have this external reason even if, because (M) is true, he also has an internal reason to do the same thing.[32]

Third, when Williams refers to *rational* deliberation, he uses 'rational', as we have seen, in a procedural sense. For our deliberation to be procedurally rational, we must avoid 'errors of fact or reasoning', and we must meet certain other conditions; but there are no substantive requirements on the motivation with which we begin. If that is the sense of 'rationally' used in (6), Externalists can deny that (4) entails (6). On that reading, the claim that (4) entails (6) assumes Internalism; so it cannot be an argument for this view. And if this entailment seems plausible, Externalists can say, that is because (6) has a different reading. (6) could be taken to mean

> (7) If Jack deliberated on the facts, and were fully substantively rational, he would be motivated to do X.

To be substantively rational, we must want, and do, what we know that we have most reason to want and do. If what (4) entails is (7), it is irrelevant whether, after informed and procedurally rational deliberation, Jack would be motivated to do X. What (4) would entail is that, if Jack were substantively rational, his awareness of this external reason would motivate him. This claim, which Externalists could happily accept, is not challenged by the argument that we are now discussing.[33]

Williams sometimes appeals to a weaker form of Internalism. On this view, for it to be true that we have a reason to do something,

---

32. As before, Williams himself notes that claims about internal reasons do not conflict with claims about external reasons (*IER* p. 108). This suggests that I am misinterpreting the first full paragraph on *IER* p. 109. Williams's argument may instead be this:

(i) Since (4) entails (6), Jack cannot have an external reason to do X unless it is true that, if he rationally deliberated, he would become motivated to do X.

(ii) Jack could not rationally become motivated to do X unless he were deliberating from some earlier motivation.

(iii) In that case, Jack would have had an internal reason to do X.

(iv) *Ex hypothesi*, however, Jack had no such reason.

Therefore

(v) Jack cannot have an external reason to do X.

As I have just implied, and shall argue further below, we can reject (ii).

33. As Williams points out, (4) could not always entail (7), since what Jack has reason to do may in part depend on facts about him that would not have obtained if he had been fully substantively rational (*WME*, p. 190).

REASONS AND MOTIVATION 117

it need not be true that, after a certain process of deliberation, we *would* become motivated to do this thing. What is required is only that, by deliberating in this way, we *could rationally* come to have such motivation.[34]

When stating this view, Williams often applies it, not to our becoming motivated, but to our deciding to act. For such a decision to be rational, as Williams notes, we must believe that we have *most* reason to act in some way. According to what we can call

> *Weak Internalism*: For it to be true that
>
> > (A) X is what we have most reason to do,
>
> it must be true that
>
> > (B) there is 'a sound deliberative route', starting from our 'existing motivations', by which we could rationally decide to do X.

According to the rival view, which we can call

> *Strong Externalism*: If it is true that
>
> > (A) X is what we have most reason to do,
>
> it must be true that
>
> > (C) we could rationally decide to do X, for this reason, *whatever* our existing motivations.[35]

In rejecting Strong Externalism, Williams calls it 'unattractive'. What objection might he have in mind?

Strong Externalists assume that, given certain ways of specifying X, (A) could be true whatever our existing motivations. Williams would reject this assumption, since he believes that, for (A) to be true, (B) must be true. But, since this belief assumes Weak Internalism, it cannot provide an argument for preferring Weak Internalism to the rival, Strong Externalist view.

34. *IER*, p. 105, and *IROB*, p. 35.

35. I take my description of these views from *WME*, pp. 186–7. The phrase 'we could rationally' here means 'it would not be irrational for us'.

Such an argument must allow us to suppose that, whatever our existing motivations, (A) might be true. The argument must claim that, even if we come to believe truly that

(A) X is what we have most reason to do,

that, by itself, would not make it rational for us to decide to do X. For such a decision to be rational, we must have reached it by a deliberative route that appealed to some motivation that we already had.[36]

There seem to be two ways to defend these claims. Weak Internalists might say that, even if (A) is true, we could not rationally come to believe (A) except by deliberating from some earlier motivation. Or they might say that even if, in some other way, we have rationally come to believe (A), that would not make it rational for us, whatever our earlier motivations, to decide to do X.

Both these claims can be plausibly denied. If it is true that we have most reason to act in some way, it could be rational to come to believe that truth by some process of deliberation that did not start from facts about our existing motivations. When we consider certain other facts or arguments, we may rationally change our view about which aims are worth achieving, and we may thus be rationally led to some new belief about what we have reason to do.[37] And, if we believe both rationally and truly that we have most reason to act in some way, that must make it rational for us, whatever our earlier motivations, to decide to act in this way. That is an understatement. If we know that we have most reason to act in some way, it would be irrational for us *not* to make that decision.

Weak Internalists might now reply that, if we decide to do X because we come to believe (A), we must have been deliberating *from* one of our earlier motivations. Williams includes, among what he counts as motivations, 'dispositions of evaluation.'[38] Since our deliberation has led us to believe (A), and to decide to do X, we must have been such that, given such deliberation, we

---

36. The argument might then claim that, if (A) doesn't entail (C), we should drop our assumption that, even if (B) is false, (A) might be true.

37. For what may be a different view, which appeals to a 'non-rational' change of mind like that involved in 'conversion', see John McDowell, 'Might there be external reasons?', (*MWE*, pp. 72–8).

38. *IER*, p. 105.

might come to reach that belief and make that decision. We must, that is, have had a disposition to reach this evaluative conclusion. And that might be held to show that, as Weak Internalists claim, any rational decision to act must be reached by deliberation from some pre-existing motivation.

Williams would not, I believe, give this reply. It would achieve nothing. No Externalist would mind conceding that, if our deliberation leads us to make some decision, we must have been such that our deliberation might lead us to make this decision.[39]

Return now to Williams's objections to the weaker form of Externalism. Williams suggests one other argument against this view. Externalists might say, he writes,

> that the force of an external reason statement can be explained in the following way. Such a statement implies that a rational agent would be motivated to act appropriately, and it can carry this implication because a rational agent is precisely one who has a general disposition... to do what (he believes) there is reason for him to do.[40]

Such a claim, Williams objects,

> merely puts off the problem... *What* is it that one comes to believe when he comes to believe that

> > [(1)] there is reason for him to do X,

> if it is not the proposition, or something that entails the proposition, that

> > [(2)] if he deliberated rationally, he would be motivated to act appropriately?

> We were asking how any true proposition could have that content; it cannot help, in answering that, to appeal to a supposed desire which is activated by a belief which has that very content.[41]

Since Williams believes that (1) could be true, and that (1) either means or entails (2), the problem that he mentions cannot be how

---

39. Suppose that we are *not* such that, if we deliberated in this way, we might come to believe (A), and for that reason decide to do X. According to Weak Internalists, (A) would then be false. According to Strong Externalists, (A) might still be true. Strong Externalism might here be claimed to violate the principle that 'ought' implies 'can'. Though I believe that this objection is unsound, I have no space to argue that here.

40. *IER*, p. 109.

41. *IER*, pp. 109–110 (I have substituted 'do X' for 'phi').

propositions with that content could be true. But his objection may be this. If we claim that (1) means (2), and we use 'rationally' in (2) in Williams's preferred procedural sense, that gives (1) a determinate content. It is an empirical question whether, if someone deliberated in this way, he would be motivated to act. But, if (2) is to give the content of a claim about some *external* reason, it would have to use 'rationally' in the other, substantive sense: the sense in which, to be fully rational, we must be motivated by our awareness of any reason. On such a view, in claiming that

> (1) someone has a reason to do X,

we would mean that

> (3) if this person deliberated on the facts, and he would be motivated to do whatever he knew that he had a reason to do, he would be motivated to do X.

This account would be vacuously circular. It would be like the view that, in claiming

> (4) We have a duty to do Y,

we mean

> (5) Y is what, if we always did our duty, we would do.

Even Kant needed to assume more than that.

Externalists can reply that, even if (1) entails (3), that is not all that (1) means. Return to Williams's imagined person who does not care about his further future, and whose indifference would survive any amount of Internalist deliberation. When we claim that such a person has reasons to care about his future, and to take the medicine that he needs, we do not merely mean that, if he were fully rational, he *would* care, and *would* take this medicine.

What, then, *do* we mean? We are back with Williams's main objection. As he later wrote: 'I do not believe... that the sense of external reason statements is in the least clear.'[42]

III

Williams's objection has great force. It is not, however, an objection to Externalism. Some Externalists hold analytically

---

42. *IROB*, p. 40.

reductive views. For example, they might say that, in claiming that this person has a reason to take this medicine, we mean that he needs this medicine, or that it would promote his well-being. Such proposed analyses are as clear as the one that Williams suggests.

Williams's objection applies to all views that are not analytically reductive. Some Internalists hold such views, since they believe that, even though claims about reasons must be supported by claims about the agent's motivation, that is not what they mean. If we hold such a view, and we were asked what 'reason' means, we would find this hard to explain. Reasons for acting, we might say, are facts that *count in favour* of some act. But 'counting in favour of' means 'giving a reason for'. Or we might say that, if we have *most reason* to act in some way, that is what we *ought rationally* to do, or—more colloquially—what we *should* do. But we could not understand this use of 'should' unless we had the concept of a reason.

These two concepts—that of a normative reason, and the concept that is expressed by this use of 'should'—cannot I believe be helpfully explained, since they cannot be explained in non-normative terms. This fact is not surprising. Normative concepts form a fundamental category—like, say, temporal or logical concepts. We should not expect to explain time, or logic, in non-temporal or non-logical terms. Similarly, normative truths are of a distinctive kind, which we should not expect to be like ordinary, empirical truths. Nor should we expect our knowledge of such truths, if we have any, to be like our knowledge of the world around us.

To defend such a view, we must answer several objections, and we must show that other views are, in various ways, inadequate. I hope to do that elsewhere.[43] I shall end, here, with some brief and oversimplified remarks.

Reductive Internalism, as I have said, is a form of naturalism. According to analytical naturalists, normative statements mean the same as certain statements about natural facts. That cannot be true, Moore argued, since we could believe the latter but intelligibly question the former. Analytical naturalists rightly reply that some definitional truths can be, because they are not obvious, intelligibly questioned.

43. In my *Practical Realism*, Oxford University Press, in preparation.

122   I—DEREK PARFIT

Non-analytical naturalists reject Moore's argument as irrelevant. Such writers often appeal to analogies drawn from science, such as the discoveries that water is H_2O or that heat is molecular kinetic energy. These identities were not implied by the existing concepts of water and heat. In the same way, these writers claim, though normative and naturalistic statements do not mean the same, some pairs of such statements may turn out to refer to the same properties, or to report the same facts.

I believe that we should reject all forms of naturalism. Though we cannot helpfully explain what normative concepts mean, we can sufficiently explain what they do not mean. And we can thereby show that, if there are normative truths, these could not be the same as, or consist in, natural facts. These two kinds of fact are as different as the chairs and propositions that, in a dream, Moore once confused.

It may seem that, by appealing to claims about normative concepts, we could at most refute analytical naturalism. Since non-analytical naturalists do not appeal to claims about meaning, their views may seem immune to this kind of argument.

That, I believe, is not so. Reductive views can be both non-analytical and true when, and because, the relevant concepts leave open certain possibilities, between which we must choose on non-conceptual grounds. But many other possibilities are conceptually excluded. Thus it was conceptually possible that heat should turn out to be molecular kinetic energy. But heat could not have turned out to be a shade of blue, or a medieval king. In the same way, while it may not be conceptually excluded that experiences should turn out to be neurophysiological events, experiences could not turn out to be patterns of behaviour, or stones, or irrational numbers.

Similar claims apply, I believe, to Reductive Internalism, and to all other forms of naturalism. Since normative facts are in their own distinctive category, there is no close analogy for their irreducibility to natural facts. One comparison would be with proposed reductions of necessary truths—such as the truths of logic or mathematics—to certain kinds of contingent truths. Given the depth of the difference between these kinds of truth, we can be confident, I assume, that such reductions fail. There is a similar difference, I believe, between normative and natural truths.[44]

44. For strong objections to both of these reductive views, see Thomas Nagel, *The Last Word* (Oxford University Press, 1996).

Compare, for example, these two claims:

(1) There are acts that maximize happiness.

(2) There are acts that are right.

According to Reductive Utilitarians, even if (1) and (2) have different meanings, they report the same fact. One objection to this view is that it makes morality trivial. We already knew that some acts maximize happiness; and it could not be significant that this fact could be redescribed by calling these acts right. For morality to be significant, it must claim that, when acts have certain natural properties, something *else* is true: these acts are *right*. These must be *different* properties, and *different* facts.[45]

Return next to Reductive Internalism. Suppose that, because my hotel really is on fire, I know that

(A) Jumping into the canal is my only way to save my life.

Given my rational desire to live, I decide to jump. According to Reductive Internalists, if I accepted their view, my practical reasoning could be this:

(B) Jumping is what, after rationally deliberating on the truth of (A), I am most strongly motivated to do.

Therefore

(C) As another way of reporting (B), I could say that I have most reason to jump.

On this view, I believe, normativity disappears. If there are normative truths, they could not be facts like (B). When I believe that I have most reason to jump, I am believing that I *should* jump, and that, if I don't, I would be acting irrationally, or making a terrible mistake. That, if true, could not be the same as the fact that, after such deliberation, jumping is what I most want to do.

Reductive Internalists, or other naturalists, might give the following reply. When we claim that we have some reason for

---

45. Note that, for this objection to be good, it need not assume that there *are* any moral truths. It assumes only that, *if* there are such truths, they could not be in this way trivial. (Nor does this objection assume that moral naturalism is trivial. If morality were trivial, that fact would not be trivial.)

124   I—DEREK PARFIT

acting, what we appeal to is very often some natural fact. Thus, in our example, my reason to jump might be the fact that

(A) jumping is my only way to save my life,

or—less plausibly—the fact that

(D) jumping is my only way to get what I most want,

or—least plausibly—the fact described by (B). If any of these facts *is* my reason to jump, that reason, naturalists might claim, is a causal or psychological fact.

Such facts can indeed be claimed to be reasons for acting. But, if that is all we say, such claims are seriously misleading. They suggest that, in believing that there are normative reasons, and normative truths, we can avoid any commitment to non-natural properties and facts. That, I believe, is not so. We must distinguish between the fact that

(A) jumping is my only way to save my life,

and the fact that

(E) the truth of (A) gives me a reason to jump.

Though (A) has *normative significance*, (A) is not a normative fact. The normative fact is (E), or the fact *that* (A) has such significance. That is not, like (A) itself, an empirical or natural fact.

Naturalists would now reply that their view sufficiently preserves normativity. Thus, when discussing Analytical Internalism, Williams writes:

> It is important that even on the internalist view, a statement of the form 'A has reason to do X' still has what may be called *normative force*. Unless a claim to the effect that an agent has a reason to do X can go beyond what that agent is already motivated to do... then certainly the term will have too narrow a definition. 'A has reason to do X' means more than 'A is presently disposed to do X'.[46]

Williams's point may here be this. When we say that you have a reason to do something, we intend to be giving you advice. If our claim merely meant that you were already disposed to do this thing,

46. *IROB*, p. 36.

that would hardly be advice. Things are different if we mean, not that you are *now* disposed to do this thing, but that you *would become* so disposed if you knew certain facts. As Williams later writes, in saying what someone has reason to do, we are allowed to correct this person's factual beliefs, and 'that is already enough for the notion to be normative'.[47]

That, I believe, is not so. On this view, if we claimed

(F) You have a reason to jump,

we would mean

(G) If you believed the truth, you would want to jump.

(G) could indeed be used to give you advice. You may rightly assume that, if (G) is true, you must have a reason to jump. But that does not make (G) normative. (G) is like

(H) This building is on fire,

which could also be used to give advice. These cannot be normative claims, since they do not even use a normative concept.

It may be said that, though (G) is not explicitly normative, this claim has normative *force*. Have I not just admitted that (G) could be used to give you advice? But this fact does not, I believe, answer this objection. In claiming (G), we may be implying that you have a reason to jump. But, for such advice to be implied, it must be able to be explicitly stated. We must be able to think about what we have reason to do, or what we ought rationally to do. To be able to think such thoughts, we must understand the normative concepts *ought* and *reason*. And, if (F) meant (G), the concept of a reason would not be normative. If we had no concepts with which we could directly state or understand normative claims, we could not imply such claims by making other non-normative claims, even ones with normative significance.

Williams's own view appeals, not to mere knowledge of the facts, but to *rational* deliberation. On his proposed account, statements about reasons are explicitly normative. But, as I have begun to suggest, they are still not *relevantly* normative. On this view, the fact that

47. *IROB*, p. 36.

126   I—DEREK PARFIT

(R) we have a reason to do something

is the same as the fact that

(M) after informed and procedurally rational deliberation,
we would be motivated to do this thing.

However we answer the normative question of which kinds of
deliberation are procedurally rational, (M), if true, is a psychological fact. Though such facts can have normative significance,
they are not normative facts. And, if these were the only kinds of
fact to which our view appealed, we could not understand their
normative significance. Similar objections apply, I believe, to all
forms of normative naturalism, including those that are not
analytically reductive.

These objections, which I shall try to defend elsewhere,[48]
assume a certain view about normativity. Many people, I should
admit, hold very different views.

One difference is this. Many people, I believe mistakenly, regard
normativity as some kind of motivating force. For example,
Korsgaard writes that, if a certain argument 'cannot motivate the
reader to become a utilitarian then how can it show that
utilitarianism is normative?'[49] Railton writes: 'there is no need to
explain the normative force of our moral judgments on those who
have no tendency to accept them and who recognize no significant
community with us. For that is not a force that we observe in moral
practice.'[50] McNaughton writes that, when externalists deny that
moral beliefs necessarily motivate, they 'deny the authority of
moral demands'.[51] Scheffler writes that, even if wrong-doing were
always irrational, that would not give morality 'as much authority
as some might wish', since it would not 'guarantee... morality's
hold on us.'[52]

48. In my *Practical Realism, op. cit.*

49. *The Sources of Normativity* (Cambridge University Press, 1996) p. 85.

50. Peter Railton, 'What the Non-Cognitivist Helps Us to See', in *Reality, Representation,
and Projection*, edited by John Haldane and Crispin Wright (Oxford University Press, 1993).
Though Railton is here describing what other people might claim, he seems to endorse this
claim.

51. *op. cit.*, p. 48.

52. Samuel Scheffler, *Human Morality* (Oxford University Press, 1992) p. 76.

REASONS AND MOTIVATION   127

Consider next some remarks of Mackie's. Since Mackie is an *error theorist*, who believes that ordinary moral thinking is committed to peculiar non-natural properties, we might expect that he at least would give a non-reductive account of the normativity that he rejects. Mackie writes that, according to some cognitivists, a moral judgment is 'intrinsically and objectively prescriptive', since it 'demands' some action, and implies that other actions are 'not to be done.' These phrases look normative. But Mackie later writes that, in response to Humean arguments for non-cognitivism, cognitivists might

> simply deny the minor premiss: that the state of mind which is the making of moral judgments and distinctions has, *by itself*, an influence on actions. [They] could say that just seeing that this is right and that is wrong will not tend to make someone do this or refrain from that: he must also *want* to do whatever is right.

If cognitivists made such claims, Mackie continues, they would 'deny the *intrinsic* action-guidingness of moral judgments', and they would 'save the objectivity of moral distinctions... only by giving up their prescriptivity.' Mackie here assumes that, in claiming moral judgments to be action-guiding and prescriptive, we mean that such judgments can, by themselves, *influence* us, or tend to *make* us act in certain ways. So, even when describing the view that he rejects—or the 'objectively prescriptive values' that he calls 'too queer' to be credible—Mackie takes normativity to be a kind of motivating force.[53]

Normativity, I believe, is very different from motivating force. Neither includes, or implies, the other. Other animals can be motivated by their desires and beliefs. Only we can understand and respond to reasons.

Internalists could accept these claims. Some Internalists believe that, when we have some reason for acting, that is an irreducibly normative truth. But, as I shall also argue, we should reject even Non-Reductive Internalism.

If we consider only reasons for acting, Internalism may seem to be broadly right, or to contain most of the truth. But the most important reasons are not merely, or mainly, reasons for acting.

---

53. J.L.Mackie *Hume's Moral Theory* (Routledge and Kegan Paul, 1980) pp. 54–5. For another discussion of this view of normativity, see Stephen Darwall, 'Internalism and Agency', in *Philosophical Perspectives*, Volume 6, *Ethics*, 1992.

They are also reasons for having the desires on which we act. These are reasons to want some thing, for its own sake, which are provided by facts about this thing. Such reasons we can call *value-based*.

Since Internalist theories are desire-based, they cannot recognize such reasons. On such theories, all reasons to have some desire must derive from other desires. Thus we might have reason to want something to happen because this thing would have effects that we want, or because we want to have this desire, or because we want the effects of having it. But we cannot have reasons, provided by the nature of some thing, to have an intrinsic desire for that thing. Such a reason would have to be provided by our wanting this thing; but the fact that we had this desire could not give us a reason for having it. So, on desire-based theories, any chain of reasons must end with some desire that we have no reason to have.

Such a view, I believe, misses most of the truth. According to many Internalists, all reasons are provided by desires. There are, I believe, no such reasons. It is true that, in most cases, we have some reason to fulfil our desires. But that is because, in these cases, what we want is in some way worth achieving. We can also have reasons that *depend* on our desires, since our having some desire may affect what is worth achieving, or preventing—as when it makes some experience enjoyable or frustrating. But the fact that we have some desire never, by itself, provides reasons.[54]

Why has it been so widely thought that all reasons must be provided by desires, since we cannot have value-based reasons to have these desires?

There are some bad arguments for this view. Thus Hume claimed that, since reasoning is entirely concerned with truth, and desires cannot be true or false, desires cannot be supported by or contrary to reason. If this argument were good, it would show that, since acts cannot be true or false, acts cannot be supported by or contrary to reason. Most Internalists would reject that conclusion. And Hume's argument is not good. Hume assumed that there is only one kind of reason: reasons for believing. He said nothing to

---

54. For defences of this view, see Warren Quinn, 'Putting Rationality in its Place', in his *Morality and Action* (Cambridge University Press, 1993), and Thomas Scanlon, *What We Owe to Each Other* (Harvard University Press, forthcoming), Chapter 1.

support the view that we cannot have reasons either for caring or for acting.

Of the other grounds for ignoring, or rejecting, value-based reasons to have desires, one is especially relevant here. On Internalist theories, the source of all reasons is something that is not itself normative: it is the fact that we have some desire, or the fact that, if we knew more, we would be motivated to act in some way. On Externalist theories, the source of any reason is something normative. These theories appeal, not to facts about our actual or counterfactual desires, but to facts about what is relevantly worth achieving or preventing. Such alleged normative truths may seem to be metaphysically mysterious, or inconsistent with a scientific world view.

The important distinction here is not, however, between Internalism and Externalism. It is between reductive and non-reductive theories. For Internalist theories to be about normative reasons, they must, I have claimed, take a non-reductive form. Even if all reasons were provided by certain motivational facts, the fact that we have some reason could not be the same as, or consist in, such a motivational fact. Internalists must claim that, because some motivational fact obtains, something *else* is true: we have a reason for acting. In making that claim, they are committed to one kind of irreducibly normative truth. That undermines their reason to deny that there can be such truths about what is worth achieving, or preventing.

According to normative Internalism:

> (A) Some acts really are rational. There are facts about these acts, and their relations to our motivation, which give us reasons to act in these ways.

According to normative Externalism:

> (B) Some aims really are worth achieving. There are facts about these aims which give us reasons to want to achieve them.

(B), I believe, is no less plausible than (A). (B) has metaphysical implications, since it implies that there are irreducibly normative properties, or truths. But the same is true of (A).

Reasons for acting, I believe, are all external. When we have a reason to do something, this reason is not provided by, and does not require, the fact that after Internalist deliberation we would want to do this thing. This reason is provided by the facts that also give us reason to have this desire. We have reason to try to achieve some aim when, and because, it is relevantly worth achieving. Since these are reasons for *being* motivated, we would have these reasons even if, when we were aware of them, that awareness did not motivate us. But, if we are rational, it will.

[11]

REASONS AND MOTIVATION

Derek Parfit and John Broome

II—*John Broome*

REASON AND MOTIVATION[1]

Derek Parfit takes an externalist and cognitivist view about normative reasons. I shall explore this view and add some arguments that support it. But I shall also raise a doubt about it at the end.

I

When we are wondering what to do, how far can reason guide us?

No doubt it can guide us in forming empirical beliefs about the acts we might do: about their nature or their effects. That is one role it can have in guiding our actions. For instance, reason can guide us in forming beliefs about which means are appropriate to our ends. Suppose the hotel is burning and you want to stay alive. Reason, in the form of inductive and deductive reasoning, may guide you to form the belief that the only way to stay alive is to jump into the canal. Once you have formed this belief, you may find you want to jump into the canal, and indeed you may actually jump.

Some philosophers think this role exhausts the contribution reason can make to action. Reason has an influence on what we do only because it can guide our beliefs. Our beliefs in turn affect the desires we have, and hence what we do. Beyond that, reason can do nothing. In particular, though our beliefs affect our desires, reason plays no part in mediating this effect. Reason does not guide our desires, because no desire can be contrary to reason—irrational, that is to say. True, we may call a desire irrational in a derivative way. We might call one of your desires irrational if it results from a belief it is irrational for you to have. In that case, reason may be able to rid you of it by ridding you of the irrational belief. But in

---

1. I am grateful to Derek Parfit, Peter Schaber, John Skorupski and Stewart Shapiro for very helpful comments and discussion.

Reason, Emotion and Will

II—JOHN BROOME

this case the irrationality is in the belief and not the desire; reason can influence the belief directly, but the desire only indirectly. Provided it results from no irrational belief, a desire cannot be irrational. For instance, suppose you rationally believe the only way to stay alive is to jump, and you want to stay alive, but suppose the desire that arises in you as a result is not to jump but to remain on the windowsill singing happily. Then this desire is not irrational even derivatively, because it results from no false belief. Reason cannot guide you away from it.

In this theory, the connection between belief and desire is purely causal. Most of us are so constituted that, when we want something, and we believe that some particular act is the only way to get that thing, then we want to do that act. This disposition is one of our natural features, and it has nothing to do with reason. Someone who does not have it is not irrational, and someone who fails to exhibit it on a particular occasion is not irrational on that occasion. Let us call a person 'together' if she has this feature. Togetherness is not a part of rationality.

I shall call this minimalist theory about the role of reason in action 'the Humean theory of reason', and the role it ascribes to reason the 'Humean' role.[2] The Humean theory claims no desire or act is contrary to reason. It follows immediately that no desire or act is required by reason either, because if it was, the opposite desire or act would be contrary to reason. We may fairly say the Humean theory denies there is such a thing as practical reason. Reason's only role in practical matters is the theoretical one of guiding people's empirical beliefs.

The Humean theory of reason is surely implausible. If you want to stay alive, and you believe that jumping is the only way to do so, and the result is that you want to remain on the windowsill and sing, this want is surely irrational. Reason surely tells you at least that.

This thought can be reinforced by realizing that the relation between means and ends is normally much more complicated than it is in the jumping example. Normally we have many ends, which conflict to various degrees. Normally we have many acts to choose

---

2. Christine Korsgaard (in 'The normativity of instrumental reason', in Garrett Cullity and Berys Gaut (eds), *Ethics and Practical Reason*, Oxford University Press, 1997) and Elijah Millgram (in 'Was Hume a Humean?', *Hume Studies*, 21 (1995), pp. 75–93) report this as Hume's own view.

amongst and normally none of these acts will have perfectly certain results; each may bring about one or more of our ends with various degrees of likelihood. Furthermore, many of our activities interact with the activities of other people, and that adds the complications of strategic planning. How to choose appropriate means to our ends is the subject matter of decision theory and game theory. Game theory suggests that strategic planning is only possible if reason governs our acts as well as our beliefs. Even in nonstrategic situations, once all your relevant empirical beliefs are settled, it is still often a complicated matter to decide what to do. You might think, for instance: 'Given the likelihood of traffic and the penalty for missing the plane, I should leave home by 6.15; even though that means I should load the car the night before, and take the risk of its being broken into.' According to the Humean theory of reason, once you had formed the relevant empirical beliefs, you would have to leave it to your natural constitution, unaided by reason, to form in you a desire to leave at 6.15 and a desire to load the car the night before. But surely we rely on reason to guide us through these complicated problems; our unaided constitution is too unreliable.

How can reason help? An obvious answer in this case is that it can bring you to believe you ought to leave at 6.15, and you ought to load the car the night before. In general, it can bring you to normative beliefs: beliefs about what you ought to want or ought to do. This is a cognitivist answer. I shall pursue it through Sections II, III, IV and V. In Section VI I shall briefly mention a noncognitivist alternative.

II

If reason is to do what the cognitivist answer suggests, there must be valid patterns of inference that can lead to normative con-clusions. I do not mean we must necessarily reason by making formal derivations. But if reason is to bring us to normative beliefs, those beliefs must be justified by valid inferences. What might these patterns of inference be? I have little positive to say about this, but in this section I shall say something negative about one particular attempt to go beyond the Humean theory in this direction.

It can be imperfectly illustrated in the jumping example. You might reason: 'I want to stay alive; the only way for me to stay

alive is to jump; therefore, I ought to want to jump.' Here you apply to yourself an inference of the pattern:

(1)   *M* wants *X*, and the only way for *M* to get *X* is for her to do *A*. Therefore, *M* ought to want to do *A*.

At first sight this seems valid; its basis is the plausible general principle that a person's desires ought to be consistent with each other. *A* is not necessarily a means to *X*; it may be *X* itself under a particular description. For instance, writing an article is a way to work, but not a means to work; it is in itself working. Nevertheless, for brevity I shall call (1) 'naive instrumentalist reasoning'. By 'instrumentalism' I mean the view that our desires gives us reasons to pursue their satisfaction. Instrumentalism is one attempt to go beyond the Humean theory of reason.

As it happens, (1) is invalid for one type of reason that I propose to ignore. Even if the premises of (1) are true, *M* may want something else more than she wants *X*, or her dislike of doing *A* may outweigh her desire for *X*, and consequently it may not be true that she ought to want to do *A*. To deal with these problems properly, instrumentalism needs to be expressed using the resources of decision theory.[3] For one thing, it needs to be expressed in terms of preferences—comparative desires—rather than monadic desires. It should not appeal to a principle that a person's desires ought to be consistent, but to the principle that her preferences ought to be consistent. This requirement of consistency is precisely specified within decision theory. But to state instrumentalism properly in this way would take too much space, so I shall stick with the simple means-end example, and ignore these particular defects. To help avoid them, I intend the wants in (1) to be all-things-considered wants, which cannot be overridden by others.

It will be useful to compare another pattern of inference that also seems valid at first sight:

(2)   *M* believes *P*, and *M* believes *P* → *Q*. Therefore, *M* ought to believe *Q*.

---

3. Jean Hampton (in 'The failure of expected-utility theory as a theory of reason', *Economics and Philosophy*, 10 (1994), pp. 195–242) assumes that decision theory is itself an instrumentalist theory, and this is a common assumption. But it is mistaken. Decision theory can help to express instrumentalism accurately because it specifies consistency requirements for rational preferences. But it is consistent with decision theory to add noninstrumentalist requirements too. For instance, we might add the requirement that a person ought to prefer one thing to another if and only if it is better.

This seems a consequence of the plausible general principle that a person ought to believe the immediate consequences of her beliefs.

Both (1) and (2) derive an ought from an is; they draw a normative conclusion from non-normative premises. Presumably that is why Hume rejected (1) as a basis for practical reasoning. And indeed neither (1) nor (2) is valid, despite first appearances. To see (2) must be invalid, think about a case where M has inconsistent beliefs, as is obviously possible. Suppose she believes all of P, $P \rightarrow Q$, R and $R \rightarrow \neg Q$. Then (2) implies she ought to believe Q and she ought to believe $\neg Q$. But this cannot be true, because she ought not to have inconsistent beliefs.

Inference (1) also cannot be valid, because it can lead to inconsistent conclusions when a person has inconsistent desires. This is obvious, but a thoroughly convincing example is hard to produce, because the idea of inconsistent desires cannot be made precise without the resources of decision theory. We should really deal with inconsistent preferences rather than inconsistent desires. But, to stick with the simple example, suppose M desires both X and not X, and these are all-things-considered desires, so they are genuinely inconsistent with one another. Then (1) will imply both that M ought to want to do A and that she ought to want not to do A. These conclusions cannot both true, because M ought not to have inconsistent desires.

Although (1) and (2) are invalid, there is evidently some truth in the idea that you should have consistent desires and that you should believe the immediate consequences of your beliefs. There must be some way of fixing (1) and (2). One possibility is to make the ought that appears in them in some way relative. If M believes both P and $P \rightarrow Q$, perhaps she ought, in some way relative to these beliefs, to believe Q. Similarly the ought in (1) might be made relative to the desire. But a relative ought cannot justifiably guide a person in forming her beliefs and desires. Even if M ought, in some way relative to her desire for X, to want to do A, it remains possible that she ought nonrelatively not to want to do A. So the relative ought cannot justify her in wanting to do A.

To be sure, you can only draw inferences from the beliefs you have, so you can at best form your desires on the basis of what you believe you ought to want. This may be different from what you actually ought to want. Still, to be justified in wanting something,

you need to believe you ought nonrelatively to want it. But (1) could only lead you to believe you ought relatively to want it. You could consistently believe this and at the same time believe you ought nonrelatively not to want it. So this belief could not justify you in wanting it.

We could directly block the self-contradictory implications of (1) and (2) by adopting these more sophisticated inference patterns:

(3)   *M* wants *X*, and all *M*'s desires are consistent, and the only way for *M* to get *X* is for her to do *A*. Therefore *M* ought to want to do *A*.

(4)   *M* believes *P* and *M* believes *P* → *Q*, and all *M*'s beliefs are consistent. Therefore *M* ought to believe *Q*.

Let us call (3) 'sophisticated instrumentalist reasoning'. But (3) and (4) are subject to a second, equally fatal, objection. In (4), substitute '*P*' for '*Q*'. We can take it for granted that *M* believes the tautology *P* → *P*. So (4) implies that, if *M* believes *P*, and all her beliefs are consistent, it follows she ought to believe *P*. But it plainly does not follow. Similarly, (3) has a plainly false implication. Take a case where *X*, the thing *M* wants, is to do something, *B* (like stay alive). Then we can replace '*X*' in (3) with 'to do *B*'. Let us also substitute '*B*' for '*A*'. We get

(5)   *M* wants to do *B*, and all *M*'s desires are consistent, and the only way for *M* to do *B* is for her to do *B*. Therefore *M* ought to want to do *B*.

It is obviously true that the only way for *M* to do *B* is for her to do *B*. So we get that, if *M* wants to do *B*, and all her desires are consistent, it follows she ought to want to do *B*. This is plainly false. Just because you want something (and have consistent desires) it does not follow you ought to want it. Sophisticated instrumentalism is little better than the naive sort.

Schema (5) could not be obtained from (3) if we required *A* in (3) to be strictly a means to *X*. But that would not be enough to rescue (3). Wanting *X* does not give you a reason to want *A* when *A* is actually *X* itself under a particular description. *A fortiori*, it does not give you a reason to want *A* when *A* is a mere means to *X*. If wanting *X* cannot give you a reason to want an act that is *X* itself, it cannot give you a reason to want an act that is more remote

from *X*. Similarly, I have been doing instrumentalism no injustice by treating it as a view about what you ought to want rather than what you ought to do. If instrumentalist reasoning cannot validly conclude you ought to want to do an act, *a fortiori* it cannot validly conclude you ought to do the act. Instrumentalism is just false: wanting something is not a reason to want it, and consequently not a reason to try and get it.

Is there an alternative pattern of inference that could lead you to the conclusion that you ought to want to do some act? Consider:

(6)   *M* ought to want *X*, and the only way for *M* to get *X* is for her to do *A*. Therefore, *M* ought to want to do *A*.

This is instrumental reasoning, but not instrumentalism as I defined it. It has the same decision-theoretic problems I mentioned earlier over conflicting ends. But setting those aside, (6) is surely valid. However, it is useless if its premise that *M* ought to want *X* cannot ever be true. According to the Humean theory of reason, it cannot be, because no want can be required by reason. Instrumentalism tries to escape the Humean theory by claiming that *M* ought to want *X* if *X* is the only way of getting something *M* wants—for instance, you ought to want to stay alive if you want to see your friends again. But I have denied instrumentalism.

So I have so far made no positive progress towards extending the role of reason beyond the Humean one. To make progress in this direction, I would need to show how, for some *X*, it could be true that you ought to want *X*. That may be possible. For instance, perhaps I could show that you ought to want to stay alive. Perhaps it is a general principle of reason that you ought to want what is good, and perhaps it could be shown that your staying alive is good. But I shall not try and make this argument here. I shall now turn round and work forwards to what follows the conclusion of our reasoning, rather than backwards to what grounds it. For the sake of argument, I shall simply assume that (6) or some other pattern of reasoning can justify the conclusion that you ought to want to jump. Without this, the cognitivist theory I am exploring would not be possible.

Having got this far, we need not hesitate to go further and conclude you ought actually to jump. To be sure, there are unusual situations where you ought to want to do something (all things considered) without its being the case that you ought to do it. These

will be situations where the reason for wanting is a property of the
want itself and not of the act. (Parfit calls this a state-based reason
rather than an object-based one.) For instance, a millionaire might
offer you a large prize for wanting to drink a toxic drink, whether
or not you actually drink it.[4] But in (6) the reason for wanting to
do A is a property of X, which M will get only if she actually does
A. So (6) is not relevant to the unusual situations, and we can
conclude M ought to do A.

III

So let us now assume that in one way or another reason can lead us
to a conclusion about what we ought to do. If this is so, it means
reason goes far beyond its Humean role. It guides us, not merely to
beliefs in empirical propositions, but to beliefs in normative
propositions. In this, however, it is still playing a role that could
fairly be called theoretical rather than practical. It works by the
usual processes of inductive and deductive reasoning, and perhaps
by other reasoning processes too, to carry us from beliefs in some
propositions to beliefs in others. This reasoning would be exactly
the same whether conducted in the first person or the third person.
We cannot plausibly call third-person reasoning—which arrives,
for instance, at the conclusion that someone else ought to jump into
the canal—truly practical, even though its conclusion is normative.
So if this was all there was to it, reason would not yet have found a
truly practical role. I shall continue to call reasoning of this type
'theoretical', even when it is reasoning about normative
propositions.

But there is more. In the Humean theory, reason, having guided
you by some process of reasoning to believe that jumping is the
only way to stay alive, guides you no further. By contrast, we are
now supposing reason guides you by some process of reasoning to
believe the normative proposition that you ought to jump. To put
it another way, you believe reason requires you to jump. Normative
propositions have the special nature that they are about what reason
requires. Consequently, theoretical reasoning about normative
propositions has as its subject matter part of reason itself. So when
the theoretical reasoning leaves off, we have not finished with
reason. We are left with a proposition about what reason requires:

4. This example is inspired by Gregory Kavka's in 'The toxin puzzle', *Analysis*, 43 (1983),
pp. 33–6.

in your case, with the proposition that reason requires you to jump—you are irrational if you do not. Reason plays a double role, then. By the ordinary processes of theoretical reasoning it guides you to a belief, and then it directs you how to act.

We might be inclined to call reason in the second role practical, but for it to be truly practical we need more. Imagine people who have normative beliefs—they believe they ought to do one thing or another—but who never do what they believe they ought to do because they believe they ought to do it. If one of them happens to do what she believes she ought to do, the explanation is always something other than her belief. We could not say these people are guided by reason in their acts, nor that reason is truly practical for them. So for reason to be truly practical, we must sometimes do what we believe we ought to do because we believe we ought to do it. Our normative beliefs must sometimes explain our acts. This is what Christine Korsgaard calls 'the internalism requirement'.[5] It is implausible that people *necessarily* do what they believe they ought to do; that would be 'belief internalism', and we may happily reject it. But for reason to be practical, it must be *possible* for people to do what they believe they ought to do because they believe they ought to do it.

Actually, for reason to be practical, we need more than this. A normative belief can explain the right act in the wrong way. Your belief that you ought to jump might perversely cause you to sing happily, so that you start to skip about on the windowsill and by accident jump into the canal. In this case, you were not guided by reason. If reason is to be practical, not only must normative beliefs sometimes explain acts, they must sometimes do so in the right way. We must add this 'right-way' requirement to the internalism requirement. What is the right way? I shall come to that in Section V.

IV

How can the internalism requirement be met? Definitely not by the definition of 'rational'. If a person fails to do what she believes she ought to do, she is by definition irrational or at least not fully rational; so rational people always do what they believe they ought to do. This explains why rational people do what they believe they

5. *Op. cit.*

ought to do. But it does not explain how, in a rational person, the belief explains the act, which is what the internalism requirement requires. Sometimes a person acts because she believes she ought to. When this happens, the person is acting rationally. But how does it happen at all? How can a normative belief explain an act?

Faced with this question, some authors proceed as follows. They start from some preconceived view about how an act can be explained. This view imposes some constraint on the sorts of things that can explain an act. We are asking how a particular belief can explain an act. This strategy will impose some constraints on the nature of the belief, or it may even lead to the conclusion that the belief itself cannot explain the act. So it may force a reformulation of the question.

An example of this strategy starts from the preconceived view known as the Humean theory of motivation. This theory says an act cannot be explained by a belief alone, but only by a belief together with a desire. Specifically, if a person does A, the explanation cannot be just that she believes something, but that she wants something and believes doing A is a way for her to get this thing. Conversely, if the person wants something and believes doing A is a way for her to get this thing, then, if she does A, her desire and belief can constitute an explanation of her act. For instance, if you jump, that can be explained by your desire to stay alive and your belief that jumping is a way to stay alive.

If you ought to jump, let us say you have a 'complete reason' to jump. Now, this argument goes, our problem was to understand how your complete reason can explain your jumping. According to the Humean theory of motivation, this reason can only explain your act if it takes a particular form: the form of a desire for something together with a belief that jumping is a way to get this thing. So this argument uses the Humean theory of motivation to put a constraint on the form of a reason. The argument may be used to give some support to instrumentalism. It says that only a desire, together with a belief, can give you a complete reason for jumping. Only a desire, with a belief, can supply a reason.

There is a mistake in this argument. Our problem was not how your complete reason can explain your jumping, but how your belief that you have a complete reason—that you ought to jump— can explain it. The Humean theory of motivation says this belief by

REASONS AND MOTIVATION 141

itself cannot explain your act. One Humean response would be to find a desire that can be added to the belief in order to explain the act; I shall explain below that this can indeed be done. But the argument above, as I intended it to be understood, offered a quite different Humean explanation: a desire together with a quite different belief—a desire for something together with a belief that jumping is a way to get it. And the argument claimed that this desire and this different belief together constitute your complete reason for jumping. But if indeed this desire and this different belief do explain your jumping, your belief that you ought to jump plays no part in the explanation. Nor can this desire and this different belief justify you in believing you ought to jump; I showed that in Section II. So this argument gives no place to the belief that you ought to jump. Yet the only role we have so far found for reason, beyond the Humean one, was to bring you to this belief. Starting from the Humean theory of motivation, then, this argument simply takes us back to the Humean theory of reason. All it can say by way of explaining your jumping is this: you are naturally constituted so that, when you want something, and you believe jumping is a way to get it, you come to want to jump, and do so. Reason plays no part in this explanation, except that it no doubt helps bring you to believe that jumping is a way to get what you want. To say the belief and desire together constitute a 'reason' to jump is only a courtesy. They bring you to jump without the participation of reason.

Put it this way. Instrumentalism is the view that desires supply reasons for action. The argument I have given supports instrumentalism to the extent of saying that *only* desires (together with beliefs) can supply reasons for action. We know from Section II that instrumentalism is false: desires do not supply reasons for action. So if this argument is sound, there are no reasons for action.[6]

Fortunately it is not sound. There is another way to explain how a normative belief can explain an act. We may suppose it is simply a feature of most people's psychology that they are disposed to do what they believe they ought to do. Let us call this feature 'general practical rationality' or 'general rationality'. Those of us who do not have it are irrational. Even those who do have it will not always

6. I think this is the correct conclusion to draw if you are persuaded by the argument in Bernard Williams's 'Internal and external reasons', in his *Moral Luck*, Cambridge University Press, 1981, pp. 101–13.

do what they believe they ought to do. Sometimes things will obstruct their general rationality, such as weakness of will or inertia. Sometimes, too, a person will try to do something and fail. But for simplicity I shall concentrate only on acts that the person can do, so this type of failure will not arise. Given that, the obstructions to general rationality will, like general rationality itself, be features of the person's psychology.

Take a particular occasion when you believe you ought to do some act. If you are generally rational and if your general rationality is not obstructed on this occasion, let us say you are 'specifically rational' on this occasion. Specific rationality is another feature of your psychology. If you believe you ought to do some specific act, and if you are specifically rational, you will do the act. Your belief, in combination with your specific rationality, explains your act. This answers our question about how your belief that you ought to do the act explains your doing it. It explains it through a natural feature of your psychology: your specific rationality.

Let us call this the 'natural disposition' account of rational action. It is consistent with the Humean theory of motivation. Specific rationality is a psychological state that disposes you to do what, on a particular occasion, you believe you ought to do. Put differently, it disposes you to do what you believe is a way to do what you ought to do. According to a common functionalist definition of desire, a state that disposes you to do what you believe is a way to do B is a desire to do B. So specific rationality is nothing other than a desire to do what you ought to do. This desire, together with a belief that some act is a way to do what you ought to do, explains your doing this act. This exactly conforms to the Humean theory of motivation.

The natural disposition account satisfies the internalism requirement: it shows how a normative belief can explain an act. It is also consistent with externalism in Parfit's sense: it allows it to be the case that you ought to do some act without its being the case that, if you went through informed deliberation, you would do it. Informed deliberation would presumably bring you to believe you ought to do this act, but it might not bring you to be specifically rational, so it might not bring you to do it. So Parfit's externalism can satisfy the internalism requirement. Can it satisfy it in the right way?

V

Does the natural disposition account satisfy the right-way requirement? I shall present a case for saying it does, and a case against, in the form of a dialogue.

Against. There must be some way of dividing the right way from the wrong way, but the natural disposition account seems not to have the resources to distinguish them. Think about someone with a strange mental sickness. Various events cause her to become fixated on particular acts, and she sets out to do these acts with mindless determination. Reasoned argument cannot turn her away from them. For example, if she sees a city mentioned on page four of a newspaper, she goes there. She keeps what she calls a 'book of acts'. Whenever she sees a greyhound, she looks up an act at random in her book, and does it. And so on. She does not believe she ought to do these things; she simply wants to do them badly. However, she does sometimes form beliefs about what she ought to do. When she does, this is one of the events that precipitates a fixation. She becomes fixated on what she believes she ought to do, and sets out to do it with the same unreasoning, mindless determination. So this person has a natural disposition to do what she believes she ought to do. Consequently, when she believes she ought to do something, that belief can explain her doing it. She is generally rational according to the definition of general rationality, and when she does what she believes she ought to do, she is specifically rational. The natural disposition account is not in a position to repudiate her claim to rationality. Yet the belief clearly explains the act in the wrong way, because the way it explains it also explains this person's definitely irrational behaviour.

How should we characterize the right way for a normative belief to explain an act? If reason is to be truly practical, the right way should somehow involve reason. By this test, the natural disposition account fails. When a person does what she believes she ought to do, what makes her do so is a feature of her natural psychology. It is not any process involving reason. True, reason leads her to her belief about she ought to do, and we can say reason directs her to do what she believes she ought to do. But what actually explains her doing what she believes she ought to do is a natural disposition to do so, which does not involve reason. The

natural disposition account is externalist in a stronger sense than Parfit's: motivation is external to reason; it comes from a person's natural constitution. We may say this account agrees with Hume that reason in perfectly inert: reason only brings us to *beliefs* about what we ought to do, not to *acts* themselves.

So far as practical reason is concerned, we have not progressed much beyond the Humean theory of reason. Within the Humean theory, I gave the name 'togetherness' to the feature of people's psychology that disposes them to do what they believe will get them something they want. Togetherness is openly conceded to be nothing to do with rationality. We have now called on a feature of people's psychology that disposes them to do what they believe they ought to do. I called that feature 'practical rationality', but it does not in fact involve reason. We seem to have two separate faculties at work. There is reason, which brings us to beliefs about what we ought to do, and in a sense directs us to do what we believe we ought to do. Then there is rationality, a natural feature that causes us to do what we believe we ought to do. Why should this rationality be considered a part of reason?

For. But now, in favour of the natural disposition account, we might ask: what more do we want? Reason brings a person to a belief about what she ought to do, and then she sometimes does what she believes she ought to do. We have explained how that happens, and the explanation fits the fact that it happens when she is rational, and not when she is irrational. We call the explanatory disposition 'rationality' because it is what brings her to do what she believes reason requires her to do. Together with the ability to reason, it is part of what makes a person rational in thinking and in acting. To ask that this disposition should itself involve reason is to ask too much. It is to suggest that reason should actually bring a person to act rationally. Of course reason cannot make you act in accordance with reason.

Moreover, there is another way to distinguish the right way from the wrong way. Reason is not *involved* in the right way, but it does *sanction* the right way: we can say you *ought* to have the natural disposition of rationality. This distinguishes the right way from the wrong way. It is not the case that the person with fixations ought to have her peculiar disposition.

REASONS AND MOTIVATION   145

This suggestion that you ought to have the disposition of rationality needs to be treated carefully. Let us ask whether, on the natural disposition account, it satisfies the internalism requirement. If you believe you ought to be rational, can that belief explain your being rational? A belief of that sort could certainly explain your being *specifically* rational on some particular occasion. For instance, suppose that today, while cool, you believe you ought to be specifically rational tomorrow, when you will have an emotional decision to make. If you are specifically rational today over this particular belief, you may take steps today to give yourself the specifically rational disposition for the appropriate occasion tomorrow. On the other hand, believing you ought to be *generally* rational could not explain your being generally rational. If the belief was to explain the rationality, it would have to make you rational when you are not. But when you are not, you are not disposed to do what you believe you ought to do. So, even if you believe you ought to become rational, that belief will not dispose you to become rational.

But why should that matter? This ought does not satisfy the internalism requirement, but that does not seem to prevent its being true that you ought to be rational. So this does seem to be a way of distinguishing the right way from the wrong way. We have simply come up against an obvious limit to the power of reason in practical matters. Reason can have no part in explaining why, ultimately, we have a rational disposition.

Against. A final response on behalf of the case against the natural disposition account. To ask that reason should be involved in bringing a person to do what she believes she ought to do is *not* asking too much. It is certainly not asking that reason should make a person do what she believes she ought to do; we need not insist that the involvement of reason should be infallible. Nor do we ask that reason should be involved in explaining our rationality. Our complaint is simply that, in the natural disposition account, the role of reason is cut off too early. It is cut off before the real decision making begins.

Still, if this is the only available account of the role of reason, we shall have to be content with it. Is there another?

146   II—JOHN BROOME

VI

At the end of Section I, I made a cognitivist assumption that has determined the direction of my argument up to now. I assumed that if reason is to go beyond its Humean role, it must do so by giving us normative beliefs. Then the question arose: once we have a normative belief, how can reason bring us to act in accordance with it? That has proved difficult to answer satisfactorily. Perhaps this is not surprising. If we start by assigning reason the job of forming beliefs, perhaps it is not surprising if we cannot see how it can go beyond beliefs to acts.

There are processes of reasoning that do not involve normative beliefs. For example, when we come to believe a proposition by theoretical reasoning, we do not normally first come to believe we ought to believe the proposition, and for that reason come to believe it. We go straight to the proposition without forming any normative belief on the way. A more controversial example appears in a case when you have a choice between two different acts A and B, where each will achieve something of value, but where the values achieved by each are incommensurable. Then it may not be the case that you ought to do A, nor that you ought to do B. If so, you cannot rationally decide which to do by first forming a belief about which you ought to do. Does this mean reason cannot be involved in your decision, once you know all the relevant empirical facts? We may think a rational faculty is involved. It is sometimes called 'judgement' (though that term is misleading because this faculty judges no fact).

Examples like this suggest practical reasoning perhaps need not involve normative beliefs. Korsgaard[7] reminds us that Kant thought practical reason is concerned directly with the will. It goes directly from willing an end to willing the means. If you will to stay alive, that commits you to willing the means of staying alive, and so to jumping. Your reasoning does not go through the normative belief that you ought to jump, so it does not have to navigate the difficult passage from this normative belief to jumping.

This idea needs to be spelt out, and it faces difficulties of its own. One is to deal with the complexity of real instrumental reasoning that I mentioned in Section I, without the benefit of normative beliefs. But it may be a live noncognitivist rival to the natural disposition account of practical reason.

7. *Op. cit.*

Part III
Desire and the Good

[12]

DESIRING THE BAD: AN ESSAY IN MORAL PSYCHOLOGY *

D ESIRING the bad and not desiring the good are ordinary features of our everyday life. Because of their solutions to the problem of weakness of will, many philosophers disagree with this, thinking it very problematic, if not incoherent. But such solutions pose at least as large a question about philosophy as that problem poses in philosophy.

Important questions have been conflated, and important and all too common psychological phenomena have been misunderstood or ignored. As Amelie Rorty argues,[1] typical discussions of that problem conflate the question of (i) how people can "fail" to do or even try to do what they decide/d or intend/ed to do, and the question of (ii) how people can "fail" to decide or intend to do what they believe good or best or right or. . . . Rorty deals illuminatingly with (i), explaining how such "weakness" is all too common, not merely possible.

In this paper, I examine (ii), explaining how this "weakness," also, is all too common, not merely possible, and that if such weakness, desiring the bad, is problematic, then so is the corresponding strength, desiring the good. I shall argue that motivation and eval-

* My thanks are owed to the many people who have discussed these issues with me; and to the philosophy departments of the following universities to which I read versions of this work: Australian National University, La Trobe University, Macquarie University, State University of New York at Stony Brook, University of Adelaide, and University of Sydney.

[1] In her unpublished "Weakness, Imagination, and the Self." I owe her my warmest thanks for discussing these issues with me.

0022-362X/79/7612/0738$01.60

uation do not stand in a simple and direct relation to each other, as so often supposed. Rather, they are interrelated in various and complex ways, and their interrelations are mediated by large arrays of complex psychic structures, such as mood, energy, and interest. Philosophical theories have ignored or misunderstood these structures and the corresponding all too common psychological phenomena. They have depicted the psyche, especially the interrelations between motivation and evaluation, as far too simple, far too unified, and far too rational.

I. SOME TRADITIONAL LiNKINGS OF MOTIVATION AND EVALUATION

Since my main concern is working toward an adequate moral psychology, I shall ignore questions of exactly how and why so many philosophers have held that, of necessity, the good or only the good attracts us. It should be sufficient merely to list some exponents and allude to various theories.

Socrates, Plato, Aristotle, and such followers as Aquinas hold this because of their "metaphysics" of psychology. Spinoza, Perry, Sartre, many contemporary social scientists, and want-satisfaction utilitarians hold this since they hold that the good is constituted by attraction. Hare and various internalists hold it since they hold that to assent to a moral principle or judgment involves being attracted to the relevant act. Various action theorists hold that this view is analytic of acting: to act involves preferring, one prefers the preferable, and 'preferable' is another name for 'better'. Leibniz holds that such a connection is a principle of reason of a normative sort:

> If the will of God did not have for a rule the principle of the best, it would either tend toward evil which would be the worst of all, or else it would be in some fashion indifferent to good and evil and guided by chance.[2]

Other philosophers see the connection between values and desires or choices as essential underpinnings to liberalism, for respect for individuals and individual moral freedom.[3]

To be sure, the psychological phenomena and structures I shall discuss have not gone entirely unnoticed by other philosophers, not even by all those mentioned above.[4] Nonetheless, it is hardly

---

[2] Quoted from *Theodice* in *Philosophische Schriften*, vi. §86 by Arthur O. Lovejoy in *The Great Chain of Being* (Cambridge, Mass.: Harvard, 1936), p. 166.

[3] See e.g., Alan Montifiore, "Goodness and Choice," *Proceedings of the Aristotelian Society*, suppl. vol. xxxv (1961).

[4] Cf. Aristotle on spite and envy, the *Rhetoric*, II, 2 and 10; Augustine on stealing the pears; Aquinas in 2a2ae of the *Summa Theologica* on anger and hatred (34, 6), on spite (*rancor*) and malice (*malitia*) (35, 4), and on envy (36, 2);

unfair, if unfair at all, to suggest that the philosophical view is overwhelmingly that the good or only the good attracts. At the least, this is how I am forced to interpret so many philosophers. This affords me no pleasure, since that view, as argued below, is clearly and simply false. I would welcome contrary interpretations.

II. SOME TERMS OF MY CLAIM

For some purposes it will be important to specify what sorts of good or bad are involved in the claims that the good or only the good attracts. It may, for example, be important to determine whose good is involved, the agent's or someone else's; whether the good is an important good or not; whether 'good' would better be replaced by 'best' or 'right'; whether what is supposedly desired is a good thing or the thing-as-good or its goodness; whether in all or some cases believed goodness, not goodness, is in question. When it is important, I shall so specify.

I shall not, however, offer an account of goodness and badness, nor of what it is to believe something good or bad, nor of the nature of motivation. My reasons for not attempting these vital tasks are, first, that my arguments are meant to be very general: to apply to any plausible accounts of evaluation and motivation, especially but not only as these figure in practical or moral reasoning and action as engaged in by us and as studied by philosophers.

Second, in order to give an adequate account of these notions, we need an adequate moral psychology. And there seem good heuristic reasons for arguments like those below to precede that psychology or those accounts. For it is unclear how successful they could be until those notions are freed from their traditional misunderstandings.

How are we to understand the relation between the good and attraction? It is too weak to require only that the attractive act or act-feature is, e.g., (believed) good in some respect or over-all or even best.[5] For unless such acts or features are (believed) absolutely

---

and at least implicitly, philosophers such as Butler, Hume, and Firth on the conditions of ideal observers and the like. But they often do not seem wholehearted about such phenomena and structures. For example, the moral psychology of the *Nicomachean Ethics* appears to preclude them. (But perhaps we should take seriously the first lines of ch. 2, Bk. II, which suggest that that work is concerned with the moral psychology of good men, with references to that of bad men only to illuminate the former. The *Rhetoric*, which recognizes those phenomena and structures, is concerned with men as found, both good and bad.)

[5] For 'good or believed good', I shall often use '(believed) good', and similarly with '(believed) bad' and the like. However, the occurrence of only the one, e.g., only 'good', should be taken as signaling exclusive import only if such intent is made clear.

good—i.e., with no aspects that are (believed) bad or neutral in any respect—they can attract because or only because they are (believed) bad or neutral in some respect or other. Thus this requirement does not give an interesting version of the thesis that the good always attracts or that only the good attracts, that we always act *sub specie boni*. These require that the (believed) goodness or the (believed) good qua good is somehow essential to the attraction: e.g., that acts or features attract because or only because they are (believed) good. It remains problematic exactly how to specify this requirement.

However, in order to show that we can "fail" to be attracted to the (believed) good and that we can be attracted to the (believed) bad, not only to the (believed) good, it is unnecessary to sort out this problem. It will be sufficient to show that there are clear and unproblematic cases where what attracts us to do an act is attractive because it is (believed) bad or in spite of its being (believed) bad, where the act or feature is not attractive because or only because it or some other relevant act or feature is (believed) good. Showing this shows neither, first, that we ever perform an act that is in no way (believed) good; nor, second, that we ever perform an act that does not attract us at least in part because it is (believed) good.[6] It is not, however, necessary to show either in order to establish that the (believed) good need not attract, that not only the (believed) good, but also the (believed) bad, can attract, and that the interrelations between motivation and evaluation are various and complex.

III. THAT THE GOOD MUST ATTRACT

Recently, I read a story of what might be taken as typical of one course of life. It was said of this political figure that, in his youth, he cared a lot about the suffering of people in all parts of the world and devoted himself to making their lives better. But now he concerns himself only with the lives and fortunes of his close family and friends. He remembers his past, and he knows that there is still a lot he could do to help others. But he no longer has any desire so to do.

We can fill out this story in any number of ways. Perhaps he calculated that he could do the most good close to home. This

---

[6] The first quickly leads to questions of absolute (believed) badness. As to the second, although the cases below do not establish such complete lack of motivation by the (believed) good, they make it extremely plausible, even if such acts would not attract were they (believed) absolutely bad, or even simply worse than they are.

completion of the story need pose no problem for the thesis that the (believed) good must attract: it must allow for choices between various goods. Variants of the thesis deal differently with such choices. For example, some hold that it is always the (believed) best that attracts or attracts most.[7] Others hold that it is merely some (believed) good or other, whether or not it is (believed) best, that must attract.[8]

Perhaps the politician is not attracted to helping those people now because he believes he has already done enough for them or because he plans to help them a very great deal in the near-enough future. Such a completion of the story does confute many variants of the thesis that the (believed) good must attract. But just as we previously allowed for synchronic choices between goods, perhaps we should allow for diachronic choices. If we do not, that thesis would require far too rigorous a dedication to the good and its increase for it to be part of a plausible moral psychology of all people at all times.

It may not be clear exactly how to state the thesis to avoid such excessive dedication—e.g., how to include a principle that allows considerations of justice to explain, and justify, non-attraction to a (believed) good. But this internal problem of the thesis need not detain us. For the thesis is clearly wrong for reasons entirely unconnected with such, or other, choices between goods.

Suppose it is because of bitterness at the way the politician was treated that he does not desire to help those people. He has ceased caring about or for them. Perhaps he dislikes them. His non-attraction—his indifference or hostility—to the (believed) good confutes the thesis that the (believed) good must attract.

Citing the politician's bitterness or dislike or lack of care might naturally suggest two claims that sustain the thesis: First, if he does not help those people because of those feelings or moods, then his reason for not helping them must be (something like) to preserve his own peace of mind and happiness, to satisfy or at least not to displease himself. Second, these "psychic states" are (believed) good. This objection, then, is that my completion of the story involves competing (believed) goods, and thus really concedes

---

[7] Cf. Donald Davidson's principle P2: "If an agent judged that it would be better to do x than to do y, then he wants to do x more than he wants to do y" ["How Is Weakness of the Will Possible?," in Joel Feinberg, ed., *Moral Concepts* (New York: Oxford, 1969), p. 95].

[8] Cf. Alan Gewirth, *Reason and Morality* (Chicago: University Press, 1978). p. 49.

the truth of the thesis. Discussing this objection should help both recapitulate and advance my argument.

The objection may pose a special problem for the claim that the (believed) better attracts more. Sustaining this variant of the thesis often requires imputing to the agent an implausible weighting of values. But here—because those states would have to be (believed) better than the good involved in helping the others—an implausibly egoistic weighting must be imputed.

This objection to my claim is problematic, however, whether the thesis is taken in a comparative or noncomparative form. Rejecting its first suggestion, I would argue for the following: what the politician wants can be simply that those people not be helped by him or that they not have that good. Dislike or bitterness or not caring for or about are all sufficient explanations of such non-attraction to the good of someone. They need not be supplemented by some other state or condition, in particular some egoistic state or condition, to make the non-attraction intelligible. To be sure, each of these replies needs further discussion. But for reasons concerning the second suggestion, we need not pursue them.[9]

The second suggestion must be considered. For it can be taken in a general way, independent of the first: if the attractive feature is avoiding displeasing himself, then that is (believed) good; but if the attractive feature is simply that those people not be benefited by him, then that is (believed) good. In its full generality, then, this suggestion is just what is in question: that the (believed) good must attract.

This evokes my original claim: the completion of the story in terms of dislike, bitterness, lack of care for or about does not involve competing (believed) goods; and, thus, it confutes the thesis that the (believed) good must attract. Since this objection need concern us only insofar as it raises again the question of whether the (believed) good attracts, I shall continue my argument that it need not.

I offered different explanations of the politician's indifference or hostility to the good of those people: he no longer cares for or about them, or he dislikes, is bitter toward them. Both can be expanded in various directions: e.g., to involve annoyance, hatred, fury, disgust, and the like. They can also be expanded in another direction,

---

[9] For a brief discussion, see my "Morally Good Intentions," *The Monist*, LIV, 1 (January 1970): 124–141, esp. pp. 125–128 and 140/1; for an extended discussion, see Roy Lawrence's important *Motive and Intention* (Evanston, Ill.: Northwestern UP, 1972).

by considering people who are training themselves not to be affected by cares or considerations of this world. If one does not care for others, or is not interested in them, why should it be imagined that one will desire to benefit them?

Lack of this desire is commonplace. Through spiritual or physical tiredness, through accidie, through weakness of body, through illness, through general apathy, through despair, through inability to concentrate, through a feeling of uselessness or futility, and so on, one may feel less and less motivated to seek what is good. One's lessened desire need not signal, much less be the product of, the fact that, or one's belief that, there is less good to be obtained or produced, as in the case of a universal Weltschmertz. Indeed, a frequent added defect of being in such "depressions" is that one sees all the good to be won or saved and one lacks the will, interest, desire, or strength.

Let us note another consideration that shows that the (believed) good need not attract. The concept of selfishness may encompass the "metaphysical" egoist who believes that something is good only if it is good for, or a good of, him/herself. Selfishness may also encompass the "evaluative" egoist who recognizes that things can be good even insofar as they affect only others, but who ignores or discounts (his/her beliefs about) what is good for, or a good of, others. Perhaps it is "lexically" discounted—i.e., any of his/her self-regarding good is desired more than any amount of others' good; perhaps it is more modestly discounted. Families, clans, friends, classes, nations, races, . . . can play the same role as the person of these egoists. A metaphysical familist would hold that if something is good, it must be good for a family member; an evaluative familist would ignore or discount the good of those not in the family.

That the believed good must attract is consistent with the metaphysically selfish, family-ish, ... Such people see no good elsewhere; nor therefore do they desire it elsewhere. But evaluative egoists, familists, . . . do see value outside their area of concern. They simply may not be attracted to it.

I have not so far discussed the egoistical claim that the agent's own (believed) good must attract. There are some special problems with this claim: e.g., we often forego good for ourselves in order to benefit others. As well, there are problems strictly analogous to those presented above. Self-abnegation and self-denial can be successfully implemented. One can feel, and be disposed accordingly, that one is of no worth, and thus not be at all moved to benefit

oneself, to get or keep self-regarding good. So too, the various maladies of the spirit, as they might be called, such as despair, accidie, weakness, tiredness can play their role even in regard to self-regarding good and even to the point of extinguishing all desire for good for oneself, even to the point of making such goods repulsive.

Another variant of the claim that the (believed) good must attract is that if people are not attracted to what they believe good, then they are, so far at least, irrational. I would suggest that the same objections apply here. Not all cases of selfishness, callousness, uncaringness, and the like are irrationalities. The case for irrationality may be stronger if the (believed) good is the agent's own. But, again, what of demands of morality requiring giving up one's own good? What of manifestations of despair, loss of will, accidie? And what of passing up innocent goods such as the goods of amusement and the like? Are all these irrationalities?

Now we may think irrational those people so sunk in despair as not even to try to get anything of value for themselves out of life. (People are, for better or worse, locked away for such.) Some care and esteem for oneself may be, *ceteris paribus*, near enough to necessary for rationality of purpose and action, at least for certain sorts of people. However, not the care suggested by any of these variants on the theme that the good attracts.

It might be suggested that some goods or great goods play one or other of the attractive roles sketched above. Perhaps Plato's view was that people could not but seek the goods constitutive of self-esteem.[10] Many medieval Christian philosophers held that God or the vision or presence of God or perhaps salvation was an irresistible good.[11] I shall leave these claims and similar claims about more mundane goods to others.

So far, then, I have argued that (believed) goods, at least some obvious and important (believed) goods, can "fail" to attract us, at least at times. One need not forget what is (believed) good, e.g., for a person, nor that it is good that a person have health, wisdom, and the like, simply because one no longer cares for that person. More generally, something can be good and one can believe it to be good without being in a mood or having an interest or energy structure which inclines one to seek or even desire it.

Let us here note a related point which sustains both my claim

---

[10] I thank Kim Lycos for this suggestion and many others.
[11] I thank Ben Gibbs for this suggestion and many others.

that the (believed) good need not attract, and my more general claim that where the (believed) good does or does not attract, this is due to complex arrays of psychic structures. It is often held that something's being good or believed good—its being rational, given the agent's values and beliefs—makes intelligible (explains) why a person seeks or desires it. If what I have said above is correct, then this is mistaken. For in at least many, if not all, of the cases mentioned, just as the person may well not seek or desire the (believed) good, so, were that person to do what would produce (believed) good, that fact might well not make intelligible why the person so acted. If I am known to be sunk deeply into despair or some other depression or to have long ago ceased caring about someone's welfare, then citing the (believed) goodness of my act will not make intelligible my act which benefits that other person.[12]

To be sure, citing the (believed) good may suggest an explanation—e.g., that the despair or depression has lifted, that I now care. But this is another way of putting my point: only against a certain assumed background of agent mood and interest does citing the (believed) good make an act intelligible. We can be as mystified by a selfish person's gratuitously benefiting a stranger as by a kindly person's gratuitously harming a stranger. Given certain assumptions about the latter's moods and interests—which do not make the harm a good or a believed good—such gratuitous malice is intelligible. So too, given certain assumptions about the former's moods and interests, such gratuitous helping is unintelligible. In all cases, the relevant moods and interest structures must be understood if the desire and act are to be intelligible.

Of course, citing the (believed) good may always be a reason in the sense of being a justifying reason. But this is only to say that what serves as a justifying reason may not help make an act intelligible, and what may help make an act intelligible may be not a justifying reason, but a "dysjustifying" one.

IV. THAT ONLY THE GOOD ATTRACTS

To establish my general contentions about the interrelations between motivation and valuation, it is insufficient to establish that the (believed) good need not attract. It is necessary to show that

---

[12] Thus, rationality in the sense of value maximization against the background of an agent's beliefs is not the form of all action, nor even all intelligible action. Nor is the correspondingly rational person the form of all people, nor even all intelligible people. Trying to understand people as if they were such rational beings involves inadequate moral psychologies and ignores or misunderstands the important and all too common psychological phenomena discussed in this paper.

not only the (believed) good attracts. Some of the examples mentioned above—e.g., gratuitous malice and repulsive goods—suggest
this; for they involve the attractiveness of the (believed) bad. I
shall now argue explicitly for this: that we have desires and appetites for the (believed) bad.

I may desire or have an appetite for this food. But it may be the
wrong amount or sort of food, it may be poisoned, spoiled. . . .
Thus, the actual object of attraction is bad. To this it might be
replied that desires and appetites are intentional, they may aim at
what could be called the "proper" object of attraction: viz., perhaps only some aspects of a concrete object, and even an object or
aspects that are mistakenly believed available. Thus, it could be
held, were I aware of the nature of that food, I would see that the
proper object of my desire or appetite is absent, and thus not be
attracted to that food.

But there seems little justification for this claim. Actual desires
and appetites may not conform to the evaluative sense of 'want' or
'lack' found in philosophers since Socrates and still in our language: "He was examined and found wanting." Given certain
moods, interest structures, energy levels, and the like—e.g., my having ceased caring about my well-being—what I want is this food,
even though, perhaps even because, I realize it is the wrong amount,
the wrong sort, . . . i.e., bad for me.

But of course, it is difficult to identify the real object of attraction. I may have wanted that food because I wanted something
else, e.g., pleasure, which other thing may be consistent with the
view that only the (believed) good attracts, that we always act *sub
specie boni*. This can be brought out by considering the following
interchange between me and supporters of that view.

To confute that view, I instanced the case of a man who wanted
to and did burn himself to see if he could emulate the famous
Roman. I suggested that whatever (believed) good there might be
in what attracted him, such (believed) good need not be the whole
or even part of what attracted him. My interlocutors said that since
the act was motivated by the desire or appetite for knowledge, perhaps self-knowledge, the feature of the actual object of attraction
which attracted him—viz., the knowledge—was wholly good. But,
I contend, some knowledge is bad or harmful, some is simply not
worth having, the desire to know some things is shameful, and so
on. (This is so even if some knowledge is good in itself.) Thus, it
seems that we can take the desire or appetite to know as having
proper objects which are (believed) good, bad, or neutral.

Consider also our desires to harm others. To save the thesis that we desire only the (believed) good, it must be maintained either that such harming is (believed) good or that it is not the direct or proper object of desire. The former is too implausible. My interlocutors maintained the latter, holding that harming others is only an intermediate desire of, say, the desire to get pleasure for oneself, power over others, showing oneself powerful, getting things to go one's way, getting revenge.

Even if they are correct, however, what reason is there to take such (instances of those) desires to be aimed at what is (believed) good—apart, that is, from saving the thesis that only the (believed) good attracts? It might be objected that, apart from my contrary thesis, I have no reason to deny that they are (believed) good. As this paper shows, that claim is false. Even if it were true, I would be content for the issue to be put: Which thesis is better able to account for important and common psychological phenomena and structures?

But I do not think they are correct. Just as helping another can be the direct and proper object of desires and appetites, so can harming others. (Arguments to the contrary are quite similar to traditional arguments for egoism.) One way to see this is that in certain loving or caring moods, helping is precisely what is desired. So too, in other moods, harming is precisely what is desired. When we feel furious, hurt, envious, jealous, threatened, frustrated, abandoned, endangered, rejected, and so on, what we often seek is precisely the harm or destruction of someone, and not always the "offending party": "If I can't have her, no one will." "So, you are leaving me after all I have done for you. Well then, take that." "You stole her from me, now it's my turn to get even." "The whole day has gone so badly, I might as well complete it by ruining the little I did accomplish." "I let him have it with the horn; he was the millionth Sunday driver who cut in front of me." "Watch out for him today, he just had an awful fight with his wife."

Given such moods and circumstances, harming another can be the proper and direct object of attraction. There is no need to posit another object, especially not an egoistic object like pleasure, power over others, showing oneself powerful, getting things to go one's own way, getting revenge.

Just as there are desires and appetites directed at harming others, there are desires and appetites directed at harming oneself. In certain moods, such as the self-directed modes of disgust, hatred, guilt, shame, I may seek to humble, abase, or harm myself.

Agents, even in the planning and doing of such acts, and certainly afterwards, can believe or know that what is desired is bad. Moods, interest structures, and the like can make us unconcerned about achieving the (believed) good. In such moods, . . . , we not only do not care, we are filled with "uncare."

Perhaps we have such moods, . . . and thus bad-seeking desires or appetites only under certain, mainly adverse, conditions. Perhaps having such moods, . . . , desires, and appetites shows some moral or psychological defect in us or some defect in our circumstances or society. This suggests what seems correct in any case: First, desiring the (believed) bad and not desiring the (believed) good raise serious practical problems about moral education and personal and social conditions, not just conceptual problems. Second, if it is irrational to have bad-seeking desires and appetites, the relevant sense of 'rational' evaluates not only the agent's means and ends and character but also the agent's situation in society and that society as well.

In conclusion, it seems at best unjustifiable optimism or complacency to accept the liberalism and relativism of values embodied in the claim that we always act *sub specie boni*, that we desire or have an appetite for only what is (believed) good.[13] "I don't know what is good, but I know what I want" contains more truth than many seem to believe. A desire for what is bad need not make it good; on the contrary, its badness may infect the desire, making it bad.

V. SOME PROGRAMMATIC CONCLUSIONS

I have argued that what is (believed) good can "fail" to attract us and that what is (believed) bad can attract us. This argument is about us, not about people with radically different psychologies from ours, like those portrayed in Kosinski's novels or like psychopaths or sociopaths.[14] Even we have moods, interest and energy structures, . . . which "allow" us not to be attracted to a (believed) good or to be attracted to a (believed) bad.

The argument was not intended to show that those moods, interest and energy structures, . . . could operate—could lead to desire, intention, action—without a background structure of evaluation, as hating may require desiring the bad for the hated. Rather, it was intended to show that value structures are only complexly

---

[13] This optimism has clear implications for social policy, education, and so on. I thank Graeme Marshall for discussing this and other issues with me.

[14] Who we are is, of course, a question. But for the present purposes, we should readily enough be able to identify ourselves.

related with those structures and other structures such as those of
motivation. To what extent moods and the like could operate without such background value structures needs discussion in any adequate moral psychology. Also needing discussion is the related
problem of the extent it is possible for people—and for what sort
of people—not to be attracted to what is (believed) good or to be
attracted to what is (believed) bad. (As Rorty argues, other reasons,
roles, group encouragement, . . . also account for such attraction
and non-attraction.)

My arguments, then, must be understood as having a limited
purview. But within that purview, it has been argued that motivation and evaluation need not point in the same direction, that they
are related only through complex structures of mood, care, energy,
interest, and the like. Upon even brief reflection, we see that those
complex structures are, themselves, not of one natural, psychic
kind. For example, desire arising from pique is very different from
desire "failing" to arise from lack of energy. But since this paper
is concerned with a role played by these disparate structures—
mediating between evaluation and motivation—treating those structures as if of one sort is not harmful.

My claims about such mediation can be divided into two sub-
claims, the first about cases that controvert, and the second about
cases that might seem consistent with, the alleged necessary connection between motivation and evaluation. This paper has been concerned almost exclusively with the controverting cases. I shall now
comment directly on the "consistent" ones. Even in them, I suggest,
motivation and evaluation are mediated by those psychic structures. This, if correct, helps show that the controverting cases are
not exceptions, aberrations, mere anomalies or mere counterexamples, but rather that they exhibit deep and general relations between motivation and evaluation.

My comments about the "consistent" cases have been and will be
brief for various reasons. To establish my contention about the
lack of simple, direct, or necessary connections between motivation
and evaluation, the controverting cases are sufficient, and more
easily handled. A discussion of the "consistent" cases requires far
more psychological, sociological, and anthropological information
than I have. To explain these cases requires an adequate moral
psychology: a brief paper like this can at best show the inadequacies of various moral psychologies and point the way toward
an adequate one.

That moods, care, interest, energy, . . . account for disconnec-

tions between motivation and evaluation would not, of course, prove that they play a similar role in accounting for connections. But it should alert us to that possibility. If we do look at cases of such connection, at least in many of them we do find moods, care, interest, energy, and the like. It is not noteworthy if a mother gives her son something (she believes) good for him. But typically, mothers stand to their sons in ways constituted by exceptionally complex arrays of mood, interest, energy, and the like. Similarly, there are complex arrays in at least many cases of a friend helping another, of people doing what they believe obligatory, and so on. (The presence of such arrays, I take it, is the subject not so much of philosophical argument as of psychological, sociological, or anthropological study.)

Of course, the mere presence of such arrays of structures does not establish that they play the same mediating role—now with a different "polarity"—between motivation and evaluation as is played by those arrays in accounting for disconnections between motivation and evaluation. But I suggest that they do, as the following, related points might indicate.

It is now a truism that men and women of our culture have different motivational "orientations" to (believed) good. Men, archetypically, seek their own good and through that the good of their families; women, archetypically, are more self-sacrificing, more altruistic, directly more eager for the good of their families. To the extent that this and similar claims are correct, such differences are explained, at least in a constitutive, if not a generative, way by the very different mood, interest, energy, . . . structures of men and women in our culture.

If this is correct and if my earlier claims are correct, then both some disconnections between motivation and evaluation and also some—e.g., sex-role-linked—connections between motivation and evaluation are mediated by arrays of structures of mood, interest, energy, and the like. It would be surprising, then, if the generalized connection between motivation and evaluation were not also so mediated. Indeed, if all people who have so far lived have had arrays of such structures mediating the particular ways their motivation and evaluation were connected, what can be made of the claim that motivation and evaluation are directly and simply connected?

This raises the second point. Very frequently at least, only what is unusual or wrong is thought to need an explanation. If our cultural archetype or ideal of a person has certain arrays of such struc-

tures, they might well go unexplained, even unnoticed. Cross-cultural studies may help us recognize and understand these structures —thus, ourselves. The point can be brought out this way: When I consider people who have been defeated by life, the wretched of the earth, those who see no hope for themselves or those they care for, who lack physical and spiritual energy, I am not at all surprised that—as political and anthropological data suggest—they may not seek even what little good they do perceive. Life may be too much for them. We, on the contrary, see the world as open to us, and more importantly, open for us. We can progress. We can make it. We see ourselves out there to be won. We have self-confidence and hope. Indeed we have more than this: we have an optimistic certainty. We have energy. We know we are worthy. We know that, barring bad luck, our enterprise will be rewarded. And so on. Such an array of structures of mood, interest, energy, . . . makes it natural, almost inevitable, that we seek the (believed) good for ourselves or others. And it seems at least arguable that such an array must be posited to give an adequate account of how, at least according to our cultural ideal, motivation and evaluation are related in us.

If this is right, then, first, even in the "consistent" cases, the connection between motivation and evaluation is mediated by those complex arrays. And, second, moods and the like cannot be understood as "deflections" from our normal—and mood-free—orientation to value, nor can values be understood as what we would desire were we not in a mood.

Four brief and interrelated points should be made. It might be argued that those who are unlike us in their orientation to the (believed) good suffer from some defective or pathological condition of their psyche or society. Certainly, were we to become like them, while still in our life and society, we would very likely be said to be in such a condition. (But were they to become like us, while still in their life and society, might they not, too, be said to be in such a condition?) However, for their being in such a condition to bear on whether motivation and evaluation can be connected without the mediation of those arrays, any array playing such a mediating role would have to be, as such, pathological or defective.

Second, it will not have gone unnoticed that in indicating "our" cultural ideal, what I sketched was the successful and striving man. It may well be no accident, as various critiques put it, that this psychology is presumed, perhaps unknowingly, to be the natural

or healthy human psychology by philosophers. For after all, to put it far too crudely and quickly, philosophers, at least those we now read, have been successful and striving—and with few exceptions—men. Current cultural critiques—e.g., by some feminists and Marxists—argue, first, that such an array is not inevitable, nor clearly desirable; and, second, that such an array does play the mediating role I have been urging, even in our culturally ideal cases where we "naturally" desire and seek the (believed) good.

Third, even within our culture and in regard to attraction to the (believed) good, there is not just one, but rather many significantly different, though interrelated, ideals and archetypes for men, and of course also for women and children. Just as our personality does not "fit" a defeated person, even in our society "exchanges of personality" would produce strange fits. Consider such exchanges between an American and English academic, or between a successful business man and a factory worker. Thus, even for only our culture, there will not be one array, but rather many arrays, of those mediating structures. We will need not one, but many moral psychologies.

Fourth, understanding these moral psychologies requires not only philosophy, but also psychology, sociology, and anthropology. We will need typological descriptions of different human psyches and also accounts of these differences. These would involve both interrelations among various moral-psychological notions and interrelations between these and class, culture, nationality, occupation, sex, status, region, religion, and the like—the subjects of psychology, sociology, and anthropology.

The implications of these last points are very large. Let me conclude on a smaller scale, by returning to the opening themes of the paper: If weakness of will, desiring the (believed) bad, is problematic, so is strength of will, desiring the (believed) good. We must replace those moral psychologies which generate the traditional philosophical problems about weakness of will. We need moral psychologies that recognize, in general, the complexities of the psyche and, in particular, those complex arrays of psychic structures of mood, interest, energy, . . . and also the complex mediating roles played by these arrays between motivation and evaluation.

MICHAEL STOCKER

La Trobe University

[13]

The Guise of the Good[1]

J. DAVID VELLEMAN
University of Michigan

The agent portrayed in much philosophy of action is, let's face it, a square. He does nothing intentionally unless he regards it or its consequences as desirable. The reason is that he acts intentionally only when he acts out of a desire for some anticipated outcome; and in desiring that outcome, he must regard it as having some value.[2] All of his intentional actions are therefore directed at outcomes regarded *sub specie boni:* under the guise of the good.[3]

This agent is conceived as being capable of intentional action—and hence as being an agent—only by virtue of being a pursuer of value. I want to question whether this conception of agency can be correct. Surely, so general a capacity as agency cannot entail so narrow a cast of mind. Our moral psychology has characterized, not the generic agent, but a particular species of agent, and a particularly bland species of agent, at that. It has characterized the earnest agent while ignoring those agents who are disaffected, refractory, silly, satanic, or punk. I hope for a moral psychology that has room for the whole motley crew.

I shall begin by examining why some philosophers have thought that the attitudes motivating intentional actions involve judgments of value. I shall then argue that their conception of these attitudes is incorrect. Finally, I shall argue that practical reason should not be conceived as a faculty for pursuing value.

One source of the view that intentional actions are aimed at the good has been a desire, on the part of moral psychologists, to reconcile two seemingly incompatible stories about how human action originates. These might be called the story of motivation and the story of rational guidance.[4]

The story of motivation says that an action is caused by a desire for some outcome and a belief that the action will promote it. The agent wants to know the time, for example, and believes that looking at his watch will result in his knowing the time; and he consequently looks at his watch.[5] The desire and belief cited in this story are conceived as propositional attitudes. That is, each is thought to

consist in the agent's grasping and being somehow disposed toward a proposition. He is, so to speak, desirous toward the proposition "I know the time" and credent toward the proposition "Looking at my watch will result in my knowing the time." These attitudes combine to cause a new attitude—a desire toward the proposition "I look at my watch." And since looking at his watch is something that the agent can just do if he wants, this desire causes him to act.

The story of rational guidance tells how an agent acts for a reason. According to this story, a reason for acting is a proposition whose truth would reflect well on, count in favor of, recommend, or in some other sense justify an action.[6] A reason for performing an action exists so long as a proposition justifying the action is true.[7] But an agent cannot act for this reason unless he has mental access to it—unless he believes the proposition or at least grasps it in some related fashion. And even if he has appropriately grasped the reason, and is therefore in a position to act for it, he doesn't ultimately act for the reason unless his grasp of it results in his being influenced or guided by its justifying force. An agent acts for a reason, then, when the action-justifying character of a proposition prompts his action via his grasp of that proposition.[8]

The apparent discrepancy between these stories lies in the relation posited between the agent's action and the propositional objects of his attitudes. In the story of motivation, the objects of the agent's attitudes are propositions that do not in themselves justify his action. They do, of course, help to determine which action he is moved to perform. The agent would not be moved to look at his watch if he didn't want, in particular, to know the time and if he didn't believe, in particular, that looking at his watch would result in his knowing the time. Yet the content of these attitudes doesn't in any way reflect well on, count in favor of, or otherwise justify looking at his watch. Indeed, the propositions "I know the time" and "Looking at my watch will result in my knowing the time" do not reflect more favorably on watch-consulting behavior than on watch-ignoring behavior. When the agent's attitudes toward these propositions move him to consult his watch, he is not responding to any action-justifying property of the propositions themselves; he is simply manifesting the valence of his attitude toward the former proposition. Because the agent has a desire toward "I know the time," he is moved to look at his watch; whereas if he had an aversion toward the same proposition, he would be moved to ignore his watch instead. The content of his attitudes is in itself neutral between these alternatives.

The action performed in the story of rational guidance is also determined in part by the nature of the agent's attitudes and not merely by their content. When the protagonist of this story acts for a reason, he acts partly because of grasping the reason in an attitude something like belief. But more than the nature of the agent's attitude toward his reason must work in favor of his action. When an agent acts for a reason, he acts not only because his attitude toward the reason is more like belief than disbelief but also because the proposition involved militates in favor of his action rather than against it. The agent's attitudes are thus con-

ceived as having propositional objects that intrinsically favor a particular action, and their favoring the action is conceived as crucial to their behavioral influence.

This aspect of rational guidance is what makes rationally guided behavior, as we conceive it, comparable to the conclusion of an inference. The premises of an inference are propositions whose truth guarantees or makes probable the truth of the conclusion; and in this sense they favor the conclusion solely by virtue of their content, antecedently to any attitude in which one might fix them. In order for a particular set of premises to become one's reasons for drawing a conclusion, one must somehow be influenced, in grasping them, by their antecedently favorable relation to the conclusion. Similarly, in order for a particular reason to become one's reason for performing an action, one must be influenced by its bearing favorably on that action. To be motivated by a desire, by contrast, is to be guided by attitudes toward propositions that do not in themselves favor anything.

This fundamental difference between motivation and rational guidance wouldn't necessarily render the two stories incompatible if neither purported to be the complete explanation of an action. One and the same action could be due to a confluence of motivation and rational guidance. Yet philosophers have tended to interpret each story as purporting to be the whole story; and they have therefore assumed that the apparent discrepancy between these stories has to be removed. They have sought to remove the discrepancy by slightly retelling one story or the other.

Noncognitivists, for example, retell the story of rational guidance in such a way that it collapses into the story of motivation. According to their version of the story, the agent's reason for acting is the proposition "Looking at my watch will result in my knowing the time," a proposition that recommends looking at his watch, not by virtue of its content, but rather because his belief in it inclines him to look at his watch, given his desire to know the time. Noncognitivists thus deny that the propositions constituting an agent's reasons for acting are intrinsically favorable to his action. Propositions recommend acting, they think, only in relation to desires that lend motivational force to the agent's belief in those propositions.[9]

Some noncognitivists may resent the suggestion that they are hereby retelling or revising anything—that there ever was any other story of rational guidance than theirs. But the noncognitivist story diverges from the commonsense story of rational guidance in one important respect: it reverses the order of explanation between justificatory and motivational force. In the commonsense story, the agent is moved toward an action because his reasons justify it; whereas in the noncognitivist story, his reasons justify the action in virtue of moving him toward it. The noncognitivist thus treats motivation as a constituent rather than an effect of justification.[10]

6   *NOÛS*

I shall not consider here whether this departure from the commonsense story
of rational guidance is defensible. What suffices for my purposes is that some
philosophers have preferred to avoid it, by adopting a different strategy for
reconciling the two stories of human action. Rather than characterize rational
guidance noncognitively, so that it collapses into motivation, they characterize
motivation cognitively, so that it amounts to something like rational guidance;
and they thereby introduce the evaluative conception of agency that interests me.

Proponents of this alternative strategy portray motivation itself as an inference,
governed in part by action-justifying content to be found in the motivating
attitudes. To this end, they incorporate the valence of desire into its content, by
describing desire, not as a favorable attitude toward the representation of some
outcome, but rather as an attitude toward a favorable representation of the outcome. The agent who wants to know the time is said, not to be favorably disposed toward "I know the time," but rather to accept a proposition such as "My
knowing the time would be good." The content of this attitude and the content of
the agent's belief, "Consulting my watch would result in my knowing the time,"
are sufficient to justify the conclusion "Consulting my watch would be good."
And the agent's accepting this favorable representation of consulting his watch is
now conceived as constituting a desire to consult his watch. Hence his transition
from a desire to know the time to a desire to consult his watch appears to be
dictated, in the fashion of an inference, by a privileged logical relation between
the contents of the attitudes involved.

The leading contemporary proponent of this latter strategy is Donald
Davidson. Consider the following passage, in which Davidson is discussing an
agent who is moved to add sage to his stew by a desire to improve the taste:[11]

> [L]et us suppose [the agent] wants to improve the taste of the stew. But what is the
> corresponding premise? If we were to look for the proposition toward which his
> desire is directed, the proposition he wants true, it would be something like: He
> does something that improves the taste of the stew (more briefly: He improves the
> taste of the stew). This cannot be his premise, however, for nothing interesting
> follows from the two premises: Adding sage to the stew will improve its taste, and
> the agent improves the taste of the stew. The trouble is that the attitude of *approval*
> which the agent has toward the second proposition has been left out. It cannot be
> put back in by making the premise 'The agent wants to improve the taste of the
> stew': we do not want a *description* of his desire, but an *expression* of it in a form in
> which he might use it to arrive at an action. The natural expression of his desire is,
> it seems to me, evaluative in form; for example, 'It is desirable to improve the taste
> of the stew,' or, 'I ought to improve the taste of the stew'. We may suppose
> different pro attitudes are expressed with other evaluative words in place of
> 'desirable'.

In this passage Davidson subjects the story of motivation to the retelling that I
have just described. He demands that the outcome of motivation—the act of

adding sage—be justified by some propositional content of the agent's attitudes, as if it were a conclusion following from premises. And he obtains the required content by incorporating the valence of the agent's attitude toward "I improve the taste" into a new proposition: "Improving the taste is desirable." The story of motivation is thus transformed into the story of an inference, in which the agent is under genuinely rational guidance.

Here, then, is one way in which rational agency comes to be conceived as a capacity for pursuing value. Desires are conceived as value judgments, with intrinsic justificatory force, so that the desire motivating an agent can be identified with the reason guiding him. The result is that all actions performed for reasons are conceived as arising from favorable value judgments, and hence as being aimed at the good.

This reconciliation of motivation and rational guidance comes under pressure from two different directions. If the cognitivist seriously means to characterize desire as an attitude toward an evaluative proposition, then he implies that the capacity to desire requires the possession of evaluative concepts. Yet a young child can want things long before it has acquired the concept of their being worth wanting, or desirable. Surely, the concept of desirability—of something's being a correct or fitting object of desire—is a concept that children need to be taught. And how would one teach this concept to a child if not by disciplining its antecedently existing desires?[12]

This problem may explain Davidson's apparent efforts to avoid saying that evaluations serve as the contents or propositional objects of desire. Davidson often favors alternative formulations, as in the passage quoted above, where he says that the relevant evaluation is "the natural expression of [the agent's] desire" rather than its propositional object.

But this qualification leaves the cognitivist open to a different objection, since it seems to undermine his attempt to reconcile the stories of motivation and rational guidance. According to the latter story, acting for a reason entails being influenced by the force of a mentally grasped justification of one's action. According to Davidson's qualified formulation, however, a proposition that's essential to the justification of the action—namely, the proposition that the action's expected consequences are desirable—is merely a proposition that would naturally be used to express the agent's desire. And the agent can be moved by his desire without either being able to express it or grasping the proposition with which it would naturally be expressed. He can therefore satisfy Davidson's story of motivation without having mentally accessed anything that justifies his action. Hence the resulting story of motivation no longer corresponds to the story of rational guidance.[13]

These two objections seem to leave no room for the cognitivist strategy. But they do not rule out a sophisticated version of cognitivism—a version that is suggested, in any case, by an important feature of propositional attitudes in

general. The feature in question is the so-called direction of fit that distinguishes conative attitudes such as desire from cognitive attitudes such as belief.[14] As we shall see, reflection on this feature naturally leads to a version of cognitivism that escapes the foregoing objections.

The term "direction of fit" refers to the two different ways in which attitudes can relate propositions to the world. In cognitive attitudes, a proposition is grasped as patterned after the world; whereas in conative attitudes, a proposition is grasped as a pattern for the world to follow. The propositional object of desire is regarded not as fact—not, that is, as *factum,* having been brought about—but rather as *faciendum,* to be brought about; it's regarded not as true but as to be made true.

There is a temptation to think that regarding something as to be brought about or made true is tantamount to holding a value judgment about it. Perhaps, then, when philosophers say that to want something is to regard it as good or desirable, they are thinking of the attitude's direction of fit—of the distinctive way in which a proposition is regarded when it's the object of desire rather than belief.[15]

I shall argue presently that the use of an evaluative term like "good" to express desire's direction of fit is a potential source of confusion. For the moment, however, I shall adopt that usage, in order to examine precisely what it might mean and where it might lead.

As for the meaning of this usage, note that even if desiring something entails making a value judgment about it, by regarding it as good, this attitude qualifies as a value judgment in only a rather unusual sense of the phrase, a sense corresponding to that in which a belief might be called a "truth judgment." The desire that p is here conceived as a value judgment in the sense that it involves regarding p as to be brought about and hence, supposedly, as good, just as the belief that p involves regarding p as true. But to say that belief in p involves regarding p as true is not to say that it consists in a judgment whose object is the proposition "p is true." That way lies a vicious regress of propositional attitudes. Similarly, to say that the desire involves regarding p as good is not to say that it consists in a judgment with an evaluative proposition as its object.

Expressions like "regarding...as true" and "regarding...as good" are intended to describe belief and desire in a way that elucidates the difference in their directions of fit. Because we conceive of belief and desire as alike in being attitudes toward propositions, and as differing in their treatment of the fit between propositions and the world, we unavoidably describe them with a common attitudinal verb ("regarding") and different predicate adjectives ("as true," "as good"). But this construction—attitudinal verb plus differentiating predicate—must not be interpreted as invoking a further attitude directed toward a proposition containing that predicate. The desire that p is not to be analyzed as an attitude toward the proposition that p is good; it must be analyzed as an attitude toward p *as* good.[16]

Even so, the resulting conception of desire does seem to allow for a reconciliation between the stories of motivation and rational guidance. For although the desire that p doesn't entail grasping a proposition that justifies action conducive to p, the desire itself may appear to constitute an attitude that justifies such action, if it consists in regarding p as good.

Once we recognize that a propositional attitude must be characterized, not only by the proposition that embodies its content, but also by a predicate expressing how that proposition is regarded—that is, whether it's regarded as *factum* or *faciendum,* as true or to be made true—we are less inclined to insist that the justificatory force influencing reason-guided behavior be lodged in the propositional objects of the agent's attitudes. When the valence of a desire that p is represented by the expression "regarding p as good," valence takes on the form of a content-like phenomenon and begins to seem like a potential bearer of justificatory force. For even if no action is justified by the fact that p, some action might well be justified by the *faciendum* that p—by p's being something to be brought about.

Thus, if an attitude combines the propositional object p with a direction of fit expressible by the predicate "good," then it would seem to harbor justificatory force—not in its propositional object alone but rather in the combination of its propositional object and its direction of fit. And the agent can be imagined as having mental access, not only to the propositions that he grasps in various attitudes, but also to the attitudes' direction of fit, as expressed by their constitutive predicates.

We may therefore be inclined to revise the story of rational guidance, by replacing its references to the agent's grasp of action-justifying propositions with references to his action-justifying attitudes. We might say, for example, that an agent is mentally in touch with a justification for looking at his watch not only if he believes that knowing the time would be good but also if he regards it as good that he know the time—an attitude that supposedly constitutes a desire. We might also say that being guided by a desire's direction of fit entails being guided by its evaluative aspect, which lends the desire its mentally accessible justificatory force. We might then conclude that being motivated by a desire can amount to acting for a reason.[17]

This version of cognitivism, like the previous version, implies that every action that's motivated by a desire—or, equivalently, performed for a reason—is guided by some favorable value judgment, and hence that intentional action is always aimed at the good. The judgment involved is no longer conceived as an attitude toward an evaluative proposition; but it is still conceived as having the recommending force of an evaluation, so that it can serve as the agent's reason for acting.

I believe that this version of cognitivism is an improvement on its predecessor, but that it is not ultimately more successful. For even if desiring

something entails regarding it as good in some sense, regarding something as good in that sense does not in fact amount to making a value judgment about it. An agent's motivating desire consequently lacks the justificatory force that the cognitivist attributes to it for the sake of identifying it with the agent's reason for acting. The cognitivist strategy for reconciling motivation and rational guidance, and the resulting conception of intentional action as aimed at the good, thus turn out to rest on a mistake.

Before I attempt to demonstrate this mistake, however, I had better define more clearly what sort of mistake it is. When I deny that desire has the justificatory force with which it is credited by the cognitivist, I am not necessarily denying that having a desire provides one with reason for acting. It often does. Yet the cognitivist doesn't merely claim that desire provides reason for acting; he claims that being moved by a desire amounts to acting for a reason. And this claim implies, as we have seen, that to fall under a desire's motivational influence is to fall under the rational influence of a mentally grasped justification.

Yet one can agree that having a desire—and *a fortiori* being moved by a desire—sometimes entail the existence of a reason for acting, while denying that they entail being in the appropriate mental rapport with that reason. Suppose, for example, that the reason generated by a desire is the fact that one has the desire, a fact to which one can be utterly oblivious even as the desire moves one to act. In that case, one can have a desire and be moved by that desire without having grasped the reason that it generates; and so one can have and be moved by a desire without being in a position to be guided by the associated reason for acting.[18]

How the fact that one has a desire might justify action, and how an agent might be influenced by this justification, are questions that lie beyond the scope of this paper.[19] I mention this view of the matter only for the sake of distinguishing the sense in which I concede that a motivating desire justifies action from the sense in which I deny it. I concede that desire can justify action objectively, by making true a proposition that could guide one's actions if one gained appropriate access to it; but I deny that desire justifies action subjectively, by constituting an evaluative attitude whose justificatory force is already available to guide one's actions. I thus deny that desire amounts to an evaluation, and that motivation consequently amounts to rational guidance, in the sense proposed by the cognitivist.[20]

The cognitivist thinks that desire provides a mentally accessible justification for acting because it harbors justificatory force in its direction of fit, as expressed by its constitutive predicate, which he takes to be a term of evaluation. But why would one think that the constitutive predicate of desire was "good" or "desirable" or some other evaluative term?

One reason, I suspect, is a tendency to psychologize various extrinsic descriptions of mental states. For example, to desire something is to be disposed toward it in a way that would be appropriate if the thing were good; and a person who desires something can therefore be said to regard or treat it *as if* it were good or, more concisely, *as* good. But this description of the person's attitude, which cites a purely extrinsic fact about it, should not be mistaken as expressing a psychological aspect of the attitude itself. That someone's attitude would be appropriate if its object were good is not something to which he has mental access simply by virtue of having the attitude; and so it's not something whose justificatory force is necessarily available to guide him. Treating something as good in this sense is no more a value judgment than treating someone like dirt is a soil-judgment.

Similarly, a person who desires something can be said to find it attractive, but this description does not necessarily mean that he makes an attractiveness-judgment about it. It may mean simply that he is attracted to the thing and thereby has an experience that's indicative of, or evidence for, its attractiveness. Although the combination of "to find" with a predicate adjective has the superficial grammar of an attitudinal verb, it doesn't necessarily express the content or valence of an attitude. Someone can find his dinner indigestible, for instance, without having any attitude toward it whatever: he may simply have a cramp. To say that he finds his dinner indigestible in this case is not to describe his cramp as an attitude; it's to describe the cramp in terms of what it indicates. Of course, the phrase "find attractive" does describe an attitude when it's applied to desire; but it may still describe the attitude in extrinsic terms, as evidence of its object's attractiveness, rather than in terms of the attitude's content or direction of fit. Hence the subject's finding something attractive may not entail that he has mental access either to a proposition about attractiveness or to an attitude that takes "attractive" as its constitutive predicate.

These subtleties in our descriptions of propositional attitudes are compounded by the fact that predicates like "attractive" and "desirable" can have both normative and nonnormative senses. Calling something desirable can have the normative meaning that the thing is correct or fitting to desire; but it can also have the purely psychological meaning that the thing tends to be desired, that it's easy or natural to desire. We must therefore be doubly careful with the observation that someone who desires something can be said to find it desirable. Desiring something may sometimes entail having an experience indicative of the thing's being easily or naturally desired; and in such a case, it entails finding the thing desirable, in some sense. But to have an experience that's evidence of something's tendency to be desired is not necessarily to think of the thing as readily desired, much less to think of it as correct to desire or worth desiring. Hence we mustn't assume that someone who finds something desirable thereby makes a desirability-judgment that would subjectively justify action.

Although I think that some such confusion is responsible for the use of "good" or "desirable" as the constitutive predicate of desire, I also think that this usage can be harmless, if properly understood. I am not opposed to describing desire as the attitude of regarding something as good, so long as this description is taken merely to express the attitude's direction of fit. Unfortunately, the description is also taken to imply that desire has the justificatory force of a value judgment; and in this respect, the description is misleading.

The resulting confusion can best be explained by analogy to a related misunderstanding about the justificatory force of belief. We are inclined to think that belief qualifies as a judgment of a proposition's truth, and carries the justificatory force of a truth judgment, simply because it entails regarding the proposition as true. Yet to say that belief entails regarding a proposition as true doesn't exhaust the relation between belief and the truth. There are many cognitive attitudes other than belief, attitudes that have the same direction of fit and consequently take the same constitutive predicate. Hypothesizing that p, assuming that p, fantasizing that p, and the like are all attitudes in which p is regarded, not as a representation of what is to be brought about, but rather as a representation of what is. The propositional object of these attitudes is thus regarded as true. Yet fantasizing that p doesn't amount to a judgment on the truth of p, and it lacks the justificatory force that would attach to such a judgment. Hence the reason why belief qualifies as a truth judgment cannot be simply that its constitutive predicate is "true."

One might be inclined to say that fantasizing and hypothesizing don't involve regarding anything as *really* true. But to say this is simply to acknowledge that there is more than one way of regarding a proposition as true. The sense in which hypotheses aren't regarded as really true is, not that they aren't regarded as true at all, but rather that they are only hypothetically so regarded. Fantasies aren't regarded as really true because it is only imaginatively, or in imagination, that they are regarded as true—not because they aren't so regarded at all. To regard something as "really" true must therefore be a particular way of regarding it as true—and, in particular, some way other than imaginatively or hypothetically.

My point here is not the purely grammatical point that imagining or assuming something entails imagining or assuming it to be true; after all, wanting something entails wanting it to be true, as well. In this construction, "true" attaches, trivially, to all propositional attitudes, simply by virtue of their being attitudes toward the bearers of truth values. My point is rather that what distinguishes belief from desired distinguishes assumption, hypothesis, and imagination from desire, too—namely, that they treat their propositional objects as reflecting antecedently fixed conditions rather than as dictating conditions to be achieved, as *facta* rather than *facienda*. To be sure, these attitudes don't treat their propositional objects as reflecting *the actual* facts. But they still treat those propositions as factual reports rather than practical dictates—as being already true of some completed, though unreal, states of affairs rather than as to be made true by the

completion of such states. These attitudes therefore share the distinctively cognitive direction of fit.

The definition that philosophers have traditionally offered for direction of fit has somewhat obscured the difference between cognitive and conative attitudes, as well as the differences among the attitudes within either category.[21] Direction of fit has traditionally been defined in terms of the locus of responsibility for correspondence between an attitude and the world. Whether an attitude has one direction of fit or the other is said to depend on whether the attitude is responsible for conforming itself to the world or makes the world responsible for conforming itself to the attitude. The difference in direction of fit between an expectation and an intention is thus supposed to entail that when an expectation isn't fulfilled, the fault lies with the expectation, whereas when an intention isn't fulfilled, the fault lies with the world.[22]

This definition doesn't accurately characterize the difference between cognition and conation. A lack of correspondence between the world and an assumption, for example, doesn't constitute a failure for which one party or the other must be to blame. If the assumption is made solely for the sake of argument, then it neither takes responsibility for fitting the world nor makes the world responsible for fitting it. Fit between such an assumption and the world is of no importance and is therefore neither party's responsibility. Yet an assumption is still like an expectation, and unlike an intention, in that what's assumed is regarded as true rather than as to be made true, as modelled after its intentional object rather than a model for it. Thus, an assumption still possesses the cognitive direction of fit, even though neither it nor the world is responsible for conforming itself to the other.

Where the traditional definition goes wrong, then, is in presupposing that whenever a proposition is regarded as true or to be made true, its truth thereby comes to constitute a success—and its falsity, a failure—for which either the attitude or the world must bear responsibility. Not every attitude of regarding something as true, or to be made true, has the thing's being or coming true as a criterion of success. I shall now argue that different criteria of success—or, as I shall now put it, different constitutive aims—help to account for the differences among attitudes with the same direction of fit.

Let us say that to regard a proposition as true, in the sense that applies to all cognitive attitudes, is to accept the proposition. We can then distinguish believing that *p* from assuming or fantasizing that *p*, for example, as follows. Assuming or fantasizing that *p* consists in accepting it irrespective of whether it is really true; whereas believing that *p* requires accepting it as if in response to its being true. Thus, belief bears a double relation to the truth. Believing a proposition entails not only regarding the proposition as true but, in addition, so regarding it in a manner designed to reflect whether it really is true.[23] The latter relation to

the truth is part of what distinguishes believing from the other cognitive attitudes, in which a proposition is regarded as true without concern for whether it really is.

The clearest way to analyze such differences between belief and the other cognitive attitudes is in terms of the subject's dispositions to regulate his acceptance of a proposition. When someone assumes a proposition, he or his cognitive faculties are disposed to regulate his acceptance of it in ways designed to promote the ends of argument or inquiry: he comes to accept the proposition when doing so seems conducive to scoring a point or making a discovery, and he is disposed to continue accepting it only insofar as doing so seems to serve such polemical or heuristic purposes. When someone fantasizes, his acceptance of propositions is regulated in ways designed to whet his appetites, stimulate his mind, or provide a substitute for the fulfillment of his wishes: he accepts whatever propositions promise to provide the appropriate excitement or vicarious satisfaction.

When someone believes a proposition, however, his acceptance of it is regulated in ways designed to promote acceptance of the truth: he comes to accept the proposition, for example, when evidence indicates it to be true, and he's disposed to continue accepting it until evidence indicates otherwise. Part of what makes someone's attitude toward a proposition an instance of belief rather than assumption or fantasy, then, is that it is regulated in accordance with epistemic principles rather than polemics, heuristics, or hedonics. An attitude's identity as a belief depends on its being regulated in a way designed to make it track the truth.[24]

Although the dispositional explication of this difference between belief and the other cognitive attitudes is perhaps the clearest, its import can be expressed, as I expressed it above, in attitudinal terms. That is, regulating one's acceptance of the proposition by the exigencies of argument can be described as accepting the proposition without regard to its truth but rather with polemical or heuristic intent. And regulating one's acceptance of a proposition by evidence of its truth can be described as accepting the proposition with an eye to its truth, or with truth as one's aim. Belief and assumption are then described as two-tier attitudes, combining the first-order attitude of acceptance with different second-order attitudes—namely, the different aims or intentions with which a proposition can be accepted.[25]

We thus arrive at the familiar dictum that belief aims at the truth.[26] Properly understood, this dictum means that belief combines the attitude of regarding something as true with the aim of regarding *as* true what really *is* true—of getting the truth right. Hence belief not only has truth as its constitutive predicate but also has correctness in matters of truth—or, as one might put it, the "real" truth—as its constitutive aim.[27]

The difference between the constitutive aim of belief and those of other cognitive attitudes can also be expressed, even less clearly, by being incorporated into the constitutive predicates of these attitudes. Once we conceive of belief

as a two-tier attitude, we tend to think of the second tier as having a constitutive predicate of its own, or as modifying the constitutive predicate of the entire attitude. Accepting a proposition is the attitude of regarding it as true; but accepting a proposition with the aim of accepting what's really true must entail regarding the proposition's acceptance as a means to that end. If one is aiming to get the truth right when one comes to regard p as true, then one must in effect regard p not only as true but also as something to be regarded as true for the sake of getting the truth right. The double relation between belief and truth can thus be expressed, somewhat obscurely, in the thought that believing a proposition entails regarding it as something that one is right to regard as true. Surely, that's what we mean when we say that believing p entails regarding p as "really" true; we mean that it entails regarding p not only as true but also as correct to regard in this way. Belief can thus be conceived as having a constitutive predicate that expresses its own correctness.[28]

The constitutive aim of belief is necessary to belief's being a judgment on the truth of a proposition, since nothing would count as judgment on p's truth if it didn't aim at getting right whether p is true. The constitutive aim of belief is also essential to the attitude's justificatory force as a premise of inferences.

Consider, for example, why my believing that p and that $p \rightarrow q$ gives me subjective justification for believing that q. The answer cannot be simply that believing these propositions entails regarding them as true, and that the truth of the premises guarantees that of the conclusion. After all, fantasizing that p also entails regarding p as true, but fantasies justify nothing whatever, not even other fantasies.

The reason why one belief has subjective justificatory force for other beliefs is that the attitude of belief involves not only regarding a proposition as true but also doing so with the aim of getting the truth right. Because my belief that p is an attempt at tracking the truth, it makes a *prima facie* claim to be on the right track; and with this claim, the belief offers itself as a guide for other attitudes, provided that they, too, aim to track the truth. One belief guides the others because the latter aim at getting the truth right and the former represents my best efforts thus far toward the same end.

Those who have noted that belief aims at the truth are often inclined to think (mistakenly, I shall argue) that desire correspondingly aims at the good.[29] What are the consequences of the assumption that desire and belief are analogous in this respect?

Well, desire is like belief in being only one of many attitudes with its characteristic direction of fit. Wishing, hoping, and the like are also attitudes in which a proposition is regarded as a pattern for the world to follow, as something

to be brought about or made true. Let us say that these attitudes are different ways of approving a proposition, just as the cognitive attitudes are different ways of accepting one. Suppose, then, that the difference between desire and other modes of approval was analogous to that between belief and other modes of acceptance.[30] In that case, wishing that *p,* for example, might entail regarding *p* as to be brought about, but so regarding it irrespective of whether it really was to be brought about; whereas desiring that *p* would entail regarding *p* as to be brought about, and doing so with an eye to whether it really was.[31] The analogy between desire and belief would thus lead to the conclusion that, just as belief aims at tracking the actual facts, so desire aims at tracking the actual *facienda.*

Such an attitude would indeed have the justificatory potential claimed for it in Davidson's theory of rational guidance. As an attempt to track the actual *facienda,* it would present itself as a guide for one's actions, representing one's best efforts to identify what really was to be brought about. What's more, the feature lending justificatory force to this attitude would also give the attitude a constitutive predicate expressing its correctness. For if desiring something entailed regarding it as to be brought about, with the aim of so regarding what really was to be brought about, then it would entail regarding the thing as correct to regard in that way—as correct to approve.

We would thus arrive in the vicinity of Davidson's claim that to desire something is to regard it as desirable.[32] This claim seems to say that to desire something is to have an attitude toward it as worthy of that very attitude. We can now see that such a claim would make sense if it rested on the assumption that desire, like belief, had correctness as its constitutive aim.

Yet when the use of an evaluative term as the constitutive predicate of desire was first introduced, it was understood merely as a way of expressing the attitude's direction of fit—as a colorful alternative to the predicates "to be brought about" or "to be made true." Now a different interpretation has emerged. The claim that to desire something is to regard it as desirable is now being interpreted to imply, not just that the propositional object of desire is regarded as something to be made true or brought about, but also that it is so regarded with the aim of getting things right.

This implication can easily infiltrate our understanding of every evaluative term used to express a desire. Whereas the word "good" in "regarding *p* as good" was initially taken as a synonym for "to be brought about," a phrase that merely expressed the attitude's direction of fit, it can easily be understood as meaning "*really* to be brought about" or "correct to approve"—phrases expressing the aim of tracking the actual *facienda.* Regarding *p* as good can thus be thought to entail a potentially action-guiding judgment as to what is worth bringing about or making true.

In order to assess the validity of this new interpretation, we must ask whether desire really has a constitutive aim analogous to that of belief. The answer, I'm

afraid, is no. When we consider how desire differs in aim from other modes of conation, we find that the difference is not analogous to that between belief and other modes of cognition. The difference in aim between desire and other conative attitudes appears to be that desire aims, not at the good, but rather at the attainable.[33]

One cannot desire something if it seems impossible or if it seems already to have come about; one can desire that *p* only if *p* seems attainable, in the sense of being a possible future outcome. Yet the obstacle to desiring what seems unattainable, or already attained, is not that such things cannot be objects of approval. One can wish that *p* even if the truth of *p* seems quite impossible, and one can hope that *p* when *p* already seems to be true. Thus, one can approve the unattainable or the attained, and what prevents one from desiring them must be something else.

The obstacle, I would suggest, is that desire has the attainable as its constitutive aim. That is, unless approval is regulated in a way designed to track what's attainable, it doesn't qualify as desire; and approval isn't being regulated in a way designed to track the attainable if it's directed at what already seems actual or impossible.[34]

Although this explanation for the limits on desire is only an hypothesis, I think that it is clearly more plausible than the alternative hypothesis about desire's constitutive aim. The grounds that I have just outlined for thinking that desire aims at the attainable are not matched by any comparable grounds for thinking that it aims, more narrowly, at what really is to be brought about. Nothing other than allegiance to the cognitivist program would tempt us to think that desire must be regulated in a way designed to track the *facienda*.

The upshot is that nothing about desire entitles us to credit it with the justificatory force of a value judgment. A judgment on something's value would be an attempt to get things right, and it would consequently have the standing to guide one's actions. But even if desiring something consists in regarding the thing as good, in a sense synonymous with "to be brought about," it isn't an attempt at getting right whether the thing really is to be brought about, and so it doesn't amount to a judgment on the thing's goodness. Desiring something consists in regarding it as to be made true only in the sense that imagining something consists in regarding it as true. Hence desire has the same subjective justificatory force as fantasy—that is, none at all.

That desire doesn't aim at correctness explains why desire can be perverse.[35] As Michael Stocker has pointed out, one can often desire things conceived as worthless, or even bad, and desire them precisely under those descriptions.[36] A tendency to desire things under negative descriptions is an essential element of various emotions and moods such as silliness, self-destructiveness, or despair. A mood of playfulness is, in part, a disposition to form desires for things conceived as having no particular value; a self-destructive mood is, in part, a disposition to

form desires for things conceived as harms; and so on. None of these desires could retain its characteristic idleness or perversity if it involved an attempt at getting things right.

After all, what makes a desire perverse is that its propositional object implies that it is inappropriate. That is, the perverse subject desires that something undesirable occur, and its being undesirable is part of the description under which he desires it. He thus holds the attitude of desire toward something under the description that it is unworthy of that attitude. This discrepancy between his attitude toward an object and his conception of the object's deserts would be impossible in an attitude whose nature was to aim at getting things right and whose constitutive predicate consequently implied the attitude's correctness. Correctness in approval simply cannot be one's aim when one approves of something under the description that it is unworthy of approval.

Consider, by way of analogy, the prospects for perversity in belief. Because belief entails not only regarding a proposition as true but, in addition, doing so with the aim of getting the truth right, belief cannot be transparently perverse. That is, one cannot believe a proposition that presents itself as false—say, the proposition "I am five inches taller than I really am."[37] The reason why one cannot believe such a proposition is not that one is incapable of accepting it. The reason is rather that the only way of accepting such a self-evident falsehood would be to accept it irrespective of its truth; and accepting a proposition irrespective of its truth wouldn't amount to believing it. If one accepts this proposition irrespective of its truth, one will then be assuming it, as one might do for the sake of reasoning counterfactually ("Let's assume that I'm five inches taller than I really am...").

In short, a proposition that presents itself as false cannot be the object of an attitude that aims at getting the truth right. Similarly, a prospect that presented itself as bad could not be the object of an attitude that aimed at correctness in regarding things as to be brought about. Thus, if aiming at correctness were constitutive of desire, as it is of belief, perverse desire would be inconceivable.

The assumption that desire aims at the good forces the cognitivist to misdescribe examples of perverse desire. Consider, for a particularly vivid example, the figure of Satan in *Paradise Lost,* who responds to his defeat with the cry, "Evil be thou my Good."[38] Satan is here resolving to desire and pursue evil, and hence—as he himself puts it—to regard evil as good. But he cannot reasonably be interpreted as adopting new estimates of what's valuable—that is, as resolving to cease judging evil to *be* evil and to start judging it to be good. If Satan ever loses sight of the evil in what he now desires, if he ever comes to think of what he desires as really good, he will no longer be at all satanic; he'll be just another well-intentioned fool. The ruler of Hell doesn't desire what he wrongly thinks is worthy of approval; he desires what he rightly thinks isn't. He thereby illustrates

my point that regarding something as good, in the sense requisite to desiring it, does not amount to making a favorable judgment on its value.

See how Satan's horns are blunted when his desires are misinterpreted as full-blooded value judgments, in this passage from Elizabeth Anscombe's *Intention:*[39]

> 'Evil be thou my good' is often thought to be senseless in some way. Now all that concerns us here is that 'What's the good of it?' is something that can be asked until a desirability characterisation has been reached and made intelligible. If then the answer to this question at some stage is 'The good of it is that it's bad', this need not be unintelligible; one can go on to say 'And what's the good of its being bad?' to which the answer might be condemnation of good as impotent, slavish, and inglorious. Then the good of making evil my good is my intact liberty in the unsubmissiveness of my will.

What sort of Satan is this? He is trying to get things right, and so he rejects the good only because he has found respects in which it is unworthy of approval. He rejects the good, that is, only because it is slavish and inglorious, and hence only because shunning the good is a means to liberty and glory. But then he isn't really shunning the good, after all, since the goods of liberty and glory remain his ultimate goals. Anscombe's Satan can desire evil only by judging it to *be* good, and so he remains, at heart, a lover of the good and the desirable—a rather sappy Satan.

Let me summarize my argument thus far by updating one of Anscombe's own devices for analyzing the difference between cognition and conation. Anscombe suggests that the difference between cognition and conation is analogous to that between an inventory and a shopping list.[40] An inventory is modelled after one's existing stock: it represents things as being on the shelves, having already been obtained. A shopping list is a model for one's stock to follow: it represents things as not yet on the shelves but to be obtained.

What I have argued, in effect, is that Anscombe's analogy neglects differences within the categories of possible inventories and possible shopping lists. When a list of items falls into our hands, we must of course ascertain whether it represents those items as having been obtained or as to be obtained. But we must also ascertain the aims with which the contents of the list have been regulated. A list of things on the shelves may have been compiled in a way designed to represent what's actually on the shelves, but it may also have been compiled in a way designed to include whatever *might* be on the shelves, as a checklist against which the actual contents of the shelves can then be compared. A checklist is also an inventory; it's just a hypothetical inventory. Similarly, a list of things to be obtained may have been compiled in a way designed to track what's actually needed, but it may also have been compiled in way designed to lend excitement

20   *NOÛS*

to one's bet on the lottery. A wish-list is also a shopping list; it's just a fantasy shopping list.

Thus, to find a list headed "Things in stock" is not yet to have grounds for any conclusions about what's available for dinner; and to find a list headed "Things to buy" is not yet to have grounds for making purchases. If the inventory is hypothetical—merely a checklist—then it doesn't embody a judgment of what's in stock and doesn't justify any conclusions about what's available; and if the shopping list is fantastical—merely a wish-list—then it doesn't embody a judgment of what to buy and doesn't justify any purchases. Judgmental and justificatory force attaches only to those lists whose entries have been compiled and regulated with the aim of getting things right.

The cognitivist conception of desire as an action-justifying value judgment thus depends on a misinterpretation of the sense in which desiring something entails regarding it as good. Properly understood, the use of "good" as desire's constitutive predicate doesn't support the cognitivist conception of desire as a value judgment of the sort that would subjectively justify action; and it therefore doesn't support identifying an agent's motivating desire with his guiding reason.

Of course, to show that desire lacks the subjective justificatory force of a value judgment is not to show that such force may be lacking from whatever else might constitute an agent's reason for acting. Indeed, one might think that my arguments thus far prove only that desire cannot be what constitutes an agent's reason for acting, precisely because his reason, whatever it may be, must somehow present his action as a good thing to do.[41] One might then continue to claim that an action performed for a reason must be aimed at the good, without assuming that the guiding evaluation is embodied in a desire.

Yet I think that one of my arguments against identifying reasons with desires suggests an argument against identifying reasons with value judgments in any form. In that argument, I explained the capacity of desires to be perverse in terms of their not being aimed at the good; here I shall contend that reasons for acting can be perverse as well. That is, an agent's reason for doing something can be that it's a bad thing to do; and so its justificatory force cannot depend on that of a favorable evaluation.

Suppose that I have suffered a profound disappointment that has cast me into a mood of bitterness and despair. In this mood, the very thought of ameliorating my condition, or the condition of the world, strikes me as a sick delusion. All attempts at constructive action seem absurd. No more earnest efforts for me, I say to myself, no more worthy endeavors: to hell with it all.[42]

Being in despair doesn't prevent me from being moved to act, however. I am moved to stay at home, refuse all invitations, keep the shades drawn, and privately curse the day I was born. I may even be moved to smash some crockery —though not in order to feel better, mind you, since trying to feel better seems just as ludicrous a project as any other. (Someone who smashes crockery in order

to feel better didn't feel all that bad to begin with.) What's more, I engage in these actions not only *out of* despair but also *in light of* and *on the grounds of* despair. That is, despair is part of my reason as well as part of my motive for acting.

But do I regard my actions, in light of my despair, as good or desirable or positive things to do? Far from it. I am determined never to do a good or desirable or positive thing again. If smashing things seemed like a good thing to do, I would pointedly avoid it; even if it seemed good only for someone in despair, I would still avoid it; indeed, it's seeming good for someone in despair would count most strongly against it, since doing things that are good for someone in my condition is exactly what, in light of that condition, makes sense for me to avoid.[43] I'm smashing things because this seems like an utterly worthless act, worthless from every perspective but especially from mine. My reason for acting thus includes not only my mood but also an unconditionally negative evaluation of the action.

To be sure, there is a kind of perversity that would preclude my acting for reasons; but the perversity that would preclude acting for reasons is not a counter-evaluative state of mind but rather a counter-rational one. That is, I cannot act for reasons if I don't care about doing what's justified or (as I would prefer to put it) what makes sense. But I can still care about doing what makes sense even if I don't care about the good. This possibility is demonstrated by my capacity to be guided by what makes sense in light of a counter-evaluative mood such as despair, since what makes sense in light of such a mood just is to do what's bad rather than what's good.

Yet pursuing the bad on the grounds of despair would be impossible if every reason for an action had to present that action as a good thing to do. The problem is not that the badness of an action could never make the action seem good. The problem is that if the badness of an action weighed with me by making the action seem good, then I would be once again engaged in pursuing the good—a pursuit incompatible with the very mood that helps to constitute my reason for acting. Just as Satan would have to shed his satanism in order to value evil *sub specie boni,* so I would have to shed my despair in order to pursue a self-destructive course under that positive guise. If I were swayed toward an action because its badness made it seem like a good thing to do, then I'd be in the business of finding silver linings, a business that's closed to me so long as I am truly acting out of despair.

If my arguments are correct, then practical reasoning is nothing like what it has traditionally been conceived to be. Desires lack the evaluative force that is thought to make them reasons for acting; and the justificatory force of reasons is not evaluative, in any case. Since reasons do not recommend an action by presenting it as a good thing to do, actions performed for reasons need not be performed under the guise of the good.

Notes

[1]The material in this paper has been presented, in various forms, at the University of Michigan, Yale University, and the University of Dayton. I am grateful to these audiences for their comments. I am also indebted to Rüdiger Bittner, Paul Boghossian, Jennifer Church, Carl Ginet, Jonathan Lear, Richard Miller, Donald Regan, Connie Rosati, Geoffrey Sayre-McCord, Sydney Shoemaker, Michael Slote, Michael Smith, and Dennis Stampe for comments on earlier drafts or discussion of related issues. Thanks are also due to Lloyd Humberstone for allowing me to read the manuscript of a paper entitled "Direction of Fit."

[2]Anscombe [1963], 70 ff.; Davidson [1978], 97, note 7; Stampe [1987], 355; Goldman [1970], 94.

[3]See De Sousa [1974]; see also Davidson [1970], 22; Pears [1984], 198.

[4]Smith [MS] refers to these two stories as the "intentional perspective" and the "deliberative perspective." I understand that Rüdiger Bittner is also working independently on the relation between these stories.

[5]I have borrowed this example from Davidson [1970], 31 ff. I shall presently discuss Davidson's own analysis of the case.

[6]I realize, of course, that some philosophers would deny that genuine propositions justify action, independently of their actually or potentially exerting some motivational influence on the agent. I discuss this view briefly below, under the name of noncognitivism.

[7]I shall avoid giving an example of an action-justifying proposition, so as to remain neutral on the precise nature of practical reason.

[8]To say that acting for a reason entails being influenced by the intrinsic action-justifying character of a belief is not to say that it requires the operative belief to have intrinsic motivational force that's independent of any desires. One may have a desire to perform actions that are justified, or to perform actions that are related to one's circumstances in particular ways, which are in fact justifying. Any belief that gains motivational force from such a desire will also owe that motivational force, in part, to its own action-justifying character, and will therefore fulfill the story of rational guidance. I thus assume that beliefs can be intrinsically justifying even if they cannot be intrinsically motivating. Here I differ with, e.g., Nagel [1970] and McDowell [1978].

[9]This approach can be traced back at least as far as Hobbes's definition of deliberation, at *Leviathan*, Part I, chapter vi.

[10]The noncognitivist cannot remove the discrepancy by pointing out that he conceives of justificatory force as a disposition to motivate, which can indeed explain particular instances of motivation. In the commonsense story, the justificatory force of a reason explains (rather than consists in) the reason's disposition to motivate as well as its motivating on particular occasions.

My remarks on the noncognitivist view echos much that is said in Falk [1963] and [1986]. Yet Falk does not ultimately reject noncognitivism, since he, too, believes that reasons "are...choice-supporting in proportion to their choice-influencing potential" ([1963], 92).

[11][1978], 86.

[12]Of course, the young child may not be susceptible to rational guidance, either; but this point hardly counts in Davidson's favor. When Davidson characterizes belief-desire motivation as equivalent to rational guidance, he leaves no room for agents who are moved by desires without being guided by reasons. The fact that children, who pursue desired ends, can nevertheless be too young for rational guidance is therefore a point against Davidson, on a par with my point that they can be too young for the concept of the desirable. (For an alternative argument against identifying desires with evaluative judgments, see Lewis [1988].)

[13]I think that Davidson sometimes betrays an uncomfortable awareness of this difficulty. He wants to avoid the implausibly strong claim that desires consist in value judgments. (See, e.g., the discussion of wanting to drink a can of paint at [1963], 4.) And yet he senses that he is committed to that claim by his strategy of equating motivation with rational guidance. (See, e.g., [1978], 102 [desires "constitute" value judgments]; [1970], 31 [desiring something is "setting a positive value" on it]; [1978], 97, note 7 [desiring something entails "holding" it to have "some positive characteristic"].)

[14]The reader will find that I use the term "direction of fit" in a somewhat different sense from others who have used the term—including, for example, Searle [1983], 7 ff.; and Platts [1979], 257. (See also Anscombe [1963], 56.) The definition offered by these authors will be explained and criticized in the text below.

15Direction of fit is clearly what Dennis Stampe has in mind in his version of this claim: "[W]hile the belief and the desire that *p* have the same propositional content and represent the same state of affairs, there is a difference in the *way* it is represented in the two states of mind. In belief it is represented *as obtaining,* whereas in desire, it is represented as a state of affairs *the obtaining of which would be good."* ([1987], 355).

16What psychological realization, if any, attends the predicates used to characterize propositional attitudes? A behaviorist might insist that regarding a proposition as true is nothing more than being disposed to behave as would be appropriate if the proposition were true. Alternatively, one might imagine that regarding a proposition as true entails having a representation of it in a particular mental compartment, which might be called the "true" box, because of its role in the mental architecture. Another alternative would be to give a phenomenological rather than functional account of the relevant mental posture toward a proposition—whatever such an account might be. The most attractive alternative, for present purposes, is a stance of neutrality among these and other models of propositional attitudes. One needn't adopt any particular model of propositional attitudes in order to adopt the descriptions whose realization is the point of contention among such models. One can thus insist that whatever believing that *p* consists in, it must be something that would appropriately be called regarding *p* as true; and whatever desiring that *p* consists in, it must be something that would appropriately be called regarding *p* as to be made true.

17This version of cognitivism is articulated by Dennis Stampe: "Desires constitute reasons for us to act because their contents are represented as states of affairs the realization of which would be good" (*ibid.*). I do not know whether Davidson accepts or would accept this formulation. His accepting it would explain why he says both that desires are and that they are expressed by value judgments.

18Davidson seems to entertain a view like this when he says, "[I]f someone acts with an intention, he must have attitudes and beliefs from which, *had he been aware of them* and had the time, he *could* have reasoned that his action was desirable" ([1978], 85, emphasis added). Here Davidson seems to suggest that the agent needs to become aware of his attitudes in order to be in a position to draw a conclusion about the desirability of his action. I do not understand, however, how this suggestion squares with Davidson's claim that an intentional action constitutes the agent's conclusion that the action is desirable ([1978], 99). For how can his action constitute a conclusion that he might not have been in a position to draw?

19But see the discussion of the issue in my [1989].

20That Davidson regards desire as justifying action subjectively is confirmed by passages such as this: "Thus there is a certain irreducible—though somewhat anaemic—sense in which every rationalization justifies: *from the agent's point of view* there was, when he acted, something to be said for the action" ([1963], 9, italics mine).

21In this paragraph and the next I have benefitted from Lloyd Humberstone's manuscript "Direction of Fit."

22See the references to Searle, Platts, and Anscombe in note 14, above.

23For an explication of this expression, see the following note. The expression gives, at most, a necessary condition of belief, not a sufficient condition. Indeed, even to call it a necessary condition may still be too strong. My suspicion is that attitudes qualify as beliefs or desires or intentions, etc., by virtue of approximating to a paradigm or ideal specimen. What are usually called the necessary conditions for belief or desire are in fact a definition of the paradigm case; and instances that fail to meet one condition may still qualify as beliefs or desires if they sufficiently resemble the relevant paradigm in other respects. (See my [1989], 136.)

24What do I mean when I describe a cognitive mechanism as "designed to track the truth"? I don't mean that it's designed in such a way that it succeeds in tracking the truth, since beliefs can be false. Rather, I mean that its design is governed by the goal of tracking the truth, although it may not attain that goal invariably or completely. And I am of course assuming that the concept of design encompasses the work of the pseudo-designer known as evolution.

In the text I have assumed that a mechanism designed to track the truth would operate in response to evidence, as it probably would if designed by evolution. But other mechanisms might also qualify as being designed to track the truth—particularly if they were designed by the subject himself, in accordance with an alternative epistemology. For example, someone who believes that the truth about something is to be found by consulting scripture or seeking revelation may regulate his acceptance of the relevant propositions by those means. The resulting attitudes will qualify as

beliefs, however, since the method of their regulation will be designed to track the truth, in the requisite sense. (I am indebted to Michael Slote for pointing out this possibility.)

[25]Note that the aim or intention with which a proposition is accepted may belong to the subject's cognitive faculties rather than to the subject himself, depending on who or what is regulating the subject's acceptance of propositions. I shall henceforth ignore this distinction. In "Direction of Fit," Lloyd Humberstone cites Urmson [1967] as offering a similar account of the difference between imagining and remembering.

[26]The notion that belief aims at the truth figures prominently in the literature on believing at will. See, e.g., Williams [1970].

[27]This aspect of belief is, I suspect, what leads Davidson to say, "Someone cannot have a belief unless he understands the possibility of being mistaken" ([1975], 168). Because believing entails aiming to get the truth right, it would seem to entail understanding the possibility of a mistake. But the soundness of this argument depends on the assumption that the constitutive aim of belief must be an attitude of the believer rather than a purpose inherent in the design of his cognitive faculties. I have suggested that a person's acceptance of a proposition can be aimed at getting the truth right— and hence qualify as a belief—so long as it is regulated by a mechanism designed to track the truth. (See note 24, above.) In that case, the believer himself might lack the conceptual resources for framing the requisite aim in an attitudinal sense.

[28]Or, more precisely, the correctness of the acceptance involved in the belief. The view that belief involves an intimation of its own correctness is similar to the view of judgment that Hannah Ginsborg attributes to Kant. Ginsborg argues that reflective judgment, for Kant, is "the capacity for taking one's states of mind in the perception of given objects to be universally valid" (MS, p 13). See also Ginsborg's [1990].

[29]See Anscombe [1963], 76: "Truth is the object of judgment, and good the object of wanting..."; De Sousa [1974], 538: "[T]ruth and good are the *targets* of belief and want."

[30]Note that the distinction developed here is different from Pears's distinction between "weak" and "strong" value judgments, even though Pears regards his distinction as defining the line between those value judgments which are and those which are not necessarily implicated in preference and noncompulsive intentional action ([1984], 196 ff.). "Weak" value judgments, in Pears's terminology, are still *judgments*; what distinguishes them from their "strong" counterparts is the set of interests on which they are based. My distinction, by contrast, divides value judgments from valuings or preferrings that aren't judgments at all.

[31]What would it mean to say that something really was to be brought about? I'm not sure. This phrase is generated when the formula describing the constitutive aim of belief is adapted for the purpose of attributing an analogous aim to desire. Since I reject the analogy, I needn't take responsibility for the language it generates.

[32]I say "in the vicinity" because to regard something as worthy of approval is not quite to regard it as worth desiring—approval and desire being slightly different attitudes.

[33]For this point I am indebted to Geoffrey Sayre-McCord.

[34]Note, as before, that an attitude's constitutive aim should be treated as a necessary but not a sufficient condition. An instance of approval must have other features—including, perhaps, actual or counterfactual behavioral manifestations—in order to qualify as a desire. Compare note 23, above, for further qualifications.

[35]Although I believe that we can indeed have perverse desires (and shall assume so in the text), I am not strictly committed to this empirical claim. I am committed only to the claim that desires can *in principle* be perverse, in the sense that there is nothing about the concept of desire that would prevent a perverse attitude from satisfying it. That is, an attitude can qualify as a desire even if it is perverse. This conceptual claim would be compatible with there being some contingent feature of human psychology that prevented us from having perverse desires.

[36]Stocker [1979]. See also Anderson [MS].

[37]The word 'really' in this proposition rigidly designates our world, so that the proposition is evidently false in this world but true in some other possible world.

[38]Book IV, line 110.

[39][1963], 75.

[40]*Ibid.*, 56 ff.

[41]For the view that evaluation is embedded in the very concept of a reason, see, e.g., Baier [1984], 202: "What I call 'cognitive' reasons are employed in the activity of examining what to

believe, and 'practical' ones are employed in the activity of examining what to do. The specific aim of the first is beliefs that are true; the second is intentions or acts that are good. We could say that the aim in the case of the first is the true and in the case of the second the good." See also Bond [1983], 2 - 3. For a persuasive attack on this view, see Anderson [MS].

[42]Again, see Stocker [1979], 745.

[43]*Ibid.*, 748.

References

Anderson, Elizabeth
MS   "Pluralism, Deliberation, and Rational Choice," Chapter II of a book in progress.

Anscombe, G.E.M.
1963   *Intention* (Ithaca, New York: Cornell University Press).

Baier, Kurt
1984   "Rationality, Reason, and the Good," in *Morality, Reason and Truth*, ed. by D. Copp and D. Zimmerman (Totowa, New Jersey: Rowman & Littlefield), 193 - 211.

Bond, E.J.
1983   *Reason and Value* (Cambridge: Cambridge University Press).

Davidson, Donald
1963   "Actions, Reasons, and Causes," reprinted in Davidson [1980], 3 - 19.
1970   "How is Weakness of the Will Possible?" reprinted in Davidson [1980], 21 - 42.
1975   "Thought and Talk," reprinted in *Inquiries into Truth and Interpretation* (Oxford: Clarendon Press, 1984).
1978   "Intending," reprinted in Davidson [1980], 83 - 102.
1980   *Essays on Actions and Events* (Oxford: Clarendon Press).

De Sousa, Ronald B.
1974   "The Good and the True," 83 *Mind* 534 - 51.

Falk, W.D.
1963   "Action-Guiding Reasons," reprinted in the same volume as Falk [1986], 82 - 98.
1986   "On Learning about Reasons," in *Ought, Reasons, and Morality* (Ithaca, New York: Cornell University Press), 67 - 81.

Ginsborg, Hannah
MS   "Kant on Judgment," unpublished
1990   "Reflective Judgment and Taste," 24 *Nous* 63 - 78.

Goldman, Alvin I.
1970   *A Theory of Human Action* (Princeton: Princeton University Press).

Lewis, David
1988   "Desire as Belief," 97 *Mind* 323 - 42.

McDowell, John
1978   "Are Moral Requirements Hypothetical Imperatives?" 41 *Proceedings of the Aristotelian Society* (supp. vol.) 13 - 29.

Nagel, Thomas
1970   *The Possibility of Altruism* (Princeton: Princeton University Press).

26   *NOÛS*

Pears, David
1984   *Motivated Irrationality* (Oxford: Clarendon Press).

Platts, Mark
1979   *Ways of Meaning* (London: Routledge and Kegan Paul).

Searle, John
1983   *Intentionality: An Essay in the Philosophy of Mind* (Cambridge: Cambridge University Press).

Smith, Michael
MS   "Valuing: Desiring or Believing?".

Stampe, Dennis
1987   "The Authority of Desire" 96 *The Philosophical Review* 335 - 81.

Stocker, Michael
1979   "Desiring the Bad: An Essay in Moral Psychology," 76 *Journal of Philosophy* 738 - 53.

Urmson, J.O.
1967   "Memory and Imagination," 76 *Mind* 83 - 91.

Velleman, J. David
1989   *Practical Reflection* (Princeton: Princeton University Press).

Williams, Bernard
1970   "Deciding to Believe," reprinted in *Problems of the Self* (Cambridge: Cambridge University Press, 1973).

[14]

The Philosophical Review, XCVI, No. 3 (July 1987)

THE AUTHORITY OF DESIRE

Dennis W. Stampe

Aristotle said that the "intellect itself moves nothing"; not even the thinker himself is moved by thought alone. But thinking which " . . . aims at an end and is practical" does issue in "choice" and rational motion. Such practical thought originates in the appetite, and such motions, therefore, begin in desire. ("Hence choice is desiderative reason or ratiocinative desire . . . " N.E. 1139b). But how is it *possible* for practical reasoning to begin in desire? That is perhaps the central question about practical reasoning. The central question about *desire* is the question how practical reasoning can begin in *it*.[1]

I. REASONS AND OBJECTS

It is in the power of reason to determine what we do, and also what we think. Reasoning from our present beliefs, we come to new ones. We reason out what we believe from what we already believe—not from our believing it, but from *what* we believe, from the "object" rather than the "act" of belief: it is in that sense that reasoning that issues in belief starts from belief. And from what we believe, and our desires, we reason out what to do. But how do we reason "from our desires"? It is not that we reason from *what* we want, as we reason

---

[1]The Aristotelian dictum that desire is the starting point of practical reasoning that ends in action can of course be denied. Its denial is a commonplace of moral theory in the tradition of Kant. But in this essay I am concerned with that issue only indirectly. I shall not contend that rational action always or necessarily does involve desire as its starting point; nor shall I deny it. My question concerns instead the *possibility* of its ever beginning in desire. For there is a question whether it is even possible for reasoning to begin in desire, a question arising from the nature of desire and its objects, which to my knowledge has not been articulated. If we can see how desire *can* provide the *arche* of action, then we can consider later, and from that vantage point, whether it is necessary that it should do so. It will, I think, be possible eventually to argue that if practical reasoning has the character it must have, if it *can* begin in desire, then its starting point can be nothing but desire.

DENNIS W. STAMPE

from what we think. *What* I *think* might be, for example, that a hat would keep my head warm, and I can reason from that *fact,* to one conclusion or another about having a hat. But *what I want* is not the kind of thing from which I can reason: *what I want* is such a thing as: a hat; or: *to have* a hat. A hat, or *to have a hat* are not the kinds of things *from* which one may reason. Even if what I want is specified with a propositional clause, I cannot reason from what I want. For then what I want is *that I have a hat,* or *that it should be the case* that I do. But these clauses are in the subjunctive, as they must be if they are to specify what I want: and in that mood my having a hat is not represented as a state of affairs that holds in fact. So even when what I want is specified by a propositional clause, it is not represented as something from which I may reason. For it is not represented as being a fact. Nor should it be. For if it is what I *want*—that is, a state of affairs I *want to be* the case—it is apt at present not to *be* the case.

At bottom, the problem is this: it is only from a fact, or what is supposed to be a fact, that one may reason—in the sense, that is, in which "what one reasons from" is itself one of the reasons one reaches the conclusion one does.[2] What one believes either is, or is something taken to be, a fact. It is, one may say, the office of belief to present the facts to the forum of reason, and its contents are accordingly presented as fact. Desire is a very different thing. The "content" of a desire (like the content of a belief)[3] is indeed a state of affairs: the desire for a hat has, as its content, the state of affairs in which one has a hat. But a state of affairs presented to the mind

---

[2]In hypothetical reasoning too, and even *reductio.* Here, while the reasoning begins with the consideration of a mere supposition, or of a state of affairs not obtaining in fact, what one *reasons from* are the facts about that supposition or state of affairs being considered: for example, facts about what would be the case if it were true, or were it to hold. Again, in the sense in question, what one "reasons from" are themselves reasons for one to reach the conclusions one does, or would be such if things were as they are believed to be. Neither the hypothetical state of affairs nor the supposition of it are *themselves* such reasons. Obviously, if my reasoning begins with consideration of the proposition *p,* and my conclusion is that *p* is false, then *p* is not my reason for concluding that *not-p.*

[3]The "content" (or "object") being what is designated by the complement clause of a sentence ascribing a belief, or a desire, to someone; thus what is designated by "*p*" in sentences of the form "S wants/believes it to be the case that *p.*"

THE AUTHORITY OF DESIRE

by desire is not thereby presented as obtaining in fact—even if it should happen that it does obtain in fact; at least, if the desire comprises a basis for *doing* something, what is wanted is a state of affairs which either does not or *might* not obtain in fact. And while I might reason from the fact that I do *not* have a hat, *that* is not what I want; the object of my desire is my *having* a hat, and that non-obtaining state of affairs cannot possibly be that from which I reason. (Thus my having a hat might better be said to be and to be presented as being a possible "objective.") But such states of affairs, not being represented as facts, cannot be what we reason from, and cannot themselves comprise reasons for us to act. For only what it is possible to reason from can constitute a reason to believe or to do something. Reasons are what we mean to reason from, and reasons are facts. What we *take* to be a reason to do or believe something, we *take* to be a fact. If we are wrong in taking it to be a fact, we are wrong in supposing that there was, in that belief—in its content, that is; in *what* we believed—a reason to do or believe that thing. Thus the sailors who, believing that the earth is flat, declined to sail with Columbus, had *in* that belief no reason to decline: since the earth is not flat, its being flat was no reason.[4]

When we reason from our beliefs it is from *what* we believe—the objects of our beliefs—that we reason: the facts as we believe them to be. (If those beliefs are true, then there are reasons therein—facts—from which to reason; and if they are false, then the belief may be counted a reason only because its content *would* comprise a

---

[4]They did of course reason it out from something, that one could not get to the east by sailing west. Indeed, it was from their belief that the earth is flat that they reasoned: and the fact that they had that belief was a reason for their refusal. We may cite the belief itself as their reason, however, only because *what* they believed, *were* it a fact, *would* be a reason for refusing to go. Whether the belief that *p* may itself be described as a reason for something, depends upon whether the *fact* that *p* would be a reason for that thing. Desire differs. The desire that it be the case that *p* may be a reason for one to do something, but its being a reason does not depend on whether the *fact* that *p* would be a reason for doing that thing—it depends more nearly on whether its *not* being a fact that *p* would be a reason for doing it. Thus my wanting it to be the case that I am immune from tetanus is a reason for me to get vaccinated, but this is certainly not because it *is* the case that I am immune, nor because *were* it the case, the fact that I was immune would be a reason to get vaccinated. (It would, in fact, be a reason not to do so.)

337

DENNIS W. STAMPE

reason, were it true.) Our beliefs, then, comprise reasons for us to
act *through* their objects. But when we reason from our desires, it is
not from what we want that we reason. Desires, then, cannot, in
that sense, comprise reasons for acting *through* their objects. How
then *can* they do so? How can practical reasoning possibly begin in
desire?

Desires do not have facts as their contents. Some writers who
would keep desire at the bottom of practical reasoning simply provide themselves, more or less by fiat, with contents that *are* facts,
and facts brought into the picture, one way or another, by desire.
There is the very fact that one wants the thing—the desire itself; or
the fact that one doesn't have it. Whatever the relevance of these
facts might be, one thing is clear: they are not the *objects* of our
desires; they are not *what* we want. Again, as Miss Anscombe said,
perhaps one who wants something must have some "desirability
characteristic" of it in mind.[5] One must think that the desired state
of affairs would meet one's needs, or be pleasant, or, in a word, that
it would be *good*. If you want a hat, you must think it would be good
in some way to have a hat; and it might be a *fact* that it would be
good to have a hat. One could take this to be the fact, introduced by
desire, from which practical reasoning proceeds, the reason one
who wants a hat has to go and get one.

But, again, these propositions that ascribe some such desirability
characteristic to a state of affairs—for example, it would be good
were it to be the case that *p*—designate neither what one wants nor
the desire for it. They might state reasons for *having* the desire. (As
might also the fact that one doesn't have the thing.) Thus they
specify the contents of *beliefs* a person might have, from which
there might arise a desire that it be the case that *p*. If practical
reasoning begins from such premises as these, then it does not

---

[5]G. E. M. Anscombe, *Intention* §37 (New York: Blackwell, 1958). Some
writers depend on the very characteristic of being desirable, representing
the beginnings of practical reasoning as "It is desirable that *p*." But reasoning beginning in "It is desirable that *p*" is not reasoning beginning in the
desire that *p*: the proposition "It is desirable that *p*" does not represent the
content of a desire. Were one to construe theoretical reasoning analogously, one would have it beginning not from, for example, "All Greeks
are mortal," but from "It is believable that all Greeks are mortal." (That, of
course, is just the content of a distinct belief.)

THE AUTHORITY OF DESIRE

properly begin in desire in any sense at all; indeed, desire plays no essential role in it. Desire drops out of the picture altogether, or is reduced to some merely auxiliary role.

Some philosophers welcome any such derogation of the role of desire in practical reasoning; reasoning dependent on desire has such an odor of contingency or self-interest, so they think, that morality cannot be founded upon it. Others might simply identify desires with beliefs of a certain kind[6] and have done with it. Desires might be identified with beliefs having a certain content—perhaps the desire that *p* is just a peculiarly efficacious belief that it would be good if *p*.

One might reason out what to do from the fact that it would be good if *p*. But could one explain thereby, by reason alone, one's doing it, or intending to? We must consider what the logic of this reasoning might be, this transition from the propositional contents of the belief to those of the intention. Starting from *It would be good if p*, and perhaps *Only my doing A will make it the case that p*, by what logic do we pass to *I will do A*? All that seems to *follow* is that *It would be good to do A*—and this neither denotes an action nor the content of an intention; further premises would yield *I ought to do A*, but to believe that is not to intend to do A. We confront a logical gap. And it cannot, it seems, be bridged by the addition of further beliefs.

We should aim for a view on which the practical reasoning concludes, by force of some sort of logic, in propositions expressing the contents not just of belief, but of intention. I shall assume, accordingly, that desires are states of mind distinct in kind from beliefs. And surely one can believe that it would be good that *p*

6Or, with some generic attitude toward a proposition common to both belief and desire. I have in mind, for example, Donald Davidson, who writes "I do not suppose that someone who wants to eat something sweet necessarily *judges* that it would be good to eat something sweet; perhaps we can say he *holds* that his eating something sweet has some positive characteristic. By distinguishing among the propositional expressions of attitudes I hope to mark differences among the attitudes." ("Intending," in *Essays on Action and Events* (Oxford: Oxford University Press, 1980; footnote, p. 97.) Mark them, may be: but of course what may serve to mark a difference may reveal nothing about the nature of that difference, and may tend in fact to conceal it. Distinguishing the attitudes as proposed will mark that difference in a way less than perspicuous if belief and desire may be attitudes regarding the very same state of affairs, as I think they may be.

without in the least way wanting it to be the case that *p*. (Neither, of course, will it do to say that desires are peculiarly efficacious beliefs with that content, for the belief that it would be good if *p* which is *not* a desire might well be a peculiarly efficacious *belief*.) The problem I am trying to state affords us a chance to penetrate the difference between belief and desire.

It is surely of the first importance in the philosophy of mind to recognize that the mind is occupied not just with states of affairs that do obtain, but with states of affairs that ideally *are* to obtain: with representations not conformed to the way the world is, but to which the world might better *be* conformed. I shall work toward a view in which reason functions to maximize the extent to which the state of the world and the state of our minds stand in conformity— both, through theoretical reasoning, by conforming the mind—in respect of what we believe—to the way the world is, or, through practical reasoning, by conforming the world to the state of our minds, as when we make things be the way we want them to be.

If desires do not represent states of affairs that obtain in fact, what they present to us are not reasons for us to act. In view of something that is *not* a fact—for example, one's having the hat one wants—practical reasoning may aim at a conclusion that would *make* it a fact. It may conclude in some intention or action intended to bring it about that one has it in fact. That is the kind of reasoning that is practical, the peculiar way it is directed upon fact.

But what can the logic of such reasoning be? Aristotle gives examples of practical reasoning that are perfectly good despite their being deductively invalid: I need a covering; I would have one if I made a cloak; so I'll make a cloak (*De motu animalium* 701ª18.) There are other kinds of coverings, so how does the conclusion follow? Anthony Kenny has maintained that this is not just good but logically *valid* reasoning, validity, in practical reasoning, consisting not in the necessity but in the sufficiency of the conclusion for the truth of the objective specified in the major premise— that is to say, that I have a covering. And he suggested that this locates the difference between practical and theoretical reasoning. But what his important discussion also suggests is a formal similarity between practical reasoning and one kind of theoretical reasoning—namely, *abduction,* in which the conclusion represents the

THE AUTHORITY OF DESIRE

explanation of the state of affairs cited in the premise.[7] For in abduction too, the conclusion represents an hypothesis the truth of which is not necessary but is rather sufficient for the truth of the premise: the streets are wet; they would be wet if it had rained; so it must have rained. There is no obvious *logical* difference between practical and theoretical reasoning of this type, and it becomes interestingly difficult to see what their basic difference might be. In both cases the reasoning aims at something that would make the state of affairs named in the first premise a fact: its having rained would make it a fact that the streets are wet; my buying a hat would make it a fact that I have a hat. The first would make the initial belief true; the second would satisfy the initial desire—make it a fact that I have a hat. Alternatively, the first (its having rained) would make something that *is* a fact (that is to say, that the streets are wet) *be* a fact; the second would make something that is *not* a fact (that I have a hat) be a fact. The rationality of the conclusion differs accordingly: it is rational to believe the conclusion of the abductive syllogism because it would explain the observed fact from which the reasoning begins. Where the conclusion is an action (my buying a hat), it is rational to *do* that thing because the act would make it a fact (this being something which is not a fact) that I have a hat; it is not rational to do it because doing it would explain

---

[7]"Practical Inference," *Analysis*, 1966. Cf. his *Will, Freedom, and Power* (New York: Blackwell, 1975). In this view, the logically operative premise of the practical syllogism must be taken to be my having a covering—what is needed (or wanted)—not the proposition that I need or want it.

Kenny's practical logic of satisfactoriness is surely a special case of the logic of *acceptability*—whether of a plan of action or of an hypothesis. The analogy between practical and abductive "inference" has been noted also by R. M. Hare and H. Simon, perhaps among others. It was perhaps not far from the mind of Aristotle himself, who remarks on the analogy between practical reasoning and the reasoning of a geometer. Practical reasoning concerns the way to get what is wanted, there being often more than one way. The relevant geometrical reasoning concerns the way some given geometrical figure might be constructed of simpler figures, there being several such ways conceivable, several hypotheses regarding its generation, as it were. Thus, he says, " . . . what is last in the order of analysis is first in the order of becoming," both in practical and in geometrical reasoning—as it is in the abductive reconstruction of the cause of some phenomenon (*Nicomachean Ethics*, 1112ᵇ23; Ross translation).

DENNIS W. STAMPE

its being a fact. If the conclusion is rational the premise must represent my having a hat as something that is not a fact. (But it is also
necessary that it be the content of a desire of mine—or of *some* state
of mind—that comprises a reason for me to do the thing.)

Here, then, against the background of their logical similarity a
difference emerges between the two kinds of reasoning. It is a
difference in the nature of their starting points, or the ways they
respectively provide reasons for their conclusions. Each begins in a
state of mind the content of which is a state of affairs that would be
made the case by the conclusion. But that from which the abductive
syllogism begins—the reason one has for concluding that it rained
—is a *fact*, the fact for example that the streets are wet: not that one
believes that to be the case, but that it *is* the case, in fact; again, the
conclusion is something that would make something that *is* a fact *be* a
fact. But the reason given in the practical syllogism—the reason one
has for making something be the case—is that one *wants* it to be the
case, not, of course, that it is the case in fact; and the conclusion is
something (an action) that would make it a fact. Beliefs, then,
comprise reasons through their objects: they are, if you will, reasons
per objectum. But it is the *desire itself* that comprises the reason one has
to act as the reasoning concludes—the desire *itself*, and not its object.
A desire, unlike a belief, is *per se* a reason for action. It must be so, if
the object of the desire that *p* be the state of affairs in which *p*, and if
a reason must be a fact. The very point of the practical reasoning,
and the rationality of the act, depends on its *not* being a fact that *p*, or
on the possibility of its not being a fact.

If we recognize the symmetry between practical and abductive
reasoning, and thus the sense in which practical reasoning can
conclude in an act, then we must at the same time recognize an
*a*symmetry in the ways desires and beliefs contribute reasons to our
reasoning.

II. The Authority of Desire

I shall begin with a declaration of "the authority of desire," and
develop its defense as we proceed.

The fact that I want something, in and of itself, is ordinarily a
reason for me to act accordingly. The desire itself therefore makes
the act a rational one, in the sense of one I have a reason to perform—not, perhaps, a decisive one, perhaps not even a good one,

THE AUTHORITY OF DESIRE

but still *a* reason.[8] I call this the *per se authority* of desire. I call it "authority" because it is not with mere force or sheer power that desire moves us, and contends with the intellect, but with a certain right. Desire confers upon action a rationality not inherited from the rationality of one's beliefs or the rationality of any others of one's attitudes. Even if one knows no reason to want the thing, and thinks there is none, the fact that one wants it may still be a reason to try to get it. Even if there is a good reason *not* to want it, the fact that one does want it may nevertheless itself be a reason to try to get it. It is not the rationality of desire that confers rationality upon action: it is the desire itself, whether it be rational or not. It is not that desire is necessarily at war with belief but that a desire is a reason in itself, and in its own right, the contrary dictates of belief notwithstanding.

Desire is an origin of rationality. It is not merely, like belief, a conduit for the authority of the facts, as we believe them to be, to determine the rationality of action, or of other states of mind. If I believe that it has rained because the streets are wet, it is the fact that the streets are wet, not the fact that I believe them to be, that comprises my reason for believing that it has rained.[9] Even if the streets are not, in fact, wet, my belief that it rained is reasonable only because were it a fact that the streets are wet, then that fact would be a reason to believe that it has rained. The authority of a

---

[8]This is not, I think, well put by saying that a desire is a *prima facie* reason to act, if that means just that a desire appears at first, or on its face, to be a reason. What a desire may appear to be, at first or upon reflection, is another matter. My claim is a claim about what a desire is, not what it appears to be. The distinction between a reason and a good reason should not be confused with the distinction between a *prima facie* reason (or what appears to be a reason) and a reason in fact.

[9]Were I to cite, as my reason for believing that it rained, the fact that I *believe* the street to be wet, I would have defended the rationality of my belief if the fact that I *have* the latter belief—that the street is wet—is itself a reason to believe that it has rained. This is conceivable. It might, for example, be the case that if anything other than its having rained had caused the street to be wet, I would not believe that it was wet. (It might be arranged that if the streets have been hosed down, etc., I will not be allowed to see that they are wet.) This, of course, would not be the ordinary state of affairs, or the way the premise would ordinarily support the conclusion. Ordinarily it is the fact itself that comprises evidence for the conclusion, not the fact that it is believed to be a fact.

DENNIS W. STAMPE

belief is in that way derivative from that of its object, which is, ideally, then a fact. The authority of a desire is not: for what is wanted is not, ideally, then a fact. And certainly, when we call the desire itself a reason for doing the action, this is not because if the state of affairs one wants to obtain *were* to obtain in fact, that fact would be a reason to do the action in question.

I must try to elicit an "intuition" of this feature of desire, mainly just by pointing it out. But an argument of sorts may help in this. Consider two people who do exactly the same thing, between whom there is no difference save that one of them did the thing because that one wanted to do it (Suppose they both spent their weekend studying German, with the intention of learning the langauge.) Beyond that neither of them has any belief about the act that would explain their curious behavior; neither believes that there is any point in his learning German. Then the one who has no desire to do this thing has absolutely no reason to do it (none in view of which he does it), and the act is utterly irrational. But the act of the one who wants to do it is not *utterly* irrational. He does at least have *a* reason—*something* of a reason, surely—to do it, for it is something that he wants to do. And if he has a reason then there *is* a reason for him to do it. What can this be but the only thing that he has that the other party lacks? That is: the desire itself. The *desire*, it may be, is irrational, but it does not follow that the act it inspires is irrational. For the action is done for a reason: the desire the agent has to do it. Desire, it seems, has an extraordinary authority: if there is no reason to do a thing, my *intending* to do it is no reason to do it, and neither is my *believing* that it would be a good idea to do it, if in fact it would not. But even then, the fact that I *want* to do it *is* a reason to do it.[10]

---

[10]Cf. David Gauthier's discussion of how "wants provide reasons for acting" in *Practical Reasoning* (Oxford: Oxford University Press, 1963), p. 45, 3.3.1; cf. p. 47. What I am asserting about the phenemenon is very different from what Gauthier says: "One has a reason to perform an action if [the desire's] objective is worth wanting." (He call this "the condition of prudential practical reasoning"; it assumes the role of a principle of practical inference.) The statement I have quoted is true enough. But my claim is that ordinarily even if the objective of the desire is *not* worth wanting, if one *does* want it, one has a reason to perform an action: the fact that one wants it. Just that.

THE AUTHORITY OF DESIRE

Philosophers have not been entirely oblivious to the feature of desire that I call its *per se* authority. But they have noted it mainly as a feature just of certain visceral desires, like the desire to scratch. The phenomenon has not, I think, been seen in its proper connection with the nature of the objects of desire, and thus the nature of desire itself, desire of every kind. Thus it is sometimes acknowledged only so as to confine it just to a certain class of desires. But we ought to be most reluctant to introduce such a dichotomy in our account of desire.[11]

Others will deny the alleged authority of desire altogether. It is a somewhat elusive thing in itself: the intuition of it waxes and wanes. Moreover, there are, I think, reasons for a certain "failure to perceive" the *per se* authority of desire—to borrow a (tendentious) phrase. There is of course the fact that we say that a person "has no reason whatever" for an action when we mean merely "no *good* reason"; a person who does something just because he wants to may, indeed, have no good reason, even though he does, to speak literally, have a reason. The statement that something is a

---

[11]Of the writers I know, Steven Schiffer recognizes this feature the most clearly, in his "A Paradox of Desire" (*American Philosophical Quarterly* 13 (1976), pp. 195–203). He describes what he calls "reason-providing desires," such as wanting to scratch one's nose. He says that should one act on that desire, the reason for which one does so " . . . is provided entirely by one's desire to do that thing," and, in a sense . . . , one's reason just is that desire"; and, he says, were he to scratch his nose because he had such a desire, "I should have a good and sufficient reason for doing it" (p. 198). Schiffer does not, however, regard this kind of thing as being generally true, of desires of any kind, as I am inclined to do. Instead, he distinguishes desires having the reason-providing feature, from another "kind" of desires, which are "reason-following"—like the desire to repay a loan. One presumably has this desire, if one has it, because there is reason to repay the loan (this being also the reason for which one wants to do so). Here the reason (as Schiffer notes) is independent of the desire, in this sense: one would have that reason to repay even if one did not have the desire to do so. My contention is that the desire would be a reason even if one did not have any reason to have it. Schiffer however takes the view that a desire, if it provides reasons, is itself a reason for one to have that desire—that such desires are "self-justifying" (p. 198). Here we disagree. (See below, Section III.) Also, I am not saying what Schiffer's remark might suggest, that desires, or reason-providing desires, are "good and sufficient" reasons for acting accordingly, but only that they are reasons. Their quality is another matter.

reason thus has an associated force of commending it as a basis for action, etc.; but that is not part of the statement's meaning, for such suggestions can readily be cancelled with consistency: "Don't do it. Granted, you do have a reason to do it, but it's not a good one."

The authority of desire may be denied owing to a failure to recognize the objectivity (or "externality") of reasons—a failure to appreciate the fact that a reason is simply a fact, and its being a reason depends on nothing more than its semantic and logical relations to that for which it is a reason—to one's thinking or wanting or feeling or doing whatever it may be. Its being a reason does not depend on what one may know about that fact, including what one may know about those relations. The fact that a tin can is bulging is a reason to think its contents are spoiled and a reason to throw it out, whether one knows it to be such a reason or not. One may see that, and grant also that the fact that one wants something may be a reason to act accordingly; still one may recoil from the claim that it remains such a reason even if one *knows* that there is no reason to want it and good reason not to want it or to act accordingly. I have pointed out that it does not follow from the fact that there is no reason to want a thing, and good reason not to want it or to act accordingly, that one's wanting it cannot *be* a reason to act accordingly. It may be suggested that the desire might be counted a reason only if one *did not know* it to be an unreasonable one, or did not know that there was better reason not to act on it. But *why* should one's ignorance or knowledge of these facts about the desire determine whether it constitutes a reason to act? To suppose that it does is to fail to see its status as a reason as a fully objective matter.

Again, the fact that a desire is unreasonable simply does not entail that the desire is not a reason for one to act in accordance with it. For the desire's being unreasonable, or irrational, is a matter of its logical relations to the subject's beliefs and other desires. (Thus it is rational for the believer to want to be baptised, but irrational for the nonbeliever to want the same thing.) And it is entirely possible for a desire which is in the relevant sense inconsistent with one's beliefs (which may be false) and other desires (which may be ill-conceived) nonetheless to constitute a reason to act accordingly. This can be argued from the existence of cases where an irrational desire constitutes a *good* reason to act accordingly. One possible case is this: there is an eating disorder ("pica") in which an

THE AUTHORITY OF DESIRE

animal or person compulsively eats "non-foods" like earth or ice or laundry starch or worse. The desire to eat a box of laundry starch is irrational, and is regarded as such by those who suffer the condition. But there is evidence that some pica is caused by specific nutritional or metabolic deficiencies, and in some of these cases it may be that the desire to eat some odd substance is in fact a *good* reason to do exactly that, notwithstanding the irrationality of the desire.[12]

Finally, I suspect the idea that the mere desire for something is a reason for acting offends against our philosopher's ideology, for we are *partisans* of reason. This idea mocks our allegiance to rationality. It takes the part of childishness: "I *do* have a reason to do it: I *want* to!" Is this not the very voice of unreason? But I think we are wrong to dismiss what we may learn perhaps even from the mouths of babes.

How then are we to account for the *per se* authority of desire? We must not, I think, abandon the point that only facts can be reasons, either for believing or for doing something. It must be, then, the *fact* that one wants something that constitutes a reason for one to act accordingly. But it will not do to make practical reasoning begin from the proposition that one *wants* a certain thing: that would be nothing more than reasoning *about* one's desires. Kinds of reasoning, including practical reasoning, are not distinguished by their subject matter.[13] Neither should we be content to say that the

---

[12]M. Blum, C. Orton, and L. Rose, *The Effect of Starch Ingestion on Excessive Iron Absorption* (New York, 1968). In a group of habitual starch eaters, the rate of absorption of iron was as much as three times as high as normal, resulting sometimes in hemochromatosis. A pronounced reduction in iron absorption was found during periods of starch ingestion. Here, the irrational desire to eat laundry starch appears to have been rather a good reason for these subjects to do so; even though, considered in relation to the other "normal" beliefs and desires they had, it was utterly irrational.

[13]Otherwise, as Anscombe decisively observed, we should have to distinguish also "mince-pie" reasoning: " . . . the peculiarity of this would be that it was about mince pies" (*Op. cit.*, p. 58). Neither, of course, is "theoretical" reasoning merely reasoning about one's *beliefs*: a theoretical syllogism begins from the premise, for example, that all Greeks are mortal, not from the premise that one believes that all Greeks are mortal—unless, of course, it is to represent reasoning about beliefs instead of Greeks.

Perhaps *deliberation*, properly so-called, does consist of such reasoning, about what one wants, and how much one wants it, and about what one

DENNIS W. STAMPE

authority of desire is inexplicable, or granted by the special logic of practical reasoning, by some *ad hoc* principle of practical inference. Not, at least, until other accounts are tried and shown to fail.

III. THREE ACCOUNTS CONSIDERED

The authority of desire is extraordinary, but perhaps it is not unique among the things that move us. It is in order at this point to look for analogies to the case of desire, in other mental states that similarly comprise, in themselves, reasons for doing things. Sensory states come to mind. The fact that I itch is in itself a reason to scratch. A pain is a reason to do what will relieve that pain, a reason in itself, not through its object—for pains, and itches, *have* no objects, no propositional or other content. Itches make it reasonable to scratch and the rationality of scratching is not derived from the rationality of itching. Such sensory states are not themselves either reasonable or unreasonable. They too are origins of rationality.

An attractively simple account, built along the lines of a classical empiricist view, is suggested by this model:

> A desire has, in its own nature and apart from its object or apparent representational character, an unpleasant, uncomfortable, or even painful character: as Locke said, a desire is "an uneasiness." (We know things more or less well, believe things more or less firmly, but want things more or less *badly*.) Any discomfiture is itself a reason to do what will relieve that discomfiture. Doing what one wants to do or bringing about the state of affairs that one wants to obtain, is what will relieve the discomfiture that is involved in wanting it. Therefore, a desire is a *per se* reason to act.

Now in such an account as this, the apparent representational qualities or "contents" of desires play no part in the rationalization

---

believes, and how firmly. But deliberation is a relatively sophisticated and self-conscious thing—not a mere "process," but often itself a deliberate act. For that reason I think deliberation, properly so-called, is not fundamental in philosophical psychology. "Deliberation" is not the name for that minimal and basic rational process the products of which are rationally formed beliefs, desires, and intentions. It is that process that I am here trying to understand, in seeking to understand the structure of "practical reasoning."

THE AUTHORITY OF DESIRE

of action by desire. It is therefore parsimonious, given such a view, to deny the representational character of a desire. It is natural, that is, to deny that that character belongs properly *to* the desire, as Hume delighted in doing.[14] It is natural therefore to go further, and simply identify desires with a kind of unpleasant sensation: a desire is, in itself, nothing more than a kind of pain. Of course, unlike other pains, desires are often caused by beliefs. The belief that it would be a good thing if I had a peach, together with the belief that I do not have one, may well cause me to have a certain desire, which desire may be identified by reference to, and described in terms of, the contents of the belief that typically causes it: thus, it is the desire, so-called, "that I have a peach." Likewise, the content of that belief will be what determines which action it takes to "satisfy" the desire—that is, to *terminate* the discomfiture caused by that belief—by removing the proximate cause of it, which is the belief that I have no peach.

This is a view of great economy.[15] I shall limit myself to raising just that objection to it that goes to its adequacy as an account of the authority of desire. On the view before us, desires are *per se* reasons

---

[14]"A passion is an original existence . . . and contains not any representative quality, which renders it a copy of any other existence or modification. When I am angry, I am actually *possest* with the passion, and in that emotion have no more a reference to any other object, than when I am thirsty, or sick, or more than five foot high" *Treatise,* II, iii (Selby-Bigge, p. 415 (Oxford: Oxford University Press, 1888)). Desires are one kind of passion, so-called "direct" ones, that "arise immediately from good or evil, from pain or pleasure" (II, i). Hume says that desire *arises* from "the good [i.e., from pleasure], considered simply"—though he also acknowledges that "hunger, lust, and a few other bodily appetites . . . produce good and evil and proceed not from them" (II, iii, 9)—which, as Schiffer notes, is an acknowledgment of the reason-providing character of those desires. But Hume's view is not the one stated above: he does not, I think, identify a desire with a painful sensation, nor does he assign the quality of painfulness to desire. Instead, he refers the action-determining powers of desire to the mind's "original instinct to unite itself with the good and avoid the evil" (II, ix; 438). While that recognizes the natural force of desire, it is, I think, precisely a refusal to recognize the rational *authority* of desire.

[15]Economy, that is, of principles. But it entails surprising complexity in the phenomenon. For surely the way pains work is by making one *want* them to stop. Pains generate desires. But then a desire will be a pain that generates another desire, that is, another pain. And that pain in turn generates another desire, or pain. And so on.

DENNIS W. STAMPE

to act accordingly, where "acting accordingly" is acting in such a
way as to bring it about that one does not have those desires. To act
so as to "satisfy" one's desire is nothing more than to act so as to
extinguish that desire—that is, that pain. Satisfaction is extermination. One way of satisfying, that is, terminating a desire, will be to
bring it about that one has what one wants. But on the present view
this works because it eliminates one cause of the desire, the belief
that one lacks the thing in question. The desire can be removed by
removing other things, including the bodily conditions or the perceptual provocations that cause it—thus by the proverbial cold
shower, or the devices of substitution, distraction, and diversion.

There is no denying that a desire often constitutes a reason to act
in some such way to rid oneself of it. But even where this is feasible,
a desire remains a reason to act in another way. It remains, ordinarily, a reason to act so as to bring it about that the state of
affairs one wants to obtain *does* obtain. And the view under discussion cannot explain why that is so. It cannot explain why, even if
one could extinguish the desire without fulfilling it, one's wanting
the thing would still be a reason to try to get that thing and *fulfill*
the desire. If for example I am hungry and want to eat, and I have
a way of getting rid of that hunger and that desire without eating, it
remains the case that I have, in the fact that I want to eat, *a reason* to
do exactly that.

If a desire is *per se* a reason for one to act so as that the state of
affairs one wants to obtain does obtain, then the desire must involve that state of affairs in its own essential nature: "involve" it,
that is, "intentionally," or by virtue of its being represented therein.
Its character as representing that state of affairs, as having that as
its object, must be essential to it. An adequate account of the authority of desire must account for it in terms of the representational quality of desire.

For contrast we may sketch a second account, one which meets
this requirement, depending crucially on the relevant (that is, the
semantic) concept of the satisfaction of desire. We begin with the
thought that what is needed to explain the *per se* authority of desire
to rationalize action, is a correlative idea of a state of affairs that is
good, and good *in itself*—this being the state of affairs determined
by the representational character of the desire. This will not however be the state of affairs one wants to have obtain—for example,

THE AUTHORITY OF DESIRE

that in which one has a hat—for this need not be good in itself. But might it not be that relational state of affairs in which the desire that it be the case that *p* is satisfied by its coming to be the case that *p*? Then the explanation of the fact that a desire is a reason to act so as to satisfy that desire may go as follows.

> The satisfaction of a desire is in itself or intrinsically a good thing. When one comes to want something, it transpires *ipso facto* that one's coming to have that thing would be a good thing, merely *in that* it would constitute the satisfaction of a desire. It is in that sense that one's wanting the thing comprises, in itself, a reason to bring it about that that desire is satisfied. Not because some discomfort would be relieved by its satisfaction, or something good accrue to it, but just because the satisfaction of the desire is in itself a good thing.

But I think it is impossible to believe that the satisfaction of a desire *is* in itself a good thing. Surely there could be a creature with faculties so malformed, wiring so scrambled, that while it nonetheless experienced genuine desire, there would be nothing good about its desires being satisfied, not even a moment's pleasure much less anything more substantial. In that case, there would then *be* nothing good in the satisfaction of its desires. The fundamental idea of this approach is wrong. It is not because satisfying a desire is a good thing intrinsically that a desire is a reason, *per se*, for acting so as to secure that satisfaction. If that were so it would be completely obscure what this "goodness" could *be*. It would make as much sense to hold that there is something intrinsically good about a belief being satisfied—that is, true—regardless whether anything good follows from its being true, and regardless what the belief might be.

Steven Schiffer's account of this matter in effect combines elements of both the approaches I have criticized. He distinguishes between "reason-providing" and "reason-following" desires, and attributes the feature in question only to the former. His view is that a reason-providing

> desire is a self-referential desire for its own gratification; [a reason-providing] desire to φ is a desire to φ to relieve the discomfort of that desire, a desire to φ for the pleasure of its own relief. So a thirst is a desire to drink, a discomforting desire to drink, a discomforting de-

351

DENNIS W. STAMPE

sire to drink which would be pleasurable to relieve, a desire to drink to
gratify itself. In this way [reason-providing] desires are self-referring
(*op. cit.*, p. 199).

It is a virtue of Schiffer's account of the matter that it depends on
the representational or semantic properties of the desire. What is
crucially represented is the desire itself (it is its own object), and
what the desire is, is a desire for it itself to be satisfied. These
desires are semantically solipsistic. But what is good about satisfying (such) a desire? Schiffer does not entertain the fatuous idea
that there is something intrinsically but inexplicably good about the
satisfaction of a desire. Instead, he finds the good of it in the relief
from discomfort or the pleasure of its satisfaction. Earlier, in criticism of similar views, I claimed that if the discomfort of the desire
could be got rid of without its being fulfilled, there would still
remain, in the fact of the desire itself, reason to act so as to fulfill it;
and if the pleasure attending the slaking of one's thirst could (by
some neural engineering) be had without actually drinking anything, the desire to drink might well remain itself a reason to drink
something. If this is so, then Schiffer's view likewise fails adequately to account for the reason-providing powers of desire. For
Schiffer says that to act on a reason-providing desire, like the thirst
for something to drink, is to act " . . . because one has that desire,
but also only because one desires the pleasure and relief of discomfort that" the action provides. But is it necessarily to act *only* because of that? Surely one can act on that *same* desire *also* because it
may indicate a need for water. Schiffer must find here two desires,
one reason-providing, and another reason-following one. But this
seemingly *ad hoc* proliferation of desires is a consequence one cannot much favor.[16] (A more general line of criticism might be devel-

---

[16]It is a danger of indulging in the distinction between two kinds of
desires, that—since no single thing can be of two contrary natural kinds—
it enforces a criterion of individuation on desires, and the results, I think,
are quite unnatural. One would not have thought that the identity of a
mental state, for example, a belief, should turn on the matter of whether
one does or does not have reason to hold it; it would seem that one could
come to have a reason to hold it, or come to have no reason to hold it, and
the belief would be the same. Should it be otherwise with desires? Schiffer
describes a case in which you have reason to drink a scotch (doing so is a
prearranged signal of something) and then come in the ordinary way to

THE AUTHORITY OF DESIRE

oped from a functionalist perspective: *why* should an organism be subject to such solipsistic states as these—these desires for the satisfaction of themselves, for the sake of the relief or pleasure of such satisfaction—states having essential reference just to themselves and justifying their own existence.)

The accounts considered here imply that every desire, or every desire of the relevant ("reason-providing") kind, is and is necessarily a reason to act accordingly. They would therefore yield the strongest version of the thesis of the *per se* authority of desire. This might be deemed a virtue, but I am inclined to regard it as a fault. I think a better—a naturalistic—account would leave room for the anomalous desire, in which the apparatus of appetition is so completely broken down that the desire comprises no reason whatever to act in accordance with it. The distinction I drew between *per se* and *per objectum* properties of mental states is not to be confused with the distinction between necessary and accidental properties. Desire has the *per se* feature of rationalizing action. This does not mean that it has that property necessarily, but rather that it has it (that is, when it *does* have it) owing to its intrinsic and essential character, and not owing to its having the object that it does.

IV. THE NATURE OF DESIRE

If it is not because desire is intrinsically unpleasant, nor because its satisfaction is intrinsically a good thing, why is it that desires are *per se* reasons for acting—that is, reasons through their own nature,

---

crave a scotch; at the appropriate time you give the signal (you drink a scotch) " . . . satisfying your [reason-following] desire for a scotch, but this barely touches your still persisting desire for a scotch. Is it really so implausible," he asks, "to suppose that during the over-lap you had two desires to drink scotch [*sic.:* not "a scotch"], one a [reasoning-following] desire, the other [a reason-providing] desire, the two having different causes and different durations?" (*op. cit.,* p. 199). It is more natural, I think, to say that you initially had a reason to want to drink a scotch, and it then came to happen that this same desire did not depend on your having that reason, but had an additional independent cause. *Either* that or that while there are two desires, one is for *a* scotch and the other for *scotch*— that is, scotch enough to satisfy your craving. But then the desires are distinguished by their objects, and that is why the latter outlives the satisfaction of the former.

DENNIS W. STAMPE

not that of their objects? To answer this question we shall have to answer, or begin to answer, the question, "What *is* a desire 'in itself'," in its own nature?

That would require us to find the essential difference between desires and beliefs. This difference does not lie in their differing contents or propositional objects, for these may be the same. One may believe it, or one may desire it, to be the case that *p*—for example, that one has a drink. The proposition is the same, in that it represents the same state of affairs—the one state of affairs that would make true the belief, or satisfy the desire. Perhaps, then, the difference lies in the functional roles of the two states. A start in this direction is provided in a formula drawn up by Robert Stalnaker:

> To desire that *P* is to be disposed to act in ways that would tend to bring it about that *P* in a world in which one's beliefs, whatever they are, were true. To believe that *P* is to be disposed to act in ways that would satisfy one's desires, whatever they are, in a world in which *P* (together with one's other beliefs) were true.[17]

These interlocking characterizations neatly express the way belief and desire jointly determine rational behavior. They are dispositions to do certain actions that they provide the agent reason for doing. But notice the difference between them. My wanting to stay dry (given my belief that it's raining) is a reason for me to take an umbrella because my doing so will satisfy that desire: that is, it will result in what I *want* to be the case *being* the case. My belief that it is raining is also a reason for me to do that thing (to take my umbrella), but *not* because my doing so will result in what I *believe* to be the case being the case. Obviously not: beliefs provide reasons to do what will satisfy one's desires, or make them come true; beliefs are

---

[17]*Inquiry* (Cambridge, Mass.: The MIT Press, 1984), p. 15. Stalnaker discusses the apparent "circularity" in these formulae, and shows that as they stand a "fatal relativity in the propositional relations" they define leaves the problem of intentionality unsolved; the causes of the states, as well as their behavioral effects, must be brought into the picture. One may agree, as I do, with that treatment of the representational contents of the states. But the specific difference between belief and desire remains elusive. I have treated all this more thoroughly in "Defining Desire," in *Ways of Desire*, ed. Joel Marks (Chicago: Precedent Publishing, 1986).

THE AUTHORITY OF DESIRE

not reasons to do what will make those beliefs themselves true. Nor is it, in general, rational to try to bring it about that one's beliefs— beliefs one already has—are true. (My believing that I am being poisoned is no reason for me to take poison.) For to believe that p is not to think it good that p.

The difference between beliefs and desires lies somehow in the differing ways in which they determine the rationality of action. To locate the difference, we must look back, after all, to the representational character of the two states: for while the belief and the desire that p have the same propositional content and represent the same state of affairs, there is a difference in the *way* it is represented in the two states of mind. In belief it is represented *as obtaining*, whereas in desire, it is represented as a state of affairs *the obtaining of which would be good*. This *modal* difference explains why the desire that p is a reason to make it true that p, while the belief that p is not. Desires constitute reasons for us to act because their contents are represented as states of affairs the realization of which would be good; this is of the essence of desire, and we can begin to see here why it is that desires are *per se* reasons for actions.

The same point explains something about the intentionality of desire. If the desire that it be the case that p is a disposition to do what will bring it about that p, it is *a fortiori* a disposition to do what will bring about the causal and logical consequences of its being the case that p. But these include consequences that are *un*wanted. (The desire to eat a burrito is not the desire to incur the heartburn that will follow, and that may be expected to follow.) The propositional identity of the desire that p is not therefore given by "the" state of affairs it would tend to cause. It is, however, given by the state of affairs that tends to cause it, or rather by a certain one of things that tends to cause it—that is, *its being good that it be the case that p*. That defines the object of the desire as being p and nothing more. For its being good that p does not entail, causally or logically, what is entailed by its being the case that p, and this confines the thing wanted to what is represented therein as being good. Roughly, the desire that p is a state of mind caused, ideally, by something's being good, and *what* is wanted is the thing the apparent goodness of which would cause it.

But this does not distinguish *all* beliefs from desires. For one can perfectly well *believe* that something would be good—that it would

355

DENNIS W. STAMPE

be a good thing, say, to take a new job—and this belief, quite as
much as the desire to do it, would ideally be caused by the fact that
it would be a good thing. And one can have this belief without
wanting to do it. If one does believe this, then that state of affairs
(one's taking a new job) is here too represented as something the
obtaining of which would be good, but now in one's belief, not in a
desire. So the question now becomes, what is the difference between one who believes *it would be good were it the case that p*, and one
who *wants* it to be the case that *p*? In either case, one and the same
state of affairs is represented "in the same way," that is, as having
the same property. The difference, we may say, is one such that it is
essential to the desire that *p being a desire* that something is represented therein as good, whereas it is not essential to the belief (that
is, that *p* would be good) *being a belief* that something is represented
therein as good (though it is essential to its being that particular
belief). But to say just this is not, I think, sufficiently explanatory.
The state of affairs represented, in one or the other state of mind
as good, is represented in a certain way, if you will, in *different* ways,
in the two states of mind; there is a difference in the modality of its
containment. But what is this difference?

Let us ask this: What is lacking in the person who simply has no
desire to take the new job, although he thinks, even knows, that it
would be a good thing were he to do so? One is tempted to describe
the difference in some such way as this: in desire, one is somehow
struck by, affected by, the merits of the thing wanted, or the prospect of having it, in a way one needn't be if one merely knows it
would be good; so one may say, "I know it would be best to take
that job, but the prospect of doing so simply leaves me cold, does
not strike me as something I want to do; it somehow doesn't *seem* to
me the good prospect I know it is." Sometimes one is thus affected
through a feeling, as in thirst; sometimes not. In either case, there
is something characteristic of desire: if one wants a thing it *seems* to
one as if the thing wanted would be good. This is not necessarily
the case when one merely believes (or knows) that it would be a
good thing: knows it, say, because one has been reliably told it, or
because one has reasoned it out. For in that case, there is, I think, a
sense in which it need not *seem* to one at all a good thing, and thus
one may say, "Although it doesn't *seem* so to me, it is my belief that
it would be good to do it" (just as one might say, consistently,

THE AUTHORITY OF DESIRE

"Although it doesn't *seem* to me to be so, the President is a great man").[18] But one may not say, "I want it, though it in no way *seems* to me as if it would be good to have it"; if one wants the thing, it must in some way *seem good*, when one wants it.

In the belief that something would be good, the thing is *held* to be good, but not necessarily because it seems to be so; rather it is represented (*conceived*) as good *via* the *predicate* "is good." I think this points to a difference between one who wants a thing and one who knows it would be good to have it but doesn't want it. If so, it points to two *ways in which* one and same state of affairs may be represented in one and the same way, as something that would be good. (Thus, perhaps, the pragmatic inconsistency in "I believe it would be good, but in fact it would be bad," is not present in "I want it, but in fact it would be bad"; this stands to reason if the latter is of the form "It seems to me as if it would be good, but in fact it would be bad"—and if the former is not of that form; notice also that "It seems to me as if it would be good, but it also seems in many ways, or all in all, as if it would be bad" is consistent.)

The way it "seems" to one as if the thing wanted would be good is cast in relief in the *onset* of desire for something already believed to be good: where for example, one knows the cheese would be good to eat and then, in time, the desire to eat it comes upon one, perhaps as one grows hungry; but not necessarily through any such feeling, as when one comes after a time to want to take the new job, without any decisive change in one's beliefs, so that now it even *seems* to one a good thing to do, as one had known it would be. To describe the advent of desire in such ways is to acknowledge the affective character of desire; it is to see it, as it traditionally was seen, even as a *passion*, not in the sense of an emotional disturbance but in the sense of a state we are moved to, *subject* to.

Thus it is to see the gulf between judgment and desire. Consider some distant war, perhaps the one currently between Iran and Iraq, the scene of untold suffering. One judges that (perhaps knows that) it would be a good thing were that war to end, but it

---

[18]Of course, the belief may be *expressed* by saying "It seems to me that it would be good if *p*," but here I think "it seems" has a merely "parenthetical" use ("It would, it seems, be good if *p*"); it need not refer to the way things genuinely seem to the speaker.

357

DENNIS W. STAMPE

does not follow and it may not be accurate to say that one *wants* that war to end. One does not lack reason to want to it to end. But one may simply not really care about it, sufficiently to arouse anything rightly called desire.[19] An end to the war is represented, in one's mind, as something that would be good, but it is not, may be, represented in that way *in the way* it would be were it something one wanted to happen. It is not represented in that way *effectively;* we are not, it may be, *moved* to desire.

Such phenomena suggest that in desire there is a certain way the prospect of the thing wanted somehow affects one, whereas one who merely believes the thing would be good is not affected in that way. Consider, then, one who feels the shape of a coin, and another who sees its shape: in either case, the shape of the coin affects one in a certain way, so that it seems to one to be round; but in the one case it *feels* round and the other it *looks* round. In either case, the coin is represented in a certain way (as having a certain property), and the difference is in the way it is so represented; it is a difference, again, in the way the coin is represented in that way. Whereas, one who knows—has been reliably told, say—that it is round, but who in no way perceives its shape, differs in that it does not *seem*, in any such way, to him to be round; its shape has no such effect on him.

This, then, is the analogy I shall pursue—the analogy between desire and perception. In desire, the prospect of the thing wanted affects one in a certain way, or ways, so that it is represented *as good*, and the difference now between the belief that it would be good, and the desire for it, is the way in which it is represented in that way, as being good. I fasten on the analogy between desire and perception not just because of its descriptive appeal—and of course there are disanalogies—but because perceptions, as I shall argue, are the prototype of mental states which comprise *per se* reasons for one to do, that is, think, what one consequently does.

---

[19]Given the power to do so, such a person would presumably choose to stop the war. It is not some disposition to act appropriately that is essentially lacking. And neither is it a matter of remoteness of the possibility of acting. In the case of another distant war (the Falkland war, perhaps), offering no more opportunities for action, one might find oneself wanting the war to go on until a certain side won it, even while one's *belief* is that it would be best were the fighting simply to stop.

THE AUTHORITY OF DESIRE

And because it will complete the account of the difference between belief and desire.

The view I shall take is this: Desire is a kind of perception. One who wants it to be the case that p perceives something that makes it seem to that person as if it would be good were it to be the case that p, and seem so in a way that is characteristic of perception. To desire something is to be in a kind of perceptual state, in which that thing seems good, this "seeming" hereafter marked by the subscript "$_d$". The term "seems$_d$" may be understood, initially, by analogy with the verbs "sound" and "look" in the contexts "it sounds, looks as if p," where these statements specify the perceptual states distinctive of hearing and seeing respectively. Analogously, we have "It seems$_d$ as if it would be good if p," which specifies the perceptual state distinctive of desire, and constitutive of the desire the propositional object of which is that it be the case that p. Its seeming$_d$ a good thing is *constitutive* of the desire, not something external to it. (This will be crucial to vindicating the notion that a desire is a *per se* reason for action.) Its seeming$_d$ a good thing is not to be construed as a reason one has for wanting the thing, nor as a cause of that desire—no more than its looking a certain way to one is a *reason* one has for being in the visual state one is in when one sees the thing that looks that way to one; nor is it a cause of one's being in that state. There too its looking a certain way is constitutive of the visual state, not something external to it.

In introducing the notion of seeming$_d$, I do not mean to suggest that desire is distinguished essentially from belief, etc., by dint of some peculiar *quale* or conscious phenomenology. The phrase *seeming$_d$ as if it would be good* is not to be understood as designating any single feeling or even a set of resembling feelings or conscious characteristics distinctive of desire.[20] What will matter is instead its

---

[20]The view I am putting forward smacks of a tired formula: the desire is the 'thought' that the thing would be good *plus* a certain something—a certain simple affective character, impossible perhaps to describe, but familiar to anyone who has ever wanted anything. We have grown skeptical of such formulae: of the ineffable *quale*, which, it seems, would not be missed, *ceteris paribus*, if it were not there; and skeptical also of the associated presumption that there must be some single thing that distinguishes desires from the relevant beliefs: particularly if it turns out that it is some peculiar mental quality that distinguishes them, all too conveniently, and

epistemic role, and its epistemic role will be construed on the model of that of perception. I do not say that desire is a mode of sensuous perception, involving a distinctive sensation, nor does my thesis require such a view. For the essential connection between perceiving and sensing is not the matter of having sensations, but that of being *sensitive to*—as to light or heat, and as even a plant may be, whether it experiences sensations or not. (Of course, sensitivity is not enough for perception; the phototropic plant is sensitive but not percipient, for things *seem* no way to it. But what it lacks is not sensation, necessarily, but a kind of awareness of its own states and of what they represent.)

Sensitivity, I suggest, is a matter of being affected by and only by the presence of certain specific properties. And the sensitivity involved in desire is a matter of such states being produced by a mental mechanism that is activated, ideally, by and only by the apparent goodness of a state of affairs. Thus what makes one's state that of something's *seeming$_d$ good*—seeming good in the desiderative way—is its etiology, not its phenomenology.

This now completes the earlier attempt to specify the nature of desire in such a way as to distinguish the desire that *p* from the belief that *p would be good*. It was suggested that the desire that *p* is a state of mind caused, ideally, by the fact that something would be

---

seems to do nothing else. For on honest introspection, the conscious agitations associated with, say, lust or with thirst, or with the desire to lose some weight, or one's longing to see an old friend, or one's desire to pay lower taxes or to get revenge—each of these is found to differ, more or less, from each of the others, if indeed one finds any desiderative feelings at all.

I do not hold that the desire that *p* involves such a feeling in addition to the *belief* that *p* would be good, for I have held that one who wants that *needn't* believe it would be good. I do suppose that the desire involves the mental representation of *p* as being good, but not that it involves this *plus* an affective character, as if this character were an added something: for the state of affairs' *seeming to one as if it would be good,* is a *modal* property of the representation of that prospect, *the way* it is represented. It is, I should think, a sort of category error to construe the *way* something exists, whether in reality or in the mind ("intentionally"), as an extra added entity, like a feeling might be.

Finally, I would dissociate myself from the procedure (Hume's, I think) of treating the question of the nature of a mental state as if it were (as it is not) the question how we intuitively *recognize* its nature.

THE AUTHORITY OF DESIRE

good, *what* is wanted being the thing the apparent goodness of which would cause it. The belief that p would be good is perhaps also caused, ideally, by the fact that p *would be good,* but it is not produced by a mechanism activated, ideally, by and *only* by *that* property of states of affairs—by something's being *good.* It is instead produced, ideally, by (and only by) *its being the case* that p, as beliefs, generally, are produced by the *obtaining* of the states of affairs that comprise their contents. The difference in the ways in which the state of affairs (p) is represented, in the desire that p and the belief that it would be good if p, may be regarded as a difference in the mechanisms reponsible for the two states of mind, the one—the Appetite, if you will—being in the nature of a perceptual mechanism, the other not.

I do not say that its seeming$_d$ as if something would be good (nor thus one's wanting it) is a matter of being in a distinctive *sensory* state, produced through the senses and involving sensations.[21] Whatever the relation may be between those desires that are bound up with sensory states (and especially with sensations, like that of thirst), there are other desires without such sensory embodiment. There are desires, certainly, which are among those "perceptions [as Descartes said] whose effects we feel as though they were in the soul itself," not felt as if they were somewhere in our bodies, or in objects external to it. (*Le passions de l'âme* I, xxv.) Some may regard "nonsensuous perception" as a contradiction in terms. Then let it be called "consciousness" or "awareness," and my thesis will be that *desire is a form of awareness.* That will suffice for the account I shall give of the authority of desire.

The crucial thing is this: there is, in any desire that it be the case that p, a certain way in which its being the case that p seems to one: to wit, *as if it would be a good thing.* Its "seeming$_d$" that way is owing to a certain actual (or "formal") property of the mental state of one

---

[21]Nor does this take us so far from the paradigm of sensuous perception as might be thought. For similarly, I think, its *sounding* a certain way to one is a matter of the etiology of the state; or so I would contend: that is, if the state is not caused by sound, through a mechanism activated by or sensitive to sound, it is not literally true that "it sounds to one thus and so," but merely that it *seems* to sound that way, the auditory quality of the experience notwithstanding.

who wants something, a property intrinsic to it, that is what makes it, or part of what makes it, a *desire* that one has, and not a state of another kind. This is the characterization of the nature of desire that will permit us to sketch an account of the authority it possesses through its own nature.

V. THE AUTHORITY OF DESIRE EXPLAINED

The hypothesis that desire is a form of perception was introduced to explain the authority of desire. How would it do so? What was to be explained was this: desires are in themselves—that is, by virtue of their own distinctive natures, and not owing to their objects or their objectives—reasons for action. I have been discussing what a desire *is* "in its own nature," and trying to distinguish desires from related beliefs, without denying the representational or intentional character of desire. The thesis offered was that a desire is a certain kind of perception or awareness. The explanation of its authority, then, is obvious.

The authority of desire is the authority of perception. Desire is an origin of rationality because it is a kind of perception. And perception is an origin of rationality—of the rationality, for example, of beliefs. Its looking, sounding, feeling as if something is the case—these are states that confer rationality on the beliefs that one forms in view of them, the belief that things are the way they look or sound or feel. The fact that it sounds as if it is raining is a reason to believe that it is, and the rationality of that belief *originates* in that fact: for one can neither have, nor lack, a reason for it to sound to one as it does. As before, the fact that it sounds that way may be *a* reason, whether it be a good one or a bad one, much less a decisive one, for believing that it is raining; *and* it would be a reason, even if there were better reason to believe otherwise, *even if one knew that it was not raining.* This is exactly parallel to what I claimed earlier about the capacity of a desire to confer rationality on actions taken in accordance with it. My desire to have a beer may be a reason for me to have one, even if there is better reason not to, and even if I know it would not be a good idea to have a beer. This is now explained, if my desire is a kind of perception—if my desire for a beer is a state wherein it seems$_d$ to me as if it would be a good thing

THE AUTHORITY OF DESIRE

to have one. The fact that it seems as if it would be a good thing, which is not something I could either have or lack a reason for, nonetheless constitutes a reason for me to act accordingly. And this would, or could, be the case, even if the desire is adjudged an unreasonable one.

But the problem, more particularly, was to explain how a desire is in itself a reason to act accordingly, *per se* and not through its object. (As it must be, again, since its objects are not facts, as reasons must be.) My suggestion is that *in itself*—that is, as distinct from its objective or object—what a desire *is* is a perceptual state, a state wherein it seems$_d$ as if some state of affairs would be good. If I want it to be the case that p, it may not be, or be going to be, a fact that p; it might not be a good thing if it *were* a fact that p. But it *is* a fact that it seems$_d$ to me as if it would be a good thing if it were. That fact is at once a thing fitted to the rôle of a reason I have, insofar as I want this thing, for acting accordingly, and also a thing definitive of and intrinsic to the *nature* of this state, this desire. For that it seems in that way as if it would be a good thing is what differentiates my desiring it from being in some other state of mind such as belief. (Analogously, that it sounds to me as if p is what differentiates my auditory from my visual state, wherein it looks as if p, and the fact that it sounds that way is a reason I have to believe that p. And the perceptual state is likewise a reason *per se* for that belief, not a reason *per objectum,* supposing that the *object* of the state in which it seems as if p is taken to be the apparent *fact that p,* not its *seeming as if p.* For it is not the fact that p, presented to me in my perception, that comprises my reason for believing that p: it is instead the fact that it seems to me that p.)

While this proposal would delineate the relevant difference between desire and belief, it does not deny that desire is a genuine propositional attitude; it does not deny its intentionality or its representational character. On the contrary. It is only by virtue of the representational character of the state, by virtue of its objective being presented to one, in the way that it is, as something that would be good, that the state of mind qualifies as a desire, and that the desire rationalizes the actions that it does.

In this way, the rationality of action may originate in desire. I hope to have reduced the mystery in this. This rationality does not

DENNIS W. STAMPE

materialize magically from the thin air inside a psychological context—from the nonactual things I may want or want to be facts. It
emerges from a fact—as it must, for only facts can be reasons. It
emerges from the fact that it seems$_d$ as if that (as it may be) nonactual thing would be good. But this fact is constitutive of the desire,
intrinsic to it, for a desire is a kind of perceptual state.

My business is to explain the authority of desire. In attempting to
do so, by advancing the thesis that desire is perception, it is not my
business to account for the authority of perception. However, I do
assume, as I think is fairly standard, that a perceptual state is a
"reliable indicator" of facts of the kind that seem therein to be
indicated. The way things look is a reliable, not to say infallible,
indicator of the way things are: that is, under certain favorable
conditions, things are the way they look. And, the way things
seem$_d$, I assume, is a reliable, not to say infallible, indicator of the
way things would be: that is, under certain favorable conditions, it
would not seem$_d$ as if it would be good if p were the case, if it would
not in point of fact *be* good. It seems to me that if it were not so—at
least, if we did not believe it to be so—then we could not describe
our state of mind, when we want something, as one in which it
seems as if it would be good to have what we want. Why should we
say—why should it be *true*—that it seems *that* way, if the state were
not one that would *indicate* that the thing would be good? Why
should we describe the state in that way, if we did not think that if it
would be good to have the thing, then it would seem to us like *this*?

Treating perceptual states, whether appetitive or sensual, as indicators fits with what we have said about them. The fact that
something *indicates* that something is the case does not entail that it
is the case; so even if it is not the case, say, that the tank is full, and
one knows that it is not, the fact that the needle in the gauge stands
at "F" may nonetheless *indicate* that it is full. And that fact constitutes *a* reason for one to think that it is full, even if one knows it is
not. In that case, of course, a reason to be ignored.

If the authority of desire is the authority of perception, the extent and limits of the one should coincide with those of the other.
And so, I think, they do. First, neither is *absolute*. There are conditions under which the fact that one is in a certain perceptual state
indicates nothing whatever about the actual facts, and constitutes

THE AUTHORITY OF DESIRE

no reason to do or believe anything. I said earlier that the fact that you want something may be a reason to try to get it, even if there is no reason to want it, even if there is better reason not to want it, and even if you know that it would not be a good thing to have it. These several "even ifs" do not add up to "no matter what." I do not say that wanting something is necessarily or always or under all conditions a reason to act accordingly, but rather that it is under certain normal conditions.

By "normal conditions" I do not mean conditions under which things are the way they seem, conditions under which if it seems$_d$ good it is good. It is entirely a normal thing sometimes to want things that would not be good, just as it is normal for white things to look yellow under yellow light, and abnormal for them not to. The conditions necessary for the proper functioning of the visual apparatus may be perfectly intact, and the perceptual faculties operating flawlessly. Here, I think, the fact that it looks yellow is a reason for you to think it is yellow, even though it is a better reason to think it is white. But should the case be that the connections between your eyes and your brain are cut, and it now looks to you as if there is something yellow before you, here I am inclined to say that the fact that it looks that way under these conditions is no reason whatever, and no indication, that it is so. Likewise, if the gas gauge is ripped from the dashboard of the car and found lying in the back seat, the fact that the needle points to "E" is no reason whatever to think, and no indication, that the tank is empty. This is different from the case where the car is parked on a hill and the gauge shows "E." Here, it may inaccurately indicate—but it does indicate—that the gas tank is empty, and its doing so is a reason for believing that it is so, even when one knows that the tank is not empty. It would seem that the apparatus has to be properly connected, and it has to be "working"—though it need not be working *well*—if it is to yield indications or representations of the way things are. Thus a watch running fast, indicates the time, but inaccurately; a stopped watch doesn't indicate the time at all.

Now I imagine these same possibilities arise in the blandishments of the appetite. That is, I imagine that there are cases in which the mechanisms of the appetite are so thoroughly broken down, the normal hook-ups severed or so badly scrambled, that the fact that it

365

DENNIS W. STAMPE

seems$_d$ to someone as if a certain thing would be good—the fact that he wants it—is no reason, not even a bad one, for him to act accordingly. Why should there not be such cases? So I do not suppose that every desire is a *per se* reason for action, nor that the authority of desire is absolute. (To assert that "desires are reasons *per se*" is to make an assertion about the "essence" of desire, rather like the assertion that fish are vertebrates: either is consistent with the occurrence of freaks.)[22]

But I shall not attempt to decide which cases should be taken as examples of such desires, or pursue this matter further. My suggestion is just that the situation is the same for indication, perception, and desire; that desire is a form of perception, that its authority is that of perception, and the authority of perception is that of indication. It is intrinsic to a desire, essential to its being a desire, that it should, radical breakdowns apart, comprise an indication that the thing wanted would be good. If, in itself, a desire is such a state, then we may understand why a desire, *through* itself, comprises a reason to act so as to get the thing one wants. A desire is in itself a state in which it seems as if something would be good. That it seems so is a fact. Only a fact can be a reason for doing something and this fact—insofar as it indicates that the thing *would* be good— is a reason to act accordingly. *In* this fact, one who has the desire, has a reason to do so. That, then, is how I propose to understand the *per se* authority of desire.

It may seem that the claim that desire is perception cannot be maintained consistently with the claim that desire is *per se* a reason for action. (I am indebted to David Shwayder here.) According to the explanation offered, it is owing to the relation a desire bears to its perceptual *object*—to the putative fact that it would be good were something to be the case—that it comprises a reason. But then is it, after all, *in itself* a reason? Is it not a reason only *insofar as it stands in*

---

[22]The claim that desire is a form of perception is (of course) an "empirical" claim. If evidence should show that desires are *not* reliable indicators of what would be good (or of anything else), then it would turn out that desires are not perceptual states. In that case, the present view would imply that the fact that someone wanted something would (presumably) *not* be a reason to try to get it, and the phenomenon with which this paper is concerned would be a mirage.

that relation? And can its relational character be an *intrinsic* character of the state?

Any account that turns on the representational character of desire will inevitably seem to fight with the view that desire is a reason *per se.* For in its representational nature it points *beyond* itself (save on a view like Schiffer's in which the desire's reference is *to* itself). But it only *points* beyond itself. The representation "relation" is intentional, and the thing represented may not exist, may not be the way it is represented as being; so the representational character must *be* wholly in the desire itself, something, in that sense, "intrinsic" to it, and not itself a genuine *relation.* My claim has been that even if there is no Fountain of Youth, and even if it would not be a good thing to find it if there *were* one, the desire to do so comprises a reason to look for it. This is the "authority" of the desire, and if this authority lay in its representational character its authority is likewise intrinsic to the state. (Of course its being a *veridical* perception or indication is relational and not an intrinsic property, but it needn't be veridical in order to be a reason.)

Now it has been suggested that the representational nature of a thing may be identified with its being such that it *would* stand in a certain genuine (not merely intentional) relation, under certain conditions, to the thing it represents. For a state to be such that, in it, it seems a certain way to one, may be for it to be such that under ideal conditions, one would be in that state only if the situation external to the state were as it seems. (Such, at least, is the view I favor.) But this does not compromise the claim that the authority of the state is *per se.* For such ideal conditions may well fail to obtain, and if the state even then possesses that property owing to which it has such authority as it may possess, then its authority is, in that sense, intrinsic to it. The authority of desire is its capacity to confer rationality on action. That capacity lay in its seeming as if the thing wanted would be good, indicating that it would be good. And it may do this even if the desire is generated under conditions less than ideal, even if the desiderative perception is not veridical. To put it slightly differently, the *explanation* of this authority—of *this* being the way it seems, or what is indicated, when one wants something—does indeed refer to the relationships between the desire and things other than it; it refers to the mental mechanism from which it must arise, and the merits of the thing wanted, which are, I

367

DENNIS W. STAMPE

have suggested, being given representation in the desire. It is *because* in the ideal case the thing would be as it seems it is, that the desire for it is a reason to try to get it, *even if* this is not the ideal case; even if those relationships are not as they ideally would be, the desire ordinarily possesses that same authority, remaining an indication that the thing wanted would be good, thus *per se* a reason to try to get it.

Misgivings may persist. I have suggested that there is a sense in which a desire is a *per se* reason for action whereas a belief, including the belief that it would be good if *p*, is not *per se* but only *per objectum* a reason. But in the sense leaned upon in the last paragraph, the representational character of the *belief*, and thus its authority, is quite as "intrinsic" as is that of a desire, although belief is supposed to be a reason *per objectum*. But the difference first observed remains: it is the object of the belief that is, or may be, a reason for acting—that is, the fact that it would be good if *p;* but the *object* of the desire—its being the case that *p*—cannot possibly be a reason for acting. The issue here turns on how the proper "objects" of the attitudes are identified. It may be suggested that if the desire that *p* is a perception, its object should be regarded as being its *perceptual* content—the fact that it would be good if *p*. Why must we be bound by the common form of ascription, rather than re-describing the object of the desire in the way the theory would suggest? My answer to this is that the proper object of an attitude is the state of affairs that it functions to introduce into reasoning, and that fundamental process of practical reasoning must begin from the state of affairs one wants to obtain, not from the perceptual content of desire. I shall return to this in the final section of the essay.

Now as only a fact can be a reason, a fact *cannot* be reasonable or unreasonable. (A *reason* cannot be reasonable or unreasonable.) And so it is that a desire can be *per se* a reason to act, whether that desire be reasonable or unreasonable. For a desire is reasonable or unreasonable not *intrinsically* (in the sense I have tried to explain, in which it is "intrinsically" a reason), but extrinsically—that is owing to the relations it bears to others of the beliefs, desires, and intentions a person might happen to have. The predicate "reasonable" applies to a desire in view of the logical relations holding among

the several propositions that express the contents of the desire and of other relevant states of mind, just as one's belief is "unreasonable" if what one believes is inconsistent with everything else one believes. So while a desire is *per se* a reason to act, it may be, relative to others of one's states of mind, utterly unreasonable. That it *seems$_d$* as if something would be good is *not* the content (not the object) of one's desire for that thing, so there is no inconsistency in saying that the desire is in itself a reason to act despite the fact that it is an unreasonable desire.

It is possible to be clearer about such unreasonableness. Suppose Jones harbors an unreasonable desire to be department chairperson—unreasonable because Jones knows perfectly well that there is nothing good about being chairperson, but nonetheless it somehow seems$_d$ to him as if it would be a good thing. The content of this desire (in view of which it *is* unreasonable) is the state of affairs that would satisfy it: Jones' being chairperson. Now Jones also wants to be happy and knows that no chairperson is happy. The states of affairs comprising the contents of these three states of mind are incompatible: a situation in which Jones is chairperson and happy and in which no chairperson is happy is impossible. Thus his desire is unreasonable.

The following objection may be raised against the thesis that a desire is a perceptual state. (1) It is not (cannot be said to be) unreasonable, or reasonable, that it *seems* to someone as if something would be good—no more than it can be said to be reasonable or unreasonable that something looks to someone as if something is green; but (2) a perceptual state is just a state in which it seems as if something is the case; therefore (3) no perceptual state can be reasonable or unreasonable. (4) But a desire can be reasonable or unreasonable, and therefore, by Leibniz's Law, (5) a desire is not a perceptual state.

Plainly I must, and I do, reject (3), for I hold that a desire is a perceptual state and agree with the other premises. But (3) does not follow from those premises. It would follow only if (2) strictly *identified* a perceptual state with the *fact* that it seems a certain way when one is in such a state. But it does not do so; that would be a category error. For no *state* is one and the same thing as any *fact*. Instead, (2) identifies perceptual states in terms of a fact that ob-

369

DENNIS W. STAMPE

tains when one is in such a state; it does not say that such states and such facts are the same things.[23] Nor do I say that one's desire is the same thing as the fact that it therein seems$_d$ to one as if something would be good. (I am indebted to William Rowe for pressing the original question about the predicability of reasonableness to desires.)

A second thing that may cast doubt on the hypothesis that desires are perceptions, is the fact that one can, so we say, *decide* what one wants. This may again suggest that there is another aspect to desire, other than the perceptual or passionate character that allegedly explains its *per se* authority—that there is a way in which it is "up to us" what we want. For we cannot, in any such way, decide or make up our minds what perceptual state we are in. But our so-called decisions as to "what we want" are really decisions about what we will *have*, or what we will *do*. When I make up my mind that "what I want" is the fish and not the fowl, I am really deciding that I will *have* the fish. In the absence of any prospect of choosing the one or the other, I can see no sense in which I can "decide" which one I want. We can make up our minds only which of the things that antecedently seem$_d$ as if they would be good, is the one we will, or would, choose to have.

In this connection I am inclined to view with skepticism the notion of the "all-things-considered desire," where this is supposed to be what we *want* as a (more or less immediate) consequence of our considering the comparative desirability of various things we wanted prior to such deliberation. Deliberation leads to conclusions about which thing would be better, decisions about what to do. But I see no compelling reason to suppose that deliberation has the power to make our desires fall in line, nor thus to generate all-things-considered desires. It *seems*, indeed, that it has no such

---

[23]There are other facts that may serve to identify (but are not identical with) the state, including facts that do so tautologically. Thus compare (2) to (2') *a desire is a state in which (it is a fact that) someone wants something*. Now the *fact* that someone wants something cannot be reasonable or unreasonable either. (No fact can be.) But the conclusion that a desire cannot be reasonable or unreasonable clearly cannot be soundly inferred from (1) and (2'). Compare also the following paralogism: "Paranoia is incurable. And (2'') paranoia is a condition in which it seems as if everyone is plotting against one. But *the fact that it seems so* cannot be said to be incurable. It follows that (2'') is false." Obviously it *doesn't* follow.

THE AUTHORITY OF DESIRE

power—no more than does thinking about the visual situation have the power to generate "all-things-considered" perceptions. Neither, surely, is the theory of how practical reasoning takes us from conflicting desires to action enhanced by supposing that it must generate intermediate desires to do things that the reasoning results in one's deciding to do.

VI. DESIRE AS PROPRIOCEPTION

If desire is a kind of perception, it is a peculiar one not just in being non-sensuous but in a more important way. For whereas what you see or hear or feel is the very thing you perceive, *what* you want cannot be identified, in general, with the thing you are perceiving (or of which you are aware). Of course you do see things sometimes that seem$_d$ as if they would be good to have and you want them. But you can also want things that do not exist or for other reasons cannot be perceived. Nor is what one desires to be the case identifiable with that which, in desiring it, one might *perceive to be the case*. Those who wanted the Baltimore Orioles to steal the pennant (—this was written in 1982—) from the Milwaukee Brewers were in no way perceiving that that was to be the case; and neither were they perceiving that it would have been, as it seemed$_d$ to them it would have been, a good thing were that to have happened. (It would of course have been a very bad thing.)

If desire is a kind of perception, it must have the features of genuine perception. What are they? First, what is perceived must be there, must actually exist, if it is to be perceived. Second, it must be capable of making some kind of appearance, capable, that is, of making it seem a certain way to the subject. And third, a genuine form of perception is a route to possible knowledge, about the things thereby perceived, and things relevantly related to them. There is, further, the usual distinction between *"nonepistemic"* (or simple, or object-) perception, and *"epistemic"* (or propositional) perception to be drawn among perceptions of any modality.[24] One

---

[24]This distinction is presented and well delineated in Fred Dretske's *Seeing and Knowing* (Chicago: Anchor Books, 1969). Cf. G. J. Warnock, "Seeing," in Robert Swartz, *Perceiving, Sensing, and Knowing* (Garden City, N.Y., 1965).

DENNIS W. STAMPE

sees the cheese, "nonepistemically," for just to see it, one needn't know what it is that one is seeing; it is sufficient just that the cheese present a visual appearance, or look some way, to one. One sees "epistemically" that the cheese is moldy (here the verb takes a *that*-clause as its complement), because if one sees that then one knows that the cheese is moldy. (And, sometimes, one can see that the cheese is moldy because one sees the cheese, and because of the way it looks to one.)

Now if a person's desire for the cheese involves a kind of perception, we must ask what it is a nonepistemic perception *of*, and what, if anything, it might be an epistemic perception of. It cannot be that the object of nonepistemic perception should be the cheese itself, the object of desire. One need not perceive *what* one wants, in any sense at all. (And only metaphorically does one see something good in the things one wants.) Neither can the propositional object of the desire—that I have the cheese—be the fact that might be epistemically perceived. I cannot see how anything can, as required, present some appearance, or make it seem to someone as if something is the case, unless it has some *effect* on that person, and what is presumably not (yet) the case cannot be appearing anyway to me. And it is difficult to see how the *goodness* even of some present state of affairs, much less the goodness of some merely prospective state of affairs, such as my having the cheese, could have any such effect, how it could appear any way at all. If the property of being good is itself inefficacious it cannot be offered as the object of appetitive perception or awareness.

The view I favor is this. The object of nonepistemic desiderative perception is some state of the desirer himself; the desirer himself is in a certain state, which I shall call Σ, which *causes* it to seem to him as if the thing wanted would be good. Desire is one's non-epistemic perception of this state of oneself, and it is one's being in that state that causes one to be in the distinct state wherein it seems$_d$ to one as if it would be good were something to be the case. This state, Σ, is a state distinct from that (normally conscious) mental state (that is, that wherein something seems$_d$ a good thing), and what it is may also be distinguished from the "objective" state of affairs in which that thing *would* be a good thing. Σ is a state of the subject, but it is not in the other sense of the phrase a subjective state; in particular, it is not one which necessarily *is* as it is perceived

THE AUTHORITY OF DESIRE

to be. Finally, Σ is not to be identified with the desire itself, as if the desire involved the perception of that very state, the desire itself.[25]

It may be, however, that Σ is a plain bodily state—for instance, a state in which the body is depleted of air or water, where one's being in that state makes it seem to one as if it would be good to breathe or drink. (And in this case, the subject's state may be identified with the objective state of affairs which is such that it would be good for him to breathe or drink.) That state, then, will be the object of nonepistemic perception. I suggest that Σ may also comprise the cognitive and larger conative state of one who has certain beliefs, aims, and other desires, where one's being in that state makes it seem to one as if something would be good—as it *may* do. Here too, I suggest, in wanting that thing one is subject to a certain kind of nonepistemic awareness of one's own state, even one's own total mental state. Traditionally, the awareness of one's own *mental* state—the perception of one's "perceptions"— is "*apperception.*" All desire is perception, and some, I suggest, is apperception.

Turning then to epistemic perception, what one may come to *know*, owing to the perception of a Σ state, is that it would be good were one for example to drink, or generally, that it would be good were the objective of the desire to obtain. For Σ is to be a state of the subject such that, ideally, if one is in such a state—a state that makes it seem$_d$ to one as if it would be good if p—then it *would* be good were one for example to drink, or generally, that it would be good were the objective of the desire to obtain. So, desire is a form

---

[25]That being the view that Descartes took of volitions (*volontez*), but not of desire (*desir*). He said that volitions are perceptions of the kind that have the soul, not the body, as a cause. They are perceptions because " . . . we cannot will anything without our perceiving by the same means that we will it (*que nous la voulons*). . . . [T]his perception and this volition are in effect one and the same thing . . ." *The Passions of the Soul*, I, xix. (The causal theory of perception is retained even here: a volition is its own cause.) Descartes's view of *desire*, however, is another matter. At II, lxxx, he said " . . . [B]y the word 'volonté' I do not here intend to speak of desire (*desir*), which is a passion apart, and one which has reference to the future." At Article lxxxvi, he defines desire as " . . . an agitation of the soul caused by the spirits, which dispose it to wish (*vouloir*) for the future those things that it represents to itself as suitable (*convenable*)." The definition would of course be circular were desires not distinct from volitions or wishes. It is not clear to me whether Descartes regarded desire as involving a *perception* of that bodily state, which he describes as an agitation of the spirits.

of *proprioception,* its direct or nonepistemic object being a state of the subject himself. It is a source of knowledge for the subject, first of the subject himself—of this Σ state he is in—and second, under further conditions, it is a source of knowledge of what would be good. That is to say, it affords the possibility of one's perceiving, knowing, that certain states of affairs would be good. (Notice, then, that the thing one may come to know is not the thing that one wants to be true. Again, while desire is a form of perception, *what* one wants is not what one therein perceives, or perceives to be true.)

Finally, Σ may be a state such that the subject *needs* something, as one depleted of water may need water. In this way it may be that a desire is a perception of a need. The causal set-up here is roughly as follows: the organism's being depleted of water causes it to be the case that it needs water, *and,* its being depleted of water also causes certain bodily sensations which cause the desire for water. The desire for water is the perception of the state of depletion, thus of a state *in which* one needs water, thus of a state such that it would be good if one had water.[26]

I have suggested that desires are reliable indicators of what would be good, and that their authority involves nothing more, and nothing less. But still it may seem to involve something distinctly

---

[26]An organism's need can affect its own satisfaction, *via* the mental representation of that need. The simplest way an organism's needs might do so is that in which the mental states representing those needs are states which have as their contents precisely the state of affairs that the organism needs to have realized; thus the need, or necessity, that *x has water at t* achieves representation in a mental state of the form ϕ (*x has water at t*). Since the content of this mental attitude is the state of affairs the organism needs, the semantic satisfaction of the attitude (its being made "true") is one and the same thing as the satisfaction of that need. Suppose there is a mechanism that works to bring about conformity between the world and the organism's representation of the world, adjusting the one to the other according to the cognitive or conative modality of the representational states. Then we would seem to have the gross outlines of the way rational action might serve to satisfy needs. The mental state that intervenes—ϕ (*x has water at t*)—is one exhibiting the form of a desire for water. It would, according to the present account, *be* a desire, assuming that ϕ is *in itself* (in its intrinsic nature) a state wherein it *seems$_d$* to *x as if it would be good* were its object to be realized—that is, *good were it to be that* x has water at t. (I explore this further in a paper called "Need," to appear in the *Australasian Journal of Philosophy*, 1987.)

THE AUTHORITY OF DESIRE

less, for this reason. I said that if you should want to learn German you have therein a reason to do it, even if there is, apart from that desire, no reason whatever to do it. But if your desire to learn German is, as I have now said, an indication that it would be good to do so, is there not a reason for *me* to learn German? But one would have thought, or even hoped, that the fact that one person wants to learn German is no reason whatever for another person to learn it. This consideration starts thoughts about the egocentricity of desire. We may, I think, say this: the fact is that it seems$_d$ to you that it would be a good thing were *you* to learn German; a good thing, perhaps, (though this is not the same thing) *for* you. Your desire may indicate just that *that* is the case. (If so then I am not threatened with the existence of a reason for me to learn German.) Maybe your situation is one such that it seems a good thing for you to do, since you are going off to live in Germany to study Hegel. Not I. My suggestion has been that when one wants something, what one is perceiving is one's own state, or situation, not the way things are in general.

This is part of the reason I say that desire is a form of proprioception. If you want a beer, in the ordinary way, it isn't that it seems to you as if it would be a good thing for *everyone* to have a beer; you are perceiving, may be, the state of your own body, not everyone's. There is, I think, a deep and inviting question here— important to ethics—about the *capacity* of desire, its limits. *Can* it seem$_d$ as if something would be good for everyone, if desire is, as I suggest, a form of proprioception? If so, *how* can it? Suppose you want everyone to learn German, not just you: it seems$_d$ as if that would be a good thing. Is that possible? It is a bit like going to the window during a blizzard and saying, "It looks as if the whole world is white." But it *doesn't* really look that way, for one is not seeing the whole world. The way things *can* look—or seem$_d$—is constrained by the objects of immediate perception. But not *just* thereby constrained, delimited, but also, it may be, enlarged, as the mirror we immediately see enlarges the range of our vision. The idea that desire is proprioception is the idea that in desire one perceives a state of oneself which state is *such that* some state of affairs would be good. But how may one human being be in a state such that it would be good were some benefit to befall someone else? What relationships of similarity, sympathy, or caring might

375

DENNIS W. STAMPE

explain this? And the way things seem is a function also of belief—
or at least the way we *think* things seem is—so that it *is* possible for
someone to want even such a thing as that everyone should know
German; or to think that that is what he wants. But if we may be
wrong about the way things seem to us, and surely we may, we may
be wrong about what we want.

I only mention these matters. I think they point to no defect in
the present conception of desire, but rather to a virtue of it. It
seems to me, that is, that while it does not solve them, the conception of desire as a form of proprioception places the hardest and
most important human problems about desire in the right light.
These are problems about the capacity and limits of desire, the
promiscuity and the hardness of the human heart. How on the one
hand can anyone *want*, almost more than anything, one baseball
team to win a game and not another? And on the other hand, how
can anyone *not* want, genuinely want, a war to stop, knowing what
wars are? Why is knowledge so impotent? Why doesn't our merely
knowing what would be good haul our desires in line? Why doesn't
one's knowing that it would be good if something were to happen
make one *want* it to happen? Why must we be shown the starving
children to make us want to feed them?

But then too, I know what the Pacific Ocean sounds like; why
can't I hear it? I know what Paris looks like. Why can't I see it? The
powers of knowledge, of belief, *are* small, in matters of perception.
And if desire is a form of perception our knowing that something is
good *would* not, of itself, make us want it.

VII. Desire, the Crux of Practical Reasoning

I began by asserting that the central question about desire is the
question how practical reasoning can begin in it, and the central
question about practical reasoning is how it can begin in desire.
The problem is that reasoning, of any variety, can begin only in
something that constitutes a reason for reaching the conclusion
that is to be reached. But only facts can be reasons, and what one
wants is not a fact.

I have tried to understand this matter as follows. It is, indeed, *not*
from what we want that we reason out what to do, but rather from
the fact that we want it. We reason from the desire itself. Accord-

THE AUTHORITY OF DESIRE

ingly, desires are reasons not *per objectum,* but *per se* reasons for acting in accordance with them. This cannot mean, however, that practical reasoning begins from premises *about* our desires, from premises like "I want a covering." This merely expresses the belief that one wants something. It is the desire itself that comprises one's reason to act. Nor is this because desires are like itches, merely brute reasons for action, but rather because desires, like perceptual states, essentially involve the representation of something as being the case. It is because they are states indicating that it would be good were the objective of the desire to be realized. There is therefore, I have argued, an epistemic warrant for the authority we attribute to a desire. Because it is a form of perception, desire is autonomous in its authority, as is any perceptual modality, not requiring legitimation by the representations of the intellect. A desire is certified a reason to act by its perceptual content;[27] being a state in which it seems$_d$ to one as if it would be good were a certain state of affairs to obtain, it is a state in which the thing wanted is represented as such that *it would be good were that state of affairs to obtain.* Ideally, the desire contains that information.

Suppose the starting point of a bit of practical reasoning is a

---

[27]On the present view, desire might be said to have a *dual* content: one perceptual (it would be good if it were to be that I have a cow), being the state of affairs that seems$_d$ to one to obtain, and one prospective (I have a cow), being the state of affairs one wants to obtain. On at least one view of content ascription, there is no reason this should not be so. (Such a view is offered in my paper, "Toward a Causal Theory of Linguistic Representation," *Midwest Studies in Philosophy: Studies in the Philosophy of Language II* (1977), pp. 42–63, Morris, Minn.) The ascription of "content" to a state of mind is nothing more than the specification of that state of mind by a specification of a state of affairs to which it stands in a certain ideal relation: a state of affairs, for example, which would cause that state of mind, under certain ideal conditions (cf. perception)— or, a state of affairs which would, under certain *other* ideal conditions, be caused *by* that state of mind (cf. intention). (This specification is notoriously constrained in certain ways, and consequently has the feature called "opacity"; but this constraint on the manner of the specification need not be taken to determine *what* is being specified.) There is no reason why there should not be a single state of mind which may be described, in a Hobbesian phrase, both as a passive power and as an active power, either in terms of its ideal cause or in terms of its ideal effect. Desire, I think, is just such a state. What I have called its perceptual content is its ideal cause, and its prospective content is its ideal effect.

desire. If a valid conclusion from it is an action that would make that premise true, then the perceptual content of the desire (it would be good if *p*) does not express that premise. Making a cloak does not make it true that it would be good to have a covering. What it makes true is that one *has* a covering, and that—which is *what* one wants—is the starting point of the reasoning. This state of affairs (one's having a covering), not being a fact, cannot be the thing—the reason—"from which one reasons." But the fact that one wants it to obtain (that is, that it seems$_d$ as if it would be good if it did) nonetheless constitutes *it*—one's having a covering—an Aristotelian fixed point, toward which reasoning aimed at making it a fact may aim.

It is from the *prospective* content of a desire, not its perceptual content, that practical reasoning begins. There is no rational step from *it seems$_d$ it would be good if p* to one's desiring that *p;* and were one to reason from the former to the conclusion that it *would* be good, or good to bring it about, that *p*, this is not yet the intention to do so. So it is not in the relevant sense *practical* reasoning. If we take the perceptual content of the desire to be its starting point, it is hard to see how the conclusion of the reasoning could be an act or an intention to act.[28] For the reasoning would then be confined to what

---

[28]From the proposition that it would be good were *p* to be the case, together with the proposition that I can make *p* the case by and only by doing A, no proposition follows to the effect that I *will* do A; nor does the proposition that I *ought* to do it follow. No such thing follows without importing other premises, such as the premise that *if it would be good if p were the case and I can make it the case by (or: only by) doing A, then I ought to do A.* But such a premise as that, even though it might be something one believes, ought not to enter into the reasoning as a premise: that would be like having, as a premise in a piece of theoretical reasoning *If I believe one thing that entails a second I should believe the second too.* One might better conceive of it as a principle of inference rather than a premise. But that seems wrong too. For in the first place, one would not wish to admit principles of inference, in the case of theoretical syllogisms, of an analogous form, concerned with mental attitudes instead of the propositions in question. Proper principles of inference should be of the form, for example, *P and if P then Q entails Q,* not of the form *If one believes if P then Q, and believes P, then one should believe Q.* In any case, a practical syllogism of such a kind will not yield the content of an intention as its conclusion. If it can be made to yield *I ought to do A,* this is still only a reason for forming an intention, and not the content of the intention I ought to form—which is

THE AUTHORITY OF DESIRE

is entailed by the putative fact that it would be good were *p* to be the case, and *via* other credible premises it could reach no further than the conclusion that one's doing something would be good; the reasoning cannot be made to yield the content of the intention actually to do it, that is, a conclusion of the form *I will do A*.

Reasoning of any kind consists in one's tracing out the way one state of affairs is involved in another one, with a view to certain ends. In practical reasoning one does this with a view to determining what to do, and the states of affairs in question comprise the contents of one's desires, beliefs, and possible intentions. To reason practically is to attend to the entailment relations between the state of affairs in which one would have what one wants—that in which one has, for example, a cow—the state of affairs in which certain of one's beliefs are true, and the state of affairs in which one does certain things. One might see, for instance, that if the situation is one in which he will have a cow if he goes out and buys one, the state of affairs in which he does so would *entail* that in which he has a cow in fact. And he might, should he think it possible to do that thing, form the intention to do it, as a causal consequence of this reasoning. That is what reasoning from the desire to a decision to do something would be. It may be represented by such a configuration as this:

desire	(a)	I have a cow tomorrow.
belief	(b)	I have a cow tomorrow if (or: if and only if) I will go buy a cow today.
intention	(c)	I will go buy a cow today.

Here propositions (a), (b), and (c) stand to one another in some logical relation: (a) and (b) imply (c); or (b) and (c) imply (a); or both. These clauses specify the contents of the states of mind respectively indicated at the left of them. That is, they specify the states of affairs one wants to obtain, or believes to obtain, or intends

---

instead *I will do A*. To derive *that* we should have to add the premise *If I ought to do A then I will do A*. But this is not the content of a *belief* anybody actually has. It might, perhaps, be construed as the content of an *intention*, but if it is implausible to suppose agents harbor so optimistic a belief about themselves, it is implausible to ascribe that intention to them.

379

to obtain; they *express* those states of mind, respectively.[29] While these states of affairs stand to one another in relationships of entailment the states of mind of which they comprise the contents stand only in a corresponding *causal* relationship. For of course the fact that one has that desire and that belief does not logically entail that one has that intention. It is rather that this desire and this belief would *cause* one to form this intention, under certain conditions. (For instance, under the condition that the desire is sufficiently strong, that there is no doubt about the possibility of one's doing the thing, and so forth.) So, this practical syllogism represents the causal (psychological) process of rational decision making, or intention-formation, by means of a configuration of logically related propositions, representing logically connected states of affairs contained in those causally related states of mind.

This is exactly parallel to the "theoretical" syllogism, in which premises and conclusion alike represent the contents of possible beliefs or judgments. The structure represents the logical relations among states of affairs, and insofar as these are the contents of possible beliefs, represents thereby the causal process of rational belief formation. The temporal order of that process need not correspond to the logical order in respect of the "direction" of implication, nor, as Aristotle observed, need it correspond to the objective temporal order in which those states of affairs may transpire. So we may include among theoretical syllogisms both the ordinary deductive syllogism and the abductive syllogism (for example, the streets are wet; they would be wet if it had rained; it has rained). In the deductive syllogism, the state of affairs represented by the final proposition is both entailed by the first two and is the content of the judgment with which the reasoning concludes. In the abductive syllogism, however, the state of affairs represented by the last proposition, together with the second, entails the first, although the content of the state of mind with which the reasoning

---

[29]The practical syllogism should require no premises *about* these states of mind, asserting, for example, that one ought to decide to do—or that one will decide to do—that which is necessary and sufficient to get one what one wants. The psychological process which the practical syllogism serves to model is one that presumably could occur in creatures that had no conception of their own mental states; or, at least, it is better not to prejudice that question by our conception of the practical syllogism. Further, the practical syllogism should, if possible, yield its conclusion without the aid of special principles of inference.

THE AUTHORITY OF DESIRE

concludes is stated by that last proposition. Thus what is last in the order of thought is first in the order of logical derivation, and first also, as Aristotle observed, in the order in which those states of affairs would come to obtain in the course of time; as its raining precedes and results in the streets' being wet. Likewise, in the practical syllogism, what is last in the order of "deliberation"—the intention—is first in the order in which the states of affairs that are the contents of that intention and that desire, would come to obtain; as my going to the cow market precedes and results in my having a cow. And this is so whether the direction of implication runs one way or the other, according to whether the belief is that this is the only way to get what I want, or merely one way (as in the cloak syllogism, and similarly in the abductive syllogism where the conclusion represents only one way in which the major premise could come to be a fact.) In the deductive cases, the premises provide a putatively *conclusive* reason for accepting the conclusion, whether as what one must believe or what one must intend to bring about. In the latter cases, they provide, putatively, merely *a* reason for doing so. In the abductive case, however, the reason one has to affirm the conclusion is the fact stated by the major premise, not the fact that one believes it to obtain. One's belief is that reason, *per objectum.* In the practical case, the reason one has to form the intention represented by the conclusion is the fact that one wants the state of affairs represented by the major premise to obtain. The desire is *per se* that reason. It is this difference that I have tried to understand in this essay, and this difference that I take to be the key to understanding the peculiarity of practical reasoning. For, as I hope to have indicated, through it all, in every case, the logic is the same. The peculiarity of practical reasoning lies not in its logic, but in the nature of its starting point, in the way in which that starting point comprises a reason for its conclusion.

Like a fulcrum, then, desire transforms the inward pressure of perception into the outward impetus of intention. Desire is the crux of practical reasoning, and around it we turn.[30]

University of Wisconsin, Madison

---

[30]I am indebted to several philosophers, at Purdue, Western Ontario, Illinois and Wisconsin for helpful discussion, and especially to Nancy Sweet Thomadsen.

[15]

THE FAINTEST PASSION*

Harry Frankfurt
Princeton University

Presidential Address delivered before the Eighty-Eighth Annual Eastern Division Meeting of the American Philosophical Association in New York City, December 29, 1991.

1. My title is from an observation by A.E. Housman. "The faintest of all human passions" he wrote, "is the love of truth."[1] There are two senses in which a passion may be faint: it may be weak, or it may only be difficult to discern. Housman certainly intended the former. But be that as it may, there is a passion that, in both senses, is even fainter than our love of truth. Surely the very faintest human passion—both the least salient and the least robust—is our love of the truth about ourselves.

The ability both to believe something and at the same time to conceal this from oneself is a bit paradoxical. Philosophers have found it difficult to explain how we do this. There is no problem, however, in understanding *why*. The facts about ourselves are often hard to take. When they move us to self-deception, it is because we find them irreconcilable with what we want to believe. We hide from the truth, it seems clear, because it conflicts with our self-love. My theme today, however, is not self-deception. I am aiming at another enemy of the truth about ourselves—one whose relation to self-love is rather more complex and uncertain. My approach will be somewhat oblique. I begin with a question about lying.

2. When we object to being the victim of a lie, just what is it that we find so objectionable? I am not asking why lying is wrong. My question has to do not with the morality of lying, but with our experience of it. What offends us when we are offended that someone has told us a lie? What accounts for how the lying affects us?

Much is often made of the notion that lying undermines the cohesion of human society. Kant says that "without truth social intercourse and conversation become valueless."[2] And he argues that because it threatens society in this way, "a lie always harms another; if not some particular man, still it harms mankind generally. . . ."[3] Montaigne makes a similar claim: "our intercourse being carried on solely by means of the word, he who falsifies that is a traitor to society."[4] "Lying is an accursed vice," Montaigne declares; and then he adds, warming rather frenetically to his subject, that "if we did but recognize the horror and gravity of it, we should punish it with flames more justly than other crimes."[5]

----

* I dedicate this address to my first teachers in philosophy—George Boas and Albert Hammond, of blessed memory.

5

Montaigne and Kant certainly have a point, but they exaggerate. Profitable social intercourse does not really depend, as they maintain, upon people telling each other the truth; nor does conversation lose its value when people lie. The actual quantity of lying is enormous, after all, and yet social life goes on. That people often lie hardly renders it impossible to benefit from living with them. It only means that we have to be careful. We can quite successfully negotiate our way through an environment full of lies, as long as we can reasonably trust our own ability to discriminate more or less effectively between instances in which people are lying and those in which they are telling the truth. General confidence in the honesty of others is not essential, as long as we are justified in having confidence in ourselves.

In any case, however, it is not because we think that lies threaten or encumber the order of society that we are upset by them in the first place. Our concern when someone lies to us is not the concern of a citizen. What is most immediately aroused in our reaction to the liar is not public spirit. The reaction is personal. As a rule, we are dismayed far less by the harm the liar may have done to others than by his conduct towards ourselves. What stirs us against him, whether or not he has somehow managed to betray all of mankind, is that he has certainly injured us.

Lying is a rather complicated act. Someone who tells a lie invariably attempts to deceive his victims about matters of two distinct kinds: first, about the state of affairs to which he explicitly refers and of which he is purporting to give a correct account; second, about his own beliefs and what is going on in his mind. In addition to misrepresenting a fact about the world, then, the liar also misrepresents various facts about himself. Each of these aspects of what he does is significant in its own way.

First of all, the liar aims at inducing his victims to regard as real a world that he himself has designed. To the extent that he is successful in this, he is the originator of what they take to be reality. How the facts appear to them is determined by what he says. Thus he arrogates to himself something like the divine prerogative of creative speech, simulating the omnipotent will by which God (according to *Genesis*) brought a world into being merely by stipulating that it should be so. This arrogance offends our pride. We are angered by the liar's insulting effort to usurp control over the conditions in which we understand ourselves to live.

Secondly, by imposing a false world on his victims, the liar excludes them from his world. Insofar as he places them within an understanding of reality that differs from his own, he separates them radically from himself. This is what leads Adrienne Rich to observe, with poetic exactitude, that "the liar leads an existence of unutterable loneliness."[6] The loneliness is precisely *unutterable* because the liar cannot even reveal that he *is* lonely without disclosing that he has lied. By hiding his own thoughts, he makes it impossible for others to be in touch with him—to understand him or to respond to him as he really is, or even to be aware that they are not doing so. This forecloses a mode of human intimacy that is both elementary and normal, and for this reason it too is insulting. Like his presuming to exercise the creative prerogative of a god, the liar's refusal to permit himself to be known is an injury to his victim's pride.

3. In certain cases, lies cause a deeper damage. Adrienne Rich says that "to discover that one has been lied to in a personal relationship leads one to feel a little crazy."[7] Here again, her observation is perspicuous and exact. When we are dealing in an important matter with someone whom we hardly know, we can be confident that what he says coincides with what he believes only on the basis of a more or less deliberate evaluation of his reliability; and ordinarily, this evaluation only covers specific communications. With our close friends, as a rule, both of these conditions are relaxed. We suppose that our friends are generally truthful with us; and we take this pretty much for granted. We tend to trust whatever they say; and we do so, mainly, not on the basis of a particular calculation that they are telling the truth, but because we feel comfortable with them. As we familiarly put it, "we just know they wouldn't lie to us."

With friends, the presumption of intimacy has become natural. It derives most immediately from our feelings—that is, from our sense of our own state, rather than from an evaluation of pertinent evidence about them. It would be too much to say that a person's inclination to trust his friends belongs to his essential nature. But it could properly enough be said that trusting them has come to be second nature to him.

This is why finding that we have been lied to by a friend engenders a feeling of being crazy. The discovery exposes something about ourselves more disturbing than that we have merely miscalculated or made an error of judgment. It reveals that our own nature (i.e., our second nature) is unreliable, leading us to count on people who cannot be trusted. Needless to say, the deception of a friend implies a fault in the one who tells the lie. But it also shows that the victim is defective too. The liar betrays him, but he is betrayed by his own feelings as well.

Self-betrayal pertains to craziness because it is a hallmark of the irrational. The essence of rationality is to be consistent; and being consistent, in action or in thought, means proceeding so as not to defeat oneself. Aristotle explains that an agent acts rationally insofar as he conforms his actions to the mean. Suppose that for the sake of good health, a person follows a diet either so meager or so indulgent that it actually leads him away from his goal of well-being. It is in this self-betrayal that the irrationality of his divergence from the mean consists. Intellectual activity is similarly undermined by logical incoherence. When a line of thought generates a contradiction, its further progressive elaboration is blocked. In whatever direction the mind turns, it is driven back: it must affirm what is has already rejected, or deny what it has already affirmed. Like behavior that frustrates its own ambition, contradictory thinking is irrational because it betrays itself.

When a person discovers that someone he had found it natural to count upon has lied to him, this shows him that he cannot rely upon his own settled feelings of trust. He sees that his sense of whom he can have confidence in has betrayed him. It has led him to miss the truth rather than to attain it. His assumption that he could guide himself by it has turned out to be self-defeating, and hence irrational. He may well feel, accordingly, a little crazy.

4. According to Aristotle, philosophy in the ancient world began in wonder.[8] In the modern world, of course, it began in doubt. These are both attitudes of uncertainty. We are moved to wonder when the phenomena are unclear. On the other hand, the uneasiness that lying may arouse in us, concerning our own cognitive capacities, is more like the mode of uncertainty that beset Descartes. What disturbed him was not how to think about the phenomena, but what to make of himself. The doubt in which his epistemological and metaphysical enterprise began was self-doubt.

The ancient philosophers, Aristotle explains, "philosophised in order to escape from ignorance."[9] Descartes was moved to philosophise less by ignorance than by anxiety, less by a lack of knowledge than by a lack of self-confidence. What worried him was that he might be by nature so profoundly defective that his intellectual ambitions would be betrayed by the very cognitive capacities upon which he needed to rely in pursuing them. "How do we know," he asked, "that we have not been made in such a way that we constantly deceive ourselves?" In other words, how do we know that rationality is possible at all? Descartes's particular fear was that we might perceive, with equally irresistible clarity and distinctness, both that certain propositions are true and that they are not true. That would show reason to be hopelessly divided. It would mean that anyone who attempted persistently to be rational would end up not knowing what to think.

Spinoza defines a condition of our affective nature that is analogous to this division within reason. The "constitution of the mind which arises from two contrary affects," he says, "is called vacillation of mind, which is therefore related to the affects as doubt is to the imagination."[10] Now I want to consider a somewhat different, but still analogous, type of psychic instability or conflict. I shall call it "ambivalence." Here what is divided is neither a person's reason nor his affects, but his will. Insofar as someone is ambivalent, he is moved by incompatible preferences or attitudes regarding his affects or his desires or regarding other elements of his psychic life. This volitional division keeps him from settling upon or from tolerating any coherent affective or motivational identity. It means that he does not know what he really wants.[11]

Ambivalence is constituted by conflicting volitional movements or tendencies, either conscious or unconscious, that meet two conditions. First, they are inherently and hence unavoidably opposed; that is, they do not just happen to conflict on account of contingent circumstances. Second, they are both wholly internal to a person's will rather than alien to him; that is, he is not passive with respect to them. An example of ambivalence might be provided by someone who is moved to commit himself to a certain career, or to a certain person, and also moved to refrain from doing so.

Conflicts involving first-order psychic elements alone—for instance, between an attraction and an aversion to the same object or action—do not pertain to the will at all. They are not volitional, but merely impulsive or sentimental. Conflicts that pertain to the will arise out of a person's higher-order, reflective attitudes. But even conflicts that do implicate a person's will are nonetheless distinct from ambivalence

if some of the psychic forces they involve are exogenous—that is, if the person is not identified with them and they are, in that sense, external to his will.

An addict who struggles sincerely against his addiction is contending with a force by which he does not want to be moved and which is therefore alien to him. Since the conflict is not wholly within his will, he is not volitionally divided or ambivalent. The unwilling addict is wholeheartedly on one side of the conflict from which he suffers, and not at all on the other. The addiction may defeat his will, but does not as such disrupt its unity.

A person is ambivalent, then, only if he is indecisive concerning whether to be for or against a certain psychic position. Now this kind of indecisiveness is as irrational, in its way, as holding contradictory beliefs. The disunity of an ambivalent person's will prevents him from effectively pursuing and satisfactorily attaining his goals. Like conflict within reason, volitional conflict leads to self-betrayal and self-defeat. The trouble is in each case the same: a sort of incoherent greed—trying to have things both ways—which naturally makes it impossible to get anywhere. The flow of volitional or of intellectual activity is interrupted and reversed; movement in any direction is truncated and turned back. However a person starts out to decide or to think, he finds that he is getting in his own way.

The extent and the severity of ambivalence nowadays are probably due in some part to conditions especially characteristic of our time. But volitional disunity itself is, of course, nothing special and nothing new. St. Augustine observed that "it is . . . no strange phenomenon partly to will to do something and partly to will not to do it." Division of the will, he believed, is "a disease of the mind" from which we suffer in punishment for Original Sin.[12] At least in his view, then, ambivalence in one degree or another is inherent in the destiny of man.

5. If ambivalence is a disease of the will, the health of the will is to be unified and in this sense wholehearted. A person is volitionally robust when he is wholehearted in his higher-order attitudes and inclinations, in his preferences and decisions, and in other movements of his will. This unity entails no particular level of excitement or warmth. Wholeheartedness is not a measure of the firmness of a person's volitional state, or of his enthusiasm. What is at issue is the organization of the will, not its temperature.

As in the case of the unwilling addict, the unity of a healthy will is quite compatible with certain kinds of virulent psychic conflict. Wholeheartedness does not require that a person be altogether untroubled by inner opposition to his will. It just requires that, with respect to any such conflict, he himself be fully resolved. This means that he must be resolutely on the side of one of the forces struggling within him and not on the side of any other. Concerning the opposition of these forces, he has to know where he himself stands. In other words, he must know what he wants.

To the extent that a person is ambivalent, he does not really know what he wants. This ignorance or uncertainty differs from straightforwardly cognitive deficiency. There may be no information concerning his will that the ambivalent

person lacks. The problem is rather that since his mind is not made up, his will is in fact unformed. He is volitionally inchoate and indeterminate.

This is why ambivalence, like self-deception, is an enemy of truth. The ambivalent person does not hide from some truth or conceal it from himself; he does not prevent the truth from being known. Instead, his ambivalence stands in the way of there being a certain truth about him at all. He is inclined in one direction, and he is inclined in a contrary direction as well; and his attitude towards these inclinations is unsettled. Thus, it is true of him neither that he prefers one of his alternatives, nor that he prefers the other, nor that he likes them equally.

Since ambivalence is not a cognitive deficiency, it cannot be overcome merely by acquiring additional information. It also cannot be overcome voluntaristically. A person cannot make himself volitionally determinate, and thereby create a truth where there was none before, merely by an "act of will." In other words, he cannot make himself wholehearted just by a psychic movement that is fully under his immediate voluntary control.

The concept of reality is fundamentally the concept of something which is independent of our wishes and by which we are therefore constrained. Thus, reality cannot be under our absolute and unmediated volitional control. The existence and the character of what is real are necessarily indifferent to mere acts of our will.

Now this must hold as well for the reality of the will itself. A person's will is real only if its character is not absolutely up to him. It must be unresponsive to his sheer fiat. It cannot be unconditionally within his power to determine what his will is to be, as it is within the unconstrained power of an author of fiction to render determinate—in whatever way he likes—the volitional characteristics of the people in his stories.

Indeterminacy in the life of a real person cannot be overcome by preemptive decree. To be sure, a person may attempt to resolve his ambivalence by deciding to adhere unequivocally to one of his alternatives rather than to the other; and he may believe that in thus making up his mind he has eliminated the division in his will and become wholehearted. Whether such changes have actually occurred, however, is another matter. When the chips are down he may discover that he is not, after all, decisively moved by the preference or motive he supposed he had adopted. Remember Hotspur's reply when Owen Glendower boasted "I can call spirits from the vasty deep." He said: "Why, so can I, or so can any man; but will they come when you do call for them?"[13] The same goes for us. We do not control, by our voluntary command, the spirits within our own vasty deeps. We cannot have, simply for the asking, whatever will we want.

We are not fictitious characters, who have sovereign authors; nor are we gods, who can be authors of more than fiction. Therefore, we cannot be authors of ourselves. Reducing our own volitional indeterminacy, and becoming truly wholehearted, is not a matter of telling stories about our lives. Nor, unless we wish to be as foolish as Owen Glendower, can we propose to shape our wills by stipulating peremptorily at some moment that now we are no longer divided but have become solidly resolute. We can be only what nature and life make us, and that is not so readily up to us.

This may appear to conflict with the notion that our wills are ultimately free. But what is the freedom of the will? A natural and useful way of understanding it is that a person's will is free to the extent that he has whatever will he wants. Now if this means that his will is free only if it is under his entirely unmediated voluntaristic control, then a free will can have no genuine reality; for reality entails resistance to such control. Must we, then, regard our wills either as unfree or as unreal?

The dilemma can be avoided if we construe the freedom of someone's will as requiring not that he originate or control what he wills, but that he be wholehearted in it. If there is no division within a person's will, it follows that the will he has is the will he wants. His wholeheartedness means exactly that there is in him no endogenous desire to be volitionally different than he is. Although he may be unable to create in himself a will other than the one he has, his will is free at least in the sense that he himself does not oppose or impede it.

6. Being wholehearted is not always warranted. There are circumstances in which it is only reasonable, no matter how uncomfortable it may be, for a person to be drawn in several directions at once. But while accepting ambivalence may sometimes be helpful or wise, it is never desirable as such or for its own sake. And to remain persistently ambivalent, concerning issues of substantial importance in the conduct of life, is a significant disability. Moral and political theorists often emphasize how valuable it is for people to have extensive repertoires of worthwhile options from which they are free to choose. The actual value to people of possessing these options depends to a large extent, however, upon their capacities for wholeheartedness.

After all, what good is it for someone to be free to make significant choices if he does not know what he wants and if he is unable to overcome his ambivalence? What is the point of offering a beguiling variety of alternatives to people who can respond to them only with irresolute vacillation? For someone who is unlikely to have any stable preferences or goals, the benefits of freedom are, at the very least, severely diminished. The opportunity to act in accordance with his own inclinations is a doubtful asset for an individual whose will is so divided that he is moved both to decide for a certain alternative and to decide against it. Neither of the alternatives can satisfy him, since each entails frustration of the other. The fact that he is free to choose between them is likely only to make his anguish more poignant and more intense.

Unless a person is capable of a considerable degree of volitional unity, he cannot make coherent use of freedom. Those who care about freedom must therefore be concerned about more than the availability of attractive opportunities among which people can choose as they please. They must also concern themselves with whether people can come to know what they want to do with the freedom they enjoy. It may be, as St. Augustine supposed, that a thoroughly unified will comes only as a gift of God. Still, the extent to which people suffer from volitional indeterminacy is not entirely independent of the social, political, and cultural

conditions in which they live. Those conditions may either facilitate or impede the development of unambivalent attitudes, preferences, and goals.

7.   So far I have provided for wholeheartedness only a brief conceptual sketch, elaborated primarily in relation to an equally sketchy account of the notion of ambivalence. Now I will try to develop a more fully articulated understanding of what it is to be wholehearted, by construing it as tantamount to the enjoyment of a kind of self-satisfaction. In speaking of self-satisfaction, I do not mean to refer pejoratively to a state of narcissistic complacency or smugness. The state I have in mind—a state of satisfaction with the condition of the self—is utterly inoffensive and benign. Clarifying its structure will actually help not only to illuminate what is involved in being wholehearted. It will also help in coping with an alleged difficulty in hierarchical analyses of the self. And I believe that, in addition, it will enhance our understanding of a rather troublesome notion—the notion of identification—that is fundamental to any philosophy of mind and of action.

Consider a person who believes something wholeheartedly, who is wholehearted in some feeling or attitude, or who intends wholeheartedly to perform a certain action. In what does his wholeheartedness with respect to these psychic elements consist? It consists in his being fully satisfied that they, rather than others that inherently (i.e., non-contingently) conflict with them, should be among the causes and considerations that determine his cognitive, affective, attitudinal, and behavioral processes.

This is compatible with his also being wholehearted with respect to other psychic elements, which contingently (i.e., due to particular circumstances) conflict with these and which are more important to him. The fact that a person is satisfied with an intention, a feeling, or a belief does not entail that he is committed to acting on it. Being wholehearted with respect to one element is consistent with assigning a higher priority to another. Someone may be satisfied to have both elements play active roles in his psychic economy, though not roles that are equally urgent or compelling. The element that is less important to him is not necessarily alien, threatening him from outside the structure of his self. It may be as much a part of him as those other elements that are more important parts of him.[14]

Now what does it mean to say of a person that he is satisfied with his psychic condition, or with some element or aspect of it? It does not mean that he considers it the best condition available to him. Some people may be so demanding that they are never willing to settle for anything less than that. But as a rule, satisfaction is not conditioned by an uncompromising ambition to maximize. People often settle gladly for less than what they think it would be possible for them to get. From the fact that someone is satisfied with his condition, then, it does not follow that no alteration of it would be acceptable to him. It goes almost without saying, of course, that he would be satisfied with an improved condition. However, he might also be satisfied even with a condition inferior to the one he is in.

What satisfaction does entail is an absence of restlessness or resistance. A satisfied person might willingly accept a change in his condition, but he has no active interest in bringing about a change. Even if he recognizes that he could be better

off, the possibility does not engage his concern: being better off is simply not interesting or important to him. This is not because he believes that becoming better off would be too costly, or because it is too uncertain. It is just that, as a sheer matter of fact, he has no ambition for improvement; he accepts the state of things as it is, without reservation and without any practical interest in how it compares with other possibilities. Perhaps his condition could be improved at no net cost, and perhaps he is aware of this, but he simply does not care.[15]

To be satisfied with something does not require that a person have any particular belief about it, nor any particular feeling or attitude or intention. It does not require, for instance, that he regard it as satisfactory, or that he accede to it with approval, or that he intend to leave it as it stands. There is nothing that he needs to think, or to adopt, or to accept; it is not necessary for him to do anything at all. This is important, because it explains why there is no danger here of a problematic regress.

Suppose that being satisfied did require a person to have, as an essential constitutive condition of his satisfaction, some deliberate psychic element—some deliberate attitude or belief or feeling or intention. This element could not be one with which the person is at all dissatisfied. How could someone be wholehearted with respect to one psychic element by virtue of being halfhearted with respect to another? So if being satisfied required some element as a constituent, satisfaction with respect to one matter would depend upon satisfaction with respect to another; satisfaction with respect to the second would depend upon satisfaction with respect to still a third; and so on, endlessly. Satisfaction with one's self requires, then, no adoption of any cognitive, attitudinal, affective, or intentional stance. It does not require the performance of a particular act; and it also does not require any deliberate abstention. Satisfaction is a state of the entire psychic system—a state constituted just by the absence of any tendency or inclination to alter its condition.

Of course, a person may make the judgment that he is well enough off; and on that basis he may decide to refrain from doing anything to improve his situation. Making this judgment or this decision does not, however, either make him satisfied or entail that he is satisfied. His decision to refrain from trying to change things is, in effect, a decision on his part to act *as though* he is satisfied. Refraining from trying to change things *simulates* the equilibrium in which satisfaction consists. But to simulate satisfaction is not the same as being satisfied. A person is actually satisfied only when the equilibrium is not contrived or imposed but is integral to his psychic condition—that is, when that condition is settled and unreserved apart from any effort by him to make it so.

Being genuinely satisfied is not a matter, then, of choosing to leave things as they are or of making some judgment or decision concerning the desirability of change. It is a matter of simply *having no interest* in making changes. What it requires is that psychic elements of certain kinds *do not occur*. But while the absence of such elements does not require either deliberate action or deliberate restraint, their absence must nonetheless be reflective. In other words, the fact that the person is not moved to change things must derive from his understanding and evaluation of how things are with him. Thus, the essential non-occurrence is neither deliberately

contrived nor wantonly unselfconscious. It develops and prevails as an unmanaged consequence of the person's appreciation of his psychic condition.[16]

8. Let me try briefly to sketch how this bears on the hierarchical approach to analysis of the self and on the notion of identification. On hierarchical accounts, a person identifies with one rather than with another of his own desires by virtue of wanting to be moved to action by the first desire rather than by the second. For example, someone who is trying to quit smoking is identified with his first-order desire not to smoke, rather than with his concurrent first-order desire for another cigarette, if he wants the desire not to smoke to be the one that effectively guides his conduct. But what determines whether he identifies with this second-order preference?

Considered in itself, after all, his desire to defeat the desire to smoke is just another desire. How can it claim to be constitutive of what he really wants? The mere fact that it is a second-order desire surely gives it no particular authority. And it will not help to look for a third-order desire that serves to identify the person with this second-order preference. Obviously, the same question would arise concerning the authority of that desire; so we would have to find an even higher-order desire; and so on endlessly. The whole approach appears to be doomed.

Hierarchical accounts of the identity of the self do not presume, however, that a person's identification with some desire consists simply in the fact that he *has* a higher-order desire by which the first desire is endorsed. The endorsing higher-order desire must be, in addition, a desire with which the person is *satisfied*. And since (as I tried to explain earlier) satisfaction with one psychic element does not require satisfaction with any other, being satisfied with a certain desire does not entail an endless proliferation of higher orders and desires. Identification is constituted neatly by an endorsing higher-order desire with which the person is satisfied. It is possible, of course, for someone to be satisfied with his first-order desires without in any way considering whether to endorse them. In that case, he is identified with those first-order desires. But insofar as his desires are utterly unreflective, he is to that extent not genuinely a person at all. He is merely a wanton.

9. Is it possible to be satisfied with ambivalence? A person may certainly come to accept the fact that he is ambivalent as unalterable. It seems to me, however, that it is not a fact with which he can possibly be satisfied. No one can be wholeheartedly ambivalent, anymore than someone can desire unequivocally to betray himself or to be irrational. That someone accepts his ambivalence can mean only that he is resigned to it; it could not mean that it satisfies him. Perhaps conditions are imaginable in which a person might reasonably regard ambivalence as worthwhile in order to avoid some even more unsatisfactory alternative. But no one can desire to be ambivalent for its own sake.

It is a necessary truth about us, then, that we wholeheartedly desire to be wholehearted. This suggests a criterion for use in the design of ideals and programs of life, and generally in determining what to regard as important and to care about.

What we care about should be, to the greatest extent possible, something we are able to care about wholeheartedly. We do not wish to work against ourselves, or to have to hold ourselves back. There are many things to which we find ourselves attracted. In trying to decide which of them is to be important to us, we must anticipate the extent to which each can be coherently elaborated in our lives.

This may be quite different than the extent to which, considered in itself, it is worthy of being cared about. The fact that something is important to us does not primarily consist in our estimate of its own value. The question of what we are to care about is not settled by arriving at judgments as to the inherent or comparative merits of various possible objects of devotion. The fact that a person cares about or is devoted to something—an ideal, or another person, or a project—means that, whatever he may *think* about it, to one degree or another he *loves* it. The problem has to do most fundamentally, then with what we are capable of loving.

What about self-love? That a person is fully satisfied with himself means that he is wholehearted in his feelings, his intentions, and his thoughts. And insofar as being wholehearted is tantamount to loving, wholeheartedness with regard to such things is the same as self-love. Now someone who is engaged in self-deception, in a matter concerning what he is or what he is doing, is conceding thereby that he is not satisfied with himself. Like everyone else, of course, he would like to be wholehearted; as all of us do, he wants to love himself. Indeed, this is his motive for self-deception. It is his desire to love himself that leads him to replace an unsatisfying truth about himself, which he cannot wholeheartedly accept, with a belief that he can accept without ambivalence.

Of course, the effort is misguided. Psychic unity obviously cannot be achieved by dividing oneself. However, the self-deceiver is in fact attempting to escape from being ambivalent. He is trying to overcome the indeterminacy of his cognitive state. What he desires, in other words, is that there be an unequivocal truth concerning what he thinks. We might even say, if we are fond of paradox, that what moves him to deceive himself is the love of truth.

10. Unfortunately it is rare, as we know, for our desire to love ourselves to be fulfilled. We are not often satisfied with our conduct or with what we are. Our lives are marred, to one degree or another, by ambivalence. St. Augustine thought that a transition to psychic unity from a state of volitional division requires a miracle. So he prayed for conversion. That is not actually such a bad approach to the problem. In any case, it seems to have worked out well for him.

I have another suggestion, however, which he appears not to have considered. I will offer it by relating a conversation I had a few years ago with a woman who worked in an office near mine. She and I did not know each other very well, but one day our talk somehow became a bit more personal than usual. At a certain point in the conversation she told me that, in her opinion, in a serious relationship only two things are really important: honesty, and a sense of humor. Then she thought for a moment, and she said: "You know, I'm really not all that sure about honesty; after all, even if they tell you the truth, they change their minds so fast, you can't count on them anyhow."

Sometimes a person is so ambivalent, or vacillates so fluidly, that there is no stable fact concerning what he thinks or feels. In cases like that, when the only truth is too limited to be helpful, meticulous honesty may not be such an important virtue. No doubt the best thing would be for the person to settle down: give up trying to have things both ways, and find some coherent order in which he can be more or less wholehearted. But suppose you are simply unable to make up your mind. No matter how you twist or turn, you cannot find a way of being satisfied with yourself. My advice is that if your will is utterly divided, and volitional unity is really out of the question, be sure at least to hang on to your sense of humor.

Endnotes

1. A.E. Housman, *M. Manilii, Astronomicon I* (London, 1903), p. xliii.
2. *Lectures on Ethics*, p. 224.
3. "On a Supposed Right to Lie from Altruistic Motives".
4. "Of Giving the Lie".
5. "Of Liars".
6. "Women and Honor: Some Notes on Lying," in *On Lies, Secrets and Silence* (New York, 1979), p. 191.
7. *Ibid.*, p. 186.
8. *Metaphysics* I, 2: 982b12.
9. *Ibid.*, 982b20.
10. *Ethics*, 3P17S.
11. There are degrees of the sort of conflict I am considering. In discussing ambivalence, I am concerned with conflict sufficiently severe that a person: (a) cannot act decisively; or (b) finds that fulfilling either of his conflicting desires is substantially unsatisfying.
12. *Confessions* VIII, 9.
13. *Henry IV, Part 1*.
14. It is only to persons that wholeheartedness and ambivalence are attributable. For this reason, wholeheartedness is not exactly equivalent to the absence of ambivalence: the fact that there is no inherent conflict among the various elements of someone's psychic state does not quite entail that he is wholehearted with respect to them. To be a person, as distinct from simply a human organism, requires a complex volitional structure involving reflective self-evaluation. Human beings that lack this structure may be free of inherent volitional conflict, but they are not persons. Therefore, they are neither ambivalent nor wholehearted.
15. A satisfied person may become dissatisfied upon realizing that things might be better. The realization may cause his expectations to rise. This does not mean, of course, that he was dissatisfied before they rose.
16. Being or becoming satisfied is like being or becoming relaxed. Suppose that someone sees his troubles recede and consequently relaxes. No doubt it is by various feelings, beliefs, and attitudes that he is led to relax. But the occurrence of these psychic elements do not constitute being relaxed, nor are they necessary for relaxation. What is essential is only that the person stop worrying and feeling tense.

Part IV
Weakness and Strength of Will

[16]

Australasian Journal of Philosophy
Vol. 58, No. 94; December 1980

WHERE DOES THE AKRATIC BREAK TAKE PLACE?

Amelie Oksenberg Rorty

When Mohammed the Mullah first accepted the sage young Fatima as a private pupil to study the Koran, he did not forsee the dangers they would run, dangers to Koranic rules that both took to form their actions. Since Mohammed had studied abroad, his worldly experience should have led him to forsee that despite Fatima's modest decorum and his precautions in assuring a chaperone, their close study together was likely to put their strictly Koranic lives in peril. In him, such a failure of imaginative foresight may well have been akratic, the akratic beginning of a series of other akratic actions. After a time, he and Fatima began to perceive one another — flashing eyes and dark brows, the curve of the head bent over the sacred text — in ways that ill accorded with their commitments to the commandments. Their akrasia was then in their perceiving, their ways of focusing and attending to one another. After the surprise of their passion, they began to form intentions that violated their judgments. Their lapses were not simply lapses between intention and action, their elaborate assignations required nested conditional qualifications: 'If your uncle is at the mosque, we'll meet here; but if he is at home, I shall see you at the oasis by the well.' Their akrasia was then in the formation of their intentions. Yet sometimes, having formed prudent resolutions, they nevertheless impulsively decided to meet. Their akrasia then fell between resolution and decision, a decision that was still at least sometimes an act of thought requiring further planning to execute. Yet sometimes, their akrasia came between decision and action: having met, and decided against passion, they sometimes acted contrary to their decisions. There is more to their story: but for the time, we have ample material for philosophical investigation.

Let us suppost that in all these cases, Mohammed and Fatima acted as voluntarily as anyone does, that their actions were intentional, falling under descriptions that on some level they took to conflict with their judgments about the preferred course for them in that situation. Let us suppose these are cases of akrasia, if ever there are any.* What has gone wrong and where?

We can distinguish:

1. A person's general beliefs about appropriate human aims, what is commanded by God, or required by morality, or conduces to human well-being:
>   (a break here is akrasia of direction or aim)

2. A person's commitment to actualise or realise those aims, to instantiate them in his actions, to attempt to be guided by them:
>   (a break here is akrasia of interpretation)

---

* (My preference for retaining the greek term *akrasia* is not an arcane taste for the esoteric; it arises from my conviction that the other expressions for the phenomena — *weakness of will* and *moral weakness* — are, as we shall see, profoundly misleading.)

3. A person's interpretation of a particular situation:
    (a) his perceptual categorisations: the structuring of what is salient in a situation, at the centre of his focused attention
    (b) his verbal descriptions and characterisations of his situation
    (c) his beliefs about that situation
    (d) his emotional responses, as they affect and are affected by, his perceptions
                 (a break here is akrasia of irrationality)
4. A person's forming an intention to act:
    (a) a person's forming an *intention* to act, where the intention is conditional on the satisfaction of some antecedents in one isolated piece of practical reasoning directed by one end. 'If it is raining, we'll meet at the porch of the mosque.'
    (b) a person's forming a *resolution* to act, where the resolution is not detached from the comparative practical reasoning that has formed priorities. 'Despite all to be said against it, we must continue to meet.'
    (c) a person's *deciding* to act according to his resolution, where the *decision* is detached from the comparative practical reasoning in which it was imbedded and from it was derived. The decision is no longer treated as a conditional.
                 (a break here is akrasia of character)
5. A person's acting according to his decision. These 'stages on thought's way to action' can be regarded as supplementing Aristotle's schema of the practical syllogism: the person's most general evaluations represent the major premise; his interpretation of his particular situation represents the minor premise; his intentions and decisions represent his forming the conclusion of the argument and his action is the consequence of his having drawn the conclusion. These distinctions allow us to locate the junctures where psychological akrasia can occur, in ways that explain the occurrence of behavioural akrasia. When a person commits himself to a major premise that violates his general ends, he might be said to suffer from akrasia of direction or aim. When the minor premise is malformed, the person suffers from interpretive akrasia. Flaws of inference in drawing the appropriate intention or decision are forms of akrasia of irrationality; failure to act from one's decision is akrasia of character.

Traditional accounts of akrasia that concentrate exclusively on behaviour often cannot explain why and how the person succumbed to akrasia. While they diagnose the difficulty as a flaw of character leading to irrationality, they do not specify the aspect of character that has failed. By distinguishing the varieties of psychological akrasia, we can get a much more detailed explanation of behavioural akrasia: we can locate the distinctive psychological and intellectual sources of (specific types of character failures that issue in) behavioural akrasia. The place where the akratic break takes place also locates the place where the self-reforming akrates can best intervene to remedy his condition.

Of course an agent does not generally *first* form general evaluations, and *then* commit himself to them, and *then* apply his general principles to particular cases, and then form an intention, then a resolution and then decision, and then

proceed to act. Moreover, his actions need not be means to realising his ends; they can constitute or instantiate those ends. Nor need ends be purposes that are realised in actions: they can give the significance or the point of acting. The thought that forms the action can be, as Aristotle said, *in* the action. The thoughts that are sometimes the reasons for, sometimes the formulations of, and sometimes the causes of actions need not be at the centre of a person's awareness; and certainly they need not be the result of conscious deliberation.

Now, types and stages of akrasia.

1. The akratic break can appear between a person's general beliefs about what is good, divinely commanded, morally desirable — his general principles and ends — and his commitment to guide his actions by those evaluations. Traditionally this form of akrasia has been characterised as a debility of the will, and has been allied to sin or vice. Because this characterisation misleadingly reifies the will as a single faculty, it might be better to describe this form of akrasia as *deflected direction or aim.* Such akrasia can consist of a person *failing* to commit himself to follow what he judges best; or it can consist in his *refusing* to follow what he judges best.

In the first sort of case, a person can allow himself to succumb to lassitude, cynicism, weariness, depression.[1] What medievals called *accidie* or *melancholia,* is — at least for some sorts of agents — voluntary. Not only is it often a predictable result of more obviously behavioural actions, but it can also consist in a series of minute psychological activities: actions of interpretation and decision. The person who fails to commit himself to a policy of following the course that would realise his general values and principles need not be radically conflicted: as a result of actions he could have, and still can avoid, he treats himself as powerless to realise his ends. His conflicts result from, rather than explain his akratic powerlessness. Like other akratic conditons, *accidie* or *melancholia* can carry other akratic actions in their wake: having failed to commit or to engage oneself to ends one judges best, a person can — as did Goncharov's Oblomov — form further akratic intentions and decisions.

The second sort of case — *refusing* rather than failing to commit oneself to follow one's general views about what is best — is the rarest and perhaps only a notional kind of akrasia. Traditionally, it is classified as vice, but it is the kind of vice where the agent knows that his secondary ends conflict with what he takes to be best. A Dostoyevskian character, Goethe's Mephistopheles, can for a time, or at least in principle, decline to serve the ends he takes to represent the Human Good. ('Non serviam.' 'Let evil be my good.' 'I will be the imp of the perverse.') Because there is standardly a psychological as well as a conceptual connection between the structure of a person's motives and his primary principles and values, someone who consistently denies his general ends and values in favour of such other goods as freedom, or self-determination, or the contemplative life, will generally tend to elevate these other goods to the status of primary ends, often incommensurate with and sometimes opposed to other

---

[1] Cf. Michael Stocker, 'Desiring the Bad: An Essay in Moral Psychology', *The Journal of Philosophy* 76 (1979) pp 738-753.

human goods. Nevertheless, someone who believes that free self-determination is superior to (say) happiness can akratically commit himself to follow the course he thinks less noble or dignified, taking what he regards as the merely human, lesser course. (In Dostoyevsky's account, the Grand Inquisitor commits himself to·the course he thinks incompatible with what Christ represents as the Word of God; he chooses to follow what he takes to be the weaker good.)

Not every radically conflicted person is akratic, and not every kind of akrasia involves radical conflict. A person whose conflicts are unresolved, and certainly a person whose conflicts are unresolvable will violate at least one of his preferences: but such a person is akratic only when he stands behind, underwrites, avows one side of the conflict, reflexively taking himself to be identified with, and judged by his commitment to that side. To be capable of this sort of akrasia, an agent must, as Frankfurt and others have shown, be capable of evaluating his motives and actions, taking second-order attitudes towards his wanton self.[2] But second-order evaluations — stirrings that present themselves as conscience — can sometimes be regarded as remnants of poor social conditioning, and a person can sometimes reflectively favour first-order motives against second-order evaluations. When evaluative attitudes are themselves in radical conflict, the strongly voluntary agent can, as Charles Taylor has suggested, take reflexive attitudes that put a stop to the indefinite regress of reflective n^{th} order evaluative attitudes.[3] By underwriting one side, he takes a reflexive stance that not only evaluates his motives and reactions, but identifies him as a certain sort of agent, defined by his primary commitments. But it is not enough for reflexive identificatory attitudes to be formed in a Gide-like journalistic way ('Ah, how interesting, *this* is the kind of person I am, fundamentally!') As Alston has argued, for someone to qualify as capable of voluntary action, there is a presumption that such attitudes can modify the person's motivational structures.[4] Ironically, akrasia is among the diseases only the strong can suffer. Among the radically conflicted, only those capable of strongly identifying themselves with one side of their conflicts, and of acting from that identification can suffer from this sort of akrasia. As long as radically conflicted agents do not primarily underwrite or commit themselves to one side of their conflicts, they suffer vacillation, indecision, vertigo, but not this sort of akrasia.

When the radically conflicted agent underwrites one side of conflicting ends or principles, say self-determination rather than the happy political life, he need not make that commitment on rational grounds; nor, having made that radical choice or commitment, need he think that following it represents the most rational course. Certainly having underwritten his preference, he will have *a*

[2] Harry Frankfurt, 'Freedom of the Will and the Concept of a Person', *The Journal of Philosophy* 67 (1971) pp 5-20.

[3] Charles Taylor, 'Responsibility for the Self' in *The Identities of Persons*, University of California Press, (1976) pp 281-299.

[4] William Alston, 'Self-Intervention and the Structure of Motivation' in T. Mischel, *The Self*, (Blackwell, 1977) pp 65-102.

reason to act consistently with his commitment; but he need not suppose *that* reason to be identical with, or justifiable by what on other grounds he takes to be the summary conclusions of rational prudence. He need not even believe that the details of the actions that would follow from his primary commitment will promote his welfare, as measured by grounds he considers both morally and rationally prudent. Of course his commitment to the preferred course can be formulated *as* a general rule, and his acting inconsistently with that course is, just so far, nominally or minimally irrational. But by the agent's criteria of prudential rationality — his criteria of benefit — the akratic alternative need not be itself irrational: it can violate his conception of what is most important and *best*, without violating his conception of what is either morally or prudentially *beneficial*.

Akrasia originally appeared problematic within the context of theories of moral psychology according to which no one willingly follows a course he takes to be bad.[5] Because such theories not only identify the best with the most rational course, but also deny that there are radical conflicts between incommensurable human ends, akrasia was characterised as a species of irrationality, a lapse from a person's best reasoning about the best course. Davidson, among others, schooled us to see that akrasia is not necessarily a problem of moral psychology, that the best or most preferable course need not be thought morally the best.[6] We can also see that although it is inconsistent with the preferred alternative, the akratic course is not in itself necessarily prudentially irrational. To say that the akrates violates his preferred judgment about what is best, is ambiguous between saying that he deviates from his judgment, *however arrived*, about the preferred course, and saying that he deviates from a preferred course which he underwrites because it is the most rational course.

Mohammed and Fatima's commitment to follow the commands of the Koran, fall the skies where they may, need not be a commitment that they regard as either rationally grounded or rationally justifiable. Whether the details of Allah's commands can be reconciled with the dictates of rational practical reasoning, whether the Koran exists for the benefit of the Faithful, whether Paradise is the promise of those who succeed in living Koranically, are, they believe, beyond anyone's powers to judge. Not only is following the Koran a principle of necessity beyond reason, neither rational nor irrational in itself, but also the details of its commands are not subject to independent rational evaluation. Let us suppose the Koranic penalty for their infraction requires the most ignoble possible death for Fatima, while for Mohammed it decrees decapitation followed by whatever consequence Allah sees fit. And let us suppose that Mohammed and Fatima live in the heart of brightest Saudi Arabia, in a wealthy but miserable village where they are the only learned, indeed the

---

[5] The Socratic formulation is to be found in the Protagoras 352A-358D; the Platonic account is advanced in *The Republic*, 439A-441C. While Aristotle modifies the Platonic account, he accepts at least part of the motivational theory. Cf. Book VII of the *Nicomachean Ethics*

[6] Donald Davidson, 'How is Weakness of the Will Possible?' in Joel Feinberg, *Moral Concepts* (Oxford University Press, 1970) pp 93-113.

only literate sages. If they accept their Koranic punishment, they endanger their brothers in Islam: there will be no one to read, let alone interpret the Law. Let us suppose the Koran is silent on the priority of the punishment for their infraction, and their implicit duties to their Islamic community. They are strict constructionists; where the Koran is silent, there is no presumption of legitimacy. Fatima must die, Mohammed must be decapitated. Having studied at Harvard and MIT, Mohammed sees that rational morality and rational prudence coincide ... but on the side he considers the akratic alternative. Although he has accepted the views of rationality he learned abroad, he considers his commitment to the Koran to have over-riding force: counter-rational though it may be, following the Koran outweighs all rational considerations of moral benefit and utilitarian prudence. Akratically, Mohammed persuades Fatima that they must not accept the punishments allotted them by the Koran. Of course, having acted inconsistently with their primary commitment, they have behaved irrationally. But both regard their akratic action as the prudentially and morally rational, yet lesser course.

2. The akratic break can take place between a person's general principles and commitment on the one hand, and his interpretation of the situation in which he finds himself on the other. This interpretive form of akrasia is, as Aristotle and some Stoics suggested, a flaw of the imagination; a person comes to see or interpret his situation and condition in a light that does not conform to his commitment to general ends or principles. His perceptions and interpretations are formed by inappropriate *fantasia*. Interpretive akrasia can take place at a number of points:

(2a) A person's *perception* of a situation can fail to accord with his summary judgments: someone who has repudiated racism might see Caucasians as crude or Orientals as sly: someone who has repudiated age-ism might see the lines of the faces of the elderly as deformations, their motions as disabled. Of course many aspects of perception are not voluntary: there are more constraints on what one sees than there are on how one can move one's body. But at least some aspects of perceptual interpretation are voluntary: and they can conflict with a person's judgment about what is best. As one can voluntarily shift one's focus on gestalt sketches, seeing now a vase, now two women, so one can see the lines on the face of an elderly person as deformations or as marks of stoic and humourous endurance. But there are more obviously voluntary aspects of perception: Mohammed and Fatima might akratically attend to one another's sexually arousing features, instead of concentrating on one another's more scholarly contributions. For some people, at least some aspects of seeing involve *looking for:* when scanning the visual field is a way of answering questions, it is possible to ask different questions; doing so allows quite different aspects of the perceptual field to emerge. One sees differently. Someone might akratically scan a landscape looking for its defensible strongholds or its potential mineral wealth, instead of looking at it — as he believes he should — for its fertility or aesthetic composition. Or someone might scan a social gathering of friends, akratically looking for occasions for advancement or the exercise of power. *Scanning, looking for, focusing* are activities in which we have (at least in part) been

schooled. To be formed by a culture or a milieu is to acquire just such habits: patterns of salience, implicit questions that direct attention. Of course patterns of perception also standardly express a person's general evaluations: it is because the two standardly go hand in hand that the person of practical wisdom can straightway act from what he sees without elaborate calculation or deduction. Because his values form or are expressed in his habitual perceptual patterning, he can act directly from his interpretations. But sometimes, a person can revise his general evaluations — the phenomena of moral and religious conversion are examples of such revisions — without straightway revising his perceptual habits. Someone who can become aware of the selective patterns of his perceptions, the ways in which his preoccupations form his interpretations is then sometimes in a position to modify those patterns to accord with his revised evaluations: he can avoid the interpretive akrasia he would suffer from the discord between his perceptions and his values or principles.

(2b) One of the ways it is possible for a person to bring his perceptions into accord with his preferred judgments is to redescribe what he sees. Verbal interpretations are, at least for some, far more voluntary than perceptual ones. For that very reason, interpretive akrasia is much more frequently verbal than perceptual. A person's descriptions of his situation can fail to accord with his evaluations and commitments. He can categorise situations in ways that form expectations which will predictably lead him to act contrary to his judgment. The verbal connotations carried by etymology, by literary and private associations, by contextual expectations naturally carry presumptive evaluations which influence action. Often in speech, more often in writing, the choice, shading and informal implications of descriptive expressions can violate a person's preferred judgment. Someone who is committed to nonsexist attitudes can describe the behaviour of men and women differentially in ways that prevents his really hearing what women say, in the same ways he would hear those words spoken by a man. What he calls self-respecting behaviour in a man, he calls manipulative or demanding in a woman. These differences can lead to different responses and actions: the man requires and deserves respect and co-operation; the woman is to be suspected and resisted. This is one of the reasons that political reformers stress revising and changing the vocabulary of the old regime: banning references to niggers, broads and old geezers can sometimes be a way of attacking more overt behavioural akrasia that sometimes originates in akrasia of description. The hope is of course, that it will not only modify the behaviour of the akrates . . . but, by modifying the behaviour, also change the beliefs of those who had been non-akratically discriminatory.

(2c) A person can akratically come to believe something against his better judgment. We do not choose to come to conclusions, and we cannot directly will to believe; but we can sometimes put ourselves in situations where, predictably, we will form specific beliefs because we have used judgments in inferences that we took to be merely provisional. While we cannot directly control the formation of our expectations, we can avoid *using* judgments that we regard as unsound, in inferences 'just for the sake of the argument', when we can predict that we are likely to detach the conclusions of such hypothetical arguments,

acquiring working beliefs that conflict with our better judgment.[7] Someone who akratically behaves rudely to Swedes may do so because he continues to use a 'belief' he regards as suspect, voluntarily licensing jokes, snide remarks and the like, in ways that will predictably affect his perceptions and actions. Or someone can akratically cut off inquiry or investigation, knowing that if he pressed on he would revise his beliefs. Or a person can direct experiments — experiments of all kinds, not only laboratory experiments but thought experiments — selecting, describing them and conducting them in ways that will predictably reinforce questionable beliefs, quite voluntarily avoiding investigations that might jeopardise such beliefs. Often akrasia works as a strategy towards self-deception: a person can be his own home sophist.

Akrasia of belief can be quite extended: it can involve sets of narratives or scenarios that form a person's expectations and strategies of explanations. So, for instance, a person can continue to make decisions by means that he does not underwrite, allowing daydreams to have more weight than he thinks they should. Or he can engage in elaborate patterns of praise and blame, exuses and expectations that do not reflect his judgments about what is praiseworthy and blameworthy. Such akrasia of belief is not limited to individuals in private life: a scientific community or a governmental and bureaucratic elite can be akratic in this way, forming judgments by procedures and habits that they do not underwrite, and that they could modify. Akrasia of belief and self-deception often go hand in hand.

Of course these cases most commonly involve conflict or hypocrisy rather than akrasia of belief. As things stand, only a relatively select part of the population is capable of the sort of self-conscious reflection that can gauge a belief to be provisional; few are capable of predicting the ways that beliefs can be secured or revised, even fewer are capable of setting about deliberately attempting to revise dispositional beliefs that no longer command assent.

(2d) A person's emotional reactions can fail to accord with his judgments about what is appropriate to a particular situation, and with his preferred judgment. He might fear someone he does not consider dangerous or hostile, knowing that if he concentrated on, or described the person in a different way, he would cease being afraid. Or he might be vengeful or envious in circumstances he thought did not warrant those reactions, when redescribing the situation could modify his responses. Because emotions are rarely under direct voluntary control, akrasia of the emotions generally follows akrasia of interpretation or akrasia of description; sometimes it follows behavioural akrasia.

It might seem improper to treat an emotional *state* as akratic: after all, emotions are generally not obviously actions or activities. Yet sometimes being in what is called an emotional state just *is* — consists in — a nexus of minute activities of interpreting, reacting in specific ways, following certain characteristic trains of thought.[8] Even when an emotion is a relatively simple

[7] Daniel Dennett, 'How to Change your Mind', *Brainstorms* (Bradford Books, 1978) pp 300-309.
[8] Cf. Leila Tov-Ruach, 'Jealousy, Attention and Loss' in A. O. Rorty, *Explaining Emotions*, (University of California Press 1980) pp 463-486.

state, the agent can be in that state as a result of voluntary actions. When the whole sequence — the action and its predictable outcome — is akratic, we can elliptically speak of the outcome — the emotional state and the actions that partially constitute being in that state — as akratic, just as, under similar conditions, we speak of someone's being drunk as akratic and consider the actions he involuntarily performs as a result of that condition as actions for which he can be held responsible when he is the sort of person who could have avoided being in that state.

That some emotions are in some circumstances voluntary does not, of course, mean that they all are, or could be. In any case, it is not an emotion type as such — vanity and disdain, or pride and hate — that is voluntary or involuntary, but a particular emotion in a particular context for a particular person. A person who is not able to evaluate or redirect his emotional reactions can suffer conflict or hypocrisy but not emotional akrasia. Nevertheless, because various types of emotions are normally typically voluntary or involuntary in standard situations, we can elliptically distinguish involuntary fears from, for instance, voluntary contempt.

Although the varieties of interpretive akrasia (perceptual, descriptive, belief, emotional) are analytically distinguishable, and although a person can be susceptible to one without being susceptible to others, they are often strongly interactive. In the 'The Idea of Perfection', Iris Murdoch describes how a person can come to change her akratic attitudes towards a daughter-in-law whose brash vulgarity irritates her by coming to think of the young woman as spontaneous rather than brash, unaffected rather than vulgar. The mother-in-law attempts to diagnose the juncture where she can most effectively intervene in the interactive psychological activities that have akratically composed and formed her attitudes. It is because we tend to bring our interpretive attitudes into consistent alignment, that we have some leeway in changing those that are less voluntary by changing those that are more voluntary. But people differ in the juncture at which such changes have optimal efficacy. These differences give us one way of distingushing types of agents by distinguishing the ways that different psychological activities function in the formation or determination of their behavioural actions.

3. The akratic break can also take place between a person's evaluation, his commitments and his interpretive stance on the one hand, and his forming a particular intention or decision to act on the other. Akrasia of irrationality involves drawing an inappropriate conclusion from a practical syllogism.

(3a) A person forms an *intention* when he proposes to take an action that, under specified conditions, is required by some end to which he is committed. The akratic break take place when the person draws a conclusion inappropriate to the premises of an *isolated* piece of practical reasoning, performedwithout comparing ends. Fatima says, 'I want to be a good physician, I want the best medical training possible. The University that has the strongest department has accepted me with a generous fellowship for next year. So I think I shall stay here and study the Koran with Mohammed.' Of course as it stands, the irrationality and irrelevance of the conclusion is so extreme that we can hardly recognise the

patterns of thought as an inference, a piece of practical reasoning. Without further embedding the iceberg tip of this practical thought, we can't identify the problem: it is not clear whether it is an enthymeme, with the crucial ruling premises suppressed; or whether the intention has been akratically formed. The oddity of the inference reveals what is often hidden and unnoticed in most philosophical discussions of practical reasoning. The considerations that are represented as an agent's practical reasoning are, even when intelligibly and validly formulated, the merest surface of a ramified structure of thought, patterns of interpretation, motives — the vast array of psychological functions required to explain the significance, the justification and the motivational power of the agent's reasoning. The practical syllogism is an elliptically formulated reconstruction of the agent's ends, perceptions — indeed his character structure.[9] When there is nothing deviant in the way that an agent formulates his intentions, we suppose that the last piece of his practical reasoning represents the whole. We implicitly supply the rest of the missing structure: introducing the standard motives and ends that are characteristic of normal voluntary agents, in those sorts of situations. When things go awry, we are at a loss because we cannot attribute the psychological structures that are standardly formative in identifying and determining that sort of action. The behavioural action is then not explicable by the psychological history that is its characteristic ground and rationale. In extreme cases, we may be unable to identify the action.

(3b) More commonly, the akratic break occurs in the formation of a *resolution* that expresses a comparative summary of the various considerations relevant to the action. The formation of an intention arises from one line of practical reasoning; the resolution is a summary of weighted comparisons. When, as is often the case, many of the considerations are incommensurable, the person forms a resolution by assigning priorities, by standing behind one set of considerations, underwriting them. But having constructed an elaborate piece of comparative practical reasoning, a person might form a summary resolution that is irrelevant or inappropriate to his reasoning, even though it is still attached to the premises that provide the conditions for acting.

(3c) The akratic break can come in detaching a decision from the practical reasoning in which it is embedded and which provides its grounds; when it is so detached, the decision is no longer treated as conditional. A person's practical reasoning can lead him to form a summary resolution that reflects his evaluation and commitments; but he can then detach an inappropriate decision. Charitable interpreters tend to suppose that the inappropriate decision is detached from (other) practical reasoning that does support it, or that the person made an involuntary error in computation. But sometimes a longer and more detailed investigation makes the charitable interpretation inplausible: it seems the person has been voluntarily irrational.

One of the reasons that akrasia of irrationality is difficult to attribute is that there are two criteria for identifying an intention or a decision. On the one

---

[9] Cf. David Wiggins, 'Weakness of Will, Commensurability, and the Objects of Deliberation and Desire' *Proceedings of the Aristotelian Society*, 79 (1978-79) pp 251-277.

hand, a decision is identified by the behavioural action which it typically initiates. When after a long time of squatting on his haunches waiting by the well for Fatima, Mohammed stretches his legs, he can be presumed to be doing so for a familiar set of psychological antecedents — perceived discomfort, beliefs and habits. His decision to stretch is generally implicit in his action. But sometimes the decision is more properly specified by the agent's practical reasoning than by the action which typically follows from it. In 'stretching' his legs, Mohammed may be really signalling Fatima that her uncle's jealous eyes are upon her. To be sure, these two criteria for identifying decisions — the agent's practical reasoning and the behavioural action typical of such reasoning — normally coincide. It is a good thing, and no accident that they do: that is how we are generally able to distinguish friends from enemies, and to undertake cooperative actions, by reading off a person's psychological dispositions from what he does. But the two criteria can diverge: and when they do, it is difficult to substantiate an attribution of akrasia, because we can't tell whether there has been an akratic break, or whether the person's action is supported by atypical practical reasoning. One of the reasons that isolated cases of akrasia are difficult to identify is that one does not know how they connect with the agent's *extended* practical reasoning, the practical reasoning that locates the action and its immediate antecedents within the larger contexts of his ends and habits, his character.

There is more akrasia of irrationality than meets the eye or ear. Even when the agent's decision or intention conforms with his preferred judgments, with his ends and commitments, he may in fact have formed his decision through a deviant chain. Although his decisions and resolutions coincide with his preferred judgments, they do so accidentally, having been formed by a series of considerations that violate his preferred judgment, the position that he underwrites.

An action can be akratic under one description but not under another. When an action is described as issuing from interpretations and decisions that are themselves akratic, it need not be nominally akratic in relation to the last bit of reasoning. The action may nevertheless be a case of submerged akrasia, if it violates the agent's primary commitments, and the preferred judgments and interpretations that he underwrites. The extent of akrasia of irrationality is often masked not only by the difficulties of opacity that are to be expected in intentional contexts, but also by self-deception.

4. For good reasons, akrasia of character that occurs between a person's decision and his behavioural actions has received the closest philosophical attention. The paradigm cases of akrasia have been taken to be those where a person has decided one way about food, sex, going to the movies — and then the hand, the body goes another way.

Because a person's character includes his interpretive and inferential habits, the varieties of psychological akrasia can be subsumed under akrasia of character, largely defined. A person's patterns of thought not only reveal and express, but also constitute part of his character. His character *is,* among other things, how he thinks, and vice versa. While cases of akrasia can be described as

character flaws that issue in inconsistency and thus in minimal irrationality, describing akrasia in that way does not explain how or why someone who is capable of voluntary action, nevertheless in this instance failed to take the course he preferred. The generality of this characterisation prevents our understanding of what has happened.

Akrasia of character arises from and is the expression of conflicts among the person's psychological and intellectual traits. Some of these — those that are represented in akrasia of direction and aim — are conflicts between basic ends. But the conflicts expressed in akrasia need not be radical conflicts: what is more interesting, they need not even be conflicts among evaluations and motives. They can involve conflicts among voluntary habits — habits of thought, perception, inference as well as behavioural habits. To be sure, sometimes conflicting habits reveal or represent conflicting ends. But not all habits are acquired because, or in the service of the agent's own ends. Some voluntary habits of thought and behaviour are acquired quite accidentally. In evaluating the ends that may sometimes be implicit in them, an agent need not make a radical choice between his ends. For instance, the bon vivant who acquired miserly puritanical habits at his parents' knees, but who successfully repudiated the principles behind his puritanical upbringing as soon as he was old enough to understand them, might now and again akratically forgo a present pleasure — buying a basket of fresh strawberries, or taking a pointless saunter by the river — in favour of a stern distant alternative he considers inappropriate. It is also revealing that the akratic alternative need not be the second best alternative: it is often a dark horse among the range of the agent's considered preferences. When Fatima's uncle prevented her meeting Mohammed, her sorrow and frustration led to bizarre akratic actions: against her better judgment, she drove her camel through a red light. But breaking the traffic laws of Saudi Arabia was by no means the thing that, next to seeing Mohammed, she most wanted to do.

The attractions of the akratic alternative are often not those they wear on their face, not evident in the intentional description of the action. The course represented by the akratic alternative sometimes has the attractions of presenting a conflicted person with an action outcome. The attractions lie not so much in *what* is done, as in the case of doing that sort of thing, for that sort of agent when he is conflicted. Far from being pathological, the various strategies and habits that pull towards the akratic alternative are standard psychological functions and activities that operate even in the most rationally considered actions.[10] Because such strategies do not require any particular motive to be brought into play, because they are habits of thought and behaviour that can operate independently of the agent's current motives, they can alleviate the condition of a conflicted agent who has no taste for conflict, and no approved means for resolving it.

Where, if anywhere, are we after running this maze of distinctions? And what is the view like from there?

---

[10] Cf. my 'Akrasia and Conflict', forthcoming in *Inquiry*, 1980; in that paper I discuss the attractions of several strategies that pull an agent towards the akratic side.

Distinguishing the varieties of akrasia enables us to distinguish the layers of psychological activities that can conflict. Disentangling the strands in the intentional components and determinations of action enables us to supplement the standard story of how beliefs and desires determine actions in ways that, according to some accounts, can be overcome by acts of rational will. The class of intentional activities that are classified together under the rubric of beliefs do not of course form a strongly homogenous class: some of them are not even propositional in form. Nor do the motivational dispositions generally classified together as desires form a homogenous class: the wishes, emotions, moral or religious commitments, wants, needs, fantasies of different types of agents enter into the formation of their actions in functionally distinguishable ways.[11]

The advantages of distinguishing varieties of akrasia by distinguishing the locations of the akratic break do not stop with providing a sharper, more precise and acute diagnosis of the character flaws of our friends. One of the conditions for akrasia is that the agent be capable of recognising that he has violated his preferences. Of course that recognition, and as Aristotle says, the regret that characteristically accompanies it, need not be made at every time and every level. Even if the akrates suffers the additional (usually unforgivable) akrasia of giving a fraudulent justification of his akratic action, he must in principle be capable of seeing that what he has done is akratic. If he were incapable of recognising that his action violates his preferred judgment, then he would not be the sort of person for whom that action is properly voluntary. This condition is a *reflexive* one. Not only does the akratic agent have preferences, but he must also be capable of recognising them *as his* preferences. If the akratic action is voluntary, the agent must be capable of avoiding it, not just accidentally avoiding it, but avoiding it because he takes it to be a violation of his preference. Someone capable of akrasia of a particular kind is capable of voluntary action in *that* domain: this means that he is in principle the sort of person who could have done otherwise. The conditions for akrasia assure the conditions for the self-reformation of akrasia; the precise location of his akrasia locates the place where intervention is optimally appropriate.

On Aristotle's account it is the agent's capacity for effectively regretting what he has done that explains why the akrates is more likely to reform than the vicious person. But while that regretful recognition may be necessary, it is not sufficient for such self-reforms. And it is just here that our distinctions between the varieties of psychological activities that enter into behavioural akrasia can help the self-reforming akrates. The usual admonitions to exercise rational will are singularly unhelpful. Like the terms *desire* and *belief, will* and even more so, *rational will,* cover a wide array of quite different activities, carried out in quite different psychological domains and in quite different ways, by different types of agents. For some, the 'reforming will' consists largely of the exercises of redescription; for others, it consists largely in more persistent and careful wary attention to inferential procedures, not cutting them short, avoiding hasty detachment of marginally relevant conclusions. For some, it consists in

---

[11] Cf. my forthcoming paper, 'Telic Desires, Psychogenic Desires and Just Hanging In There.'

acquiring new habits of attentive focusing; for others it consists in avoiding situations where certain sorts of action-guiding emotions can predictably be aroused. It is just here that the distinctions between types of akrasia that can help the self-reformer. The particular juncture where the akratic break has taken place — the location of person's characteristic psychological akrasia — reveals the optimal leverage for change. Akrasia can take place only where there is voluntary action: locate the precise point of akrasia, and you have located at least one place where there is scope for alternative action.

Livingston College, Rutgers University   Received June 1980

[12] This paper was delivered as an invited address at the December, 1979 meetings of the APA. I am greatly indebted to the commentator, Georges Rey, for extremely valuable suggestions. I also benefitted from discussions with Robin Jackson, Mark Johnston, Graeme Marshall, Michael Stocker and Genevieve Lloyd.

[17]

Weakness of Will and Practical Judgment

ROBERT AUDI

UNIVERSITY OF NEBRASKA, LINCOLN

Weakness of will is a common phenomenon of human experience. But what is it? It has proved highly resistant to analysis,
and even the accounts that seem to capture our intuitions
about what weakness of will is raise problems about how it is
possible. This is because these accounts seem inconsistent with
some highly plausible principles about action. My aim here is
to propose a new account of weakness of will and its relation to
practical judgment, and to explain how weakness of will so
conceived is possible.

I

Let us start with some examples. Imagine a person reading in
a lounge chair under a maple tree on a fine spring afternoon.
He has planned to write some letters after reading for an
hour. He considered putting them off another day, but
judged that it would be best not to delay. As the end of the
hour approaches, he feels a certain discomfort and quickens
the pace of his reading. When the end of the hour comes, he
thinks momentarily of the letters; he is enjoying his reading
and again considers putting them off, but he again realizes
that he should not do so. He leans forward to get up, but
pauses as he feels the inertia of his comfortable position. He
looks at the book still open in his hands; his eyes fall on the
paragraph he left; and he settles back to his reading without
ever laying down the book. When he gets up for dinner, he
feels guilty about failing to write the letters and resolves to do
them tomorrow. Now consider a different case. A teacher is
grading papers. He comes to one which seems to deserve
about a C-plus or a B-minus. Conscious of grade inflation, he
reviews it. After looking back through it he judges that he
should give it a C-plus, but as he turns to the last page it occurs

NOÛS 13 (1979)   173

to him that he has been giving a lot of C's. The prospect of the students' soon evaluating him also crosses his mind. When he reaches the last page he recalls that it is after all a close case and writes a B-minus with a long dark minus sign. Feeling a little cowardly, he hurries to the next paper.

In both cases the action exhibiting weakness of will is also against the agent's better judgment. What is the relation between actions exhibiting weakness of will and actions against one's better judgment? It is plausible to hold, as some philosophers have, that these are equivalent.[1] In asking whether they in fact are equivalent, I shall suppose that

(1) An agent, S, acts against his better judgment in doing A at t if and only if, at t, (i) S does A intentionally or knowingly, (ii) there is another action, A' (possibly just abstaining from doing A), such that S has judged, or makes or holds the judgment, that it would be better to do A', (iii) S has not abandoned this judgment, and (iv) S is aware of (ii) and (iii).

Three points should be made immediately. First, S's being aware of (ii) and (iii) requires (at least) that he know them and not have temporarily forgotten them, but it does not require that he be entertaining them. Second, we must take (ii) broadly: S's judging that it would be better to do A' must encompass both unconditional judgments, e.g. that he ought to do, or that it would be best to do, A', and relativized judgments, e.g. that A' is the thing to do, all things considered, or that A' is preferable to A, given the available information. Clauses (ii) and (iii) are meant to express the idea that S's current practical judgment *favors* A' over A, and (ii) imposes no restrictions on the form or basis of the judgment. The judgment may arise from moral, prudential or other considerations, or from a combination of kinds of considerations. Third, (iii) requires not that S *never* have abandoned the judgment, but only that if he has, he holds it again at t. We could require simply that S *judge* at t that it would be better to do A', but that would blur the distinction between making and holding a judgment. It is easily read as requiring that acting against one's better judgment at t requires making a judgment at t. But as our examples show, all that is required is holding, and being aware that one holds, the judgment, which may have been made earlier. This is not to say that nothing need

occur in S's consciousness at the time he acts against his better judgment; the point is that whatever must occur does not entail S's making, at t, the judgment against which he acts.

How shall we characterize actions exhibiting weakness of will? Following Davidson, I shall call these incontinent actions for short, though 'incontinent' suggests that the agent is dominated by passion, which need not be so with weakness of will. For the time being, let us suppose that incontinent actions (i.e., actions exhibiting weakness of will) are definable as Davidson initially characterizes them:

(2) S does A incontinently at t if and only if, at t, (i) S does A intentionally, (ii) S believes that there is an alternative A' open to him, and (iii) S judges that, all things considered, it would be better to do A' than to do A. ([4]: 94. Davidson's variables have been altered to correspond to mine.)

If incontinent actions and actions against one's better judgment are construed as in (1) and (2), then whether they are equivalent depends in part on at least two questions: whether (1) and (2) presuppose different degrees of conceptual sophistication, and how 'judging' is to be understood in (2). Let us take these in turn.

It initially appears that (1) presupposes more conceptual sophistication on the part of S than (2), since (1) requires S to have concepts of judging, making a judgment, etc., whereas (2) seems to require nothing comparable. But how much conceptual sophistication is needed to believe that there is an alternative *open* to one, and to judge that, all things considered, it would be better to do A' than A? If this judgment requires a conception of *relevant* considerations, it is arguable that (2) presupposes at least as much conceptual sophistication as (1). It is typically very difficult to determine how much conceptual sophistication is required for understanding a notion, but fortunately we need not decide whether (1) and (2) differ on this count. Even if they do, it is important to know whether, *for* normal adults, who can instantiate both, acting incontinently is equivalent to acting against one's better judgment. (I doubt whether very small children just learning to speak can instantiate either (1) or (2), but that seems perfectly appropriate.) This brings us to the question of how 'judging' is to be taken in (2).

It will help to start with a minimal interpretation of (2): Suppose S's judging that p to be equivalent to his holding it and suppose this to be equivalent to his believing it. Incontinent actions would not then be equivalent to actions against one's better judgment. Imagine that S judges, in the minimal sense that he simply believes, that it would be better not to eat any caviar at the party. Suppose that he then intentionally but very unselfconsciously eats some offered him on a platter, and that because he is absorbed in conversation, he does so without *at the time* judging that it would be better not to, or even being actively aware that he holds this, as he would be if it occurred to him that he is committed to refusing such things. He would be acting incontinently according to (2) read with 'judge' equivalent to 'believe'; but he would not satisfy (1), since he has never actually judged that it would be better not to eat any caviar. One might conclude that (1) should not require, at least in cases like this, that S be aware of having judged that it would be better to do A' than A. But however we analyze 'judging', we need such a requirement to distinguish acting *against* one's better judgment from merely acting *inconsistently* with it. S may act inconsistently with a judgment or belief, even in acting unintentionally. By contrast, acting against one's better judgment, like acting against persons, policies, and at least many other sorts of things, requires some kind of awareness of what one is acting against. The awareness requirement in (1) also enables us to distinguish acting against one's better *judgment* from acting, even intentionally, merely against a *standing belief* about what one ought to do. The caviar example would illustrate the latter if we imagine that though S never judges that it would be better not to eat any caviar, he is appropriately aware, as he eats it, that he believes it would be better not to. S would be strongly disposed to make the corresponding judgment, and this makes the case look like incontinence. But note that he might still be such that if he were to make this judgment, he would act in accordance with it. Moreover, his standing evaluative belief remains merely that; hence it is at no time *affirmed* in S's judgment. The will is given no *directive*, one wants to say. We have *imprudence*, not incontinence. Neither entails the other, though they often coincide.

In order to preserve these distinctions and to maintain the intuitive idea that acting incontinently entails acting against one's better judgment, we should construe 'judging' in (2) as in (1), so that judging cannot be merely believing; and we

should give judging the same role in (2) as in (1), substituting (ii)-(iv) of (1) for (iii) of (2). Incontinent action will then require *making* or having made a judgment, e.g. by sincerely affirming, silently or orally, that one ought to do A' rather than A, or by concluding this through practical reasoning. If judging is so construed and given the same role in (2) as in (1), it may again appear that incontinent actions are simply actions against one's better judgment. It might be objected that an incontinent action need not be against S's better judgment, because it may be merely against S's *judgment of the moment*, yet accord with S's "better" judgment: one he previously adopted on reflecting about the situation. S might cooly judge that he ought to stay with his shrewish wife, then, in anger, judge instead that he should leave her. He might now act incontinently in failing to do so, yet thereby act in accord with his previously adopted, better judgment. I agree that the act is incontinent, but it would also be against one's better judgment in what seems the standard sense and is in any case the sense that concerns me: acting against a present (overall) judgment of what it would be better to do. That S would be acting consistently with a previous judgment better than his present one shows at most *vacillation of intellect*, not action against his better judgment or incontinence. Similarly, suppose that at t S *decides* to do A at t', e.g. speak out against a rival, yet does not do it when he knows t' has come. Couldn't this be incontinent even if S has never judged that he should do A? To say so would conflate weakness of will with *irresolution*. The conflation is natural because the latter is typical of people who often exhibit the former. But irresolution, though consistent with incontinence, does not entail it. Since it is important to avoid conflating vacillation of intellect and irresolution with incontinence, let me suggest some reasons why neither example shows that incontinence does not entail acting against one's better judgment in the sense of (1).

In the first example, S has changed his mind, apparently unwisely. But if we conclude that because the change was unwise he did not act against his better judgment when he acted against his present overall judgment, what will be our standard for the occurrence of weakness of will? Why say S exhibited it if he acted in accord with his better judgment? On the view I am imagining, the reply would be that acting against one's better judgment is something like acting against what one takes to be a more *reasonable* judgment one has made on

the relevant alternatives, and incontinence *does* entail acting
against one's better judgment in this sense. But then whether
S exhibits weakness of *will* must often depend on his resolution of such *intellectual* questions as which of his judgments
about a situation is more reasonable. Yet surely whether the
will is weak does not depend on the intellect's discernment, or
on whether it vacillates. In our second example, though *S* fails
to carry out his decision, he might be such that if he *had* judged
he should speak out, he would have. And even if this were not
so, we surely want to distinguish between a mere change in *S*'s
will and his exhibiting weakness of will. If he had judged at *t'*
that he should now speak out and failed to, this would (typically) be a case of both irresolution and incontinence. But
when he at no time makes this judgment, his not speaking out
could stem from a perfectly reasonable change of will based
on, say, a natural, usually justified disposition to avoid attacking people. We should not, then, infer weakness of will from
mere irresolution, any more than from vacillation of intellect.
For reasons I shall introduce in Section II, whether one's will is
weak at a given time should be determined in relation to the
practical judgments one holds at that time. It does not depend
on which of one's judgments about a given option is better,
nor does it ever depend simply on what decisions one has
made (and not abandoned) prior to the time in question.

So far, then, we have seen no decisive objection to construing incontinent action (at least for normal adults) as action
against one's better judgment. However, (1), unlike (2), allows
actions against one's better judgment to be non-intentional,
provided they are done knowingly, in the broad sense that *S*
knows that he is, or at least that he may be, doing them. For (1)
must accommodate cases like this: *S* knows that by nominating
Hal he will offend Sam and believes that though Hal would do
the job best, nominating him is not worth offending Sam. *S*
judges that it would be best not to offend Sam and thus better
not to nominate Hal even though in every other respect
nominating him would be good. But *S* wants to nominate Hal
and when Hal looks at him as nominations are opened, *S*
nominates him, thereby offending Sam. Since *S* has no desire
to offend Sam nor to bring about anything to which he believes offending Sam would contribute, and indeed *S* offends
Sam only as an unwanted by-product of something *S* does
intentionally, *S* does not offend him intentionally. This is not
to imply that *S* offends him *un*intentionally. That is not so; the

action is not, e.g., accidental or inadvertent. But *S* surely does offend Sam against his better judgment. If doing so were not against his better judgment, we could not explain why nominating Hal is against it. In the light of this it is reasonable to say that *S*'s offending Sam is incontinent and qualify the idea that incontinent actions must be intentional. Note also that since *S* is aware that offending Sam is against his better judgment and that nominating Hal will do it, *S* can be expected to exercise *will power* to avoid offending Sam, as well as to avoid nominating Hal. That makes it reasonable to say, as I believe we should, that *S*'s failure to avoid offending Sam is also incontinent. Thus, it may again appear that incontinent action, at least for normal adults, is simply action against one's better judgment.

It can be shown, however, that even if incontinent action coincides with the most common kind of action against one's better judgment, we should not construe incontinent action and action against one's better judgment as equivalent. Suppose that a post-hypnotic suggestion or a manipulation of *S*'s brain induces in him a truly irresistible desire to do *A*, which is against his better judgment. *S* may still do *A* knowingly—even intentionally, since he may perfectly well *mean* to do it. He could also satisfy the other conditions for acting against his better judgment. Would the action then be incontinent? Granted, if the instilled desire were such that a normal person in *S*'s circumstances could reasonably be expected to resist doing *A* if he judged that it would be better not to do it, then *S*'s doing it presumably *is* incontinent. But we are imagining a desire which is irresistible. Here it would be a mistake to call *S*'s doing *A* incontinent. *S*'s will is overwhelmed, one might say. It may also be overwhelmed by sufficiently strong desires that are *not* externally imposed, e.g. certain desires arising from paranoiac fears.

What such cases suggest is that incontinent actions cannot be compelled. I see no way to prove that incontinent actions cannot be compelled, but the plausibility of this idea can be seen through at least two considerations. First, weakness of will is surely a normative phenomenon in at least this sense: if *S* does *A* incontinently, then *S* is in some way criticizable for doing *A*; e.g., if *A* is wrong, whether morally, prudentially, or in some other way(s), *S* is criticizable (morally, prudentially, etc.) for doing it. Now suppose we add the widely believed premise that if *S* does *A* under compulsion, he is *not* criticizable

for doing it. It would follow that incontinent actions are never
compelled. I have argued in [2], however, that in very special
cases S would be criticizable for doing A even if S did it under
compulsion; so I reject this argument. Nevertheless, I believe
that in these special cases S acts under so much pressure that it
is unreasonable to say his doing it is incontinent (see, e.g., [2]:
3-5). To be sure, if S is criticizable at all for doing A, then there
is a degree of will power possible for at least some agents in the
relevant situation such that had he exercised his will to this
degree, he would not have done A. But if we consider S's doing
A incontinent whenever such a degree of will power is *possible*
for agents in the relevant situation, we shall surely have to call
a huge proportion of compelled acts incontinent. That would
weaken—perhaps destroy—the contrast between incontinent
action and action under compulsion. Admittedly, the existence of this contrast does not entail that incontinent acts
cannot be compelled. But the contrast is most easily explained
on this hypothesis, and the hypothesis in turn is supported by
a second consideration: compelled actions are in a sense involuntary; they are not done of one's own free will. Intuitively,
such actions occur because the will is not free, not because it is
weak.[2] The notion of compulsion is problematic and controversial, but it is well enough understood to help us understand
incontinence,[3] and anyway no plausible view of compulsion
seems inconsistent with the idea that incontinent actions must
not be compelled.

If we are to preserve the contrast I have drawn between
incontinent action and action under compulsion, we must go
yet another step beyond (2), which entails at most that S *believe*
he is free to do something other than A, and is consistent with
his doing A under compulsion. I propose, then, that we
conceive incontinent action as uncompelled action that is
against one's better judgment in the sense specified by (1):

(3) S does A incontinently at t if and only if, at t, S does A
     intentionally or knowingly, (ii) there is another action
     A', such that S believes he can (or at least that he
     probably can) do it, and has judged, or makes or holds
     the judgment, that it would be better to do A', (iii) S has
     not abandoned this judgment, (iv) S is aware of (ii) and
     (iii), and (v) S does not do A under compulsion.[4]

II

Supposing that (3) is a correct account of actions exhibiting weakness of will, is weakness of will exhibited *only* by incontinent actions? Some writers characterize weakness of will in a way that suggests they think this,[5] and certainly incontinent action is the typical subject of discussions of weakness of will. But it does not exhaust the subject. Suppose *S* judges that he should not take a drink and quite consciously tries to resist doing so. He may still form the intention to take one. May he not have thereby exhibited weakness of will? Even if he is not able to take one because the bottle is empty, he has already failed in the kind of inner struggle that often precedes incontinent action. Since the intention arises as it does out of his failure in this struggle, it is surely reasonable to say that his forming it manifests weakness of will. Similarly, if *S* makes the judgment at *t* that it would be better to do *A* than anything incompatible with doing it, then provided he believes he can do it, his *failure* to form, at (approximately) *t*, an intention to do *A* would manifest weakness of will. For here too there is the same kind of failure of will.

It is a more difficult question whether *S* exhibits weakness of will when he is simply unable to prevent himself from forming a predominant want (a want on balance) to take a drink, i.e., a want stronger than any set of wants *S* has for things he believes incompatible with taking one, e.g. pleasing Mary and driving safely. He could want it on balance without forming the intention to take it. He might believe the bottle is empty, or the want might not generate a corresponding intention until *S* decides to take a drink. But it is a conceptual truth that *S*'s having a predominant want to do *A* creates a strong tendency for him to form the intention to do it; and surely "the will" may exhibit weakness if it fails to prevent the formation of a predominant want at odds with *S*'s practical judgment that it would be best to do *A'*. In saying that a want of *S*'s is at odds (or does not accord) with a practical judgment of his I mean that the object of the want is an action such that *S* judges it would be better to do something else. Note also that *S*'s forming a predominant want does not entail his coming to want something he did not already want. It may be formed when a standing want simply becomes stronger than any set of "competing" wants, whether because the latter loses strength or the former gains it, or both.

These examples suggest a conception of will which it is important to understand in some detail. Let me start by suggesting that philosophers and others who have written on the will used to think of it as a faculty and often imagined it (usually unwittingly) as an inner agent. The job of the will was taken to be mainly to keep one's actions in accord with one's practical judgments, which in turn were typically conceived as deliverances of practical reason. These constituted directives for the will. The will may have been conceived less explicitly as having the derivative function of keeping one's decisions, resolutions, intentions, and certain other motivational elements in accord with one's practical judgments. But whether anyone thought of the will as having this derivative function or not, it clearly would be natural to attribute this function to it *given* the main job it was conceived to have on the model I am sketching. Will power, on this model, was measured by the will's success in carrying out its job in the face of inclinations that conflict with practical judgment, and weakness of will consisted in its failure to override certain such inclinations.

Philosophers now generally do not believe there is an entity, the Will. Talking of the will, weakness of will, etc. is apparently a way of talking about agents. But if my historical speculations are even roughly correct, it should not be surprising if the central uses of will-locutions parallel their uses on the model I have sketched (which seems by no means dead today). To a large extent this is surely so. For instance, S has *will power* when he ("his will") can resist certain inclinations that are against his better judgment; he exhibits *weakness of will* when he fails to resist certain such inclinations; and he performs an *act of will* when he performs a mental act appropriate to get himself to carry out an intention. (At least typically we speak of acts of will only when the intention accords with S's practical judgment, e.g. that he should refrain from losing his temper.) Thus, instead of speaking of S's will's carrying out its function, we may speak of his adequately controlling himself in the relevant ways, chiefly by keeping his actions, intentions, and predominant wants in accord with his practical judgments. By including predominant wants I may be slightly extending what is implicit in "the tradition" (or even in the use of will-locutions in current philosophical or other discourse); but even if I am, I think that predominant wants should figure as I propose in an adequate account of incontinence.

In the light of the suggested conception of will, we can see why it is not reasonable to regard as incontinent just any want of *S*'s that is at odds with his practical judgment. *S*'s want to do *A* may be too weak to be at all likely to bring him to do or even intend to do it; hence, even if doing *A* is against *S*'s practical judgment, his wanting to do it does not imply that his will has failed in its function. But what if the want, though not predominant, is "strong"? Certainly *S*'s having a great many such wants may be a *sign* of a weak will, but it does not follow that having one of them, or even the whole set, is incontinent. For though we may reasonably conceive as incontinent the formation of predominant wants at odds with one's practical judgment, we do not and should not assume that one ought not to want, even strongly, things whose realization is against one's practical judgment. For one thing, we regard it as quite natural to want, even quite strongly, certain things which we judge we ought not to have, e.g. sweets. Another reason is that non-predominant wants can usually be expected to be prevented, by stronger wants, from bringing about actions. Still another is that a strong want for something is widely known to lead, often, to contemplating what realizing that thing would be like, and if we expected people *not* to have strong wants for things against their better judgment we could not reasonably expect them to reflect as often or as much as they now do on what they take to be their alternatives. That would be an unfortunate loss.

A natural direction to take in accounting for weakness of will exhibited by non-actions is to extend the notion of compulsion. Thus, at least when *S* cannot help forming the intention or a predominant want to do *A*, let us speak of his forming it under compulsion. If, e.g., he is ordered to withdraw his savings to ransom his child, he cannot help forming, and may be said to form under compulstion, the intention to withdraw them. Speaking of intentions and predominant wants as formed under compulsion may initially sound odd, but it presents few if any theoretical difficulties beyond those raised by the notion of compelled action. Moreover, if 'free will' and 'coercing the will' mean any more than 'free action' and 'coercing an action', as they certainly seem to, then applying 'compulsion' to intentions and predominant wants, which are among the most important "acts of will," is not only intelligible but likely to help us explicate the concepts of the freedom and coercion of the will. Failure to form intentions may seem

harder to handle along these lines. Can one be compelled not
to form an intention? Imagine that S's doing A is unthinkable
for him; it makes sense to say that he cannot bring himself to
do or even form the intention to do A, or that he cannot bring
himself even to want to do A. With his child's life at stake, e.g.,
S cannot form the intention not to withdraw his savings, any
more than he can bring himself not to withdraw them. The
compulsion under which he withdraws them is the same compulsion preventing him from intending not to.

The 'could not' here is not that of causal impossibility. It is
not implied that S's forming the intention or want would
violate a law of nature. Rather, a compulsion prevents his
forming it. Though I cannot offer an analysis of the relevant
kind of compulsion, it will help to note a necessary (but not
sufficient) condition: if, under compulsion, S forms the intention to do A, then it is not the case that he is in circumstances such that it would be reasonable to expect a normal
person in those circumstances *not* to form the intention to do
A. Here being in S's circumstances includes (among other
things) holding the same practical judgments and having the
same wants, though the wants should not be assumed to be of
the same relative strengths (since then we could not in general
reasonably expect different conduct). I believe the same holds
if, in place of forming the intention to do A, we substitute
forming a predominant want to do A. Note that the principle
does not apply where we cannot conceive a normal person in
S's circumstances, e.g. because S is insane, or driven by a
pathological fear such that he is at least temporarily abnormal,
or afflicted with brain damage that causes him to do apparently inexplicable things. Often, however, we can reasonably
expect a normal person in S's circumstances not to form an
intention or a predominant want against his better judgment;
and if we can, it is reasonable to say that in forming the
intention or predominant want against his better judgment S
is incontinent.

The examples of incontinent action given so far would all
be cases of forming incontinent intentions if we altered them
by simply substituting the intention to do A for doing A. By
contrast, consider an addict with his heroin beside him and
withdrawal sysmptoms coming upon him. We cannot reasonably expect him not to form the intention to take some heroin,
even if it is against his better judgment; and if we assume a
normal person can be in these circumstances, our principle

does not require us—indeed it disinclines us—to call the intention incontinent. Construing compulsion as I propose introduces a normative element into our account: the notion of what can reasonably be expected of a normal person. But surely what counts as weakness of will depends on some *standard* of how much will power a normal person may be reasonably expected to have and exercise in the relevant circumstances.

Weakness of will, then, manifests itself not just in action but at the level of intending and wanting. To accommodate these instances of weakness of will, we may speak of *S*'s exhibiting incontinence in general or, more specifically, of *S*'s exhibiting weakness of will *with respect to an action* (not merely in performing it). The broad conception of weakness of will I want to propose, then, is this:

(4)   *S* exhibits weakness of will with respect to *A* at *t* if and only if, at *t*, either (a) *S* does *A* incontinently, in the sense of (3); or (b) *S* forms the intention or a predominant want to do *A*, where doing *A* is against his better judgment, and he does not form the intention or want under compulsion; or (c) *S fails* to form the intention to do *A*, where he believes that he can do *A*, makes the judgment that he ought to do *A* (or some other practical judgment favoring *A*), and his failure to form the intention does not occur under compulsion.[6]

Analysis (4) does not mention decisions, resolutions, plans, or other motivational elements whose formation may be incontinent, because these presumably entail intentions or predominant wants or both. Note also that (4) does not apply where *S has* exhibited weakness of will, for instance by forming (or failing to form) an intention, but does not now (at *t*) satisfy (4). We may often speak in such cases of *S*'s being in a *state* that exhibits weakness of will; for often in such instances he *would* satisfy (4) if, e.g., he judged at *t* that he should do *A*, since he would again fail to form the intention to do it. Let us say that *S* is in a state that exhibits weakness of will after he has exhibited weakness of will in the sense of (4), so long as his motivation remains at odds with his practical judgment in the way (4) specifies. We then have a dispositional as well as an occurrent notion of exhibiting weakness of will.

The remainder of this section will take up some problems raised by (4): Does it do justice to certain cases of extraordinary will power? Does it posit incontinent intentions and wants to explain phenomena understandable in terms of incontinent action alone? And how is it related to what we might call a volitional theory of incontinence?

Consider the possibility that someone who usually resists a degree of temptation which the normal person cannot be expected to resist, will sometimes act against his better judgment in yielding to it.[7] If S usually resists seduction to which the normal person would yield against his better judgment, what should we say about a case of the same degree of temptation in which, against his better judgment, S gives in? It may be that this time S is compelled. He might be temporarily debilitated, e.g. by depression, so we could not reasonably expect him or any normal person in his circumstances to withstand that degree of temptation (where degree of temptation is understood partly in terms of the strength of desire created). But suppose S is not compelled. One may then resist the implication of (4) that he acts incontinently; for one may imagine someone of ordinary will power in the situation and realize that he *would* be compelled to yield. But surely what compels one person (or most) should not be expected to compel us all; and even if a normal person in S's circumstances could not reasonably be expected to do otherwise, it does not follow that S acted under compulsion, nor that *no one* in the circumstances could reasonably be expected to do otherwise. One man's temptation may be another man's aversion. And just as an action incontinent relative to one agent's practical judgments may be continent relative to another's practical judgments, incontinence is relative to factors determining whether the agent is compelled. There is not some one degree of will power such that failure to exhibit that degree is to exhibit weakness of will; rather, there is a kind of balance, achievable in many ways, among one's practical judgments, motivational states, and actions, and weakness of will consists in failing to achieve or maintain that balance. It is a merit of the account expressed in (4) that it does justice to these points.

The next objection I want to take up is that (4) assimilates incontinent acts of omission to the motivational states whose occurrence the ommitted acts should have prevented. On this view, it may be incontinent to omit to do something to prevent one's forming an intention, but forming an intention cannot

be incontinent. I agree that such acts of omission may be incontinent, but this fact does not make the notion of incontinent intentions dispensable. First, there may *be* no action S believes would or might prevent him from (say) incontinently intending to drink, hence no act of omission on which to pin the incontinence we feel the formation of that intention exhibits. Second, the very same exercise of will required to get oneself to do something one finds hard produces the intention to do it; and the same exercise of will that enables one to resist temptation produces the intention not to do the tempting thing, or at least prevents one's forming the intention to do it. Thus, if S exhibits weakness of will when he manifests, in action, a failure to exercise enough will power, it is surely reasonable to say that he exhibits weakness of will when he manifests, in motivation, the same failure we criticize when it is manifested in action. It is not as if there were different kinds of exercises of will to produce action and to produce the intention to act: these exercises are of the same kind, and they usually coincide when S's forming the intention to do *A* is approximately simultaneous with his intentionally doing *A*, or the action flows from the intention without "prodding" by the will. Failures in such exercises are instances of weakness of will.

Since volitions have figured prominently in many traditional and some contemporary discussions of will, one may wonder how they are related to my account. Among the contemporary writers on action who have made significant uses of a notion of volition are Sellars ([16]), Castañeda ([3]), McCann ([12]), and perhaps Goldman ([7]) (under the description, 'occurrent want'). To cite one of the most explicit characterizations available,

> A volition is an endorsingly rehearsing thinking of an intention, i.e., the fully endorsing episode of thinking of a thought-content of the form *I shall do A*, which is *not* a proposition . . . the activation of the practical action schema by a volition need *not* be effective . . . But when they [volitions] are [realized] we *do* something . . . If the reader wants to speak of mental acts, then volitions are acts, but they are still not doings ([3]: 309-310).[8]

Not all action theorists would hold just this, but the characterization expresses most of the common content of the main views of volition and will in any case serve my purpose. I simply want to suggest how appeal to volitions might help us,

and to explain how (4) would square with a volitional account
of incontience. The core of a plausible version of such an
account might be this: Incontinence occurs if and only if (1) S
has a practical judgment such that (a) he fails to have any
volition in accord with it, or (b) S has at least one volition in
accord with it, yet fails to act (or intend) accordingly; and (2)
neither (a) nor (b) essentially results from compulsion (I
ignore subleties that do not affect my point, but a number of
the needed additions are suggested by our previous discussion).

Something like this could be true, and it is consistent with
(4). But I doubt that we need to *analyze* 'incontinence' this way.
Whether such an analysis could be correct depends heavily on
what else we say about volitions. Perhaps a plausible volitional
account of incontience would be at least roughly equivalent to
(4). The most obvious difference is that the former requires
something quite specific—a volition—to occur in consciousness in at least the typical cases of incontinence, whereas (4)
entails simply that S be appropriately aware of his holding the
relevant practical judgment. However, (4) allows that the
required kind of awareness be just the kind one would have
when one has a volition, and indeed I think it sometimes is this
kind. Moreover, perhaps the non-occurrence of a volition can
help explain *why* the incontinent agent fails to act in accord
with his practical judgment. But supposing volitions can
partially explain how incontinence actually occurs, it of course
does not follow that they must enter into its analysis. In the
light of these and other points, I conclude that volitions may
help us understand incontinence and that a plausible volitional account of incontinence might very well turn out to be at
least roughly equivalent to the one I have proposed. But I see
no need to supplement (4) with any explicit appeal to volitions.

It should now be apparent how my account is unified by
the idea that the logic of will-locutions strongly reflects the
view that the chief function of the will is to keep our actions,
intentions, and predominant wants in accord with our practical judgments. If this idea is correct, it explains why acting
incontinently entails acting against one's better judgment,
why S may exhibit weakness of will even without acting, and
why it is that actions, intentions, or predominant wants are not
incontinent when, though against one's better judgment, they
are compelled (for in these cases the will is in some sense
coerced). Conceiving of will as I suggest also enables us to

explain why, as Kant saw (e.g. in [10]: 10 and 53), at least one ground for attributing *good will* to a person is what intentions he has or fails to have. For if one function of will is to exercise at least some control over one's intentions, then how good one's will is depends in part on how well one exercises this control. Thus, the conception of weakness of will expressed in (4) helps us both to understand incontinent action and to unify such diverse phenomena as action against one's better judgment, forming intentions to do things which are against one's better judgment, failing to form intentions to do things which are required by one's better judgment, having a good will, and coercion of the will.

III

I want now to consider how weakness of will is possible. The difficulty of explaining this is brought out cogently by Davidson. He says that all the following "seem self-evident":

P$_1$ If an agent wants to do x more than he wants to do y and he believes himself free to do either x or y, then he will intentionally do x if he does either x or y intentionally.

P$_2$ If an agent judges that it would be better to do x than to do y, then he wants to do x more than he wants to do y.

P$_3$ There are incontinent actions. ([4]: 95.)

If P$_3$ is taken, as it normally would be, to entail that there are incontinent actions which are both intentional and such that there is an alternative S believes he is free to do and judges it would be better to do, then P$_1$, P$_2$, and P$_3$ cannot all be true.

The most common way out is to deny P$_2$, the Socratic Principle, as we might call it. It is thus surprising that Davidson does little to defend P$_2$. Perhaps this is because he believes that

> It is easy to interpret P$_2$ in a way that makes it false, but it is harder to believe there is not a natural reading that makes it true. For against our tendency to agree that we often believe we ought to do something and yet don't want to, there is also the opposite tendency to say that if someone really (sincerely) believes he ought, then his belief must show itself in his behaviour (and hence, of course, in his inclination to act, or his desire). ([4]: 99.)

But as Davidson seems to grant in the same paragraph, P_2 is not entailed by the fact that we tend to say that if someone really believes he ought, his belief must show itself in his behavior or wants.

Hare appears to accept P_2; but even if he would not accept it without qualification, he seems to hold at least equally strong internalist principles. He says, e.g., that "typical cases of 'moral weakness' are cases where a man *cannot* do what he thinks he ought" ([9]: 68); and

> If a man does what he says he ought not to, though perfectly able to resist . . . there is something wrong with what he says, as well as with what he does. In the simplest case it is insincerity . . . In other cases it is self-deception . . . There are endless possible variations upon this theme, but until one is produced which really does run counter to prescriptivism, the prescriptivist need not be concerned. ([9]: 82-3.)

No doubt what looks like incontinence may be compulsion, self-deception, or other things. But to point this out does nothing to show that there is no incontinence in the sense of (3). Hare's strategy seems to be not to argue directly for any internalist principle, but to rebut apparent counterexamples and suggest there are none. But there surely are counterexamples.

Consider a case of adultery with the following features. 1. S might at the time be disposed to say sincerely that it would be better to abstain from it; he might even utter this judgment and momentarily back away as he says the words. 2. He might be disposed to make the inferences we would expect from a person who judged that he ought not to perform the act, e.g. that now it will be hypocritical to talk as if he had maintained fidelity. 3. He might be disposed sincerely to advise and criticize others in just the ways expectable from a person who judged this. 4. He might be disposed to do things he believes would reduce his desire for his companion, e.g. dwelling on her faults and on the attractions of his spouse, hoping thereby to reverse his direction. 5. The judgment might cohere well both with S's other moral beliefs and with his prudential beliefs; e.g., he might believe in keeping solemn promises, and be aware that he has solemnly promised fidelity. 6. S might carry out the act only with considerable guilt and might also feel guilt and regret later. In the light of 1.- 6., I believe it would be at least unreasonable to maintain P_2 or any equally strong internalist principle.

A likely internalist objection would be Hare's claim that "the person who accepts some moral judgment but does not act on it is actually giving commands to himself, but is unable to obey them because of a recalcitrant lower nature or 'flesh'." ([9]: 81.) Let us first notice an underlying suggestion here: that whenever one apparently fails, through incontinence, to act on a moral judgment that one holds, one is "giving commands" to oneself. If we accept this, we are already granting Hare too much. As our previous examples show, even when incontinent action also exhibits moral weakness, S need not make the judgment, at the time he does A, that he ought not to do A (or that he ought to be doing A', etc.). And even when S does make such a judgment at t, he need not be doing anything plausibly called giving a command to himself. The picture Hare suggests is one of someone repeatedly commanding an action, yet failing thereby to bring it about. Whether we imagine self-command or, more naturally, commanding someone else, it is indeed plausible in *this* case to conclude that either the commander cannot bring about the action, or is using at least some prescriptive term in an "off-colour" way such that he is not really prescribing. But supposing Hare is right about cases like this, as I believe he may be, he gives us no reason to regard all apparently incontinent actions as instances of psychological inability, and in our examples of incontinence this seems clearly absent. In the adultery case, for instance, it is not as if the temptress used hypnotic powers, or even pressed the incontinent husband on that Achilles heel, the fear of failing to be masculine. Both may be imagined with considerably less than irresistible passion, or indeed with such largely non-passional motives as ego needs. And note that S himself does not believe he is *unable* to resist; he considers himself morally responsible, as he surely seems to be.

Is self-deception possible in our example? It seems very unlikely, given 1.- 6., particularly since S has tried to reverse his direction, exhibited genuine guilt during and after the act, and holds (and has confirmed by much previous behavior that he holds) principles which he is aware rule out the act. Might we deny that S really judges it would be better not to do the thing? This is especially easy to do if we take incontinence to involve actively "giving commands to oneself." But as I have argued in the light of many examples, this would give us too narrow a conception of incontinence. Moreover, in the case we

are examining S *is* imagined as sincerely saying it would be
better not to do the deed. Though I do not take this to entail
his judging that it would be better not to, that he does indeed
judge this seems clear and is part of what would be easily the
best explanation of his saying it. Surely the voice of conscience
can speak authentically even while S is doing the deed; and we
may imagine its authenticity reflected in S's pangs of conscience temporarily inhibiting his carrying the action out.
Similarly, the context (as specified by points 2. - 6.) is such that
it is quite implausible to suppose S judges only that, say, what
he is doing is *considered* wrong. On balance, then, while 1. - 6.
perhaps do not entail the falsity of P_2, they at least make it
unreasonable to maintain P_2 or any equally strong internalist
principle.

   Let us now consider the issue more explicitly from the
point of view of developing the best theory we can of the
nature of the concrete phenomena we have been considering
as incontinence. If we maintain P_2 or an equally strong
internalist principle, then it is not clear how certain kinds of
incontinence, of which we have seen apparent examples, are
possible at all. For though we might reject P_1 as it stands,[9] it can
be refined so as to seem clearly true, and the problem will
persist if we retain P_2 or any principle entailing that our
motivation always accords with our better judgment.[10] Davidson in particular has sought to resolve this problem. Why not
explain the possibility of incontinence as he does? He first
proposes what he calls a plausible modification of the characterization of incontinence given in (2): Now S's doing x is
incontinent when "he does x for a reason r, but has a reason r'
that includes r and more, on the basis of which he judges some
alternative to be better than x." ([4]: 111.) Still, how can P_1 and
P_2 allow for incontinence in this sense? By P_2, if S judges, on
the basis of r', that it would be better to do A' than A he would
presumably *want* to do A' more than A and would, by P_1, do A'
if he did either intentionally. But Davidson holds that even
though r' "includes" r, S's judging, on the basis of r', that it
would be better to do A' than A does *not* entail either S's
judging simply that it would be better to do A', or his wanting
more to do A' than to do A. For despite appearances, 'S's
judging, on the basis of r' that it would be better to do A' than
A', is not to be analyzed as the conjunction of

(i)   *S* judges that it would be better to do *A'* than *A*

and

(ii)   The basis on which *S* judges this is *r'*,

but rather into an attribution to *S* of the *prima facie* judgment

(iii)   *pf*(*A'* is better than *A*, *r'*).

I believe (iii) provides a correct analysis of the form of the judgment attributed in some uses of '*S* judges, on the basis of *r'*, that it would be better to do *A'* than *A*', whereas (i) and (ii) together do the same for other uses of it. In any case, surely some incontinent agents judge simply that it would be better to do *A'* than *A*, yet intentionally do *A*. To *these* cases Davidson's account of how incontinence is possible does not apply.

One might deny that we ever make such judgments, on the ground that every practical judgment is relative to some ground. But this premise is ambiguous between

(iv)   For every practical judgment there is a ground on the
        basis of which the person makes it, in the sense that he
        holds the judgment *because* he accepts that ground

and

(v)   Every practical judgment is *prima facie*, i.e., relativized,
        in the manner of (iii), to a ground.

Statement (v) does not follow from (iv) (as I think Davidson would agree): the ground of a judgment, in the sense of 'ground' relevant in (iv), need not be reflected in its form or content. Moreover, an internalist may grant that we sometimes judge simply that *A'* would be better than *A*, and Davidson himself seems to allow this:

> Intentional action, as I have argued in defending P$_1$ and P$_2$, is geared
> directly to unconditional judgements like 'It would be better to do *a*
> than to do *b*'. Reasoning that stops at conditional judgements such as
> (C$_a$) [*pf*(*a* is better than *b*, *e*), where *e* is all that *S* considers relevant] is
> practical only in its subject, not in its issue. ([4]: 110.)

On the other hand, Davidson clearly allows that *S* may incontinently do *A* where *S* "believes it would be better, all

things considered, to do another thing." ([4]: 112.) This is possible because this judgment is *prima facie* and *S* "sometimes holds that all he believes and values supports a certain course of action when at the same time those same beliefs and values cause him to reject that course of action." ([4]: 111.) This may indeed happen to *S* and may explain some cases of incontinence, such as some in which *S* does not make an unconditional judgment. But it does not render P_1 and P_2 consistent with those cases of incontinence—the most full-blooded, I believe—in which *S* does *A* intentionally though he judges simply that it would be better to do *A'*. We can deny that such cases are possible, and allow only those in which the relevant judgments are *prima facie*; but this seems to go against our experience, as I have argued in the light of a number of examples of incontinence; and I have tried to show that the reasons for saying it, mainly those supporting P_2, are far from compelling.

To be sure, even if we give up P_2 we still need to explain how weakness of will actually takes place and how practical judgments favoring an action are related to motivation to perform it. There is at least a *tendency* for one's motivation to accord with one's practical judgments, and nothing I have said precludes *some* kind of "non-contingent" relation between the two. Perhaps it is implicit in the concept of practical judgment that such judgments create a tendency to do the thing judged best. There is something strange about doing *A* when one is aware that one holds the judgment that it would be best to do *A'*. The problem is particularly acute if, as Hare seems to (e.g. in [9]: 81), we imagine *S saying* to himself, at the time he does *A*, things like 'I ought not to do this', for then the words tend to sound hollow, though logically they may still express a judgment of *S*'s. But these facts can be explained on the principle, far weaker than P_2, that practical judgments necessarily create a tendency to act accordingly; and in any case weakness of will can occur without *S*'s rehearsing all the while the practical judgment he is failing to live up to. Presumably, in the typical cases enough must go on in consciousness at the time of weakness to make it plausible to assume that "the will" struggles for control and fails, or fails to struggle at all where *S* sees he should. But however weakness of will occurs, it is surely possible, even when *S* judges unconditionally that it would be best not to do the thing in question. My account of inconti-

nence and of its relation to practical judgment explains this possibility. The account also encompasses not only incontinent action but other phenomena plausibly called weakness of will; and I believe it provides some of the materials needed to understand how the various kinds of weakness of will actually take place.[11]

REFERENCES

[1] Audi, Robert, "Intending," *Journal of Philosophy* 70(1973): 387-403.
[2] _____, "Moral Responsibility, Freedom, and Compulsion," *American Philosophical Quarterly* 11(1974): 1-14.
[3] Castañeda, Hector-Neri, *Thinking and Doing: The Philosophical Foundations of Institutions* (Dordrecht and Boston: D. Reidel, 1975).
[4] Davidson, Donald, "How is Weakness of the Will Possible?", in Joel Feinberg (ed.), *Moral Concepts* (New York: Oxford University Press, 1970): 93-113.
[5] Duggan, Timothy, and Bernard Gert, "Voluntary Abilities," *American Philosophical Quarterly* 4(1967): 127-35.
[6] Gert, Bernard, "Coercion and Freedom," *Nomos* 14(1972): 30-48.
[7] Goldman, Alvin I., *A Theory of Human Action* (Englewood Cliffs: Prentice-Hall, 1970).
[8] Griffiths, A. Phillips, "Acting With Reason," *Philosophical Quarterly* 8(1958): 289-99.
[9] Hare, R. M., *Freedom and Reason* (Oxford: Oxford University Press, 1963).
[10] Kant, Immanuel, *Foundations of the Metaphysics of Morals*, Trans. by Lewis White Beck (New York: The Liberal Arts Press, 1959).
[11] Matthews, Gwynneth, "Weakness of Will," *Mind* 75(1966): 405-19.
[12] McCann, Hugh, "Volition and Basic Action," *Philosophical Review* 83(1974): 451-73.
[13] Mortimore, G. W. (ed.), *Weakness of Will* (London: Macmillan, 1971).
[14] Rapaport, Elizabeth, "Explaining Moral Weakness," *Philosophical Studies* 24(1973): 174-82.
[15] Santas, Gerasimos, "Plato's *Protagoras* and Explanations of Weakness," *Philosophical Review* 65(1966): 3-33.
[16] Sellars, Wilfrid, "Fatalism and Determinism," in Keith Lehrer (ed.), *Freedom and Determinism* (New York: Random House, 1966).
[17] Smith, M. B. E., "Indifference and Moral Acceptance," *American Philosophical Quarterly* 9(1972).

NOTES

[1] Among the philosophers who seem to take these notions to be equivalent are Donald Davidson ([4]: 93-5 and 111); Gerasimos Santas ([15]); A. Phillips Griffiths ([8]); and perhaps Gwynneth Matthews ([11]).

[2] It seems clear that if S could not have done otherwise than A (so that it is "strictly unavoidable"), then S is not criticizable for doing A. Thus S's doing A is incontinent *only if* it is not strictly unavoidable. (See [2] for an account of strict unavoidability). It might be argued that strict unavoidability should be substituted for compulsion in (3); after all, where an intentional action is strictly unavoidable S does not even have the "ability to will" otherwise, so of course his doing A does not exhibit weakness of will. (See Duggan and Gert [5] and Gert [6] for an account of ability to will). I find this argument plausible, but do not think (3) need be weakened accordingly. To adopt the revision, however, would be in the spirit of my overall account.

[3]In [2] I have developed an analysis of compelled action.

[4]One might argue that since the judgment specified in (ii) is practical, our requiring that S believe he can (or that he probably can) do A' is redundant. This overlooks the possibility (which is not implied in any of my examples in the paper) that S's judgment favoring A' is not practical in what seems the most common sense, in which a practical judgment is one's "best," so there is no *other* action S judges to be better still. This is appropriate, since incontinence may occur even if there is no action S judges, at t, would be best. Thus, (i) allows that, e.g., S judge A" to be still better than A', and one ground he might have for this is that it does not seem likely that he can do A', whereas he is sure he can do A". There may still be a redundancy: perhaps S's judging just that it would be better (not best) to do A' entails his believing he can (or that he probably can) do A'. But if so, the redundancy is harmless.

[5]For instance, Santas [15], Griffiths [8], and perhaps also Davidson [4]. The impression is confirmed by other papers in [13].

[6]One might construe as weakness of will cases in which (a) S forms a predominant want for a state of affairs φ, where φ is *not* an action of S's but S judges that its non-occurrence is possible and would be better than its occurrence, or (b) S *fails* to form a predominant want for φ, where he judges that the occurrence of φ is possible and would be better than its non-occurrence. For if S satisfies (a), then if he believed doing A would realize φ, he would tend to do A; and if S satisfies (b), he is *not* so disposed that if he believed this, he would tend to do A. In both cases what S wants on balance does not accord with an *evaluative* judgment which under certain conditions would give rise to a practical judgment such that if S held it he would exhibit weakness of will in the sense of (4). But in part because wants that are not to perform an action might conflict only quite indirectly with practical judgments, it seems preferable not to regard their formation (or non-formation) as incontinent. Note, by contrast, that (4) entails incontinence where, though S does form a predominant want to do A (which is required by his practical judgment), he fails to form the intention to do it. The failure of will here is admittedly quite minor, but I think it is genuine.

[7]This example was suggested to me by Michael Bratman.

[8]Cp. Sellars: "A volition is an inner episode, a mental act, which is, in the absence of paralysis and granted the existence of favorable circumstances, the cause of the corresponding action" ([16]: 150).

[9]In [1] I have argued that temporary forgetting may falsify such principles as P_1, and it also appears to need revisions on other counts.

[10]For other objections to P_2 and similar internalist principles, see [14] and [17].

[11]For helpful comments on one or another earlier version of this paper I want to thank readers for *Noûs*, especially Hector-Neri Castañeda, and Michael Bratman, Lawrence Davis, David Gerber, Hardy Jones, Hugh McCann, Elizabeth Rapaport, Richard Reilly, and M. B. E. Smith.

[18]

Mind (1984) Vol. XCIII, 1–18

Weakness of Will

FRANK JACKSON

There is a long tradition which views the problem of weakness of will as the problem of how agents can intentionally do what they consider wrong. And given that intentional acts are ones in accord with wants and desires, the problem becomes how we can simultaneously judge something wrong and yet want to do it. Some say, 'Nothing easier—unfortunately.' Suppose they are right; that is, that there is no *philosophical* problem about desiring to do what you judge to be wrong. Would there then be no philosophical problem of weakness of will at all?

In this paper I argue that there would still be a problem, and seek to solve it. I start, in §1, by locating the problem and distinguishing it from the problem (if any) about desiring to do wrong. Donald Davidson, in 'How is Weakness of Will Possible?',[1] separates out the problem of weakness of will from the problem of intentionally acting contrary to one's judgement of the *morally* best thing to do. In his view, that is only a special case of the general problem of intentionally acting contrary to one's judgement of what is best *simpliciter*. The aim of §1 is to justify taking the extra step of entirely separating out the problem of weakness of will from that of acting contrary to what is judged best. I should, however, point out that the arguments of the later sections do not depend crucially on §1. I have, naturally, largely formulated them on the assumption that the conclusion of §1 is correct, but they can be reformulated without this assumption.

§2 is concerned with certain essential preliminaries, principally about how the objects of desire can be viewed; and with how this view solves some puzzles about desiring and wanting, quite apart from its role in our solution to the problem of weakness of will. In §3 I derive from the central idea of §2, an account of how desires can evolve in accord with the agent's reason: weak-willed behaviour being behaviour springing from desires that do not evolve in this way.

1   Reprinted in his *Essays on Actions and Events*, (Oxford: Oxford University Press, 1980).

1. *Separating out the problem*

Cases of intentionally acting against one's judgement of what is
right can be divided into many sub-cases. In particular, a contrast
can be drawn between those we naturally describe in terms of a
conflict between reason on the one hand, and passion, bodily
appetites and the like on the other; and those where appetite *et al.*
have no special role. My contention is going to be that we can
identify a problem about understanding conflict between reason
and appetite, independently of whether one or the other (reason
most likely) is directed towards what is judged good. Here is an
example where appetite *et al.* have no special role. While backing
out of a parking bay I dent the bodywork of someone else's car,
causing what I estimate to be $200 worth of damage. My car is
unmarked. No-one sees me. I know that I ought to leave my name
and address under the windscreen wiper of the damaged car; but I
also know that if I don't no-one will know that I haven't. I succumb
to temptation and drive away quickly. In this case I intentionally do
what is wrong because I want to hold on to my $200 more than I
want to do what is right. I was not, though, overwhelmed by
appetite, passion, emotion, feeling, or anything like that. I wanted
to hold on to my $200, but I (perhaps unlike some misers) do not
thirst or *lust* after money.

The contrast is with cases where agents are led to act against their
better judgement by something that can be broadly classed as a
bodily feeling. Cases of this kind are only too familiar to those who
have struggled to give up smoking, or to stay on a diet. What leads
me to succumb to a cigarette or a chocolate is different from what
leads me to succumb to the temptation to hold on to my $200. It is
the cases essentially involving feelings, bodily appetites, and so on
that we will concentrate on.

Why is there a philosophical problem about them, regardless of
whether there is one about desiring to do what is judged wrong? We
naturally describe cases of weakness of will as cases where appetite
plays an unduly significant role in causing action. The problem is to
specify *undue*. Appetite can play *a* causal role without the action
thereby being incontinent; otherwise everyone who drinks because
they are thirsty acts incontinently. Of course it is a good thing that
on the appropriate occasions one feels thirsty to the appropriate
degree. But that is not why drinking because one feels thirsty is,
typically, not incontinent. Plenty of smokers decide that the

WEAKNESS OF WILL   3

unpleasantness associated with resisting their desire to smoke outweighs the improved chance of long life if they stop. (I have in mind smokers who face up to the issues honestly, not those who pretend—maybe half-successfully—that the chances of early death are less than they are.) Perhaps they make the decision to continue smoking after their family tells them just how unpleasant they were to live with the last time they tried to give up. These smokers need not be acting incontinently in smoking; yet they smoke because of the craving, and grant that it would be better if they did not have the craving; and, no doubt, wish that they didn't have the craving, and so wish that they did not want to smoke. Nevertheless, their smoking need not be incontinent. They may simply have concluded, continently, that the increased chance of long life is not worth the certainty of increased misery for themselves and their family.

Also, undue influence cannot be analysed as influence over and above the ordinary. We may suppose that Casanova was influenced over and above the ordinary by sexual appetite, without thereby supposing him to be incontinent. For (as has been widely recognized) there is a distinction between being passionate or intemperate and being weak-willed. Two hypotheses about Casanova (as we are supposing him) are possible. According to one, he experienced greater sexual urges than most of us; according to the other, his urges were the same as ours, but he valued their satisfaction more highly than most of us by comparison with other things. Similarly, an overweight gourmet may be overweight because he experiences greater pleasure when eating than most of us; or because, though his pleasure is the same as ours, he values it more highly than, say, we value remaining slim. On neither hypothesis does it *follow* that our Casanova or our gourmet are weak-willed. Neither their strength of appetite nor their difference in values is sufficient for their being weak-willed. They may be weak-willed, but if they are, something else is involved as well.

At this stage one may be tempted to declare the attempt to identify a problem about weakness of will separate from the whole question of desiring what is wrong, a failure. 'It is obvious what the required sense of "undue" influence is: it is influence that leads agents to intentionally act contrary to their *better* judgement.' But, on the contrary, it seems that causing agents to act contrary to better judgement is neither necessary nor sufficient for weak-willed action.

4   FRANK JACKSON:

Firstly, it is not sufficient, because there are *three* kinds of case
where appetite leads to acting contrary to better judgement, only
one of which is the case of weakness of will. Consider someone
offered 'one for the road' at the end of a party, and suppose that he is
in no doubt that the best thing for him to do is to say 'No'—he has to
drive home, he needs to be up bright and early next morning, and so
on. We distinguish three cases, which shade into each other, where
he nevertheless says 'Yes'. The first is where he simply does not care
enough about the dangers to others of driving home under the
influence or about his duties on the morrow. He doesn't care
enough about what he acknowledges to be what it is best to do. The
second kind of case is the weak-willed. He gives in because his will is
weak in this particular case (and perhaps in general as well). The
third case is where the desire for a drink is irresistible; his behaviour
is neither reckless nor weak-willed, but rather is compulsive. In
each of these three cases the agent intentionally acts against better
judgement because of the influence of appetite; but only in one, the
second, do we have weak-willed behaviour—the first is reckless-
ness, and the third is compulsion.[1]

Secondly, it is not necessary. Weakness of will can be the
explanation of your failure to follow out a course of action you judge
to be the *wrong* one. It does not have to be a course of action you
judge to be right, though typically it is. Imagine a committed
catholic who is raped and becomes pregnant. She is certain that it
would be wrong for her to have an abortion, but she determines
nevertheless to have one. When the time comes, however, her
feelings of guilt overcome her resolve to have the abortion. Cannot
such a case be one of weakness of will? Had she been more strong-
willed, she would have gone through with the abortion; hence her
failing must count as one of weakness of will. She acts incontinently,
while doing what she judges best.

I have sought to raise our problem about weakness of will by
pointing to the problem about specifying the undue influence we
intuitively assign feeling in cases of weak-willed action. We have
seen that the undue influence definitive of incontinence does not
amount to some influence, nor to influence that is not desired, nor to
influence above the norm, and nor to influence that leads to acting
intentionally against better judgement. These difficulties may
engender scepticism about the viability or significance of our

1   I am indebted to Gary Watson, 'Skepticism about Weakness of Will',
      Philosophical Review, LXXXVI, **3** (July 1977), pp. 316–339.

WEAKNESS OF WILL 5

ordinary concept of weakness of will. After all we invoke weakness of will as an explanation in conflict situations. Something about a contemplated course of action appeals; something else about it repels. If our intuitions about undue influence prove so hard to clarify, perhaps the right response is to abandon weakness of will as a possible explanation of how the agent comes to choose as he does. Perhaps all there is to say is that if the agent adopts the course of action, this proves his desire for the appealing feature is greater than his desire to avoid the unappealing feature; while if he refrains, this proves his desire for the appealing feature is less than his desire to avoid the unappealing one.

The attraction of such a procrustean position is obvious: explanation solely in terms of relative strength of competing desires is explanation in comparatively well-understood terms; and so invoking weakness of will as a possible factor can be seen as muddying the waters with pre-scientific and pre-Humean notions about the existence and relative independence of various faculties of the mind. What are Reason and Desire? And, supposing we have clear answers to this question, how can they conflict, given Hume's dictum about reason being the slave of the passions?[1]

Nevertheless, I think that clear sense can be made of weakness of will in terms of agents' acting against the dictates of their reason; and that this can be done without becoming enmeshed in the faculties of the mind, and without denying what is right about Humean views about reason and desire. My starting point is, in fact, a Humean position about reason and desire.

2. *Preliminaries concerning wanting*

Hume said that 'Reason alone can never be a motive to any action of the will . . .'[2] I am going to assume what I take to be a non-controversial element in this and related views of Hume's about action. According to the non-controversial element, every action (or at least every action of the kind we are concerned with—maybe idle tongue clickings and the like are exceptions) involves *both* beliefs and something like wants or desires. When I sign a cheque,

---

1   A subtle sceptical position is put by Watson, ibid.; also Davidson, ibid., rightly points out how reflection on weakness of will can easily lead to 'absurd' pictures of what is going on.
2   *Treatise of Human Nature*, Bk II, Pt III, §3.

6   FRANK JACKSON:

there is something I want or desire—say, to pay a bill—and also something I believe about how what I am doing will achieve what I want; and both are involved.

There are a whole host of terms—'want', 'desire', 'preference', 'value', 'pro- and con- attitudes', to name a few—used for the thing which is not belief, but which must be involved along with belief, in intentional action. I am going to assume that there is some unified notion lying behind all these terms; and I will use the various terms more or less interchangeably for it, but without, I hope, making controversial presumptions about how it is to be analysed, and without presuming that in other, related contexts, it might not be important to distinguish one from another. Also I will, a little later, assume that we can measure an agent's wants, desires, etc. with a *value function* which takes a higher positive value the more something is wanted, and a lower negative value the more something is disliked; and which is such that if A is wanted as against an alternative B, $V(A) > V(B)$. This last assumption is one of convenience, considerable convenience admittedly, but dispensible nevertheless. The calculation sketches given later could all have been replaced by a purely qualitative and comparative discussion entirely in English.

There is one respect in which what I will be assuming is weaker than Donald Davidson's thesis in 'Actions, Reasons and Causes'.[1] I will *not* be assuming that wants cause actions. For all I assume, it might be the case that it is (always or sometimes) beliefs alone among psychological states that do the causing; the reason that wants are always involved being that wanting in the relevant sense is a consequence of the fact that belief does the causing. According to such a position, what made it true that I wanted to pay my debts may have been nothing more than the fact that my belief that a certain action would have that result was what caused the action. The want did no causing, rather that I had it followed from the fact that the belief did the causing.[2] Alternatively, for all I need, you might hold that wants do the causing, and the fact of belief follows from that. All I need is the common ground that both wants and beliefs are involved.

The main preliminary concerns how I will treat the objects of

1   Reprinted in his *Essays on Actions and Events,*
2   A position of this kind is put by Don Locke, 'Reasons, Wants and Causes', *American Philosophical Quarterly,* **11**, 3 (July 1974), pp. 169–179; and Tom Nagel, *The Possibility of Altruism* (Oxford: Oxford University Press, 1970).

WEAKNESS OF WILL 7

wanting, valuing, *et al.* I am going to borrow from the treatment characteristic of decision theory (though not from those parts embroiled in the dispute over Newcomb's paradox). I will talk of states of affairs as being what is wanted, desired, valued, and so on, and regard them as propositional in that they are subject to the standard logical operations—conjunction, negation, and so forth. (One way of articulating this treatment is by identifying a state of affairs with the set of possible worlds in which it obtains and treating, for instance, conjunction as intersection.) We will be discussing such questions as how the value placed on a state of affairs A relates to that placed on $A\bar{B}$ and AB; and we will be treating A as one and the same as AB or $A\bar{B}$, and as one and the same as ABC or $A\bar{B}C$ or . . .; and so on. Incorporated in this treatment of wanting, desiring, *et al.* is the intuitively appealing idea that how much I want something depends in part on what I think is likely or probable if that something obtains. I want a holiday in the sun. I know that one way this might obtain is by my having a holiday in the sun along with my getting skin cancer obtaining; another is by my having the holiday along with returning refreshed to work obtaining. It is clearly vital to my wanting a holiday in the sun that I judge the second much more likely than the first, if I take that holiday.

The justification for this treatment is partly that it leads naturally to my account of weakness of will, but also that it enables a relatively straightforward account of features of wanting that otherwise are hard to understand. I think that this fact has not received the publicity it deserves. I will consider, briefly and in turn, the account we get of the distinction between derivative and ultimate desires, of why certain inference patterns involving desires are invalid, and of the relationship between conditional and unconditional desires.

(a) Suppose I come to believe that having cold showers will strengthen my moral fibre; then, assuming I am not a masochist, the value I give having cold showers will derive from that I give having them *and* strengthening my moral fibre. (And if I am a masochist, the value will still be derivative, but on the value I give suffering.)

(It can be tempting to say that I don't want, *really* want, to have a cold shower, C, at all. What I really want is the moral uplift, M. I don't want C, I do want M. But this is to restrict one's use of 'want'—or of 'really want'—to what one wants as an ultimate end. And this will not serve the purpose of understanding our ordinary talk of wanting, valuing, *et al.* For the vast majority of things we cite as desirable, including those cited in potential cases of weakness of

8   FRANK JACKSON:

will, are not ultimate ends. And, after all, *derived* value is derived
value.)

   What makes it true that the (positive) value I give C derives from
that I give CM? The answer seems to be the combination of the
following facts: (i) I value CM—the state of affairs of having both
cold showers and strengthened moral fibre. It would not be enough
just to value M; the game has to be worth the candle. (ii) I *dis*value
C$\bar{\text{M}}$. The cold shower without the uplift is of no interest to me. (iii) I
judge CM much more likely than C$\bar{\text{M}}$, given C. In sum, the value of
C derives from that of CM because—although C can obtain by
either CM or C$\bar{\text{M}}$ obtaining, and I disvalue C$\bar{\text{M}}$—I value CM, and
I judge it to be much the most likely given C; to be, that is, much the
most likely way of C's obtaining.

   In general, we can use any mutually exclusive and jointly
exhaustive set of states of affairs $\{B_1, \ldots B_n\}$—(exactly one B_i
obtains at every possible world)—to partition a state of affairs, A,
into $\{AB_1, \ldots, AB_n\}$. And where P is the agent's probability
function, the value of A is related to that of its sub-cases AB_i by

$$(P) \quad V(A) = \sum_i V(AB_i) . P(AB_i/_A) = \sum_i V(AB_i) . P(B_i/_A).$$

Intuitively, $\{AB_i\}$ is *a* set of ways of realizing A, and the value of A is
the value of each of the ways weighted by how likely it is to be the
actual way given A obtains.[1] What we have just been doing, in
effect, is looking at a particular instance of (P), namely V(C)
$= V(CM). P(M/_C) + V(C\bar{M}). P(\bar{M}/_C)$; and noting that the derived
nature of C's value is reflected in the high values of V(CM) and
$P(M/_C)$, together with the low values of V(C$\bar{\text{M}}$) and $P(\bar{\text{M}}/_C)$.

   (A variant on (P) which also is intuitively appealing is

$$(P^*) \qquad V(A) = \sum_i V(AB_i). P(A \,\square\!\!\rightarrow AB_i).$$

However a discussion of the relative merits of (P) and (P*) would
involve inessential complications: the points I wish to make could
be made with either. We will work with (P) as—for reasons related
to the example about blood types to be given shortly—it happens to
be the one I accept.[2])

---

[1]   I have taken (P) from Richard Jeffrey, *Logic of Decision*, New York: McGraw-
      Hill, 1965; see also David Lewis, 'Causal Decision Theory', *Australasian
      Journal of Philosophy*, **59**, 1 (March 1981), pp. 5–30, §2.
[2]   Incidentally the choice between (P) and (P*) is a separate matter from the
      choice between classical and causal decision theory—see Lewis, ibid.

WEAKNESS OF WILL 9

The information about the structure of an agent's values that a partition yields and explicates varies. Partitioning having cold showers into CM and CM̄ told us that my value for C derived from my value for CM. But partitioning can equally reveal—and explicate—irrelevance. Consider a utilitarian who holds that ultimately value is nothing but a matter of the total amount of happiness. Any and every way of partitioning the state of affairs of the total happiness equalling n will give sub-cases all having exactly the same value, because for her everything else is irrelevant when set beside total happiness. For instance, her V (total happiness = n & the happiness is distributed equitably) = her V (total happiness = n & the happiness is not distributed equitably). And if she balks at this, she reveals herself as a lamb in wolf's clothing, as one who tempers utilitarianism with a principle of justice. Ultimate value is a matter of $V(AX) = V(AY)$ for any X, Y. There are, of course, complications. For instance, the value of many states of affairs is neither ultimate nor wholly derivative. Thus, the value I give being happy now derives partly from the fact that I believe happiness breeds happiness, that is, from the fact that I think the most likely way that happiness now will be realized is by happiness now and later being realized; but also the value I give happiness now and later partly derives from that I give happiness now. Also, a person may have a number of ultimate values, which may or may not form a hierarchy.[1] In such a case, the fact that, say, A, B, C are all the states of affairs that are ultimately valued, will be reflected in facts like that $V(ABCX) = V(ABCY)$, $V(\bar{A}\bar{B}\bar{C}X) = V(\bar{A}\bar{B}\bar{C}Y)$, and so on, for any X, Y. But, without going into these complications, I trust enough has been said to show how a decision-theoretic approach can illuminate the nature of derived versus ultimate value.

Incidentally, although what value derives from is often a causal result—we pretended that I believe cold showers *cause* strengthened moral fibre—this is not essential. Suppose I read in a medical journal that a certain blood type is highly correlated with long life, not because it causes long life but because it is a reliable sign of genes which cause long life. Then I would want to have that blood type, and my valuing having it would derive from my wanting long life. (Of course, what I would want would be to have that blood type, not to bring it about that I have it: bringing that about, even if

---

[1]   As in certain *prima facie* duty theories.

it were possible, would achieve nothing, because it wouldn't change my genes.[1]

(b) Donald Davidson in 'Intending'[2] raises the problem that you can desire something sweet yet not desire something sweet and poisonous. How so—after all, eating something sweet and poison-ous is a sure-fire means to eating something sweet. Our answer is that the relationship between the desirability of a state of affairs and its sub-cases is mediated by probability. Provided that eating something sweet and poisonous is a very improbable way of realizing the eating of something sweet, the undesirability of the former does not make the latter undesirable.

Of course, we frequently argue on the pattern: A is desirable, B is a known sure-fire means to A, therefore B is desirable. (And 'desirable' may be replaced by 'ought to be', *et al.*) Now we have, from (P), $V(B) = V(AB). P(A/_B) + V(\bar{A}B). P(\bar{A}/_B)$. If B is a known sure-fire means to A, $P(\bar{A}/_B) = 0$ and $P(A/_B) = 1$, so $V(B) = V(AB)$. Therefore, provided only that B does not unduly detract from A, so that $V(AB)$ and $V(A)$ are close, B must be desirable if A is. This is typically the case when we use the pattern in question: not getting polio is desirable, taking the Sabin vaccine is a known virtually sure-fire means for avoiding polio; therefore, taking the Sabin vaccine is desirable. We ought to be able to vindicate this inference. And we can, because the value of avoiding polio and taking the vaccine is nearly as high as that of avoiding polio.

As well as wanting A without wanting AB, you can want AB, yet not want A. I don't want to smoke, but only because of the risk to health (let's say). That is, I do want to smoke *and* have a long life; my reason for not wanting to smoke is only that I believe it is not that conjunctive state of affairs which would most likely obtain if I smoked, but rather the highly undesirable one of smoking and short life. Hence I want smoking and long-life, but not smoking.

Perhaps the failure of wanting AB to entail wanting A is most transparent when looked at in terms of the contrapositive. It is clear that not wanting A does not entail not wanting AB. Take most things you do not want, can't they be conjoined with something—a million dollars, two million dollars, . . . to give something you do

1   This distinction between wanting A to be the case, and wanting to bring about
    A will be familiar to any 'two-boxer' about Newcomb's paradox. Two-boxers
    want it to be the case that they choose one box, but do not want to bring it about
    that they choose one box. See Lewis, ibid.; and Brian Skyrms, *Causal Necessity*
    (New Haven: Yale University Press, 1980), p. 128 f.
2   Reprinted in his *Essays on Actions and Events*.

want? (You may want the money by itself more, but we are talking about wanting, not most wanting.)

Clearly we can explain the failure of wanting AB to entail wanting A in the same sort of way we explained the failure of wanting A to entail wanting AB. From (P), it is perfectly possible for V(AB) to have a high value while V(A) has a low one; either due to the effect of a low $p(A/_B)$ diminishing V(AB)'s contribution to V(A), or due to V(A$\bar{\text{B}}$) having a significant negative value, or to a combination of both. Intuitively, the typical case will be where AB is an unlikely way for A to obtain, and A$\bar{\text{B}}$ is bad. In the same general sort of way, we can explain why wanting A and wanting B is not equivalent to wanting A-and-B. (Wanting neither agglomerates nor distributes.)

The theme for the past few paragraphs has been that whether a person wants $\bar{\text{A}}$, or wants A more than $\bar{\text{A}}$, depends in part on what they hold likely to be the case if A is the case; and that when you bear this in mind, you can see why the various inference patterns are invalid. It might be objected that what is desirable depends not at all on the person's opinions, but rather on the facts. Smoking was as undesirable before the health risks became known, as it was afterwards. The facts alone, be they known or not, are enough. It would be absurd to say, 'What a pity we know about the health risks; for it is only the knowledge, not the risks themselves, that makes smoking undesirable.' But this is more the making of a distinction than the making of an objection. I am talking about wants, desires, *et al.* in the sense in which they feature in explaining choice, decisions, *et al.*; and in that sense they do depend in part on opinions—or, more exactly, subjective probabilities. Before the health risks became known, I *did* desire to smoke, and that fact is important in explaining my choosing to smoke. I do not, though, deny that there is another notion, for which terms like 'desir*ability*' or '*objective* value' might be used; and I grant that this is independent of opinion, and consequently that a discussion of, for example, whether 'AB is objectively desirable, therefore A is objectively desirable' is valid would have to follow different lines from those above.

(c) Also in 'Intending', Davidson raises a problem about how conditional intentions relate to unconditional ones.[1] A similar problem can be raised for wants and desires. For just about anything I want, it will be true that I do *not* want it if . . .. I want breakfast tomorrow, but I don't want breakfast tomorrow if I'm not

[1] Ibid., esp. p. 100.

hungry. Similarly, I value telling the truth, but not if it leads to World War III. The only wants, desires, values, obligations, intentions, *et al.* for which this is not true, are the ultimate ones. Provided she did not backslide, our utilitarian wanted an increase in total happiness, *be it equitably distributed or not*. The temptation, then, is to hold that all the non-ultimate wants are conditional. It is literally false that I want breakfast tomorrow; all that is literally true is that I want breakfast if I'm hungry.

We need a way of resisting this conclusion, for consider the following sequence: I want breakfast; I do not want breakfast if I am not hungry; I do want breakfast if I am not hungry but need nourishment; I do not want breakfast if I am not hungry but need nourishment though not of the kind provided by breakfast; . . .. If the second member shows that the first is not strictly true, then equally the third must show that the second is not strictly true, and the fourth must show that the third is not strictly true, and so on and on. We won't only lose a host of unconditional wants, but a host of conditional ones as well.

The observations already made show us how to resist the undesirable conclusion. We are dealing with derived wants, for, as we saw, the problem of wanting A but not wanting A if C, does not arise with ultimate ones. Let $\{AB_i\}$ be a partition that reveals (at least in part, whether it goes 'all the way down' to the ultimate wants does not matter) the derivative nature of my want for A. From (P), we have $V(A) = \sum_i V(AB_i) \cdot P(B_i/_A)$. Now the obvious treatment of my want for A if C is to look at what happens to this expression for $V(A)$ if we conditionalize the probabilities in it on C; we look, that is, at $\sum_i V(AB_i) \cdot P(B_i/_{AC})$. Hence I can want A yet not want A if C, in exactly the same way A can be probable yet not be probable given C. It follows that if C is certain according to me, my want for A if C must be the same as my want for A; because if C is certain, conditionalizing on C cannot change the probabilities. This is the right result. The more sure I am that I will be hungry tomorrow, the closer my want for breakfast will be to my want for breakfast if I am hungry.[1]

3.   *The dynamics of value*

The previous section was about the *statics* of value, about how a person's wants at a time for various states of affairs are inter-related;

1   As Davidson, ibid., in effect observes in the case of intention.

but the discussion naturally suggests *one* way that a person's wants may evolve over time. (P) yields a whole host of truths (one for each way of partitioning) of the form $V(A) = \sum_i V(AB_i) \cdot P(B_i/_A)$, about a person's values at a time. When the value an agent gives A changes, these sums will have to change too. The obvious speculation is that *sometimes*, for *some* of these summations, the change will be in the probability terms alone. More specifically, it is that sometimes the value an agent gives A changes on acquiring new information, I, due *not* to any change in the $V(AB_i)$ for some sets of AB_i, but due to the change in the probabilities from $P(B_i/_A)$ to $P(B_i/_{AI})$. (I'm going to assume, for concreteness, that probabilities evolve by conditionalization; and I will sometimes describe the evolution of value consequent upon change in probability alone, as evolution by conditionalizing.)

I think exactly this often happens. At the beginning of 1967 I wanted to smoke more than not smoke, and so did smoke (when I felt like it, not all the time, of course). During 1967 the health risks associated with smoking were drawn to my attention. By the end of 1967 I no longer wanted to smoke more than not smoke, and accordingly stopped smoking. My pro-attitude towards, my preference for, my desire for, the value I gave, . . . smoking went down sharply; and the job was done *entirely by information*—by my reason, if you like. How?

The explanation, in simplified form, can be represented as follows. The state of affairs of my smoking, S, can be partitioned into my smoking and dying young, SD, and my smoking and not dying young, S$\bar{\text{D}}$. My attitude towards each sub-case remained unchanged throughout 1967. The high value of S$\bar{\text{D}}$ remained constant, as did the low value of SD; the information acquired did not change these values. The crucial changes were in my opinion about the chance of D given S—that went up sharply; and in my opinion about the chance of $\bar{\text{D}}$ given S—that went down sharply. Now, from (P), we have $V(S) = V(SD) \cdot P(D/_S) + V(S\bar{\text{D}}) \cdot P(\bar{\text{D}}/_S)$. My $V(SD)$ and $V(S\bar{\text{D}})$ remained as before, and the change in my $V(S)$ was due solely to those in my $P(D/_S)$ and $P(\bar{\text{D}}/_S)$ to, respectively, $P(D/_{SI})$ and $P(\bar{\text{D}}'/_{SI})$, where I is what I learnt about the dangers of smoking.

This change in value, therefore, was determined by my reason alone. Nothing but a change in my probabilities was called for. Let's say, then, that a change in an agent's value, want, *et al.*, for A on learning I is *in accord with the dictates of an agent's reason* if there

is a partition of A (in general, if there is one, there will be many) by
$\{B_i, \ldots, B_n\}$ such that each $V(AB_i)$ is the same before
and after, the change in $V(A)$ being due to the change in the $P(B_i/_A)$
to $P(B_i/_{AI})$; that is, his wants evolve by conditionalization. The
germ of this paper will now be clear. There is a long tradition
according to which weak-willed action is action *not* in accord with
the agent's reason—'passion pushes reason from its throne';[1] thus
my suggestion is that weak-willed action is action arising from
wants and desires that have *not* evolved according to the dictates of
the agent's reason, as just defined.

It may be objected that thirst leads people to want water, and so to
drink water, yet thirst is not a change in subjective probability; it is a
bodily feeling. Hence it may seem that I am forced to judge anyone
who drinks water because he is thirsty as thereby acting incontinently, because he is not acting from a want evolved in accord with
the dictates of reason. This would be directly contrary to our earlier
observation that you can act out of bodily feeling, passion, appetite
and so on, without it having to be the case that you are displaying
weakness of will; and would anyway be absurd.

Thirst can, however, make your wants change so that you choose
to drink, and it still be the case that your wants have evolved in
accord with reason alone. For although thirst is not a belief
(*simpliciter*, anyway), *it typically changes belief*. When I get thirsty, I
acquire beliefs like that my body has a physiological need for water,
and that I am experiencing a vaguely unpleasant feeling. Given
what I know about how drinking meets the need and removes the
feeling, these beliefs in themselves can be more than enough to
explain why my wants change so that I come to want to drink, and so
choose to drink. For simplicity I will just detail this for the impact
of acquiring the belief that I have a need for water.

Let D stand for my drinking in the near future, and U for my
having an unsatisfied need for water; then, from (P), we have:

$$V(D) = V(DU) \cdot P(U/_D) + V(D\bar{U}) \cdot P(\bar{U}/_D),$$
$$V(\bar{D}) = V(\bar{D}U) \cdot P(U/_{\bar{D}}) + V(\bar{D}\bar{U}) \cdot P(\bar{U}/_{\bar{D}}).$$

Suppose that $V(DU)$, $V(D\bar{U})$, $V(\bar{D}U)$, $V(\bar{D}\bar{U})$ all remain the same,

---

1   After writing this paper I read David Pears, 'How Easy is Akrasia', *Philosophia*,
    11, 1–2 (Feb. 1982), pp. 33–50. In setting up the problem he says, 'The idea is
    that your *thoughts* ought to control your actions and akrasia occurs when they
    do not control them. In a case of akrasia the action fails to fit the *preparatory*
    thoughts and is therefore irrational', ibid., p. 33, my emphasis.

WEAKNESS OF WILL 15

before and after I get thirsty; what I have to show is that information consequent on becoming thirsty may change the probability factors in a way which is in itself sufficient to explain why I want to drink in the near future. Before I get thirsty, I know that I don't have an unsatisfied need for water, whether I drink or not. Thus, $P(U/_D)$ and $P(U/_{\bar{D}})$ will be almost nought, and so $P(\bar{U}/_D)$ and $P(\bar{U}/_{\bar{D}})$ will be almost one. Hence, before I get thirsty, $V(D)$ $\simeq V(D\bar{U})$ and $V(\bar{D}) \simeq V(\bar{D}\bar{U})$. As a result $V(D)$ and $V(\bar{D})$ will be much the same. After I get thirsty, I know that I will have an unsatisfied need for water unless I drink in the near future; thus $P(U/_{\bar{D}})$ will be close to one and $P(\bar{U}/_{\bar{D}})$ close to nought. $P(U/_D)$ will remain near nought, because I know that water will relieve the need, and so $P(\bar{U}/_D)$ will stay near one. Consequently, after I get thirsty, $V(D)$ stays near $V(D\bar{U})$, but $V(\bar{D})$ drops to the low value I give $V(\bar{D}U)$—for it is bad to have unsatisfied physiological needs. Hence we have the desired explanation of how probability changes alone can make $V(\bar{D})$ less than $V(D)$, and so make me want to drink water in the near future.

The crucial point here is, put very simply, that agents may value removing thirst—in itself and by virtue of the undesirability of not satisfying physiological needs—even when they are not actually thirsty. Not every traveller in the desert is experiencing thirst when he packs his water bag. At some *fundamental* level, the evaluations of the strong-willed are not changed by the onset of feeling, appetite, emotion, or whatever. Delve deep enough, and you will find a relevant set of evaluations unchanged by the onset of feeling. The change appears on the surface, so to speak, by virtue of changes in the probabilistic way that evaluations of more specific states of affairs feed into evaluations of more general states of affairs.

This treatment of how thirst can change your wants so that you choose to drink, without departing from the dictates of reason, confirms our observation at the very beginning that feelings may have some influence without thereby having the undue influence characteristic of weak-willed behaviour. Similarly, the influence may be greater than normal without being undue in the relevant sense. According to our account, it is irrelevant to weakness of will whether or not the agents' values, wants, *et al.* are like ours or are close to the norm. What matters is, rather, whether feelings and the like have influence over and above that which the change in probability they cause has.

Consider another example, smoking—where weakness of will is

notoriously prevalent. Suppose, for simplicity, that what value
smoking, S, has derives entirely from its role in eliminating a
craving, C. (I understand that this has come to be its only attraction
for some.) From (P), we have

$$V(S) = V(SC) \cdot P(C/_S) + V(S\bar{C}) \cdot P(\bar{C}/_S),$$
$$V(\bar{S}) = V(\bar{S}C) \cdot P(C/_{\bar{S}}) + V(\bar{S}\bar{C}) \cdot P(\bar{C}/_{\bar{S}}).$$

Now consider smoker Fred's situation when he is not experiencing
the craving. Given plausible assumptions, both $P(C/_S)$ and $P(C/_{\bar{S}})$
will then be negligible, both $P(\bar{C}/_S)$ and $P(\bar{C}/_{\bar{S}})$ close to one; hence
$V(S) \simeq V(S\bar{C})$, $V(\bar{S}) \simeq V(\bar{S}\bar{C})$, and so $V(S) \leq V(\bar{S})$. And this, of
course, is the right answer. Smokers don't want to smoke when they
are not experiencing the craving (given our simplifying assumption). What happens when the craving comes on? $P(C/_{\bar{S}})$ will jump
to nearly one, $P(\bar{C}/_S)$ will stay near one (smoking always works to get
rid of the craving), and $P(C/_S)$ and $P(\bar{C}/_{\bar{S}})$ will be near nought.
Hence, if Fred's prior $V(S\bar{C})$ is enough above his prior $V(\bar{S}C)$, we
can explain his $V(S)$ rising above his $V(\bar{S})$, and so his choosing to
smoke, without supposing any change in $V(S\bar{C})$ or $V(\bar{S}C)$. He is
following the dictates of his reason, and so not displaying weakness
of will. On the other hand, his prior $V(S\bar{C})$ may not be enough
above $V(\bar{S}C)$. *When the craving is not on him*, he may value $S\bar{C}$ less
than $\bar{S}C$ (presumably because of the health risks associated with
smoking). In this case, the explanation for his choosing to smoke
when the craving is on him, lies not just in the craving's effect on his
probability function but in its effect on his value function too. The
craving must have lifted $V(S\bar{C})$ above $V(\bar{S}C)$. In this case he is
weak-willed; the mark of his incontinence being the disparity
between his prior and his posterior underlying values consequent
upon the craving.

We can express the difference between the strong-willed smoker
and the weak-willed one in terms of the distinction between
conditional wants (discussed earlier) and conditionals about wants.
Neither smoker has the conditional want to smoke if he has no
craving; both are such that if they have the craving, then they want
to smoke. But they differ in that when they have no craving, the
strong-willed smoker nevertheless has the conditional want to
smoke if he craves to (because his wants evolve by conditializ-
ation), whereas the weak-willed smoker does not. He wants *not* to
smoke if he craves to—although when the time comes, he will want
to smoke.

This joint consequence of our account of weakness of will and of our earlier account of conditional wants seems plausible. Isn't it characteristic of dieters who fear that their wills may not be up to the task, that they are clear that they want not to eat cheesecake when the urge is upon them, while at the same time fearing that when the urge is upon them, they will want to eat cheesecake? They want not to eat when the testing time comes; but fear that when the testing time comes, they will want to eat.

All this assumes that we can talk of how much an agent values eliminating a craving, avoiding thirst, and so on when he is not actually experiencing them. But I don't think there is any real problem here. People usually buy aspirin in anticipation of a headache, not while they are actually experiencing one; picnic hampers are packed before hunger sets in; and so on and so forth. People's behaviour now can indicate the attitudes they take *now* to experiences in the future (and the past), which attitudes may or may not remain the same when the time comes. Consider the behaviour characteristic of dieters who fear that they will be weak-willed. At a time when they are not feeling hungry, they take steps to make it hard to get fattening food when they are hungry—they throw out the cheesecake, they arrange to lunch at special restaurants, they make sure they won't have time to stop at the cakeshop. These actions indicate their attitudes when not hungry. They are doing things which they know will ensure that a state of affairs of their being hungry and slim rather than one of being not hungry and fat, will obtain. Hence, at the time, they value the former more than the latter. But these actions also indicate their knowledge about how these attitudes may change later, when they get hungry; about their tendency to weakness of will. For if their underlying attitudes remained constant, there would be no need to throw out the cheesecake or whatever; if when the hunger struck, they still valued being hungry and slim over being not hungry and fat, then their wants would not be such as to lead them to choose eating.

We can summarize our problem and our answer, as follows. Before the onset of appetite, passion, craving, yearning, or whatever, Fred does not want to smoke, eat, drink, make love, or whatever. After the onset, he does; and does. In saying just this much, I have not said enough to determine whether Fred was weak-willed. The problem is what to add to my description in order to make it true that the explanation of Fred's action is that his will was weak. Our answer is that it depends on what Fred's values were

before the onset. If his prior values, when taken along with the change in his subjective probabilities consequent upon the onset, are enough—as revealed by some suitable instance of (P)—to make him want to smoke, or want to smoke more than not smoke, his action is not a manifestation of weakness of will. On the other hand, if the onset does more than can be got from prior values and posterior probabilities, he is rightly said to succumb to passion or whatever, in the way characteristic of weakness of will.

Thus we explain why it is right to say that the weak-willed act against their reason, and show how to meet the sceptical challenge mooted early in this paper. Consider a fairly typical someone who values remaining slim and also satisfying hunger. The sceptical challenge was what more is there to say than that such a person will frequently find themselves in a conflict situation where one or the other value—not necessarily the same one on different occasions—will prove itself stronger by winning out. What more there is to say concerns the agent's values when not hungry.[1]

DEPARTMENT OF PHILOSOPHY,
MONASH UNIVERSITY,
CLAYTON,
VICTORIA,
AUSTRALIA 3168

1   I am indebted to David Lewis, Elizabeth Prior, and Peter Singer for forcing changes to earlier versions of this paper; but I fear the changes may not be as great as they should be.

[19]

SKEPTICISM ABOUT WEAKNESS OF WILL*
Gary Watson

Two kinds of skepticism

Although it occurs with deplorable frequency, weakness of will has seemed to many philosophers hard to understand. The motivation of weak behavior[1] is generally familiar and intelligible enough: the desire to remain in bed, or the desire for another drink are ordinary examples. Nevertheless, our common ways of describing and explaining this phenomenon have been thought to involve serious difficulties. These descriptions and explanations can, upon reflection, seem incoherent.

Accordingly, weakness of will has given rise to various forms of skepticism. The most notorious form is socratism, which denies the possibility of such behavior. Another form of skepticism admits its possibility but casts doubt upon a complex of distinctions and moral attitudes involved in the common view. Briefly, it argues that no one who acts contrary to his or her better judgment does so freely, that weakness of will cannot be significantly distinguished from psychological compulsion[2], and that therefore certain moral distinctions implicit in the common view cannot be justified.

My concern in this paper will be to explore and develop a version of nonsocratic skepticism. In my view, socratism is incorrect, but like Socrates, I think that the common understanding of weakness of will raises serious problems. Contrary to soc-

---

* Many people have contributed to my thinking on this topic. I am especially grateful to Robert Audi, Charles Kahn, Ruth Mattern, the editors of the *Philosophical Review,* and Michael Slote.
    [1] Weakness of will occurs only if one knowingly does something contrary to one's better judgment. We will see that this condition does not distinguish between weakness and compulsion.
    [2] I shall assume throughout that if someone is psychologically compelled to do something, he or she is unable to refrain from doing it (though not necessarily conversely). The compulsive's motivation is literally irresistible. This concept is discussed further on page 323.

GARY WATSON

ratism, it is possible for a person knowingly to act contrary to his or her better judgment. But this description does not exhaust the common view of weakness. Also implicit in this view is the belief that actions which are contrary to one's better judgment are free in the sense that the agent could have done otherwise. The grounds for skepticism about this belief will be my theme.[3]

To clear the way and to introduce some important distinctions, it will be helpful to begin with a discussion of socratic skepticism. Then I will set out what I take to be the crucial elements in the common account of weakness, and consider the apparent emptiness of that account as an explanatory model; it is said that one takes the drink *because* one's will is weak, for example, and this explanation is supposed to contrast with the compulsive case in which one takes the drink because one's desire is too strong. Finally, I will discuss and compare the merits of an alternative way of drawing the distinction between weakness and compulsion.

Socrates and Davidson

A brief look at Donald Davidson's essay, "How is Weakness of Will Possible?",[4] will help us to isolate the errors of socratism. His paper is worth considering because, among other reasons, it contains an excellent formulation of some principles which have caused much of the traditional philosophical trouble. Although I believe his own solution to have difficulties of its own, I wish rather to examine the way in which he generates the problem.

Davidson sees the problem of "incontinence" as arising from the apparent incompatibility between two principles which connect judgment, motivation, and action, and the belief that

---

[3] In the socratic dialogues of Plato, the view that Socrates denies is often formulated as the view that people often, *freely and voluntarily,* act contrary to their better judgments. This position will be rejected by both forms of skepticism. But the focus of Socrates' arguments is the weaker proposition that one can knowingly act contrary to one's better judgment. Hence I call "socratic" only this version of skepticism.

[4] In *Moral Concepts,* edited by Joel Feinberg, Oxford University Press, 1970.

SKEPTICISM ABOUT WEAKNESS OF WILL

incontinence (possibly) exists. He characterizes incontinence in this way:

In doing *x* an agent acts incontinently if and only if: (*a*) the agent does *x* intentionally; (*b*) the agent believes there is an alternate action *y* open to him; and (*c*) the agent judges that, all things considered, it would be better to do *y* than to do *x* (p. 94).

The principles with which the belief in the existence of incontinence is at odds are these:

P1. If an agent wants to do *x* more than he wants to do *y* and he believes himself free to do either *x* or *y*, then he will intentionally do *x* if he does either *x* or *y* intentionally.

P2. If an agent judges that it would be better to do *x* than to do *y*, then he wants to do *x* more than he wants to do *y* (p. 95).

As Davidson says, P1 connects "wanting" with "acting intentionally," whereas P2 connects "judging better" with "wanting." He insists that the tension cannot be alleviated by modifying these principles to make them both true and consistent with the belief in incontinence—not that P1 and P2 are crystal clear and unambiguous as they stand: but "the problem will survive new wording, refinement, and elimination of ambiguity" (p. 96).

Since Davidson accepts these principles and believes incontinence exists, he must deny that these principles logically conflict with this belief. The main burden of his paper is to show how we may accept them and still maintain weakness to be possible. The first point to notice, then, is that with the appropriate addition of the phrase "all things considered" to P2, the principles and the belief in incontinence clearly are contradictory. The incontinent are supposed to act against their all-things-considered judgments; but P2 is stated in terms of judgment *simpliciter*. It is this apparent difference that Davidson exploits. What he thinks happens in incontinence (so defined) is that one acts contrary to one's all-things-considered judgment; but in so acting one acts in accordance with one's "unconditional" or "unqualified" judgment, or with one's judgment *simpliciter* (pp. 110-113).

Several questions arise about Davidson's position. First, is the distinction between a judgment all-things-considered and an unqualified or unconditional judgment sound? It might well be supposed that an all-things-considered judgment is precisely an unqualified judgment made on the basis of all considerations thought relevant by the agent. Second, even if this distinction were made out, is there not equally good reason to think that people act contrary to their unqualified or unconditional judgments, as there is to think that people act contrary to their all-things-considered judgments? Davidson's theses entail that this is impossible. Third, are *P*1 and *P*2 true?

Davidson's remarks on practical reasoning are certainly novel and interesting; but it is this last question that will concern me here, for the problem lies with these socratic principles. Aside from the fact that *P*1 and *P*2 lead to a denial of what intuitively seems to exist, there are strong general reasons for rejecting them. To see this, recall the reasoning in Plato's *Protagoras* which led Socrates (or the early Plato) to deny the possibility of *akrasia*. In this work, Socrates denied the common account, according to which agents may knowingly fail to do what they believe best in the situation, because they yield to temptation, or short-term pleasure, or are overcome by appetite. Socrates denied this account because he believed that human beings always most desire, and hence pursue, what is (thought to be) best (compare *P*1 and *P*2). On this supposition, in acting weakly they would have to be pursuing what they believe to be best, believing it not to be best.

Instead, Socrates insisted that what is called weakness of will (*akrasia*) is really a species of ignorance. The weak agent suffers from a kind of evaluation illusion, very like an optical illusion—the nearer, more immediate good looks the greater. The so-called weak agent lacks the art of measurement, the art of correctly weighing nearer and farther goods, and to have this art is to have knowledge of good and evil. (Hence the thesis that virtue is a kind of knowledge, to which I shall return.)

Despite the ingenuity of this appeal to evaluational illusions (which I think in fact occur), the later Plato came to see this matter differently. He came to realize that we are generally susceptible to motivation which is independent, in strength and origin, of our

SKEPTICISM ABOUT WEAKNESS OF WILL

judgments concerning how it is best to act. Plato's distinction between the rational and nonrational parts of the soul may be taken as a distinction between sources of motivation. The rational part of the soul is the source of evaluations—judgments as to the value or worth of a particular course of action or state of affairs. The nonrational part of the soul is the source of such desires as arise from the appetites and emotions. These desires are blind in the sense that they do not depend fundamentally upon the agent's view of the good. Since these sources of motivation differ, they may conflict, and in certain cases, the desires of the nonrational soul may motivate the agent contrary to his or her "desires" for the good. In some such way, Plato tried to account for motivational conflict and for the possibility of both self-mastery and its opposite.[5]

On the basis of this distinction, then, Plato rejected Socrates' (or his own earlier) view that a person's desires are always desires for the "good" and that what a person most desires is what is (thought) best. Elementary as these points are, they suffice to show the possibility of weakness of will. The desires of hunger and sex, the desires of anger and fear, do not depend upon one's assessment of the value of doing what one is thereby inclined to do. But if such desires exist, as they surely do, then it is possible that they are strong enough to motivate one contrary to one's judgment of what is best; it is possible that one's evaluations and desires diverge in certain cases in such a way that one is led to do things which one does not think worth doing, or as much worth doing as some available option. Hence socratism is false. There are no good theoretical grounds for denying *akrasia*.

To bring these points to bear on Davidson's principles: let us distinguish two senses of "wants more" or "wants most," an evaluational sense and motivational sense.[6] In the first sense,

---

[5] I develop this distinction, and apply it to the concept of free action, in "Free Agency", *Journal of Philosophy,* April 24, 1975.

An interpretative point: Plato appears to have held that the distinction between knowledge and belief is relevant in some way I fail to appreciate. Hence he may still have denied the possibility of acting contrary to one's *knowledge.*

[6] The distinction between the language of motivation and the language of evaluation is clearly drawn by G. Santas, in "Plato's *Protagoras,* and Explanations of Weakness", *The Philosophical Review,* 1966. His discussion of weakness

GARY WATSON

if one wants to do *x* more than one wants to do *y*, one *prefers x* to *y* or ranks *x* higher than *y* on some scale of values or "desirability matrix." In the second sense, if one wants to do *x* more than *y*, one is more strongly motivated to do *x* than to do *y*. Thus, *P2* may be true if understood in the language of evaluation, but false if understood in the language of motivation; whereas *P1* is true if understood in the language of motivation, but false if understood in the language of evaluation. If a person judges *x* to be better than *y*, then he or she values *x* more than *y*. But as we have seen, it does not follow that the agent's desire or want for *x*, rather than for *y*, will motivate the agent to act (if either does). But this must follow if *P1* and *P2* are jointly to have the consequences that Davidson accepts. There is no univocal interpretation of the key phrases of *P1* and *P2* on which these principles turn out to be true, or even very plausible.

Thus, even though Davidson wishes to allow the existence of "incontinence," in these principles we encounter the socratic viewpoint once again. It is important to note in addition that the above principles also rule out the possibility of being compulsively motivated to act contrary to one's practical judgment. Once we are disabused of the idea that the strength of one's desire is necessarily proportional to the degree to which one values its object, there is conceptual room for compulsion as well as weakness.[7] The real problem, as we shall see, is not to admit but to distinguish them. But first it will be instructive to look at some related distortions implicit in the socratic theory of virtue.

Self-control and the socratic theory of virtue

Consider the virtue of courage, and how this virtue is misconceived by the socratic view. Courage is a virtue which it is in the

---

is one of the best that I know of. In insisting upon this distinction, I do not wish to assert a semantical ambiguity of "want." The point is rather that there are different, and noncoincident criteria for whether someone wants to do one thing *more than* another.

[7] The existence of weakness of will, or generally the divergence between evaluation and motivation, reveals one kind of limitation on decision theory, conceived as an explanatory theory of behavior. Decision theory will be correct only on the assumption (often unjustified) of "continence." Explaining weak action will require a different branch of psychology.

SKEPTICISM ABOUT WEAKNESS OF WILL

interest of everyone to have, and is in this respect like continence. Now for Socrates, courage is, as it should be, the virtue which applies to situations of danger. But for him it applies in the following eccentric way: courage is the knowledge of what is really dangerous or not. Since Socrates thought that the only danger is evil, or doing evil, all that it takes to possess the virtue of courage, and to act courageously in appropriate circumstances, is the knowledge of what is good and evil. (This is the keystone of his doctrine of the unity of the virtues: each virtue is a special case of wisdom (knowledge of good and evil) applied to particular contexts: courage is wisdom about danger, temperance is wisdom about what is really pleasant, justice is wisdom applied to social relationships and statecraft, and so on. If you have wisdom in general, then you will have the other virtues, and if you lack one of these, you will lack wisdom). Hence the coward is one who has a false view of what is really dangerous. The courageous person is one who is able to distinguish apparent from real dangers.

But surely courage is not like this. Courage is the capacity to deal with one's fear in contexts where one is thereby spontaneously inclined to actions which are contrary to one's view of what should be done. The virtue of courage has a role only because we are not as Socrates says we are; it is needed because of the irrational part of the soul, because our inclinations do not always harmonize with our judgments of the good. Socrates thinks that the courageous person's virtue is that he or she sees there is nothing really to fear, whereas the coward is benighted about this. But the truth appears to be that courage is needed precisely where there *is* something to fear, but where this emotion would lead one to act contrary to one's better judgment.

Courage is thus a special type of self-control; it is self-control in situations of personal danger. Consequently, self-control has a broader application than to pleasure and temptation. If human psychology were as Socrates assumes, such a virtue would have no use. Self-control is a virtue only for beings who are susceptible to motivation which is in potential conflict with their judgments of what is good to pursue; only to beings like ourselves who have

322

GARY WATSON

appetites and emotions which may incline them contrary to their better judgments.[8]

In passing, it is worth noting that possessing the capacity to make one's practical judgments effective in action is generally in the interest of every being with some sort of view of how to live, and does not presuppose a particularly austere or "rationalistic" ethic. Even those who favor spontaneity and propose to follow their inclinations should want the virtue of self-control. To use an example of Thomas Nagel,[9] even those who favor a spontaneous life will want to be able to resist the sudden urge to join the Marine Corps—or more generally, to resist those inclinations the satisfaction of which would render them unable to act impulsively in the future.

As I see it, then, the virtue of self-control is the capacity to counteract recalcitrant motivation, that is, motivation which is contrary to one's better judgment. It is this virtue that the weak agent lacks, or at least fails to exercise; and for this virtue, knowledge in the ordinary sense is clearly insufficient. Now both compulsion and weakness of will involve a failure of self-control. In the next section, I want to consider some common ways of distinguishing these types of failure.

Weakness and compulsion

Suppose that a particular woman intentionally takes a drink. To provide an evaluative context, suppose also that we think she

---

[8] The appetites and emotions are not the only sources of such motivation. Perhaps appetites (like hunger, thirst, sex) may be distinguished from emotions (like anger, fear, resentment) in that the latter essentially involve beliefs (that something is dangerous, that one has been wronged, that another is obstructing one), whereas appetites do not. But the following examples do not seem to fit clearly into either category—the inclinations arising from pain, the inclination to excrete, the inclination to sleep (arising from sleepiness)—and these surely belong to the "nonrational" part of the soul. Why isn't sleepiness, like hunger, an appetite?

Let me hasten to add that, as Ruth Mattern has pointed out to me, self-control should not be conceived as a unified capacity, such that if one has it in one area, one will have it in all areas. A person may be "soft" with respect to pain, but never yield to temptation, or one may be perfectly courageous, but continually give in to the desire to drink.

[9] In *The Possibility of Altruism,* Oxford, The Clarendon Press, 1970.

SKEPTICISM ABOUT WEAKNESS OF WILL

ought not to have another because she will then be unfit to fulfill some of her obligations. Preanalytically, most of us would insist on the possibility and significance of the following three descriptions of the case. (1) the reckless or self-indulgent case; (2) the weak case; and (3) the compulsive case. In (1), the woman knows what she is doing but accepts the consequences. Her choice is to get drunk or risk getting drunk. She acts in accordance with her judgment. In (2) the woman knowingly takes the drink contrary to her (conscious) better judgment; the explanation for this lack of self-control is that she is weak-willed. In (3), she knowingly takes the drink contrary to her better judgment, but she is a victim of a compulsive (irresistible) desire to drink.

These variations reveal the leading features of the common conception of weakness. On this model, the weak drinker is like the compulsive drinker in that she acts contrary to her better judgment,[10] but she is like the reckless drinker in that she is able to resist the drink. Accordingly, she is placed morally somewhere "in between" the others. Since she acted contrary to her judgment, she is not, like the reckless drinker, just morally "bad"— her values and judgment are not in question. But unlike the compulsive, she is not a victim of irresistible desires. She shares with the reckless the ability to resist, and for this reason we hold her responsible.

The common account, then, insists that the weak person has, but fails to exercise, the capacity of self-control. It is this requirement that nonsocratic skepticism challenges. Before posing the challenge, I will illustrate and clarify the concept of motivational compulsion, and then raise some preliminary difficulties in distinguishing it from weakness. Subsequently, I will argue that this common way of making the distinction is untenable, and will propose an alternative way that does not rest upon this requirement.

The notion of psychological or motivational compulsion is probably an extension of the ordinary notion of interpersonal

---

[10] Acting contrary to one's better judgment is not, however, a necessary condition of compulsion; one's desire might be compulsive and happen to accord with one's judgment.

compulsion, in which one person is forced by another to act
"against his will." Although psychological compulsion may not
be widely recognized in ordinary life, I think that the concepts of
mania, phobia, and addiction imply its possibility.[11] I shall
assume that when an action is literally compelled motivationally,
the agent is motivated by a desire (or "impulse" or "inclination")
that he or she is unable to resist. In illustration, a man might have
a dread fear of spiders or rats so overwhelmingly strong that, even
when it is urgently important for him to do so, he is literally unable to handle one. Or a starving woman may be driven by her
hunger to do such acts as she would rather die than perform. Or a
drug addict, because of his or her unconquerable craving for the
drug, may be unable (at least over a span of time) to refuse the
opportunity to obtain and consume some heroin.

It is not true that manic and phobic actions are necessarily
compulsive; the motivations may raise the cost of alternative
actions prohibitively, and thus "coerce" rather than compel. If
I give in to my fear of flying, recognizing all the while that this
fear is baseless, it does not follow that I was compelled to remain
grounded. It may rather be that the difficulties and anxieties involved in my overcoming my admittedly irrational fear make
doing so too costly. (Nor would this be a case of weakness of will;
here I act on my judgment that flying is not worth the suffering.)
However, there may be circumstances in which I am unable to
overcome my phobia, even when it is practically urgent for me
to fly. Nevertheless, even though manic or phobic desires do not
necessarily compel, they are potentially compulsive in that their
strength is to a large degree independent of the person's will.

In what follows, I wish to exclude from consideration cases of
unconscious or "semi-conscious" or self-deceptive actions. Where
one deceives oneself about what is best, or about one's situation
of action, one does not act contrary to one's better judgment, but
rather in accordance with one's self-deceptive judgment. Or
perhaps in such cases, it is radically unclear what the real judgment *is*. Self-deception is itself philosophically troublesome, and

---

[11] See the leading psychological study, *Fears and Phobias*, by Marks. In his
discussion of "obsessive-compulsive" neuroses, Freud also speaks of being unable to resist certain "impulses".

SKEPTICISM ABOUT WEAKNESS OF WILL

as a matter of fact many actions we call weak may involve self-deception of some sort. But no philosophical reasons drive us to redescribe the phenomenon in this way, and certainly the common view insists on the possibility of "clear-headed" action contrary to better judgment. Furthermore, the problems raised by weakness of will differ distinctively from the problems raised by self-deception. The former problem is how a judgment can fail to lead to appropriate action. The latter problem concerns the way in which beliefs and judgments can be influenced by desires. Consequently, I will restrict my attention to actions involving failures of the former kind.[12]

Preliminary difficulties

It is important to emphasize that "weakness of will," in ordinary usage, purports to be an explanatory concept; weakness of will is not just any sort of action contrary to the agent's judgment. To identify behavior in this way is to offer a minimal kind of explanation: one acts contrary to one's better judgment *because* one is weak; one *yields* to temptation, *allows* oneself to give in to appetite, and so forth.

Now the force of this explanation is quite unclear, especially if it is supposed to contrast with an explanation in terms of compulsion. For the present, the problem of distinguishing weakness from compulsion may be expressed in the following way. In those examples given earlier, what is most striking, and leads naturally to the invocation of the notion of compulsion, is that the agents' actual motivation is independent of any conception that they have of the worth of their actions. Their motivation is in this way

---

[12] On a larger view, this distinction may prove to be superficial. If, as I suggest, self-control or strength of will is the capacity to ensure that one's practical judgment is effective in action, then presumably it would be part of this capacity to maintain clarity of judgment in the face of temptation. In a significant sense, one's practical judgment is ineffective in self-deceptive action, and one can yield to bad reasoning as well as directly to temptation. But I shall adhere in the text to this characterization of weakness as action contrary to one's conscious and immediate practical judgment, both for simplicity and because this case is conceptually most problematic for my concerns.

326

GARY WATSON

"alien" to them. In some significant sense, they seem motivated contrary to their own wills. Clearly, the "will" here cannot be the *strongest* motive; for compulsives do not act contrary to their strongest motive. They act contrary to their judgments of the worth of their actions. It is plausible, then, to identify the "will" with practical judgment. This suggests that the mark of a compulsive desire is its capacity to motivate the agent contrary to practical judgment. But it follows that the weak agent acts contrary to his or her judgment in exactly the same sense, and therefore acts under compulsion.

This consequence is admittedly counterintuitive. Surely if it is plausible in some circumstances to say that a starving person is unable to resist taking the bread, that in general compulsives are driven ineluctably to acts beyond their control, it is quite implausible to say this of the well-nourished who capitulate to their fondness for bagels.

Similarly, we are inclined to contrast weakness and compulsion like so: in the case of compulsive acts, it is not so much that the will is too weak as that the contrary motivation is too strong; whereas, in weakness of will properly so-called, it is not that the contrary motivation is too strong, but that the will is too weak.

There is, I think, something correct in this contrast; but the following difficulty remains. This talk of strength of desires is obscure enough, but insofar as it has meaning, there does not appear to be any way of judging the strength of desires except as they result in action. For why is it said that the compulsive's desires are too strong? Isn't it just because these agents are motivated contrary to their wills? Isn't the only relatively clear measure of strength of desires the tendency of those desires to express themselves independently of the agent's will? If this is so, the desires which motivate the weak contrary to their judgments are "too strong" as well, and explanations of weakness and compulsion come to the same thing. We are left again with the conclusion that weakness is a case of compulsion.[13]

---

[13] A few remarks on internalism may be in order here. I am supposing, as I think we ordinarily do, that when one acts weakly, one wants to some degree to do what one judges best. Weakness of will is marked by conflict and regret. However, this supposition does not entail a commitment to a general internalist

SKEPTICISM ABOUT WEAKNESS OF WILL

We have seen why socratism is to be rejected, but a real problem remains. If a sufficient condition of compulsive motivation is that the motivation be contrary to the agent's practical judgment, then weakness of will is a species of compulsion. And if compulsive behavior is involuntary and unfree, weak behavior is involuntary and unfree. In any case, weakness and compulsion are on a par. The intuition that the agent's will is too weak, whereas in the other case, the contrary motivation is too strong, appears to rest on an illusion.

One way to avoid this conclusion—that all weak actions are compulsive—would be to argue that no actions are compulsive, since no desires are irresistible. One philosopher who is skeptical about the idea of an irresistible desire is Joel Feinberg. "There is much obscurity in the notion of the strength of a desire," Feinberg writes, but he thinks several points are clear:

The first is that strictly speaking no impulse is irresistible; for every case of giving in to a desire, I would argue, it will be true that, if the person had tried harder he would have resisted it successfully. . . . Nevertheless, it does make sense to say that some desires are stronger than others and that some have an intensity and power that are felt as overwhelming.[14]

Feinberg's confidence on these points puzzles me. One may well be dubious in practice about particular pleas of irresistibility. And, if one is in the dark about the notion of strength, one may well have blanket doubts about such claims. But if it is granted

---

view that a person necessarily wants what he or she judges best. (Note that even this general view is a weaker internalism than Davidson's *P2*.) For even if it is possible not at all to want what one judges best, it would be a distortion to describe such a case as weakness of will. For such an externalist agent would have a strong and undivided will—and what he or she lacked certainly would not be self-control. I think one trouble with Davidson's discussion (op. cit.) is that it leaves untouched the way in which weakness of will is supposed to involve weakness; "incontinence" turns out to be a "surd" noncompliance with the "principle of continence," and hence is construed as merely practical irrationality. (Compare Nietzsche's remark: "When the mind is made up, the ear is deaf to even the best arguments. This is the sign of a strong character. In other words, an occasional will to stupidity." [*Beyond Good and Evil*, sec. 107] Consider also a cartoon I recently saw. On his way to the local bar, the character encounters his priest, who asks him, "Have you no self-control?" He replies, "Yes, Father, I have, but I will not be a slave to it.")

[14] "What is So Special about Mental Illness?", in *Doing and Deserving*, Princeton University Press, 1970, pp. 282-283.

GARY WATSON

that desires may be *hard* to resist, on what grounds can it be denied that sometimes desires may be *too* hard to resist? Why must the feeling that some desires are overwhelmingly "intense and powerful" be mistaken? What puzzles me is how the possibility of irresistible desires can be rejected a priori unless the notion of strength here is altogether empty.

Not only do many psychologists assume this possibility, the common view of weakness seems committed to it as well. For it insists that the weak person has but does not exercise the capacity to resist. This insistence presupposes the intelligibility of lacking this capacity. In any case, even if it is true, as Feinberg believes, that in all cases, "if the person had tried harder, he would have resisted," this does not show that no desires are irresistible. For a person may be unable to try harder and for this reason be unable to resist.

Therefore, it seems unjustified to hold that no desires are too strong for an agent to resist. In fact, we very frequently compare the strengths of desires, both when they are those of a particular individual at a given time, and when the desires belong to different persons or the same person at different times. (*P*'s desire to lounge in bed is stronger than his desire to keep appointments; *Q* has stronger sexual desires than most, or than she herself had when she was fifteen.) It is not clear what criteria we invoke in such comparisons, but two obvious criteria are clearly unhelpful. Motivational efficacy will not do because on this measure any desire which motivates would thereby be the strongest.[15] And this measure would not allow for significant interpersonal comparisons. Nor, once again, will independence of the agent's will or better judgment do, for then the desires of the weak and the compulsive will be equally strong.

---

[15] This needs some qualification. The motivational efficacy of desire could be understood counterfactually. For example, it may be that a woman is motivated by her thirst rather than her hunger, even though the latter is stronger than the former in this sense: if she had thought she could satisfy her hunger, that desire rather than her thirst would have motivated her. But the statement in the text seems to hold for *competing* desires, where two desires are competing if the agent believes it is now possible to satisfy either but not both. I owe this notion of a competing desire to Robert Audi.

SKEPTICISM ABOUT WEAKNESS OF WILL

Strength and resistibility

It might help at this point to return to my earlier description of self-control as the capacity to resist recalcitrant desires; such desires are strong to the extent to which they *need* to be resisted. For again, not all actual desires which one does not in the end act upon are therefore resisted. To resist cannot simply be to refrain from acting upon some desire one has. As Aristotle observed (*Nicomachean Ethics,* 1152a1 ff.), there is a difference between the "continent" and the "temperate" person which rests upon the notion of strength. For both types, "choice" regulates action— both act upon their evaluations—but while the temperate person has moderate appetites, the continent person acts rightly *despite* strong contrary inclinations. A person's desires are moderate to the degree to which they do not require resistance.

The important point is that practical conflict may assume both a decision-theoretic and a psychological form. When the conflict takes the first form, it arises from the question of what to do. But motivational conflicts may persist after this question is settled. Here the strength of desires is revealed and the need for resistance emerges. The temperate are less susceptible than others to this motivational conflict. Their souls are harmonious. The continent are so susceptible, but manage to resist. The weak fail.

Why then do the continent manage successfully to resist, whereas the weak do not? The answer cannot be that the weak are subject to stronger desires than the continent, for this would not explain why they are weaker; nor would it enable us to distinguish weakness from compulsion. The proposal I now wish to entertain is the following. The weak and the strong may be subject to desires of exactly the same strength. What makes the former weak is that they give in to desires which the possession of the normal degree of self-control would enable them to resist. In contrast, compulsive desires are such that the normal capacities of resistance are or would be insufficient to enable the agent to resist. This fact about compulsive desires is what gives substance to the claim that they are too strong. The fact that weak agents' desires would be controlled by the exercise of the normal capacities of resistance gives point to the claim that these agents are weak.

330

GARY WATSON

Something like this distinction is suggested by a passage of Aristotle. He remarks that the difference between weakness and what we have called compulsion might depend on the fact that the desires which defeat the weak person are such that most people could have resisted:

> . . . if a man is defeated by violent and excessive pleasures or pains, there is nothing wonderful in that; indeed we are ready to pardon him if he has resisted [is overcome while offering resistance—Ostwald] . . . But it is surprising if a man is defeated by and cannot resist pleasures and pains which most men can hold out against, when this is not due to heredity and disease . . . (*Nicomachean Ethics,* 1150*b*7 ff., Ross trans.).

This way of expressing the point is unfortunate; for it may suggest that desires are like barbells which most people can or cannot lift. Whatever the ontological status of desires, it does not seem intelligible to say of an inclination that a particular person has on a particular occasion, that most others would be able to hold out against that very inclination. It makes better sense to ask not whether other people could have resisted that particular motivation—but whether the individual would have been able to hold out had he or she possessed and exercised the kinds of capacity of self-control normally possessed by others, or whether persons of normal self-control would resist similar desires of the same strength. Such a counterfactual is no doubt formidable to establish, but at least it is intelligible. I suggest that when we believe it, or something like it, to be true of people who do not resist, we think them weak (the fault is with them, not with the opposing desires); when we believe that they could not have resisted even so, then we think of them as victims of compulsion (the fault is not with them, but rather their desires are too strong). (Perhaps this way of looking at the matter also presupposes that we believe weak persons both could and should possess and exercise those skills—otherwise it would not be their *fault.*) In this manner, we can distinguish among "temperance" and "continence" (in Aristotle's sense), weakness and compulsion. And we can avoid saying either that no desires are irresistible or that weakness is a case of compulsion.

In summary, then, there are capacities and skills of resistance which are generally acquired in the normal course of socialization

SKEPTICISM ABOUT WEAKNESS OF WILL

and practice, and which we hold one another responsible for acquiring and maintaining. Weak agents fall short of standards of "reasonable and normal" self-control (for which we hold them responsible), whereas compulsive agents are motivated by desires which they could not resist even if they met those standards. That is why we focus on the weakness of the agent in the one case (it is the agent's fault), but on the power of the contrary motivation in the compulsive case. And this view allows explanations in terms of weakness of will to be significantly different from explanations in terms of compulsion. In the case of weakness, one acts contrary to one's better judgment *because one has failed* to meet standards of reasonable or normal self-control; whereas, this explanation does not hold of compulsive behavior.

Let us now note some of the implications of this proposal. One obvious point is that, on this account, a desire is compulsive (irresistible) or not only relative to certain norms of self-control; only relative to the capacities of the normal person, and this probably means the typical adult in our society. It may be true, for example, that having undergone from childhood an intensive program of discipline, such as yoga, would have enabled a person to resist certain desires now. But this fact would not incline us at all to withdraw the claim that the individual was suffering from compulsive desires. Hence the fact that one would be a weak person in a community of yogis does not mean that one would not be compulsive among us. (It does not follow from this account, however, that weak agents are those with less self-control than most others in their society *in fact* have. Weakness is relative to expectations and norms, and it is conceivable that a whole community could fall short of these.)

The relativity of this viewpoint may conflict with our ordinary view of weakness; perhaps prior to reflection we think that a desire is either resistible or it isn't. Even so, it seems to me that this relativity is a desirable feature of the present account. We could define an absolute concept of compulsion in something like the following manner: an agent is motivated by a compulsive desire if *no* degree of training and discipline would have enabled him or her to resist. But it is an open question whether *any* desires are compulsive on this definition, and it does not seem to apply in

332

the right way to the cases we think of as compulsive. Relativity is in any case a feature of the concept of weakness in general—for example, the concept of physical weakness. The possible existence of races of creatures who could lift 500-pound weights, or of training programs which would enable most of us to do so, would not mean that those of us who cannot lift this weight were physically weak.[16]

This doctrine accords fairly closely with typical moral attitudes toward weakness as well. In contrast to "bad characters," we do not criticize weak agents for their principles or values but for their failure to develop or maintain the capacities necessary to make those values effective in action. The appropriate blaming attitudes toward the weak, by themselves and others, are shame and (if one goes in for this sort of thing) contempt, not guilt and indignation. For the fault is not injustice, but lack of control. And since they have (or may have) the right values, they are as much an object of pity as reproach—from any point of view, *especially their own,*[17] they are in a bad way. Since shame characteristically involves falling short of shared standards of excellence in conduct, shame will often be appropriate in the case of weakness in a way in which it will not be for compulsion.[18]

The proposed account versus the common account

The proposed account entails that the desires of weak agents are resistible in the sense that had they developed and maintained

---

[16] Note, however, that on this account I could easily be mistaken about whether my action was weak or compulsive, because I could be mistaken about what the relevant standards were. Indeed, in the absence of shared expectations and norms the distinction might come to lose its force altogether.

[17] For one's "point of view" includes preeminently the values which determine one's better judgment.

[18] To say that there is generally a moral contrast between weak and compulsive behavior is neither to deny that a compulsive may sometimes be blameworthy, nor to imply that a weak person always is. Just as compulsive agents may sometimes be responsible and blameworthy for having allowed themselves to become or remain compulsive, so the failure of the weak agent might be excusable, as Aristotle intimates, if it were due to "disease." Perhaps we would not or should not classify such a person as weak of will; we would not call a person negligent who was subnormally careless due to disease. If so, weakness of will differs in this respect from physical weakness, which carries no implication of responsibility.

SKEPTICISM ABOUT WEAKNESS OF WILL

certain normal capacities of self-control, they would have resisted them. And to the degree to which we judge such agents blameworthy and responsible for their weak behavior, we believe they could and should have developed and maintained these capacities. So the weak must be constitutionally capable of meeting these standards. But these implications are consistent with their being unable at the time of action to resist. Hence, this account differs significantly from the common one. On the latter the ability to resist at the time of action is a distinguishing feature of weakness.

Morally, the proposed account likens weakness to negligence in its emphasis on the point that blameworthiness does not require that one be able to resist or that weak behavior be fully under voluntary control. For negligence is a paradigm case of blameworthy but nonvoluntary behavior. Engrossed in an interesting conversation, a man forgets to look both ways at the intersection and therefore collides with another vehicle. He does not do so voluntarily, or even intentionally, and yet we may judge him blameworthy for failing to meet standards (or the "duty") of reasonable care. (To be sure, the man is engaged in numerous voluntary actions at the time of the collision, but colliding, for which he is blamed, is not among them.) Could he have remembered? It is not at all clear that he could have. Remembering is not in this case even an action. What we believe is that he should have remembered to look and because of this, that he falls short of standards of reasonable care. The accident is explained by his fault (just as weak behavior is explained by the agent's fault). [19]

Perhaps to think him blameworthy we must also believe that he could have been or become the kind of person who exercises reasonable care. But these beliefs do not entail that he was able, at the time of action, to avoid the accident. On the proposed account, the case of weak behavior is quite parallel. The weak person may be seen as negligent for failing to acquire the relevant

---

[19] I do not suppose that the phenomenon of negligence is well understood; it poses some hard questions for the theory of responsibility. I would claim, however, that weakness resembles negligence in this respect, that both are nonvoluntary behavior thought to be open to blame. The important point is that the responsibility of weak agents is no more (or less) problematic than the responsibility of negligent agents.

GARY WATSON

capacities. And like the standard of normal self-control, the standard of reasonable care (and thus what counts as negligence) is relative to social norms and particular contexts. Moreover, like the weak person in the above example, the negligent person is not criticized for his values and judgments (he is not bad or unjust) but for failing to ensure that his behavior is informed by, and conforms to, those values and judgments. (However, unlike the negligent person, but like the compulsive, the weak person does of course act intentionally.)[20]

Therefore, the fact that on the proposed account weak agents may be no more able at the time of action to conform their behavior to their judgments than compulsives does not rob the distinction between weakness and compulsion of its moral significance. That distinction can be significantly drawn without requiring ability. I shall now argue that, furthermore, there are strong reasons for doubting that this requirement can be satisfied, and thus for rejecting this central feature of the common account. By the common account, the culpability of the drinker in our earlier example is located not in her failure to develop or maintain the normal capacity of resistance, but in her failure to exercise the capacity she possesses. The challenge to this account is to find a pertinent explanation of this failure.

Generally, people fail to perform some action for a combination of the following kinds of reason: (*a*) they are unaware of the action as an option; (*b*) they do not want or choose to do it; or (*c*) they are unable to do it. Given awareness, nonperformance indicates lack of "power" or lack of "will" or both.[21] This is

---

[20] Some may wish to deny that compulsive behavior is, or can be, intentional if it is not free. This denial seems to me unjustified. For one thing, on leading views of intentionality, both compulsive and weak action will count as intentional. Both the compulsive and the weak person act on a "primary reason" (in Davidson's sense: "Actions, Reasons, and Causes", *Journal of Philosophy*, 1963.) Their behavior is consciously motivated; hence both may have "practical knowledge" and be able to answer a certain kind of question "Why?" (See E. Anscombe, *Intention.*) More decisively, compulsive and weak behavior both involve at least a minimal form of practical reasoning: the person with a dread fear of spiders may reason about how best to escape, a weak person about how best to obtain some cigarettes. To deny intentionality here is unjustifiably to conflate intentional with free action.

[21] This theme is pursued in Chapter 2 of Stuart Hampshire's *Freedom of the Individual.*

SKEPTICISM ABOUT WEAKNESS OF WILL

why inquiries into capacities and knowledge are relevant in contexts of moral appraisal. For instance, if you know that the curtains are burning, and you are able to extinguish the fire, I infer from your nonperformance that you did not want or choose to put the fire out. I thereby learn something important about your values and priorities. On the other hand, of course, if you did not choose to let the curtains burn, or did not even do it knowingly, you would not necessarily be exculpated, for your action or omission may be explained by your culpable ignorance or carelessness. Generally, then, culpable failures or omissions are explained either by lack of choice, or by culpable lack of care, knowledge, or ability.

The proposed account fits weakness into a scheme of this kind. Weak agents fail or neglect to meet certain standards of self-control, and their culpability does not require choice or ability at the time of action. The explanation of the weak agent's failure to act upon practical judgment involves attributing this failure to another culpable failure to develop or maintain the relevant capacities.

The challenge to the common account is to provide a similarly pertinent explanation of the weak person's failure. This failure is due neither to lack of knowledge nor, putatively, to lack of ability or negligence. To return to the case of the weak drinker, the woman judges that she should resist and therefore, by her own lights, has sufficient reason for exercising her alleged capacity. What might explain her not doing so?

There seem to me only two possible explanations. (1) She *chooses* not to. (2) Her *effort* to resist is culpably insufficient. Both of these explanations will be found inadequate.

(1) First, the notion of choice (and also decision) seems to me to involve the notion of applying one's values to the perceived practical options. (Aristotle is close when he speaks of choice as desire in accordance with deliberation.) In this sense, it is of course generally true that one may choose not to exercise some capacity that one has. But the capacity of self-control is special in this respect. For the capacity of self-control involves the capacity to counteract and resist the strength of desires which are contrary to what one has chosen or judged best to do. The weak drinker's

GARY WATSON

failure to resist her desire to drink is a failure to implement her choice not to drink. To choose not to implement this choice would be to change her original judgment, and the case would no longer be a case of failure to implement judgment. Therefore, the weak agent's failure to resist the drink cannot intelligibly be explained by her choice.

Equally important, even if it made sense to explain her failure in this way, doing so would result in the moral assimilation of the weak case to the reckless case. The common account rightly wishes to distinguish these, but the difference would collapse if both involved choice.

(2) Second, it might be supposed that the drinker's failure is to be explained by her culpably insufficient *effort*. Sometimes we attribute a person's failure, not to absence of ability or choice, but to lack of sufficient effort.[22] I may try and fail to throw a coin across the Schuylkill River even when I wanted very much to do so and was able to do so. The explanation may be that I misjudged either the amount of effort required or the distance across. Or in a basketball game, my failure to make a jump-shot from the free-throw line might be explained by insufficient concentration rather than lack of capability or will. Using "effort" to include both physical exertion and psychological factors such as concentration and "keeping one's head," in both cases, we may suppose, I not only would have succeeded with greater effort, but could have made the requisite effort.

Perhaps weakness of will is commonly viewed as involving insufficient effort. In order to help here, an explanation of this kind must be conjoined with the assumption that the weak person is able to make the requisite effort to resist. For obviously, if effort of a certain kind and degree is necessary to successful resistance, it will be true that the drinker is able to resist only if she has the capacity to make an effort of that kind and degree to resist. Our focus is thus shifted to her failure of effort, and everything now turns on why she does not make *it*. But it is far from clear what explanation is forthcoming.

---

[22] I owe my appreciation of this point to the editors of *The Philosophical Review*.

SKEPTICISM ABOUT WEAKNESS OF WILL

The explanation cannot be that making the effort is not thought to be worth it. For once again, implicit in the judgment that it is best not to drink is the judgment that it is best to resist contrary desires. If the drinker really judges that it is not worth that much effort, she either changes her mind or originally only made a conditional judgment of the form: it is best not to drink unless not doing so requires too much effort.

The explanation cannot be that she misjudged the amount of effort required. I may have underestimated how much exertion would be required to throw the coin across the Schuylkill, or how much concentration was necessary to make the basket. But it is not clear what the analogue to this in the case of resisting a drink would be. And even if misjudgment were involved, that would be a different fault from weakness of will.

So we do not seem to have a pertinent explanation of why the weak drinker fails to exert adequate effort. No doubt her failure has something to do with the relative strengths of her desires to resist and to drink. But *this* is not enough for the common account, since it is consistent with her being unable to make the effort. Inasmuch as she has the same good reasons for making the effort to resist as for not drinking, we need an explanation which makes it clear that she is able to resist. For even if some (further) effort would enable her to resist, the desire to drink may generate desires not to make this effort (in the way that desires frequently cause other desires for the means to their fulfillment) and these may be irresistibly strong.

Given her strong motive for making an effort (namely, her considered practical judgment), and in the absence of a special explanation for her not making it (such as "I didn't think it was worth it", or "I didn't think it was necessary"), we are entitled to be skeptical about the common view, and to conclude that the person was unable to resist.

Conclusion

Socrates found the common conception of weakness of will to be confused. However, his reasons for rejecting that account are unsound. They deny the morally and psychologically important

338

GARY WATSON

complexity of human motivation, and in particular the potential divergence between certain kinds of desire and judgments of the good. This divergence is what makes room for the virtue of self-control and, obversely, the vice of weakness of will.

Just the same, I have offered doubts of a nonsocratic sort about the common account of weakness. To take seriously the possibility of acting contrary to one's better judgment is at the same time to raise problems about the distinction between weakness and compulsion. I have argued that the common view, according to which the differentiating feature is that the weak are able to conform their behavior to their practical judgments, is unjustified. Instead, I have proposed that weakness of will involves the failure to develop certain normal capacities of self-control, whereas compulsion involves desires which even the possession of such capacities would not enable one to resist.

University of Pennsylvania

[20]

The Philosophical Review, XCIII, No. 2 (April 1984)

WILL POWER AND THE VIRTUES
Robert C. Roberts

I

A number of authors in the past twenty-five years have tried to answer the general question "What is a virtue?" or as G. H. von Wright says, to "shape a concept of a virtue." This project has thrown light on the nature of the virtues, but has sometimes tended to raise the expectation that they must all be the same kind of trait.[1] One proposition which has enjoyed general consent is the denial that virtues are skill-like dispositions or powers. I shall argue here that one group of virtues, which might be called the moral strengths or virtues of will power, are to a large extent skill-like.

Some theorists have proposed that moral virtues are all determinations of the good *will*. A broad-ranging list of traits having moral relevance will probably include some that are not easily corralled into this pen. For example, foresight and psychological insight are characteristics of an ideally moral person, yet it seems wrong to call them determinations of the will. And gentleness, politeness, and friendliness, in some people at least, are unwilled and nonwilling styles of behavioral demeanor. So probably not all morally relevant traits are matters of the will. Yet it is clear why philosophers might make this mistake, for many of the virtues most central to the moral life, such as honesty, courage, justice, compassion, and self-control, *are* determinations of the will.

But this observation is not very clarifying unless we know what will is. There are broadly two ways in which we employ 'will' or its cognates. In the first kind of case we designate inclinations and disinclinations, desires and aversions, motivations. If I go willingly to a horse race, I go gladly or at least with a minimum of distaste. A willful person is one who does just whatever he wants to, without

---

[1]Important essays in which this tendency is evident are Chapter VII of von Wright's *The Varieties of Goodness* (London: Routledge, 1963); R. B. Brandt's "Traits of Character: A Conceptual Analysis," *American Philosophical Quarterly* 7, (1970): pp. 23–37; Phillippa Foot's "Virtues and Vices" in *Virtues and Vices* (Berkeley: University of California Press, 1978); and John McDowell's "Virtue and Reason," *Monist*, 62 (1979): pp. 331–350.

ROBERT C. ROBERTS

regard for the rights or concerns of others. To lose the will to live is
no longer to care much about living. In the second kind of case
'will' designates not motivations, but a family of capacities for *resisting* adverse inclinations. When we say someone has a "strong will"
we are often referring to the presence in her of such virtues as
perseverance, resoluteness, courage, patience, and self-control.
When we speak of "efforts of will," we refer to the acts or activities
which correspond to such virtues: fighting boredom, controlling
one's emotions, resisting temptation, persevering in the face of
discouragement, overcoming the impulse to flee, fighting anxiety,
forcing oneself to the magnanimous gesture, and the like.[2] That
this use of 'will' is distinct from its use to designate motivation is
suggested by the oddity of the expression "an effort of wanting."

Where people make efforts, there exist human capacities. A person can make a muscular effort because in general he has muscular
powers, and an effort to pay attention because in general he can
pay attention. (Obviously, it doesn't follow that he has the power to
do the particular act he tries to do; efforts can fail in many ways,
and some of these involve a failure to possess, or to possess enough
of, the relevant capacity.) So if people do make efforts of will—that
is, efforts to resist adverse inclinations—it follows that there exist
human capacities by which to resist adverse inclinations. It will be
my contention in this paper that the virtues of will power are indeed largely capacities, and that these are more like skills than like
other kinds of capacities. But first it will be enlightening to discuss
the relations between the virtues of will power and other virtues.

II

The most important distinction between kinds of virtues is that
between the virtues of will power and those that are substantive
and motivational. I call virtues like honesty, compassion, justice,

---

[2]When I call a virtue a "virtue of will power" I do not suggest that every
action exemplifying it is an exercise of will power. There are acts of courage and patience and perseverance (I am less sure about self-control) that
do not require will power, much less an effort of will. I use this name to
indicate a salient, but not necessary, feature of these virtues. Also, will
power is probably, as a matter of psychological fact, always needed in the
acquisition of these virtues.

WILL POWER AND THE VIRTUES

generosity, promise-keeping, and kindness "substantive" because they are the psychological embodiment of ethical rules—the substance of the ethical patterns of behavior and judgment and emotion. To be honest is to be disposed to tell the truth in appropriate situations, to judge well which situations demand telling the truth, to be "alive" to dishonesty in oneself and others, and to feel uneasiness, guilt, indignation, sadness, and other emotions upon encountering dishonesty in oneself and others. Compassion is the disposition to help others who are suffering, to notice and recognize sufferers as sufferers, to judge them to be in some fundamental way similar to oneself, and to be sad to see suffering and glad to see it relieved.

By contrast, patience does not imply any characteristically ethical patterns of behavior, judgment, or emotion. Racists, cheats, sadists, and thieves may well be persevering, resolute, and self-controlled; and indeed they will be more likely to succeed in their chosen style of life if they are. Whether courage is equally lacking in moral substance has been questioned.[3] Philippa Foot has noted that we are disinclined to call particularly heinous acts, such as "a murder done for gain or to get an inconvenient person out of the way,"[4] courageous, even if they are done in circumstances which would require courage. But our disinclination here can be accounted for by the *associations* that 'courage' has for us: we do associate courage with the substantive moral virtues, and there are important anthropological reasons for this association, which in turn give courage its moral importance. And Foot admits that it is only the attribution of courage to the *act* that troubles us; we find no difficulty in calling a murderer courageous, nor in saying that his act "took courage."

By saying the substantive virtues are "motivational," I mean what I think Aristotle is talking about when he says

---

[3]Lester Hunt has argued that all virtues are dispositions to act on principles (see his "Character and Thought," *American Philosophical Quarterly,* 15, no. 3 (1978): pp. 177–186, and has thus sought the principle which courage is the disposition to act on. He comes up with the following: courageous acts "are ones which are done from the principle that one's own safety, in general, has no more than a certain measure of importance." ("Courage and Principle," *Canadian Journal of Philosophy,* 10, no. 2 (1980): p. 289). But this principle is clearly not a moral one.

[4]*Op. cit.,* p. 15.

ROBERT C. ROBERTS

> We may even go so far as to state that the man who does not enjoy
> performing noble actions is not a good man at all. Nobody would call a
> man just who does not enjoy acting justly, nor generous who does not
> enjoy generous actions, and so on (*Nicomachean Ethics* 1099a).

To be just is to want just states of affairs to prevail and consequently, in the appropriate circumstances, to want to do what will
bring about such states of affairs. Thus the just person takes satisfaction ("pleasure") in the performance and beholding of such
actions, and feels frustration ("pain") at failure in them. But Aristotle seems to have missed the difference between the kinds of virtues
that I am pointing out. The following words ring strange:

> A man who abstains from bodily pleasures and enjoys doing so is self-
> controlled; if he finds abstinence troublesome, he is self-indulgent; a
> man who endures danger with joy, or at least without pain, is cou-
> rageous; if he endures it with pain, he is a coward (*Nicomachean Ethics*
> 1104b).[5]

Enjoying the activity of abstaining from bodily pleasures is not a
criterion of self-control. There may be a psychological connection
between a person's achieving self-mastery and his taking pleasure
either in the activity itself or in the fruits of it. But the quality of a
person's self-mastery cannot be called into question on the account
of his failing to enjoy it. Whereas the idea of a person who possesses the virtue of justice, and yet hates doing just actions or is
indifferent to their fruits, is a contradiction.

A person who enjoys enduring dangers is better called dare-
devilish than brave. A particularly bizarre illustration of what courage would be like if it were a motivational virtue has been collected
by William James:[6]

---

[5]But compare 1117b.

[6]*The Varieties of Religious Experience* (Garden City, New York: Doubleday
1978), pp. 266–267, note. H. A. Prichard finds another way of making
courage a passional virtue: for him it is not an enjoyment of dangers, but
"the desire to conquer one's feelings of terror arising from the sense of
shame which they arouse." *Moral Obligation* (New York: Oxford University
Press, 1950), p. 13. While some courageous actions are motivated by shame
of fear, the most typical moral examples are motivated in other ways (see
below). But the essential point is that there is *no* motive that always goes
with courageous actions.

WILL POWER AND THE VIRTUES

> I believe, says General Skobeleff, that my bravery is simply the passion for and at the same time the contempt of danger. The risk of life fills me with an exaggerated rapture. The fewer there are to share it, the more I like it . . . a meeting of man to man, a duel, a danger into which I can throw myself head-foremost, attracts me, moves me, intoxicates me. I am crazy for it, I love it, I adore it. I run after danger as one runs after women . . . my entire nature runs to meet the peril with an impetus that my will would in vain try to resist.

If joy in enduring danger were a mark of courage, General Skobeleff would appear to be an exceptionally courageous man. And no doubt a casual observer of his exploits might call him courageous. But this peek at the General's interiority shows that his disposition is not courage. For whatever else courage may be, it is a virtue; but the disposition he describes is a vice. Even the courage of the thief elicits our admiration; for though his disregard for property rights is despicable, still he possesses a trait without which one leads a crippled life. But there is nothing admirable about the General's lust for dangers; and we can guess that people who possess it tend to be a menace both to society and to themselves. For positions of leadership we want courageous persons, but not daredevils. We do not want our generals to be enthusiasts for military exploits.

Unlike justice, compassion, generosity, and friendship, courage and self-control are not in themselves moral motives. A person can feed the poor out of compassion, struggle on behalf of the oppressed out of concern for justice (i.e., out of concern for people who are being treated unjustly), and perform sacrifices out of friendship. But actions exhibiting courage and self-control are not done *out of* courage and self-control.[7] Actions done out of moral

---

[7]Though they are sometimes done for the sake of courage and self-control, as when you "do every day or two something for no other reason than that you would rather not do it, so that when the hour of dire need draws nigh, it may find you not unnerved and untrained to stand the test" (William James, *Principles of Psychology,* vol. I, p. 126), or as when, like G. Gordon Liddy, you eat a rat as an exercise in mastering your fear of rats (*Will: The Autobiography of G. Gordon Liddy,* p. 24). But this kind of case is untypical, the typical case being that of acting courageously or self-controlledly for the sake of some other end. If someone always acted courageously *only* to exhibit courage or to train herself in it, and never out of friendship, justice, compassion, etc., her action would not be moral. And to

231

ROBERT C. ROBERTS

motives may, however, be done *in virtue* of courage and self-control and patience, if the circumstances, psychological and environmental, demand such virtues.[8]

I think Plato is on the right track when he calls courage a "preservative."[9] A preservative is in the service of something other than itself that is cherished, and needed because this cherished thing is in some way threatened. Courage, self-control and patience are in the service of the moral and prudential life, and needed because this life is beset with trials. These trials, which are part of the everyday context in which we exercise the virtues, are functions of our desires and aversions. The virtues of will power are the capacities by which a person copes with these trials in the interests of the moral and prudential life.

Philippa Foot has noticed this "corrective" character of the virtues of will power:[10]

> As things are we often want to run away not only where that is the right thing to do but also where we should stand firm; and we want pleasure not only where we should seek pleasure but also where we should not. If human nature had been different there would have been no need of a corrective disposition in either place. . . .

But she mistakenly generalizes this characteristic to all the virtues:

---

the extent that acting courageously out of the desire to be courageous is morally praiseworthy, this is because courage is in aid of the actions characteristic of the substantive moral virtues.

[8]Aquinas seems to be aware of the distinction I am pointing to when he says, "By its nature virtue is concerned with the good rather than the difficult," and "A man exposes himself to mortal danger only to preserve justice. Therefore the praise accorded to courage derives in a sense from justice" (Summa Theologiae 2a2ae 123.12). But he is not consistent in this observation that courage and similar virtues do not supply a motive, for he assimilates courage and charity by saying, "Charity does prompt the act of martyrdom as its first and most important moving force by being the virtue commanding it, but courage does so as the directly engaged moving force, being the virtue which brings out the act" (2a2ae 124.2). But unless the martyr is acting not just courageously, but for the sake of courage (which is not the typical case and certainly not necessary for martyrdom), it seems wrong to say that courage "prompts" the act in any sense. In the normal case courage *enables* the act, but only motives *prompt* it.

[9]*Republic* 429c-e.

[10]*Virtues and Vices*, p. 9.

WILL POWER AND THE VIRTUES

> There is . . . a virtue of industriousness only because idleness is a
> temptation; and of humility only because men tend to think too well of
> themselves. Hope is a virtue because despair is a temptation. . . .

Her mistake is that of confusing the existence of something with
the existence of its name or concept. If people were never led
astray by fears and pleasures, it is plausible that courage and self-
control themselves would not arise. For courage and self-control
are (in large and basic part) the capacities to manage our inclinations, when they are wayward, to flee dangers and seek pleasures.
But industriousness is needed not basically because people are
prone to laziness, but because work is a good thing. Industriousness could exist in a world in which no one suffered from
laziness, and hope in a world where no one ever despaired, and
honesty in a world where no one lied—though it is likely that in
such a world these virtues would not be named or much noticed.
The substantive virtues are "corrective" in the trivial sense that
there are vices which correspond to them; the virtues of will power
are corrective in the significant sense that, in our present psychological condition but not in every imaginable one, they are needed
to keep us on the path of virtue and our higher self-interest.

III

But this is not the whole story. In assessing the degree to which
an action reflects moral credit on its agent, we often feel two contrary tendencies. On the one side, like Kant, we are inclined to give
greater credit for actions (or character traits) which result from
moral struggle. We might call this the hero assessment: just as
running a mile in under four minutes is praised not as a speedy
mode of transportation, but as an extraordinary feat for legs and
lungs and spirit, so some acts are morally praised not just because
they are good, but also because they are difficult. Why do we tend
to think a moral achievement greater if more difficult? Not, I
think, just because we have confused morality with athletics. One
obvious reason is that morally difficult actions display some virtues—namely the virtues of will power. But I think a deeper basis
for our feeling here is that the greater the moral obstacles (that is,
contrary inclinations) a person has overcome in doing something,

233

the more his action seems to be his own *achievement*, his own *choice*, and thus to reflect credit on him as an *agent*. It seems to show that his action is *his* in a special way.

But the moment we make the hero assessment we may have some doubts and think: the very fact that somebody *has* those fears and lusts and countermoral impulses which make right action difficult for him reflects discredit on him; an action is the more praiseworthy the more it is done purely out of moral inclinations and in the absence of contrary inclinations—that is, the more it is done *without* moral struggle. This we might call the purity of heart assessment. Here the emphasis is not on the agent as an achiever or chooser, but rather, I should almost say, as a personal *artifact*. Here we assess the individual not with respect to how he brought off the act or how he got to be the kind of person he is, but just with respect to what he *is* in the sense of the configuration of his cares and un-cares. The ideally moral person is one who is concerned about important things and relatively unconcerned about relatively unimportant things, and so he does not have to struggle with himself to do what is right.

These kinds of assessments correspond to the kinds of virtues I have distinguished. When we make the hero assessment, we are demanding of an action or character trait that its accomplishment require one or more of the virtues of will power. If we make the purity of heart assessment, it is because we are laying emphasis on the motivational virtues. The virtues of will power are needed on the road to purity of heart because in most of us the moral inclinations are so weak and the road is so strewn with psychological obstacles. But unlike the motivational virtues, these are not the substance of the moral life and their "corrective" function is no longer needed when full sainthood has been attained.

But as I have suggested the virtues of will power are needed not only for their "corrective" function, but also because they are essential to the development of the agent's agenthood. Struggles are an important part of the way we become centers of initiation of actions and passions. They are the contexts in which the shape of our personality takes on that toughness and independence which we call "autonomy," and which seems to be a basic feature of mature personhood. Could a person gain autonomy without struggle,

WILL POWER AND THE VIRTUES

and thus without the capacities necessary to win in struggles? In a famous letter John Keats wrote,[11]

> The common cognomen of this world among the misguided and su-
> perstitious is 'a vale of tears' from which we are to be redeemed by a
> certain arbitrary interposition of God and taken to Heaven—What a
> little circumscribe [d] straightened notion! Call the world if you Please
> "'The vale of Soul-making" Then you will find out the use of the
> world. . . . I say '*Soul making*' Soul as distinguished from an Intel-
> ligence—There may be intelligences or sparks of the divinity in mil-
> lions—but they are not Souls . . . till they acquire identities, till each
> one is personally itself. . . . Do you not see how necessary a World of
> Pains and troubles is to school an Intelligence and make it a soul?

We might generalize Keats's "World of Pains and troubles" to "a World of temptations" (psychological adversities). We can guess that it will never be possible to give a person a moral "identity"—a tough and abiding passion for justice or a stable and focused desire to relieve suffering—by injecting him with a drug or giving him a brain operation or fiddling with his genes. But the impossibility of giving somebody moral character in this way seems to be more than psychological. For even if we could in this way produce a being who was indistinguishable, in terms of his present dispositions, from a saint, still I think we would have no inclination whatsoever to cano-nize him. For the praise for his saintliness, and thus for his deeds, would not be due *him*. If it were due anyone, the pharmacologist or brain surgeon would seem more likely candidates. So the idea of somebody acquiring moral character without struggle seems not only psychologically, but logically amiss. Such a person does not have an appropriate moral *history*. Thus, if powers of will are those powers by which moral struggles are prosecuted, then they may be more than just "corrective." They may be a logically and psycholog-ically necessary part of our development as persons.

The relation, then, between the virtues of will power and the substantive virtues is mutual need: neither kind can exist as moral virtues without the other kind. Without the virtues of will power, the moral motives would too often be sabotaged by counter-moral

---

[11]*The Letters of John Keats* (Cambridge, Mass.: Harvard University Press, 1958), vol. II, p. 101f.

ROBERT C. ROBERTS

impulses and the relative weakness of the substantive virtues; nor
would these latter be gained in a morally appropriate way. On the
other hand, the character of a person who had only the virtues of
will power would be empty of moral content.

IV

I want now to consider the view of the virtues of will power which
I take to be the strongest alternative to my suggestion that they are
capacities. In "Traits of Character: A Conceptual Analysis"[12] Richard Brandt argues that moral character traits are "the kind of
dispositions that wants and aversions are" (p. 27). They are inclinations which can be called into activity by features of a subject's
environment or thoughts and which, when they have become active, issue in behavior of a type corresponding to the inclination.
Thus a person with the trait of sympathy, if he sees a child in
distress from falling off his bicycle, will go to the child and help or
comfort him, if some other, competing and stronger, inclination is
not presently active in him. For example, if what knocked the child
from his bike is a bag of $100 bills falling off a truck, which are now
floating up the street in the wind, the active trait of sympathy may
start to be challenged by that of avarice. Assuming the sympathetic
and avaricious individual judges the wind strong enough to render
the fulfillment of the one desire incompatible with that of the
other, then his behavior at that moment will be determined by the
relative strength of these two inclinations. Brandt generalizes: the
motivation theory of character traits

> holds that, under conditions not fully understood, they become active
> and generate "force vectors" in the psychological field of the person,
> their direction and degree depending partly on the person's beliefs;
> what the person actually does is a function of the force vectors in his
> psychological field at the moment of action (p. 31).

This account, like Aristotle's, begins to fidget when courage and
self-control are mentioned. Unlike Aristotle and Prichard, Brandt
does not treat courage and self-control as though they are themselves passional virtues; but he does treat them as nothing but a

---

[12]*American Philosophical Quarterly*, 7 (1970), pp. 23–37.

WILL POWER AND THE VIRTUES

function of passions, among which are to be found some moral ones. These virtues, though not themselves tendencies of the desire/aversion sort, must be understood as the relative weakness, vis-á-vis some passional virtues, of desires/aversions which stand in opposition to virtuous behavior. Thus the courage of the rat-phobic who crawls under the house after a child is simply the weakness, relative to his desire to free the child, of his desire to avoid the company of rats. On this analysis a *generally* courageous or self-controlled person is just one who has sufficiently intense moral and prudential desires and aversions that they override, generally, his morally and prudentially aversive passions.

Some cases of courage, etc., fit Brandt's analysis. We do sometimes ascribe courage to a person whose impulse to act virtuously is strong enough, by itself, to override his impulse to flee. Maybe this is typical of the courage of the saints: in them the passional virtues are so strong that in a sense they do not need courage. That is to say, in them courage is not a function of will power. But most of us would not have much courage or patience if we didn't have will power, so we are led, like James D. Wallace, to feel that Brandt's analysis has neglected something. These virtues are not just "privative states," but some kind of "positive capacity."[13]

V

If desires and aversions (duly shaped by our beliefs) were the only kind of element contributing to our psychological "force vectors," the virtues of will power would not be capacities or powers, but only patterns of relative strength among our desires and aversions. However, our desires and aversions are not the only psychological factors contributing to our actions and the course of our

---

[13]*Virtues and Vices* (Ithaca, NY: Cornell University Press, 1978), p. 61. Wallace suggests that the "positiveness" of virtues like courage is their capacity to preserve us in the course of practical reason. But as A. O. Rorty has pointed out, the *akrates* need not consider the course in which he fails to take the more rational of the choices which conflict in him ("Where Does the Akratic Break Take Place?" *Australasian Journal of Philosophy*, 58, no. 94 (1980): p. 336f). Just as *akrasia* cannot be defined as a form of irrationality, so courage and other virtues which are the opposite of *akrasia* cannot be defined as capacities to preserve rationality. Their "positiveness" lies not here, but in their being capacities.

ROBERT C. ROBERTS

lives; for there is also such a thing as our *management* of our desires and aversions; and these capacities of self-management are an important aspect of the virtues of will power. People are capacitated in numerous ways. We have bodily powers like food and oxygen assimilation; physical strengths (muscles and bones); faculties (sight, hearing, smell); and aptitudes (mathematical, musical, linguistic). But the capacity to resist adverse inclinations seems to be learned. Since learned capacities are called skills, I propose that powers of will are skills of self-management.

Skills may be more or less completely mental, like the ability to focus attention at will, or motor, like riding a bicycle. But most skills have both motor and mental aspects. Riding a bike in traffic requires a combination of motor skill and knowledge of rules of the road, attentiveness to events occuring in the traffic, judgment about the speed of cars relative to their distance from oneself and one another and one's own speed or potential for speed, etc. It is characteristic of skills in both their mental and motor aspects that they become in large part "automatic" and unnoticed by their practitioners. Many skills combine procedures governed by rules which can be (though by no means always are) formulated, patterns of such "automatic" physical and mental behavior, and a certain element of creativity in the application of the rules and the "automatic" behaviors to new challenges. Most sports and games, and activities such as weaving, producing portrait photography, doing algebra, speaking a language, cooking, getting dressed, and cabinet building would be skills falling under this last description.

People can be more or less skilled in the management of their own inclinations, and these skills are an important part of the virtues of will power. We can be more and less "good at" breaking bad habits and forming new ones, at "deferring gratification," at resisting cravings and impulses; and we can be trained and/or train ourselves in the control of emotions like anxiety, fear, disappointment, anger, and hatred. I want to illustrate and partially analyse these truths in a moment. But before I do, let me consider four *a priori* objections to the proposal that virtues can be skills.

Three such arguments are found in James D. Wallace's book, *Virtues and Vices*, pp. 44–47. The first is this:

> 1. Courage and patience are capacities to overcome difficulties arising from inclinations contrary to right action.

238

WILL POWER AND THE VIRTUES

2. Inclinations contrary to right action are not technical difficulties, but skills are always capacities to overcome technical difficulties. So courage and patience are not skills.

The crux of the argument is the word 'technical'. It certainly sounds right to say that, of the various kinds of difficulties standing in the way of acting compassionately towards a rebellious and abusive teenage son, the difficulty of overcoming one's feelings of resentment towards him (which might be met by possessing the virtue of patience) is not a *technical* one. (We might say, "Not technical, but *moral!*") "Technical" difficulties in this situation might be questions of psychological strategy: What is in the son's best interest? To confront him and have it out? To assert some authority over him? To use benign neglect? To shower him with affection? Or some combination of these? To answer a "technical" question like this, one might consult a professional, thus perhaps increasing one's skill in handling rebellious sons. But one would not (so suggests Wallace's argument) seek such "technical" guidance as to, or training in, how to handle one's *own* feelings of resentment towards the son. *That* is a matter not of "technique," but of morality.

But why not seek such "technical" help in handling one's own emotions? One reason we are inclined to accept the "not technical, but moral" disjunction, is a failure to distinguish virtues like courage and patience from the substantive moral virtues like caring for one's children. But if somebody already has a moral motive, and then finds that bad habits and adverse emotions are getting in the way of acting lovingly, the psychologist has a potential role, and though we would not normally call this role "technical," what the psychologist may supply here is precisely information and training of a "how to" sort. I suggest that when this "how to" knowledge has become assimilated, the person will have gained in the virtue of patience.

Here is Wallace's second argument:

1. If any trait is a skill, then it can be inculcated through instruction in techniques and by practice that leads to proficiency.
2. But no virtue can be so inculcated.
   So no virtue is a skill.

But the second premise is false. As Aristotle points out,

239

ROBERT C. ROBERTS

by abstaining from pleasures we become self-controlled, and once we
are self-controlled we are best able to abstain from pleasures. So also
with courage: by becoming habituated to despise and endure terrors
we become courageous, and once we have become courageous we will
best be able to endure terror (*Nicomachean Ethics* 1104a-b).

In the next section I shall illustrate how the virtues of will power
can be inculcated through instruction and practice.

In his third argument Wallace adapts an insight from Gilbert
Ryle, namely that it is logically amiss to say someone has *forgotten*
the difference between right and wrong. Wallace's argument is
this:

1. If any trait is a skill, it can be forgotten.
2. But courage, self-control, and patience cannot be forgotten.
   So these traits are not skills.

Both premises are questionable. In general it is only more complicated skills that are forgettable, and even here it is unlikely that a
skill, well-learned, will be completely forgotten. Someone who has
played the piano well, and then lets twenty years elapse without
practicing, will get rusty indeed. But that she has not lost all her
skill will be evident from how quickly it comes back with practice. A
total loss of the skill would require more than forgetting; it would
take some kind of injury or illness or aging process resulting in
neurological or muscular deterioration. But simpler skills are virtually unforgettable: one does not forget how to swim, or ride a
bike, or walk. It is possible that courage and self-control are simple
enough to be as unforgettable as bike-riding. (Though maybe, like
biking, they are susceptible to considerable development and
sophistication.)

It seems to me that courage, etc., cannot be flat forgotten; but if
we allow that getting "rusty" is a sort of forgetting or partial forgetting, it is not so obvious that one cannot forget courage. See the
autobiography of Gordon Liddy, who in prison felt it necessary to
exercise himself in withstanding pain, to make sure that he hadn't
gone "soft."

Unlike Wallace, Ryle nowhere claims it is logically amiss to say
someone has forgotten a *virtue*, but only to say that someone has

WILL POWER AND THE VIRTUES

forgotten the difference between right and wrong.[14] Ryle explains this impossibility by the fact that to know the difference between right and wrong is a matter of *caring* about right and wrong, and ceasing to care is not a sort of forgetting. In my terms, Ryle is only claiming the impossibility of forgetting the substantive and motivational virtues—because only these "tell us," as it were, the difference between right and wrong.

Wallace is clear enough about the difference between the substantive virtues and the virtues of will power not to explain the supposed unforgettability of self-control and patience by the supposition that they are modes of caring.

> The reason is not that there is a motivational component to these things that cannot be lost by forgetting. The reason why one cannot forget how to be brave or honest is like the reason why one cannot forget how to see or how to be strong: there is no "how to" to these things (p. 47).

But as we shall see in the next section, this supposition too is false.

A fourth argument that no virtue is a skill has been presented by Philippa Foot. Following Aristotle and Aquinas she notes that when a person's action bespeaks a lack of a skill (let us say he misspells a word), he can defend himself against the implication by saying "I did it intentionally." But when his action bespeaks a lack of virtue (let us say he tells a lie), he does not exculpate himself by saying "I did it intentionally." Thus no virtue is a skill.[15]

This argument overlooks that virtues relate in more than one way to morality. It is of course true that an action does not become any the less immoral by being intentional; and so where doing the moral thing (say, being compassionate) requires the exercise of a skill virtue (say, patience), the fact that one's failure of patience was intentional is no *moral* exculpation. But claiming that the failure to exercise patience was intentional *would* defend against the accusation of lacking patience. But patience is a virtue. So it is false that one cannot defend against the implication of failure to possess a virtue by claiming that failure to exercise it was intentional.

---

[14]Gilbert Ryle, *Collected Papers* vol. II (London: Hutchinson, 1971), pp. 381ff.

[15]See Foot, *op.cit.*, p. 7f.

241

ROBERT C. ROBERTS

VI

I shall now indicate sketchily some ways people manage their adverse inclinations, and draw attention to the skill-likeness of these ways. Like other skills, some of these "ways" are strategic, like the duck hunter's knowledge of the precise moment when to rise in the blind, while others are more basic, like his ability to squeeze the trigger without disrupting his aim. My argument is not that because there are strategies for *developing* courage, courage must be a skill. (One might develop compassion by the strategy of meditating on the lives of compassionate people.) It is rather that being courageous is *in itself* (often subtly and sub-consciously) in part strategic, and so is formally like those many skills that have strategic dimensions. Nor is my argument that merely because the exercise of these virtues can develop them, they must be skills. (Performing compassionate actions can perhaps cause a person to become more compassionate.) Instead, I shall try to describe the exercises leading to the acquisition of the virtues of will power in such a way as to highlight *specific* similarities between these exercises and ones which issue in skills. I shall speak first of the management of cravings and impulses, then of emotions.

Cravings and Impulses. Søren Kierkegaard depicts a gambler struggling against his compulsion:[16]

> Imagine that he . . . said to himself in the morning, "So I solemnly vow by all that is holy that I shall nevermore have anything to do with gambling, nevermore—to-night shall be the last time." Ah, my friend, he is lost! Strange as it may seem I should venture to bet rather on the opposite, supposing that there was a gambler who at such a moment said to himself, "Very well, thou shalt be allowed to gamble all the rest of thy life, every blessed day—but tonight thou shalt let it alone," and so he did. . . . For the resolution of the first man was a knavish trick of lust, but that of the other is a way of hoaxing lust. . . . Lust is strong merely in the instant. . . .

The more normal development of this aspect of self-control might occur as follows: parents teaching their children to defer gratification would begin with small stretches of time. They would

---

[16]*For Self-Examination and Judge for Yourselves!* translated by Walter Lowrie, (Princeton: Princeton University Press, 1968), p. 69.

WILL POWER AND THE VIRTUES

say not "Here is your Easter basket, and you may eat your chocolate bunny the day after tomorrow," but instead, "after dinner, you
may bite off his ear." (And, by the way, they will not set the temptation out of the child's reach until the appointed time, nor keep a
nervous eagle eye out so as to slap the hand that reaches for the
bunny, but will let the child develop her *own* ability to resist the
impulses she may feel.) If the parents are wise in engineering settings for gratification-deferment which are manageable for the
child, she may grow up with an unreflective tendency to pick for
herself deferment goals that are realistic given her own powers of
resistance, and thus put herself in for a minimum of discouragement. It is imaginable that this skill of self-management might
develop without any explicit discussion of its rules or reflection on
them, and might be as natural as speaking one's native language. A
cabinet builder follows a dictum which might be expressed, "He
who starts a project square and level has less need of compensating
exercises in ensuing stages." When he was a novice his teacher
perhaps had to voice the dictum a few times, but after he had built
some cabinets himself the dictum became integrated into the practice, sinking to the status of a mentally unrehearsed policy or rule
of skill founded on the ineluctible geometric properties of cabinets,
floors and walls. The remark that "lust is strong merely in the
instant" is an easily accessible piece of psychological wisdom, one
which can become as integral a part of a person's dealings with
himself as the carpenter's dictum is of his dealings with boards and
nails. The more self-mastering person knows, either intuitively or
perhaps expressly, such things as that committing oneself to long-
term abstention from the fulfillment of a strong impulse is probably either self-deceptive or likely to overwhelm and discourage.
Skill at the management of impulses and cravings must take this
fact of human nature into consideration, just as carpentry must
take geometric truths into consideration. (I am told that "one day
at a time" is one of the basic rules of Alcoholics Anonymous.)

We can imagine that at first, upon hearing or formulating for
himself this dictum, the weak-willed gambler might succeed in
"hoaxing his lust" by explicitly telling himself that he is not promising to abstain for life, after all, but only for the next twenty-four
hours. Then when the next day comes, he renews his commitment,
assuring himself that it is only for the day, etc. But after the rule

243

ROBERT C. ROBERTS

has been successfully applied a few times, the "hoaxing" may gradually change to a habit, a sub-conscious policy of choosing manageable time-parameters for one's choices of self-denial. When this happens, the individual is beginning to gain a stronger will.

The way of mastering impulses that I have just discussed is "strategic": In its more self-conscious (though not in its deeper and more usual) forms it involves considering what one is up against, and then in the light of this figuring out a way to meet the challenge. But there may also be an aspect of impulse-mastery that is more basic. Boyd Barrett[17] proposes a number of exercises by which a person can increase his ability to resist impulses. These involve doing such "useless" things as standing on a chair for ten consecutive minutes and trying to do so contentedly; listening to the ticking of a clock and making some definite movements at every fifth tick; and replacing in a box, slowly and deliberately, one hundred matches. In all these activities one is almost certain to get impulses to quit: boredom, physical discomfort, thoughts of things one would rather be doing. We might speculate that here one does not necessarily resist the impulse by some "method" such as hoaxing the lust or re-construing the impulse. Maybe one resists the impulse to discontinue the activity by simply continuing the activity. If this interpretation is correct, then there would seem to be a power to resist impulses which is a *basic* ability—basic not in the sense that it is unlearned, but in the sense that one does not exercise it by exercising some *other* ability. It would be like some people's ability to look cross-eyed or wiggle their ears.

Emotions. Some impulses are emotions, as when fear is the impulse to flee, or boredom the impulse to quit an activity. But others are not: for example, physical pain, and "lusts" for sex, money, gambling, and philosophic discussion. Conversely, not all adverse emotions are impulses: an impulse, it seems, has to be directed at *doing* something, and when I experience an adverse emotion such as malicious joy, I may not have an inclination to do anything at all. In such cases the emotion is "adverse" not because of what it may *lead* to, but because it is itself unfitting, morally or from the point of view of psychological health or happiness.

---

[17]In a book called *Strength of Will and How to Develop It* discussed in Robert Assagioli, "The Act of Will" (New York: The Viking Press, 1973), pp. 39ff.

WILL POWER AND THE VIRTUES

There are two senses in which we may "control" an emotion: if it is an impulse to some undesirable behavior such as fleeing a danger which should be faced, or emitting some angry behavior that will have untoward consequences, then "controlling" it may just mean resisting the impulse to act in such ways. But it may also mean the reshaping of the emotion itself: mitigating the anger or fear, or eliminating them altogether. For the sake of brevity I shall focus here on the control of emotions in the second sense.

Any of the virtues of will power may involve power over emotions. Self-control can be, among other things, a mastery of anger, resentment, malicious joy, scorn, hatred and envy. Where patience is directed to a task, the emotion with which it typically has to do is boredom. (A related virtue is tenaciousness or perseverance, whose emotional adversary seems to be primarily discouragement or some degree of hopelessness.) Where patience is used in dealing with people, emotions typically mastered are anger and resentment and boredom. The emotions that courage relates to are fear and anxiety.

In some cases anger diminishes with oblique behavioral "expression." Thus a man may diminish his anger at an oppressive boss by kicking pasteboard boxes around in the privacy of his garage and cursing loudly. It may help to imagine the boss's face or backside in the boxes and to go through the procedure in a somewhat ritualistic and comical manner. Similar activities may have the effect of increasing one's anger at the boss, so knowing when this sort of thing will work and prescribing to oneself and carrying out appropriate rituals is clearly a skill-like ability.

One can often alter an emotion by behaving in a way that conflicts with it. Thus if I am afraid of someone, one way to handle the fear is to stand up straight, look him in the eye, and speak clearly in an even, strong voice. The fear may not disappear entirely, but it will certainly be less than if I shrink back, speak in a weak mumble, and generally present myself to myself as one who is in an oppressive situation.[18] I think that courageous people are typically aware, intuitively, of the influence that their bodily dispositions and voice and speech have on their anxiety and fear, and practice this kind of

---

[18]For an explanation of why techniques like this work, see my "Solomon on the Control of Emotions," *Philosophy and Phenomenological Research*, (March, 1984).

ROBERT C. ROBERTS

self-management. It is far from obvious that courageous people typically feel fears and anxieties less intensely than cowardly people. But through practice in facing up to threatening situations, they have learned how to manage and mitigate their fears.

Skillful self-talk is another way of controlling emotion. I am becoming impatient with my four-year-old's bedtime delaying tactics, and so I talk to myself: "I did the same when I was four," or "Notice how ingenious his tactics are—bright little guy, huh?" or "Just relax and bear with it a moment longer; it *will* soon be over." Such self-talk often mitigates or even dispels the welling anger, along with the urges to be abrupt, to behave punishingly, and generally to lose my cool. Perseverance may also involve self-talk making use of "the power of positive thinking," as well as the tactics of reading "encouraging" literature (e.g., to help one persevere in a diet or a language-learning program) and associating with "encouraging" people. But self-talk and these more external self-management tactics are crude forms of this aspect of self-control: the experienced self-controller just flashes the strategic thoughts across her mind at the appropriate moments, the way a basketball player moves intelligently but without deliberation in the split-second of court action.

VII

Before I end, I must put the thesis of this paper in perspective. I have argued that the virtues of will power are in an important aspect skills or skill-like powers. But I have nowhere claimed that this is the whole story of these virtues.

There may be saints whose patience and courage do not involve any exercise of will power, in the form either of efforts of will or of an effortless mastery of adverse impulses and emotions. The reason their goodness involves no exercise of will power is what makes them saints: they don't *have* any adverse impulses or emotions to which will power might be directed. Whether there are any saints in this sense I don't know; but there are certainly particular acts of courage and perseverance that involve no exercise of will power. Some acts of heroic courage are performed so spontaneously that there can be no question of the individual overcoming his fears; he just doesn't have any fears at the moment.

246

WILL POWER AND THE VIRTUES

But even when skills of self-mastery are still needed there are two other kinds of feature typical of people with the virtues of will power. First, they *care* intensely about something. I have argued that the virtues of will power, when they are moral, derive their moral import from the concerns in the interest of which they are exercised. But the virtues of will power are never exercised apart from any motivation whatsoever; and generally speaking, the more intense the concerns, the more likely that the skills of self-mastery will be exercised and their power increased. So where courage does have moral import, it will be generally true that the deeper the courage the more powerful the moral concerns of the individual. Not all passionate people are courageous, but it is typical of courageous people that they are passionate.

The third aspect of the virtues of will power is self-confidence. There is a correlation between people's ability to handle their adverse inclinations and the confidence of their belief in their ability to determine their own destiny. Of course it is typical of skilled people in general that they are confident of themselves in respect of the skill in question. And so, since self-mastery is so fundamental to the successful conduct of a human life, it might seem that self-confidence is a by-product of the virtues of will power rather than an element of them. But while self-mastering skills clearly cause self-confidence, it is equally true that self-confidence grounds the exercise of self-mastery skills. When an athlete loses his self-confidence, he loses some of his ability to exercise his skill, even though his skill *per se* (so to speak) is not at all diminished. Similarly in a situation of testing the individual who has ceased to believe that he can persevere will show himself as weak, even though he possesses all the necessary skills to see him through his difficulty. An athlete needs three things for success: the requisite skills, an enthusiasm for the game, and a belief in his own powers. And the virtues of will power are the athletic side of the moral life.

Western Kentucky University

Part V
Shame, Guilt, Remorse

[21]

Subjective Guilt and Responsibility [1]

P. S. GREENSPAN

Several recent authors on guilt and related notions apparently allow for the rationality of guilt feelings in at least some cases of unavoidable wrong. Their views yield different decisions on some troubling real-life cases ranging from cases of survivor's guilt and vicarious or collective guilt to a case often brought up in the literature involving feelings of guilt after a car accident that without any fault on the part of the driver results in the death of a child. I want to take a new look at these cases and others—and a critical look at some of the views proposed—in an attempt to work out an understanding of the content of guilt and the grounds for its appropriateness that will better support the general conclusion that detaches grounds for guilt from grounds for blame.

This project rests on a rejection of the standard view of the emotion as involving a corresponding evaluative judgment that we find, most notably, in Rawls (1971, p. 482). On this "judgmentalist" account emotional guilt—what we may distinguish as "subjective" guilt—requires a judgment (in the sense of a belief) that one actually *is* guilty, a judgment of "objective" guilt of the sort that implies moral responsibility. Views differ on whether this requirement is to be imposed only on appropriate instances or rather on all genuine instances of the emotion, as Rawls apparently has in mind. At any rate, there is a way of accommodating guilt for the unavoidable that remains within the judgmentalist framework but weakens the content of the requisite judgment to an attribution of *causal* responsibility that extends to cases like the accident case while apparently ruling out survivor's guilt and other disputed cases as impossible.

What I want to defend here in opposition to this account is a *non*judgmentalist view of guilt that makes out the subjectively guilty agent as feeling *as if* he were *morally* responsible. On my own view guilt amounts to discomfort with a certain evaluative propositional object and hence may be said to correspond to a judgment—though one can undergo the feeling without holding the judgment. Indeed, I shall go on to argue elsewhere (see Greenspan forthcoming) that one can even undergo it appropriately (with "appropriate" taken to mean "rationally

[1] This paper was written while I was a fellow of the National Humanities Center during 1990-91; I owe thanks to the National Endowment for the Humanities and the University of Maryland for providing funding for the year. The paper extends an earlier essay written while I was on leave from Maryland during Autumn term 1988; I am particularly grateful to then Acting Dean James Lesher for arranging for the research time. For comments on the upshot let me also thank Conrad Johnson, Walter Sinnott-Armstrong, and Michael Slote along with audiences at Indiana University and the University of Rochester and students in my 1991 "Moral Psychology" seminar at Maryland, especially Scott Gelfand and Stephen Tighe.

acceptable", not "compulsory").[2] My view will allow us to interpret survivor's guilt and other disputed cases as having the same sort of content as moral instances of guilt; and it will also give us a framework for finer-grained consideration of questions of emotional appropriateness in application to the full range of cases. However, in this paper I want to narrow attention to the question of content. I shall in effect be arguing that the simplest ways of responding to the cases under discussion are *too* simple: Either they rule out guilt as something other than the emotion it appears to be or they accept it as unproblematically rational in a way that seems equally counterintuitive.

As a way of understanding the reasons for judgmentalism we might begin with the general question: How should we analyze emotional guilt? The feeling would seem to rest on self-blame, but we should note first that it does not always have the active or aroused quality of *anger*. Following the rough lines of Aristotle's definition I take anger—meaning personal anger, the variant of the emotion that amounts to other-directed emotional blame as opposed to mere frustration—to involve a desire to inflict some sort of punishment on its object for a wrong (see Greenspan 1988, especially pp. 48-55).[3] I would analyze the emotion further into affective and evaluative aspects by taking the desire for punitive action as involving discomfort at an unfulfilled action requirement—at the thought that the agent, or the subject of emotion, ought to punish its object, meaning that action on his part is still needed to effect punishment.

Anger is thus seen as an aroused feeling at least partly because of its essential orientation towards action—its threat of continuing discomfort unless and until the agent does punish the object—even though it may sometimes be satisfied without action, or without action on the part of the agent, perhaps by an apology from the object. An apology might be seen as a kind of *self*-punishment in so far as it involves self-abasement; so it seems to count as an active expression of guilt. For that matter, emotional guilt involves a kind of self-punishment where the agent has some control over whether he experiences that unpleasant feeling. But it is important that, if anger is thought of as originally grounded in an animal urge to attack, guilt comes out not as a self-directed version of the urge—an urge to

---

[2] Cf. Greenspan (1988, especially pp. 83-107), for a fuller account of the notion of emotional appropriateness; cf. especially pp. 15-80 on judgmentalist vs. nonjudgmentalist analyses of emotion. It is important to note that appropriateness and other terms of rational assessment applied to emotions in this paper are intended as notions of "backward-looking" or noninstrumental justification. I mark off "forward-looking" or instrumental justification (which I take to influence appropriateness, but only in general terms, by affecting the standard of evidence a given emotion type requires) with the term "adaptiveness". The two are clearly distinct. For instance, guilt too overwhelming to act on but warranted by the horror of a crime the agent has committed would be a possible case of appropriateness without adaptiveness; and on the other hand, someone manipulated into unwarranted guilt that leads him to behave better might be exhibiting an emotion that is adaptive albeit inappropriate.

[3] On the connection between anger and guilt see Greenspan (1988, p. 188, n. 3); cf. Gibbard (1990, esp. pp. 126-50). I attempt a fuller treatment of guilt in relation to general foundational questions about the role of emotion in ethics in *Practical Guilt: Moral Dilemmas, Motivational Force, and the Psychological Bases of Ethics* (in progress).

attack oneself—but rather as a less aggressive counterpart of it, requiring in the first instance *reparation*, or some way of making amends. Guilt may thus involve self-punishment as a form of reparation along with the readiness to submit to attack or to other punishment from others; but in developed form it is not simply inwardly directed anger.

One might say, however, that the different desires for action essential to guilt and (personal) anger both have the same general end: a state of affairs in which the perpetrator somehow "pays for" a prior wrong. They differ in where they place the burden of active responsibility for accomplishing that end, each assigning to a different agent a requirement of action enforced by discomfort until the job is done. This difference of course amounts to a limited structural similarity: The agents in question here are different in relation to the prior wrong, but they are both subjects of the relevant emotion. On the other hand, anger has a personal *object*, viewed as the perpetrator of the wrong, whereas guilt also assigns this prior sort of responsibility to the subject. Still, insofar as they both hold some such guilty party to account, both emotions ultimately rest on the attribution of responsibility for a wrong. On the assumption, then, that emotional evaluations amount to *judgments*—the assumption I call "judgmentalism"—one might look for the basic content of both emotions in a judgment of responsibility. The judgment yields emotional guilt and blame as different specifications of the urge to right a wrong depending on the agent's practical standpoint.

In what follows I want to consider problems with this view and ways of defending it in application to some familiar cases of guilt where we do not seem to have a judgment of *moral* responsibility: cases of guilt without fault (§1). I shall work with the case of guilt for an unavoidable car accident and construct a variant of it that seems to involve guilt without *agency* in order to show the inadequacy of a recent attempt to defend judgmentalism by framing the account of guilt in terms of *causal* responsibility (Taylor 1985, p. 91). I think we can see that this move commits the agent in such cases to a counterintuitive degree of irrationality. I shall attempt to show that a *non*judgmentalist account that preserves the reference to moral responsibility would square better with intuition, particularly as extended to more standard cases of guilt without agency (§2) that another recent author (Morris 1987) makes out as rational but nonmoral. I shall end by extracting from the cases some features of the practical role of the emotion that seem to yield a rational basis for cases of guilt without blame.

1. Guilt without fault

1. Naive judgmentalism.
On the view of the content of guilt just sketched the emotion is *sui generis*, though its evaluative structure links it closely to anger, with differences in desire content but the same evaluative basis for desire in a judgment of responsibility for a wrong. It seems natural to think of the latter as a judgment of moral respon-

sibility,for a version of this view that I shall call "naive judgmentalism". A naive judgmentalist analysis of guilt makes feeling guilty rest on a straightforward belief that one *is* guilty, a judgment simply spelling out the evaluative content of the emotion. But this analysis seems immediately to be called into question by cases of guilt without fault—clear-cut cases in which the agent may be assumed to be aware that he is not at fault (an assumption I shall often take for granted in what follows)—such as guilt at causing the death of a child in an unavoidable car accident. Even if the feelings in such cases are irrational, it seems undeniable that they occur—and *almost* undeniable that they amount to guilt feelings.

However, the denial that they do amount to guilt is suggested by the responses of naive judgmentalists to another sort of case, where the agent does not believe that some act of his was *wrong*, though he does accept full responsibility for it. A standard example, found in Rawls (1971, p. 482), involves the violation of a religious taboo in a religion the agent was taught as a child but now rejects. What the agent now feels when he violates the Sabbath, for instance, may be a feeling of discomfort persisting from childhood experiences of guilt, but on this view it cannot be a genuine case of the emotion.

It may seem that we need some view of this sort to distinguish guilt from various other emotions that might be confused with it such as fear of punishment or other forms of anxiety that might be thought of as its childhood predecessors. Even as supplemented by a desire to head off or appease the punishment—to perform some act of the sort that amounts to reparation where we do have guilt—this feeling needs to be conjoined with a view of the punishment as somehow *justified* to amount to (subjective) guilt. Built into the notion of guilt, that is—as distinct from, say, fear of persecution—is a kind of acknowledgment of *grounds* for punishment as given in the corresponding judgment of fault.

In general, it seems that emotions have an evaluative content that determines their classification—distinguishing guilt from fear and various other unpleasant reactions that may not always be so distinct from it in affective quality. I take this to be the main point in support of a judgmentalist analysis, though I think it can also be used to construct an evaluative view that does not insist that the content of an emotion be an object of strict belief. But before we abandon judgmentalism we might try making room within it for cases of "emotional inertia", or the lag of feelings behind their corresponding beliefs, as in taboo cases of the sort just illustrated.

2. Weak judgmentalism.

In an attempt to accommodate taboo cases within a version of judgmentalism Gabriele Taylor seems briefly to bring together *two* such strategies (1985, p. 86). First of all, the naive judgmentalist analysis of guilt might be retained by simply weakening the notion of judgment or belief, taking it to cover any thoughts that come to mind, even if they are immediately rejected by "considered judgment". Thus, Taylor says that the act forbidden by a taboo retained from childhood still "presents itself" as wrong in the circumstances of action, though not when the agent considers it "from a more rational point of view". Her introductory remarks

on emotions and belief (p. 1) indicate that she would interpret the notion of belief to include the sort of mental state suggested by "presents itself" in this passage: what is sometimes called an "as if" feeling. An agent's residual feelings from childhood religious belief would still count as involving beliefs on this account as long as they have the thought content required for feelings of guilt.

Secondly, however, one might also allow for taboo cases by weakening that evaluative content, the content of the judgment in question, allowing for something like a conventional interpretation of "justified" punishment. Punishment might be thought to be justified in some sense, that is, as long as it is imposed for violating an authoritative rule, meaning one whose authority is generally accepted, even if the agent questions the reasons for it himself. What one feels guilty *for*, on this view, *is* just the violation of a taboo—not necessarily a moral wrong and hence not enough to satisfy the naive judgmentalist analysis. Though Taylor apparently combines a move of this sort (I have restated her version of it to apply more clearly to rules) with the weakened notion of belief that was just noted, it would seem to be sufficient on its own to allow for guilt in taboo cases.

Both of these two general judgmentalist strategies—weakening the notion of belief or the evaluative content of *the* belief required for a guilt feelings—may be extended to the cases we are concerned with. Here the agent's responsibility is in question rather than the moral evaluation of his act, or whether it amounts to a wrong in the sense of something forbidden as in the taboo cases. A different version of the second strategy, yielding what might be called a "weak" judgmentalist analysis of guilt, stands behind Taylor's own treatment of such cases. I want to consider it here at some length, since it represents a possibility intermediate between naive judgmentalism and my own view.

Taylor interprets emotional guilt in terms of a weaker sort of judgment of responsibility than that involved in ordinary judgments of fault: causal rather than moral responsibility (p. 91). As applied to the accident case this notion apparently would make guilt feelings unproblematic—though it would also leave one puzzled as to how their rationality could even be called into question. If subjective guilt implies only the self-attribution of *causal* responsibility, feelings of guilt at causing the death of a child, however unavoidably, would seem to be clearly appropriate as well as authentic.

3. A variant case.

Of course it is not unthinkable that the analysis of such complex emotions as guilt might yield a few conceptual surprises. But the only advantage of the weak judgmentalist analysis seems to be its straightforward treatment of such putatively *rational* cases of emotion as cases of rational belief. For an idea of the problems it faces in application to *ir*rational cases we might compare the usual version of the accident case with one not even involving causal responsibility. Consider what Taylor's account would have us say about the distinction between the usual version of the case, where harm results from something the agent does (albeit unavoidably), and a case where the chain of causation leads back without interruption to some prior cause. For instance, what if the agent's car had simply been

propelled into a nearby child by another vehicle that hit it—and that would have hit the child, had his car not been there—so that the accident in no way resulted from his agency? Here Taylor would have to dismiss guilt as unintelligible, it seems—at any rate, in an agent assumed to be basically rational—since the emotion could not have even the weaker belief content required by her suggested modification of its standard judgmentalist analysis.

Intuitively speaking, however, I think we have to say that such cases are possible. We can imagine someone going over in memory the sequence of events leading up to the crash, pulling out a subset of them to focus on that is compatible with the usual scenario, the one that does involve responsibility, and feeling guilty. His reason need not be uncertainty about what happened but rather, say, some irrational tendency to fix on the worst possible interpretation of events from the standpoint of self-esteem. Perhaps he was taught to blame himself excessively as a child. I take this sort of tendency to be compatible with "basic" rationality: The agent one has in mind here is not *cognitively* confused in the usual sense—his system of settled beliefs is not disrupted—but instead is subject to a relatively localized disruption of the normal response tendencies. However, in order to accommodate such cases within judgmentalism—to preserve a foothold for real but *irrational* guilt feelings—we apparently need to bring in a version of Taylor's first strategy for handling emotional inertia in taboo cases, with a notion of belief weak enough to allow for cognitive delusion.

Further weakening the *content* of belief would make the case come out as *rational*, that is; so in order to explain it as a case of irrational emotion on this account we apparently have to ascribe to its agent an irrational causal belief. We have to grant that the agent in the case believes himself causally responsible for the accident. The agent clearly feels *as if* he were responsible—at any rate, off and on, or at those times when he focuses on the subset of his memories that suggests that interpretation of events—even though he knows he is not and dismisses the feeling as deluded. But the judgmentalist account of the case insists that the feeling implies a deluded belief.

If we have to allow for this much cognitive delusion, however, why not attribute to the agent a deluded belief in *moral* responsibility? The strategy of weakening the naive judgmentalist analysis of guilt—the strategy that yields weak judgmentalism—might seem to be unnecessary, in other words, when one considers the weak sense of "belief" that the analysis still has to rely on. We might extract a similar point from the taboo cases: An agent might sometimes feel lingering guilt about the violation of a religious rule that is not actually accorded much authority in his adult life even in conventional terms, though it was in force during his childhood. Particularly clear-cut examples might be drawn from rules of conduct meant to be limited to children such as prohibitions on naughty words and the like to show that the weakening of belief content to handle irrational cases does not really represent a distinct alternative to the reliance on a weak notion of belief.

At most the weak judgmentalist strategy serves to contain the *extent* of the cognitive delusion that the naive judgmentalist strategy attributes to basically rational agents in such cases. It makes out the first version of the accident case as *un*deluded, that is, and hence as clearly rational; but on the other hand, it seems to yield a treatment of the second version of the case as involving a deeper *kind* of delusion: delusion as to the facts. Rather than merely being confused about the standards for moral responsibility the agent must on this account mistakenly believe that he somehow caused the accident after all.

Or rather, he must both believe this and believe it to be false, either at the same time or with no good reason for a change of mind, since on our hypothesis he knows he is *not* responsible for the accident, though he feels compelled to dwell on the subset of events that suggests that he is. The case thus requires logical conflict; so the extent of delusion required by weak judgmentalism still seems excessive. It is minor only if one considers how little may be built into the notion of belief on either version of judgmentalism: Any stray thought would seem to have to qualify, if all of the cases in question here are to count as cases of guilt.

4. The nonjudgmentalist analysis.

On the assumption that belief interpreted in any reasonably strict sense is governed by a principle of logical charity, I would turn instead to a *non*judgmentalist analysis of emotion. Whereas the weak judgmentalist analysis of guilt allows for a weaker *judgment* than the judgment of moral responsibility required by the naive analysis, my approach would allow for something weaker *than* a judgment but still framed in terms of moral responsibility. In general, instead of claiming that emotions entail evaluative beliefs I take it that they sometimes just involve evaluative thoughts held in mind by intentional states of comfort or discomfort. Thus, when an agent feels guilty about the death caused by an accident he was involved in, he need not actually *assent to* the evaluative basis of his emotion—the thought of himself as responsible for a wrong—but he does have to be discomfited by it in a sense that involves entertaining the thought as an object of discomfort.

This is not to say that the agent merely "entertains" such a thought; its status as an object of discomfort (with discomfort taken as a general state of feeling of a sort one would naturally want to get out of) is essential to the motivational cast of my account. Nor do I want to say, on the other hand, that the agent has to entertain such a thought explicitly. Let me very briefly try to cancel out some misleading suggestions of my account and to indicate the general rationale for it before considering its application to cases. First, the agent's discomfort *about* a certain evaluative thought is understood to be directed towards the propositional *content* of the thought, the state of affairs it concerns, not the fact that it occurs to him or some logical or other feature of it as an object of contemplation. But secondly, my analysis is meant to allow for *unconscious* emotions as involving conscious states of affect (comfort or discomfort) but with evaluative objects that the agent cannot identify correctly (cf. Greenspan 1988, pp. 25-30).

Further, though the analysis is understood to be limited to *occurrent* emotions, so that guilt amounts to occurrent discomfort at a certain evaluative thought, the thought content of an emotion need not itself be taken as occurrent. There need be no episode of mental utterance corresponding to an unconscious thought; and even on the conscious level talk of thoughts might ultimately be replaceable by hypotheticals about relations among objects of attention. The claim that an agent's discomfort in a case of guilt, say, is occurrently directed towards a thought of himself as responsible might be replaced by a claim that attention to his discomfort *would* lead to awareness of that thought in the absence of various barriers to attention—including barriers of the sort that presumably make guilt unconscious.

It is tempting to equate a dispositional mental state of attention to a proposition of the sort here in question with a belief. However, I take the relevant disposition to be tied in a special way to pre-reflective features of "mental set", as part of a preparatory form of practical reasoning that sometimes turns on remaining subliminal, immune from the intellectual criticism that belief is expected to withstand (cf. Greenspan 1988, especially pp. 153-62). Emotional evaluations, in short, amount to patterns of *attention*, without the stability we expect of beliefs. That belief implies a degree of logical coherence is suggested by some recent treatments of more straightforwardly cognitive influences on behavior. Stich (1978) makes out the less logically structured behavioral dispositions of nonhuman animals as "subdoxastic states"; and in a treatment of developed practical reasoning Bratman (1992) marks off as "acceptance" a state of taking some proposition for granted without belief relative to a given practical context.

What Bratman has in mind is the sort of assumption it is rational to make in some contexts and not others (depending, for instance, on the practical costs of error) in deliberating about what to do. It would *not* be rational on Bratman's account to let *belief* vary with the context—an instance of the principle of logical charity, I take it, based on the primary tie of belief to theoretical contexts. I want to suggest, further, that what I have called "as if" feelings in my argument above may be picked out on the model of Bratman's states of acceptance by their role in practical reasoning. Their role is of course somewhat different; but like Bratman I shall be content to characterize them in terms of it—in terms of a kind of idealized or normative functional role, in effect—without attempting to say anything about their nature in themselves except that they otherwise resemble beliefs.

The role of emotion is a complicated matter; I shall discuss some of its intricacies in relation to disputed cases of guilt at the end of this essay. But generally speaking, emotion adds motivational force to our explicit reasoning from judgments insofar as it directs attention to certain thoughts by loading them with discomfort. The usual point of guilt, after all, is to motivate action on a moral ought-judgment by inflicting emotional punishment for the failure to act. But the mechanism can operate in advance of action as applied to the mere anticipation of moral failure: the thought of oneself as already responsible for a wrong, even

where this does not amount to a belief. What it amounts to is a momentary object of (dispositional) attention, held in mind and allowed to influence thought and behavior *as if* it were believed, though unlike belief it would be discarded upon a moment's reflection.

The point is to generate a readiness to act that resists reflection—and the ability to ignore or explain away the practical urgings of judgment. Emotional motivation on this account reinforces the usual model of practical reasoning with the need to discharge discomfort as a reason for action beyond what is provided by the evaluative content of emotion, which may or may not be an object of belief. Like Bratman's "acceptance" an emotional evaluation is treated temporarily or for certain purposes *as if* it were believed; and this means that in discussing cases of the sort here at issue we cannot take at face value the various thoughts that might occur to an agent: Some mental contents that could be seen as self-ascriptions of responsibility—the agent's reflection that he should never have gone out that night, for instance—would be most charitably interpreted on that account as nonjudgmental. They may sometimes just amount to questions the agent puts to himself or thoughts he considers and rejects; or they may be held in mind on something other than a literal reading as responsibility ascriptions.

On some such assumptions, at any rate, we may say that guilt does involve a thought of oneself as morally responsible but that it need not always involve the corresponding belief. The nonjudgmental analysis will therefore allow for guilt without cognitive delusion even in the second version of the accident case, where the agent feels guilty just as a result of passive causal involvement in a child's death, though he knows he lacks even causal responsibility for it. In effect the analysis limits his disturbance to the level of emotion by detaching emotion from belief. It also has the advantage, as I shall argue, of allowing for guilt in some cases where one might be tempted to detach the emotion even from a *thought* of moral *or* causal responsibility.

2. Guilt without agency

1. Guilt for what one is.
A crucial test of my nonjudgmentalist analysis will be its ability to provide a foundation for some defensible distinctions on the issue of emotional appropriateness. For present purposes, however, let us just attempt to use the analysis to accommodate some apparent cases of guilt. First I want to show how it allows for clearly irrational cases like the one just discussed (but without defending their classification *as* irrational). Then I shall go on to apply it to some arguably rational cases that even the weak judgmentalist analysis in terms of causal responsibility would seem to rule out. In effect, in this section I shall be extending my defence of the nonjudgmentalist analysis to a widening circle of cases—and to another possible way of weakening the notion of responsibility—with implications for the justificatory question of guilt versus blame.

My analysis differs from the judgmentalist analyses considered so far in allowing guilt to take on objects other than the agent's acts—or things he does, if that should be taken more broadly; or even, perhaps, *events* involving him—for a less clear-cut dividing line than is usually drawn between objects of guilt and *shame*. On the usual view only shame applies to personal traits, thought of as distinct from conformity to rules. But if there are norms imposed on children's personal development that a child might be expected to come to live up to without necessarily doing anything, then one might very well grow up to feel guilty about violating them. An example might be guilt about not being very bright or ambitious—not having what it takes to succeed in the way that one's parents had in mind. The object of guilt here amounts to something over and above any definite omissions one might be said to have performed—omissions sufficiently localized in time to count as objects of guilt on the usual account. It need not be seen as reducible, say, to a failure to go through some particular stage in development that was supposed to involve doing something—perfecting one's talents, working hard, or the like. Intuitively speaking it seems possible, whether or not it is rational, to feel guilt, not just shame, about all sorts of uncontrollable inadequacies, inabilities, and traits of character or temperament discouraged by parents and others but extending as far back in one's history as the claim to a distinct personality or self.

This means, I take it, that the objects of guilt in certain cases will violate the assumptions of Taylor's analysis by failing to allow for reasonable causal attribution to the agent in terms of either event-causation of the usual (Humean) sort or an indeterministic notion of "agent-causation" (cf., e.g., Donagan 1977, p. 45). I shall come back to these two alternatives for making out causal responsibility in a moment; but first let me introduce another sort of case that might tempt us just to abandon reference to responsibility or at any rate to weaken the sense of the term further—the approach taken by Herbert Morris (1987) in his defense of "nonmoral" guilt.

Morris marks off as nonmoral a subtype of guilt that does not involve culpability; he explains it instead in effect as a form of what one psychoanalyst (Modell 1965) calls "separation guilt", based on the severing of personal ties to members of a group with which one identifies. Morris' argument focuses directly on the notion of appropriate guilt rather than starting from an analysis of the content of the emotion. But it is relevant to my discussion here insofar as it yields a kind of opposite pole from Taylor's account in application to cases of guilt without agency. Unlike my own view it does not require even the thought of oneself as somehow in the position of an agent.

The cases just cited of guilt for personal shortcomings might indeed seem to involve another sort of responsibility besides the sort at issue in moral blame. A child growing up is more or less held accountable by his parents for living up to their expectations of him. I would treat this as giving rise to a tendency (short of belief) to think of himself *as if* he had done something to make his personality what it is; but Morris would say that moral responsibility is not necessary even in

thought for a genuine (or even an appropriate) case of guilt. By failing to conform to the norms of the family group the child is in a certain sense breaking away from the group independently of anything it does, just in virtue of its basic personality; and this is all that a judgment of nonmoral guilt asserts on Morris' account.

2. Undeserved benefit.

Morris does not apply his view to cases of guilt for traits. However, these may not be the strongest cases in favor of either Morris' view or my own. One might object that their intuitive plausibility as cases of guilt rather than shame seems to depend on whether they involve *behavioural* shortcomings—as opposed to the failure to meet norms of attractiveness and the like—and hence on a kind of general reference to agency. But there is another set of examples among those discussed by Morris, of guilt for an undeserved benefit (pp. 232-7)—ranging from survivor's guilt to guilt at being favored economically over others—to undercut the suggestion that an object of guilt must at least be manifested in behavior.

An agent might know that there was nothing he could have done, for instance, to keep from being favored over a sibling in his childhood—and nothing he omitted then or since in attempting to make up for the inequality. But the inequality itself seems to be a possible object of guilt. Taylor has a puzzling comment about the parallel sort of economic case:

> If I feel guilty about my privileged position in society due to circumstances of birth then I see myself as an agent causally involved: it is *my* birth which has brought about the state of affairs which is my privileged position. (1985, p. 91)

The object of guilt in such cases at most seems to involve a passive event, something that happens *to* the agent as in the second version of the accident case. The agent's *birth* is no less passive; it just is less easily distinguished from the person it happens to. It is questionable, though, how this could yield the requisite sort of causal responsibility on Taylor's account without an implausible attribution of delusion to the agent. Presumably what is in question is causation *by* the agent in some sense—if not through his act or agency then at least through some other form of activity on his part. But surely birth does not qualify. Responsibility for something caused by what happens *to* the agent, though, would seem to shift back to the causes of *that* event, whether or not these are agent-causes.

3. Guilt for states of mind.

In any case, it will not be easy to find an event involving the agent that may serve even as part of a causal chain leading to the object of guilt in such cases, if we follow Hume's insistence on logically distinct cause and effect. It may not even be possible to pick out any very definite event in some cases. Consider, for instance, guilt for one's beliefs: Common talk of guilt feelings for a failure of religious belief would seem to apply to a case where the agent discovers that he never did have the kind of faith that is required of him. But then his guilt will not be attributable to an event of *ceasing* to believe—or even, given the sort of belief that is in question here, to a failure of belief *formation* at some particular time

when belief was called for. Perhaps he might see himself as involved in some sort of ongoing act of omission of belief formation throughout his life. But although some move of this sort might serve to locate within the agent's history a Humean event-cause of his lack of faith, it could not give us the *two* events we need for a Humean claim of causal connection. That is, a second application of the move would not seem to pick out a *distinct* event to serve as the object of guilt in this case. What the agent feels guilty *about*, if it does amount to an act, seems to amount to the same act: that lifelong omission of belief. But then he would not come out as causally responsible for it in Humean terms; so the case would still pose a problem for Taylor's account.

Similar cases are brought up by Morris under the heading of guilt for thoughts, as reasons against requiring culpability (pp. 226-32). By "thoughts" Morris has in mind mainly *wishes;* but it is worth noting that the strength of such cases depends on assigning them something like the dispositional structure of belief in the cases just considered. Actively *entertaining* a wish, that is—an occurrent thought of the sort that typically involves an act of attention—may be voluntary and hence avoidable. At any rate, it is subject often enough to *some* voluntary control that my nonjudgmentalist interpretation of guilt as involving an "as if" attribution of responsibility seems to fit. But on the other hand, the sort of evil wish about someone that an agent might discover in himself—perhaps as something he has carried around for years— may also be an object of guilt, whether or not harm actually befalls the other. Since the problem just noted about distinguishing cause from effect would seem to apply to it, though, it would seem to count against Taylor's causal account in the way sketched for beliefs.

4. Vicarious and collective guilt.

An alternative strategy for handling the various cases of guilt without agency that have surfaced so far might involve appeal to a notion of substantial *self*-causation that is broader than agent-causation. Agent-causation is supposed to be limited to free acts; but perhaps some other things about me are importantly attributable to *me* in a sense that appeals *neither* to some distinct event involving me nor to my agency. To say this would not be to deny that there are event-causes to be found for character traits, beliefs, and dispositional wishes—any more than for our status in relation to other members of the various groups that define us. But just because of the way such notions as character are constructed, this consequence of determinism might be held to be compatible with the view that certain traits are attributable in a special sense to the self (see Greenspan 1987; cf. Adams 1985). They serve to define its individual nature, one might say—in contrast to passive events like birth or even complex processes like the workings of the digestive tract that admit of indirect causal control but are not taken to express some basic property of the one who undergoes them.

This move beyond agent-causation would not solve all problems for the judgmentalist view that Taylor wants to maintain, however. Despite her occasional use of "as if" language, Taylor's commitment to judgmentalism is underlined by her exclusion of cases of *vicarious* guilt in the contrast she draws between guilt

and shame (pp. 91-2). On Taylor's causal version of weak judgmentalism, that is, only shame, not guilt, makes sense in response to acts ascribed to others—for the behavior of one's children, say, or of one's fellow citizens. And it is important to note that the view entails not just that vicarious guilt is irrational but rather that it is conceptually *impossible* without at least a deluded judgment of indirect causal responsibility—the belief that one's failings as a parent, for instance, must have been responsible for a child's later misdeeds. However, such cases seem to be more common, if anything, than those resembling the accident case I began with. Whether rationally or not, we sometimes feel *as if* we were responsible for the acts of others whose doings would be said to "reflect" on us just by virtue of common group membership, without really acknowledging any causal connection. A case in point might be white American guilt about slavery—or guilt for various national misdeeds that occurred before one's birth.

At least sometimes, moreover, such feelings seem to be accepted as appropriate or reasonable. Morris devotes considerable attention to cases of guilt felt in response to the acts of one's nation as cases in favor of his own account, which might be set up as an alternative version of weak judgmentalism (pp. 237-40). In place of a judgment of responsibility in the sense that involves culpability Morris appeals to our identificatory ties to other group members. But even without a judgment about the latter, if we allow for emotional reactions based on imaginative identification with others, we can make out vicarious guilt as no more problematic than a host of vicarious emotions, including the empathetic reactions to harm done to others that underlie ordinary guilt (cf. Hoffman 1982).

Taylor's contrast between guilt and shame on this question actually seems to rest on a misunderstanding of the notion of vicarious emotion. Shame is commonly felt *for* acts of others in a way that is not true of guilt. But strictly vicarious shame would amount to shame from the other's imagined standpoint; it is "for" another *agent* in the sense of being felt on his behalf. If I feel shame in response to the misdeeds of my brother, say, normally my feeling will *not* be vicarious; what I am ashamed of is something connected to myself in real-life terms. My own status is assumed to be diminished by what my brother does even without the assumption that I am responsible for it but just by virtue of the fact that status is partly a product of interpersonal ties.

Identification of course plays a role in determining interpersonal ties. Whether I feel shame, for instance, at the misdeeds of a colleague in ethics depends in part on the importance others assign to our common category but also on my own tendency to group myself with colleagues in my field. However, a similar point applies to guilt in cases where one feels guilty about activities attributable to a group to which one belongs: family, profession, nation, race, or world. In fact, there is a further way of generating vicarious guilt in such cases that is worth distinguishing from the usual mechanism of identification with other individuals. On the assumption that responsibility can sometimes be assigned to a group considered as a whole, not just to its other members, what one feels may depend on a general kind of group-identification, or imagining oneself as participating in the

300   *P. S. Greenspan*

group's collective actions. *Collective* guilt in this sense amounts to the feeling of guilt for involvement in a case of collective responsibility (cf. Feinberg 1970, p. 233).[4] It is a prime case, though not the only case, of vicarious guilt; but it seems to rest on the same general identificatory mechanism that can also operate in extending the bases for shame.

What is the function of guilt in such cases? It can sometimes just amount to an unavoidable cost of basing individual identity on group membership, as Morris wants to say (pp. 239-40). However, one can often manage to drop out of a group in imagination. Particularly when the group acts in ways one is fundamentally opposed to, it might seem unclear what the point is of feeling guilty on its behalf. Why should I punish myself for something I would never do—for wars and witch trials I know I would have resisted? Does the pride or other pleasure I take in group involvement generally somehow *commit* me to feeling guilty in a case where the group goes astray—as a matter of emotional "logic" or perhaps as a kind of recompense for the benefits of group membership?

Morris' comments elsewhere suggest grounds of general moral solidarity (cf. pp. 232 and 237); but it is important to note that the acceptance of guilt as appropriate in such cases falls short of a strict requirement to feel guilty. I may be obligated to feel *something*, say, for the American internment of Japanese civilians during World War II, and perhaps my feeling should in some way reflect my membership in the group that committed the crime; but it is unclear why its very content must reflect that fact. Assuming that I am myself unlikely to participate in such collective acts or even to allow them, it might be enough just to feel sympathy and outrage, perhaps to a degree augmented by my ties to the event. The point is to *detach* myself, after all.

However, I think we can make out vicarious guilt as having a point, even if not as obligatory, in just such terms. In cases where the identificatory bases of the emotion admit of control it can be seen as a way of clearing oneself of involvement and at the same time expiating the deed on behalf of others by a kind of ritual self-punishment. One identifies with the perpetrator, whether a group one belongs to or some other member of it, just in order to distance oneself and the group as a whole symbolically from the deed by taking on in emotional terms the punishment the deed merits.

Identification with the victims, that is, does represent an alternative way of exhibiting moral solidarity in response to the case. What distinguishes the function of guilt is its self-punitive aspect as a negative self-directed emotion. Though sympathy and outrage may involve an initial layer of negative feeling, they need not feel bad overall in the way that guilt does. I take it, then, that my nonjudgmentalist account serves to supplement Morris' appeal to identificatory ties in explaining the distinctive role of guilt in such cases. The "as if" feeling that one

---

[4] Taylor apparently misses this distinction when she cites Feinberg's point that vicarious *objective* guilt is impossible in support of her own view that "feelings of guilt... cannot arise from the deeds or omissions of others" (1985, p. 91; cf. n. 5 and Feinberg 1970, p. 231 and p. 237).

is morally responsible for a wrong and therefore deserves punishment—at any rate, the emotional *self*-punishment of guilt feelings—seems to make more sense here in intuitive terms, moreover, than Morris' denial that guilt in such cases counts as moral. Morris' distinction between moral and nonmoral guilt allows for a univocal account of the emotion just insofar as moral guilt is understood on his account to rest on separation from the moral community (p. 226). But by a kind of transitivity of identification this would seem to make vicarious cases of moral guilt come out as moral too.

5. Self-referential guilt without blame.

My suggested moral-but-nonjudgmental account of the various cases Morris considers seems to me to be compatible with the substance of his view; it rejects only his classification of separation guilt as necessarily nonmoral. I do recognize cases of nonmoral guilt—guilt about going off one's health regimen and similar examples—where the rules the agent violates are in fact nonmoral, though he treats them in emotional terms *as if* they had moral force. But this distinction of course does not turn on the issue of culpability. The hardest cases to make out plausibly as moral might seem to be cases of survivor's guilt. These may involve an "undeserved benefit" that the agent clearly did nothing to gain and can do nothing to make up for; so on the assumption of basic rationality one might want to question how he could he see himself even in "as if" terms as *morally* responsible. But Morris in fact suggests something of the sort himself when he subsumes these and similar cases under guilt about "unjust enrichment" (p. 232).

My own proposal for handling such cases can be strengthened by appeal to the *self-referential* character of guilt. In so far as guilt functions as a kind of emotional self-punishment, that is, it goes some way towards fulfilling its own characteristic desire for reparation. But in that case the failure to feel guilty counts as a possible object of guilt itself. This effectively redoubles the motivational force of anticipatory guilt—guilt about one's failure (so far) to make up for a wrong, as the basis for a "forward-looking" variant of the emotion that Morris also wants to recognize (see 1988, p. 66). On my account of it in terms of an "as if" feeling the emotion is sometimes self-generating in anticipatory form: One feels as though one *already* has done something wrong simply by failing to feel guilty (or guilty enough) *yet*.

This way of compounding guilt may seem a fiendish trick. In fact, I think it helps explain some of the pitfalls of the emotion, in particular its obsessive or unappeasable quality in many cases. But can it serve as a *foundation* for guilt or must one assume a more basic negative self-evaluation as a reason for the emotion? In cases of guilt for an undeserved benefit I think we might well begin with anticipatory self-referential guilt, if we appeal to a demand for *leveling*: a requirement that the agent bring himself down to the level of others in a group he identifies with, if only by subjecting himself to emotional self-punishment. What he should punish himself *with* according to this suggestion is discomfort at the thought that he has done something to deserve punishment—though all he has really done is to fail to inflict it so far. Indeed, some demand of the sort—requir-

ing in the first instance unconscious self-referential guilt, which then may be masked by guilt with some other (perhaps indefinite) object—may seem on occasion to be imposed by others as a condition of participation in the groups to which we are bound by mutual identification. Breaking away from the family, for instance—whether by one's own efforts or by the death of parents or other misfortunes of family members that do not befall oneself—is a prime source of separation guilt and can sometimes be encouraged by parents and other family members on a familiar picture.Morris' discussion brings up resentment and indignation as appropriate reactions on the part of others (along with self-reproach on the part of the agent as involved in feelings of guilt) only in connection with *moral* guilt (p. 226). But others' reactions in nonmoral cases may also include other-directed forms of blame of the sort that demand guilt of the agent—sometimes in no less fiendish forms than the one suggested. Part of showing that one identifies with others in a way that makes inequalities unwelcome involves the willingness to make up for inequalities by way of self-inflicted emotional distress. But this is an unachievable aim in many cases; and according to the account I have offered it is based on an illusory feeling of responsibility. On the issue of appropriateness, however, I would suggest (what I elsewhere shall argue at length) that we have reason to detach subjective guilt—even clearly moral cases of it—from the variants of other-directed blame.

Once we understand the practical function of guilt, that is, we can see that a demand that someone undergo the emotion need not be taken to depend for its justification on the sort of judgmental basis we require for blame. In the normal sort of moral case there is reason to be cautious in allocating blame, as an emotion that effectively punishes another agent by making him the object of negative attention. Appropriate blame, then, is plausibly taken to rest on a judgment of moral responsibility, or blame*worthiness*. However, I hope to have paved the way here for an asymmetrical treatment of guilt and blame by arguing with reference to guilt that no such judgment is implied by the content of emotion. Requiring less to justify guilt may be said to make sense in practical terms on the assumption that an agent has a right to inflict on himself what he could not legitimately inflict on others—as a goad to moral perfection, perhaps, beyond what morality requires. What he *may* inflict on others compatibly with this is the demand for guilt—and blame if they fail to satisfy that demand—at least where the object of guilt is something reasonable to forbid. But in cases of separation guilt we may question whether this last condition is satisfied.

Department of Philosophy   P. S. GREENSPAN
University of Maryland
College Park
MD 20742
USA

REFERENCES

Adams, R. M. 1985: "Involuntary Sins". *Philosophical Review*, 94, 1, pp. 3-31.

Bratman, M. E. 1992: "Practical Reasoning and Acceptance in a Context". *Mind*, 401, pp.1-15.

Donagan, A. 1977: *The Theory of Morality*. Chicago: University of Chicago Press.

Eisenberg, N. 1982: *The Development of Prosocial Behavior*. New York: Academic Press.

Feinberg, J. 1970: "Collective Responsibility", in his *Doing and Deserving: Essays in the Theory of Responsibility*. Princeton, N. J.: Princeton University Press, pp. 222-51.

Gibbard, A. 1990: *Wise Choices, Apt Feelings: A Theory of Normative Judgment*. Cambridge, Mass.: Harvard University Press.

Greenspan, P.S. 1987: "Unfreedom and Indeterminism", in Schoeman 1987, pp. 63-80.

——1988: *Emotions and Reasons: An Inquiry into Emotional Justification*. New York: Routledge, Chapman and Hall.

——forthcoming: "'Perspectival' Guilt", in Sinnott-Armstrong *et al.*, forthcoming.

Hoffman, M. L. 1982: "Development of Prosocial Motivation: Empathy and Guilt", in Eisenberg 1982, pp. 281-313.

Modell, A. H. 1965: "On Having the Right to a Life: An Aspect of the Superego's Development". *International Journal of Psychoanalysis*, 46, pp. 323-31.

Morris, H. 1987: "Nonmoral Guilt", in Schoeman 1987, pp. 220-41.

——1988: "The Decline of Guilt". *Ethics*, 99, 1, pp. 68-76.

Rawls, J. 1971: *A Theory of Justice*. Cambridge, Mass.: Harvard University Press.

Schoeman, F. 1987: *Responsibility, Character, and the Emotions: New Essays in Moral Psychology*. Cambridge: Cambridge University Press.

Sinnott-Armstrong, W., Raffman, D., and Asher, N., forthcoming: *Meaning, Modality, and Morality: A Festschrift for Ruth Marcus*.

Stich, S. P. 1978: "Beliefs and Subdoxastic States". *Philosophy of Science*, 45, 4, pp. 499-518.

Taylor, G. 1985: *Pride, Shame, and Guilt: Emotions of Self-Assessment*. Oxford: Clarendon Press.

[22]

Shame and Self-Esteem: A Critique*

John Deigh

Twenty-five years ago the psychoanalyst Gerhart Piers offered what remains the most influential way of distinguishing shame from guilt. Reformulated without terms special to psychoanalytic theory, Piers's distinction is that shame is occasioned when one fails to achieve a goal or an ideal that is integral to one's self-conception whereas guilt is occasioned when one transgresses a boundary or limit on one's conduct set by an authority under whose governance one lives. Succinctly, shame goes to failure, guilt to transgression. Shame is felt over shortcomings, guilt over wrong-doings.[1]

More recently, writers who have addressed themselves to the way shame differs from guilt, notably, among philosophers, John Rawls, have characterized shame as an emotion one feels upon loss of self-esteem and have analyzed self-esteem and its loss in a way that bears out Piers's influence.[2] Rawls plainly is in Piers's debt. He explains self-esteem in terms of the goals and ideals one incorporates into one's life plans, and he makes this explanation central to his account of our moral personality, in particular, our capacity to feel shame.

A characterization of shame like Rawls's, when set in the context of distinguishing shame from guilt, we are likely to find intuitively appealing. And we may feel a further pull in its direction when we think of shame in comparison with other emotions to which it is thought similar—for instance, embarrassment. For we associate both shame and embarrassment with an experience of discomfiture, a sudden shock that short-circuits one's composure and self-possession; yet we would agree, I think, that

* I am indebted to Herbert Morris for helpful comments on an earlier draft of this article.

1. Gerhart Piers and Milton B. Singer, *Shame and Guilt: A Psychoanalytic and a Cultural Study* (Springfield, Ill.: Charles C. Thomas, 1953), pp. 11–12.

2. John Rawls, *A Theory of Justice* (Cambridge, Mass.: Harvard University Press, 1971), pp. 440–46. For similar views see Helen Merrell Lynd, *On Shame and the Search for Identity* (New York: Harcourt Brace & Co., 1958), pp. 23–24; Robert W. White, "Competence and the Psychosexual Stages of Development," in *Nebraska Symposium on Motivation 1960*, ed. Marshall Jones (Lincoln: University of Nebraska Press, 1960), pp. 125–27; and David A. J. Richards, *A Theory of Reasons for Action* (Oxford: Oxford University Press, 1971), pp. 250–59.

Ethics 93 (January 1983): 225–245

embarrassment is an experience of discomfiture that, unlike shame, does not include a diminishment in one's sense of worth. An experience of shame, by contrast, strikes at one's sense of worth. Here we may be reminded of times when things were going well and we were somewhat inflated by the good opinion we had of ourselves, when suddenly, quite unexpectedly, we did something that gave the lie to our favorable self-assessment, and we were shocked to see ourselves in far less flattering light. Such are the circumstances for shame, and the positive self-image that disappears in these circumstances and is replaced by a negative one spells loss of self-esteem.

These contrasts between shame and guilt and shame and embarrassment present the bare outlines of a characterization of shame, which, when filled out, appears rather attractive. It is the topic of this article. My thesis is that this characterization, though attractive at first appearance, is unsatisfactory. It represents, I contend, a dubious conception of shame. In particular, I mean to call into question its central idea that shame signifies loss of self-esteem.

The paper is divided into three parts. In the first I lay out what I shall call the Rawlsian characterization of shame, Rawlsian in that I retain the controlling thesis and overall structure of Rawls's account but do not concern myself with its specifics, an exact rendering of Rawls being unnecessary for my purposes. Though my approach here is largely uncritical, my aim is to set up a well-defined target for subsequent criticism. In the second, then, I begin that criticism. I set forth a case of loss of self-esteem and some cases of shame that pose problems for the characterization. By themselves these cases stand as counterexamples to it, but my hope is that they will have a more illuminating effect, that they will produce a sense or spark an intuition that its central idea is problematic. Accordingly, in the third part I complete the criticism. I draw from the cases two lessons about shame intended to give definition to the intuition I hope will already have been sparked. Each lesson points to a key feature of shame that the characterization leaves out or misrepresents, its central idea being implicated as the source of these failures. Thus, while the criticism of this third part is aimed at the target set up in the first, the force of the criticism should lead us to consider rejecting the idea at the target's center.

I

We need at the start to fix our understanding of self-esteem, since the concept is at the base of the Rawlsian characterization. To this end I shall present some considerations leading up to a definition of self-esteem, from which an explanation of its loss will follow directly. This will then yield the characterization of shame we seek. Let us begin with the general idea that self-esteem relates to what one makes of oneself or does with one's life. One has self-esteem if one's spirits are high because one believes that one has made or will make something of oneself, that one has been

or will be successful in one's life pursuits. Conversely, one lacks self-esteem if one is downcast because of a judgment that one has failed to make or never will make something of oneself, that one doesn't or won't ever amount to much. Something of this idea is suggested in William James's equation that sets self-esteem equal to the ratio of one's successes to one's pretensions.[3]

The first thing to note in this general idea is that self-esteem connects up with the condition of one's spirits. We speak of vicissitudes of self-esteem: highs and lows. One's self-esteem can plummet. It can also be boosted or bolstered. Indolence and languishing in doldrums are signs that one's self-esteem is at a low ebb. Enthusiasm for and vigorous engagement in activities in which one chooses to participate are signs of an opposite condition. We also describe persons in these conditions as having or lacking self-esteem. And though subtle differences may exist between a person's having self-esteem and his self-esteem's being high and between his lacking self-esteem and his self-esteem's being low, I shall treat the two in each pair as equivalent.

A second point of note, which is corollary to the first, is that self-esteem goes with activity. But to assert that having self-esteem requires that one be active would be an overstatement. We should allow that the esteem a person has for himself is relative to that period in his life with which he identifies for the purpose of self-assessment. Thus, a person may retain his self-esteem after having retired from active life if he looks back on his endeavors and accomplishments with pride while content to take it easy. He maintains a high opinion of himself while leading a rather leisurely and unproductive life because his self-assessment proceeds from recollections of an earlier period when he was active and successful. Or, to take the viewpoint of a youth looking forward in time, he may have esteem for himself in view of the life he aspires to lead if he believes in the accuracy of the picture he has of his future. He identifies, for the purpose of self-assessment, with the person he believes he will become, his present self having little bearing. Consequently, he may even at the time be leading an altogether easygoing and frivolous life while exuding self-esteem. I mention these possibilities only to set them aside. We simplify our task of explaining self-esteem if we restrict the discussion to self-esteem had in view of one's current doings and development.

Besides this simplifying restriction, we must also add a qualification to the statement that being active is a condition of having self-esteem. As a third point, then, one's actions, if they are signs of self-esteem, must have direction. They must be channeled into pursuits or projects and reflect one's goals and ideals. A wayward vagabond does not present a picture of someone who has self-esteem. Nor do we ascribe self-esteem to someone who, having no settled conception of himself, tries on this

---

3. William James, *The Principles of Psychology*, 2 vols. (1890; reprint ed., New York: Dover Publications, 1950), vol. 1, p. 310.

228 *Ethics   January 1983*

and that trait of personality, as he would sunglasses of different styles, to see which gives him the most comfortable look. Self-esteem is had by persons whose lives have a fairly definite direction and some fairly well-defined shape, which is to say that self-esteem requires that one have values and organize one's life around them.

One's values translate into one's aims and ideals, and a settled constellation of these is necessary for self-esteem. Specifically, we may take this as a precondition of self-esteem. For, arguably, someone who had no aims or ideals in life, whose life lacked the direction and coherence that such aims and ideals would bring, would be neither an appropriate object of our esteem nor of our disesteem. We would understand his behavior as the product of primitive urges and desires that impelled him at the time of action. Having given no order or design to his life, he would act more or less at random or for short-lived purposes. We should recognize in him a figure who frequents recent philosophic literature on human freedom: the man assailed by a battery of desires and urges, who is helpless to overpower them because he lacks a clear definition of himself.[4] Such a man is impelled in many directions at once but moves in no particular one for any great distance. Frustrated and disoriented by inner turmoil, he lapses into nonaction. He would, were we ever to encounter his like, properly evoke in us pathos indicating abeyance of judgment rather than scorn indicating low esteem for him.

By contrast, when a person has aims and ideals that give order and direction to his life, counterpoint between primitive forces that impel him and his wanting to fulfill those aims and ideals becomes possible. Thus, at those times when he acts in conflict with his aims and ideals, he may declare that he was caught in the grip of some emotion or was overpowered by some urge or desire. He would then convey the idea that he had been acted upon or compelled to act as opposed to doing the act or choosing to act. Undeniably, the emotion, urge, or desire is attributable to him; but by such declaration he disowns it and so disclaims authorship of the act it prompted. Authorship, not ownership, is the key notion here, that is, authorship in the general sense of being the originator or creator of something. When one has a settled constellation of aims and ideals, then one distinguishes between the acts of which one is the author and those in which one serves as an instrument of alien forces.[5] Without any such constellation, one is never the author of one's actions, though many times the instrument of alien forces that act on one, triggered by external events.

4. See Joel Feinberg, "The Idea of a Free Man," in *Educational Judgments: Papers in the Philosophy of Education*, ed. James Doyle (London: Routledge & Kegan Paul, 1975), pp. 148–49; Harry Frankfurt, "Freedom of the Will and the Concept of a Person," *Journal of Philosophy* 68 (1971): 5–20; Wright Neely, "Freedom and Desire," *Philosophical Review* 83 (1974): 32–54; and Gary Watson, "Free Agency," *Journal of Philosophy* 72 (1975): 205–20.
5. I have drawn here from Harry Frankfurt, "Identification and Externality," in *The Identities of Persons*, ed. Amélie Rorty (Berkeley: University of California Press, 1976), pp. 239–51.

It is in view of this contrast that I suggest we take one's having a settled constellation of aims and ideals as a precondition of self-esteem: when one is the author of one's actions, one is an appropriate object for esteem or disesteem; when one is only an instrument of alien forces, one is not. We can then look to this precondition for the defining conditions of self-esteem. So while we would have said, loosely speaking, that self-esteem came from one's having a good opinion of oneself, we may now say more strictly that it comes from a good opinion of oneself as the author of one's actions, more generally, one's life. Accordingly, this opinion comprises a favorable regard for one's aims and ideals in life and a favorable assessment of one's suitability for pursuing them. Lacking self-esteem, one would either regard one's aims and ideals as shoddy or believe that one hadn't the talent, ability, or other attributes necessary for achieving them. Either would mean that one lacked the good opinion of oneself that makes for self-esteem, and either would explain the dispirited condition that goes with one's lacking self-esteem.

These considerations then yield an understanding of self-esteem as requiring that two conditions jointly obtain. This we can formulate as a definition. Specifically, one *has self-esteem* if, first, one regards one's aims and ideals as worthy and, second, one believes that one is well suited to pursue them.[6] With reference to the first we say one has a sense that one's life has meaning. With reference to the second we speak of a confidence one has in the excellence of one's person. And this combination of a sense that one's life has meaning and a confidence in one's ability to achieve one's ends gives one impetus to go forward.

Turning then to loss of self-esteem and, in particular, the sudden loss taken on the Rawlsian characterization to be explicative of shame, we obtain immediately from the foregoing definition an account of this experience. One loses self-esteem if, because of a change in either one's regard for the worthiness of one's aims and ideals or one's belief in one's ability to achieve them, a once favorable self-assessment is overturned and supplanted by an unfavorable one. The loss here is the loss of a certain view of oneself. One had self-esteem and correspondingly a good opinion of oneself: one viewed oneself as having the attributes necessary for successfully pursuing worthy ends around which one had organized one's life. The change in judgment about the worthiness of one's ends or the excellence of one's person destroys that view. One's good opinion of oneself gives way to a poor one. This constitutes loss of self-esteem.

The Rawlsian characterization has it that shame is the emotion one feels when such loss occurs. Moreover, shame is to be understood as signifying such loss. Shame on this characterization is the shock to our sense of worth that comes either from realizing that our values are shoddy or from discovering that we are deficient in a way that had added to the confidence we had in our excellence. Either is a discovery of something

6. The definition matches Rawls's (see p. 440).

false in the good opinion we had of ourselves, and such self-discovery spells loss of self-esteem.

Of course, self-discovery of this sort does not figure in every experience of shame, for a person who has a poor opinion of himself is nonetheless liable to feel shame when the very defect that is his reason for the poor opinion is brought to his notice. Thus, as a last point, we must say something about shame felt by someone whose self-esteem is already low. While a schoolboy, Philip Carey, in Maugham's novel *Of Human Bondage*, feels shame innumerable times over his clubfoot. His feelings do not involve loss of self-esteem, since his self-esteem is low to begin with, nor, obviously, do they reflect any act of self-discovery. But it would be uncharitable to object to the Rawlsian characterization on the ground that it does not cover such cases, for they can be treated on analogy with cases it does cover. Philip does not always have his crippled foot on his mind; there are plenty of times when he is forgetful of it. On these occasions, especially when he is comfortable with himself, he is liable to feel shame when made conscious of his "freakish" condition, when, as it were, he rediscovers it. Then, while he does not lose any self-esteem, his being comfortable with himself is certainly lost to him.

II

In this section I shall set forth a case of loss of self-esteem and some cases of shame that present real problems for the Rawlsian characterization. I begin with the former. The case itself is quite straightforward. We have only to think of someone who suddenly loses self-esteem because he discovers that he lacks the ability to achieve some aim he has set for himself, who is crestfallen, dispirited, and deeply disappointed with himself, but owing to circumstances or a philosophical temperament, does not feel shame. And such a case is not hard to construct.[7]

Imagine, for example, some youth who is indisputably the best tennis player in his community. He defeats all challengers; he wins every local tournament; and he has recently led his high school team to a first-place finish in a league consisting of teams from the high schools of his and the neighboring towns. His coach rates him the most promising player to come along in a decade, and he is highly touted by other tennis enthusiasts in the area. Quite naturally, he comes to have a high opinion of his ability and visions of winning tournaments on the professional tour. At some point early in his high school years, he makes professional tennis a career goal and devotes much time to improving his game. In truth, though, the grounds for his high opinion of his ability and for his decision to make tennis a career are shaky. The competition in his and the neighboring towns is rather poor, these being rural and isolated from urban centers. And the aging coach's hopes have distorted his judgment

7. Examples similar to this first case were suggested to me by Herbert Morris and Rogers Albritton.

of his star player's talents. Thus, when this young player enters his first state tournament, he quickly discovers that his skills are below those of the top seeded players. His first defeat need not be humiliating, just convincing. And though he will surely lose some self-esteem, we need not suppose that he feels any shame.

One explanation of his losing self-esteem but not feeling shame is this. The first defeat is sufficiently convincing that it alters his view of himself as a tennis player, and given his aims, this means loss of self-esteem. But just as others close to him would respond that his defeat is nothing to be ashamed of, so his own attitude toward it may reflect such judgment. Accordingly, he would be deeply disappointed with himself but not ashamed. This possibility becomes even more vivid if we suppose that he has gone to the tournament alone or with friends who, unlike him, have only a passing rather than an abiding interest in tennis. For then he does not find himself having to face someone like his coach before whom feeling some shame would be natural, though even here the presence of the coach does not necessitate the emotion. This case thus broaches the question what distinguishes those cases of loss of self-esteem whose subjects feel shame from those whose subjects feel disappointment but no shame. The inability of the Rawlsian characterization to answer this question implies that the understanding of shame it gives is, at best, incomplete.

Let us next take up cases of shame. The first comes from an observation, made by several writers, that shame is commonly felt over trivial things. One writer instances experiences of shame had on account of "one's accent, one's ignorance, one's clothes, one's legs or teeth."[8] Another, to illustrate the same point, mentions shame felt over "an awkward gesture, a gaucherie in dress or table manners, . . . a mispronounced word."[9] To be sure, none of these examples poses a threat to the Rawlsian characterization, since each of the things mentioned could be for someone a shortcoming the apprehension of which would undercut the confidence he had in the excellence of his person. This would certainly be true of someone who consciously subscribed to ideals the achievement of which required that he not have the shortcoming. For then, though others would disparage these ideals as superficial or vulgar and accordingly think the shortcoming trivial, to him it would still appear as a serious flaw in himself. Naturally, the more interesting case is that in which the subject also thinks the shortcoming trivial and is surprised at having felt shame on its account. This case too can be understood as coming under the Rawlsian characterization. For one need not fully realize the extent to which one places value on certain things, and one may even deceive oneself about one's not being attached to certain ideals. We need, then,

8. Stanley Cavell, *Must We Mean What We Say?* (Cambridge: Cambridge University Press, 1976), p. 286.
    9. Lynd, p. 40.

232   *Ethics   January 1983*

to distinguish between, on the one hand, what one would declare were one's aims and ideals and would list as one's important attributes if one were asked to describe oneself and, on the other, one's self-conception as it is reflected by one's behavior apart from or in addition to any explicit self-description. By one's self-conception I mean the aims and ideals around which one has organized one's life together with the beliefs one has about one's ability to pursue them. And what we understand is that these aims, ideals, and beliefs can guide one's behavior without one's being conscious of having subscribed to them. Consequently, a person who feels shame over crooked teeth or the slurping of soup, though he would have thought himself unconcerned with appearance and proper form, shows by his emotion that a pleasant-looking face or good table manners are important to him, that he subscribes to ideals of comeliness or social grace. Hence, we can easily understand his shame as signifying loss of self-esteem.

At the same time, such examples invite us to look for things over which someone might feel shame though he did not believe they made him ill suited to pursue his ends. Shame one feels over something one could not believe affected one's excellence, say, because one could not regard it as a fault in oneself, would present a problem for the Rawlsian characterization. Thus, consider shame felt over a humorous surname. The example comes from Gide. He describes to us the experience of a young French girl on her first day of school, who had been sheltered at home for the first ten years of her life, and in whose name, Mlle Péterat, something ridiculous is connoted, which might be rendered in English by calling her Miss Fartwell. "Arnica Péterat—guileless and helpless— had never until that moment suspected that there might be anything laughable in her name; on her first day at school its ridicule came upon her as a sudden revelation; she bowed her head, like some sluggish waterweed, to the jeers that flowed over her; she turned red; she turned pale; she wept."[10]

With this example we move from attributes that one can regard as minor flaws and insignificant defects to things about a person that leave him open to ridicule, though they do not add to or detract from his excellence. The morphemes of one's surname do not make one better or worse suited for pursuing the aims and ideals around which one has organized one's life. Hence, shame in this example, because it is felt over something that lies outside its subject's self-conception, opposes the Rawlsian characterization.

The second case of shame is cousin to the first. One finds oneself in a situation in which others scorn or ridicule one or express some deprecatory judgment of one, and apprehending this, one feels shame. Given only this general description, such a case presents no real problem

---

10. André Gide, *Lafcadio's Adventures*, trans. Dorothy Bussy (New York: Alfred A. Knopf, 1953), p. 100. The rendering of her name in English is suggested by the translator.

for the Rawlsian characterization. It serves to remind us that one's self-esteem depends to some extent on the esteem others accord one—certain others, anyway—and the greater that dependency the more readily one will feel shame in response to any deprecatory judgments they express. This can be understood by way of the amount of confidence one has in one's own independent judgments about the worthiness of one's aims and one's ability to fulfill them, for this, we might say, varies inversely with the strength of the dependency of one's self-esteem on the esteem of others. That is, the greater that dependency, the less one's confidence will be in independent judgments one makes about oneself and, concomitantly, the more accepting one will be of the judgments others make about one. Consequently, given a strong enough dependency, if they criticize or ridicule one for some fault, one accepts their criticism and thus makes the same judgment about oneself, where before one did not notice the fault or it did not much matter to one. This arouses shame inasmuch as the judgment issues in an unfavorable self-assessment that replaces a favorable one, that is, in loss of self-esteem. We have then an account of the case that is fully in line with the Rawlsian characterization.

But we must also admit cases of shame felt in response to another's criticism or ridicule in which the subjects do not accept the other person's judgment of them and so do not make the same judgment of themselves. And these cases do present a problem for the Rawlsian characterization. Consider Crito and his great concern for what the good citizens of Athens will think of him for failing to deter Socrates from meeting his demise. "I am ashamed," he says in vainly trying to argue Socrates out of accepting his fate, "both on your account and on ours your friends'; it will look as though we had played something like a coward's part all through this affair of yours."[11] And though Crito is in the end convinced that Socrates' course is the right one and knows all along that he has done everything one can expect of a friend, we still have, I think, no trouble picturing this good-hearted but thoroughly conventional man feeling ashamed when before some respectable Athenian, who reproaches him for what he believes was cowardice on Crito's part. Examples like this one demonstrate that shame is often more, when it is not exclusively, a response to the evident deprecatory opinion others have of one than an emotion aroused upon judgment that one's aims are shoddy or that one is deficient in talent or ability necessary to achieve them.

The third problematic case of shame is this. We commonly ascribe shame to small children. Shaming is a familiar practice in their upbringing; "Shame on you" and "You ought to be ashamed of yourself" are familiar admonishments. And, setting aside the question of the advisability of such responses to a child's misdemeanors, we do not think them nonsensical

11. Plato, *Crito* 45d–e. Quoted from the Hugh Trednick translation, *The Collected Dialogues of Plato*, ed. Edith Hamilton and Huntington Cairns (Princeton, N.J.: Princeton University Press, 1961), p. 30.

or incongruous in view of the child's emotional capacities. Furthermore, close observers of small children do not hesitate to ascribe shame to them. Erik Erikson, writing about human development, observed that children acquired a sense of shame at the stage when they began to develop muscular control and coordination.[12] Charles Darwin, writing about blushing, noted that small children began to blush around the age of three and later remarked that he had "noticed on occasions that shyness or shamefacedness and real shame are exhibited in the eyes of young children before they have acquired the power of blushing."[13]

But it would certainly be a precocious child who at the age of four or five had a well-defined self-conception, who organized his life around the pursuit of certain discrete and relatively stable aims and ideals and measured himself by standards of what is necessary to achieve them. In other words, a child at this age, though capable of feeling shame, does not have self-esteem. Hence, the shame he experiences does not signify loss of self-esteem.

Finally, a fourth problematic case of shame emerges once we juxtapose the orientation of an aristocratic ethic and that of an achievement ethic. The Rawlsian characterization with its emphasis on making something of oneself, being successful in one's life pursuits, is tied to the latter. The experiences of shame it describes are at home in a meritocratic society, one in which social mobility is widespread, or, at any rate, the belief that it is constitutes a major article of faith. On the other hand, some experiences of shame reflect an aristocratic ethic; one feels shame over conduct unbecoming a person of one's rank or station. The experiences are better suited to a society with a rigidly stratified social structure like a caste society. And, as we shall see, they stand in marked contrast to experiences the Rawlsian characterization is designed to fit.

The contrast is this. With shame reflective of an achievement ethic, the subject is concerned with achieving his life's aims and ideals, and he measures himself against standards of excellence he believes he must meet to achieve them. So long as he regards his aims and ideals as worthy, they define for him a successful life, and accordingly he uses the standards to judge whether he has the excellence in ability or of character necessary for success. He is then liable to shame if he realizes that some of his aims and ideals are shoddy or that he has a defect portending failure where previously he had ascribed to himself an excellence indicating success. And this fits nicely the idea that shame signifies loss of self-esteem. On the other hand, with shame reflective of an aristocratic ethic, the subject's concern is with maintaining the deportment of his class and not necessarily with achieving aims and ideals that define success in life. He is concerned with conforming to the norms of propriety distinctive of his class, and

12. Erik Erikson, *Childhood and Society*, 2d ed. (New York: W. W. Norton & Co., 1963), pp. 251–54.
13. Charles Darwin, *The Expression of the Emotions in Man and Animal* (1872; reprint ed., Chicago: University of Chicago Press, 1965), p. 331.

conformity to these is neither a mark of achievement nor an excellence that forecasts achievement. In the usual case one is born into one's class and conforms to its norms as a matter of course. Failure to conform, that is, failure to deport oneself as becomes a member of one's class, invites comparison to persons of lower classes on whom the members of one's class look down. Thus, someone from a social class beneath which there are other classes may be liable to shame over such failure: someone wellborn may be liable to shame if he behaves like the vulgar. And such shame does not fit the Rawlsian characterization. For the subject neither realizes that his aims and ideals are shoddy nor discovers a defect in himself that makes him ill suited to pursue them. In other words, given the analysis we have laid out, he does not lose self-esteem.

But, one might ask, can't we say of someone who feels shame over conduct unbecoming a member of his class that he too has ideals that regulate his actions and emotions? After all, with his class we associate a way of life, and this implies an ideal or set of ideals. To feel constrained to act as becomes a member of one's class is to feel pressed to conform to its ideals, and conduct unbecoming a member is, in other words, conduct that falls short of an ideal. Granted, one doesn't so much achieve these ideals as conform to them, which shows perhaps that the conception of self-esteem on which the Rawlsian characterization is built must be modified. But supposing we make whatever modification is needed, isn't it sufficient to bring the experience under the Rawlsian characterization that we can redescribe it as shame felt over one's falling short of an ideal?

Something, however, gets lost in this redescription. When we redescribe the experience as shame felt over falling short of ideals around which one's life is organized, our focus shifts from who one is to how one conducts one's life. The subject's identity as a member of a certain class recedes into the background. We see it as the source of his ideals but do not assign it any further part. This, I think, is a mistake. In this experience the subject has a sense of having disgraced himself, which means he has an acute sense of who he is. We do not have an understanding of shame otherwise.

It is revealing that on the Rawlsian characterization this shift in focus does not register. For the characterization recognizes no distinction between questions of identity and questions of life pursuits, between who one is and how one conducts one's life. From its viewpoint, a person says who he is by telling what his aims in life are and what ideals guide him through life.[14] This makes it an attractive characterization of the shame felt by persons who are relatively free of constraints on their choice of life pursuits owing to class, race, ethnic origins, and the like. For such persons tend more to regard their aims and ideals as constituting their identity and their ancestry, race, class, and so forth as extrinsic facts about themselves. So the characterization explains the shame they feel as including

14. See Rawls, p. 408.

236   *Ethics*   *January 1983*

an acute sense of who they are. But because it restricts a person's identity
to his aims and ideals in life, it fails to explain as including this sense the
shame someone, living in a rigidly stratified society, feels when he does
not act as befits a member of his class or the shame someone, living in
a multiethnic society, feels when he acts beneath the dignity of his people.
Granted, such a person recognizes that his conduct falls short of ideals
members of his class or culture are expected to follow, but these ideals
do not constitute his identity. Another, a pretender for instance, could
have the same ideals as he but not the same identity, just as a tomboy
has the ideals of a boy but not the identity of one. Hence, we fail to
account for such shame if we describe it as being felt over one's having
fallen short of ideals that regulate one's life.

Thus, about the following experience, which Earl Mills, a Mashpee
Indian, relates, a defender of the Rawlsian characterization will insist
that sometime during the episode Mills must have embraced the ideals
of an Indian way of life or, alternatively, that he must have realized,
though he nowhere suggests this, that the ideals he was then pursuing
were shoddy. But ignoring the Rawlsian characterization, we can explain
Mills's feeling shame without importing either of these assumptions: his
having, in the circumstances he describes, to acknowledge his ignorance
of Mashpee traditions disgraced him as an Indian, made him betray, as
it were, his Indian identity, and this aroused shame. This explanation
accepted, his experience directly opposes the Rawlsian characterization,
for it suggests that, despite the aims and ideals around which a man
organizes his life, circumstances may arise that make him, because of an
identity he has that is independent of those aims and ideals, liable to
experience shame.

> When I was a kid, I and the young fellows I ran around with couldn't
> have cared less about our Indian background. We never participated
> in any of the tribal ceremonies, we didn't know how to dance, and
> we wouldn't have been caught dead in regalia. We thought anyone
> who made a fuss about our heritage was old-fashioned, and we even
> used to make fun of the people who did. Well, when I came back
> from the Army in 1948, I had a different outlook on such matters.
> You see, there happened to be two other Indians in my basic-
> training company at Fort Dix. One of them was an Iroquois from
> Upper New York State, and the other was a Chippewa from Montana.
> I was nineteen years old, away from Mashpee for the first time in
> my life, and, like most soldiers, I was lonely. Then, one night, the
> Iroquois fellow got up and did an Indian dance in front of everyone
> in the barracks. The Chippewa got up and joined him, and when
> I had to admit I didn't know how, I felt terribly ashamed.[15]

15. Paul Brodeur, "A Reporter at Large: The Mashpees," *New Yorker* 54 (November
6, 1978): 62–150, p. 103.

III

Before drawing any lessons about shame from the discussion of Part II, I should say something to allay doubts about the import of the cases of shame presented there. Such doubts naturally arise because one might think that some, if not all, of those cases exemplify experiences of the emotion the subjects of which one could criticize for being irrational or unreasonable. That is, while agreeing that many persons are liable to such experiences, one might wonder whether they ought to be so liable and then note that a case's force as a counterexample lessens if it only describes an experience of irrational or unreasonable emotion. The first and last cases of shame are especially in point. To feel shame over one's surname and because of conduct unbecoming a person of one's class seem good examples of shame one ought not to experience. For one is not responsible for one's parentage and thus ought not to judge oneself according to facts wholly determined by it. Inasmuch as shame in these cases reflects such judgment, they exemplify experiences to which one ought not to be liable.

These doubts arise under the assumption that, in giving a characterization of an emotion, one specifies those conditions in which the emotion is experienced reasonably or rationally. Such an approach to characterizing an emotion requires that one regard as its standard cases those in which the subjects are fully rational individuals and not at the time of the experience in any irrational frame of mind. But we ought to question this requirement. Why should we restrict the class of standard cases to these? While there is, for instance, something absurd in the familiar picture of an elephant terrified at the sight of a mouse, why should this absurdity lead us to regard the elephant's terror as any less important a case to be considered in characterizing that emotion than the terror a lynch mob strikes in the person on whom it takes revenge? To be sure, the elephant is not a creature capable of bringing its emotions under rational control, whereas a human being, if sufficiently mature, is. And for this reason there is a point in criticizing the emotional experiences of human beings, whereas making similar criticisms of an elephant's emotional experiences is altogether idle. But this provides no reason to regard the class of rational or reasonable experiences of a given emotion as privileged for the purposes of conceptual inquiry. To have brought one's emotions under rational control means that the range of one's emotional experiences has been modified through development of one's rational capacities: one no longer responds with, say fear, to certain sensory stimuli that before the development provoked fear, and conversely. But far from instructing us to discount the elephant's or the toddler's emotions in our conceptual inquiries, this bids us to examine emotional experiences had in response to sensory stimuli unmediated by rational thought as well as experiences the occurrence of which we explain by reference to rational thought.

Similar points then apply to characterizing shame. To focus primarily on cases the subjects of which one would not criticize for being irrational or unreasonable is to risk introducing distortion into the characterization. Indeed, one might be well advised to examine closely those cases in which such criticism is forthcoming on the grounds that they may display more prominently than others certain characteristic features of the emotion. Thus, one might be well advised to examine closely the shame typical of *homo hierarchicus*, even though one thought that rigid, hierarchical social structures lacked rational foundations (i.e., even though one thought that the emotion indicated an irrational attachment to social class), on the grounds that in such shame one sees more clearly than in shame typical of persons living in an egalitarian society those parts of the subject's self-conception in virtue of which he is liable to the emotion. Moreover, though the resultant characterization rendered shame an emotion that, from the perspective of an egalitarian or meritocratic ethic, one never had good reason to feel, this would not in itself show the characterization to be faulty: no more than that gentlefolk like the Amish, because of certain theistic beliefs, regard resentment as an emotion one never has good reason to feel shows that they harbor misconceptions about resentment. Since we are capable of bringing our emotions under rational control, we may regard our feeling a specific emotion as incompatible with our moral principles and so try to make ourselves no longer liable to it. Alternatively, we may regard this emotion as essential to our humanity and so revise our principles. The conflict makes evident the importance of having a correct understanding of such emotions; at the same time we should see that altering the understanding one has in order simply to avoid such conflict or the criticism of irrationality would be misguided.

Turning then to lessons that come out of our discussion of the problematic cases, I shall draw two. The first is that a satisfactory characterization must include in a central role one's concern for the opinions of others. This is really a lesson in recall. From Aristotle onward, discussions of shame have focused attention on the subject's concern for the opinions others have of him.[16] Aquinas, Descartes, and Spinoza each incorporated this concern into his definition of shame.[17] And latter-day writers, Darwin and Sartre in particular, took the experience of shame before another as key to an understanding of the emotion.[18] Thus, we should not be surprised to find that the Rawlsian characterization founders, since it regards such concern as not internally related to shame.

Its failure, however, is not due to neglect. The characterization, through emphasis on the dependency of one's self-esteem on the esteem of others, can accord the concern an important role in an overall un-

16. For Aristotle's view see *Rhetoric*, bk. 2, chap. 6.
17. For Aquinas's definition see *Summa Theologiae* 1a2ae, 41,4. For Descartes's see *The Passions of the Soul*, pt. 2, article 66. For Spinoza's see *The Ethics*, pt. 3, definition 31.
18. See last chap. of Darwin. Sartre's view is found in *Being and Nothingness*, trans. Hazel E. Barnes (New York: Philosophical Library, Inc., 1956), pp. 252–302.

derstanding of shame.[19] But this makes the concern part of a mechanism that induces shame rather than part of our conception of shame. A mechanism exists which, when put into operation, transforms high self-esteem into low; part of that mechanism is the concern one has for the opinion of others; and one way in which the mechanism gets going is when others on whose good opinion one's self-esteem depends deprecate one and one apprehends this. In this way, the characterization gives one's concern for the opinion of others an important role. But it is only a supporting role and not the central one I think it deserves. And this is one reason for its failure.

Each of the first three problematic cases bears out this last point. It is evident in the second and third cases, where the subjects feel shame but do not lose self-esteem. In the third case shame is felt directly in response to another's scorn or reproach. Thus, an expressed low opinion of the subject induces in him shame without affecting his self-esteem. In other words, the mechanism is not engaged, though the subject's concern for the opinion of another is clearly operative. In the second, Mlle Péterat, even apart from the context in which she feels shame, jeering classmates, feels the emotion because of something about herself that is laughable. It invites deprecatory responses. Thus, she may feel ashamed because of it, even though it is not a deficiency. It is not a ground for reassessing her excellence, though, of course, the whole experience could cause her to think less of herself. Here, too, there is shame reflecting a concern for the opinion of others without the mechanism's being engaged.

We can also mine the first case to bring out the point that the Rawlsian characterization has misconstrued the role one's concern for the opinion of others has in shame. Consider again our young tennis phenom. In the circumstances described, he loses self-esteem, is disappointed with himself, but does not feel shame. On the other hand, as we noted, if the circumstances had been different, if he had had, say, to face his coach after the defeat, then his feeling shame would have well been imaginable. There would then have been someone at courtside whose look he could not meet. He would have averted his eyes, lowered his head, gulped to fight back tears. That the coach's presence could spell the difference between disappointment and shame cannot be explained by reference to the player's losing self-esteem, for the loss occurs in either case. The mechanism would be in operation whether or not the subject felt shame, so it would not account for the role his concern for the coach's opinion would have had in his experiencing shame. We can thus conclude from these three cases that one's concern for the opinion of others has a role in shame apart from the way in which their opinion can support or bring down one's self-esteem.

19. See, e.g., Rawls's discussion of the companion effect to the Aristotelian principle, pp. 440–41.

The second lesson is about our sense of worth. The Rawlsian characterization yields an understanding of a person's sense of worth according to which it has two sources. One is the person's conviction that he has given meaning to his life. The other is the confidence he has in his own excellence as a person. The first comes from his regarding his aims and ideals in life as worthy. The second comes from his belief that he is well suited to pursue them. Thus, according to the Rawlsian characterization, shame, since it is felt either upon a judgment that one's aims or ideals are shoddy or upon a judgment that one is deficient in a way that makes one ill suited to pursue them, is aptly described as a shock to one's sense of worth. One experiences a diminishment in one's sense of worth since either one's sense of having given meaning to one's life or one's confidence in one's excellence has been struck down.

There is difficulty in this, however, because, while the description of shame as a shock to one's sense of worth is apt, the account of the various ways in which the sense gets shocked is, at best, too meager. The reason for this is that the characterization omits important sources of our sense of worth. The point is directly evident in our last two cases. The child of four who feels shame over some misdemeanor has not given meaning to his life and does not have confidence in his excellence as a person. Hence, he has a sense of worth the source of which the characterization does not acknowledge. Similarly, we recognize in an aristocrat who feels shame over behaving like a plebian or in an American Indian who feels shame over betraying his Indian identity a sense of worth the source of which is neither a conviction about the worthiness of his ends nor a belief about his suitability to pursue them. A sense of worth that comes from knowledge that one is a member of the upper class or a noble people also lies beyond the sight of the Rawlsian characterization. To put the point generally, the Rawlsian characterization fails to recognize aspects of our identity that contribute to our sense of worth independently of the aims and ideals around which we organize our lives.

We should note here the structural, as well as the substantive, difference between the sense of worth the Rawlsian characterization recognizes and the one it excludes. We can get at this structural difference by looking at the theory of worth that underlies the characterization. That theory is based on a conception of us as the authors of our actions. We are authors in the sense discussed in Part I, that is, in virtue of having a constellation of aims and ideals according to which we live our lives. We have worth on this theory in accordance with the value of our lives, such as they are and such as they promise to be. An author has worth in view of his work, completed or in progress, and our lives, so to speak, are our work. This analogy can be pressed. Our work has value to the degree that it is the kind of thing that when well made has value and is itself well made. So we have worth to the degree that we produce such things or have directed our energies toward producing them and possess the talents and skills that augur successful production. Our lives, conceived

as our work, thus have value to the degree that the ends that give them order and direction define a kind of life that has value and those ends have been realized. And we have worth as authors of our lives to the degree that we live lives of value or have directed our energies toward living such lives and possess the attributes that promise success.

In capsule form, what might be called the auteur theory of worth is that what a person does with his life, how well he directs it, determines his worth. On this theory, then, we attribute different degrees of worth to someone depending on how valuable we deem the kind of life he lives and how successful we think he has been in living it or how suitable we think he is for it. In other words, we attribute to him more or less worth according to how well or badly he conducts his life. Contrast this with attributions of worth made because of one's class or culture. Judging from these attributions, we might say that a person's worth is determined by his status in the context of some social hierarchy. The salient feature here is that one's status, and so one's worth, is fixed independently of one's conduct. To be sure, one can change classes through marriage or cultures through immigration, but short of this the general conduct of one's life, that is, however well or badly one conducts it, does not increase or decrease the worth that is attributed to one because of one's status. And pretty much the same holds of worth that is attributed to human beings because of their species or to persons because of the kind of beings they are conceived to be: rational ones, say, spiritual ones, or autonomous ones. That is, worth attributed to one because of one's essential nature is, like worth attributed to one because of one's status, fixed independently of how one conducts one's life.

Consequently, the dynamics of the sense of worth that comes from knowing the worth that goes with one's status or essential nature, that is, the understanding we give to augmentations and diminishments in that sense, are altogether different from those of the sense of worth the auteur theory recognizes. Statically, both kinds of sense correspond to the degree of worth one attributes to oneself. But an augmentation in one's sense of worth, as is experienced in pride, or a diminishment in it, as is experienced in shame, is not, if this sense originates in a recognition of one's status or essential nature, to be understood in terms of an attribution to oneself of greater or lesser worth than one attributed to oneself before the experience.[20] A college boy who wears his fraternity pin with pride does not regard himself as having greater worth for having worn it, and a man who feels ashamed of having eaten like a pig does not regard himself as having less worth than is attributed to human beings as such. This contrasts with the way the auteur theory would have us understand augmentations and diminishments in one's sense of worth. In particular, it would have us understand a diminishment in one's sense

20. Of course there are exceptions to this, e.g., the white supremecist who discovers he has a black ancestor.

242   *Ethics   January 1983*

of worth, as is experienced in shame, as amounting to loss of self-esteem
and so corresponding to an assessment of oneself as having less worth.

On the auteur theory, a sense of worth reflects concern with one's
real worth, and one takes one's conduct and appearance as evidence of
or, more strongly, as the grounds for attributing to oneself that worth.
By contrast, a sense of worth that comes from knowing one's status or
essential nature reflects concern with the congruency between one's conduct
or appearance and one's real worth. Here, we could say, one's concern
is with the relation between appearance and reality. If one's status is high
relative to that of others or one's nature is noble, then behavior that is
congruent with one's worth and so displays it is occasion for pride, and
behavior that is at variance with it and so gives appearance of lesser
worth is occasion for shame.

This model better accommodates the idea that to have a sensibility
to shame means that one is prepared to restrain oneself when one verges
on the shameful and to cover up the shameful when it comes into the
open. We speak in this regard of having shame as opposed to having no
shame, and we connect this with modesty, particularly sexual modesty,
which involves a sensibility to shame in matters of decorum. Having
shame, that is, having a sensibility to shame, can be understood here as
self-control that works to restrain one from giving the appearance of
lesser worth and self-respect that works to cover up shameful things that,
having come to light, give one such appearance.[21]

This suggests that we should conceive shame, not as a reaction to a
loss, but as a reaction to a threat, specifically, the threat of demeaning
treatment one would invite in giving the appearance of someone of lesser
worth. Its analogues then are, not grief and sorrow, but fear and shyness.[22]
Like fear, shame serves to protect one against and save one from unwanted
exposure. Both are in this way self-protective emotions. Fear is self-
protective in that it moves one to protect oneself against the danger one
senses is present or approaching. From fear one draws back, shields
oneself, or flees. Of course, it may also render one immobile, thereby
putting one in greater danger, so the point does not hold without qual-

21. On these points, see Carl D. Schneider, *Shame, Exposure and Privacy* (Boston:
Beacon Press, 1977), pp. 24–27.

22. Whether to pattern shame after grief and sorrow or after fear and shyness is an
issue a review of the literature reveals. One often finds in the writings of those offering
definitions of shame use of one or the other of these emotions as analogues, sometimes
even as a generic emotion of which shame is defined as a specific type. For definitions of
shame as a type of grief or sorrow see Hobbes (*Leviathan* chap. 6) and Descartes (pt. 3,
article 205) (though the passage is equivocal since he also says there that shame is a species
of modesty). For definition of shame as a type of fear see Aquinas; it is also suggested in
Plato's *Euthyphro* 12a–d. In connection with this issue see Havelock Ellis's "The Evolution
of Modesty," in *Studies in the Psychology of Sex*, 2 vols. 3d ed. (New York: Random House,
1942), vol. 1, p. 36, n. 1. Ellis himself appears to hold that shame is a kind of fear (see pp.
36–52, 72).

ification.[23] Still, the general idea is clear. Shame, too, is self-protective in that it moves one to protect one's worth.[24] Here the general idea is not so clear, though a trope may be useful. Shame inhibits one from doing things that would tarnish one's worth, and it moves one to cover up that which through continued exposure would tarnish one's worth. Less figuratively, we might say that the doing or exposure of something that makes one appear to have less worth than one has leaves one open to treatment appropriate only to persons or things that lack the worth one has, and shame in inhibiting one from doing such things and in moving one to cover them up thus protects one from appearing to be an unworthy creature and so from the degrading treatment such appearance would invite.

This idea that shame is a self-protective emotion brings together and explains two important features: first, that a liability to shame regulates conduct in that it inhibits one from doing certain things and, second, that experiences of shame are expressed by acts of concealment. The second is crucial. Covering one's face, covering up what one thinks is shameful, and hiding from others are, along with blushing, the most characteristic expressions of shame. Students of shame commonly note them. A quote from Darwin is representative, "Under a keen sense of shame there is a strong desire for concealment."[25] Moreover, etymology reinforces the point. According to many etymologists, a pre-Teutonic word meaning 'to cover' is the root of our word *shame*.[26]

Now the Rawlsian characterization, since it conceives shame as a reaction to a loss, can explain, on the model of fear of loss, how one's liability to shame regulates one's conduct. Where it has trouble is in explaining shame's moving one to cover up and hide. For it does not have in itself the materials needed to construct such an explanation. Because it conceives shame as a reaction to the loss of something one prizes, it yields an account of the emotion as at first giving way to low spirits and dejection and eventually moving one to attempt to recover what one lost, that is, to regain through self-improvement one's good opinion of oneself and so one's self-esteem.[27] Acts of concealment, however, are nowhere implicated in this account. Hence, if one adheres to the characterization, one must make use of supplementary materials to explain them. One must go outside the characterization by, say, citing certain fears associated with shame: fear of ridicule or rejection by those upon

23. I owe this point to John T. MacCurdy, "The Biological Significance of Blushing and Shame," *British Journal of Psychology* 21 (1930): 174–82.

24. The idea is one of the central themes of Max Scheler's essay "Über Scham und Schamgefühl," in *Gesammelte Werke*, ed. Maria Scheler and M. S. Frings, 11 vols. (Berne: Franke Verlag, 1954), vol. 10, pp. 65–154.

25. Darwin, p. 320.

26. See *Oxford English Dictionary*, s.v. "shame"; also Ernest Klein, *A Comprehensive Etymological Dictionary of the English Language* (Amsterdam: Elsevier, 1967).

27. See Rawls, p. 484; Lynd, pp. 50–51; and Richards, p. 256.

whose good opinion of one one's self-esteem depends.[28] But such an explanation would not be adequate, for it fails to explain acts of concealment as expressions of shame. Instead, it takes these as expressions of fears associated with shame. And the same objection would hold for any explanation one constructed from materials found outside the characterization. The characterization, in other words, is unable to explain, as expressions of shame, these acts. And this should tell us that something has gone wrong.

The adherent to the Rawlsian characterization thus appears to be in an untenable position. We would dismiss any suggestion that covering up and hiding were not really among shame's natural expressions. Reflection on shame, particularly shame concerning sexual improprieties, alone suffices to rule this out. And we should reject any characterization of an emotion that misrepresents its natural expressions. Faced with these objections, the adherent might retreat to a weaker thesis by proposing that the characterization gives an adequate account of some, but not all, experiences of shame. But this thesis is no more defensible than the original. For our adherent, as we saw from the first problematic case of Part II, has the burden of showing how the emotion the characterization describes is distinguishable from disappointment with oneself. Since he admits on this weaker thesis that some experiences of shame elude the characterization, he has, in other words, the burden of showing that the experiences of emotion the characterization captures are classifiable with these as shame. What reason could he give to show this? That they have the same feeling-tone is itself questionable, insistence on the point being question begging. That they involve a shock to one's sense of worth is insufficient. For the characterization identifies this shock with one's suffering loss of self-esteem, and this by itself does not qualify an experience as one of shame. The trouble with this proposal, I think, is that it would, in effect, divide shame into disparate kinds, one kind having fear as its analogue, the other grief. That is, we should suspect of any conception of shame the proposal spawned that it covered a mismatched set of experiences.

We can trace the characterization's problems back to the understanding it gives to the sense of worth that makes one liable to shame and ultimately to the auteur theory of worth, which grounds that understanding. On that theory one attributes to oneself worth according to how one conducts one's life, and so perceptions of that conduct determine one's sense of worth. Shame then, since it is felt upon discovery of shortcomings in oneself that falsify the worth one thought one had, includes a sense that one lacks worth. And this proves problematic because it leaves unexplained how shame motivates acts of concealment. By contrast, when we conceive shame as including a sense that one has worth, we can readily explain

---

28. See Piers and Singer, p. 16; and Rawls, p. 445. White, however, expresses reservations against connecting shame to such fears (pp. 125–27).

its motivating such acts: one covers up because one senses that the worth one has is threatened. This speaks in favor of the understanding of the sense of worth the idea that shame is a self-protective emotion entails, which understanding is grounded on a conception of worth that opposes the one the auteur theory yields. Consequently, we should suspect that the conception of worth the auteur theory yields is the wrong one for explaining the sense of worth that makes one liable to shame, and, because the Rawlsian characterization presupposes that conception, we should give up the view of the emotion it represents.

IMPERSONALITY, CHARACTER, AND MORAL EXPRESSIVISM*

E ven if morality recommends that we take an objective view of ourselves, and in our deliberations each consider ourselves as but one person among many, this is not an unambiguous demand. It is not obvious, for example, what kind of impersonality is asked for in the context of moral deliberation that includes deliberation about oneself. For although our relations toward ourselves and to others are similar enough for us to use the same moral and psychological vocabulary for our first- and third-person attitudes, they are also systematically different in both ethical and epistemological contexts. Self-deception is only the most familiar case of an attitude or stance that raises very different moral and conceptual questions from those concerning its third-person cousin. Even for its most experienced practitioners, self-deception is not something one can succeed in by modeling it, in an impersonal manner, on one's relations to others.

The call for impersonality in ethics can mean various different things, and problems with certain forms of it are not confined to the difficulties concerning the *demands* of morality on the agent, which have been the focus of recent attention by theorists of "agent relativity" in ethics.[1] Some earlier writers, such as Jean-Paul Sartre,[2] for instance, saw the role of impersonality in ethics as problematic because it construed the first-person position of the deliberator as *less* demanding than he saw it as being. According to him (on one reading, anyway), if I consider myself impersonally, as someone with a certain character and history, with certain beliefs and desires that then enter into my moral deliberation along with the character and desires of others, I leave out of consideration the fact that I am *responsible* for that character and those desires. But these cannot be for me a set of data that I must simply make room for in my delibera-

* Earlier versions of this paper have benefited from audiences at Amherst College, Yale University, Princeton University, and Johns Hopkins University; and comments from Richard Farr, Harry Frankfurt, Beverly Gallo, Mary Mothersill, Jerome Schneewind, and Jonathan Vogel.

[1] Some of the initiating discussions are in Derek Parfit, *Reasons and Persons* (New York: Oxford, 1984); Samuel Scheffler, *The Rejection of Consequentialism* (New York: Oxford, 1982); and Bernard Williams, *Ethics and the Limits of Philosophy* (Cambridge: Harvard, 1985).

[2] See *Being And Nothingness*, Hazel Barnes, trans. (New York: Philosophical Library, 1956); esp. pt. I, ch. 2 ("Bad Faith") and pt. IV, ch. 1 ("Being and Doing: Freedom").

0022-362X/93/9011/578–95

tions, as I may have to accommodate the empirical fact of other people's beliefs and desires. For in my own case, I remain responsible for their *justification* and continued role in my life, and this determines whether or not they are to have any place at all in my deliberations. My reflection on the problem before me may lead me to abandon some of the beliefs or desires that led me into it. Hence they cannot enter into my thinking as the fixed beliefs and desires of some person or other, who happens to be me. Here, then, a certain form of impersonality is construed not as an oppressive, alien demand on the self but rather as a form of moral *evasion.*

It should not be surprising if a better understanding of the different senses of impersonality at stake in these contexts requires attention to what is distinctive about first-person discourse generally. The basic idea of asymmetries between first- and third-person stances toward mental life is a more or less familiar feature of contemporary philosophy of mind. A person knows his own mind in a way that is quite different from how he knows the mind of another, and he speaks with a different authority about his own beliefs and other attitudes. These considerations (e.g., first-person authority and the like) have normally been discussed in isolation from the broader issues in moral psychology, however, where one might think some of the deeper consequences of such self/other asymmetries would be played out. One general area for such connections to be drawn is in the examination of modes of appraisal which seem reserved for our relations to others, but which may have some sort of problematic application to oneself (here again one may think of the philosophical problem of self-deception). Here I want to investigate what the appropriate claims of impersonality with respect to oneself may be, but primarily by looking at certain ways in which the appeal may be misapplied or where acting on it has a self-undermining tendency. Specifically, I shall discuss a number of cases where a type of character assessment that seems unproblematic when applied to others appears to have something objectionable about it when applied to oneself. And I shall suggest that a variety of self/other asymmetries are inescapable features of human action and reflection, in ways that complicate and qualify what we can expect from an appeal to impersonality.

I

There are general issues in moral theory, concerning problems of possible tension between first-person and third-person views of oneself, which provide some context for the particular phemonenon to be discussed here. One set of problems that brings together some of these issues in epistemology and moral psychology is found in recent

discussions of the possible conflict between what a moral theory may tell us about the moral good, and what it recommends that we *believe* about the moral good. So, for instance, the question of what Derek Parfit calls the possible "self-effacement" of a moral theory —the possibility that it may recommend disbelief in itself as the attitude most conducive to the moral good, by its own lights (*op. cit.*) —has brought attention to such things as the contrast between the reasons for believing some theory to be true and reasons there may be for someone's being a believer of that theory; and the difference between the reasons a theory has for recommending certain dispositions of character, and the judgments of what is good (including judgments of good character) that will be made by people with just such dispositions of character. In considering virtues of character, the moral theorist may sometimes, then, be faced with what, in *Ethics and the Limits of Philosophy,* Bernard Williams refers to as the possible "conflict between the view the theorist has of these dispositions and the view of the world he has from those dispositions" (*op. cit.,* p. 110). A truly self-effacing moral theory would require a split between one's conception of value and justification, on the one hand, and the types of reason one is actually disposed to appeal to in one's deliberations, on the other. There would then be systematic differences between what another person may believe about my attitudes and dispositions (i.e., that they may be in some way deluded, but still, in another sense, the right ones for me to have) and what I myself may believe about them. And within the person, such disunity would thus appear to impose limits on the possibilities for moral self-consciousness.

It is a matter of some debate just what the consequences for the acceptability of a moral theory would be if it were shown to be self-effacing in this sense. But the significance of these self/other asymmetries for the virtues of character is not limited to contexts involving a moral theory that is actually self-effacing. Outside of the context of moral theorizing, there are situations involving the virtues of character, in which self-consciousness appears to have some kind of destabilizing effect on the virtues or dispositions that are its object. Williams himself suggests just such a difference between first- and third-person possibilities with respect to the virtues of character in the early pages of *Limits.*

> [I]t is rarely the case that the description that applies to the agent and to the action is the same as that in terms of which the agent chooses the action. [. . .] [A] courageous person does not typically choose acts as being courageous, and it is a notorious truth that a modest person does not act under the title of modesty. The benevolent

or kindhearted person does benevolent things, but does them under other descriptions, such as "she needs it," "it will cheer him up," it will stop the pain (*op. cit.*, p. 10).

He goes on to say how the deliberate *cultivation* of the virtues, while very familiar in its third-person form, "has something suspect about it, of priggishness or self-deception" as a first-personal exercise (*op. cit.*, p. 10). And he suggests that the reason for this is that the appraising function of the virtue terms has its primary home in their application to *others,* and not in the context of first-person moral reflection.[3]

There are, however, two quite distinct claims at issue, one concerning the role of virtue concepts in moral deliberation, and another concerning the deliberate cultivation of the virtues. As to the latter, it is hard to see what should be wrong with someone's, say, working to overcome his cowardice, and consciously trying to have a bit more courage in certain situations. And if self-deception is supposed to be involved here, it is not at all clear just what it is that the person is supposed to be deceived *about.* In any case, this is different from the former claim that there is something wrong in the idea of having, say, the manifestation of courage or modesty be one's primary motive in action. If there is a defensible criticism of such a motive, it must nonetheless allow for relevant differences between the virtues in this regard. For some are intrinsically tied to the *expression* of certain responses, like those of gratitude or remorse, in which case taking their manifestation as one's direct aim does not seem contrary to their spirit. There must also be room for historical and cultural variation here, when we recall that someone like Achilles, for example, might well be said to "choose acts as being courageous." Nonetheless, those cases where we do find something to criticize suggest moral as well as epistemological asymmetries between the first- and third-person cases. If "self-effacement" can apply to aspects of moral character as well as to possible moral theories, then there will be limits to the extent to which one can or should model one's moral estimation of oneself, in a "person-neutral" way, on the estimation of others.

---

[3] This is how I understand his diagnosis of what seems wrong in such cases. The problem, he says, is not that thought is directed at oneself, but that one's thought is, in a sense, not self-directed enough. "Thinking about your possible states in terms of the virtues is not so much to think about your actions, and it is not distinctively to think about the terms in which you could or should think about your actions: it is rather to think about the way in which others might describe or comment on the way in which you think about your actions, and if that represents the essential content of your deliberations, it really does seem a misdirection of the ethical attention"(*op. cit.*, p. 11).

In considering this possibility, it is important to recall that the virtues and vices of character involve *attitudes* as well as characteristic ways of behaving. Williams's examples of courage and modesty, for instance, involve characteristic patterns of thought and feeling as well as of behavior. In general, a person's attitude toward himself makes a difference to how we feel about him, and an attitude *we* take toward his character may depend on facts about just what attitude *he* takes toward it. Naturally, this is not to say that such attitudes must always match, our attitude toward him corresponding to his own attitude toward himself, and often they will not. A person's attitude of smug self-satisfaction does not normally lead one to feel well satisfied with *him;* and, oddly enough, the apprehension of someone's self-pity, far from inspiring pity in others, will not infrequently drive out whatever genuine pity one might have begun to feel for the person before discovering that he too felt the same way. But is this because we feel here that pity from one person is plenty enough and we can now leave that job in reliable hands? Or do we feel that however justified an attitude of pity toward someone may be, the person himself is for some reason uniquely barred from taking this up, even if he is the only person around in a position to appreciate the facts of his situation? It may well be true that, in considering myself as but one person among others, I am obliged not to privilege myself in certain ways. But, it might be thought, I ought not to be obliged for that reason to *dis*advantage myself in special ways either.

This sort of case can be internalized in a way that displays some of the features of self-effacement. We saw that a person's attitude toward himself may inspire a different attitude, perhaps a directly contrary one, in another person. And we can now see the possibility of cases where it is one and the same person responding in these contrary ways. What initially raises questions about such cases is that they need not involve the person's changing his mind, if by that we understand finding his previous attitude to be unjustified or unwarranted in some way. Rather, as in the case of responses to someone's self-pity or self-congratulation, this reversal may take place without any sense that the general attitude type is unjustified or inappropriate as applied to this person; that is, without denying that the person is indeed in some sense to-be-pitied or to-be-congratulated. This, of course, puts the person himself in an unstable situation. For in spite of the recognition of the value of ordinary moral self-examination, it will appear as if the very awareness of his attitude (and the character it expresses) causes it to be undermined, even if it is no part of his reflection that the original attitude is unjustified. This, in any case, is the possibility which has occurred to

a number of writers, and which I mean to explore in the following
examples.

II

When Samuel Johnson[4] says that "All censure of a man's self is
oblique praise. It is in order to show how much he can spare," we
need not think of this only in the context of public utterance, censure of oneself before witnesses. Such self-criticism is something
that can take place in the privacy of one's own mental tribunal, and
so can the estimation of what the making of this judgment *demonstrates* about the person in question. In that case, what one can *spare*
is measured by the distance between the character being judged so
severely and the character strong enough to make such a judgment;
the character strong enough to be confident that he can withstand
the censure, outdistance it. The praise comes from reflection on the
implications for character of the fact of his *making* the original
assessment of himself. The double movement, then, results from the
interplay between the content of the judgment and the fact of someone's making it. What is dubious about the resultant praise is that it
depends on an attitude of censure, which it then deflects.

Something very much like this same structure lies behind Sartre's
insistence on the inherent double-mindedness in any such estimation of oneself. I stand toward my character as toward some fixed,
objective, psychological datum; but at the same time the very act of
judgment itself demonstrates that I am not in thrall to this "character," for I can judge it from a standpoint superior in both clarity
and freedom. There is a sort of deliverance of myself in the assessment of my character as "just the way I am," for it absolves me of a
kind of responsibility for it. At the same time, there is another kind
of deliverance involved in feeling that my very act of naming and
judgment demonstrates that I am really superior to this given character, not determined by it. Thus, I claim for myself the best of both
worlds: I am absolved of responsibility for I am bound to express my
"nature," and at the same time I am *not* bound to my nature, for in
so judging it I express my freedom with respect to it.

> The man who confesses that he is evil has exchanged his disturbing
> "freedom for evil" for an inanimate character of evil; he *is* evil, he
> clings to himself, he is what he is. But by the same stroke, he escapes
> from that *thing*, since it is he who contemplates it, [. . .] A person frees
> himself from himself by the very act by which he makes himself an
> object for himself (*op. cit.*, p. 65).

As with Johnson, I think we need to interpret this as making implicit

---

[4] In Boswell's *Life of Johnson*, April 25, 1778.

reference to the distinction between the fact represented in the content of a judgment, and the fact of the making of the judgment. Although both facts are about the same person, the latter is not a logical consequence of the former. Rather, the former judgment makes the latter judgment "available" to me, similarly to how my judgment that it is raining makes available to me the judgment that I believe that it is raining (without facts about my belief being *inferable* from facts about rain).

Where Johnson speaks of the person judging as showing "what he can spare" of the person judged, Sartre speaks of "expressing one's freedom" with respect to the person judged. And the expression of such facts through one's self-censure is in both cases felt to impugn the authority of the original judgment. As with Williams's remarks on the role of virtue terms, however, it seems that while there *is* something unstable or reproachable in the vicinity, it appears persistently misidentified. For it is not *only* the priggish who may act under the title of some virtue of character, and the censure of one's own self is not *inherently* a calculated act, performed *in order* to show what one can spare. And similarly here, with Sartre, it ought not to be assumed that any and every act of reflection on one's own character involves making oneself an object for oneself, or not in any criticizable sense anyway. At the least, there ought to be a way for us to distinguish between those cases where such reflection has some such self-undermining quality, and those where it does not. To this end, I shall consider a very brief story in some detail, and the suggestion I want to follow is that we can understand what is sometimes paradoxical, and sometimes morally dubious in such cases by seeing them as unsuccessful attempts to adopt a stance toward oneself which is only a stable or coherent one when adopted toward some other person. We can thus see how even the legitimate demands of impersonality in reflection can be distorted to serve the ends of a kind of moral narcissism.

There's a well-known line from a novel by Kingsley Amis,[5] which concerns a married man with family, who at one point in the story spends an evening at a nightclub with another woman he knows from work. As he sneaks back home after the encounter, he describes himself in his guilty reflections as "feeling a tremendous rakehell, and not liking myself much for it, and feeling rather a good chap for not liking myself much for it, and not liking myself at all for feeling rather a good chap" (*ibid.*, ch. 7, p. 93). What has gone wrong in this man's reflections? And, more importantly, what is the implied criticism of himself he makes at the end, when he is "not

[5] *That Uncertain Feeling* (New York: Penguin, 1956).

liking himself at all"? One problem we can see right off is that the
chain of reversals of his previous assessment of himself could easily
proceed indefinitely, each current exoneration followed by an even
harsher condemnation *ad infinitum.* At the stage at which we encounter him he has just got himself to feel bad for feeling good
about feeling bad; and there seems no reason why he should stop
there, especially since with one more step he could be feeling good
again. Now, the apparent arbitrariness of his resting point here is
not his *founding* problem, of course, but it is not easy to say what
that problem is. Rightly or wrongly, he *censures* himself for something at the end. Whatever it is, it is something that occurred in the
previous train of thought, something that would make sense of his
"not liking himself at all."

There is something in the purely theoretical, or spectator's stance
he takes toward his original censure of himself which supports the
illusion that he can boot-strap himself out of that original judgment.[6] Such a purely theoretical attitude is one that is perfectly
possible with respect to others, but is less than rational when
adopted toward oneself. For we can notice right away that there
would be nothing odd in this line of thinking if more than one
person were involved. Feeling (better) about someone else for their
hard (though justified) judgment of themselves need not lead to the
collapse of either of the judgments of the two people. His deflation
and remorse may produce an improved opinion of his character in
the eyes of others, and this situation may be a perfectly stable one.
But for the rakehell in the story himself, there seems to be something wrong in his treating his first judgment of himself as simply a
kind of psychological *fact* about himself, like an action that is praiseworthy in much the same way that his original action was blameworthy, a fact about himself that indicates that he is not so bad
after all.

In the first stage of his thought, we find him with the belief that
he has acted shamefully, which is distinct from, although obviously
in close connection with, the fully experienced *attitude* of being
ashamed with himself. He then offers himself an expressive interpretation of his being ashamed according to which it indicates that
he is really rather a good chap after all. The sense in which the
expressive interpretation involves his feeling better about himself
naturally mitigates his original feeling of shame. At this point, however, he blames himself all the more for the previous train of
thought and what he now sees as its shameless exploitation of his

---

[6] An earlier account of such a theoretical attitude is given briefly in my "Making
Up Your Mind: Self-Interpretation and Self-Constitution," *Ratio* NS, I, 2 (December 1988): 135–51.

attitude. If we could say what exactly was *wrong* with the first stage of thought, up to the adoption of the new attitude of pleasure with himself, then we may have the reason for the rebuking conclusion he reaches at the end. One thing to consider at first is that there is something seriously wrong in using your awareness of some fact as a reason to disbelieve that very fact. It might be denied, however, that this is in fact what is going on here. For the new and more favorable attitude toward himself is not strictly speaking the denial of the straight belief that he did something shameful; rather, it is only the denial of, or at any rate the supplanting of, the actual experienced *attitude* of shame toward himself, the entire emotional configuration. Now, this *does* seem cutting it rather close; but there *is* nonetheless an important sense in which the truth of his original belief about the blameworthiness of what he did is not challenged at all. What happens instead is that he realizes that he has the appropriate attitude toward the facts represented in that belief, and this realization causes him to come to a more favorable assessment, not about what he did, but about himself. Still, although he does not repudiate his original belief, we could speak in terms of the replacement of one attitude by a contrary one, as a *response* to one's awareness of the first attitude, and this would be paradoxical enough. This interpretation obliges us to account for the sense of paradox as something other than a tension among beliefs, and later on we shall encounter reasons against construing the situation as a clash of beliefs in the first place.

Nonetheless, the paradoxical quality will stand out more clearly if we first consider the situation from the perspective of plain beliefs. In that case, the objection just mentioned would run (in the crudest possible terms): his awareness that he believes that he is bad cannot be his reason for no longer believing that he is bad. This would involve his adopting a kind of third-person stance toward his own attitudes, in that he takes a belief of his and regards it purely for what his having the belief says or expresses about him. This is what happens when he makes the transition from his belief about his shamefulness to the saving interpretation according to which he is quite a decent sort after all. And in so doing, his attention to the *fact* of his belief eclipses attention to what that belief is about. Thus, his awareness of his belief is not functioning as awareness of the propositional *object* of the belief (his shamefulness), even though he still takes that belief to be *true*. Now, there is nothing fishy per se in a person's reflecting on his belief as a psychological fact about himself, from which certain conclusions about himself may be drawn. What causes concern in the case of the rakehell, however, is the appearance that his attention to the fact that he (truly) believes *P*

brings him, through that recognition, to abandon that very belief.
The sense of paradox lies in the fact that he gives up the belief about
his shamefulness even though there is no stage in this whole train of
thought at which he sees that belief as unjustified. In fact, it is his
seeing it as *justified* which supports his giving it up, for there is
nothing to admire or commend in an *un*justified sense of shame. He
has to continue to take the original attitude to be justified and appropriate for his reflection upon it to issue in the contrary attitude.

One very general consideration that makes for misgivings here is,
I think, the sense that facts about what having a certain attitude
toward X *expresses* about you, ought not to enter into the reasoned
formation of your attitude toward X, just as facts about being a
person who believes X ought not to play a role in the course of
deliberating about what to believe. Philosophers may be more familiar with the problems involved in succumbing to instrumental or
consequentialist motives in one's belief (that is, adopting a belief
solely for the sake of its effects, or the consequences of believing
it—including motivated irrationality of various kinds), but we can
see now that very similar problems apply to what might be called
expressive or "symptomatic" thinking about what being a believer
of X says about one, what it *expresses* about the believer.

The rakehell himself naturally makes us doubt the genuineness of
his original feeling of shame, since he makes it seem so easy, and so
willful, when he rids himself of it. You feel shame, attend to what the
fact of your feeling it implies about you, and then you stop feeling
(so) ashamed. From the point of view from which we see the shame
and the relief from it as absolute, unqualified states, this makes it
seem as if no one could ever rationally feel ashamed: since if you do,
then rational reflection on the meaning of your feeling will make
your shame unnecessary. And all of this can be known in advance.
Thus, only someone incapable of shame ought to feel it, or, the only
proper object of shame is one's own shamelessness. Shame can seem
oddly self-canceling then; the reason for this being that it is an
emotion that refers to oneself, and is (often) a "commendable"
emotion. It is about the same person who is commended for having
it, and yet it seems incompatible with feeling commendable.[7]

It is worth noting at this point that much depends on one's atti-

---

[7] What is wrong here, however, does not depend on construing the attitudes in
question in absolute or all-or-nothing terms. For similar objections would apply to
the person's attempt to iterate this process until he reduces his degree of shame
down to zero. That is, once he has concluded that he is not so bad, it seems he
could reflect on the fact of the residual degree of shame that he may still feel, and
he might conclude that this feeling is itself commendable as well, leading him to
feel (even) less ashamed of himself; and so on.

tude toward particular attitudes and their types. Friedrich Nietzsche,[8] for instance, often writes in praise of the attitude of contempt, and it is clear that he thinks of the capacity for this feeling as something admirable, the sign of a strong nature; in other words, something worthy of respect. *Self*-contempt then, is for him an inherently unstable attitude. So he writes: "Whoever despises himself still respects himself as one who despises," thus claiming a sort of self-limiting character for this attitude (*ibid.*, § 78). Thus, a kind of *absolute* contempt, without remainder of respect for its object, is not a possible attitude toward oneself. (Incidentally, this is one case where the asymmetries in possible moral attitudes systematically would disadvantage *others* rather than oneself. Only toward another can one feel pure undiluted contempt without any redeeming remainder.) Nietzsche does not note, however, that, at best, this will only be true for those who share his special view of this and other attitudes. A different person, even if self-conscious enough to reflect on the fact of his self-despising, might be additionally ashamed of *that* fact. Hence his self-reflection would spiral downward, as opposed to Nietzsche's, which has the potential to raise one up out of despising altogether.

So the recuperation represented in the rakehell's expressive interpretation of his shame depends on his *endorsing* the judgment of shamefulness, being committed to it, and this ladder cannot be kicked away once he reaches the conclusion that he is rather a good chap. No commendation follows from an *un*justified sense of shame, after all. And this redeeming judgment depends on his continuing to maintain the initial belief that what he did was shameful, for as long as he sees himself in this new and favorable light. For his recognition of this fact about himself, i.e., the fact that he *takes* himself to be disgraceful, is not something like a momentary *spur* to his reinterpreting that sense of disgrace as meaning he is really a rather *good* person. Rather, it is his *basis* for believing that about himself; without it he has no particular reason to believe this at all. Continuing to endorse the original judgment of shamefulness is therefore necessary, and that means that he must continue to see himself and his actions through that belief, and not abandon it in favor of something else.

As before, however, one might say that, strictly speaking, he satisfies this condition, for he does *not* abandon the belief represented in the original self-censure, but only supplants the experienced or felt attitude of shame with another one. So he is not involved in outright

---

[8] *Beyond Good and Evil*, Walter Kaufmann, trans. (New York: Random House, 1966).

self-contradiction, and it is the difference between the straight *belief* about oneself or one's action, and the unaffected total *attitude* of shame that provides him with his room to maneuver. For ceasing to be ashamed or to feel ashamed is not the same thing as ceasing to believe that one did something shameful. A person is not obliged to continue feeling ashamed of himself forever, after all; but at the same time he should not give up the original belief about himself without some reason to think it untrue. And a reason to think it untrue is what he does not have here. Even giving it up in the sense of *forgetting* it may be blameable if it all takes place within a few minutes or a few days. Beliefs are not episodic like emotions; they do not typically run their natural course and then fade out like a burst of anger or relief.

So then, if he is not using his awareness of some belief of his (which he takes to be justified) as a reason to abandon that very belief, then it looks like he can maintain the expressive interpretation of the merit of his being ashamed without falling immediately into inconsistency. For, on this reading, he *does* maintain the original *belief* about his shamefulness throughout, and does not contradict himself by his later attitude. This interpretation of what he is doing is available to him by distinguishing beliefs (whose objects are propositions) and general emotional attitudes toward such things as persons and actions. But now at this point we have to ask whether the mere *belief* alone is enough to get him to the character judgment and the new attitude toward himself from which he now commends the appropriateness of his response of shame. That is, it is not clear that his simply believing that what he did was shameful, without any *feeling* or absorbing attitude of shame, provides any basis for even a limited commendation of him. But if it does not, then it is the same difference that saves him from inconsistency in maintaining the judgment of character without the actual experience of shame that now prevents him from justifiably reaching the approbation of the expressive interpretation. And this difference concerns the experiential aspect of emotions as opposed to beliefs, and the fact that an emotional attitude constitutes something closer to a total orientation of the self, the inhabiting of a particular perspective.[9]

---

[9] The sense in which a certain moral attitude may involve something like total perspectives on its object is crucial to David Hume's account of pride and humility, and relevant to the oscillating quality of the rakehell's reflections. In the *Treatise,* Hume says: "'Tis impossible a man can at the same time be both proud and humble; and where he has different reasons for these passions, as frequently happens, the passions either take place alternately; or if they encounter, the one annihilates the other, as far as its strength goes, and the remainder only of that, which is superior, continues to operate upon the mind" (*Treatise on Human Nature,* bk. II, "Of the Passions"; pt. I, "Of Pride and Humility"; sect. II).

For suppose that long after some action of his, long after the time for any occurrent feelings of shame about it, he judges, as he does here, that what he did was shameful. The cool, affectless appraisal of some long distant action of his, of a "past self" whose shameful actions do not shame *him,* would not provide the same reason for commending him, assuming that commendation had any place in our original case. At best, it would provide much *less* reason for this. And since the bridge from his original sense of disgrace to the new attitude toward it as expressive of a kind of virtue was a fragile one to begin with, weakening it now by removing from consideration the distinctive aspect of the actual emotional attitude of shame will likely make impossible any passage across to a new attitude toward himself. What matters to the success or legitimacy of the expressive interpretation, it seems, is the shame itself, the fact that it is something hard to undergo, and what *experiencing* it implies about the quality of the person's attitude toward what he did as well as his attitude toward the future. So, to gather together some of these threads, it looks as though he needs his actual sense of shame, at least initially, to get to whatever esteem he reaches at the end. And he needs the original belief that what he did was shameful *not* just initially but throughout the whole train of thought. So even if he does not flatly contradict his original judgment about what he did, there is still something wrong with his using the awareness of his proper *feeling* of shame to supplant that very attitude with a contrary one. Nonetheless, the temporal and experiential aspect of attitudes such as feeling ashamed allows room for some grey area here. After all, we say, at some point enough is enough and it is time to get over one's feeling ashamed and move on in one's life. And it may be that there is a time somewhat prior to this point when it is legitimate for the person to reflect on his response as a present psychological phenomenon rather than as an attitude toward his past action, in a way that has the effect of mitigating that very feeling.

III

If what is paradoxical in this case is a peculiarly first-person phenomenon, it must still be distinguished from another class of cases with which it is superficially similar, cases where someone's awareness of some fact alters our attitude toward the fact itself. Consider the following passage from Pascal's *Pensées*.[10]

> The greatness of man is great in that he knows himself to be miserable.
> A tree does not know itself to be miserable. It is then being miserable
> to know oneself to be miserable, but it is also being great to know that

[10] W. F. Trotter, trans. (New York: Dutton, 1958).

one is miserable. [. . .] He is therefore wretched because he is so; but
he is really great because he knows it (*ibid.*, § 397, 416).

What is paradoxical in the reasoning here lies in drawing a conclusion from someone's justified attitude toward himself (man and
his wretchedness) which seems incompatible with that very attitude.
(Although it seems clear that it is not Pascal's own point that they
are in direct contradiction.) In this example, as in the original case
of the rakehell, the sense that the original attitude is justified must
be maintained in order to reach the estimation that clashes with it.
But what is paradoxical in Pascal's inference is not, in fact, an essentially first-person phenomenon. It *does* require that the original attitude be an attitude toward oneself, otherwise there will be no clash
between the original belief and the conclusion drawn from its being
believed. But it is just as paradoxical in the third-person case to infer
from anyone's justified belief that *P*, to the conclusion that *P* is not
true. Pascal is indeed including himself in this passage, so it is a
first-person expression to that degree, but his statement can also be
read in a third-person manner. He looks at man in his wretchedness,
but concludes on the basis of man's awareness of his wretchedness
that he is "really great." This is paradoxical whether applied to
oneself or to others.

What makes for a peculiarly first-person problem in the rakehell
story is the effect on the emotion of shame of one's own judgment
of its significance for one's character. The effect of the judgment
and the conclusion drawn from it can undo the emotion itself, and
this *is* a specifically first-person phenomenon. This part of the story
has to do not only with paradoxes of drawing conclusions from a
person's beliefs which conflict with them, but also with the effect of
second-order beliefs on first-order attitudes and emotions in the
first-person case. For the rakehell does not overturn the judgment
(1) "What I did was shameful," rather the clash is with (2), the sense
of being ashamed of himself. It is this aspect of the reversals which
has no third-person equivalents. For when another person approves
of someone else's justified sense of shame, he may then draw the
Pascalian paradoxical conclusion that the person himself is not really shameful. But he does not, and could not, draw the conclusion
that this person is not in fact ashamed of himself, or that he is no
longer so ashamed of himself (the overturning of (2)). The original
paradox thus has to do with *both* the effects of a person's second-
order attitudes on his first-order attitudes (including responses like
shame) *and* with the Pascalian problem of drawing conclusions from
someone's (in this case one's own) justified belief which then conflict
with that very belief. It is also important to the chain of reversals

that emotions, such as shame, are mutable and sensitive to our attitudes toward them in ways that our plain beliefs are not. The rakehell's attitude toward his shame diminishes it, even though he has not changed his mind about the import of what he did.

In what we may call a spectator's stance toward oneself, one's attention is shifted from the object of one's intentional state to the state itself, and it is treated as a psychological phenomena with various effects and implications for the person. Having the intentional attitude in the first place, however, commits one to viewing the world from that perspective; either that or else changing one's mind about what it is that the attitude is directed upon. Neither of these facts applies to our awareness of other people's intentional states. The rakehell as described seems to attempt a relation to his original shame which does not involve viewing the world through it (in this case, himself and his actions) but treats it as an opaque psychological fact about himself that he *has* this attitude, a fact from which he can draw certain conclusions; conclusions that in this case conflict with the original attitude itself. But such a stance may involve a misplaced attention to the self even when this does *not* produce an overturning of the original judgment: the person focuses on the fact or experience of his shame rather than on that which is supposed to be its object. Indeed, normally such focusing of attention on one's own response is a retreat from the more painful attention to the actions and results which precipitated the response and which are its presumed intentional object.

For instance, we can see that, with characteristic stringency, George Eliot tracks down the erring self even when it finds the safe haven of guilty self-absorption. In *Middlemarch,* when Fred Vincy loses the money he had borrowed from the Garths, he is genuinely sorry, though somewhat removed both from the action and its effects:

> Curiously enough, his pain in the affair beforehand had consisted almost entirely in the sense that he must seem dishonourable, and sink in the opinion of the Garths: he had not occupied himself with the inconvenience and possible injury that his breach might occasion them, for this exercise of the imagination on other people's needs is not common with hopeful young gentlemen. Indeed we are most of us brought up in the notion that the highest motive for not doing a wrong is something irrespective of the beings who would suffer the wrong (ch. 24).

Fred Vincy is assessing the moral significance of what he did by reference to how it may reflect on his character, rather than by reference either to the consequences for others or even to any im-

personal deontological considerations. His attention to how he is to
be esteemed interferes with reflection on the significance of what he
did. There will be something both morally and psychologically amiss,
then, when self-reflection on the issue of the virtues of character
inhibits or distorts one's moral response to what one has done. And
I take it that this is the sort of thing Williams has in mind when he
says that the trouble with the first-person exercise of cultivating the
virtues is that such thought is not self-directed *enough,* focusing
instead on "the way in which others might describe or comment on
the way in which you think about your actions" (*op. cit.,* p. 11).

There are indeed questionable aspects of the application of virtue
terms to oneself when this is undertaken for purposes of prediction,
for example. The statement, 'Given my generous nature, I am likely
to loan him the money if he needs it', is odd-sounding because it
presents itself as a prediction when it is hard to see how such a
statement could be anything other than a declaration of intention.
And it is doubly suspicious, because, first, the reliance on a more or
less probable prediction presents the person as less than fully *committed* to loaning the money. And, second, it is this very *absence* of
full commitment that is expressed by his availing himself of terms of
self-*praise* rather than a straightforward declaration of intention
that would omit any mention of his own character. It is as if he wants
to be congratulated for being presently only half-heartedly inclined
to loan the money, but confidently predicting that his better self will
prevail, in spite of his current lack of resolve or full endorsement.
The curious distancing of oneself from one's actions in such a case is
paralleled by the sense in the rakehell case of his failure to assume
responsibility for his attitudes and dispositions, just at the moment
when he turns his attention to the question of what sort of person
they show him to be. And this, I think, is where we find the peculiarities in the *appraising* function of virtue terms when applied to oneself, as noted by Williams and others in this paper. For both the
predictive and appraising functions rest on holding the psychological facts fixed and focusing on them rather than on their objects.
Naturally, if the dispositional facts of character are taken to be so
fluid and unfixed that it is an entirely open question whether I shall
(now or ever) act out of my supposed trait of generosity, then ascribing it to me is useless as a prediction and empty as an appraisal. But
the kernel of truth in Sartre's insistence on "positing one's freedom," as quoted earlier, is that keeping the psychological facts fixed
in this way is just what the stance of practical self-reflection does *not*
involve.

A person's traits as well as his intentional states cannot be just
psychological facts for him, for they are constitutive of his relation

to the world, and subject to revision, adjustment, and inhibition in the course of his deliberation. Reflecting on them is for that person reflecting on the world, and answerable to the independent facts. The stance from which one either justifies or fails to justify one's beliefs, attitudes, or emotional responses cannot be abandoned in favor of one from which they are subject only to explanation and expressive (including moral) assessment. By contrast, Fred Vincy's guilty consciousness of himself blocks his attention to the actual object of his guilt: his actions and the beings who suffered the wrong. His indulgent self-blame, or even his concentration on the general issue of how he is now to be appraised, rests on holding the psychological facts about himself fixed. And fixed they remain, without changing into other world-directed attitudes more appropriate both to the situation, and to his original first-order feeling of remorse.

Even if the virtue-terms he uses are not reserved for relations with others,[11] it remains true that the rakehell of our story exploits the difference between beliefs and other attitudes in order to commend himself for an attitude for which he is unwilling to pay. For the *attitude* of shame is not the same as either the plain belief that he did something wrong or this belief combined with painful feelings of some kind. As an attitude it is only thought appropriate or commendable for how it *focuses the attention* and makes one receptive to considerations of a particular kind. (This is, for instance, what someone else who wanted this attitude from him would be demanding.)

But when he moves from reflection on what he did to reflection on the meaning of his feeling ashamed for the quality of his character, it is precisely a shift in the focus of his attention, in the point of view he takes upon himself. This may seem like an innocent move because it involves no change of *belief*. But beliefs are not what centrally matter to the revaluation toward which the expressive interpretation is heading. And once he has made this shift of attention toward the meaning of his shame, it can seem more blameless still for him to draw whatever conclusions this fact may suggest to him. It is not as if he is to be barred from making certain inferences, after all. What he concludes about his sense of shame here may perfectly well be true. But the shift in perspective amounts to a change of attitude, and a change in his total orientation toward the importance of what he did. And the combination of the change of orientation and the conclusions he then draws annuls whatever value for the

---

[11] As Sartre, for instance, sometimes suggests. See *Being and Nothingness*, pt. III, ch. 2, sect. 2: "Character has distinct existence only in the capacity of an object of knowledge for the Other."

interpretation of character there may have been in his original feeling of shame. And yet the "expressive" conclusions about his character are entirely dependent on the value of such feelings. That is why it can seem that the very act of reflection on himself makes it impossible for such reflection to reveal to him what his feeling appropriately ashamed means for the quality of his character. Once he decides to draw such conclusions, he no longer has any right to them, for he has relinquished claim to the proper attitude in question, which would demand that his attention be directed elsewhere. Better understanding of the peculiarities of relations to oneself requires better understanding of the range of what are called "attitudes" in the nonphilosophical sense, as opposed to beliefs. Such attitudes have every right to be considered cognitive, but they are primarily attitudes toward individuals (e.g., people, events, and situations) rather than attitudes toward propositions.

The situations of self-reflection discussed here represent one class of cases where a more realistic and detailed moral psychology reveals tensions in interpreting and living up to a common-sense appeal to impersonality. Although it is in many ways a natural and reasonable appeal (it is not only moral philosophers who may enjoin us to "see ourselves as others see us"), it is also a complex and ambiguous one, open to multiple interpretations. There are special complexities and ambiguities in the attempt to accommodate it to some of the basic asymmetries between first-person and third-person perspectives. At the same time, the complexities discussed here do not themselves discredit the claims of impersonality, and genuine concerns about what might be seen as pathologies of "self-objectification" ought not themselves to contribute to losing sight of the distinction between the idea that one should judge of one's action and character as one would that of any other person, and the idea of conceiving of one's action and character *as* that of another person. But such phenomena do suggest that we need to pay attention to the fine grain of systematic first-person/third-person differences if we are to be able to draw such distinctions in a principled way. A central aim of this discussion has been to make a start at showing how some of these seemingly remote matters from philosophy of mind have a genuine role to play in accounting for aspects of the structure and phenomenology of moral experience.

RICHARD MORAN

Princeton University

[24]

IS IT REASONABLE TO REGRET THINGS ONE DID?*

W e all know regret. Whether we take ourselves to be moral persons or immoralists, and, if the former, whether we have an Aristotelian, Kantian, or utilitarian understanding of morality (or no clear understanding at all), sometimes we regret what we did. The object of the following is not to demarcate what it is to regret things one did, to describe how it feels, or to state the precise conditions under which regret does and does not appear.[1] A rough explanation should suffice: regret is a painful feeling about something we did which we think was bad. More specific kinds of phenomena falling under this explanation, like remorse, repentance, feeling of guilt, will not be discussed in particular. Nor is the diversity of reasons for thinking it was bad of interest here: one can regret a purchase because it was too expensive, one can regret having behaved incorrectly because it diminishes one's standing, one can regret a mean remark because it hurt the other person; though it is the last kind of case, regret over something taken to be wrong for moral reasons, which will be in the foreground in what follows. The question is this: Given that we did something bad, is it reasonable for us to regret that we did it? The word 'reasonable' is to be understood here in its everyday sense, roughly equivalent to phrases like 'it's a good idea', 'it makes sense', 'it is recommendable'. Thus, the question can also be expressed as follows: Should we regret bad things we did?

It will be wondered whether the question itself is a reasonable one. After all, you feel regret, and what you feel is not up to you. To ask whether something is reasonable, however, makes sense only if it is up to you to do it or not. So the question whether regret is reasonable is mistaken right from the start. You might as well ask whether it is reasonable to have a headache.

This raises a large problem: How is what we feel related to the rest of our mental life, and how is it related to action, in particular to

* For helpful criticism of previous versions of this text I am grateful to Celène Abramson, Thomas Pogge, Amélie O. Rorty, Nancy Schauber, and an audience at the University of Bielefeld, Germany.

[1] See Amélie O. Rorty, "Agent Regret," in Rorty, ed., *Explaining Emotions* (Berkeley: California UP, 1980), pp. 489–506; Gabriele Taylor, "Guilt and Remorse," in Taylor, *Pride, Shame, and Guilt: Emotions of Self-assessment* (New York: Oxford, 1985), pp. 85–107.

moral action?[2] Without addressing this large question, a preliminary answer to the objection at hand may be given as follows. To ask whether something is reasonable makes sense not only in those cases where doing it or not is up to you in the sense that you can do it right on the spot. It is true that in this sense it is not up to us to regret things we did. We cannot at any given moment turn off the regret we feel about something we did, nor can we turn on a regret we do not feel. Yet over longer periods of time we learn to feel a certain way, and we learn not to feel a certain way any more, on this or that sort of occasion. This holds for individuals and for groups of people. For example, a feeling of reverence has passed out of use in my life. I did feel reverence for some people when I was much younger. Now I do not; and it seems this is due, not to a scarcity of suitable objects, but to my having outgrown this feeling altogether. I have lost this language; I do not just fail to find people with whom to speak it. Similarly, over the last few centuries people in the Western world have lost the feeling of awe. It still has a prominent place in Hobbes (and there is no reason to think that he is archaic on purpose here), but it has dried out since. The massive violence of the twentieth-century state inspires terror, not awe: there is nothing sacred about it. Now, it would be a long story, both in the individual and in the larger case, to explain how it happened that these feelings fell into desuetude. But it is very unlikely that a convincing story could be told, in either case, without referring to what people came to think, to see, to recognize in the process. People do not learn, or unlearn, to feel something *just* by being pushed around; it is also a matter of what they think about what happens to them.[3] For example, it was precisely Hobbes' own construction of an awe-producing political mechanism which, among numerous other influences, contributed to awe's becoming obsolete. And it is clear that I did not lose reverence for people like a key from my pocket. It was part of a whole process in which I came to have a different view of people who were important to me, and of myself, too. So in this sense some of our feelings are indeed up to us: whether some kind of feeling is available in a situation or not depends on what we have become and

---

[2] There is a large literature on these topics. To mention only a few titles: Rorty, *op. cit.;* William Lyons, *Emotion* (New York: Cambridge, 1980); Ronald de Sousa, *Rationality and the Emotions* (Cambridge: MIT, 1987); Patricia S. Greenspan, *Emotions and Reasons: An Inquiry into Emotional Justification* (New York: 1988).

[3] The point here is the positive version of Epictet's famous line that what confuses people are not the things, but what they think about the things.

how we see things. In particular, then, it will depend, among other things, on whether we judge that feeling to be reasonable or not. Again, it is not that a feeling judged to be unreasonable is thereby and in that moment annihilated.[4] What sometimes happens is rather that a feeling judged to be unreasonable slowly recedes and eventually dies out, just because it makes no more sense to us. To be sure, this happens only sometimes: some feelings live on stubbornly in the face of better judgment. But sometimes they yield. Feeling is not in principle insensitive to insight. Perhaps it is here that the moral philosopher's task lies. He is not particularly effective in reforming action right on the spot in accordance with better insight. But he may, in the longer term, help people in learning to find sense, or to find no sense, in what they feel. Thus he may help in reaching a more sensible way of feeling and so in the end, perhaps, a more sensible way to act.

Spinoza raised the suspicion in his *Ethica* that to regret what one did is not reasonable: "Repentance is not a virtue, i.e. it does not arise from reason. Rather, he who repents what he did is twice miserable, i.e. impotent" (pt. IV, prop. 54). It is not the claim expressed in this sentence, however, which is under discussion here. That Spinoza speaks about repentance rather than regret does not make an important difference: his point, if he has one, applies to the latter phenomenon as well. The important difference lies in the concept of reason. For Spinoza, reason consists in the possession of adequate ideas about how things are.[5] This is a much narrower concept than the everyday notion indicated above. His claim that repentance, or regret, is not reasonable thus becomes uninterestingly weak. That we do not feel regret insofar as we entertain adequate ideas about ourselves and people and things around us, that is, insofar as we consider everything from the viewpoint of eternity (*ibid.*, prop. 44, corollary 2). is easy to grant. The interesting question is whether regret has a place in the broader field of what a reasonable human being does and feels, with 'reasonable' being understood in its ordinary sense. Spinoza's proposition does not address this question, but invites the reader to ask it.

Moreover, Spinoza suggests an argument for a negative answer. 'To regret what one did is to be twice miserable' means: a person is

---

[4] Hume seems to be supposing something as strong as this: "The moment we perceive the falsehood of any supposition, or the insufficiency of any means our passions yield to our reason without any opposition"; *A Treatise of Human Nature*, L. Selby-Bigge and P. Nidditch, eds. (New York: Oxford, 1978), p. 416.

[5] *Ethica*, Pt. II, prop. 40, scholium 2.

first miserable because he did something bad, and he is miserable a second time because he is in pain over what he did. 'To be miserable' must be understood here in an objective sense, not as 'feeling bad', but as 'being in a bad way'. This is so because the first misery is not a case of feeling bad. It is not, for otherwise it could not be distinguished from the second one. Rather, feeling bad is one kind of being in a bad way, which is why both the first and the second misery can indeed be called "misery." (Spinoza hints at this in adding the phrase 'i.e. impotent'.) What is under discussion is the state of an organism that is objectively 'low'. Still, one way for an organism to be low is to feel low. So what Spinoza is saying is this. The person who regrets what he did is in a bad way twice. Whoever did something bad is thereby, independently of how he feels about it, badly off. The pain he feels about what he did is for him to be badly off a second time. Thus, Spinoza's argument is: it is not reasonable, because one did something bad, to go and make things worse. But that is what regret is, double misery, the second for the sake of the first. So, regret is not reasonable. The same argument, incidentally, occurs in Nietzsche: "Never give room to repentance, but tell yourself at once: this would mean to add a second piece of stupidity to the first."[6]

The argument also gives a clearer idea of the nonregretting person Spinoza has in view. It is not because this person never goes wrong or never admits to having gone wrong that he does not regret. Accordingly, Spinoza is not uselessly advising never to have grounds for regret. The reasonable person without regret has done something bad, and for the sake of the present argument it should be supposed that we all agree with him on this. So he is not one of those famous people who decline to regret because they do not recognize the law under which they appear guilty, from Don Giovanni's "No!" when the Commendatore asks him to repent, to Edith Piaf's "Non, je ne regrette rien." Unlike them, Spinoza's reasonable person is indeed once miserable. He is not immoral, nor is he bound to be heartless. He sees that what he did was wrong and he may be perfectly aware of the suffering he inflicted on others. He just does not grieve. Thomas Aquinas[7] held that the saints in the new life after judgment will be displeased by their earlier sins, but "without any

---

[6] *The Wanderer and His Shadow*, 323. A similar sentiment is expressed in Ralph Waldo Emerson's essay "Self-reliance," as quoted by Rorty in "Agent Regret," p. 501.

[7] *Summa Theologiae*, III, qu. 84, art. 8.

sadness." These are sensible saints, Spinoza is saying, let us be like them, right now in this life.

The opposite view has been put forward by Bernard Williams:[8] "it would be an insane concept of rationality" which insisted that a rational person would never experience sentiments of agent regret (*ibid.*, p. 29). In fact, here and in other passages Williams has a stronger claim in mind than the one under discussion here, and what he says is not specifically directed against the Spinozistic view just sketched. Williams holds that regret is sometimes appropriate not only with regard to intentional actions, but also with regard to consequences of action which the agent did not intend and could not even foresee, so that the field of potential regret extends to "almost anything for which one was causally responsible in virtue of something one intentionally did" (*ibid.*, p. 28). Williams holds this partly because it allows him a respectable concept of tragedy. It is true that tragedy presents us with extreme cases.[9] Still, what is central to tragedy is central to our life, too: the acceptance of things that just happened as part of what one has done and, thereby, of what one is.[10] Neither accident nor the machinations of the gods lead Oedipus into disaster, but rather what he did. It is what he did, for in the important sense "it was him," even though he did it unwittingly and unwillingly. This, evidently, is a far-reaching and quite doubtful thesis. Williams asks rhetorically: "Could we have, and do we want, a concept of agency by which what Oedipus said [namely, that he did not do it] would be simply true, and by which he would be seeing things rightly if for him it was straight off as though he had no part in it?" (*ibid.*, p. 30 fn.) But that is just to frighten the children. The answer to this question should simply be, "yes." Agency requires intentionality. In any case, what is under discussion here is not the strong thesis that regret is in order even with respect to unintended consequences of actions, but the weaker one that there are some cases where regretting what one did is reasonable. Given Spinoza's challenge, the thesis needs reasons.

Williams does not state his reasons explicitly, so an argument has to be constructed. The most natural consideration may be this: to regret something bad that one did is reasonable because it makes it more probable that one will do better in the future. There may be

---

[8] "Moral Luck," in *Moral Luck* (New York: Cambridge, 1981).
[9] Williams, "Ethical Consistency," in *Problems of the Self* (New York: Cambridge, 1973), p. 173.
[10] Williams, "Moral Luck," pp. 29f.

some hints in this direction in Williams's texts,[11] but it does not seem
to be the reason on which his claim is based. Nor would it be a good
reason. Regret does not in fact make doing better in the future
more probable. The impression that it does arises from a confusion
of Spinoza's reasonable person who does not regret with an immoral
or heartless one. No doubt somebody who does not see anything
wrong in what he did or has no sense for the suffering he caused is
likely to do similar things again. That is not the case of the reasonable person who does not regret, however. He understands what he
did, he knows that it was bad, it just does not pain him. And there is
no reason to assume that it is simply being pained by what one did
which makes doing better in the future more likely. Failure to learn
from what went wrong comes in many forms. In moral matters there
is the self-complacency of feeling terrible about what one did and
leaving it at that, as well as the impassiveness of going on with business as usual. There are cases in all four fields of the two distinctions: there is regret with improving and without improving, and
there is absence of regret with improving and without improving.
That the ratio of improving to not improving is higher under regret than under absence of regret is not a plausible or justified
assumption.

Second, regret could be defended with the idea of atonement. He
who did evil must suffer evil, otherwise things will not return to
order. Since the normal course of the world cannot be relied upon
to make this happen, it is a good thing for the agent himself to pay
for what he did by grieving about it. If he only registers that what he
did was bad and even does everything he can to prevent his doing it
again, he seems to get off the hook too easily. This leads to the idea
of a regret that cleanses the heart: sincere grief can balance, and
thereby remove, the agent's guilt. In this way, regret promises liberation. Suffering through what he did, the agent becomes free of the
burden of the deed and can start afresh.

This defense has no chance to succeed, nor is there any indication
that Williams would want to use it. Atonement is itself not a reasonable idea and cannot show regret to be reasonable. That he who did
evil should suffer evil is neither required nor even desirable. However deeply it may have been inculcated in us that it ought to be the
case that the good be happy and the evil suffer, the truth is that, if
anything, it ought to be the case that everybody, good and evil alike,

[11] "Ethical Consistency," p. 175; "Politics and Moral Character," in *Moral
Luck*, p. 62.

be happy. The suffering of him who did evil is only a further evil; it does nothing to remove the first. That the agent should, if possible, repair the damage he caused or recompense for it is another matter. Atonement is taken to eliminate, not the damage, but the guilt incurred in causing the damage. But this is a mythical idea. That we did what is bad cannot be undone. The promise of liberation through regret is a false promise. We should free ourselves, not of the burden of the deed, but of the idea that the deed is a burden.

The arguments considered so far have parallels in the discussion of punishment, in the attack on punishment as a mere duplication of suffering, in the defense of punishment as a way to make betterment more probable, in the defense of punishment as atonement. Not so the following consideration, which probably comes closest to being the argument on which Williams's thesis is based. Having made the point, as quoted several paragraphs back, that a concept of rationality which excludes regret over what one did would be an insane one, Williams continues as follows:

> To insist on such a conception of rationality, moreover, would, apart from other kinds of absurdity, suggest a large falsehood: that we might, if we conducted ourselves clear-headedly enough, entirely detach ourselves from the unintentional aspects of our actions, relegating their costs to, so to speak, the insurance fund, and yet still retain our identity and character as agents.[12]

This statement is meant to support Williams's stronger thesis that regret is appropriate even with regard to unintended consequences of actions. The reasoning is: not to regret the unintended consequences of actions is to detach oneself from them, but in detaching oneself from them one fails to retain one's identity and character as an agent. The reasoning should apply with all the more force to the core area of action, intentional action, which is what is under discussion here. Not to regret what one did, Williams is saying, is to detach oneself from one's actions, but that is to lose one's identity and character as an agent.

So the reasoning is not: failure to regret would amount to a detachment from what one did, but that is impossible, so it makes no sense to try. Detachment is possible. What is wrong with it, according to Williams, is only that it is too costly; morally costly, that is. You pay detachment with your identity and character as an agent.

---

[12] "Moral Luck," p. 29.

The present argument, then, like the previous ones, tries to defend regret by indicating a benefit of it which is overlooked in Spinoza's challenge. Regret, the first argument said, makes better action in the future more likely. That did not appear plausible. Regret, the second argument said, obliterates the wrongdoing. That appeared false. Regret, now the third argument is saying, allows us to retain our identity and character as agents. This is unclear. We need to know three things. What is meant by 'retaining our identity and character as agents'? Why is it desirable to retain them? And why does it take regret to retain them?

The expression 'our identity and character as agents' cannot mean "our character of being agents." On this reading, Williams would claim that by not regretting one ceases to be an agent altogether, which is quite implausible. On the other hand, 'our identity and character as agents' cannot mean what is normally simply called "character," our individual qualities as they are manifested in how we act. On this reading, Williams would claim that failure to regret leads to the loss of one's character traits. That again is implausible. A generous, courageous, or short-tempered person does not stop being any of these things just by not regretting what he did. Rather, what is meant must be something like this. We are the agents we are not just by having done what we did. We are the agents we are by accepting these doings as ours. This is what the person who does not regret fails to do. He sheds what he did rather than identifying with it. He steals away out of his own deed. He does not doubt that he did it; rather, the point is that he does not positively take it on as his. What he thereby loses is after all, in one sense and to a certain extent, his character of being an agent. He loses it not in the sense that henceforth he is barred from agency. He loses it with respect to the past. He loses it in the sense that something he actually did gets cut out from what he is as an agent, given that what he is as an agent depends in part on what he accepts as his. "Where It was, there I shall become," Freud wrote. Where I was to be, there It is—this is what failure to retain one's identity and character as an agent means. It is an agent's crippling himself as an agent, by surrendering something he did to the realm of what just happens through him, rather than incorporating it in what he is as an agent. So what Williams is saying about the person who does not regret is that, in a specific sense, he lacks character. Not that he is characterless, i.e., bland. He lacks character the way a person does who, on encountering any sort of resistance, abandons people and projects to which he was committed: the person without regret abandons his deeds.

In short, Williams is Polonius: "This above all; to thine ownself be true."[13]

Why, really? This is the second of the questions distinguished above, about the desirability of retaining your identity and character as an agent. If failure to identify with what you did is held to make lack of regret morally costly, indeed on Williams's view prohibitively costly, it needs to be explained what is good about identifying with what you did. Why not throw your identity and character, in this sense, to the winds? There seems to be only one answer. You should identify with what you did because you did it after all. It is the truth about you that you realize in acknowledging agency. To thine own self, expressed in your actions, be true, for that is what you really are.

This is not a good answer, given the terms of the question. If your identity and character as an agent is something you may retain or fail to retain, then the option of retaining cannot be recommended on the grounds that thereby you acknowledge the truth about you. About this purported truth you are just called upon to decide, or else the question about retaining or not does not arise. If you are in the position to retain or not, then you are not in the position to stay true to yourself by either retaining or not retaining. "You must become who you are," Nietzsche said,[14] but the pathos of truth to oneself rests on an assumption, namely, that there is such a self to be true to, which it precisely undercuts, namely, by understanding truth to oneself as merely one option among others.[15] Thus, Williams's warning that by not regretting we fail to retain our identity and character as agents turns out to be another case of frightening the children. There is nothing detectably wrong with a failure to retain one's identity and character as an agent, in the sense of failing to identify with what one did. There is nothing detectably wrong with simply walking away from it. To be sure, we are not talking here about denying that one did it, in the ordinary sense. The person without regret and his opponent are agreed on the facts of what happened. The latter only claims that there is, beyond the trivial knowing that one was the doer of this deed, an acceptance of one's having done it as part of what one is, as part of one's identity, as this

---

[13] William Shakespeare, Hamlet, I 3.
[14] *The Gay Science*, 270.
[15] Alexander Nehamas's discussion of Nietzsche's idea does not resolve this paradox; see his *Nietzsche: Life as Literature* (Cambridge: Harvard, 1985), ch. 6.

is often expressed;[16] and that such acceptance is what is required of agents. This claim is what is unfounded. We can live, and perhaps live better, without identity and character in this sense. Sure, we will have identity and character in the ordinary sense. We will be the individual agents we are, with these particular features manifesting themselves in action. The fact that we have identity and character in this sense, however, lends no support to the demand expressly to retain identity and character, in the special sense, through identification with what we did. Identity and character in the ordinary sense we will have in any case, so we may identify or not with what we did as we please. And sometimes it will make sense not to identify, and to say: "True, I did that, I even did it intentionally. But I am no more in it. You cannot find me there. That is history. It does not cast a shadow over what I do now." No doubt, somebody talking like that may be deceived and may, by anxiously denying the shadow, rather confirm its presence. The point is that this need not be the case. He may truly be free.

Suppose, for the sake of the argument, that all of that is wrong. Suppose, that is, that there is a sense of "our identity and character as agents" which makes the demand to retain our identity and character neither unjustified nor superfluous. That leaves us still without an answer to the third question, namely, why the retaining needs regret about the bad things one did. Why should not remembrance and understanding suffice, remembrance of what was done and understanding of what was bad about it? Why grieve in addition?

The best answer in defense of regret may be this: there is no understanding that the thing was wrong without the grief about having done it. This is not the cynical wisdom that "they won't remember what hasn't been beaten into them." The point is: to know that one did it and that it was bad is by itself painful. Spinoza may be right in saying that he who regrets is twice miserable. What he overlooks is the fact that the second misery is linked to the experience of the first. Thus, the only alternative to regret is simply to be blind to one's failings, and that this is not a desirable attitude is obvious. "Suffering we recognize that we did wrong," Antigone says.[17] The thought here is: only in suffering we recognize it. This is not evident.

---

[16] See again Williams, "Moral Luck," pp. 29f.: "if one attaches importance to the sense of what one is in terms of what one has done and what in the world one is responsible for, one must accept much that makes its claim on that sense solely in virtue of its being actual."

[17] Sophocles, *Antigone,* 1. 926.

It is not evident that one could not see, in full clarity but without grief, what one did wrong. In fact, the contrary may be true: that with grief one could not see in full clarity what one did wrong. After all, to see such a thing is itself an achievement and, hurt, torn, and dejected by regret, we may not be capable of doing it. However this may be, the case for the necessity of regret for recognizing one's failing has not been made.

"Aren't you really returning now," it may be objected, "to Spinoza's understanding of reason, instead of staying with the ordinary one, as promised? Full clarity about what one did wrong, unclouded by grief, looks suspiciously like considering things from the point of view of eternity, not like something which it is a good idea to reach." Maybe this is what Spinoza meant by a consideration of things from the point of view of eternity: without pain just to get clear about matters. (Though 'eternity' speaks against this reading and suggests, rather, that this point of view lies beyond the human field.) If he meant that, then it is true, we are back with Spinoza's understanding of reason here. But it is not true that this is to quit the ordinary one. To look things straight in the face, unburdened by grief, is just a very good idea, and a good idea in the same sense in which it is a good idea, say, to have the snow tires mounted before the first snowfall. True, there is this difference: some people do mount their snow tires in time, but few people are likely to take in their failings without regret. Still, this shows only that some forms of unreason are more common and harder to eradicate than others. As discussed earlier, it does not show that this is a form of unreason we are stuck with once and for all.

"Your argument proves too much," it will be said. "This reasoning can be applied not only to regret of things done, but also to regret of things lost and above all to grief and mourning over people who are no longer with us, whether they died or went away. Let us not quarrel about whether it is possible to do without these emotions. Let us grant your point for now that a suitable *éducation sentimentale* may in the end eliminate them. But is that a desirable state? Imagine a man saying: 'Yes, it is a bad thing, we broke up, even though I had loved her from my heart; but it does not hurt me, I am alive and well as ever'. Isn't this a terribly cold, cruel, inhuman reaction? Something must be wrong with an idea of being reasonable which recommends such brutishness." There need not be anything cruel or brutish here. True, we often take such a reaction rightly as evidence that he did not love her so much after all or that, if he did, he now has lost, or indeed destroyed, his sense for why he

loved her. But it need not be so. We may know independently that
he did love her deeply and that his present reaction is not owed to
his being blind to her. Also, a man speaking like this will often be
speaking falsely, either hiding his pain from others or deceived
about it himself. Again, this need not be so, however. And if everything is as he says it is: love, loss, and no wound, then so much the
better. ("If you were the woman with whom he broke up, would you
still say that?" Yes, especially then, I hope.) We do grieve about
separations, but there is nothing recommendable or praiseworthy in
grieving. If you can do without it, do not think you rather ought to
grieve.

Or somebody may argue *ad hominem:* "I gather you are German.
So obviously you are engaged in a little whitewash. Stripped of the
philosophical disguise, your message is that Germans should stop
doing penitence for what they did under the Nazis. We should all
forget about the past, wipe the slate clean and turn to the business at
hand as if nothing had happened. Alexander and Margarete Mitscherlich[18] lamented an inability to mourn, as they called it, in the
German attitude to their past. You just give that defect a good
name." There is a misunderstanding here. I am saying that penitence, in the sense of grieving over what one did, and mourning are
not recommendable attitudes. I am saying that the Nazi who did the
most horrendous things would still be wise to try, undejected by
what he did, to do what now is right. To speak against penitence and
mourning, however, is not to say that the events which penitence
and mourning are about are any less bad. Nor is it to recommend
forgetting them. On the contrary, it is with mourning and regret left
behind that we may come to see what we did in the sharpest light.
We should not suffer from what we did, we should face it.

RÜDIGER BITTNER

University of Bielefeld

[18] Alexander and Margarete Mitscherlich, *Die Unfähigkeit zu trauern*
(München: Piper, 1967).

[25]

The Decline of Guilt

Herbert Morris

With over thirty years of psychoanalytic reflection behind him, Freud observed in the concluding chapter of *Civilization and Its Discontents* that it was his "intention to represent the sense of guilt as the most important problem in the development of civilization and to show that the price we pay for our advance in civilization is a loss of happiness through the heightening of the sense of guilt."[1] This sense of guilt to which Freud refers, and to whose influence he assigns so significant and baneful an effect, generally becomes activated because of a belief that one is or would be, if one were to act in a certain way, in fact, guilty. This concept of guilt plays, of course, a major role in our moral life. Without it our morality would significantly differ from that with which we are now familiar. But the idea of one's being guilty, though integral to morality as we know it, seems even more central to law. We can imagine moral forms of life without guilt, but deep puzzlement confronts us when we make this attempt with the idea of law. In law, guilt clearly assumes its most systematic, its most recurrently public deployment.

While central to our idea of law and while a concept with the most serious legal and social implications, guilt remains, quite surprisingly, little examined. To be sure, much scholarly attention has been bestowed upon concepts closely linked with it, concepts such as responsibility, causation, and culpability, but guilt itself has largely escaped notice. In this paper I hope to go some way toward remedying this neglect. I first describe in some detail the nature and role of guilt and the sense of guilt in law, and I compare this with the situation in morality. I then set out a variety of theoretical critiques of guilt, each of which has in some way disturbed the comfort of mind of many who employ the concept, and I also draw attention to certain forces at work within society that I believe may slowly be transforming guilt's role. These critiques and these forces, reinforcing each other, strike at the very heart of law and create a crisis for guilt, posing what we might describe as "the problem of guilt in law." I intend to represent this problem, to echo Freud's formulation, as "the most important problem" presently before us in the development of law.

---

1. S. Freud, *Civilization and Its Discontents*, in *The Standard Edition of the Complete Psychological Works of Sigmund Freud* (London: Hogarth, 1961), vol. 21, p. 134.

Ethics 99 (October 1988): 62–76

Finally, I argue—and here my position contrasts sharply with Freud's though not in its speculative character—that the erosion of guilt within law, coupled with a narrowed and weakened compass for our sense of guilt, both with respect to law and more generally, may carry a cost comparable to the lost happiness which Freud attributes to guilt.

Let us now turn to the first issue: the nature and role of guilt within law. While it may be impossible to imagine law without guilt, its role there has always been circumscribed. Judgments of guilt should neither be identified with, nor thought of as implied by, judgments of invalidity or judgments of liability. A marriage or a will, or, for that matter, a verdict of guilt itself, might be invalid, but this implies nothing about one's guilt in failing to satisfy the conditions required for a valid marriage or will or verdict. And in a civil action, judgment rendered for plaintiff and against defendant, establishing defendant's liability, implies nothing by itself about defendant's guilt, and this is so regardless of defendant's fault. Verdicts of guilt are rendered within and restricted to criminal proceedings or other proceedings, such as court-martials, which are criminal in character.

What, then, does legal guilt imply? No simple answer to this apparently simple question will suffice. I divide my discussion as follows: I first set out those conditions which legal systems generally require—exceptions will be addressed later—for a person to be guilty. With these conditions satisfied and the person in, what I shall label, "the state of guilt," I then attempt to answer the question, What is implied by being in that state? I then turn attention to those general beliefs about the world presupposed by application of the concept. I conclude this first major section of my discussion by offering an analysis of the sense of guilt that differs significantly from Freud's, and I offer for consideration some contrasts between law and morality.

What conditions characteristically must be satisfied if one can truthfully be said to be legally guilty? These are quite familiar. I shall enumerate them briefly, though the meaning of each, of course, deserves fuller discussion as does the respect accorded them by actual legal systems. First, legal guilt requires conduct. This means several things: first, a person must do something rather than merely, for example, desire or intend to do it; second, a person must do something rather than merely have something happen that involves one's body that results in harm— causing damage, for example, as a result of being lifted up by the wind; and, third, a person must do something rather than simply have a status of a certain kind such as being a member of a certain race. Each of these conditions is, of course, consistent with guilt attaching to omissive conduct. A second point is this: guilt requires conscious conduct; consequently, conduct while asleep precludes guilt. Third, legal guilt requires fault or culpability with respect to wrongdoing, what criminal lawyers refer to as a "guilty mind" or "the mens rea of an offense." The absence of a requisite culpability state or one's fair opportunity to behave otherwise than one

did, precludes guilt. Fourth, legal guilt is individual, never vicarious, and requires a culpable relationship of the guilty person to the wrongful conduct. If guilty because of what another has done, some culpable relationship to that other's conduct must be present. Fifth, one must possess the capacity to appreciate the significance of the norms applicable to one. Immunizing, as we do, animals and infants from guilt reflects this requirement as does exculpation of at least some individuals suffering from mental illness. Sixth, legal guilt requires legal wrongdoing. Even the most egregious moral wrong, if unaccompanied by legal wrongdoing, does not incur legal guilt. Finally, "guilty" is a predicate that attaches to acts, states of mind, and persons. To be a guilty person (the particular focus of my concern in this study) requires satisfaction of all of the above conditions and a further condition that one be the self-same person as the one who satisfied all the above conditions. Puzzlement felt over guilty verdicts returned against those suffering severe amnesia at the time of conviction, or suffering any other condition that deprives them of a sense of continuity with the person who has committed the offense, would reflect one's attachment to this condition for guilt.

Important issues for my purposes arise if, within a system of criminal law, legal guilt is incurred when one or more of these conditions do not obtain. I shall address these issues shortly, but I want now to suppose that a particular person satisfies all these conditions. It would then be true to say of such a person that he or she was, to use a rough summary description, "culpably responsible for legal wrongdoing." And as such, the person would be legally guilty. But for an understanding of guilt, one must, I believe, keep in mind the distinction between two closely related, and therefore easily confused, concepts. To say of a person that he or she is "culpably responsible for legal wrongdoing" implies only that those conditions I have listed bearing on wrongdoing and culpability and causation have been satisfied, while to ascribe guilt to someone, though presupposing these conditions, implies more.

First, a guilty person is in a state deserving of some negative attitude, condemnation appearing the most apt term for this attitude, and the delivered verdict of guilt provides a formal expression of this attitude by an authoritative social organ. In declaring people guilty, we label them, perhaps more accurately, "brand" them, and thereby transform their status into that of the legally condemned. Second, being in the state of guilt implies that one has, through one's guilty act, set oneself apart from the community, membership in which we partly define by commitment to communal norms. Again, the verdict of guilt, with its branding one as guilty, reflects this fact of separateness, mirroring, through its setting the guilty apart from others, their having set themselves apart. Third, the state of guilt implies a special kind of separateness, for persons in this state have arrogated to themselves that to which they are not entitled, thereby placing themselves in a position of superiority to others who have complied with the norms. Thus, being guilty, one deserves a

response that operates to cancel this improper arrogation. Again, branding one "guilty" supplies some of this, and the actual visiting of punishment upon the guilty provides more. Next, nothing seems more fundamental to guilt than the idea that being guilty one owes something. Of course, within law no formal legal obligation necessarily attaches to guilt, but we nevertheless believe that we are entitled to take from the guilty something they owe. It is from this that the imagery of "a debt owed to society" derives. Next, closely connected with this is the idea that the guilty are subject to a sentence of punishment and to its imposition which constitutes the "exacting of the debt." Any legal practice restricted to establishing one's liability to make reparations or restitution or to providing compensation would differ fundamentally from a legal practice involving guilt. None of these alternative practices implies that wrongdoers are deserving of condemnation, that they are insufficiently committed to the norms or that their conduct has caused injury to society, not just to a particular person. Finally, guilt admits of degrees, some persons being more, some less, guilty, and each of the above responses is guided by concepts of proportionality or fittingness or both.

If this analysis has validity, certain quite general beliefs would seem to be held by those who internalize this practice. There would appear to be, for example, beliefs in an established order of things where limits are respected and relationships among people are as they ought to be, beliefs in an imbalance to that order caused by the guilty, beliefs in individuals being together and apart, determined to some significant degree by their conduct with respect to norms, beliefs in the possibility of restoration—matters in the world of guilt may, after all, be righted—beliefs in one's being tainted because of one's guilt, and even beliefs, perhaps, residues from times when the conception of pollution was dominant, of society remaining itself not quite right, somewhat unclean, until through punishment purification is achieved.

Punishment, while certainly having other explanations as well is, on this conception, highly overdetermined, at once a means of righting wrongs, correcting imbalances, reordering disturbed relationships, promoting restoration, and cleansing both the criminal and society. As a response to guilt, punishment must be seen, then, as freighted with rich symbolic significance, and in considering what might justify punishment we risk, I believe, incompleteness in our theories if we neglect this symbolic baggage.

For the above to hold true, for there to be in effect a practice of the kind I have described, it would also appear necessary that there exist throughout society a general commitment to norms established by law, to the values they support and to the legitimacy of the practice that has been established to determine violations and guilt. Widespread disaffection among the populace from the norms or lack of belief in the legitimacy of tribunals established to judge people would transform the legal practice into one in which individuals with power merely enforced their will upon

others. In such circumstances, the normative basis of the practice would crumble; condemnation would inevitably fall upon deaf ears and lose its point; punishment would become merely a matter of pain inflicted or freedom limited. Our conduct might be, in such circumstances, much as it presently is, but we should be going through the motions only—our world would have dramatically changed. If this is correct, a certain correspondence exists within society—and this hardly seems surprising—between being guilty and feeling guilty. Among the matters that seem presupposed by the practice would appear a generally pervasive vulnerability within the population covered by the legal norms to having their sense of guilt activated when contemplating or engaging in violative conduct. It is but the flip side of the disposition to feel indignation when others violate the law. To imagine that it was generally otherwise would throw into question central elements in the practice. But, if this is so, something needs to be said about the nature of our sense of guilt and its principal mark—one's feeling guilty.

Our sense of guilt reveals itself in our feeling inhibited from doing what we believe wrong and feeling guilty when we do it. Thus, it operates in a forward-looking and backward-looking manner. Freud's views about guilt are most thoroughly formulated in *Civilization and Its Discontents.* He there concentrates upon the sense of guilt as it operates in a forward-looking manner, conceiving of guilt as internalized anxiety, the incorporation or internalization by children of a threat of loss of love or attack embodied in parental attitudes. This view reduces guilt to anxiety, and clouds, I believe, our understanding of the former.[2] Let us see why this is so by looking first at what it is to feel guilty and then at the sense of guilt as inhibiting conduct.

A person who feels guilt holds to beliefs of a certain kind, feels a certain way, and is disposed to feel and act in certain specific ways. I believe we come at a clearer view of what it is to feel guilty by focusing on the distress that is intimately connected with it. It cannot—we shall then see—be reduced to anxiety, though if one experiences guilt, anxiety might accidentally be associated with it. A person feels such distress because of a unique set of beliefs, none of which implies either fear or anxiety. First, one has internalized norms and, as such, is committed to avoiding wrong. The mere fact that wrong is believed to have occurred, regardless of who bears responsibility for it, naturally causes distress. When we are attached to a person, injury to that person causes us pain regardless of who or what has occasioned the injury. But just as a special satisfaction attaches to thinking of oneself as the creator of what is valuable—we feel a special pleasure in our being the source of a loved

2. The fullest treatment of which I am aware of this topic is to be found in Michael Friedman, "Toward a Reconceptualization of Guilt," *Contemporary Psychoanalysis* 21 (1985): 501–45. For an early essay of mine setting out views that correspond to Friedman's, see "Guilt and Suffering," *Philosophy of East and West*, vol. 21 (1971), reprinted in *On Guilt and Innocence* (Berkeley: University of California Press, 1976).

one's pleasure—so thinking of oneself as responsible for wrongdoing arouses a special dissatisfaction. Further, in feeling guilt one turns on oneself the criticism and hostility that one would have visited upon others had they done wrong. Still another aspect of one's distress is one's feeling apart from those with whom one was attached. Indeed, another element of the distress derives from one's sense of fragmentation. Finally, in feeling guilty one feels burdened until steps are taken. One feels obliged to confess, to make amends, to repair, and to restore.

The painful feelings, then, associated with feeling guilt belong to those attendant upon damaging what we value, and not to anxiety, whether it be internalized or not. The impulse, for example, to confess reveals attachment and a desire to restore bonds. This must be kept distinct from any fear attendant upon the thought of not confessing. Likewise, to turn briefly to guilt as inhibiting wrongdoing, as a motive it derives from a desire to remain attached to what one values (with conscience, e.g., it is one's integrity). This should not be confused with the desire to avoid pain for oneself that would be attendant on damaging or betraying that to which one is attached. I am suggesting, then, that guilt is a nonegoistic motive, more like love than fear. Just as, when considering love, we should avoid confusing acting out of love for another with acting out of a desire for our own pleasure (easily confused because in achieving love's aim we derive pleasure), so we should avoid confusing guilt with a desire to avoid pain for ourselves.

This concludes my examination of the nature of guilt within law and our sense of guilt. I want now to return to an issue I raised a short while ago, namely, the status of the conditions I listed for one to be guilty, what I summarized in the phrase "culpably responsible for legal wrongdoing." Legal systems, however unjust, insist generally upon proof that these conditions obtain before judging one guilty. But we also know that our own law occasionally allows for a finding of guilt without proof in a particular case of any mens rea, and ignorance of law, which certainly bears upon culpability as I have defined it, is commonly not recognized as a defense. In these cases, though we might feel a pull to say of an individual without the requisite state that he or she was not "really guilty," we also seem prepared to affirm the existence of legal guilt if the person has been found guilty under the applicable rules. In what sense, then, are these conditions required if systems disregard them in making determinations of guilt?

To be sure, these conditions appear to embody constraints that justice places upon law and so their disregard may ground judgments of injustice. But there is still another sense in which the conditions may be viewed as required. This sense may be captured by putting the following question, How far might legal systems go in disregarding these conditions when making determinations of guilt and still be concerned with guilt?

Just so far, I would say. A system could, imaginably, impose suffering upon individuals just because of their racial characteristics. Or the law

might, for example, treat relatives of escaped felons harshly in an attempt to reduce the number of escapes. In these cases, basic conditions for guilt do not obtain, the practices are unjust, and, in addition, we should find talk of guilt, talk of punishing because of guilt, talk of verdicts of guilt as entirely inappropriate. Determinations of fact, not judgments of guilt, underlie the visiting of pain upon people in these circumstances, and puzzlement would result from any insistence upon claiming that legal guilt attaches to such persons. Some criteria for legal guilt would appear, then, to connect with the idea of guilt so tightly that failure to satisfy them would imply inapplicability of the concept.

But the examples suggested above are extreme. What shall we say about the more common instances presented to us of legal disregard of conditions for guilt? For guidance on this issue, we must turn attention to some connections between legal guilt and our moral conception of guilt.

No mere linguistic oddity lies behind the fact that the same term 'guilt' applies in these spheres of human life, and it would be surprising if within law and morality the rules governing the term's application differed markedly. No formal, depsychologized analysis of legal guilt, of the sort some legal positivists might offer, will capture its nature. As we have seen, guilt has special significance. Individuals who are guilty are viewed as justifiably condemned, justifiably punished, as having set themselves apart from the community through insufficient attachment to its values. If this is so, a number of conditions for being morally guilty— among them conditions related to a fair opportunity to behave otherwise than one did—must be presuppositions of legal guilt as well, for we should be at a loss otherwise to understand what it meant to speak of justifiable condemnation, justifiable punishment, and the like. Scattered exceptions to this might exist, and where they do, it deserves noting, we deploy justifications that commonly invoke "presumptions" that a person must, say, know the law or in fact be culpable. By doing this, we reveal our attachment to one's being guilty as a basis for one's being legally guilty.

My claim, then, is that a system that generally allowed for findings of guilt in conflict with basic moral constraints on the concept of guilt would be one that used existing institutions of the criminal law in a way fundamentally at odds with certain of its basic presuppositions. As with marked alienation by the community from the norms applicable to them, significant disregard of the conditions for guilt would transform the practice. Prevention and social control would replace crime and punishment as these are now understood.

I want now to address the question, Supposing the existence of a practice of the kind I have described, what functions does it perform in the lives of people who have internalized it? The universal fascination with crime and punishment, the mystery, illumination, conflict, the pain and suffering and violence there to be found, betray a deep emotional

need satisfied by this recurrently enacted drama. I shall draw attention to certain familiar facts and engage in some psychological speculation.

First, determinations of guilt and the infliction of punishment upon the guilty, vividly communicate, in a way no other social practice can, the community's values, serving both to instruct and to reinforce. Among law's clearest lessons are that norms exist and that they are to be taken seriously. These in turn provide reassurance that our social world is orderly and not chaotic, that it is a structured space in which not everything is permitted, where there are limits to conduct, a role for rational argumentation over who has crossed these limits, and, equally important psychologically, that closure exists as a possibility once these limits have been breached. When issues of guilt and innocence arise outside the law, we commonly meet with complexity and ambiguity. Law reduces life's murkiness, making matters somewhat neater than elsewhere. Law repeatedly enacts a compelling drama in which a person is either guilty or not guilty, in which light, so often sought and so generally elusive, is shed upon initial mystery, and in which conflict meets with resolution and guilt with its just deserts. Life, of course, is quite unlike that—indeed this is an idealized picture of law—but law, because of its relative definiteness and its institutionalized means of closure, nicely allows our indulging in this gratifying illusion. The world of guilt, then, contrary to Freud's suggestion, would appear to reduce rather than promote anxiety. This is so for still another important reason.

Guilt, perhaps more than any other concept, serves our need to believe ourselves capable of some effectiveness in the world, a need all the more insistent as conditions of modern life promote feelings of helplessness. Intimately involved as it is with responsibility, guilt testifies to human freedom and agency and, as such, it may serve to counteract one's sense of victimization. It is for this reason, I would suggest, that guilty feelings may operate for a person defensively, serving to hide from one something felt to be far more distressing than guilt.[3]

Something more needs to be said about how moral and legal guilt relate to one another. There can, of course, be moral guilt without legal guilt, legal guilt without moral guilt, and a range of instances in which the two overlap. Many lies and broken promises find no legal redress, and nothing is more evident than moral evil outside the law's compass. That legal guilt might exist without moral guilt is equally evident. Here one need only point to the moral rightness of violating an iniquitous law. That the two overlap is evident because of crimes such as murder where the legally guilty must commonly be morally guilty as well.

I earlier suggested that a conceptual connection also existed between the two kinds of guilt, with law constrained to some extent, if guilt is our concern, by moral considerations. While connected, moral and legal guilt

---

3. For a similar view, see W. R. D. Fairbairn, "The Repression and the Return of Bad Objects," in *Psychoanalytic Studies of the Personality* (London: Routledge & Kegan Paul, 1952).

also differ in significant ways. Legal systems may, and obviously frequently do, lay down norms devoid of moral justification. Just so long as there exists general societal acceptance of the procedures that generate those norms and commitment to acting in accord with them, the moral credentials of any particular norm are not an issue in determining guilt. There also remains, as we have seen, some latitude within law in specifying the circumstances under which violation of legal norms incurs guilt. But with moral guilt, the norms and the conditions to be satisfied for incurring guilt by violating them are immune from deliberate human modification. It would not follow, for example, that a society's acceptance of the authority of legal organs and the enactment by these organs of a morally iniquitous law converted a morally innocent wrongdoer into a morally guilty one because the criteria for legal guilt had been satisfied. Further, for the most part, guilt within moral situations arises when one has violated the rights of another individual, and society is not viewed as having an interest in the affair. Thus, those in a position to condemn or forgive are those whose rights have been violated and no others. Neither is there within morality the connection between punishment and guilt that one finds in law. Within morality one may criticize and resent, but commonly with moral guilt—think of guilt arising in close personal relationships—punishment would be viewed as inappropriate and entirely inconsistent with restoring the damaged relationship. Within the moral sphere essential for restoration are emotions and attitudes such as guilt, contrition, and repentance. Law and morality also differ through the objects taken for scrutiny. Maxims such as "the law aims at a minimum; morality at a maximum" and "law is concerned with external conduct; morality with internal conduct" draw attention to contrasting moral and legal emphases.

This richly textured practice of guilt, whose nature I have made an attempt to depict, did not instantaneously appear fully appareled in its customary garb in human culture. Ideas such as value and the wrongful had first to enter and assume their present hegemony in human consciousness. The story of Adam and Eve's scandalous flirtation with dreams of glory and inevitable horrifying fall condenses into a few vivid and chilling moments a long period of human development. Again, Ezekiel, signaling a shift toward the individualization of guilt, collapsed into a single edict, "the righteousness of the righteous shall be upon him, and the wickedness of the wicked upon him," a truth we now take for granted but whose acceptance surely evolved gradually. With Christianity we can record still another dramatic change, for the inner life of the moral agent assumed an importance it earlier did not have. But the words of Jesus, and the radical thoughts they embodied, fell upon receptive ears, suggesting a ground slowly tilled and made ready for the seed that flowered into a central tenet of the way in which we presently think.

I mention these few moments in guilt's history because, as I have suggested in my introductory remarks, we may ourselves be in the midst of a transformation—ironically guilt's slow demise after its slow ascendancy.

Through a confluence of factors—philosophical determinism, the development of the behavioral sciences, the ideology of sickness and therapy—the truth, indeed the rationality, of conceptions undergirding the practice of guilt have been thrown into question. And powerful social forces and an accommodating social ideology are also, even more influentially, at work, adding to the instability produced by the above views. Guilt is in the eye of a storm.

The assault on the rationality of the practice of guilt has moved along a number of parallel fronts. First, some challenge the presuppositions upon which guilt rests. Here we encounter either metaphysical lines of argument or more empirically grounded theories which claim that behind any instance of wrongdoing lie causative factors that should exempt wrongdoers from blame. Connected with these lines of argumentation are tendencies toward viewing antisocial conduct as pathological, a matter for therapy, not punishment. Sickness in our modern ways of thinking gradually occupies territory formerly governed by moral categories. Further, some have urged, taking a more epistemological than metaphysical line, that, even were we to acknowledge the possibility that people were sometimes guilty, we cannot have reasonable grounds for such belief. After all, when guilt is at issue, we make determinations about mental states and about the past, each of which presents its own epistemological difficulties, difficulties compounded when the factors are conjoined. Skepticism of this kind naturally inclines its adherents to urge forgoing concern with culpability at the time of the offense charged. Barbara Wootton's views nicely illustrate such thinking.[4] She has proposed a two-stage process in which attention would focus initially and exclusively upon what was in fact done, something observable. With this determined, focus would then shift to the responsible party's condition at the time of conviction and our concern limited to the most effective disposition of the offender. Moves to abolish the defense of insanity, a defense requiring inquiry into the state of the defendant's mind at the time of the wrongful act alleged, often reflect such a viewpoint.

These, then, are some familiar themes of discontent with guilt. It is not always evident what would practically follow from taking a particular critique seriously. For example, those who deny the existence of free will do not customarily advocate abandoning the criminal law and its distinction between those who act voluntarily and those, say, because of an epileptic seizure, who do not. It also deserves noting that these critiques have not gone unanswered; they have, in fact, mobilized tenacious defenses of customary ways of thinking about human beings. If this accumulation of critiques distinguishes the modern age so, too, do the number of defenses of human freedom and guilt made by those who have insisted that humans are free and that they often choose their own enslavement.

---

4. Barbara Wootton, *Crime and the Criminal Law* (London: Sweet & Maxwell, 1963).

What importance, then, outside of philosophy, do these various critiques of guilt possess? Sometimes, of course, they may directly influence the law, as when they serve to support abolition of the insanity defense or, to an entirely contrary purpose, when they serve to support exculpation on grounds of early and formative childhood experiences. They are also, of course, so to speak "in the air," elements in the intellectual climate, available to those who might seek support for the common human disposition to flee guilt with some justification or excuse. If there is merit in this speculation, critiques of guilt might occasionally be drawn upon to quiet an aroused sense of guilt. This is a powerful motivation with which to be aligned, and we should be cautious before discounting the potential this combination of theory and motivation has for fundamentally altering the ways in which we view ourselves and others.

Still, allowing that these negative views about guilt may have seeped into our consciousness and already even to some degree altered our practices, it seems evident, if change is occurring, that more powerful factors would have to be at work. Ideas may indeed ignite change, but to do so they obviously require combustible social conditions upon which to operate. Before entering upon some personal speculation, in no way grounded I must confess on careful empirical study, as to what other factors might be present and more effective, I should delay no further in indicating what I view as some noteworthy exceptions to the model of guilt within law.

I have in mind the following types of phenomena: (1) the practice of plea bargaining and the exercise of prosecutorial discretion more generally which operate to avoid inquiry into and determination of guilt with respect to particular offenses; (2) the employment of excessive punishments, violating the principle of proportionality that is tied to concern over degrees of guilt; (3) doctrines of strict and vicarious liability interpreted in such a way that an individual's culpability with respect to a particular matter ceases to be a material element in determining guilt; (4) constriction of or abolition of the defense of insanity; and (5) the proliferation of laws and regulations whose connection with wrongdoing, as generally conceived, is attenuated.

I must immediately acknowledge that the aspects of law to which this list draws attention have for a considerable period of time been familiar parts of the legal landscape. Our own law has always, of course, in some of its principal doctrines diverged in striking ways from basic principles governing attribution of guilt. I have in mind, to provide some greater specificity than the above list, the unavailability of certain defenses, such as reasonable ignorance or mistake of law, the pockets of strict liability with regard to certain sexual and regulatory offenses, the employment of objective standards to ground a finding of culpability, and the existence of narrow definitions of the defense of insanity which assure the conviction of those who are in fact not guilty. Those who believe that the criminal law should in its determinations of guilt reflect a person's actual guilt, that to disregard such a constraint implies injustice, have

always subjected these doctrines to criticism. Their views have at least occasionally altered practice, witness the influence of the American Law Institute's *Model Penal Code* upon the criminal law of a number of jurisdictions. If there has been some movement away from guilt, it cannot be regarded as without powerful reactive tendencies, reflecting the grip of this concept upon our thinking.

If I claim, then, that something novel may now be underway, I can hardly rest my case upon the presence of new doctrines and practices. It must rather be, as is so often the case, a question of degree, a result of a conjunction of influences promoting different emphases and because of that, a drift, a tendency to assign less importance to guilt. What might these influences be? I have already referred to certain theoretical views that question the rationality of guilt. To these must now be added a familiar and seductive mode of thinking with far more evident impact upon law and our attitudes toward it than metaphysics and epistemology. To put it most succinctly, it is an approach that subordinates principle to the realization of social goals, a mode of thinking that focuses, not upon exculpation of the innocent and conviction of the guilty, that is, upon justice, but upon keeping social disruption at an acceptable level. It promotes the slow transformation of law into administration. Such an ideology provides the justification for conviction of the innocent, non-prosecution of the guilty, and disregard for principles of proportionality. It smacks of Wilde's cynic knowing the price of everything and the value of nothing. But this, too, is hardly novel. Coupled with certain contemporary social conditions, however, I believe it may be bringing about significant change.

What are some of these social conditions? First, I would list the pervasively held belief that crime has increased. It is a belief that also corresponds to reality, for while the rate of crime proportionate to the population may have varied only slightly over the last one hundred years, more laws on the books and more people in existence to violate them inevitably result in more crime. Again, whatever the reality might be, people generally believe that mass murders and crimes involving sadism and gratuitous violence are more prevalent today than ever before. The consequence of this is evident—increased fear. Another factor of importance enters in, feeding fear—growth of the news media and instantaneous coverage of events. Were there not more crime, such coverage would create the contrary impression. But, of course, along with this sense of more crime are media focus and elaboration upon it and upon particular kinds of crimes. Commonly, either crimes of violence or crimes perpetrated by governmental officials receive widest publicity. This phenomenon must be conjoined with a major growth in the entertainment industry and the obvious marketability of crime. It hardly deserves comment that our social consciousness is immersed in crime.

I would next draw attention to the enormous increase in the number of laws and legal regulations, that familiar accompaniment to a heavily populated modern industrial society. These laws result in more offenders

and offenders whose crimes often diverge from traditional instances of wrongdoing. A consequence of legal wrongdoing diverging from accepted conceptions of wrongdoing is the dilution of respect for the law's norms generally. A consequence, of course, of many more laws and many more offenders is that those charged with responsibility for investigating crime, for finding, trying, and punishing wrongdoers, become burdened beyond their capacity to effectuate tasks assigned to them. Reported offenses commonly go uninvestigated for want of resources, and those individuals arrested, more often than not, go through a speedy, automated-like process bearing only the most distant resemblance to a solemn determination of guilt or innocence. The increase, then, of the number of laws tends, as inflation generally does, to devaluation of the currency of law generally.

Along with these familiar phenomena must be included the common belief that a sizable number of individuals within society are alienated from its values, that they do not accept the norms, that they are predators, more like enemies within than wayward citizens who have given into temptation. This perception may not accord with reality, but its source, again, lies in media focus upon such offenders, for they often excite greater interest, and incidentally stir up more intense feelings of helplessness, than one's common variety wrongdoer. What in the past has allowed for identification with wrongdoers seems, then, less operative today.

I shall only add one further speculation. It is a familiar truth that there is a pull to banalize evil. It is an effective, understandable way to survive. Almost each day, bombarded by horrifying evil and alive in a century where the scope of evil lies beyond true comprehension, we naturally defend ourselves from full emotional awareness. But in adopting this defensive maneuver, in understandably not experiencing its full impact, we cease to see new occurrences of evil for what they are. We become jaded, for we have, after all, seen everything. And so, tragically, we may purchase relief by sacrificing some of our humanity, that essential part of it that consists in emotional responsiveness to evil. But then we also run the risk that evil attendant upon departure from principles of justice, the violation, say, of the rights of a single innocent person, particularly when justified by minimization of social harm, has for us a rather banal character. The ideology of cost-effective analysis then reinforces these powerful defensive forces. And so just as the significance of violating any law may become less as there are so many laws, including morally suspect ones, around to violate, so the frequency of evil, our knowledge of it, our desensitizing ourselves to it, our attention to efficiency, lessens the seriousness of any particular instance of evil, including what we or our representatives perpetrate.

Now these factors—increased anxiety, increased crime, diminished capacity for identification with criminals, alienation, devaluation of law, and devaluation of justice—all put pressure upon guilt and pull us pow-

erfully toward responding to wrongdoing and wrongdoers from the perspective of social efficiency and social control. This is, of course, a familiar
disposition with respect to the procedural safeguards embodied in the
Bill of Rights to the U.S. Constitution. Those who initially proposed the
rights embodied in that document easily imagined that they might one
day directly benefit from their invocation. As this capacity for identification
lessens, as anxiety intensifies, support for the rights weakens. My hypothesis
is that a similar process occurs with guilt.

All this also, of course, has relevance to the vitality of our sense of
guilt with respect to law. When law begins to be viewed as a system of
social control, intent upon keeping costs down and increasing gains,
rather than a system of rules to effectuate justice, the risk is inevitably
run that one's sense of guilt with regard to law becomes less a factor in
one's conduct. One feels less the constraints of justice in responding to
wrongdoers, less the constraint, indeed, in responding to the innocent
whom we might see as justifiably sacrificed to the greater good. As those
in authority with greater frequency act to further policy rather than
promote justice, their moral authority diminishes, respect for the institutions
generating norms and implementing them lessens, and in its train there
is a lessened regard for complying with law because it is law. Further,
where the criminals focused upon, as is frequently the case, are themselves
officials, we can anticipate some erosion in respect for law. Commitment
to law compliance becomes strained when noncompliance appears in our
interest, and rationalization is readily available. And, if anything goes in
law, why not elsewhere.

If these speculations have merit, if we are witnessing lessened respect
for guilt and a lessening of our sense of guilt, we must then go on to
ask whether good or evil attend the change.

At the beginning of this paper, I suggested that the lessened role
for guilt in law and the erosion of our sense of guilt might have consequences equal in seriousness to those Freud associated with the heightening of our sense of guilt. I shall mention several such possible consequences. First, departing from the model of guilt I have set out, we
do offense to principles of justice, and we do offense by punishing the
innocent, disregarding the constraint of proportionality in punishment,
and disregarding the guilt of the guilty. Second, departures from the
practice of guilt, because they imply indifference to individual responsibility, carry an inevitable and heavy cost, for individuals come to be both
looked upon and treated as justifiably serving some higher social goal
rather than in response to choices they have made. Added to injustice,
then, is the evil of objectifying human beings.

Finally, I offer this speculation. A powerful force at work in putting
pressure on our customary ways of responding to alleged and actual
wrongdoers is anxiety. We are prepared to sacrifice elements of the practice
of guilt to allay it. An irony lurks in this. I have suggested that guilt
functions in society to provide a sense of order. Limits are set; rules are

followed in determining violations; some closure is achieved. Guilt is hardly pleasant, but there is some comfort in it. Now departures from this practice, inevitably, I believe, reintroduce into our social world a sense of disorder. A world governed by principles and respect for individual choice is transformed into a world with no fixed limits where anything goes provided some conception of a socially optimal result is foreseen. But this can only increase, not diminish, our feelings of helplessness and attendant anxiety. I believe that in our rush to quiet our fears we may be acting so as, in fact, to increase them.

To return to Freud. Because guilt constrained the instinctual, he saw it diminishing happiness. He had sex and aggression in mind when formulating his view. And, indeed, it has superficial appeal. What he failed adequately to note—and maybe it was because sex was rather too much on his mind—were the important respects in which guilt and our sense of guilt mark our attachment to others, to values outside ourselves, and how bleak life would be were these absent. He did not sufficiently note that happiness would be thrown into jeopardy in any world given over to the free play of the instinctual. Guilt also, as often as not, reduces rather than promotes anxiety. Returning to my theme, I have suggested that much is lost in any world given over to the dominance of social policy unregulated by respect for persons embodied in the idea of guilt. Pulled toward social policy and away from guilt, because we flee our anxiety, we shall end up facing a monster more fearful than the one from which we have fled.

Name Index